Molecular Imaging in Oncology

Molecular Imaging in Oncology

Edited by

Martin G. Pomper
Johns Hopkins University School of Medicine
Baltimore, Maryland, USA

Juri G. Gelovani
MD Anderson Cancer Center
Houston, Texas, USA

Section Editors

Benjamin Tsui
Johns Hopkins University School of Medicine
Baltimore, Maryland, USA

Kathleen Gabrielson
Johns Hopkins University School of Medicine
Baltimore, Maryland, USA

Richard Wahl
Johns Hopkins University School of Medicine
Baltimore, Maryland, USA

S. Sam Gambhir
Stanford School of Medicine
Stanford, California, USA

Jeff Bulte
Johns Hopkins University School of Medicine
Baltimore, Maryland, USA

Raymond Gibson
Merck Research Laboratories
West Point, Pennsylvania, USA

William C. Eckelman
Molecular Tracer, LLC
Bethesda, Maryland, USA

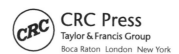

CRC Press
Taylor & Francis Group
Boca Raton London New York

CRC Press is an imprint of the
Taylor & Francis Group, an **informa** business

CRC Press
Taylor & Francis Group
6000 Broken Sound Parkway NW, Suite 300
Boca Raton, FL 33487-2742

First issued in paperback 2019

© 2008 by Taylor & Francis Group, LLC
CRC Press is an imprint of Taylor & Francis Group, an Informa business

No claim to original U.S. Government works

ISBN-13: 978-0-8493-7417-3 (hbk)
ISBN-13: 978-0-367-40348-5 (pbk)

Library of Congress Cataloging-in-Publication Data

Molecular imaging in oncology/edited by Martin G. Pomper, Juri Gelovani.
   p. ; cm.
  Includes bibliographical references and index.
  ISBN-13: 978-0-8493-7417-3 (hardcover : alk. paper)
  ISBN-10: 0-8493-7417-0 (hardcover : alk. paper)
   1. Cancer—Imaging. 2. Molecular probes—Diagnostic use. I. Pomper, Martin G. II. Gelovani, Juri.
  [DNLM: 1. Neoplasms—diagnosis. 2. Diagnostic Imaging. 3. Molecular Biology—methods. 4. Molecular Diagnostic Techniques. 5. Neoplasms—therapy. 6. Radioimmunotherapy—methods. QZ 241 M7187 2008]
  RC270.3.D53M64 2008
  616.99′4075—dc22

                                           2008019422

Visit the Taylor & Francis Web site at
http://www.taylorandfrancis.com

and the CRC Press Web site at
http://www.crcpress.com

Foreword

Molecular imaging can be traced back to France in 1896, when Henri Becquerel discovered that certain materials emitted energetic "rays," a physical process that his graduate student, Marie Curie, later called radioactive decay. In 1929, American physicist Ernest Lawrence built the first cyclotron and was able to produce positron-emitting radionuclides. In 1931, the British physicist, Paul Dirac, had postulated the existence of positrons, based on an equation he developed in quantum mechanics. He postulated the existence of the positron as an antiparticle having the same mass as an electron but with a positive rather than negative charge. The proof of the existence of the positrons was proved in cosmic radiation by another Nobel prize winner, Carl Anderson, in 1932. That same year French physicists Irene Curie (Marie's daughter) and Frederick Joliot (Irene's husband) announced their discovery of artificial radio-activity. They showed that many different atoms could be made radioactive. With the Curie/Joliot publication, Lawrence immediately recognized the enormous potential value of being able to make "radioactive tracers" that made possible medically important as well as chemical and physical measurements. Subsequent pioneers recognized the great biological importance of the radioactive elements that a cyclotron could produce, including oxygen-15 and carbon-11. In the 1930s, chemist Martin Kamen, working with Lawrence, made the key discovery that the oxygen produced by the process of photosynthesis, and so important for living organisms, came from water, not from carbon dioxide, as had been previously assumed.

In the spring of 1945, the U.S. government made the decision to produce radioisotopes for civilian use. In June 1946, President Truman signed an executive order that made iodine-131 available from Oak Ridge National Laboratory to qualified physicians throughout the United States. The first shipment of carbon-14 was on August 2, 1946, to Martin Kamen at Berkeley, California. The shipment was kept secret because Kamen was falsely thought at the time to be a communist. The first announced shipment to a civilian institution was subsequently to the Barnard Free Skin and Cancer Hospital at Washington University in St. Louis. On December 7, 1946, the revolutionary announcement was made by an internist, Sam Seidlin and colleagues that radioiodine could not just ameliorate but cure metastatic cancer. According to Marshall Brucer at Oak Ridge, within days, every Congressman had heard from his constituency, and on Jan 1, 1947, the Atomic Energy Commission (AEC) took over the distribution of radioisotopes from the supersecret Manhattan District Project of World War II that had developed the atomic bomb.

In 1946, George Moore, a neurosurgeon at the University of Minnesota, used iodine-131-labeled iodofluorescein to localize brain tumors using a Geiger-Muller detector in 12 patients during surgery. In 1950 the FDA recognized iodine-131 as the first "radioactive new drug". By 1950, 3250 publications had been published on the use of radionuclides in medicine. Molecular imaging was not accepted immediately. Marshall Brucer wrote: "Surgeons poo-poohed any thought of treating hyperthyroidism with some kind of fake iodine. Hematologists laughed at the P32 trials in the treatment of leukemias. Medical societies had no room on their agendas for radioactive isotopes."

The public was excited by news of the use of radioiodine not only in the diagnosis of hypo- and hyperthyroidism, but in the treatment of thyroid diseases, in many patients eliminating the need for surgery. It was the first example of defining disease on the basis of a measured regional molecular process, that is, the accumulation of radioactive iodine.

"Radioisotope scanning" was the name given to imaging of the distribution of radioactive tracers in the living human body at various times after injection of a radioactive "tracer." New "radiopharmaceuticals" were developed in the 1950s and 1960s as a means of "visualizing" previously invisible organs, such as the liver, that could not be examined effectively by conventional X-rays.

A tremendous boost to molecular imaging, then called "atomic medicine," and subsequently "nuclear medicine" was given by a speech delivered by President Dwight Eisenhower before the 470th plenary meeting of the United Nations in New York on December 8, 1953. He said:

"The more important responsibility of a new (atomic energy) agency would be to devise methods whereby fissionable material would be allocated to serve the peaceful pursuits of mankind. Experts would be mobilized to apply atomic energy to the needs of agriculture, medicine and other peaceful activities. I would be prepared to submit to the Congress of the United States, and with every expectation of approval, any such plan that would, first, encourage world-wide investigation into the most effective peacetime uses of fissionable material, and with the certainty that the investigators had all the material needed for the conducting of all experiments that were appropriate."

President Eisenhower's speech led to the creation of the International Atomic Energy Agency (IAEA), which made possible research with radioactive tracers all over the world. The types of studies include measurement of regional blood flow to organs and lesions, measurement of the regional bioenergetics, and molecular processes involved in intercellular communication.

Since the 1950s molecular imaging has encompassed much more than the peaceful use of radioactivity. Although radiopharmaceutical-based techniques tend to dominate clinical molecular imaging presently, molecular imaging is not really about any specific modality. It is about uncovering physiology noninvasively by probing specific cellular and molecular processes in vivo. What has made molecular imaging so exciting now is the introduction of efficient, high-sensitivity devices for preclinical (animal model) as well as clinical imaging. Hybrid imaging devices, which combine the high resolution of anatomic imaging with the physiologic techniques, are also becoming standard in clinical practice and enable determination of a metabolic or receptor defect with pinpoint accuracy within minutes. Increasingly relevant imaging targets are being uncovered due to protein arrays and high-throughput methods by which to interrogate human biopsy specimens. Mice that can be genetically manipulated not only help validate those targets but also provide excellent models in which to test new molecular imaging probes. The introduction of current molecular biological techniques—as they evolve in real time—to imaging science will only make molecular imaging increasingly relevant to study physiology and disease in the coming years.

Oncology is perhaps the most fruitful domain of molecular imaging at present, particularly because of the information provided in measuring the energy supply of lesions, the abundance of unexploited tumor markers, and intra- and intercellular communication pathways amenable to imaging. This book describes the development, principles, and uses of molecular imaging in answering the questions raised in the practice of medicine, with an emphasis on oncology: (1) What is the problem? (2) Where is the problem? (3) What is going to happen? (4) What is the best course of action and treatment? (5) Is the treatment effective? A graded approach is taken whereby there will be a brief introduction to basic principles in biology and molecular imaging, then to the modalities available on through clinical molecular imaging of cancer. Medicine has moved from whole body to organs to tissues to cells and now to molecules. We are indeed in a revolutionary time in the history of medicine.

Henry N. Wagner, Jr., MD

Preface

Although a relatively new aspect of imaging science and practice, molecular imaging is beginning to make its presence felt. It has done so because it involves the collaboration between two rapidly evolving fields, namely, molecular biology—including genomics, proteomics, and the use of transgenic animal models—and high-sensitivity imaging devices to probe cellular and molecular phenomena in vivo. Those two fields are powerful in their own right, but together they can generate considerable new knowledge about normal cellular processes and disease and, in particular, cancer.

This volume is dedicated to the molecular imaging of cancer, taking a graded approach to the subject by first introducing concepts of basic molecular biology (sect. 1) and the operation of the various imaging modalities (sect. 2). We felt it was necessary for the reader to understand the challenges in the development of imaging probes (sect. 3) and in performing imaging in animal models—the mainstay of current molecular imaging research (sect. 4). More directly germane to the molecular imaging of cancer are chapters dedicated specifically to molecular-genetic imaging (sect. 5), imaging cellular migration and other processes (sect. 6) and clinical translation (sect. 7), where examples from several key clinical challenges are provided (sect. 8). The final chapters highlight imaging in anticancer drug development and how to move into the future through collaboration with industry and the government (sect. 9).

Although molecular imaging is evolving rapidly, due to the incorporation of nanobiotechnology, microfluidics, and other rapidly advancing fields, we have tried to maintain relevance for the practicing clinician—who will be the ultimate arbiter as to whether molecular imaging will actually prove useful for and adopted into clinical practice. Nevertheless, sufficient detail is provided so that graduate students and established practitioners in allied fields, e.g., chemistry, imaging physics, and cell biology, can become acquainted with molecular imaging in cancer and begin incorporating imaging beneficially into their work, likely generating new ideas previously unseen by dedicated imaging scientists.

Martin Pomper, MD, PhD

Contents

Contributors

Paul D. Acton Johnson & Johnson Pharmaceutical R&D, Spring House, Philadelphia, Pennsylvania, U.S.A.

Mian M. Alauddin Department of Experimental Diagnostic Imaging, Center for Advanced Biomedical Imaging Research, The University of Texas M.D. Anderson Cancer Center, Houston, Texas, U.S.A.

Dmitri Artemov JHU ICMIC Program, Russell H. Morgan Department of Radiology and Radiological Science, Johns Hopkins University School of Medicine, Baltimore, Maryland, U.S.A.

Glenn Bauman Department of Oncology, Schulich School of Medicine & Dentistry, The University of Western Ontario, London, Ontario, Canada

Bohumil Bednar Imaging Department, Merck Research Laboratories, Merck & Co, Inc., West Point, Pennsylvania, U.S.A.

Ambros J. Beer Department of Nuclear Medicine, Technische Universität München, Munich, Germany

T. Z. Belhocine Department of Diagnostic Radiology and Nuclear Medicine, St. Joseph's Hospital, London, Ontario, Canada

Zaver M. Bhujwalla JHU ICMIC Program, Russell H. Morgan Department of Radiology and Radiological Science, and Sidney Kimmel Comprehensive Cancer Center, Johns Hopkins University School of Medicine, Baltimore, Maryland, U.S.A.

Alexei A. Bogdanov Jr. Departments of Radiology and Cell Biology, University of Massachusetts Medical School, Worcester, Massachusetts, U.S.A.

Mark A. Borden Department of Chemical Engineering, Columbia University, New York, New York, U.S.A.

Jeff W. M. Bulte Russell H. Morgan Department of Radiology and Radiological Science, Division of MR Research, and Cellular Imaging Section, Institute for Cell Engineering, Johns Hopkins University School of Medicine, Baltimore, Maryland, U.S.A.

Robert D. Cardiff   Department of Pathology, School of Medicine, University of California, Davis, California, U.S.A.

Thomas L. Chenevert   Department of Radiology, University of Michigan, Ann Arbor, Michigan, U.S.A.

Steve Y. Cho   Division of Nuclear Medicine, Russell H. Morgan Department of Radiology and Radiological Science, Johns Hopkins University School of Medicine, Baltimore, Maryland, U.S.A.

Barbara Y. Croft   Cancer Imaging Program, National Cancer Institute, National Institutes of Health, Bethesda, Maryland, U.S.A.

Paul A. Dayton   Joint Department of Biomedical Engineering, University of North Carolina at Chapel Hill and North Carolina State University, Raleigh, North Carolina, U.S.A.

Surajit Dhara   Russell H. Morgan Department of Radiology and Radiological Sciences, Johns Hopkins University School of Medicine, Baltimore, Maryland, U.S.A.

Chaitanya R. Divgi   Department of Radiology, Division of Nuclear Medicine and Clinical Molecular Imaging, University of Pennsylvania, Philadelphia, Pennsylvania, U.S.A.

William C. Eckelman   Molecular Tracer LLC, Bethesda, Maryland, U.S.A.

William B. Eubank   Department of Radiology, University of Washington and Puget Sound VA Medical Center, Seattle, Washington, U.S.A.

Jeffrey L. Evelhoch   Imaging Sciences, Medical Sciences, Amgen, Inc., Thousand Oaks, California, U.S.A.

Peter Gabra   Department of Medical Biophysics, Schulich School of Medicine & Dentistry, The University of Western Ontario, London, Ontario, Canada

Kathleen Gabrielson   Department of Molecular and Comparative Pathobiology, Johns Hopkins University School of Medicine, Baltimore, Maryland, U.S.A.

Craig J. Galban   Department of Radiology, University of Michigan, Ann Arbor, Michigan, U.S.A.

Sanjiv Sam Gambhir   Molecular Imaging Program at Stanford, Department of Radiology, Stanford School of Medicine, Stanford, California, U.S.A.

Juri G. Gelovani   Department of Experimental Diagnostic Imaging, Center for Advanced Biomedical Imaging Research, The University of Texas M.D. Anderson Cancer Center, Houston, Texas, U.S.A.

Ahmed M. Gharib   Diagnostic Radiology Department, National Heart, Lung and Blood Institute (NHLBI), National Institutes of Health (NIH), Bethesda, Maryland, U.S.A.

Raymond E. Gibson   Imaging Department, Merck Research Laboratories, West Point, Pennsylvania, U.S.A.

Assaf A. Gilad   Russell H. Morgan Department of Radiology and Radiological Science, Division of MR Research, and Cellular Imaging Section, Institute for Cell Engineering, Johns Hopkins University School of Medicine, Baltimore, Maryland, U.S.A.

Tracy L. Gluckman   Department of Molecular and Comparative Pathobiology, Johns Hopkins University, Baltimore, Maryland, U.S.A.

Kristine Glunde   JHU ICMIC Program, Russell H. Morgan Department of Radiology and Radiological Science, Johns Hopkins University School of Medicine, Baltimore, Maryland, U.S.A.

David M. Goldenberg   Garden State Cancer Center, Center for Molecular Medicine and Immunology, Belleville, New Jersey, U.S.A.

Brett M. Hall   Department of Pediatrics, Columbus Children's Research Institute, The Ohio State University School of Medicine, Columbus, Ohio, U.S.A.

Laurence W. Hedlund   Center for In Vivo Microscopy, Department of Radiology, Duke University Medical Center, Durham, North Carolina, U.S.A.

Julie Heroux   Diagnostic Radiology Department, National Heart, Lung and Blood Institute (NHLBI), National Institutes of Health (NIH), Bethesda, Maryland, U.S.A.

Edward H. Herskovits   Department of Radiology, University of Pennsylvania, Philadelphia, U.S.A.

Andreas H. Jacobs   Laboratory for Gene Therapy and Molecular Imaging at the Max Planck Institute for Neurological Research with Klaus-Joachim-Zülch-Laboratories of the Max Planck Society and the Faculty of Medicine of the University of Cologne, Cologne, Germany

Michael A. Jacobs   JHU ICMIC Program, Russell H. Morgan Department of Radiology and Radiological Science, Johns Hopkins University School of Medicine, Baltimore, Maryland, U.S.A.

Kimberly A. Kelly   Harvard Medical School, Massachusetts General Hospital, Boston, Massachusetts, U.S.A.

Hisataka Kobayashi   Molecular Imaging Program, Center for Cancer Research, National Cancer Institute, NIH, Bethesda, Maryland, U.S.A.

Kelly R. Kristof   Harvard Medical School, Massachusetts General Hospital, Boston, Massachusetts, U.S.A.

Vikas Kundra   Departments of Diagnostic Radiology and Experimental Diagnostic Imaging, University of Texas M.D. Anderson Cancer Center, Houston, Texas, U.S.A.

Steven M. Larson   Memorial Sloan-Kettering Cancer Center, New York, New York, U.S.A.

Roger Lecomte   Sherbrooke Molecular Imaging Center, Department of Nuclear Medicine and Radiobiology, Université de Sherbrooke, Sherbrooke, Quebec, Canada

Kuei C. Lee   Department of Radiology, University of Michigan, Ann Arbor, Michigan, U.S.A.

Jean H. Lee   Department of Radiology, University of Washington and Seattle Cancer Care Alliance, Seattle, Washington, U.S.A.

Ting-Yim Lee   Imaging Program, Lawson Health Research Institute; Imaging Research Laboratories, Robarts Research Institute; and Departments of Medical Imaging and Medical Biophysics, Schulich School of Medicine & Dentistry, The University of Western Ontario, London, Ontario, Canada

Jason S. Lewis   Department of Radiology, Memorial-Sloan Kettering Cancer Center, New York, New York, U.S.A.

David A. Mankoff   Departments of Radiology and Medicine, University of Washington and Seattle Cancer Care Alliance, Seattle, Washington, U.S.A.

Frank C. Marini   M.D. Anderson Cancer Center, University of Texas, Houston, Texas, U.S.A.

Michael T. McMahon   Russell H. Morgan Department of Radiology and Radiological Science, Division of MR Research, Johns Hopkins University School of Medicine, Baltimore, Maryland, U.S.A. and F.M. Kirby Research Center for Functional Brain Imaging, Kennedy Krieger Institute, Baltimore, Maryland, U.S.A.

Ronnie C. Mease   Russell H. Morgan Department of Radiology and Radiological Sciences, Johns Hopkins University School of Medicine, Baltimore, Maryland, U.S.A.

Anne E. Menkens   Cancer Imaging Program, National Cancer Institute, National Institutes of Health, Bethesda, Maryland, U.S.A.

Charles R. Meyer   Department of Radiology, University of Michigan, Ann Arbor, Michigan, U.S.A.

Seng Peng Mok   Department of Radiology, Johns Hopkins University, Baltimore, Maryland, U.S.A.

Noriko Mori   JHU ICMIC Program, Russell H. Morgan Department of Radiology and Radiological Science, Johns Hopkins University School of Medicine, Baltimore, Maryland, U.S.A.

Britney L. Moss   Molecular Imaging Center, Mallinckrodt Institute of Radiology and Department of Molecular Biology and Pharmacology, Washington University School of Medicine, St. Louis, Missouri, U.S.A.

Snehal Naik   Molecular Imaging Center, Mallinckrodt Institute of Radiology and Department of Molecular Biology and Pharmacology, Washington University School of Medicine, St. Louis, Missouri, U.S.A.

Arvind P. Pathak   JHU ICMIC Program, Russell H. Morgan Department of Radiology and Radiological Science, and Sidney Kimmel Comprehensive Cancer Center, Johns Hopkins University School of Medicine, Baltimore, Maryland, U.S.A.

Bradley E. Patt   Gamma Medica-Ideas, Inc., Northridge, California, U.S.A.

Marie-France Penet   JHU ICMIC Program, Russell H. Morgan Department of Radiology and Radiological Science, Johns Hopkins University School of Medicine, Baltimore, Maryland, U.S.A.

David Piwnica-Worms   Molecular Imaging Center, Mallinckrodt Institute of Radiology and Department of Molecular Biology and Pharmacology, Washington University School of Medicine, St. Louis, Missouri, U.S.A.

Andrea Pichler-Wallace   Molecular Imaging Center, Mallinckrodt Institute of Radiology, Washington University School of Medicine, St. Louis, Missouri, U.S.A.

Martin G. Pomper   Division of NeuroRadiology, Russell H. Morgan Department of Radiology and Radiological Science, Johns Hopkins University School of Medicine, Baltimore, Maryland, U.S.A.

Vladimir Ponomarev   Department of Radiology, Memorial Sloan Kettering Cancer Center, New York, New York, U.S.A.

Daniel A. Pryma   Department of Radiology, Division of Nuclear Medicine and Clinical Molecular Imaging, University of Pennsylvania, Philadelphia, Pennsylvania, U.S.A.

Venu Raman   Department of Radiology, Johns Hopkins University School of Medicine, Baltimore, Maryland, U.S.A.

Alnawaz Rehemtulla   Department of Radiation Oncology, University of Michigan, Ann Arbor, Michigan, U.S.A.

Fred Reynolds   Harvard Medical School, Massachusetts General Hospital, Boston, Massachusetts, U.S.A.

Brian D. Ross   Department of Radiology, University of Michigan, Ann Arbor, Michigan, U.S.A.

Markus Schwaiger   Department of Nuclear Medicine, Technische Universität München, Munich, Germany

George Sgouros   Russell H. Morgan Department of Radiology and Radiological Science, Johns Hopkins University School of Medicine, Baltimore, Maryland, U.S.A.

Khalid Shah   Massachusetts General Hospital, Harvard Medical School, Boston, Massachusetts, U.S.A.

Robert M. Sharkey   Garden State Cancer Center, Center for Molecular Medicine and Immunology, Belleville, New Jersey, U.S.A.

Rajendra K. Singh   Department of Radiology, Washington University School of Medicine, St. Louis, Missouri, U.S.A.

Bryan Ronain Smith   Molecular Imaging Program at Stanford, Department of Radiology, Stanford School of Medicine, Stanford, California, U.S.A.

Teresa Southard   Department of Molecular and Comparative Pathobiology, Johns Hopkins University School of Medicine, Baltimore, Maryland, U.S.A.

Errol Stewart   Department of Medical Biophysics, Schulich School of Medicine & Dentistry, The University of Western Ontario, London, Ontario, Canada

Daniel C. Sullivan   Cancer Imaging Program, National Cancer Institute, National Institutes of Health, Bethesda, Maryland, U.S.A.

Lavanya Sundararajan   Department of Medicine, University of Washington and Seattle Cancer Care Alliance, Seattle, Washington, U.S.A.

Cyrille Sur   Imaging Department, Merck Research Laboratories, Merck & Co, Inc., West Point, Pennsylvania, U.S.A.

Oleg M. Teytelboym   Division of Nuclear Medicine, Department of Radiology and Radiological Sciences, Johns Hopkins University, Baltimore, Maryland, U.S.A.

Benjamin M. W. Tsui   Department of Radiology, Johns Hopkins University, Baltimore, Maryland, U.S.A.

Peter C. M. van Zijl   Russell H. Morgan Department of Radiology and Radiological Science, Division of MR Research, Johns Hopkins University School of Medicine, Baltimore, Maryland, U.S.A. and F.M. Kirby Research Center for Functional Brain Imaging, Kennedy Krieger Institute, Baltimore, Maryland, U.S.A.

Henry F. VanBrocklin   Department of Radiology and Biomedical Imaging, University of California, San Francisco, California, U.S.A.

Wynn A. Volkert   Department of Radiology and the Radiopharmaceutical Sciences Institute, University of Missouri and H.S. Truman Memorial Veterans Administration Hospital, Columbia, Missouri, U.S.A.

Yannic Waerzeggers   Laboratory for Gene Therapy and Molecular Imaging at the Max Planck Institute for Neurological Research with Klaus-Joachim-Zülch-Laboratories of the Max Planck Society and the Faculty of Medicine of the University of Cologne, Cologne, Germany

Douglas J. Wagenaar   Gamma Medica-Ideas, Inc., Northridge, California, U.S.A.

Richard L. Wahl   Division of Nuclear Medicine, Department of Radiology and Radiological Sciences, Johns Hopkins University, Baltimore, Maryland, U.S.A.

Piotr Walczak   Russell H. Morgan Department of Radiology and Radiological Science, Division of MR Research, and Cellular Imaging Section, Institute for Cell Engineering, Johns Hopkins University School of Medicine, Baltimore, Maryland, U.S.A.

Yuchuan Wang   Department of Radiology, Johns Hopkins University, Baltimore, Maryland, U.S.A.

Michael J. Welch   Department of Radiology, Washington University School of Medicine, St. Louis, Missouri, U.S.A.

Alexandra Winkeler   Laboratory for Gene Therapy and Molecular Imaging at the Max Planck Institute for Neurological Research with Klaus-Joachim-Zülch-Laboratories of the Max Planck Society and the Faculty of Medicine of the University of Cologne, Cologne, Germany

Eugene Wong   Department of Physics, The University of Western Ontario, London, Ontario, Canada

Yi Xu   Department of Molecular and Comparative Pathobiology, Johns Hopkins University School of Medicine, Baltimore, Maryland, U.S.A.

Jim Xuan   Department of Surgery, London Health Sciences Centre, London, Ontario, Canada

Cynthia J. Zarsky   Technology and Acquisition and Outlicensing, Merck Research Laboratories, Rahway, New Jersey, U.S.A.

Guo-Jun Zhang   Imaging Department, Merck Research Laboratories, Merck & Co, Inc., West Point, Pennsylvania, U.S.A.

Jason M. Zhao   Russell H. Morgan Department of Radiology and Radiological Science, Division of MR Research, Johns Hopkins University School of Medicine, Baltimore, Maryland, U.S.A. and F.M. Kirby Research Center for Functional Brain Imaging, Kennedy Krieger Institute, Baltimore, Maryland, U.S.A.

A Word on "Molecular Imaging"

There have been several definitions published on the term "molecular imaging" (1–5), but in this volume we will conform to the definition provided by the Definitions Task Force[a] of the Molecular Imaging Center of Excellence of the SNM:

> Molecular imaging is the visualization, characterization, and measurement of biological processes at the molecular and cellular levels in humans and other living systems.

- Molecular imaging typically includes two- or three-dimensional imaging as well as quantification over time.
- The techniques used include radiotracer imaging/nuclear medicine, MRI, MRS, optical imaging, ultrasound, and others.

REFERENCES

1. Thakur M, Lentle BC. Report of a summit on molecular imaging. AJR Am J Roentgenol 2006; 186(2):297–299.
2. Jaffer FA, Weissleder R. Molecular imaging in the clinical arena. JAMA 2005; 293(7): 855–862.
3. Weissleder R, Mahmood U. Molecular imaging. Radiology 2001; 219(2):316–333.
4. Massoud TF, Gambhir SS. Molecular imaging in living subjects: seeing fundamental biological processes in a new light. Genes Dev 2003; 17(5):545–580.
5. Herschman HR. Molecular imaging: looking at problems, seeing solutions. Science 2003; 302(5645):605–608.

[a]Task-force members include Barry Shulkin, Albert Sinusas, Michael Stabin, Mathew Tahkur, Benjamin Tsui, Ronald Van Heertum, David Mankoff (chair), Bennett Chin, William Eckelman, Jerry Glickson, Craig Levin, and Chester Mathis.

1

Tumor Biology

SURAJIT DHARA

Russell H. Morgan Department of Radiology and Radiological Sciences, Johns Hopkins University School of Medicine, Baltimore, Maryland, U.S.A.

INTRODUCTION

Cancer is a disease of "chaos," a breakdown of existing biological order and rules of tissue homeostasis. In the human body, normal healthy organs obey a tightly regulated homeostatic mechanism that has evolved through millions of years of refinement. This fine balance between cellular growth and apoptosis (programmed cell death) is the key to normal tissue homeostasis. Every cell's life and death "program" is "hardwired" in its genome in the form of DNA that is packaged into 30-nm chromatin fiber within the nucleus. A cell's response to any internal or external stimuli depends on this hardwired program. Any adverse alteration of this program, such as DNA damage by either exogenous or endogenous factors, could lead to apoptosis. This is the normal defense mechanism of the body to rid itself of "bad" cells. In the process of malignant transformation, cells harbor a series of alterations that are carried through their daughter cells by mitotic inheritance. These inheritable alterations initiate the process of transformation by conferring a growth advantage to the transformed cells over other neighboring normal or non-transformed cells and make these cells capable of escaping the normal process of apoptosis. As a result, transformed cells proliferate without attenuation, expanding clonally. Several such clonal pools of highly aggressive cells then form tumor masses at the primary tissue of origin. Progressively, a

small fraction comprised of the most aggressive cells of these clonal populations leave their original site, spread through blood or the lymphatic circulation, colonize to other organs to form multiple secondary lesions, and continue to grow until the whole system collapses. All healthy metazoan systems, especially humans, are a complex harmony of cellular networks. All the cells of the body compensate for each other's needs, and live and die for each other to maintain an intricate balance overall. Epithelial cells interact with their basement membrane, the underlying stromal cells, and other cells at distant sites for cellular signaling. This "interaction" or signaling helps them to maintain the harmony of normal growth and apoptosis. In contrast, during the process of development of malignancy, cancer cells breach many if not all of the barriers of this cellular network. They become self-sufficient for growth and survival, and act independently of the signals from the tissue microenvironment. They create their own micromilieu inside the human body for their own means of survival. Therefore, in the context of cell biology, cancer holds a unique position and the knowledge gained in the field of cancer biology extends far beyond the limit of the disease alone.

The purpose of this chapter is to give an overview of the current understanding of cancer biology, the current view of the process of tumorigenesis, and the therapeutic and imaging implications of this biology translated into clinical applications. Experimental cancer research in the laboratory started more than a century ago, and our knowledge in understanding the biology of cancer has expanded hugely in the last three decades. Therefore, today it has become nearly impossible to be encyclopedic, enlisting tens of thousands of pertinent contributions to the field that uncovers different aspects of this disease. Thus, our approach in the present chapter will be to present a brief overview of the current understanding of cancer biology and discussion of some basic underlying concepts.

TYPES OF CANCER

The different types of cancer have been classified based on their clinical behavior and origin in different cell types. Histopathology is the conventional and the most reliable method of classifying tumors, by visualizing them under a microscope. Microscopic examination of thin tumor sections prepared from patients' tumor tissues serves as a powerful tool to both characterize and categorize tumors. Based on various microscopic features, it is possible to understand the clinical behavior of tumors, which enables pathologists to segregate them into two broad categories. Those that grow locally without invading the adjacent tissues are generally harmless and classified as benign tumors. Others that invade adjacent local tissues and spread through the blood and lymphatic circulation to distant organs by metastasis are the most lethal and are classified as malignant tumors.

Generally, three major cellular compartments of a given healthy, normal organ are seen under the microscope, namely, epithelial, stromal, and endothelial compartments. The epithelial compartment comprises structurally similar types of cells, called epithelial cells. A thin layer of such cells lines the cavities or lumens, or the outer surface of the skin. A thin layer of basement membrane separates the epithelial compartment from the underlying stromal compartment, which is a thicker layer of supporting connective tissue comprised of fibroblast cells embedded in the matrix. A third compartment is the endothelial compartment, comprised of endothelial cells lining the capillaries and large blood vessels within the stroma. Figure 1 shows a few examples of the three cellular compartments of different organs and their origins from the three distinct layers of embryo. Tumors may arise from all of the cellular compartments (as shown in Table 1) with varying frequencies of occurrence and degrees of aggressiveness.

A majority of tumors arise from epithelial cells and are termed carcinomas. Carcinomas are responsible for more than 80% of cancer-related deaths. Largely, carcinomas fall into two categories. Squamous cell carcinoma is a tumor originating from the epithelial cells that mainly serve as a protective layer of an organ. An example is the epithelial lining of the esophagus and oral cavity. The second category is the adenocarcinoma, which originates from the secretory epithelial cells. Secretory epithelial cells secrete products to protect organs. The lung and stomach epithelium secrete mucus, which protects the lungs from airborne particles and the stomach from gastric acid, respectively.

Tumors of the connective tissues are termed sarcomas. This type of cancer constitutes only about 1% of total tumors. Sarcomas originate from cells that are mesenchymal in origin, for example, fibroblasts secrete collagen and other extracellular matrix components, adipocytes store fat; osteoblasts form bones, and myocytes form muscles. A very rare type of tumor, called angiosarcoma, arises from endothelial cells lining the blood vessels.

Other major non-epithelial tumors derived from cells in the central and peripheral nervous systems are often termed neuroectodermal tumors. Although they comprise only 1.3% of all diagnosed cancers, they are responsible for about 2.5% of all cancer-related deaths. Neuroectodermal tumors include glioma, glioblastoma, neuroblastoma, schwannoma, and medulloblastoma.

The tumors discussed above are mostly "solid tumors" as they form visible solid masses. There are cancers of the circulating blood cells, which generally do not form visible solid masses. Leukemias are tumors arising from the hematopoietic system, comprised of cells that constitute blood. Leukemias originate from precursor cells of leukocyte lineages, and flow freely within the circulation. Although lymphomas originate from the cells of lymphoid lineages, unlike leukemias that are free-flowing, B and T lymphocytes often aggregate to form solid masses frequently found in the lymph nodes.

TUMORIGENESIS

Cause of Cancer: Carcinogens and Tumor Viruses

The incidence of different types of cancer varies between populations deriving from different ethnic and cultural backgrounds. Epidemiological studies have revealed that rates of cancer death and risk of onset of cancer in different organs vary with geographical location in which the victims reside. As an example, the United States is the country at highest risk of pancreatic cancer as compared to India, which is at the lowest risk of the same disease (Table 2). So lifestyle has also been strongly associated with the risk of development of certain kinds of cancer among different ethnic and cultural backgrounds, along with different geographical locations (1,2).

By the end of the nineteenth century, studies had closely associated the risk of cancer with the level of exposure to environmental chemical mutagens and

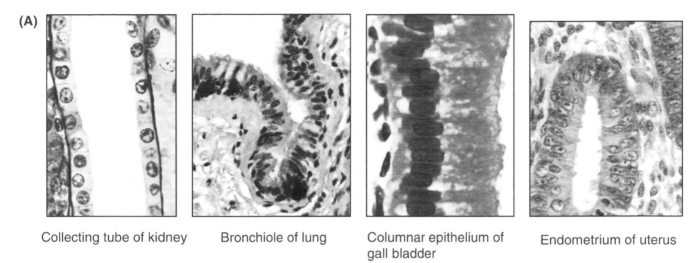

Collecting tube of kidney   Bronchiole of lung   Columnar epithelium of gall bladder   Endometrium of uterus

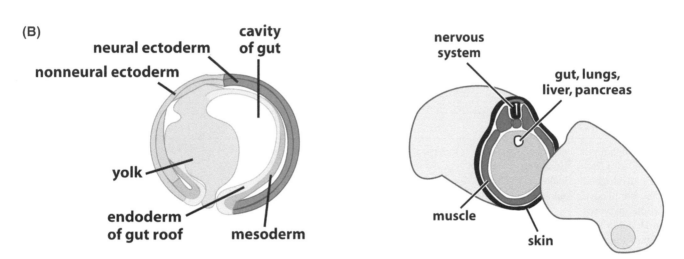

Figure 1 Architecture of normal tissues. (**A**) In kidney, lung, gall bladder, and uterine endometrium, the epithelial lining protects the underlying stroma. The basement membrane separates the epithelial and stromal layers, which are not visible under light microscope. The endothelial cells lining capillary blood vessels are visible as embedded into the stroma under light microscope. (**B**) The tissues of metazoans develop from three embryonic cell compartments—ectoderm, mesoderm, and endoderm. Each of the three embryonic cell layers is precursor to distinct types of differentiated cells. The skin and nervous system develop from the ectoderm, while the connective tissues, including bone, muscle, and blood-forming cells develop from the mesoderm. The gut and outpouchings, including lung, pancreas, and liver, develop from the endoderm.

radiation (as summarized in Table 3). At the beginning of the twentieth century, Katsusaburo Yamagiwa (1915) first reported experimental evidence of developing carcinoma in rabbits by repeated painting of the inner surface of the ear with coal tar. By 1940 British chemists purified the cancer-causing chemical components or carcinogens present in coal tar. There were certain chemicals that could induce skin cancer when applied to the skin of experimental mice (3). Compounds like 3-methylcholanthrene, benzo[a]pyrene, and 1,2,4,5-dibenz[a, h]anthracene were common products of combustion, and some of these hydrocarbons were subsequently found in the condensates of cigarette smoke as well. The chemical structures of some of these carcinogenic hydrocarbons are shown in Figure 2 (4). These findings suggested that certain chemical species entering the body could perturb the tissues and cells ultimately to cause cancer. The original compounds, which are converted to carcinogens, were called procarcinogens. Additionally, many naturally occurring foodstuffs contain carcinogenic compounds. Bruce Ames and colleagues (1983) cataloged a list of such compounds found in naturally occurring foodstuffs as listed in Table 4 (5).

Contemporary to the discovery of carcinogens, early twentieth century studies in *Drosophila* (fruit fly), showed

Table 1 Types of Tumors

Common carcinomas

Tissue sites of more common types of adenocarcinoma	Tissue sites of more common types of squamous cell carcinoma	Other types of carcinoma
Lung	Skin	Small cell lung carcinoma
Colon	Nasal cavity	Large cell lung carcinoma
Breast	Oropharynx	Hepatocellular carcinoma
Pancreas	Larynx	Renal cell carcinoma
Stomach	Lung	Transitional cell carcinoma (of urinary bladder)
Esophagus	Esophagus	
Prostate	Cervix	
Endometrium		
Ovary		

Types of sarcoma

Osteosarcoma
Liposarcoma
Leiomyosarcoma
Rhabdomyosarcoma
Malignant fibrous histiocytoma
Fibrosarcoma
Synovial sarcoma
Angiosarcoma
Chondrosarcoma

Types of lymphoid malignancies

Acute lymphocytic leukemia
Acute myelogenous leukemia
Cronic myelogenous leukemia
Cronic lymphocytic leukemia
Multiple myeloma
Non-Hodgkin's lymphoma[a]
Hodgkin's disease

[a]The non-Hodgkin's lymphoma types, also known as lymphocytic lymphomas, can be placed in as many as 15 to 20 distinct subcategories, depending on classification system.

Table 2 Countries Showing Highest and Lowest Incidence of Specific Types of Cancer[a]

Cancer site	Country at highest risk	Country at lowest risk	Relative risk H/L[b]
Skin (melanoma)	Australia (Queensland)	Japan	155
Lip	Canada (Newfoundland)	Japan	151
Nasopharynx	Hong Kong	United Kingdom	100
Prostate	United States (African American)	China	70
Liver	China (Shanghai)	Canada (Nova Scotia)	49
Penis	Brazil	Israel (Ashkenazic)	42
Cervix (uterus)	Brazil	Israel (non-Jews)	28
Stomach	Japan	Kuwait	22
Lung	United States (Louisiana, African American)	India (Chennai)	19
Pancreas	United States (Los Angeles, Korean American)	India	11
Ovary	New Zealand (Polynesian)	Kuwait	8

[a]Excerpted from Ref. 52.
[b]Relative risk: age-adjusted incidence or death rate in highest country or area (H) divided by age-adjusted incidence or death rate in lowest country or area (L).These numbers refer to age-adjusted rates, for example, the relative risk of a 60-year-old dying from a specific type of tumor in one country compared with a 60-year-old in another country.

Table 3A Environmental and Lifestyle Factors Known or Suspected to Be Etiological for Human Cancers in the United States

Type	Percentage of total cases[a]
Cancers due to occupational exposures	1–2
Lifestyle cancers	
Tobacco-related (sites: e.g., lung, bladder, kidney)	34
Diet (low in vegetables, high in nitrates, salt) (sites: e.g., stomach, esophagus)	5
Diet (high fat, lower fiber, broiled/fried foods) (sites: e.g., bowel, pancreas, prostate, breast)	37
Tobacco and alcohol (sites: mouth, throat)	2

Table 3B Specific Carcinogenic Agents Implicated in the Causation of Certain Cancers

Cancer	Exposure
Scrotal carcinomas	Chimney smoke condensates
Liver angiosarcoma	Vinyl chloride
Acute leukemias	Benzene
Nasal adenocarcinoma	Hardwood dust
Osteosarcoma	Radium
Skin carcinoma	Arsenic
Mesothelioma	Asbestos
Vaginal carcinoma	Diethylstilbestrol
Oral carcinoma	Snuff

[a]A large number of cancers are thought to be provoked by a diet high in calories acting incombination with many of these lifestyle factors.
Source: From Ref. 53.

that X-ray irradiation could cause genetic mutation or changes in genetic information in the genome. Like X-ray irradiation, a series of chemicals called alkylating agents could also cause mutation in the drosophila genome. Mustard gas, a chemical that was used in World War I, could cause such mutations. These compounds, capable of causing mutation in the DNA that could possibly lead to cancer, were termed mutagens. However, not all carcinogens are mutagens. Only about 40% of all the carcinogens studied by Ames were found to be mutagens. The rest were non-mutagenic and termed tumor promoters. Two examples of tumor-promoting non-mutagenic carcinogens are TPA (*12-O*-tetradecanoylphorbol-*13*-acetate) and PMA (phorbol-*12*-myristate-*13*-acetate). TPA alone cannot initiate a tumor, but it can promote the induction of skin adenomas via repeated painting of an area on the mouse skin that has been previously exposed to DMBA (*7,12*-dimethylbenz[*a*]anthracene), a tumor initiator carcinogen. Hence, TPA potentiated the function of DMBA in tumor formation. Figure 3 shows a schematic diagram of how a tumor initiator and a tumor promoter carcinogen could contribute to tumorigenesis (papilloma) in laboratory mice.

Chemically induced tumorigenesis by environmental or occupational hazard is a well-known phenomenon. However, the discovery of tumor viruses by Peyton Rous and others at the beginning of the twentieth century revolutionized the field of cancer research. Researchers started believing that cancer was also a viral disease like mumps, influenza, and small pox. Rigorous research in this field for the next few decades resulted in the identification of a number of tumor-causing viruses. A comprehensive list of transforming viruses is presented in Table 5. Rous sarcoma virus (RSV) was the first to be discovered. Rous

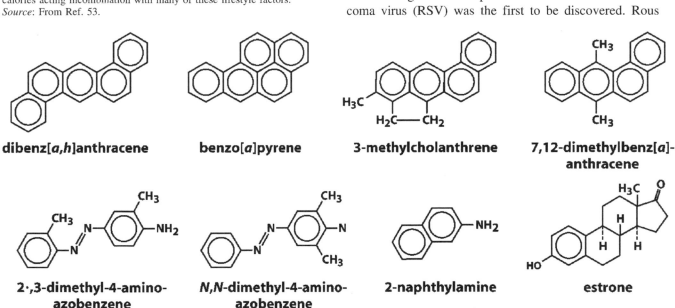

dibenz[*a,h*]anthracene   **benzo[*a*]pyrene**   **3-methylcholanthrene**   **7,12-dimethylbenz[*a*]-anthracene**

2·,3-dimethyl-4-amino-azobenzene   **N,N-dimethyl-4-amino-azobenzene**   **2-naphthylamine**   **estrone**

Figure 2 Structures of carcinogenic hydrocarbons. These chemical species arise from the incomplete combustion of organic (i.e., carbon-containing) compounds. Each of the chemical structures shown here, which were already determined before 1940, represents a chemical species that was found, following purification, to be potentially carcinogenic. *Source*: From Ref. 4.

Table 4 Ames's[a] List of Naturally Occurring Carcinogens

Foodstuff	Compound	Concentration in foodstuff
Black pepper	Piperine	100 mg/g
Common mushroom	Agaritine	2 mg/g
Celery[b]	Furocoumarins, psoralens	1 μg/g, 0.8 μg/g
Rhubarb	Anthraquinones	Varies
Cocoa powder	Theobromine	20 mg/g
Mustard, horseradish	Allyl isothiocyanate	Varies
Alfalfa sprouts	Canavanine[c]	15 mg/g
Burnt materials[d]	Large number	Varies
Coffee	Caffeic acid	11.6 mg/g

[a]Ames has cited 37 naturally occurring compounds that have been registered as carcinogens in laboratory animals; one or more have been found in each of the following foodstuffs: absinthe, allspice, anise, apple, apricot, banana, basil, beet, broccoli, Brussels sprouts, cabbage, cantaloupe, caraway, cardamom, carrot, cauliflower, celery, cherries, chili pepper, chocolate, cinnamon, cloves, coffee, collard greens, comfrey herb tea, coriander, corn, currants, dill, eggplant; endive, fennel, garlic, grapefruit, grapes, guava, honey, honeydew melon, horseradish, kale, lemon, lentils, lettuce, licorice, lime, mace, mango, marjoram, mint, mushrooms, mustard, nutmeg, onion, orange, paprika, parsley, parsnip, peach, pear, peas, black pepper, pineapple, plum, potato, radish, raspberries, rhubarb, rosemary, rutabaga, sage, savory, sesame seeds, soybean, star anise, tarragon, tea, thyme, tomato, turmeric, and turnip.
[b]The levels of these carcinogens can increase 100-fold in diseased plants.
[c]Canavanine is indirectly genotoxic because of oxygen radicals that are released, perhaps during the inflammatory reactions associated with elimination of canavanine-containing proteins.
[d]On average, several grams of burnt material is consumed daily in the form of bread crusts, burnt toast, and burnt surfaces of meats cooked at high temperature.
Source: From Refs. 54, 55.

(1911) discovered this virus from a sarcoma of chicken breast muscle. The filtered extract from chicken sarcoma could cause similar sarcoma in other chickens when injected, and also could be transmitted to the next chicken and so on (6–8). So cancer then appeared similar to an infectious disease, and the disease-causing agent was identified as a virus that could pass through the small pores of the filter. Later it was discovered that a small part of the viral genome, the viral oncogene (e.g., *src* sequence of RSV, frequently called "sark"), could be integrated into the genome of mammalian (or avian) cells as a typical viral infection, which could initiate cancer in those cells. The viral genome consists of either DNA or RNA. The RNA viruses are called retroviruses. RSV is an example of a retrovirus. The viral RNA is converted to DNA by the enzyme reverse transcriptase present in the virus, and then the resulting DNA becomes integrated into the host genome like other DNA viruses. A schematic diagram of a retrovirus virion, such as that of RSV depicting its RNA genome, is presented in Figure 4.

In 1974, Michael Bishop and Harold Varmus at the University of California, San Francisco discovered the presence of an endogenous form of the *src* sequence in uninfected mammalian cells (9,10). Eventually, it was discovered that all normal mammalian cells contain a group of such genes resembling viral gene sequences. They were termed proto-oncogenes. These proto-oncogenes are activated when their viral counterparts are integrated into the host genomes. As an example, the proto-oncogene *c-src*, the cellular counterpart of the *src* gene, was activated when the viral counterpart, called *v-src*, was integrated immediately upstream of *c-src*. Another example is the chicken retrovirus MC29- myelocytomatosis virus, which causes bone marrow malignancy in chicken. The virus contains the *v-myc* gene, and the avian or mammalian cellular counterpart of this gene, *c-myc,* is a potent proto-oncogene. The normal regulatory function of the *c-myc* gene in the mammalian cell is disrupted when, after infection, the viral oncogene *v*-myc is physically integrated immediately upstream of *c-myc*, as shown in Figure 5. Instead of being controlled by its own native promoter, *c-myc* comes under the control of the viral promoter that leads to constitutive activation. Potent oncogenes like *H-ras* and *K-ras* were discovered in the same way from Harvey and Kirsten sarcoma viruses, respectively. To date more than 30 proto-oncogenes have been discovered in this way.

In addition to activating the proto-oncogenes by genomic integration, tumor viruses can also transform a cell in a completely different way, by inactivating the function of the tumor suppressor proteins. The tumor suppressor proteins control the cell growth by acting as cell cycle checkpoints and by inducing apoptosis. The two most well studied and bona fide tumor suppressors are retinoblastoma protein (pRb) and p53. The tumor suppressor pRb acts as a cell cycle checkpoint by sequestering the E2F family of transcription factors, thereby controlling the proliferation of cells. On the other hand, p53 is a transcription factor that activates cell cycle inhibitors like p21 and many other tumor suppressor genes. Both pRb and p53 regulate apoptosis in normal cells by regulating mitochondrial apoptotic pathways. Loss of function of *Rb* or *p53* genes is a hallmark of many cancers. The adenoviral oncoproteins, E1A and HPV E7, inactivate pRb, while HPV E6 inactivates p53.

Only 15% of all cancers are caused by viruses. Common examples of cancer caused by tumor viruses include liver cancers mainly occurring in Southeast Asia, cervical cancers occurring all over the world, and Burkitt's lymphoma occurring in southern China and West Africa. The other major modes of genetic alterations found in most cancers are discussed in the following sections. However, research in the field of tumor-causing viruses has been gradually waning due to lack of evidence establishing virus as the sole cause of cancer. Nevertheless, the significant contributions of tumor virology and viral genetics

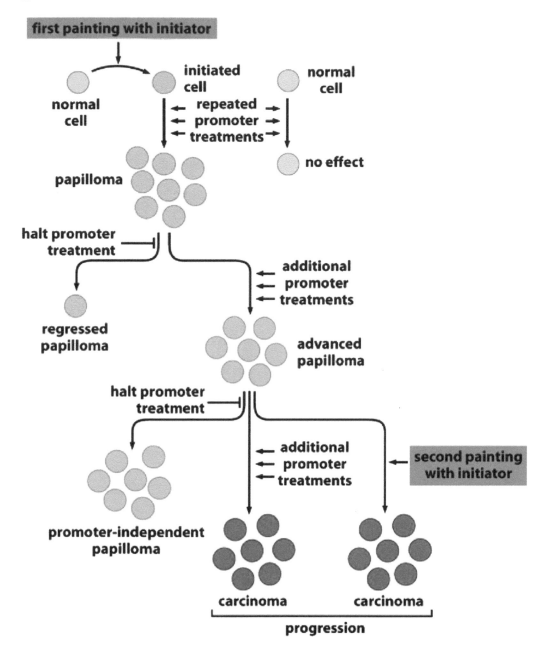

Figure 3 Scheme of initiation and promotion of epidermal carcinomas in mice. The initiating agent converts a normal cell (*gray, top left*) into a mutant, initiated cell (*top middle*). Repeated treatment of the initiated cells with the TPA promoter generates a papilloma (*cluster of cells*), while TPA treatment of a normal, adjacent cell (*gray, top right*) has no effect. Further treatment of the initially formed papilloma can be halted (*middle left*), in which case, the papilloma regresses. Alternatively, further repeated treatment of the initially formed papilloma can yield more progressed papilloma (*cluster of cells, middle*), which persists even after promoter treatment is halted (*cluster of cells, bottom left*); further repeated treatment of this more progressed papilloma with TPA eventually yields, with low frequency, a carcinoma (*bottom middle*). Alternatively, exposure of the initially formed papilloma to a second treatment by the initiating agent yields doubly mutant cells that also form a carcinoma (*bottom right*). *Abbreviation*: TPA, 12-O-tetradecanoylphorbol-13-acetate.

have provided many tools for cancer researchers who can now experimentally manipulate cellular DNA, in turn providing insight into details of cancer genetics. Therefore, tumor virology of the 1970s has created a foundation for the study of cancer genetics in the modern era.

Cancer Genetics

Since the discovery of cancer-related genes, proto-oncogenes and tumor suppressor genes, the field of cancer genetics has been a major subfield within cancer research.

Table 5 List of Transforming Viruses

Name of virus[a]	Viral oncogene	Species	Major disease	Nature of oncoprotein
Rous sarcoma	*src*	Chicken	Sarcoma	Non-receptor TK
Y73/Esh sarcoma	*yes*	Chicken	Sarcoma	Non-receptor TK
Fujinami sarcoma	*fps*[b]	Chicken	Sarcoma	Non-receptor TK
UR2	*ros*	Chicken	Sarcoma	RTK; unknown ligand
Myelocytomatosis 29	*myc*	Chicken	Myeloid leukemia[c]	Transcription factor
Mill Hill virus 2	*mil*[d]	Chicken	Myeloid leukemia	ser/thr kinase
Avian myeloblastosis E26	*myb*	Chicken	Myeloid leukemia	Transcription factor
Avian myeloblastosis E26	*ets*	Chicken	Myeloid leukemia	Transcription factor
Avian erythroblastosis ES4	*erbA*	Chicken	Erythroleukemia	Thyroid hormone receptor
Avian erythroblastosis ES4	*erbB*	Chicken	Erythroleukemia	EGF RTK
3611 murine sarcoma	*raf*[e]	Mouse	Sarcoma	ser/thr kinase
SKV770	*ski*	Chicken	Endothelioma	Transcription factor
Reticuloendotheliosis	*rel*	Turkey	Immature E-cell transcription	Lymphoma factor
Abelson murine leukemia	*abl*	Mouse	Pre-B-cell lymphoma	Non-receptor TK
Moloney murine sarcoma	*mos*	Mouse	Sarcoma, erythroleukemia	ser/thr kinase
Harvey murine sarcoma	*H-ras*	Rat, mouse	Sarcoma	Small G protein
Kirsten murine sarcoma	*K-ras*	Mouse	Sarcoma	Small G protein
FBJ murine sarcoma	*fos*	Mouse	Osteosarcoma	Transcription factor
Snyder-Theilen feline sarcoma	*fes*[f]	Cat	Sarcoma	Non-receptor TK
McDonough feline sarcoma	*fms*	Cat	Sarcoma	CSF-1 RTK
Gardner-Rasheed feline sarcoma	*fgr*	Cat	Sarcoma	Non-receptor TK
Hardy-Zuckerman feline sarcoma	*kit*	Cat	Sarcoma	Steel factor RTK
Simian sarcoma	*sis*	Woolly monkey	Sarcoma	PDGF
AKT8	*akt*	Mouse	Lymphoma	ser/thr kinase
Avian virus S13	*sea*	Chicken	Erythroblastic leukemia[g]	RTK, unknown ligand
Myeloproliferative leukemia	*mpl*	Mouse	Myeloproliferation	TPO receptor
Regional poultry lab virus 30	*eyk*	Chicken	Sarcoma	RTK; unknown ligand
Avian sarcoma virus CT10	*crk*	chicken	Sarcoma	SH2/SH3 adaptor
Avian sarcoma virus 17	*jun*	Chicken	Sarcoma	Transcription factor
Avian sarcoma virus 31	*qin*	Chicken	Sarcoma	Transcription factor[h]
A542 sarcoma virus	*maf*	Chicken	Sarcoma	Transcription factor
Cas NS-1 virus	*cbl*	Mouse	Lymphoma	SH2-dependent ubiquitylation

Abbreviations: CSF, colony-stimulating factor; EGF, epidermal growth factor; G, GTP-binding; PDGF, platelet-derived growth factor; RTK, receptor tyrosine kinase; ser/thr, serine/threonine; SH, src homology segment; TK, tyrosine kinase; TPO, thrombopoietin.
[a]Not all viruses that have yielded these oncogenes are indicated here.
[b]Ortholog of the mammalian *fes* oncogene.
[c]Also causes carcinomas and endotheliomas.
[d]Ortholog of the mammalian *rai* oncogene.
[e]Ortholog of the avian *mil* oncogene.
[f]Otholog of the avian *fps* oncogene.
[g]Also causes granulocytic leukemias and sarcomas.
[h]Functions as a transcriptional repressor.
Source: From Refs. 56, 57.

The last three decades of research in this area has lead to an explosion of knowledge. Consequently, modern cancer research has been revolutionized by advances in the genetics and molecular biology of cancer. Today it is firmly believed that "cancer is a genetic disease" (11). Thousands of genes have been identified to be related to cancer, as alterations of such genes contribute to the development of tumors. An interesting point about cancer genetics is that no single gene defect causes cancer, unlike other genetic diseases such as cystic fibrosis or muscular dystrophy. Rather, it is a series of alterations in the genome that leads to tumorigenesis. Categorically, alterations of three types of genes are responsible for tumorigenesis: oncogenes, tumor suppressor genes, and stability genes. The group of genes whose overactivity promotes tumor formation are termed oncogenes. The second group

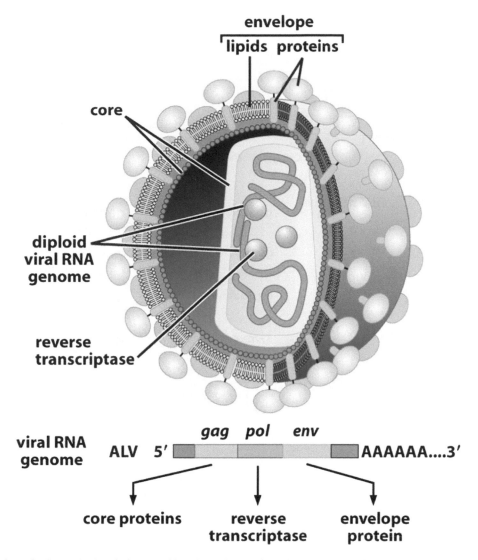

Figure 4 The virion of RSV and related viruses. This schematic drawing of the structure of a retrovirus virion, such as that of RSV, indicates three major types of viral proteins. The glycoprotein spikes (encoded by viral *env* gene) protrude from lipid bilayer that surrounds the virion; these spikes enable the virion to attach to the surface of a cell and to introduce the internal contents of the virion into its cytoplasm. These include a complex protein coat formed by the several core proteins encoded by viral *gag* gene. Within this protein shell are found two identical copies of the viral genomic RNA and a number of reverse transcriptase enzyme molecules specified by the viral *pol* gene. *Abbreviation*: RSV, Rous sarcoma virus.

of genes, which normally protect the cell from tumor formation and are often inactivated in cancers, are termed tumor suppressor genes. The third group of genes, the stability genes, repair the subtle mistakes made in DNA during the normal course of replication. Balanced action of these three types of genes maintains normalcy in the cells, whereas their functional misbalance causes malignancy (12).

Although a very small fraction of certain cancers displays an obvious hereditary influence (i.e., inherited genetic mutations), the majority of cancer is caused by sporadic genetic alterations. Interestingly, the sporadic alterations also exactly recapitulate the same genetic alterations as the inherited ones. As an example, approx-

imately 0.5% of colorectal cancer patients inherit a defective adenomatous polyposis coli (*APC*) tumor suppressor gene from one of their parents, and the rest (> 99%) do not inherit this gene. More than 90% of sporadic cases of colon cancer are also detected with the same loss of function of the *APC* gene as an early genetic alteration in this disease. In the western world, hereditary influence accounts for cancer in the range of 0.1% to 10%, depending on tumor type. However, this inherited mutation is not sufficient to initiate tumorigenesis. Further mutations are needed to develop a tumor. As an example, for patients who have "loss of function" of *APC* in both of their alleles, every cell of the colon is "at risk" for acquiring a second mutation. Two mutations of the "right type" are

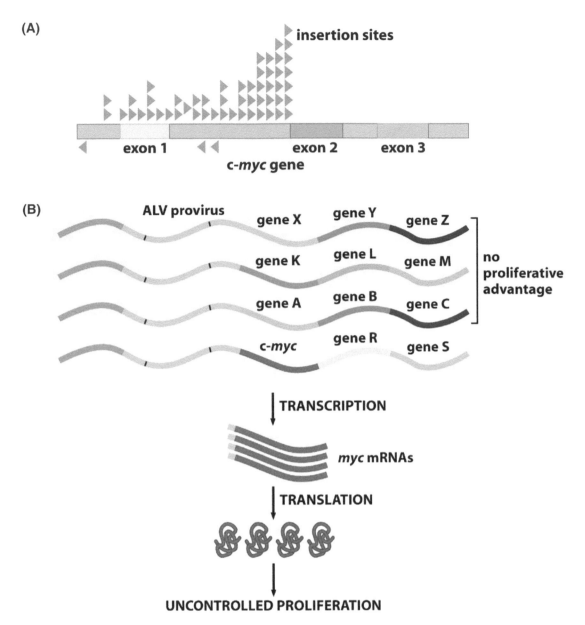

Figure 5 Insertional mutagenesis. (**A**) A large proportion of the ALV proviruses were integrated into the chromosomal DNA segment carrying the *c-myc* proto-oncogene; the majority were integrated between the first noncoding exon of *c-myc* and the second exon, in which the *myc* reading frame begins. The integration sites are shown in the figure (*filled triangles*). As indicated, most but not all of the proviruses were integrated in the same transcriptional orientation as that of the *c-myc* gene. (**B**) In the course of ALV infection of the chicken lymphocytes, ALV proviruses become integrated randomly at millions of different sites in the chromosomal DNA of the lymphocytes. On rare occasions, an ALV provirus becomes integrated (by chance) within the *c-myc* proto-oncogene. This may then cause transcription of the *c-myc* gene to be driven by the strong, constitutively acting ALV promoter. Because high levels of the Myc protein are potent in driving cell proliferation, the cell carrying this particular integrated provirus and activated *c-myc* gene will now multiply uncontrollably, eventually spawning a large host of descendants that will constitute a lymphoma. *Abbreviation*: ALV, avian leukemia virus.

believed to be sufficient for initiation of tumorigenesis. Also, the "gain of function" of an oncogene and "loss of function" of a tumor suppressor gene are often coupled together in many tumors. Colon cancers are frequently found to have "loss of function" of tumor suppressor genes *APC* (>90% cases) and *p53* (60% to 70% of cases) coupled with mutated (constitutively active) *ras* oncogene (40% to 50% cases). Another example is pancreatic cancer in which more than (~90–95%) of cases have been identified with a "gain of function" mutation of the *ras* oncogene coupled with deletion (loss of function) of the *p16* tumor suppressor gene (~90% of cases).

The following major mechanisms of genetic alterations could account for tumorigenesis:

1. *Point mutations*: Point mutations in the coding sequence of some oncogenes result in the substitution of one specific amino acid for another in the primary protein sequence. These alterations make the oncoprotein constitutively active. As in the case of *ras*, a point mutation in either codon 12, 13, or 61 of the gene encoding the Ras enzyme makes the enzyme constitutively active. Mutation of codon 12 results in glycine being substituted by valine (commonly designated as *ras*^{G12V}), which is the most frequent gain-of-function mutation in many cancers. Ras is a GTP-binding protein, a monomeric GTPase that functions as a switch, cycling between two distinct conformational states. It is active when bound to GTP and inactive when bound to GDP. Normally, the guanine nucleotide exchange factors (GEFs) stimulate the dissociation of GDP and subsequent uptake of GTP from the cytosol, thereby activating Ras. Conversely, GTPase-activating proteins (GAPs) stimulate the hydrolysis of the bound GTP by Ras, thereby inactivating Ras. Mutated Ras is resistant to GAP-mediated GTPase stimulation and therefore remains permanently in the GTP-bound active state. Table 6 shows a list of common tumors with their proportions detected with mutations in the *ras* gene.

Similar to the "gain of function" point mutation, there can also be a "loss of function" point mutation. An example of such a point mutation is in the p53 tumor suppressor protein–encoding gene, which disables its function. The primary protein sequence of p53 contains 393 amino acid residues. The central region, between 100 and 300 amino acid residues, is the DNA-binding domain. The protein p53 binds to the DNA as a homotetramer. The coding regions of the *p53* gene are hot spots for frequent mutations in cancer, which disable its DNA-binding activity, as explained in Figure 6. More than 50% of all types of cancer have been identified with inactivation of p53.

Table 6 Ras Mutations in Various Tumors

Tumor type	Proportion (%) of tumors carrying a point-mutated *ras* gene
Pancreas	90 (K)
Thyroid (papillary)	60 (H, K, N)
Thyroid (follicular)	55 (H, K, N)
Colorectal	45 (K)
Seminoma	45 (K, N)
Myelodysplasia	40 (N, K)
Lung (non–small cell)	35 (K)
Acute myelogenous leukemia	30 (N)
Liver	30 (N)
Melanoma	15 (K)
Bladder	10 (K)
Kidney	10 (H)

Abbreviations: H, human H-ras gene; K, human K-ras gene; N, human N-ras gene.
Source: From Ref. 58.

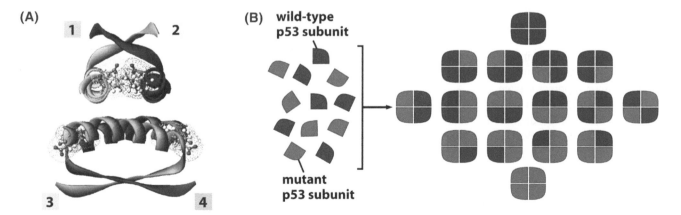

Figure 6 Mechanism of *p53*-dominant negative mutations. (**A**) The tetramerization domain of p53, composed of an α-helix as revealed here by use of X-ray crystallography. This domain usually remains intact in the mutant p53 proteins found in tumor cells, enabling these mutant proteins to form tetramers with other mutant or wild-type p53 proteins. The four helical domains illustrated here (*1–4*), each in a different color, are assembled in two pairs, the pairs assembling right angles to one another. (**B**) The p53 protein normally functions as a homotetrameric transcription factor. However, in cells bearing a single mutant *p53* allele that encodes a structurally altered protein, the mutant protein may retain its ability to form tetramers but may lose its ability to exert normal p53 function. Consequently, mixed tetramers composed of differing proportions of wild-type and mutant subunits may form, and the presence of even a single mutant protein subunit may compromise the functioning of entire tetramer. Therefore, in a cell that is heterozygous at the *p53* locus, 15/16 of the subunits may lack fully normal function.

Although there are other means of inactivation of p53 in cancers, the biallelic loss of function of the *p53* gene contributes significantly to tumor development.

2. *Chromosomal deletion*: Somatic or germline loss of a chromosome is frequently observed in cancers. It may be the loss of the whole chromosome (aneuploidy) or loss of a particular fragment of DNA in the chromosome, for example, homozygous or hemizygous deletion of exon 2 of INK4/ARF locus at chromosome 9p21, which has been detected in more than 90% of acute lymphoblastic leukemias (ALL) in children.

3. *Loss of heterozygosity (LOH)*: Aneuploidy is a common event in most cancers that results in the change of chromosome numbers ranging from subdiploid to supradiploid. However, karyotypic detection of aneuploidy is an underestimation of the degree of gross chromosomal abnormalities that occur in cancer cells. Even if the cells appear to have two normal copies of chromosomes, molecular studies have revealed that both of the chromosomes are often from the same parent. Thus, instead of one maternal and one paternal chromosome copy per cell, both copies of the same chromosome may come from paternal origin with no chromosome from maternal origin. This LOH often affects more than half of the chromosomes in an individual cancer cell, which cannot otherwise be detected in conventional karyotypic analyses. LOH provides an efficient way for cancer cells to inactivate genes. If an inactivating mutation occurs in one allele of a chromosome containing tumor suppressor gene(s), the other, still-intact wild-type allele can take over the function and prevent abnormalities in the phenotype, unless it is functionally lost by LOH. Most of the tumor suppressor genes are inactivated by two-step mechanisms: first, by an inactivating mutation and second, by LOH, which completely abrogates the function of the tumor suppressor gene.

4. *Amplifications*: Overactivity of one or more oncogenes at a time can be the result of a five- to a hundred-fold amplification of a small region of chromosome (0.3 to 10 Mb). As an example, amplification of chromosome 12 is very common in many cancers. Chromosomal amplification results in overexpression of the oncogenes residing within the amplified region due to increase in copy number, such as oncogene mouse double minute 2 (*mdm2*) residing in chromosome 12q13-15, which has been found commonly in sarcomas (>40% of sarcomas). This part of the chromosome commonly appears as extrachromosomal "double minutes"—the small segments of chromosome that have broken loose from their original site and have been replicating as extrachromosomal elements. The double minutes are frequently amplified

in many cancers, increasing the copy number of the oncogenes residing within it. Table 7 shows some frequently amplified oncogenes and their chromosomal locations.

5. *Chromosomal translocations*: Chromosomal translocation is an important genetic alteration in cancer in which a part of one chromosome is cleaved and integrated into another chromosome. In solid tumors, the translocations are random; there is no site specificity for the break points or point of insertion. On the other hand, liquid tumors such as leukemia and lymphoma generally contain characteristic translocations. For example, in acute promyelocytic leukemia (PML), there is virtually always a characteristic translocation of t(15;17) resulting in the fusion of a *retinoic acid receptor* gene on chromosome 17 with the *PML* gene on chromosome 15. In chronic myelogenous leukemia (CML), there are always t(9;22) translocations resulting in fusion of the *abl* oncogene on chromosome 9 with the *BCR* gene on chromosome 22.

Cancer Epigenetics

In addition to genetic abnormalities as discussed above, epigenetic alterations in cancer also play an important role in tumorigenesis. Epigenetics is defined as heritable changes in gene expression that do not involve any changes in the DNA sequence (13). Epigenetic alterations (e.g., gene silencing) mostly involve the covalent modifications of histones and other chromatin components. Epigenetic silencing plays a very important role in the normal growth and development of metazoans. It influences the processes of cellular proliferation, differentiation, and stem cell maturation at various stages of development. Many genes in the mammalian genome are silenced as part of their normal functioning. As an example, the X chromosome is silenced epigenetically over the lifespan of a female mammal. In another example, the series of gene inactivations during the normal process of aging are mediated through epigenetic silencing. These silencing pattern(s) or epigenetic modification(s) of chromatin are inherited through both somatic (inherited to the daughter cells through mitotic divisions) and germline inheritance (inherited through the offspring). Dysregulation of the silencing patterns leads to the development of many disease states including cancer. Several modes of epigenetic silencing in cancer that have been characterized to date are as follows:

1. *Promoter hypermethylation*: Promoter hypermethylation silences several tumor suppressor genes in cancer, which is probably the best studied epigenetic silencing mode in this disease. The process of DNA methylation is a normal epigenetic modification of the human genome. It is observed at the specific

Table 7 Examples of Some Commonly Amplified Oncogenes

Name of oncogene[a]	Human chromosomal location	Human cancers	Nature of protein
ErbB1	7q12-13	Glioblastomas (50%); squamous cell carcinomas (10%–20%)	RTK
cab1-erbB2-grb7	17q12	Gastric, ovarian, breast carcinomas (10%–25%)	RTK, adaptor protein
k-sam	7q26	Gastric, breast carcinomas (10%–20%)	RTK
FGF-R1	8p12	Breast carcinomas (10%)	RTK
met	7q31	Gastric carcinomas (20%)	RTK
K-ras	6p12	Lung, ovarian, bladder carcinomas (5%–10%)	Small G protein
N-ras	1p13	Head and neck cancers (30%)	TF
c-myc	8q24	Various leukemias, carcinomas (10%–50%)	TF
L-myc	1p32	Lung carcinomas (10%)	TF
N-myc-DDX1	2p24-25	Neuroblastomas, lung carcinomas (30%)	TF
akt-1	14q32-33	Gastric cancers (20%)	Ser/thr kinase
cyclin D1-exp1-hst1-ems1	(11q13)	Breast and squamous cell carcinomas (40%–50%)	G1 cyclin
cdk4-mdm2-sas-gli	12q13	Sarcomas (40%)	CDK, p53 antagonist
cyclin E	19q12	Gastric cancers (15%)	cyclin
akt2	(19q13)	Pancreatic, ovarian cancers (30%)	ser/thr kinase
AIB1, BTAK	(20q12-13)	Breast cancers (15%)	Receptor co-activator
cdk6	(19q21-22)	Gliomas (5%)	CDK
myb	6q23-24	Colon carcinoma, leukemias	TF
ets-1	11q23	Lymphoma	TF
gli	12q13	Glioblastomas	TF
FGFR2	10q26	Breast carcinomas	RTK

[a]The listing of several genes indicates the frequent co-amplification of a number of closely linked genes; only the products of the most frequently amplified genes are described in the right column.
Abbreviations: AIB1, Amplified in Breast Cancer-1; CDK, cyclin dependent kinase; FGFR1/2, fibroblast growth factor receptor1/2; G, GTP-binding; ser/thr, serine/threonine; RTK, receptor tyrosine kinase; TF, transcription factor.
Source: From Ref. 57.

regions of the promoters approximately 200 base pairs upstream of the transcription start site rich in the repeated sequence of cytosine-guanine (>45% rich C-G sequences, called the "CpG islands"). The DNA methylation reaction always occurs asymmetrically (i.e., one of the two DNA strands at a time) by covalent addition of a methyl group at the $5'$ carbon of the cytosine ring in the C-G repeat sequences, resulting in $5'$-methyl cytosine residues at the CpG islands. These added methyl groups bulge into the major grove of DNA and efficiently inhibit the binding of the transcription factors to the putative promoter regions. This results in the inhibition of gene transcription. The methylation reaction is catalyzed by DNA methyltransferase enzymes. It has been reported that more than 95% of human genomic methylation is mediated through two DNA methyltransferases, DNMT1 and DNMT3β (11). In cancer the alterations of the entire genomic methylation pattern or "global methylation mark" results in the silencing of a whole host of tumor suppressor genes. A typical example of tumor suppressor gene silencing is the inactivation of p16 in colon cancer by promoter

hypermethylation of its encoding gene at the *INK4/ARF* locus (14–17).

2. *Histone modification*: Covalent modifications of the specific lysine residues of histones by acetylation/deacetylation/methylation lead to global epigenetic alterations in the genome. As an example, loss of acetylation at lysine 16 and trimethylation at lysine 20 of histone H4 is a common hallmark of many human cancers. The global histone modification pattern or "histone mark" can predict the risk of prostate cancer recurrence.

3. *Physical modification of chromatin structure*: Nucleosomal positioning (the "open" or "closed" chromatin structures) greatly influences the transcription of that particular part of the genome, which then determines the expression levels of several genes. Nonhistone chromatin architectural proteins such as the high mobility group (HMG) family of proteins play a pivotal role in nucleosomal positioning by means of histone displacement from the chromatin (18,19).

4. *MicroRNAs*: Certain noncoding short RNA sequences, the microRNAs, are involved in silencing a number of important tumor suppressor genes in

cancer. The growing list of specific microRNAs interfering with gene expression patterns in several cancers suggests an existence of an entire "micro RNome," which is altered in certain cancers and results in the alterations in gene expression pattern in these cancers.

Epigenetic changes are more frequent in altering gene expression patterns in cancer than genetic mutations. Alterations in gene expression pattern induced by epigenetic events give rise to a cellular growth advantage selected by the host organs that contributes to tumorigenesis. However, growing evidence suggests that it is not a single gene silencing or a single histone "mark" that develops tumor, but rather, it is the whole group of genes that may be inactivated as a part of the abnormal "program." Moreover, epigenetic changes collaborate with genetic abnormalities. Together they confer a selective advantage to cancer cells and are also important for complementing each other in the development of malignancy.

Theories of Tumorigenesis

Tumors originate from the normal cells of the body. Several lines of evidence suggest that tumorigenesis is a multistep process. The genetic/epigenetic alterations drive the progressive transformation of normal cells into highly malignant derivatives. It is not yet clear whether this multistep transformation occurs randomly in any somatic cell of the body or whether a special pool of progenitor cells within the organ (stem cells) harbor these genetic/

epigenetic alterations to produce cancer cells in a hierarchical fashion contributing to tumorigenesis. Stochastic theory explains that the mutations (or epigenetic changes) could take place in any cell of the body because of any physical/chemical mutagens from environmental factors or deregulation of the endogenous machinery of the cell. The first set of mutations confer on the cells a growth advantage over the other normal cells. This growth advantage, with an accelerated replication, may lead to clonal expansion of a pool of immortalized cells. As a result of accelerated replication, these cells become increasingly susceptible to further mutations. The end result is the transformation into highly heterogeneous subpopulations of clonally expanded tumor cells. On the other hand, the hierarchical theory suggests that the mutations are more likely to occur in the adult stem cells as these cells have a prolonged life span with much more replicative potential than the normal somatic cells. The genetic/epigenetic changes may alter the phenotype, transforming the adult stem cells into "cancer stem cells" (CSCs). These CSCs eventually give rise to the heterogeneous pools of clonally expanded cancer cells simultaneously maintaining their own clonal population through typical "stem cell–like propagation." Figure 7 represents a schematic diagram explaining the stochastic and hierarchical models of tumorigenesis (20).

Multistep Tumor Progression Model

It is believed that cancer is the end result of a complex sequence of events. Most cancers require an extended

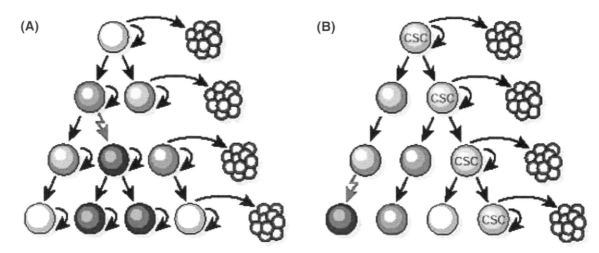

Figure 7 Stochastic and hierarchical model of tumorigenesis. Two general models of heterogeneity in solid cancer cells. (A) Cancer cells of many different phenotypes have the potential to proliferate extensively, but any one cell would have a low probability of exhibiting this potential in an assay of clonogenicity or tumorigenicity. (B) Most cancer cells have only limited proliferative potential, but a subset of cancer cells consistently proliferate extensively in clonogenic assays and can form new tumors on transplantation. The model shown in A predicts that a distinct subset of cells are enriched for the ability to form new tumors, whereas most cells are depleted of this ability. Existing therapeutic approaches have been based largely on the model shown in a, but the failure of these therapies to cure most solid cancers suggests that the model shown in B may be more accurate. *Abbreviation*: CSC, cancer stem cell.

period of time for their final onset or development as malignant. The insight or "clue" for the notion that cancer is a multistep process comes from the fact that most cancers are diagnosed in people at an older age. In the United States, the risk of dying from colon cancer is 1,000 times greater in a 70-year-old man than in a 10-year-old boy. The multistep tumor progression model has been best described in the example of the epithelia of the intestine. The normal intestinal epithelial layer facing the lumen is only one cell thick in most places of the intestine. Cells of the intestinal epithelium are in constant flux. Each minute, 20 to 50 million cells in the duodenum and at least 2 to 5 million cells in the colon die, and equal numbers of cells are replenished by newly forming cells. This epithelial layer is the major site for the pathological changes associated with colon carcinoma. Histopathological analysis of various colon biopsies reveals a variety of tissue states with degrees of abnormalities that range from mildly deviant tissue barely distinguishable from the normal histology to the chaotic jumble of cells forming highly malignant tissue that are clearly distinguishable under the microscope by their shape and size. A little hyperproliferation of cells showing almost normal histology appearing as "thicker-than-normal epithelia" is termed hyperplastic. When epithelial cellular abnormality reaches an extent at which it no longer follows an orderly growth of the epithelial layer, it is termed dysplastic. A thicker dysplastic epithelial layer with a more deviant growth pattern is termed a polyp or adenoma. In the colon, cellular transformation up to the formation of polyps is considered benign. Polyps are mostly formed in the crypts of the colon, and some sporadic polyps can be attached to the wall. These small growths or precancerous lesions consist of cells that are not yet fully transformed. A more advanced growth that ultimately breaches the underlying basement membrane into the stroma and further metastasizes to distant organs is called malignant (3).

Three lines of evidence strongly support the multistep tumor progression model in colon cancer. First, on rare occasions, an outgrowth of carcinoma from an adenomatous polyp is visible. Secondly, in clinical studies performed with large cohorts of patients, there was almost an 80% reduction of incidence of colon carcinoma in patients whose polyps were removed, as compared with the patients whose polyps were not removed after detection by colonoscopy. Finally, in the disease familial adenomatous polyposis (FAP), individuals inherit a mutant form of the *APC* tumor suppressor gene and are prone to develop from dozens to more than one thousand polyps in the intestine. Some polyps spontaneously progress into carcinoma explaining the higher risk of colon cancers in these patients.

Colon cancer is the best studied model for stepwise progression of tumorigenesis for the following reasons: it is the most common cancer in the United States. The colon is a relatively accessible organ; therefore, a large number of samples can be collected from different clinical stages of premalignant and malignant growths as determined by colonoscopy of the patients. Researchers at Johns Hopkins University, led by Bert Vogelstein, have contributed extensively to understanding the genetic basis of this disease (21). The genetic analysis of colonic epithelial tissues ranging from normal through different stages of preneoplastic to aggressive high-grade malignancy paralleled progressive accumulation of genetic alterations. The first genetic alteration found in the hyperplastic colonic epithelium was the loss of function of the *APC* gene, located at the chromosome 5q21, a common target of LOH in colonic preneoplasia. In the next stage of early to late adenomas, mutated *ras* is common (40% to 50%). Finally, the loss of function of p53 (chromosome 17p13) transforms them to aggressive carcinoma. Figure 8A represents a schematic diagram explaining the multistep tumor progression model of colon cancer, and Figure 8B represents a histological section of colon showing different stages of tumor formation, from normal epithelium through malignant adenocarcinoma.

Similarly, breast, prostate, and pancreatic cancers also progress through multistep preneoplastic condition to frank neoplasia. Breast carcinoma in situ (BCIS), prostate intraepithelial neoplasia (PIN), and pancreatic intraepithelial neoplasia (PanIN) progress to an advanced stage of malignant carcinoma with progressive accumulation of genetic alterations typical of each stage of preneoplastic and neoplastic diseases (22).

Darwinian Model of Evolution and Cancer Progression

An interesting speculation that tumor development could be better understood in terms of the biological processes resembling Darwinian evolution has been strongly supported by recent results of genetic analysis of cancers, especially colon cancer. We can consider the individual cancer cell as an evolving unit competing with other cells in a population of cells in the tumor microenvironment, analogous to individual species in nature competing with each other for survival. A random mutation in a cell confers a growth advantage of that particular cell over the other neighboring cells, which results in the domination of a clonal expansion of that particular cell. When the number of cells in that privileged clone reaches at least a million, a second mutation (considering a probability of one in a million per generation) may occur in any cell within that clonal population. If the second mutation is of the "right type," the resulting doubly mutated cell will proliferate even more than the rest of the million cells in the first selected clone. Eventually the expansion of the

(A)

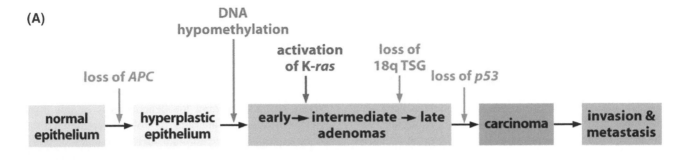

(B) normal mucosa

dysplastic mucosa

adenocarcinoma

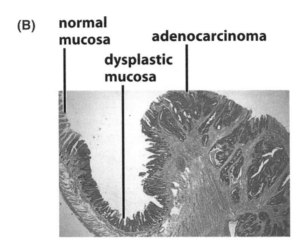

Figure 8 Multistep tumor progression model of colon cancer (**A**) Each of the chromosomal regions that underwent loss of heterozygosity was considered to harbor a TSG whose loss provided growth advantage to evolving preneoplastic colonic epithelial cells. Eventually two TSGs were identified—*APC* on chromosome 5q and p53 on chromosome 17p. The identity of the inactivated TSG or TSGs on chromosome 18q remains unclear. In addition, as indicated here, about half of the colon carcinomas were found to acquire mutant, activated alleles of K-*ras* gene, and the genomes of most evolving, preneoplastic growths were found to suffer hypomethylation (loss of methylated CpGs). The precise contribution of hypomethylation to tumor progression remains unclear; some evidence suggests that it creates chromosomal instability. (**B**) This histological section of the lining of ileum in the small intestine, viewed at low magnification, reveals the continuity between normal and cancerous tissues and also supports the multistep tumor progression model. To the left is the normal epithelial lining, termed the mucosa. In the middle is mucosal tissue that has become highly abnormal, being termed "dysplastic." To the right is a frank tumor—an adenocarcinoma—which has begun to invade underlying tissues. *Abbreviation*: TSG, tumor suppressor gene.

second clone may dominate over its precursors by over-shadowing or even obliterating the precursor clone from which it arose. A third mutation may repeat this process of another clonal selection. Therefore, it is possible that a sequence of four to six such clonal successions, each triggered by a specific mutation, suffices to explain how cancer progression occurs at the cellular or genetic level as explained in Figure 9.

Stem Cell Model of Tumorigenesis

Growing evidence suggests the existence of CSCs and strongly supports a hierarchical theory of tumorigenesis. This model is at odds with the Darwinian model of clonal selection. The Darwinian model explains the clonal succession triggered by sporadic or randomly occurring muta-

tions in a randomly selected cell from a whole population. The assumption here is that all cells in a selected clone have equal possibility to harbor the genetic alterations and are thereby equally capable of developing tumor. Recent evidence suggests that only a small fraction of cells isolated from human tumors are capable of developing a tumor. The major bulk of tumor cells lack tumorigenic potential. The tumor cells isolated from a single tumor were separated into two distinct subclasses with different biological properties. Tumor cells from the subclass that had tumorigenic potential were termed tumor progenitors or CSCs. In breast cancer (Fig. 10), a specific, small pool of cells with specific "surface markers $CD24^{low}CD44^{high}ESA^+$," as isolated from the tumor, are responsible for malignancy but not the other cells, which do not possess these surface markers. Tumor arising from this thin fraction showed a similar

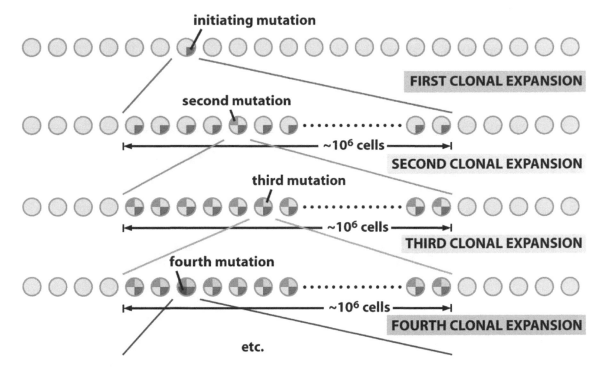

Figure 9 The Darwinian model of tumorigenesis. The Darwinian evolution involves expansions of organisms that are endowed with advantageous genotypes and thus phenotypes; a similar scheme seems to describe how tumor progression occurs. One cell amid a large cell population sustains an initiating mutation that confers on it a proliferative and/or survival advantage compared with those cells lacking this mutation. Eventually the clonal descendants of this mutant cell dominate in a localized area by displacing the cells that lack this mutation, resulting in the first clonal expansion. When this clone expands to a large-enough size (e.g., 10^6 cells), the occurrence of a second mutation that strikes with a frequency of 10^{-6} per cell generation may occur, resulting in a doubly mutated cell that has even greater proliferative and/or survival advantage. The process of clonal expansion then repeats itself, and the newly mutated population displaces (succeeds) the previously formed one. This results once again in a large descendant population, in which a third mutation occurs, and so forth.

pattern of distribution as the two distinct subpopulations. This indicates that these cells have self renewal capacity as well as the capacity to generate other tumor cells with no or less tumorigenic potential. The origin of these tumor progenitors is not clear, but it is believed that they result from the genetic or epigenetic alterations in the very thin population of normal stem cells. Even though cells produced from the "CSCs" may carry the same genetic or epigenetic imprints inherited from their precursor cells, they cannot continue to survive infinitely and therefore cannot develop a tumor when separated from the minority stem population.

TUMOR BIOLOGY

The Six Hallmarks of Cancer

In 2000, Hanahan and Weinberg summarized the biology of tumor cells and categorized six distinct hallmarks of cancer (23). Though highly heterogeneous, phenotypes of cancer cells could be grossly cataloged into six essential

alterations in cell physiology that collectively dictate malignant growth.

1. Self-sufficiency in growth signals
2. Insensitivity to growth-inhibitory (antigrowth) signals
3. Evasion of programmed cell death (apoptosis)
4. Limitless replicative potential
5. Sustained angiogenesis
6. Tissue invasion and metastasis

These six capabilities (as schematically presented in Fig. 11) are acquired in cells during tumor development and are perhaps common in all types of human tumors.

Self-Sufficiency in Growth Signals

Normal epithelial cells depend on growth factor signals from adjacent epithelial cells, basement membrane, stromal cells underneath the basement membrane, or secretory cells from distant sites. No normal cell can proliferate in the absence of such stimulatory signals. The tumor cells achieve autocrine independence by several mechanisms,

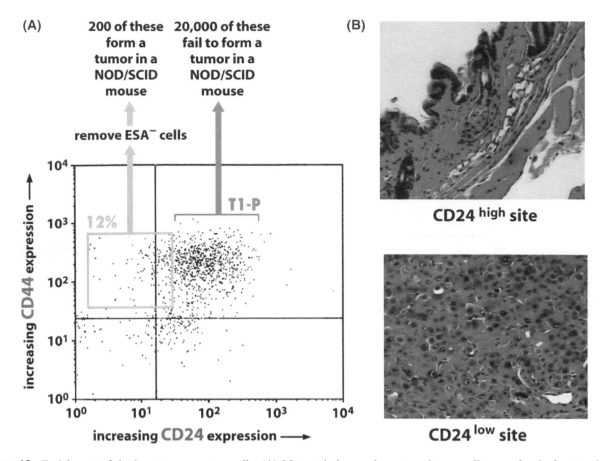

Figure 10 Enrichment of the breast cancer stem cells. (**A**) Metastatic human breast carcinoma cells were freed of contaminating noncancerous (stromal) cells and separated from one another in a fluorescence-activated cell sorter. The expression of two distinct cell surface antigens—CD24 and CD44—was gauged simultaneously, each being detected with a specific monoclonal antibody linked to a distinct fluorescent dye. The intensity of staining is plotted logarithmically on each axis. Each black dot in the graph represents the detection of a single cell. In this experiment, a 12% subpopulation of cells that expressed low CD24 and high CD44 antigens (*green box*) were separated from cells (T1-P) that showed high CD24 expression and high CD44 expression (*blue bracket*). The cells in 12% minority population were further enriched by sorting for those that expressed ESA, which resulted in the elimination of contaminating cells that did not express this antigen. (**B**) Two hundred of resulting enriched CD24^{low}CD44^{high}ESA^{+} cells were able to form a tumor following injection into a NOD/SCID immunocompromised mouse (CD24^{low} site, *below*), while 20,000 of the CD24^{high}CD44^{high} cells failed to do so (CD24^{high} site, *above*). The upper image shows a section through the subcutaneous site of cell implantation, in which relatively normal skin and underlying muscle wall are apparent; the lower image shows a section through the tumor that is formed. *Abbreviations*: ESA, epithelial surface antigens; NOD/SCID, non-obese diabetes/server combined immunodeficiency. (*See Color Insert*).

but first, by generating many of their own growth factors and thereby reducing their dependence on the stimulation from their normal tissue microenvironment. Examples are the production by many cancer cells of ligands such as platelet-derived growth factor (PDGF), tumor growth factor α (TGFα), and sonic hedgehog. Secondly, the overexpression or constitutive activation of the receptors for these ligands may confer on them independence or at least reduce the dependence on the availability of ligands. For example, the epidermal growth factor receptor (EGF-R/*erbB*) is upregulated in stomach, brain, and breast tumors, while the HER-2/*neu* receptor is overexpressed in stomach and mammary carcinomas making them hyperresponsive to the epidermal growth factor (EGF). Third, the structural

alterations of the membrane receptor molecules result in constitutive activity of the receptors, which in tern can confer independence. One example is the truncated versions of the EGF receptor lacking much of its cytoplasmic domain, which is activated constitutively. Another example is loss of function of cell membrane receptor Patched resulting in constitutive activity of hedgehog signaling pathway. Because of a mutation or promoter hypermethylation of the *PTCH* gene, it becomes dysfunctional, and releases its inhibitory influence on another cell membrane receptor Smoothened, which finally results in the constitutive activation the hedgehog signaling pathway in many cancers. Finally, an intermediate component of a signaling pathway can also become constitutively active because of

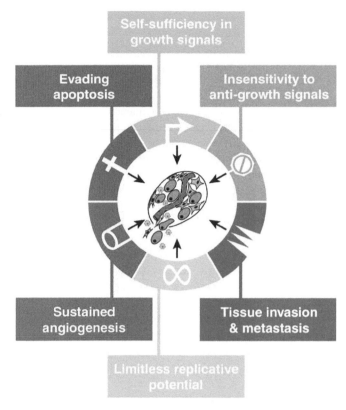

Figure 11 Six hallmarks of cancer. Most, if not all, cancers have acquired the same set of functional capabilities (as expressed in different colors and signs in the figure) during their development.

a specific mutation within the coding sequence. As in the case of Ras GTPase, which is an intermediate intracellular signaling component of several receptor tyrosine kinase signaling pathways, it can become constitutively active upon a specific mutation (codon 12, 13, or 61) of the coding sequence of its gene. *Ras* mutation is very common in many cancers as discussed above. However, this liberation from dependence on exogenously derived signals disrupts a critically important homeostatic mechanism that normally operates to ensure proper behavior of the various cell types within a tissue.

Insensitivity to Growth-Inhibitory (Antigrowth) Signals

In normal tissue, growth-inhibitory (antigrowth) signals are also transmitted through the cell membrane receptors in the same way as growth promoting signals. Antigrowth signals can block proliferation by two distinct mechanisms. First, by growth arrest, cells are forced out of the active proliferative cycle into the quiescent (G_0) state. Secondly, by inducing differentiation, cells permanently relinquish their proliferative potential with acquisition of specific differentiation-associated traits. At the molecular level, most of the antiproliferative signals are funneled

through the pRb and its two relatives p107 and p130. As mentioned before, pRb is a tumor suppressor protein. When in a hypophosphorylated state, it blocks proliferation by sequestering and altering the function of the E2F family of transcription factors, which control the expression of a battery of genes essential for cell cycle progression from G1 into S phase. Loss of function of pRb either at the gene level or at the protein level (phosphorylated state) relieves the E2F transcription factors that in turn trigger proliferation.

As an antigrowth signaling mechanism, tumor growth factor β (TGFβ) is the best documented pathway. It works in a number of ways. First, it prevents the phosphorylation events that inactivate pRb thereby blocking proliferation. Secondly, it induces synthesis of tumor suppressor proteins p15^{INK4B} and p21, which block cyclin, a cyclin dependent kinase complex responsible for pRb phosphorylation.

The TGFβ pathway is disrupted in many cancers in various ways. First, transcriptional downregulation and loss of function mutation of TGFβ receptors are common in many cancers. Secondly, the downstream protein Smad4 is eliminated through loss of function mutation of its encoding gene. Thirdly, the genetic deletion or promoter hypermethylation causes downregulation of p15^{INK4}. And finally, loss of function of pRb either by mutation or through sequestration by viral oncoproteins, such as the E7 oncoprotein of human papillomavirus, results in the disruption of this antigrowth pathway as a hallmark of cancer.

Evasion of Programmed Cell Death (Apoptosis)

The third hallmark of cancer is evasion or escaping the process of apoptosis. Virtually all cells in our body are capable of programmed cell death or apoptosis. After a finite time period, all normal cells undergo death by inducing apoptosis, which is triggered by various physiological signals. The apoptotic process goes through a very precise series of steps. Cellular membranes are disrupted, the cytoplasmic and nuclear skeletons are broken down, the cytosol is extruded, the chromosomes are degraded, and the nucleus is fragmented, all in a span of 30 to 120 minutes. In the end, the cell remnants are engulfed by nearby cells in tissue, typically within 24 hours.

Apoptosis can be initiated either through a "cell extrinsic pathway" or through a "cell intrinsic pathway." The cell extrinsic pathway involves the death receptors in the cell membrane. Fas receptor when bound to Fas ligand, or TNFα receptor when bound to its TNFα ligand, can initiate the cell extrinsic pathway of apoptosis. Whole hosts of integrin receptors present at the basal surface of epithelial cells are attached to the basement membrane underneath and can induce apoptosis when they are not bound to their ligand. These phenomena in epithelial cells are called "anoikis"—detachment-induced cell death. The cell intrinsic pathway involves the mitochondrial apoptotic pathway initiated by a DNA damage signal from the nucleus. Exposure to chemical genotoxins or radiation results in the blockage of DNA replication, which leads to collapse of replication forks and DNA double strand breaks (DSB) formation. These DSBs are thought to be crucial downstream apoptosis–triggering lesions. DSBs are detected by ataxia telangiectasia-mutated (ATM) and ataxia telangiectasia- and Rad3-related (ATR) proteins, which signal downstream to CHK1, CHK2 (checkpoint kinases), and p53. p53 induces transcriptional activation of proapoptotic factors such as FAS, p53 upregulated modulator of apoptosis (PUMA), and BCL-2 associated X protein (BAX). Many tumors harbor mutations in p53. There are p53 backup systems that involve CHK1- and/or CHK2-driven E2F1 activation and p73 upregulation, which in turn transcribes BAX, PUMA, and NOXA. The end point of the mitochondrial pathway of apoptosis is release of cytochrome C.

The ultimate effectors of apoptosis include an array of intracellular proteases termed caspases. Two "gatekeeper" caspases, caspase 8 and caspase 9, are activated by death receptors such as FAS or by the cytochrome C released from mitochondria, respectively. These proximal caspases trigger the activation of a series of more effector caspases that execute the death program, through selective destruction of subcellular structures and organelles and the genome. The most prominent effector caspase is caspase 3, the final executioner.

Modulation of the key elements of apoptosis signaling directly influences tumor cell death.

The most important example of such a modulation is through inactivation of the p53 protein. More than 50% of human cancers have been detected with the loss of function mutation of the *p53* gene. Loss of function could be either by point mutation of its encoding gene or overexpression of oncoprotein Mdm2 or human double minute 2 (Hdm2), which sequester p53 protein for degradation thereby resulting in the functional loss of p53. Transmission of antiapoptotic survival signals is achieved through the phosphoinositol-3 kinase (PI3 kinase)–AKT pathway as triggered by insulin-like growth factor-1/2 or interleukin-3 ligands binding to their cognate receptors. Signal transducers and activators of transcription-3 is also known to prevent apoptosis by transcriptional upregulation of antiapoptotic Bcl2, downregulation of proapoptotic BAX or death receptor FAS, or inhibition of NF-kB-mediated apoptosis. These were few examples of how the cancer cells evade the process of apoptosis.

Limitless Replicative Potential

Normal adult human cells carry an intrinsic, cell-autonomous program that limits their multiplication. Observations of cultured cells indicate that various normal human cell types have the capacity for 60 to 70 doublings; then they stop growing and undergo replicative senescence. Shortening of telomeres in the nucleus is an important determinant of replicative senescence. Telomeres located at the end part of chromosomes are composed of several thousand repeats of a short six base pair (bp) sequence element. Fifty to 100 bp of this repeat DNA sequence gets eroded in every doubling of cells. Because of the continuous loss of telomeric DNA, at a certain point, DNA polymerase fails to completely replicate the $3'$ ends of the chromosomal DNA during each S phase of the cell cycle. The progressive erosion of telomeres through successive cycles of replication eventually causes them to lose their ability to protect the ends of chromosomal DNA. The unprotected chromosomal ends participate in end-to-end chromosomal fusions, yielding the karyotypic disarray associated with crisis and resulting, almost inevitably, in the death of the affected cell.

Over 85% to 90% of malignant cells overexpress telomerase enzyme, which prevents the shortening of their telomeres. Therefore, malignant cells do not reach the point of replicative senescence; rather, they continue to grow without attenuation. Ectopic overexpression of hTERT (human telomerase reverse transcriptase) in normal fibroblasts immortalizes them without affecting the pRb or p53 pathway in these cells. This is a direct experimental demonstration of the importance of telomerase in the limitless replicative potential of cancer cells.

Sustained Angiogenesis

All living cells need oxygen and nutrient supply for their survival. Tissue bed vasculature serves this purpose. Growing solid tumors require the constant supply of nutrients, so new vasculature is formed in solid tumors triggered either by various tumor-induced proangiogenic factors or by downregulation of antiangiogenic factors. Foremost among all proangiogenic factors are vascular endothelial growth factor (VEGF) and acidic and basic fibroblast growth factors (FGF1/2). A prototypical angiogenesis inhibitor is thrombospondin-1, which binds to CD36, a transmembrane receptor on endothelial cells, to inhibit angiogenesis. Many tumors show evidence of increased expression of VEGF and/or fibroblast growth factors (FGFs) compared to their normal tissue counterparts. In others, expression of endogenous inhibitors such as thrombospondin-1 or β-interferon is downregulated.

When a solid tumor lesion grows beyond the oxygen diffusion limit (100 to 150 μm) of the nearest blood vessels, generally the core of the solid tumor develops hypoxia. Hypoxia stabilizes the transcription factors hypoxia inducible factor (HIF)-1α and HIF-1β. HIF-1α dimerizes with HIF-1β and induces VEGF gene expression, which results in initiation of angiogenesis in tumor. Von Hippel-Lindau (VHL) protein, a tumor suppressor, inhibits function of HIF-1, often inactivated in many cancers. This results in an elevated level of HIF-1 and thereby sustained angiogenesis mediated through VEGF. Experimental evidence for the importance of inducing and sustaining angiogenesis in tumors is extensive. Antibody against VEGF and VEGF receptor 2 (VEGF R2) (flk1) could impair neovascularization and growth of subcutaneous tumors in mice. It is also important here to mention that the tumor vasculature is not well organized like normal tissue vasculature. The vessels are tortuous, which prevents the efficient delivery of chemotherapeutic drugs. Therefore, angiogenesis inhibitory agents like anti-VEGF R2 (flk1) antibody (bevacizumab) helps to "normalize" the blood vessels within the tumor to improve the delivery of chemotherapeutic drugs to the tumor tissue bed. The area of tumor angiogenesis has become an increased focus of attention in cancer research.

Tissue Invasion and Metastasis

Metastasis is the final step of the adult neoplastic progression. Lethality of a solid tumor generally depends on its metastatic ability. It remains the sole cause of deaths from solid tumors, accounting for over 90% of cancer deaths. In order to establish metastasis, the tumor cells have to undergo several sequential events of progressive growth under selection pressure to gain metastatic competence. *Intravasation* (escaping *anoikis* and entry to the circulation), *embolization* (clumping with the platelets for better survival in the circulation), *extravasation* (leaving the circulation and entering into the host organ), and *colonization* (forming lesions in the host organ) are the four steps to a successful metastasis. The success of the process depends both on the properties of the tumor cells (the "seed") and the compatibility (or response) of the specific host organs (the "soil") (24). The healthy tissues in the host organs are generally hostile to the invading tumor cells from distant sites because of their tightly regulated tissue homeostatic mechanisms. Tumor cells with metastatic competence must therefore evade or co-opt these homeostatic barriers to colonize to a distant organ (25). Millions of cells might be released every day in circulation, but only a thin fraction of them are capable of colonizing in the distant organs (26). Therefore, metastatic potential of a cancer is correlative of the number of competent cells present in the tumor microenvironment or the number of cells becoming competent for metastasis.

The selective pressures that could confer an aggressive phenotype to the metastatic tumor may also come from the tumor microenvironment as "cell extrinsic" factors. One example of such strong selective pressure is hypoxia. In tumor, the cellular response to hypoxic stress involves

stabilization of HIF-1, a transcription factor that regulates the genes responsible for angiogenesis, anaerobic gycolysis, cell survival, and invasion.

The prerequisites of the metastatic *intravasation*, the first step of metastasis, are the acquired motility of the cells and resistance to anoikis. Acquired motility is an essential phenotype in metastatic cells called Epithelial-mesenchymal transition (EMT). EMT is a process by which the epithelial cells lose their polarity, undergo extensive cytoskeleton remodeling, and acquire a mesenchymal gene expression pattern manifesting migratory phenotype. The selective pressure in the primary tumor microenvironment could lead to genetic and/or epigenetic alterations of certain genes finally conferring EMT to the tumor cells of epithelial origin. Loss of function of cadherin 1 encoding E-cadherin, a cell adhesion receptor, is a hallmark of EMT. Several signaling pathways have been involved in the process, TGF-β pathway playing a key role. Other signaling pathways include PI3 kinase, mitogen-activated protein kinase pathway, and also activation of transcription factors like Twist, Snail, and Slug.

EMT portends a profound impact in understanding the biology of metastasis. It was originally recognized as a process critical to metazoan embryogenesis, during gastrulation and subsequent formation of the neural crest and musculoskeletal and peripheral nervous system. Interestingly, adult cells originating from neural crests retain the migratory behavior throughout their life, as in melanocytes, where their developmental program predisposes them to metastasis after neoplastic transformation (27). The "tissue of origin model of metastasis" explains how some cells in the primary tumor microenvironment could have different mutational spectra due to their developmental origin that may confer on them an advantage over other cells in acquisition of metastatic ability under the same selection pressure. Although, at the present time, experimental evidence is not sufficient to substantiate the "tissue of origin model of metastasis," it does not rule out its potential importance. Most aggressive tumors are dedifferentiated to an extent at which it is impossible to determine their tissue of origin based on standard histological examination. The fact that 5% of all cancers are diagnosed as having unknown primary origin suggests that the metastatic proclivity of certain pools of cells could also be influenced by tissue of origin.

Resistance to anoikis is a hallmark of malignancy, a fundamental prerequisite for metastatic cancer cells to survive in the primary tumor bed as well as in the circulation. The term "anoikis" (Greek meaning "homelessness") refers to a universal phenomenon in normal epithelial cells by which they undergo apoptosis when detached from their basement membrane (28). Normal epithelial cells possess a whole host of integrin receptors anchoring them to their basement membrane. The ligands for these receptors are arginine-glycine-aspartic acid (RGD) sequences of the basement membrane proteins. In the absence of these ligands bound to their corresponding receptors, apoptosis signals are induced in normal epithelial cells. Malignant cells overcome this barrier of the *anoikis* phenomena.

The Seventh Hallmark, Aerobic Glycolysis— the Warburg Effect

The abovementioned six hallmarks of cancer constitute a summary of solid tumor biology in a nutshell. In addition to these six hallmarks, another phenomenon in cancer, the Warburg effect, has recently drawn attention. Virtually all cells in our body depend on glucose metabolism (as explained schematically in Fig. 12) as the primary source of energy (ATP). Glucose is broken down to pyruvate generating two molecules of ATP for each molecule of glucose. In the presence of oxygen, the pyruvate is utilized in the mitochondrial electron transport chain to produce 36 molecules of ATP. In the absence of oxygen, pyruvate produces lactate generating only two molecules of ATP in normal cells. In the case of cancer cells, they invariably utilize the anaerobic pathway to produce lactate even in the presence of oxygen to produce only two molecules of ATP. Adaptation of cancer cells to such an inefficient mode of generating energy by aerobic glycolysis is called "the Warburg effect," named after German scientist Otto Warburg. He described this "glycolytic shift" in tumor cells more than 80 years ago and hypothesized it as the cause of tumorigenesis. However, his idea did not receive much attention at the time probably because of lack of proper experimental evidence. More recently, cancer biologists have realized the importance of this phenomenon, and it is currently being revisited extensively. Recent experimental evidence has suggested that this metabolic shift in cancer cells from an efficient system to an inefficient system may be due to an adaptation of these cells to grow (survive) under hypoxic conditions. Therefore, to meet their energy needs, cancer cells must increase their glucose uptake, and indeed radio imaging studies with ^{18}F-2deoxy-glucose, a glucose analog {in ^{18}2-[^{18}F]fluoro-2-deoxy-D-

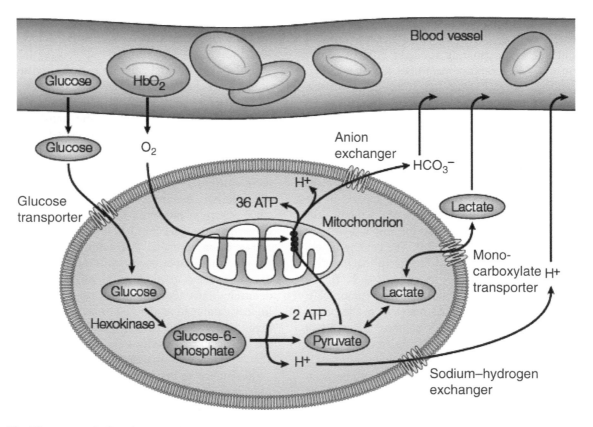

Figure 12 Glucose metabolism in mammalian cells. Afferent blood delivers glucose and oxygen (on hemoglobin) to tissues, where it reaches cells by diffusion. Glucose is taken up by specific transporters, where it is converted first to glucose-6-phosphate by hexokinase and then to pyruvate, generating two ATP per glucose. In the presence of oxygen, pyruvate is oxidized to HCO_3, generating 36 additional ATP per glucose. In the absence of oxygen, pyruvate is reduced to lactate, which is exported from the cell. Note that both processes produce hydrogen ions (H^+), which cause acidification of the extracellular space. *Abbreviation*: HbO_2, oxygenated hemoglobin.

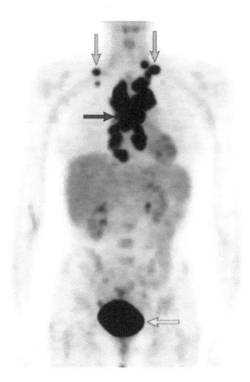

Figure 13 Positron emission tomography imaging with FdG of a patient with lymphoma. The mediastinal nodes (*arrow*) and supraclavicular nodes (*arrows*) show high uptake of FdG, showing that tumors in these nodes have high levels of FdG uptake. The bladder (*arrow*) also has high activity, because of excretion of the radionuclide.

glucose-positron emission tomography (^{18}FDG-PET)}, have substantiated the significantly higher glucose uptake by the cancer lesions as compared to their neighboring normal cells (as shown in Fig. 13 and discussed in more details in the following section). Moreover, this typical "glycolytic switch" appears to be inherited in the cancer cells through mitotic inheritance. Cancer cells in culture show the same preference for aerobic glycolysis as their ancestor cells even when they are out of their hypoxic microenvironment. Therefore, this phenomenon is also believed to be another hallmark, the seventh hallmark of cancer. Currently this phenomenon is being explored as an attractive therapeutic target in cancer (29).

Exclusive Signaling Pathways in Cancer, an "Achilles Heel"—The Primary Basis of Mechanism-Based Cancer Chemotherapy

The concept of "oncogene addiction" or "Achilles Heel" in cancer was proposed by I. B. Weinstein in the year 2002 (30). As discussed above, cancer cells produce their own ligands and also overexpress the receptors for these ligands, which in turn confer on cancer cells self sufficiency in growth signaling for their own survival. All cancer cells overexpress many of the signaling pathways that normal cells do not. Interestingly, it has been noted that blocking of any one of such signaling pathways in cancer can induce apoptosis, rather than a need to block several or all of them together. The first convincing example of this comes from the antibody trastuzumab (herceptin), which specifically targets the membrane-associated receptor tyrosine kinase Her-2 in breast cancers. Twenty to thirty percent of breast cancer cells overexpressing this receptor at their cell surface induce apoptosis upon blocking by this specific antibody. A second example is imatinib or gleevec, which specifically blocks the tyrosine kinase domain of BCR-ABL protein in leukemia. It is very effective in killing the leukemic cells and reducing the tumor burden in patients. Therefore, it has been proposed that cancer cells become "addicted" to the oncogenes or the oncogenic pathways. Therefore, blocking one oncogenic pathway could induce apoptosis in the cells that overexpress it. An oncogenic pathway may play a more essential role in cancer cells for their survival than the same pathway does in normal cells. Evidence of this strongly supports the idea of "mechanism-based chemotherapy" in cancer, that is, differentially killing cancer cells by blocking an oncogenic pathway without affecting the other normal cells in the body.

Tumor Recurrence—Targeting the CSCs

Despite the success of specific mechanism-based anti-cancer drugs (gleevec, imatinib) in reducing the tumor burden in patients, there is disappointment in the fact that the cancer (leukemia) treated with imatinib often recurs. Recurrence of solid and liquid tumors is a property mainly attributable to CSCs. The specific therapy may kill the "bulk" tumor cells, but the CSCs are often resistant to these drugs. Therefore, even if the tumor burden is significantly reduced, the cancer recurs as explained in Figure 14 (20,31). Targeting of CSCs is now being seriously considered in cancer therapy. As the stem cells are a minority population in cancer, it is very hard to detect them for experimental therapeutic studies. Prospective identification of a few surface markers for CSCs in different solid and liquid tumors has revealed that these cells possess a few specific signaling pathways, namely, hedgehog, Wnt, and notch—which are designated as "stem cell signaling pathways." In experiments, blocking the hedgehog signaling pathway by a specific inhibitor such as cyclopamine abrogated metastatic solid tumors nonrecurrently (32–34). We are almost at the beginning of a new era of identifying CSCs in different tumors. Understanding their nature will help us to detect them in vivo, and also help design better strategies to kill them successfully.

To summarize, the chapter was a brief overview of cancer biology. We have discussed the different types of

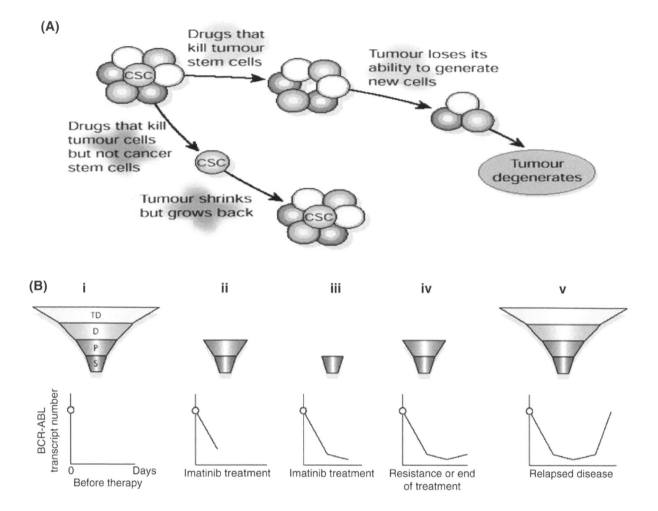

Figure 14 Cancer stem cells and chemotherapeutic drug resistance. (**A**) Conventional therapies may shrink tumors by killing mainly cells with limited proliferative potential. If the putative cancer stem cells are less sensitive to these therapies, then they will remain viable after therapy and reestablish the tumor. By contrast, if therapies can be targeted against cancer stem cells, then they might more effectively kill the cancer stem cells, rendering the tumors unable to maintain themselves or grow. Thus, even if cancer stem cell–directed therapies do not shrink tumors initially, they may eventually lead to cures. (**B**) (**i**) A mathematical model of CML as four "compartments" based on stages in the normal development of blood cells. These compartments are leukemic stem cells (*S*), which are the most immature cells and can continuously renew themselves, leukemic progenitor cells (*P*), which have developed to the extent that they can no longer self-renew, differentiated leukemic cells (*D*), which have begun to develop into specialized cell types, and terminally differentiated cells (*TD*), which are fully mature specialized cells. (**ii**) Treatment of CML with imatinib, which inhibits the BCR-ABL enzyme that causes CML, results in an initial rapid reduction of BCR-ABL gene transcript copy number, corresponding in the model to the depletion of the more differentiated cells (*TD* and *D*). (**iii**) With continued therapy, there is a slower decline in BCR-ABL transcripts, which corresponds to a reduction in the leukemic progenitor cell population, but the leukemic stem cell compartment is preserved. (**iv**) Stopping therapy or the development of resistance in the leukemic stem cell compartment allows an initial slow rate of rise of BCR-ABL transcripts corresponding to an increase in the leukemic progenitors, fueled by the leukemic stem cells. (**v**) There is a rapid rate of rise in BCR-ABL transcripts, which corresponds to relapse of disease. Monitoring of the rate of decline of progenitor cell pools may aid the development of agents to target the progenitor and leukemic stem cell compartments in CML and other cancers. *Abbreviations*: BCR-ABL, breakpoint cluster region-Abelson protein; CML, chronic myeloid leukemia.

tumors and their tissues of origin, as described by pathologists, based on the appearance of tumor sections under microscope. Epidemiological studies on the causes of cancer have associated the onset of tumors with both lifestyle and geographical locations, and also with exposure to environmental carcinogens and tumor viruses. Cancer research took a new turn after the discovery of proto-oncogenes in the 1970s. Thereafter, the genetic basis of cancer has been the main theme of cancer research in the last three decades. As a result, the rigorous research in cancer genetics and molecular biology has established the current concept of "cancer as a genetic disease." Present-day advanced knowledge of genetics and molecular biology has uncovered the major modes of genetic/epigenetic alterations that directly contribute to the process of tumorigenesis. The process of tumorigenesis is still illusive. Counterintuitive theories of tumorigenesis still leave a wide-open field for cancer researchers to explore and uncover the truth. Current knowledge of cancer biology has been distinctly categorized into six or seven hallmarks. This knowledge has been translated into the clinic in the forms of developing new therapeutic strategies or imaging tools to understand and combat this disease. In the following sections, we will discuss a brief summary of imaging in cancer, the area of research that has progressed exponentially in the recent past.

IMAGING IN CANCER

Visualization of cancer by noninvasive methods was initiated with the discovery of X-rays in the late nineteenth century by Wilhelm Roentgen (35–37). In cancer, noninvasive imaging has traditionally played a critical role in detecting and staging the disease. It has progressed through the development of new technologies, more sensitive instruments, and novel imaging probes. Present-day imaging technology has been literally revolutionized by integrating advanced knowledge in biology, molecular biology/genetic engineering, and chemistry. It has given birth to a new era of molecular and functional imaging, making the application of imaging in cancer for drug discovery, development, and basic cancer research more exiting than ever (38). Molecular imaging in cancer utilizes the functional uniqueness of cancer cells. Now it has become possible to probe them with single or multimodal imaging devices capable of detection with an appreciable resolution. The hallmarks, or the existing knowledge in biology of cancer, which have been utilized in developing molecular imaging tools are mainly the following:

Self sufficiency in growth signals in cancer cells, as mentioned before, is the result of overexpression of receptors or the ligands that are probed by molecular imaging tools. For example, HER-2/neu receptor overexpressed in breast and other cancers is imaged by a novel two-component gadolinium-based magnetic resonance (MR) contrast agent. Tumors cells are pre-labeled *in vivo* with a biotinylated anti-HER-2/neu antibody, and specific binding of avidin-gadolinium complexes to biotin moieties on these tumor cells follows, thus generating T_1 contrast in MR images (39). Another example is imaging metastatic prostate cancer with prostate-specific membrane antigen (PSMA). PSMA is overexpressed on the cell surface of androgen-independent and metastatic prostate cancer cells and provides a useful target for prostate tumor imaging and therapy. In the clinic, radiolabeled monoclonal antibodies, such as ^{111}In-capromab pendetide (ProstaScint™), are currently available to detect prostate cancer (40). The feasibility of imaging PSMA receptor expression with low-molecular-weight, high-affinity PSMA ligands labeled with $[^{11}C]CH_3I$ for positron emission tomography (PET) and $[^{125}I]NaI$/Iodogen for single photon emission computed tomography (SPECT) was recently demonstrated in studies with a prostate tumor model. These small-molecule agents gain access to their target sites more easily than monoclonal antibodies and bind to the extracellular active site of PSMA (41). In addition, imaging the cancer-specific signaling pathways with the help of different pathway-specific single- or multimodality reporter systems is underway in the laboratories.

Evasion of programmed cell death, or apoptosis, as mentioned before, is a hallmark of almost every human tumor, and pathways causing apoptosis are being targeted for cancer chemotherapy. Apoptosis is a frequent outcome of radiation therapy as well as several chemotherapies, making noninvasive imaging of apoptosis in tumors a useful pharmacodynamic end point for anticancer therapies. Radiolabeling of annexin V with radioiodine was recently evaluated for noninvasive assessment of apoptosis in tumors. Annexin V is a protein that specifically binds phosphatidylserine (PS) residues externalized to the outer surface of apoptotic cells. In an animal tumor model, binding of the $[^{124}I]$N-succinimidyl-3-iodobenzoic acid (SIB) derivative of annexin V increased after apoptosis was induced by treatment with 5-fluorouracil (42). On the basis of this proof-of-principle study, $[^{124}I]$SIB-annexin V shows promise for future noninvasive PET imaging of apoptosis induced by chemotherapy.

Telomerase reverse transcriptase (TERT) or telomerase enzyme overexpression confers limitless replicative potential to more than 85% of cancer cells as mentioned before. The expression pattern of telomerase promoter fragments in mice has been measured in vivo with PET imaging. Recombinant adenoviruses in which promoter fragments from the telomerase genes drove the expression of the sodium iodide symporter (NIS) PET reporter gene were generated. These constructs resulted in cancer-selective expression of the NIS transgene, as visualized by PET imaging (43).

Sustained angiogenesis in tumor can be imaged by probing the receptors expressed by tumor neovasculature, such as $\alpha_v\beta_3$ integrins. Because $\alpha_v\beta_3$ is highly expressed on activated endothelial cells during angiogenesis, $\alpha_v\beta_3$-detecting antibodies, such as LM609, have been used for MRI-based molecular imaging of angiogenic vasculature. Recent studies have also demonstrated the feasibility of $[^{19}F]$Galacto-RGD, a glycosylated cyclic pentapeptide binding to $\alpha_v\beta_3$, for PET imaging in tumor models and cancer patients (44,45).

Imaging tissue invasion and metastasis in cancer has been most challenging of all molecular imaging approaches, particularly imaging the metastatic potential of a cancer. Metastasis is the culmination of the entire process of tumorigenesis. It causes more than 90% of cancer-related deaths. Therefore, determination of metastatic potential of a tumor is more useful for better prognosis than the detection of an already established, full blown metastasis. Molecular imaging techniques utilize the functional biology of metastasis to anticipate the metastatic potential of a cancer. For example, the proteases cathepsin B and gelatinase are overexpressed in several cancers and have been associated with aggressive metastatic tumors and poor clinical outcomes. Imaging of protease activity in tumors is a way to detect metastatic potential. This has been primarily performed with near infrared (NIR) optical imaging of protease-activated probes. These probes are based on the principle that fluorophores in close proximity with each other are quenched, and it is only after cleavage of the probe by an enzyme that the fluorophores are released from the carrier and a fluorescent signal can be detected. This approach has been used for matrix metalloproteinase-2 detection and NIR optical imaging of cathepsin B–sensitive probes in breast tumor models (46,47). Lysosomes are the organelles that carry multiple proteases, including the different types of cathepsins, and therefore play a key role in cancer invasion and metastasis. Noninvasive optical imaging of 6-O'-glucosamine-labeled fluorescent probes, which accumulate in lysosomal proteins as a result of their high degree of glycosylation, was recently developed for the imaging of lysosomes in breast tumor models (48).

The seventh hallmark of cancer, as mentioned before, is aerobic glycolysis, "The Warburg effect" in cancer cells. Adaptation of cancer cells to an inefficient pathway for glucose metabolism results in significant increase in glucose utilization by these cells. This phenomenon is itself probed for imaging in FDG-PET, which has been a standard method for cancer imaging since long (49). 2-Deoxy-D-[^{14}C]glucose (DG)—formed by replacing the OH-group in position 2 of D-glucose with a hydrogen—was developed in the early 1950s as a drug to block accelerated rates of glycolysis in cancer, and hence tumor growth. However, it also blocked glycolysis in the brain, so it could not be used as a drug. Over 20 years later, in 1977, Sokoloff and coworkers developed a new use for DG in imaging glycolysis, by labeling DG with carbon-14 and using autoradiography, which requires the animal to be killed (50). This use was extended when 2-[^{18}F]fluoro-2-deoxy-D-glucose (FDG) was synthesized to image living subjects specifically and noninvasively with PET. FDG was first used to study tumors in the 1980s by Di

Chiro and others, who showed that the degree of malignancy of cerebral tumors was correlated with their FDG uptake (51). Tumors have a higher rate of glucose use, therefore, FDG accumulation also increases. In the early 1990s, FDG-PET started to be used in conjunction with whole-body imaging protocols. The first applications of FDG-PET outside neuro-oncology were primarily in the detection of lung cancer. At present, the vast majority ($\sim$95%) of all clinical PET studies use FDG.

REFERENCES

1. Pisani P, Parkin DM, Bray F, et al. Estimates of the worldwide mortality from 25 cancers in 1990. Int J Cancer 1999; 83(1):18–29.
2. Parkin DM, Pisani P, Ferlay J. Estimates of the worldwide incidence of 25 major cancers in 1990. Int J Cancer 1999; 80(6):827–841.
3. Weinberg RA. The Biology of Cancer. New York: Garland Science, 2007.
4. Miller EC. Some current perspectives on chemical carcinogenesis in humans and experimental animals: Presidential Address. Cancer Res 1978; 38(6):1479–1496.
5. Ames BN. Dietary carcinogens and anticarcinogens. Oxygen radicals and degenerative diseases. Science 1983; 221 (4617):1256–1264.
6. Huggins CB. Peyton Rous and his voyages of discovery. J Exp Med 1979; 150(4):733–734.
7. Peyton Rous: father of the tumor virus. J Exp Med 2005; 201(3):320.
8. Rous P. Landmark article (JAMA 1911;56:198). Transmission of a malignant new growth by means of a cell-free filtrate. By Peyton Rous. JAMA 1983; 250(11):1445–1449.
9. Newmark P. Nobel for oncogenes. Nature 1989; 341 (6242):475.
10. Varmus HE, Heasley S, Bishop JM. Use of DNA-DNA annealing to detect new virus-specific DNA sequences in chicken embryo fibroblasts after infection by avian sarcoma virus. J Virol 1974; 14(4):895–903.
11. Rhee I, Bachman KE, Park BH, et al. DNMT1 and DNMT3b cooperate to silence genes in human cancer cells. Nature 2002; 416(6880):552–556.
12. Vogelstein B, Kinzler KW. Cancer genes and the pathways they control. Nat Med 2004; 10(8):789–799.
13. Jones PA, Baylin SB. The epigenomics of cancer. Cell 2007; 128(4):683–692.
14. Herman JG, Merlo A, Mao L, et al. Inactivation of the CDKN2/p16/MTS1 gene is frequently associated with aberrant DNA methylation in all common human cancers. Cancer Res 1995; 55(20):4525–4530.
15. Myohanen SK, Baylin SB, Herman JG. Hypermethylation can selectively silence individual p16ink4a alleles in neoplasia. Cancer Res 1998; 58(4):591–593.
16. Toyota M, Ahuja N, Ohe-Toyota M, et al. CpG island methylator phenotype in colorectal cancer. Proc Natl Acad Sci U S A 1999; 96(15):8681–8686.
17. Wiencke JK, Zheng S, Lafuente A, et al. Aberrant methylation of p16INK4a in anatomic and gender-specific

subtypes of sporadic colorectal cancer. Cancer Epidemiol Biomarkers Prev 1999; 8(6):501–506.

18. Reeves R. Molecular biology of HMGA proteins: hubs of nuclear function. Gene 2001; 277(1–2):63–81.

19. Reeves R, Nissen MS. Interaction of high mobility group-I (Y) nonhistone proteins with nucleosome core particles. J Biol Chem 1993; 268(28):21137–21146.

20. Reya T, Morrison SJ, Clarke MF, et al. Stem cells, cancer, and cancer stem cells. Nature 2001; 414(6859):105–111.

21. Vogelstein B, Kinzler KW. The Genetic Basis of Human Cancer. 2nd ed. New York: McGraw-Hill, Medical Publishing Division, 2002.

22. Von Hoff DD, Evans DB, Hruban RH. Pancreatic Cancer. 1st ed. Sudbury, MA: Jones and Bartlett Publishers, 2005.

23. Hanahan D, Weinberg RA. The hallmarks of cancer. Cell 2000; 100(1):57–70.

24. Fidler IJ. The pathogenesis of cancer metastasis: the 'seed and soil' hypothesis revisited. Nat Rev Cancer 2003; 3(6):453–458.

25. Nguyen DX, Massague J. Genetic determinants of cancer metastasis. Nat Rev Genet 2007; 8(5):341–352.

26. Sporn MB. The war on cancer. Lancet 1996; 347 (9012):1377–1381.

27. Gupta PB, Kuperwasser C, Brunet JP, et al. The melanocyte differentiation program predisposes to metastasis after neoplastic transformation. Nat Genet 2005; 37(10):1047–1054.

28. Frisch SM, Francis H. Disruption of epithelial cell-matrix interactions induces apoptosis. J Cell Biol 1994; 124(4): 619–626.

29. Gatenby RA, Gillies RJ. Why do cancers have high aerobic glycolysis? Nat Rev Cancer 2004; 4(11):891–899.

30. Weinstein IB. Cancer. Addiction to oncogenes–the Achilles heal of cancer. Science 2002; 297(5578):63–64.

31. Huntly BJ, Gilliland DG. Cancer biology: summing up cancer stem cells. Nature 2005; 435(7046):1169–1170.

32. Karhadkar SS, Bova GS, Abdallah N, et al. Hedgehog signalling in prostate regeneration, neoplasia and metastasis. Nature 2004; 431(7009):707–712.

33. Berman DM, Karhadkar SS, Maitra A, et al. Widespread requirement for Hedgehog ligand stimulation in growth of digestive tract tumours. Nature 2003; 425(6960):846–851.

34. Feldmann G, Dhara S, Fendrich V, et al. Blockade of hedgehog signaling inhibits pancreatic cancer invasion and metastases: a new paradigm for combination therapy in solid cancers. Cancer Res 2007; 67(5):2187–2196.

35. Cohen M, Trott NG. Wilhelm Conrad Rontgen, 1845–1923. Br J Radiol 1973; 46(542):81–82.

36. Wicke L, Taylor KC, Firbas W, et al. Atlas of Radiologic Anatomy. 6th English ed. Baltimore: Williams & Wilkins, 1998.

37. Bleich AR. The story of X-rays, from Rontgen to isotopes. New York: Dover Publication; 1960.

38. Glunde K, Pathak AP, Bhujwalla ZM. Molecular-functional imaging of cancer: to image and imagine. Trends Mol Med 2007; 13(7):287–297.

39. Artemov D, Mori N, Ravi R, et al. Magnetic resonance molecular imaging of the HER-2/neu receptor. Cancer Res 2003; 63(11):2723–2727.

40. Ponsky LE, Cherullo EE, Starkey R, et al. Evaluation of preoperative ProstaScint scans in the prediction of nodal disease. Prostate Cancer Prostatic Dis 2002; 5(2):132–135.

41. Foss CA, Mease RC, Fan H, et al. Radiolabeled small-molecule ligands for prostate-specific membrane antigen: in vivo imaging in experimental models of prostate cancer. Clin Cancer Res 2005; 11(11):4022–4028.

42. Collingridge DR, Glaser M, Osman S, et al. In vitro selectivity, in vivo biodistribution and tumour uptake of annexin V radiolabelled with a positron emitting radioisotope. Br J Cancer 2003; 89(7):1327–1333.

43. Groot-Wassink T, Aboagye EO, Wang Y, et al. Noninvasive imaging of the transcriptional activities of human telomerase promoter fragments in mice. Cancer Res 2004; 64(14):4906–4911.

44. Beer AJ, Haubner R, Sarbia M, et al. Positron emission tomography using [18F]Galacto-RGD identifies the level of integrin alpha(v)beta3 expression in man. Clin Cancer Res 2006; 12(13):3942–3949.

45. Haubner R, Weber WA, Beer AJ, et al. Noninvasive visualization of the activated alphavbeta3 integrin in cancer patients by positron emission tomography and [18F]Galacto-RGD. PLoS Med 2005; 2(3):e70.

46. Bremer C, Bredow S, Mahmood U, et al. Optical imaging of matrix metalloproteinase-2 activity in tumors: feasibility study in a mouse model. Radiology 2001; 221(2):523–529.

47. Bremer C, Tung CH, Bogdanov A Jr., et al. Imaging of differential protease expression in breast cancers for detection of aggressive tumor phenotypes. Radiology 2002; 222 (3):814–818.

48. Glunde K, Foss CA, Takagi T, et al. Synthesis of 6′-O-lissamine-rhodamine B-glucosamine as a novel probe for fluorescence imaging of lysosomes in breast tumors. Bioconjug Chem 2005; 16(4):843–851.

49. Gambhir SS. Molecular imaging of cancer with positron emission tomography. Nat Rev Cancer 2002; 2(9):683–693.

50. Sokoloff L, Reivich M, Kennedy C, et al. The [14C] deoxyglucose method for the measurement of local cerebral glucose utilization: theory, procedure, and normal values in the conscious and anesthetized albino rat. J Neurochem 1977; 28(5):897–8916.

51. Di Chiro G. Positron emission tomography using [18F] fluorodeoxyglucose in brain tumors. A powerful diagnostic and prognostic tool. Invest Radiol 1987; 22(5):360–371.

52. DeVita VT, Rosenberg SA, Hellman S. Cancer, principles and practice of oncology. 6th ed. Philadelphia:Lippincott, Williams & Wilikins, 2001.

53. American Cancer Society. Cancer facts and figures. New York: American Cancer Society, 2008.

54. Ames BN, Profet M, Gold LS. Dietary pesticides (99.99% all natural). Proc Natl Acad Sci U S A. 1990; 87(19):7777–7781.

55. Ames BN, Gold LS. Dietary carcinogens, environmental pollution, and cancer:some misconceptions. Med Oncol Tumor Pharmacother 1990; 7(2–3):69–85.

56. Flint SJ. Principles of virology:molecular biology, pathogenesis, and control. Washington, D.C.: ASM Press, 2000.

57. Cooper GM. Oncogenes. Boston: James and Bartlett Publishers, 1990.

58. Downward J. Targeting RAS signaling pathways in cancer therapy. Nat Rev Cancer 2003; 3(1):11–22.

2

Introduction to Molecular Biology

JULIE HEROUX and AHMED M. GHARIB

Diagnostic Radiology Department, National Heart, Lung and Blood Institute (NHLBI), National Institutes of Health (NIH), Bethesda, Maryland, U.S.A.

INTRODUCTION

Within the past few years, the field of molecular biology has emerged as a powerful tool in medical and clinical research and also opened many exciting possibilities for the understanding, treatment, and imaging of a variety of diseases. Since the discovery of deoxyribonucleic acid (DNA) structure half a century ago (1), enormous advances in this field have been made. The progress led to the sequencing of the whole human genome, but the number of genes contained in the human genome is still fluctuated and under evaluation. The first human chromosome to be completely sequenced was chromosome 22 in the year 1999 (2). In 2000, the completion of a "working draft" of the entire human genome closed an important chapter in the field of genetics but opened huge avenues in medical research (3). Finally, the year 2003 marked not only the 50th anniversary of the discovery of the double-strand DNA helix but also the final step and completion of the human genome sequence, with further analysis still being published (4).

From there, research groups and pharmaceutical companies have been trying to study and identify potential targets among many families of genes that could be involved in diseases such as atherosclerosis, diabetes, and cancer. Moreover, scientific efforts have been made to elucidate the molecular mechanisms inside the cells that lead to these pathological conditions. As a result of this effort, many genes or proteins have been characterized and evaluated for a potentially differential expression in the context of specific diseases. Furthermore, a constantly growing number of new disciplines have emerged including functional genomics, proteomics, metabolimics, or pharmacogenomics, each one related to the study of a specific area in biology.

One of the areas that have become increasingly important among the field of molecular biology is molecular imaging. This discipline combines expertise in several domains, which include molecular biology, physics, chemistry, biomedical engineering, and pathology, to obtain precious information about the development of a specific disease and to allow imaging of various pathological conditions. Therefore, it is important for a molecular imager to understand the basics of molecular biology in order to exploit this growing and evolving new field. Thus, the purpose of this chapter is to introduce these basic concepts.

MOLECULAR STRUCTURE

DNA Structure

Discovery

In 1865, Gregor Mendel, an Austrian monk, was the first to publish a theory about genetic rules that govern inheritance (5). By conducting crossbreeding experiments on pea plants, he was able to propose a generalized set of rules, now known under the name of Mendel's law of heredity or Mendelian inheritance. He postulated that the transmission of hereditary characteristics from parent organisms to their progeny are governed by discrete units that are transmitted from generation to generation, even if some of these units are not expressed as visually observable trait in every generation. These units were the first report of the discovery of what we now call genes. He also postulated that for each characteristic, an organism inherit two alleles, one from each parent. Unfortunately, the results of Mendel's work were initially very controversial and neglected by the scientific community until the "rediscovery" of the theory in 1900, by three European scientists Hugo de Vries, Carl Correns, and Erich von Tschermak.

After the publication of Mendel's law of inheritance, it took nearly a century to finally elucidate the double helix structure of DNA, as first described by Watson and Crick (6). The proposed double helix structure of DNA was based on X-ray crystallography studies. In 1962, Francis Crick, Maurice Wilkins, and James Watson were awarded the Nobel Prize in Medicine and Physiology for this pioneering discovery. Their findings described how DNA is arranged into genes that are contained within the chromosomes, which is the primary genetic material. Additional findings described mitosis and meiosis processes, where cell division by mitosis maintains the parental chromosome number while cell division by meiosis reduces the parental chromosome number.

Structure

DNA is a long polymer of simple structural units called nucleotides with a backbone made of sugars (2-deoxyribose) and phosphate groups joined by ester bonds. Attached to the sugar is one of the four types of molecules called bases. The four bases present in DNA are classified into two differents subtypes: purine and pyrimidine. The purine class includes adenine (A) and guanine (G), while the pyrimidine class is represented by cytosine (C) and thymine (T) (Fig. 1). Nucleotides are linked together by phosphodiester bonds to form polynucleotides. Usually, in living organisms, DNA exists not as a single-strand molecule, but rather as a pair of strands that entwine like a vine to form a double helix. In this double helix, the two stands of DNA are in an antiparallel arrangement, whereby the direction of the nucleotides in one strand is opposite to the direction of the nucleotides in the other strand. The ends of a single DNA strand are referred to as the 5' (five prime) and 3' (three prime) ends. The segment constituting the backbone of the DNA (sugars and phosphate groups) holds the chain together while the bases (adenine, cytosine, guanine, and thymine) are responsible for the interactions with the other strand of the double helix (Fig. 2). These

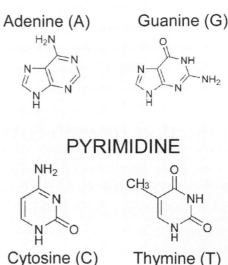

Figure 1 The four bases present in DNA. Adenine (A) and guanine (G) are purine class bases while cytosine (C) and thymine (T) are pyrimidine class bases.

interactions are achieved through hydrogen bonds and are responsible for stabilizing the double helix. Each base on one strand forms a link with just one specific base on the other strand by the process of complementary base pairing (Fig. 3). For the base pairing, purines form hydrogen bonds with pyrimidines, where A bonds only to T and C bonds only to G. These two types of base pairs form different numbers of hydrogen bonds: AT pair forms two bonds, while CG pair forms three bonds and is therefore stronger. Other forces like hydrophobic interactions can also hold the double-strand helix together.

Chromatin and Chromosome

In eukaryotes, the nucleus contains long double-stranded DNA molecules tightly packed and bounded to chromosomal proteins to form chromatin. Chemically, chromatin consists primarily of DNA associated with proteins and a small amount of RNA. The proteins inside the chromatin structure belong to two different classes: (*i*) basic proteins (positively charged at neutral pH) called histones and (*ii*) acidic proteins (negatively charged at neutral pH) called nonhistone chromosomal proteins. Nonhistone proteins are very heterogeneous and are involved in the regulation of expression of specific genes. Histone proteins play a major role in the structural integrity and the packaging of the DNA. Histones belong to five different groups: H1, H2a, H2b, H3, and H4. Histones and DNA are associated in a complex structure that forms small ellipsoidal beads called nucleosomes, which constitute the basic structural

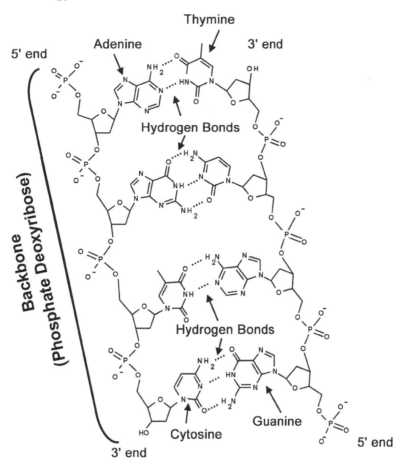

Figure 2 Chemical structure of DNA with its two asymmetric ends 5′ and 3′. The backbone segment of the DNA (sugars and phosphate groups) holds the chain together and the bases (adenine, cytosine, guanine, and thymine) interact with the other strand of the double helix. Hydrogen bonds stabilize the double helix.

subunits of chromatin (Fig. 4). The nucleosome core is 146-nucleotides pairs in length and is wrapped around an octamer of histones (two molecules each of H2a, H2b, H3, and H4). The complete chromatin subunit comprises the nucleosome core, the linker DNA associated with one molecule of histone H1, and some nonhistone proteins. The different levels of chromatin compaction are clearly visible in cells. In nondividing cells, there are two types of chromatin refered to as euchromatin and heterochromatin. A euchromatin is a relatively relaxed form of chromatin allowing for the transcription and expression of the genes in this segment of DNA. On the other hand, the DNA segment in a hetrochromatin is more tightly packed and therefore is inaccessible to transcription. The interconversion between the euchromatin and heterochromatin form is called chromatin remodeling. Chromatin undergoes various forms of structural remodeling, mainly by acetylation and methylation. Acetylation (protein modification) results in the loosening of chromatin and lends itself to replication and transcription. Methylation (DNA and protein modifi-

cation) strongly holds DNA together and restricts access to various enzymes.

In the early stages of mitosis or meiosis, the chromatin strands become more and more condensed. The chromosome becomes visible as a pair of sister chromatids attached to each other at the centromere, forming the classic four arm structure. Eukaryotic chromosomal DNA is also characterized by another feature called telomere. Telomeres are highly repetitive specialized DNA sequences protecting the end of a linear chromosome from degradation and gradual shortening. Without telomeres, a cell will lose a small piece of one of its strands of DNA at each division, which can quickly result in a loss of vital genetic information. For this reason, it is believed that telomeres are implicated in the aging process.

RNA Structure

The RNA structure is very similar to the DNA structure, except that the sugar in the backbone is a ribose instead of strand form. Instead of forming a double-strand helix like DNA, RNA forms double-strand structure either with another DNA strand during the replication process or within itself by means of intramolecular hydrogen bonds. The types of RNA secondary structures define various types of RNA.

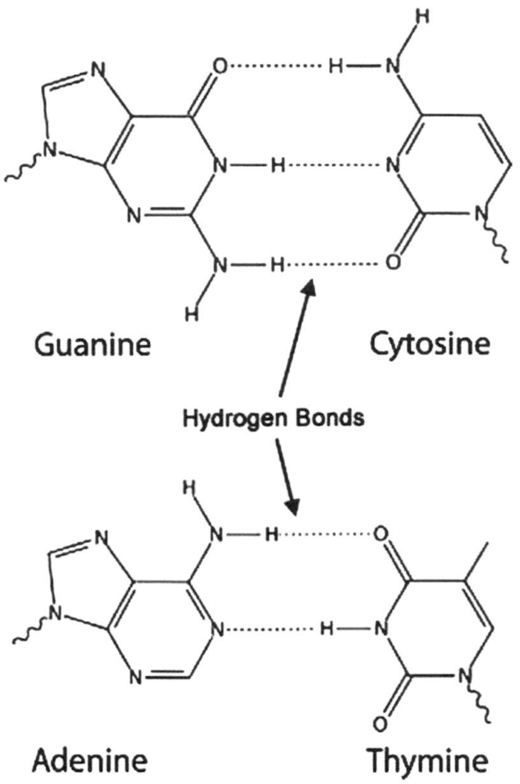

Types of RNA

Messenger RNA

Messenger ribonucleic acid (mRNA) is a molecule of RNA encoding a chemical "blueprint" for a protein product. mRNAs are intermediary molecules that carry genetic information from DNA in the cell nucleus to ribosomes in the cytoplasm for protein synthesis. After the translation process, the mRNA will be degraded. On average, between 10,000 and 20,000 different mRNA species can be observed in each cell at a given time. Despite this large number, mRNA composes only 3% to 5% of the total cytoplasmic RNA.

Transfer RNA

Transfer RNA (tRNA) is a small (73–93 nucleotides) RNA molecule folding into a cloverleaf-shaped structure as a result of intramolecular base pairing (Fig. 5). Each tRNA functions as an adaptor between a specific amino acid and its corresponding codon in mRNA. Basically, it delivers amino acids, one by one, to the growing polypeptide chain at the ribosomal site. In a typical eukaryotic cell, there are 32 different types of tRNA and each one carries one of the 20 amino acids existing in proteins at its 3′ end. It also contains a three bases region called anticodon, which can base pair to the corresponding three bases codon region on mRNA.

Figure 3 Complementary bases pairing in DNA. GC base pair forms three intermolecular hydrogen bonds, while AT base pair forms two intermolecular hydrogen bonds.

a 2-deoxyribose. Additionally, in RNA, a uracil (U) replaces the thymidine base. The other major difference between DNA and RNA is its secondary structure. While in living organisms DNA is rarely found in a single strand, the majority of RNA molecules are found in a single-

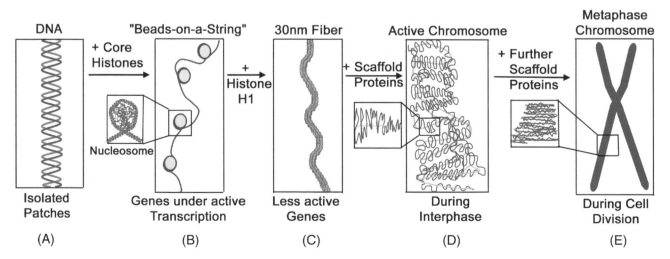

Figure 4 The major structures in DNA compaction: (**A**) DNA, (**B**) the nucleosome, (**C**) the 10 nm "beads-on-a-string" fiber, (**D**) the 30 nm fiber, and (**E**) the metaphase chromosome.

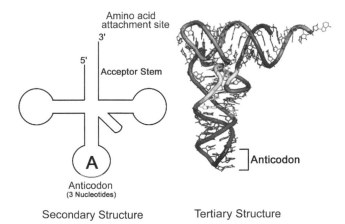

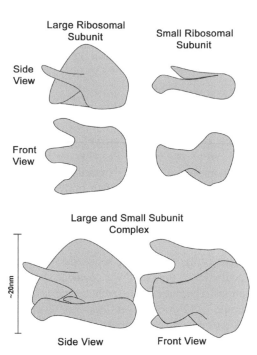

Figure 5 Secondary and tertiary structure of a transfer RNA (tRNA). The secondary structure is usually visualized as a cloverleaf structure, with an anticodon loop (A) that will base pair with the codon in the mRNA and an acceptor stem, which contains the 3′-hydroxyl attachment site for the amino acid. The tertiary structure is L-shaped and allows the tRNA to fit into the P and A sites of the ribosome.

Ribosomal RNA

Ribosomal RNA (rRNA) is the structural component of the ribosome, which is the intricate cytoplasmic machine translating nucleotide sequence of mRNAs into amino acid sequence of polypeptides (Fig. 6). The ribosome can be viewed as protein manufacturing machinery in all living cells. The rRNAs interact with more than 50 different ribosomal proteins to produce the complex tridimensional structure of the ribosome. Eukaryotic ribosomes are very complex machinery and contain four rRNA molecules and about 80 different proteins. The four eukaryotic rRNAs are designated 5S (the S represents Svedberg units), 5.8S, 18S, and 28S rRNA and are approximately 120, 160, 1900, and 4800 nucleotides in length, respectively. The small subunit of the ribosome is constituted of the 18S rRNA along with about 30 different proteins, whereas the large subunit is composed of the 28S, 5.8S, and 5S rRNA along with some 45 different proteins. In prokaryotes, these subunits are different in size and numbered 23S, 16S, and 5S rRNA.

Small nuclear RNA and small nucleolar RNA

Small nuclear RNAs (snRNAs) are a class of small RNA molecules (ranging from 100 to 215 nucleotides) that are present in spliceosomes (described later in this chapter) and play a key role in the excision of noncoding sequences (introns) from the transcripts of nuclear genes. Unlike the other types of RNA, snRNAs never leave the nucleus of the cells. snRNAs are always associated with specific proteins and beside their role in RNA splicing, they are also involved in regulation of transcription factors and maintaining the telomeres.

Figure 6 Ribosomes are small and dense structures that assemble proteins during the translation process. They are about 20 nm in diameter and are composed of 65% ribosomal RNA and 35% ribosomal proteins. Ribosomes consist of two subunits that fit together and work as one to translate the mRNA into a polypeptide chain during protein synthesis.

Small nucleolar RNAs (snoRNA) are a large group of snRNAs located in the nucleus and the cajal bodies of eukaryotic cells. These are small RNA molecules that play an essential role in RNA biogenesis, particularly in ribosome formation by splicing the 45S rRNA precursor into 28S, 18S, and 5S molecules. snoRNAs also guide chemical modifications of nucleotides in rRNAs and other RNA genes.

MicroRNA, small temporal RNA, and small interfering RNA

MicroRNAs (miRNAs) are tiny RNA molecules that appear to regulate the expression of mRNA. miRNAs and small temporal RNAs (stRNAs) are single-stranded noncoding RNA molecules of about 21 to 23 nucleotides in length that regulate gene expression. miRNA and stRNA molecules are partially complementary to one or more mRNA and function as silencers of gene expression.

Small interfering RNA (siRNA), sometimes known as short interfering RNA or silencing RNA, are a class of 20- to 25-nucleotide long, double-stranded RNA molecules. siRNA is involved in the RNA interference (RNAi) pathway where the siRNA interferes with the expression of a specific gene through a mRNA degradation pathway.

XIST RNA

Xist RNA is a spliced, polyadenylated, noncoding RNA that is expressed exclusively to deactivate one of the

X chromosomes in females. The silencing is achieved by wide alteration in X chromosome chromatin structure, a conversion of active euchromatin into inactive heterochromatin.

Protein Structure

Proteins constitute 15% of the wet weight of cells and about 50% of its dry weight. Proteins are by far the most prevalent component of living organisms and are considered building blocks of the human body. They also play many roles vital to the survival of all cells.

Primary Structure

Proteins are composed of long sequences of monomers of amino acids linked together by a covalent bond and called polypeptides. There are 20 different amino acids (Table 1). Each amino acid contains at least one carboxyl group (COOH) and one α-amino group (NH$_2$), but differs from others by a side chain. This side chain can be anything from a hydrogen atom to a complex ring. These highly variable side groups provide the structural diversity of proteins. The side chains are classified into four types: (*i*) hydrophobic or nonpolar groups, (*ii*) hydrophilic or polar chains, (*iii*) acidic or negatively charged groups, and (*iv*) basic or positively charged chains. This chemical diversity among side groups is responsible for the phenomenal versatility of proteins.

Table 1 The Name of the 20 Different Amino Acids, Their Abbreviations, and Side Chain Properties

Amino acid	3-Letters	1-Letter	Side chain polarity/ acidity or basicity
Alanine	Ala	A	Nonpolar/neutral
Arginine	Arg	R	Polar/basic (strongly)
Asparagine	Asn	N	Polar/neutral
Aspartic acid	Asp	D	Polar/acidic
Cysteine	Cys	C	Polar/neutral
Glutamic acid	Glu	E	Polar/acidic
Glutamine	Gln	Q	Polar/neutral
Glycine	Gly	G	Nonpolar/neutral
Histidine	His	H	Polar/basic (weakly)
Isoleucine	Ile	I	Nonpolar/neutral
Leucine	Leu	L	Nonpolar/neutral
Lysine	Lys	K	Polar/basic
Methionine	Met	M	Nonpolar/neutral
Phenylalanine	Phe	F	Nonpolar/neutral
Proline	Pro	P	Nonpolar/neutral
Serine	Ser	S	Polar/neutral
Threonine	Thr	T	Polar/neutral
Tryptophan	Trp	W	Nonpolar/neutral
Tyrosine	Tyr	Y	Polar/neutral
Valine	Val	V	Nonpolar/neutral

Three-Dimensional Structure

Proteins have four different levels of organization namely the primary, secondary, tertiary, and quaternary structures (Fig. 7). The primary structure of a protein is its amino acids sequence. The secondary structure refers to the special interrelationships of the amino acids within a segment of the polypeptides. The most common forms of secondary structures, which were discovered by Linus Pauling and Robert Corey in 1940 (7), are α-helices and β-sheets. Whereas the secondary structure refers to the spatial organization of adjacent amino acids, the tertiary structure or conformation of a protein is defined by the overall folding of the complete polypeptide. Finally, the quaternary structure is the association between two or more polypeptides in a multimeric unit.

MECHANISMS

Replication

DNA replication is the process of copying double-stranded DNA molecules and it takes place during the S phase of cell cycle for eukaryotes. This process is extremely important for all living organisms. The fidelity of DNA replication is astounding, with an average of only one mistake per billion nucleotides incorporated. With an estimated 40,000 genes and three billion base pairs, the human genome needs to be replicated every time before a cell divides: DNA replication must work very fast, but more importantly, with great precision. Proofreading and error-checking mechanisms ensure the accuracy of the whole process. In eukaryote, several hours are needed to complete the DNA replication process despite the synthesis rate of 30,000 nucleotides per minute. Due to the complexity of eukaryotic genome, DNA replication on a strand is started simultaneously at several origins.

Semiconservative Replication

At the end of the replication process, two DNA molecules identical to each other and identical to the parental molecule are produced. Since a single strand of the DNA helix holds the same genetic information in the complementary strand, both strands can serve as templates for replication. The template strand is preserved in its entirety and the new strand is assembled from nucleotides that are pairing with the base in the template. This process is called semiconservative replication because each of the individual parental DNA strands is preserved as part of the two newly formed DNA duplexes (Fig. 8).

Replication Process

Although knowledge of the structure of the replication machinery in eukaryotes is still limited due to its

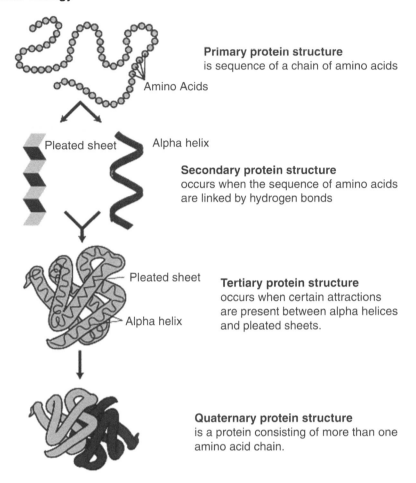

Primary protein structure
is sequence of a chain of amino acids

Amino Acids

Pleated sheet   Alpha helix

Secondary protein structure
occurs when the sequence of amino acids
are linked by hydrogen bonds

Pleated sheet

Alpha helix

Tertiary protein structure
occurs when certain attractions
are present between alpha helices
and pleated sheets.

Quaternary protein structure
is a protein consisting of more than one
amino acid chain.

Figure 7 Different levels of protein conformation, from its primary structure to its quaternary structure.

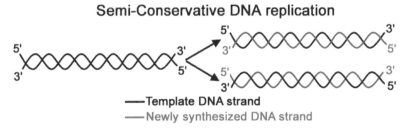

Semi-Conservative DNA replication

——Template DNA strand
——Newly synthesized DNA strand

Figure 8 Semiconservative replication process. In this process, the template strand is preserved in its entirety and the new strand is assembled from nucleotides that are pairing with the base in the template.

complexity, there are many similarities with the simpler prokaryotes DNA replication process. In eukaryotic cells, DNA exists in the nucleus as a very compact and condensed structure. In order to begin the replication process, this structure must be opened up, so the DNA polymerase enzyme can copy the DNA template. The replication process takes place at a specific site called origin of replication, which is rich in AT content. The first step in DNA replication begins with the binding of the origin recognition complex (ORC) to the origin of replication. ORC complex is a hexamer of related proteins that

function as a replication initiation factor that promotes the unwinding or denaturation of DNA. Following the binding of the ORC complex, other proteins (Cdc6/Cdc18 and Cdt1) will bind and coordinate the recruitment of the minichromosome maintenance function (MCM) complex to the origin of replication. The MCM complex is a hexamer and is thought to be the major DNA helicase in eukaryotic organisms. Once the binding of MCM occurs, a fully licensed pre-initiation replication complex (pre-RC) now exists. This process occurs during the G1 phase of the cell cycle and therefore, cannot initiate the replication.

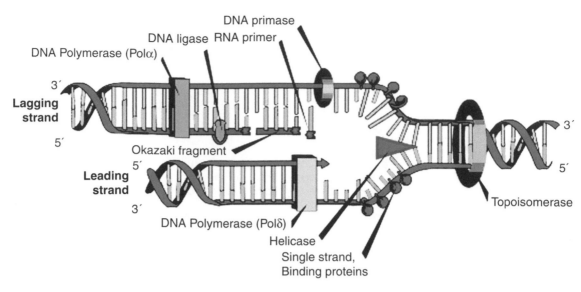

Figure 9 Schematic representation of a DNA replication fork with the key features of transcription process and its several enzymes.

Replication only occurs during the S phase. Thus, separating the licensing and activation is a mechanism that ensures only one replication per origin in a cell cycle.

After the unwinding of the double helix, a new DNA strand is synthesized in the 5′ to 3′ direction for each parental strand by an enzyme called DNA polymerase. The synthesis of the new strand at the replication fork is bidirectional (Fig. 9), with two different DNA polymerases in function. One is for the leading strand and the other is for the lagging strand. In the leading strand, the DNA polymerase catalyzes the formation of a phosphodiester bond between the 5′-phosphate on an incoming nucleotide and the free 3′-hydroxyl group on the growing polynucleotide. Thus, the growing DNA fragment is synthesized by complementary base pairing with the parental DNA template. By this mechanism, the DNA polymerase moves along the template and adds nucleotides in the 5′→3′ direction. This is true for the parental strand in 3′→5′ orientation, which is called leading strand. However, it works differently for the second strand with the 5′→3′ orientation, which is called lagging strand. The replication fork moves only in one direction and DNA replication goes only in the 5′→3′ direction, so how can this replication process be bidirectional? The paradox was solved by the discovery of Okazaki fragments (8). Instead of the continuous replication as in the leading strand, the lagging strand is produced in a discontinuous manner, which is accomplished by the synthesis of short DNA sections called Okazaki fragments. These fragments are produced from short RNA primers synthesized by an enzyme called RNA polymerase or primase. Thus, the free 3′-hydroxyl group of the RNA primer can be used by the DNA polymerase to extend the DNA. In eukaryotes, the lagging strand synthesis is carried out by the DNA

polymerase α-primase complex and the primers are later removed by enzymes like ribonucleases and endonucleases. The gaps created by excised RNA are filled out by the DNA polymerase and then linked by DNA ligase to form a continuous strand of DNA.

Transcription

Transcription is the process by which a DNA template is copied to form an mRNA by a RNA polymerase. This results in the transfer of the genetic information from DNA to RNA. This is the first step in gene expression. The transcription mechanism is situated in the nucleus of the cell. The resultant mRNA will be processed and transported into the cytoplasm for the translation process. A segment of DNA that is transcribed to form one molecule of RNA is called transcription unit. In most mammalian cells, it is estimated that only 1% of the DNA sequence will be transcribed into functional mRNA. The transcription process can be divided into three important steps: (*i*) initiation of RNA chain, (*ii*) elongation of the chain, and (*iii*) termination of the transcription that results in the transcript release.

Initiation

Unlike prokaryote, eukaryotes require transcription factors to initiate transcription process. The transcription factors must bind the promoter region in DNA and form an appropriate initiation complex before the initiation of the transcription. In eukaryotic cells, three types of RNA polymerases (RNA polymerase I, II, and III) are involved in this process. The promoter region is constituted of

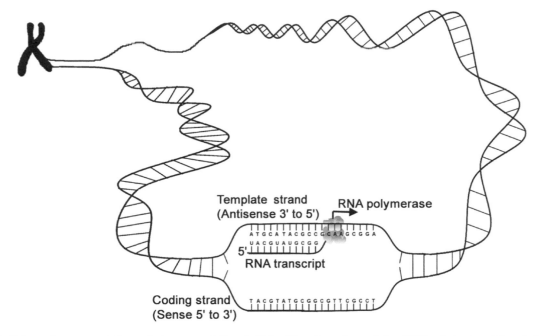

Template strand
(Antisense 3' to 5') RNA polymerase

A T G C A T A C G C C G C A A G C G G A
U A C G U A U G C G G
5'
RNA transcript

Coding strand
(Sense 5' to 3') T A C G T A T G C G G C G T T C G C C T

Figure 10 Schematic representation of the transcription bubble. The elongation of the RNA chain is catalyzed by the RNA polymerase on the template strand (3′ to 5′) of the DNA.

specific nucleic acid sequence recognized by the polymerase. There are various types of promoters, such as the TATA box or the CATT box promoter regions, but all of them contain the specific sequence referred to as the starting site of transcription. In the vast majority of eukaryotic genes, the RNA polymerase II is responsible of the initiation of transcription. For the correct initiation of the transcription, the transcription factors must interact with the promoter region in a specific order. For example, in order to bind to the promoter region and initiate transcription efficiently, the DNA polymerase II (Fig. 10) requires transcription factors: TFIID, TFIIA, TFIIB, TFIIF, and TFIIE (**T**ranscription **F**actor for Polymerase **II**). After the arrival of the transcription factors, the polymerase II can bind to the promoter region and begin the transcription. Usually, the promoters for the genes transcribed by the RNA polymerases are situated upstream from the transcription start points, with some exceptions such as the genes transcribed by the RNA polymerase III.

For sustained transcription in eukaryotes, the promoter needs additional short regulatory sequences that are also located at varying distances from the starting point. Some of these elements are close to the core promoter and called proximal elements, while some others are situated several kilobases upstream or downstream and called enhancers or repressor sequences. The binding of these transcription factors to the DNA promoter regions causes local unwinding of the double helix, like in DNA replication, which allows the transcription to start.

Elongation

The elongation process is accomplished by base-pairing mechanism as is DNA replication. However, unlike in replication, there is only one transcript and the base pair are RNA-DNA instead of DNA-DNA. While in replication, either DNA strand can serve as a template, in transcription, the polymerase proceeds only along a strand in 3′ to 5′ direction. In other words, the synthesis of the mRNA is 5′→3′ directed on the 3′→5′ oriented template DNA strand. Thus, the mRNA molecule produced is complementary to the DNA template (3′→5′ or antisense) strand and identical to the DNA nontemplate (5′→3′ or sense) strand. For the complementary base-pairing process, the same rules are applied, but the AT coupling in DNA-DNA duplex is replaced by an AU coupling in RNA-DNA duplex. The elongation of the RNA chain is catalyzed by the RNA polymerase enzyme, which produces covalent link between each ribonucleoside triphosphate. RNA polymerase contains both unwinding and rewinding activities, so the process forms a structure called transcription bubble that moves along the DNA during the transcription process (Fig. 10).

Termination

In prokaryotes, the transcription termination mechanisms are very well defined. There are two processes leading to the termination of the transcription. One is Rho independent and the other Rho dependent. In the Rho-independent type, RNA transcription stops when the newly synthesized RNA molecule forms a hairpin loop and sequence of many Us, which makes it detach from the DNA template. In the Rho-dependent process, a protein called "Rho" destabilizes the RNA-template DNA complex allowing for the release of the mRNA. Unlike prokaryotes, the termination process in eukaryotes is poorly understood. It involved the endonucleolytic cleavage of the RNA transcript rather than the termination of the transcription. This cleavage event that produces the 3′ end of the transcript usually occurs downstream a conserved consensus sequence AAUAAA, which is located near the end of the transcript unit.

Posttranscriptional Modifications

After the transcription process, the population of primary transcripts in the nucleus is called heterogeneous nuclear RNA (hnRNA). This population of RNA molecules is highly varied in sizes. Likewise, the primary transcript product is called pre-mRNA, because it will undergo three major modifications prior to its transport to the cytoplasm for translation. These modifications include 5′ capping, 3′ polyadenylation, and splicing.

Capping

The first processing step for the mRNA is the 5′ capping. This process referred to the addition of a 7-methylguanosine cap at the 5′ end of the primary transcript. This residue is linked to the initial nucleoside of the transcript by a 5′–5′ phosphate linkage. This 5′ cap addition stabilizes the mRNA as it undergoes translation and plays a role in the initiation of translation.

Polyadenylation

The addition of poly (A) tails at the 3′ end of the transcript is called polyadenylation. This process takes place in the nucleus of the cell after transcription. After the polyadenylation signal has been transcribed, an endonuclease complex cleaves the mRNA chain and 50 to 250 adenosine residues are added to the free 3′ end at the cleavage site by the poly (A) polymerase. The polyadenylation process initially depends on the existence of the AAUAAA sequence for the first 10 nucleotides, but then is simply dependent on the preexisting poly (A) tail for the remaining 50 to 250 nucleotides. The poly (A) tails of eukaryotic mRNAs enhance their stability and facilitates their transport from the nucleus to the cytoplasm.

RNA splicing

RNA splicing is the process by which introns (the regions of RNA that do not code for proteins) are removed from the pre-mRNA and the remaining exons (regions that carry the code needed for protein synthesis) are connected to reform a single continuous RNA molecule. In 1989, Tom Cech won the Nobel Prize for his works on the mechanism of RNA splicing (9), prize that he shared with Sidney Altman for his work on RNA. Although the splicing occurs after the complete pre-mRNA synthesis and end-capping, some primary transcripts with many exons can be spliced during transcription. The splicing process needs to be very accurate, because an error in only one nucleotide (removal or addition) can cause a complete shift in the open reading frame of the code. This shift will, therefore, result in a new sequence of codons that will end in a completely different amino acid sequence or possibly insert a stop codon for the termination of the synthesis of the peptide. This kind of error in the splicing process accounts for about 15% of the genetic disease. The machine responsible for the RNA splicing is called spliceosome and is composed of a large enzymatic complex, which includes 145 different proteins (snRNPs or small nuclear ribonucleoproteins) and several snRNAs. This complex recognizes specific splice sites in the introns of pre-mRNA sequences. A pre-mRNA can be spliced in many different ways, thus producing different mature mRNAs that encode for different protein sequences. This process is called alternative splicing and it allows the production of a large amount of proteins from a limited amount of DNA.

An intron in the pre-mRNA molecule often begins with nucleotides GU and finishes with AG, which is preceded by a pyrimidine-rich sequence called polypyrimidine tract. The splicing reaction occurs in two steps, (Fig. 11) in a region called branchpoint sequence, which is situated 10 to 40 nucleotides upstream of the polypyrimidine tract. The first step is the attack of the G residue in the 5′ splicing site by the 2′-hydroxyl of the A residue in branchpoint. It results in the formation of a lariat and a free exon. In the second step, the 3′ end G residue of the intron is cleaved, which brings the two exons together and release the intron in a lariat form. This process generates a mature mRNA molecule that can further be exported into the cytosol for the translation process.

Translation

Translation refers to the process by which the genetic information stored in an mRNA is translated into the amino acid sequence (protein), according to the specification of the genetic code. Unlike transcription, which takes place in the nucleus of the cell, the translation process is effectuated in the cytosol. This process is extremely complex, requiring numerous macromolecules including over 50 polypeptides, at least 20 amino acid–activating enzymes, from 40 to 60 tRNA molecules and a large number of soluble proteins involved in the polypeptide chain initiation, elongation, and termination. With

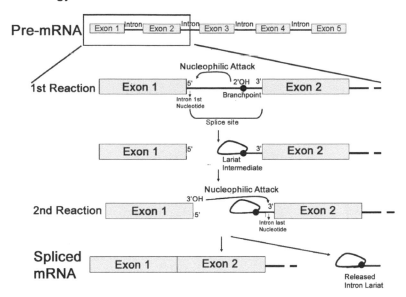

Figure 11 Diagram illustrating the two-step biochemistry of splicing. The first step is the formation of a lariat and free exon and the second one is the cleavage of the 3′ end of the intron, which brings the two exons together and release the intron in a lariat form. The resultant mature mRNA can be transported in the cytosol for translation.

this enormous complexity, it is not surprising that the process is highly regulated and guided by a combination of rules, called genetic code.

Genetic Code

The first elucidation of a codon was done by Marshall Nirenberg and Heinrich J. Matthaei in 1961 at the National Institutes of Health (10). The genetic code contains a total of 64 different codons derived from four different nucleotides bases: 61 codons specify amino acids while 3 others specify a STOP signal. The rules of the genetic code (Table 2) can be grouped into seven important properties, which are as follows:

1. The genetic code is composed of nucleotides triplets, in other words, an amino acid in the peptide is specified by three nucleotides in the mRNA called codon.
2. The genetic code is nonoverlapping, with each nucleotide in the mRNA belonging to just one codon except in rare exceptions.
3. The genetic code is coma free, which means that during the translation, the codons are read consecutively without any forms of punctuation.
4. The genetic code is degenerate, with more than one codon specifying one amino acid (61 codons for 20 amino acids).
5. The genetic code is ordered, which means that codons for similar amino acids or multiple codons for the same amino acids are closely related, usually with a difference of only one nucleotide.
6. The genetic code contains start and stop codons.
7. The genetic code is nearly universal and all the codons have the same meaning in all living organisms, with minor exception.

This combination of rules is applies for the transfer of information from an mRNA into amino acids sequence of a protein and translation can be divided in three processes: initiation, elongation, and termination.

Initiation

In eukaryotes, the initiation of the transcription begins with the binding of a protein called cap-binding protein (CBP) to the 7-methylguanosine cap at the 5′ end of the mRNA, followed by the binding of other initiation factors and the recruitment of the 40S subunit of the ribosome. The ribosome scans the mRNA in the 5′ to 3′ direction until it encounters the first methionine starting codon (AUG).

The 40S subunit contains two tRNA-binding sites in its cleft, called P site for peptidyl tRNA site and A site for aminoacyl tRNA site. When the ribosome arrives to the starting codon, an initiator tRNA charged with a methionine binds to the ribosomal complex. The Met-charged initiator tRNA is brought to the P site of the small ribosomal subunit by eukaryotic Initiation Factor 2 (eIF2). The hydroxylation of a GTP then signals the dissociation of several factors from the small ribosomal subunit, which results in the association of the large subunit (or the 60S subunit) to the transcription complex. The complete ribosome (80S) is now formed. The

Table 2 Genetic Code Showing the 64 Codons and the Amino Acid Specified for Each Codon

First Base	Second Base: U	Second Base: C	Second Base: A	Second Base: G	Third Base
U	UUU, UUC: Phenyl-Alanine (Phe/F) UUA, UUG: Leucine (Leu/L)	UCU, UCC, UCA, UCG: Serine (Ser/S)	UAU, UAC: Tyrosine (Tyr/T) UAA, UAG: **(Stop)**	UGU, UGC: Cysteine (Cys/C) UGA: **(Stop)** UGG: Tryptophan (Trp/W)	U C A G
C	CUU, CUC, CUA, CUG: Leucine (Leu/L)	CCU, CCC, CCA, CCG: Proline (Pro/P)	CAU, CAC: Histidine (His/H) CAA, CAG: Glutamine (Gln/Q)	CGU, CGC, CGA, CGG: Arginine (Arg/R)	U C A G
A	AUU, AUC, AUA: Isoleucine (Ile/I) AUG **(Start)**: Methionine (Met/M)[a]	ACU, ACC, ACA, ACG: Threonine (Thr/T)	AAU, AAC: Asparagine (Asn/N) AAA, AAG: Lysine (Lys/K)	AGU, AGC: Serine (Ser/S) AGA, AGG: Arginine (Arg/R)	U C A G
G	GUU, GUC, GUA, GUG: Valine (Val/V)	GCU, GCC, GCA, GCG: Alanine (Ala/A)	GAU, GAC: Aspartic Acid (Asp/D) GAA, GAG: Glutamic Acid (Glu/E)	GGU, GGC, GGA, GGG: Glycine (Gly/G)	U C A G

Triplet nucleotide sequence or codon refers to the sequence in mRNA, not DNA. The direction is 5′ to 3′.
[a]The codon AUG both codes for methionine and serves as an initiation site; the first AUG in an mRNA's coding region is where translation into protein begins.

Met-charged initiator tRNA is the only tRNA to first bind the P site, as all the others tRNA have to enter the A site first. Even if many proteins start with the amino acid methionine, in some cases it is cleaved after by a protease.

Elongation

Once the initiation complex is complete, the elongation process begins (Fig. 12), which is carried out by a set of elongation factors. The addition of each new amino acid

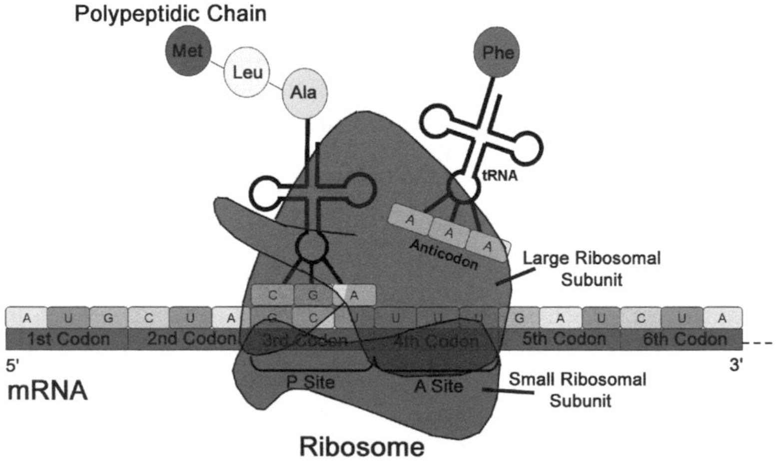

Figure 12 Elongation step in translation process. Each aminoacyl-tRNA, except the first one, first enters into the A site of the ribosome. The amino acids in the A site is then connected to the polypeptide chain in the P site with a peptide bond. As the ribosome moves along the mRNA in the 5′→3′ direction, the now uncharged tRNA is translocated into the P site and the next aminoacyl-tRNA enters the A site. Thus, the ribosome and tRNA molecules translate the genetic code contained in the mRNA into an amino acid sequence, to produce a protein.

within the growing polypeptide occurs in three steps: (*i*) the binding of an aminoacyl-tRNA into the A site of the ribosome, (*ii*) the formation of a new peptide bond, and (*iii*) the translocation of the ribosome to the next three nucleotides (next codon) along the mRNA chain. In the first step, the specificity of the tRNA binding is provided by the mRNA codon located on the A site. In other words, the anticodon on the incoming tRNA must pair with the mRNA codon present in the A site. The binding of the tRNA into the ribosome complex requires GTP hydrolysis. After both P site and A site are occupied, the two proximal amino acids are joined together to form a peptide bond by the catalytic activity of an enzyme called peptidyl transferase. This enzymatic activity is situated on the ribosome and no energy is expended at this stage. During this step, the ribosome uses the energy from GTP hydrolysis to move three nucleotides toward the 3′ end of the mRNA. As the ribosome moves, the peptidyl-tRNA present in the A site is translocated in the P site with the aid of translocase enzyme and GTP, while the uncharged tRNA in the P site is translocated to the E site. The A site is now unoccupied and ready for the next tRNA molecule complementary to the mRNA codon. These three steps will be repeated in a cyclic manner during the whole elongation process until the termination happens.

Termination

The polypeptide chain elongation process undergoes termination when the ribosome comes across a stop codon in the A site, for which there is no tRNA. There are three different stop codons: UAA, UAG, and UGA. In eukaryotes, each of these three codons can be recognized by a releasing factor called eukaryotic release factor (eRF). The release factor induces a nucleophilic attack of the C-terminus of the nascent peptide by water. This process releases the polypeptide from the tRNA, triggering the translocation of the tRNA from the A site to the P site, the dissociation of the small and large subunit of the ribosome and the release of the mRNA. Ribosomal subunits are now ready for the next round of protein synthesis, while the mRNA can be either retranslated or degraded. All mRNAs are eventually degraded when the synthesis of a protein in no longer required.

Posttranslational Modifications

In mammalian cells, there are different compartments called organelles, which include the rough endoplasmic reticulum (ER), the smooth endoplasmic reticulum, the Golgi apparatus, the lysosomes, and the peroxisomes. In these cells, most proteins destined for secretion are targeted to the ER by a signal sequence at the amino end of the peptide, called signal peptide. This sequence is recognized by a signal recognition particle (SRP), which binds to the signal peptide. The protein-SRP complex can therefore bind to the SRP receptor on the target ER membrane. Proteins destined for other compartment are initially directed into the ER and will then follow the secretory pathway with similar signal peptides. This process is posttranslational and the proteins are packaged into vesicles as they move between the lumen of different organelles. After its synthesis, a protein can undergo some other posttranslational modifications while in these compartments. Basically, a protein is a simple chain of a combination of 20 different amino acids, but the posttranslational modifications of these amino acids can extend the range of functions of this protein. A large variety of posttranslational modifications exists for proteins, including addition of functional groups by the processes of biotinylation, glycosylation and/or phosphorylation. Other forms of posttranslational modifications include the addition of other peptides, changes in the chemical nature such as deamidation, or structural changes such as addition of disulfide bridges. All these modifications will allow the production of the vast complexity of different protein types, from enzymes that catalyze fundamental reactions to antibodies participating in the immune response.

SUMMARY

The field of molecular biology is extremely vast, involving numerous processes and biological molecules. The impressive machinery by which a progenitor cell can transmit its genetic information to daughter cells, or by which it can synthesize the various macromolecules necessary for its survival, is precisely and accurately regulated. However, all this complexity could be resumed by a general theory called the central dogma of molecular biology. According to this central dogma, genetic information is stored in DNA and flows from DNA to DNA during the transmission from generation to generation, or from DNA to protein during its phenotypic expression in an organism. The transfer of genetic information from DNA to proteins is a two-step process, beginning with the transcription of the DNA in an mRNA (DNA-RNA transfer) and finishing by the translation of this mRNA into a protein (RNA-protein transfer). The central dogma also states that unlike the transcription that can be sometimes reversible, the translation process that transfer genetic information from RNA to protein, is irreversible. This central dogma of molecular biology is largely responsible for the ability of a cell to maintain its order in a chaotic environment. Understanding the processes involved in the central dogma is important for studying both hereditary and nonhereditary diseases. Additionally, grasping the concepts of these biological processes is crucial for the application of the different molecular biology methods discussed in the next chapter.

REFERENCES

1. Watson JD, Crick FH. Molecular structure of nucleic acids; a structure for deoxyribose nucleic acid. Nature 1953; 171 (4356):737–738.
2. Dunham I, Shimizu N, Roe BA, et al. The DNA sequence of human chromosome 22. Nature 1999; 402(6761):489–495.
3. Venter JC, Adams MD, Myers EW, et al. The sequence of the human genome. Science 2001; 291(5507):1304–1351.
4. International Human Genome Sequencing Consortium. Finishing the euchromatic sequence of the human genome. Nature 2004; 431(7011):931–945.
5. Mendel JG. Versuche über Plflanzenhybriden. Verhandlungen des naturforschenden Vereins Brünn, Bd. IV für das Jahr 1865; Abhandlungen:43–47.
6. Watson JD, Crick F. Molecular structure of nucleic acids; a structure for deoxyribose nucleic acid. Nature 1953; 171(4356):737–738.
7. Pauling L, Corey RB, Branson HR. The structure of proteins; two hydrogen-bonded helical configurations of the polypeptide chain. Proc Natl Acad Sci U S A 1951; 37(4): 205–211.
8. Okazaki R, Okazaki T, Sakabe K, et al. Mechanism of DNA chain growth. I. Possible discontinuity and unusual secondary structure of newly synthesized chains. Proc Natl Acad Sci U S A 1968; 59(2):598–605.
9. Zaug AJ, Cech TR. In vitro splicing of the ribosomal RNA precursor in nuclei of Tetrahymena. Cell 1980; 19(2):331–338.
10. Martin RG, Matthaei JH, Jones OW, et al. Ribonucleotide composition of the genetic code. Biochem Biophys Res Commun 1962; 6:410–414.

3

Methods in Molecular Biology

JULIE HEROUX and AHMED M. GHARIB

Diagnostic Radiology Department, National Heart, Lung and Blood Institute (NHLBI),
National Institutes of Health (NIH), Bethesda, Maryland, U.S.A.

INTRODUCTION

There is a vast diversity of methods in molecular biology. These range from the simple techniques used for DNA or RNA extraction, to the more complex methods utilized for the production of transgenic animals. All of these techniques constitute very valuable tools essential for understanding the pathogenesis of various diseases and for the development of new treatments. Moreover, understanding these techniques is important for the development of image-guided therapeutic methods and molecular imaging. Here, we will emphasize and revisit the basic principles behind various molecular biology protocols, which should allow multidisciplinary imaging specialists to better understand the techniques. With this in mind, the description of these methods will be presented not so much as a technique, but more as an approach focusing on the molecular level of biological events.

BASIC CLONING TECHNIQUES

The mammalian genome contains about 3×10^9 nucleotides pairs, with a single gene averaging 3000 nucleotide pairs (many are larger). Thus, isolation of a single gene is a meticulous process requiring rigorous methods that will be discussed in this chapter. Most techniques used for analyzing genes require significant amount of the gene

sequence in a relatively pure form. The development of recombinant DNA and gene cloning technologies has allowed for the isolation, the replication and the study of chromosomes by different techniques, such as nucleic acid sequencing, electron microscopy, and other analytical techniques. There are two essential steps in the gene cloning procedure: (*i*) incorporation of the gene into a small self-replicating chromosome called cloning vector and (*ii*) amplification of the structure by its replication in an appropriate host. The first step involves the in vitro production of recombinant DNA by fusing one or more DNA fragments (gene) of interest with the vector. The second step is gene cloning, where the recombinant vectors transfect an appropriate host cell line and replicate, thereby producing many copies of the cloned gene.

Restriction Endonucleases

Due to the immense size of genomic DNA, any gene or DNA fragment of interest first needs to be cleaved out or separated into smaller more manageable fragments before it can be cloned or sequenced. This is achieved using a special group of bacterial enzymes called restriction endonucleases. Thus, one of the most powerful tools for molecular biologists, in conjunction with polymerase chain reaction (PCR), was the discovery of these

Table 1 Some Important Restriction Endonucleases from Different Organisms Showing the Preferential Cleaving Site for Each Enzyme and the Resultant DNA Fragment with Blunt or Cohesive Ends

Enzyme	Source	Recognition sequence	Cut
EcoRI	Escherichia coli	5′GAATTC 3′CTTAAG	5′—G AATTC—3′ 3′—CTTAA G—5′
BamHI	Bacillus amyloliquefaciens	5′GGATCC 3′CCTAGG	5′—G GATCC—3′ 3′—CCTAG G—5′
HindIII	Haemophilus influenzae	5′AAGCTT 3′TTCGAA	5′—A AGCTT—3′ 3′—TTCGA A—5′
NotI	Nocardia otitidis	5′GCGGCCGC 3′CGCCGGCG	5′—GC GGCCGC—3′ 3′—CGCCGG CG—5′
HinfI	Haemophilus influenzae	5′GANTC 3′CTNAG	5′—G ANTC—3′ 3′—CTNA G—5′
SmaI[a]	Serratia marcescens	5′CCCGGG 3′GGGCCC	5′—CCC GGG—3′ 3′—GGG CCC—5′
HaeIII[a]	Haemophilus aegyptius	5′GGCC 3′CCGG	5′—GG CC—3′ 3′—CC GG—5′
AluI[a]	Arthrobacter luteus	5′AGCT 3′TCGA	5′—AG CT—3′ 3′—TC GA—5′
EcoRV[a]	Escherichia coli	5′GATATC 3′CTATAG	5′—GAT ATC—3′ 3′—CTA TAG—5′
KpnI	Klebsiella pneumonia	5′GGTACC 3′CCATGG	5′—GGTAC C—3′ 3′—C CATGG—5′
SacI	Streptomyces achromogenes	5′GAGCTC 3′CTCGAG	5′—GAGCT C—3′ 3′—C TCGAG—5′
SalI	Streptomyces albus	5′GTCGAC 3′CAGCTG	5′—G TCGAC—3′ 3′—CAGCT G—5′
ScaI	Streptomyces caespitosus	5′AGTACT 3′TCATGA	5′—AGT ACT—3′ 3′—TCA TGA—5′
SphI	Streptomyces phaeochromogenes & badrii	5′GCATGC 3′CGTACG	5′—G CATGC—3′ 3′—CGTAC G—5′
XbaI	Xanthomonas badrii	5′TCTAGA 3′AGATCT	5′—T CTAGA—3′ 3′—AGATC T—5′

[a]Blunt ends.

restriction enzymes. In 1970, Hamilton Smith (1) and Daniel Nathan (2) first discovered the existence of this type of enzyme and later, in 1978, won the Nobel Prize in Physiology and Medicine for their work. Now, more then 200 different endonucleases isolated from different organisms are commercially available. The name given to each enzyme reflects its origin with the first letter for the genus, next two letters for the species, and a letter for strain specificity if applicable (EcoRI: Escherichia coli, strain RY13, was first discovered in this strain). The biological function of these restriction endonucleases is to protect the host against invasion by foreign DNA. Unlike the other types of endonucleases that cut randomly into a DNA sequence, restriction endonuleases cleave into very specific nucleotide sequences, which are called restriction sites and the resulting double-stranded DNA fragment is hence called restriction fragment. Usually, restriction endonucleases recognize DNA sequences that are four to eight nucleotides long and called palindromes. Palindromes are nucleotides pair sequence (in a double-stranded DNA segment) that can be read the same from 5′ to 3′ for each strand as seen in this example:

5′-GGATCC-3′
3′-CCTAGG-5′

Some enzymes cut directly in the middle of the sequence, generating "blunt ends," while others cleave both strands at different points, generating staggered ends called cohesives or "sticky" ends (Table 1). The off-staggered cleavage produces segments of DNA with complementary single-stranded ends that can be joined together again by DNA ligase. This enzyme catalyses formation of 3′ → 5′ phosphodiester bond between the 3′-hydroxyl end of one restriction fragment strand and the 5′-phosphate end of another during the time that the cohesive ends are transiently base paired. These cohesive or sticky ends are very useful for "cutting and pasting" DNA from different origin to create recombinant molecule with the aid of a DNA ligase. Therefore, a hybrid combination of two fragments is called recombinant DNA molecule.

Vectors and Plasmids

In 1972, Cohen et al. developed a recombinant DNA technology that allowed DNA from one organism to be cloned into a carrier DNA molecule and be replicated and expressed in a new host (3). This technique, called molecular cloning, has revolutionized the field of molecular biology. DNA molecule used to carry a foreign DNA fragment into a bacterial or eukaryotic host organism is called cloning vector. There are several different types of vectors. The simplest and most commonly used DNA vector is derived from viral chromosomes and called plasmid. Plasmids are extrachromosomal, doubled-stranded circular molecules of DNA present in microorganisms, especially bacteria. They range from about 1 kilobase (kb) to over 200 kb in size, with an average 15 kb, and replicate autonomously. Other types of cloning vectors include cosmids, bacteriophages, bacterial artificial chromosomes (BACs), and yeast artificial chromosomes (YACs).

A cloning vector has three essential components (Fig. 1): (*i*) an origin of replication; (*ii*) a dominant selectable marker gene, usually conferring drug resistance to the host cell; and (*iii*) at least one unique restriction endonuclease cleavage site, which is present only once in the vector. Usually, a cloning vector contains unique cleavage site for several different restriction enzymes. This cluster of unique restriction sites is called polylinker or multiple cloning sites (MCS). In addition to these features, a vector may contain a promoter inserted in front of the polylinker site. This promoter drives the expression of the DNA fragment inserted into the polylinker site. The insertion of a DNA fragment into a cloning vector is carried out by treating both vehicle and foreign DNA with the same restriction enzyme, then ligating the fragments with a DNA ligase.

Transformation and Transfection

Transformation is the genetic alteration of a cell resulting from the uptake and expression of foreign genetic material (DNA). Transformation of eukaryotic cell is usually called transfection.

Transformation

In nature, transformation does not occur in every species of bacteria. Instead, it takes place only in the species possessing proteins and enzymatic machinery necessary to bind free DNA molecules and transport them into the cytoplasm. Only cells that secrete a competence factor, competent cells, are considered able to serve as recipient cells in transformation. This natural capability of taking up DNA is called natural competence. However, there are mechanisms that can force passive incorporation of a plasmid into an artificially permeabilized cell; this is called artificial competence. For example, cell wall permeability to DNA can be induced by chilling cells in the presence of divalent cations such as Ca^{2+} or heating them. Electroporation is another way to make holes in bacterial (and other) cells, by briefly shocking them with an electric field of 10 to 20 kV/cm. If the plasmid is present when the shock is applied, it can enter the cell through these holes and natural membrane repair mechanisms will then close these holes.

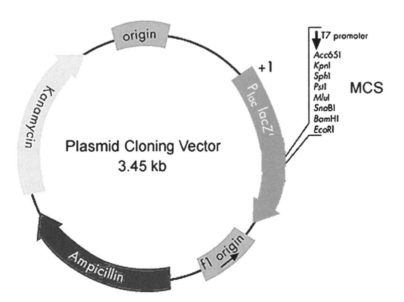

Figure 1 Schematic representation of a typical plasmid with (*i*) an origin of replication, (*ii*) a selectable marker gene conferring ampicillin and kanamycin drug resistance, and (*iii*) a multiple cloning site (MCS). Additionally, features are also presents, like a T7 promoter for the expression of the inserted gene.

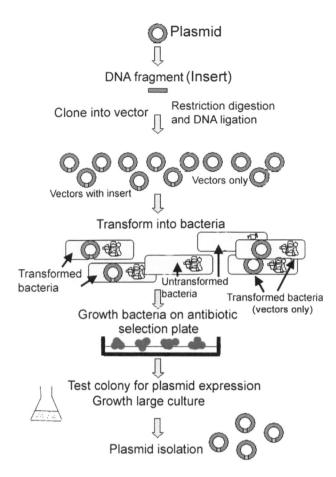

Plasmid

DNA fragment (Insert)

Clone into vector   Restriction digestion
                     and DNA ligation

Vectors with insert   Vectors only

Transform into bacteria

Transformed
bacteria   Untransformed
                  bacteria   Transformed bacteria
                                   (vectors only)
Growth bacteria on antibiotic
selection plate

Test colony for plasmid expression
Growth large culture

Plasmid isolation

Figure 2 An overview of DNA cloning in bacteria, using a plasmid vector. The target insert is first cloned into a vector, and the construction is then used to transform bacteria. Bacteria with incorporated vectors are selected by growing them on antibiotic plate and finally, plasmid are purified from large culture preparation.

Only one type of recombinant plasmid can transform a single bacterial cell. In other words, multiple different types of vector molecules cannot replicate in a single bacteria. This provides a powerful tool for isolating a clone of interest (Fig. 2).

Transfection

Like transformation process, transfection typically involves opening transient pores or holes in the cell plasma membrane, to allow the uptake of material. There are various methods of introducing foreign DNA into a eukaryote cell. They fall into three categories, namely, (i) biochemical methods using calcium phosphate, diethylaminoethyl (DEAE)-dextran, and several cationic liposome-based transfection agents; (ii) physical methods including electroporation and direct injection; and (iii) transduction mediated by viruses. In the liposome-based transfection technique, lipid-based agents (Lipofectamine 2000, Superfect, FuGEN6, Poly-l-lysine) form complexes with DNA. The resultant lipid-coated DNA is taken into the cell using nonreceptor-mediated endocytosis.

Transfection efficiency is variable and can be affected by the cell line, DNA quality, and the nature of transfection, whether stable or transient. In transient transfection, the transfected DNA is not integrated into the host chromosomal DNA, and foreign DNA is lost at the later stage when the cells undergo mitosis. If the transfected gene integrates into the genome of the cell, a stable transfection occurs. To accomplish this, another gene has to be cotransfected into the cell, which gives the cell a selection advantage, such as drug resistance.

Complementary DNA

A large percentage of DNA sequence in eukaryotes is not expressed. Thus, expressed sequences can be identified more easily by working with complimentary DNA (cDNA). Additionally, cDNA sequences are smaller in size and can be cloned more efficiently into a variety of vectors. The first step of cDNA synthesis depends on an enzyme called RNA-dependent DNA polymerase or reverse transcriptase (Fig. 3). Reverse transcription exploits a characteristic of mature mRNAs known as the 3′-polyadenylated region, commonly called the poly (A) tail, as a common binding site for poly (T) DNA primers. These primers will anneal to the 3′ end of every mRNA in the solution, allowing 5′ to 3′ synthesis of cDNA by the reverse transcriptase enzyme. Gene-specific primers or random hexamer primers can also be used to generate the cDNA. The mRNA is subsequently removed by treatment with RNase H. The second strand of the cDNA is usually synthesized by a combined action of both DNA polymerase 1 and T4 DNA polymerase, which used the RNA fragments as amorces. DNA polymerase I is used since the 5′ → 3′ exonuclease activity is needed to remove RNA in front of the enzyme. DNA polymerase I also removes the RNA primer from the 5′ lagging strand and fills in the recessed 3′ end. T4 DNA ligase then joins the various fragments together into a continuous strand of DNA. The final products are cDNA molecules with blunt ends, which can be further ligated to linkers containing restriction sites using T4 DNA ligase. The cDNA molecules are ultimately cleaved at the restriction site of the linker and ligated into a compatible vector for the formation of a cDNA library. The ligation mixture is transformed into a bacterial or phage host. A cDNA library can be used for different purposes. There is a broad diversity of cDNA libraries that are available commercially. As cDNA sequences differ in each library, comparison between libraries constructed from cells derived from different organisms can provide useful information.

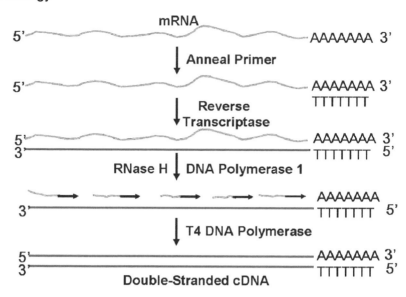

Figure 3 Schematic description of the principal steps of double-stranded cDNA synthesis from an mRNA template. *Source*: From Ref. 4.

DNA, RNA, AND PROTEIN ANALYSIS

Gel Electrophoresis

Electrophoresis was discovered by Reuss, in 1809, and is defined by the motion of dispersed particles relative to a fluid under the influence of an electric field that is space uniform (5). Gel electrophoresis is the process by which biological macromolecules such as DNA, RNA, or proteins are separated on the basis of their electrophoretic mobility, into a gel, from the cathode (negatively charge) toward the anode (positively charge) of an electrical current. DNA and RNA molecules have a relatively constant negative charge per unit mass, so they migrate naturally toward the anode on the basis of their size and conformation. However, for the separation of proteins, an anionic detergent sodium dodecyl sulfate (SDS) is used, which applies a negative charge to each protein in proportion to its size. By this process, and because size is closely proportional to the mass, proteins (similarly to nucleic acid) migrate according to their molecular weight toward the anode. The gel refers to the matrix used for containing and separating the target molecules, and is a cross-linked polymer with different composition and porosity. The composition of the gel used depends on the target molecules. For example, acrylamide is preferred for proteins and small DNA or RNA, while agarose is generally used for large (greater than a few hundred bases) DNA and RNA. The matrix created by the polymerization of the gel creates molecular sieves, retarding the passage of large molecules more than small molecules. After the migration, different techniques of staining can be used to visualize the separated bands. The most common stains are Coomassie Brilliant Blue or silver stain for proteins and ethidium bromide or ^{32}P radioactive isotope for DNA and RNA. There are other methods of band visualization, including photograph under ultraviolet light for fluorescent molecules or autoradiogram for molecules with radioactive atoms.

Gel electrophoresis is usually used for analytical purposes, but may also be used as a preparative technique for partial purification of molecules prior to the application of other methods, such as cloning, PCR, mass spectrometry, or DNA sequencing.

DNA Analysis by Southern Blot Hybridization

This technique was developed by the British biologist Edwin Southern (6) in 1975. The method utilizes a radioactive or chemiluminescent probe to visualize genes and others DNA fragments that have been previously separated by electrophoresis (Fig. 4). First, restriction endonucleases are used to cleave high–molecular weight DNA into smaller fragments. After the digestion, these fragments are separated by agarose gel electrophoresis and then transferred onto a nitrocellulose or nylon membrane. The DNA is denatured either prior to or during the transfer using alkaline solution to produce single-stranded DNA. After the complete transfer, the DNA is immobilized on the membrane by high temperature drying or ultraviolet irradiation. This process creates an exact replicate of the gel on the nylon or nitrocellulose membrane. The membrane is now ready to be hybridized or annealed with a DNA or RNA probe containing the sequence of interest. This hybridization is based on the complementary

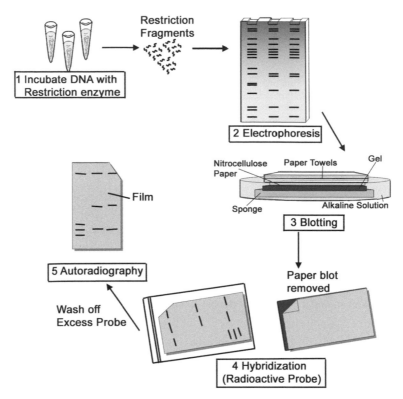

Figure 4 Schematic representation of a Southern blot analysis, showing DNA preparation (enzymatic digestion), electrophoresis, Southern blot transfer, and revelation by autoradiography. *Source*: From Charles Mallery, Department of Biology, University of Miami, Coral Gables, Florida, U.S.A. (last updated November 11, 2001).

nucleotide sequences between the probe and the DNA molecule on the membrane. Radioactive or chemiluminescent probes are visualized with autoradiography or color development of the membrane, respectively.

RNA Analysis by Northern Blot Hybridization

RNA, like DNA, can be similarly transferred from agarose gels to nitrocellulose or nylon membranes for hybridization studies. The procedure is very similar to the Southern blot hybridization and is called Northern blot. However, in Northern blot technique, care should be taken to prevent RNases contamination, because RNA is extremely sensitive to degradation. Also, formaldehyde should be applied to keep RNA molecules denatured during electrophoresis, because of the presence of secondary structure inside RNA molecules.

Protein Analysis by Western Blot

Western blot as opposed to Southern and Northern blots involves the transfer of proteins from polyacrylamide gels, instead of agarose gels, to nitrocellulose membranes. Unlike the capillary action of the Southern or Northern

blot technique, Western blot requires an electrical current for moving the proteins from the gel to the surface of the membrane. Another major difference between these techniques is the use of antibodies instead of probes for the detection of the protein of interest. These antibodies are designed to bind specifically and exclusively to the protein or a fragment of the protein of interest. There are various methods used for the identification of a specific protein with antibodies, including radioactive isotopes, fluorescent, colorimetric, or chemiluminescent detection. In all of these techniques, the antibody is labeled by conjugation with a reporting molecule. The detection can be achieved either in a one-step or a two-step process. Depending on the detection method, sensitivity is extremely variable. The so-called "enhanced chemiluminescent" (ECL) detection is considered to be among the most sensitive detection methods for blotting analysis.

GENES AND CHROMOSOMES ANALYSIS

Polymerase Chain Reaction

PCR technologies are fundamental to many other molecular biology techniques. By amplification of a selected DNA sequence, PCR allows other techniques to be performed, even when a very small amount of DNA is available. PCR reactions such as in DNA fingerprinting, are largely used in forensic cases and paternity testing. They also provide shortcuts for many cloning and sequencing applications. Another major application is in diagnosis of inherited human diseases, especially in prenatal diagnosis, where only limited amount of DNA is available. It may also be used as an amplification step for the genetic analysis of various nonhereditary neoplasms.

PCR was invented by Kary Mullis (7), who won the 1993 Nobel Prize for this work. Basically, PCR allows in vitro cloning of a given sequence, with only a small amount of DNA (few molecules) and without the need of living cells. However, to apply this technique, the nucleotide sequence of a short segment on each side of the region of interest needs to be known.

The PCR proceeds in three steps, which are repeated multiple times (Fig. 5). The first step is the heat

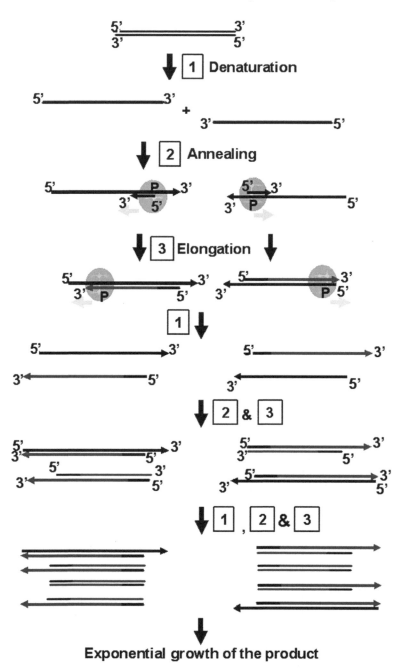

Exponential growth of the product

Figure 5 Schematic drawing of the polymerase chain reaction (PCR) cycle with its three important steps: (1) denaturing at 96°C, (2) annealing at 68°C, and (3) elongation at 72°C (P = polymerase). After, the completion of the first cycle, the two resulting DNA strands make up the template DNA for the next cycle, thus doubling the amount of DNA duplicated for each new cycle.

denaturation (94°C) of the DNA to be amplified. The second step is the annealing of the complimentary stands of the target using two short sequences of single-stranded DNA called primers. Annealing temperature is usually between 50°C and 60°C, but varies according to the primers. In the third extension step, an enzyme called Taq DNA polymerase covalently extends the primers at the 3'-hydroxyl end, using target DNA as a template for the incorporation of nucleotides. This process creates a DNA strand complementary to the strand of the primers annealed. This denaturation, annealing, and extension cycle is repeated many times (usually 30–40), which leads to the exponential amplification of the targeted DNA product. Normally, a few kilobases products can be amplified, but some PCR reagents (Elongase tag) can amplify up to 40-kb products.

Reverse Transcription-Polymerase Chain Reaction

Reverse transcription-polymerase chain reaction (RT-PCR) is the process by which an RNA strand is first reverse transcribed into a cDNA, followed by amplification of the resulting DNA using PCR. The first step is the same as the one in cDNA synthesis whereby the target mRNA is extended by a reverse transcriptase with the use of oligo-dT primer, random hexamer primer, or gene-specific primer. The generated cDNA is then amplified by PCR using gene-specific primers. This method is very sensitive for the amplification of low copy number RNA molecules. It is widely used in diagnosis of genetic diseases or as a measure of the gene expression levels by real-time PCR.

Real-Time PCR

Real-time PCR, also called quantitative real-time PCR, is based on the same principle used in PCR, but it allows quantification of the target product after each round of amplification. In other words, instead of the qualitative nature of the PCR, the real-time PCR technique is quantitative. In this technique, commercially available fluorescence detecting thermocyclers are used to amplify specific nucleic acid sequences while simultaneously following the concentration of the products. There are two common methods of RT-PCR product quantification. One utilizes fluorescent dyes, such as SYBR green (asymmetrical cyanine dye), that intercalate with double-strand DNA. Another uses modified DNA oligonucleotide probes that fluoresce when hybridized with a complementary DNA as in Taqman technique (Fig. 6). This method involves the use of an oligonucleotide reporter probe where the fluorophore is quenched by another molecule. After annealing into the complementary DNA strand, the fluorophore inside the probe is still quenched. However, during PCR reaction, the probe is degraded by the $5' \rightarrow 3'$ Taq polymerase activity and the reporter is then unquenched resulting in emission of fluorescence. The major advantages of real-time PCR are its high sensitivity and the ability to process many samples simultaneously.

DNA Sequencing

The term DNA sequencing encompasses biochemical methods for determining the order of the nucleotide bases in a DNA oligonucleotide. Modern sequencing is derived from the chain-termination method developed by

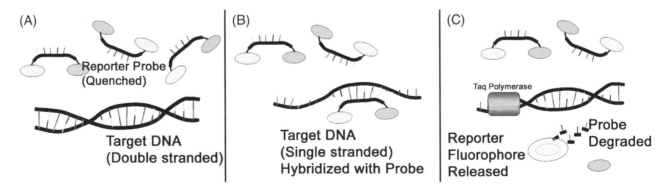

Figure 6 Principle of Taqman technique: (**A**) In intact probes, reporter fluorescence in quenched. (**B**) Probes and the complementary DNA strand are hybridized while reporter fluorescence is still quenched. (**C**) During the PCR, the probe is degraded by the Taq polymerase and the fluorescent reporter is released.

Sanger and coworkers (8) in 1977. From 1976 to 1977, Allan Maxam and Walter Gilbert (9) developed a DNA sequencing method based on chemical modification of DNA, which rapidly becomes more popular, since purified DNA could be used directly, while the initial Sanger method required production of single-stranded DNA. However, with the development and improvement of chain-termination method in combination with the technical complexity (hazardous chemicals, difficulties with scale-up) of Maxam-Gilbert sequencing, the Sanger method has regained popularity. The key feature of this method is the incorporation of dideoxynucleotides triphosphates (ddNTPs) as DNA chain terminators. Briefly, the technique requires a single-stranded DNA template, a DNA primer, a DNA polymerase, labeled nucleotides, and modified nucleotides lacking the 3′-hydroxyl group necessary for the formation of a phosphodiester bond between two nucleotides. The DNA template is divided into four separate sequencing reactions, each one containing only one of the four dideoxynucleotides (ddATP, ddGTP, ddCTP, or ddTTP). Thus, incorporation of these nucleotides into the nascent DNA strand terminates the elongation process and creates fragments of different length. The dideoxynucleotides are added at lower concentration than the standard deoxynucleotides to allow strand elongation sufficient for sequence analysis. The DNA fragments are then denatured and separated by gel electrophoresis, creating a ladder of DNA fragments, each one differing in length by one single base. DNA bands can be subsequently visualized by autoradiography or ultraviolet light allowing the sequence to be read (Fig. 7).

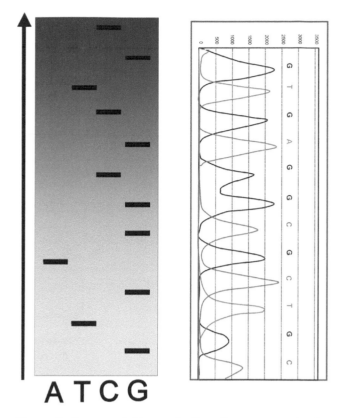

Figure 7 Sequence ladder results from Sanger sequencing by radioactive sequencing compared with fluorescent peaks.

DNA Microarrays

Microarrays are often used for expression profiling studies, where the expression of thousands of genes can be monitored simultaneously using DNA to DNA hybridization and fluorophores detection. The level of gene expression is based on the amount of mRNA translated by the cells, which is usually correlated to the level of protein production. In fact, DNA microarray is a collection of microscopic DNA spots called probes (cDNA, oligonucleotides, or small fragment of PCR products corresponding to mRNAs), arrayed on a solid surface by covalent attachment to chemically suitable matrices. cDNA from two samples to be compared (e.g., diseased vs. healthy tissue) can be affixed onto two different matrices or a single matrix, but in the latter case, samples should be labeled with two different fluorophores (Fig. 8). This technique is used in various applications, including foren-

sic science, assessment of genetic susceptibility to disease (single nucleotide polymorphism microarray), or identification of DNA-based drug candidates.

Microarray techniques are always coupled with statistical analysis and bioinformatics. To be able to decipher the enormous amount of information in a single microarray (Fig. 9), many software and normalization techniques are necessary. Even with these advanced analysis techniques, DNA microarrays pose a large number of statistical problems, because of the biological complexity of gene expression. Thus, experimental designs are of critical importance if statistically and biologically valid conclusions are to be drawn from the data.

With the great advances in sequencing techniques and the existence of technical variations of chain-termination sequencing, the goal of sequencing the complete human genome was achieved. Modern sequencers now use multiple capillary electrophoresis and sequencing techniques that are applied in a variety of fields such as diagnostic and forensic research.

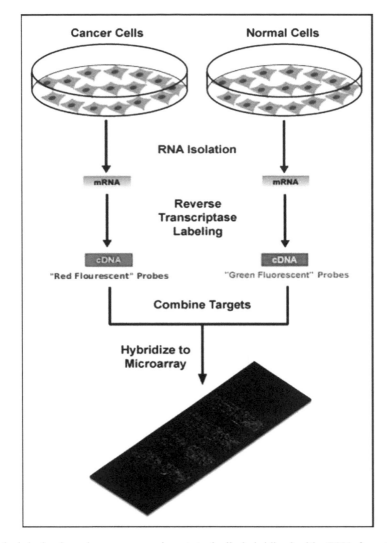

Figure 8 Diagram of typical dual-color microarray experiment, typically hybridized with cDNA from two samples to be compared (diseased tissue vs. healthy tissue) that are labeled with two different fluorophores.

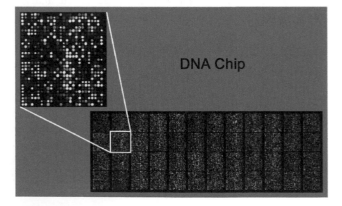

Figure 9 Example of an approximately 40,000 probe spotted oligo microarray with enlarged inset to show detail and complexity of the analysis.

SUMMARY

Since the late 1950s and early 1960s, molecular biologists have learned to characterize, isolate, and manipulate the molecular components of cells and organisms. These components include DNA, RNA, and proteins, which are all related and interconnected. The modern molecular techniques have proved to be extremely useful in a vast diversity of fields, such as biological process characterization, forensic analysis and treatment, and characterization of disease. These techniques are increasingly being incorporated in many molecular imaging laboratories. They are not only important for the understanding of disease processes, but also for developing imaging probes that are visualized by imaging devices, such as magnetic resonance and positron emission tomography scanners. Therefore, understanding such methods is vital for the progress of the field of molecular imaging.

REFERENCES

1. Orkin SH, Alter BP, Altay C, et al. Application of endonuclease mapping to the analysis and prenatal diagnosis of thalassemias caused by globin-gene deletion. N Engl J Med 1978; 299(4):166–172.
2. Kelly TJ Jr., Smith HO. A restriction enzyme from Hemophilus influenzae. II. J Mol Biol 1970; 51(2):393–409.
3. Cohen SN, Chang AC, Boyer HW, et al. Construction of biologically functional bacterial plasmids in vitro. 1973. Biotechnology 1992; 24188–192.
4. Pandit SD, Li KC. A primer on molecular biology for imagers. Acad Radiol 2004; 11(suppl 1):S42–S53.
5. Reuss FF. Mem Soc Imperiale Naturalistes de Moscow 1809; 2:327.
6. Southern EM. Long range periodicities in mouse satellite DNA. J Mol Biol 1975; 94(1):51–69.
7. Mullis K, Faloona F, Scharf S, et al. Specific enzymatic amplification of DNA in vitro: the polymerase chain reaction. 1986. Biotechnology 1992; 2417–27.
8. Sanger F, Nicklen S, Coulson AR. DNA sequencing with chain-terminating inhibitors. Proc Natl Acad Sci U S A 1977; 74(12):5463–5467.
9. Maxam AM, Gilbert W. A new method for sequencing DNA. Proc Natl Acad Sci U S A 1977; 74(2):560–564.

4

The Analysis of Complex Data Sets: Challenges and Opportunities

EDWARD H. HERSKOVITS

Department of Radiology, University of Pennsylvania, Philadelphia, U.S.A.

INTRODUCTION

Although molecular imaging promises profound changes in the nature of information, we can obtain from patients noninvasively, this promise will not be realized in the absence of parallel developments in data analysis. Most advanced imaging techniques yield enormous quantities of data, sometimes at great expense, and often representing complex spatiotemporal associations across experimental groups. Based on the example of microarray data, this chapter delineates the challenges inherent to the analysis of such complex data, and presents several analytic approaches that address these challenges.

EXAMPLE: MICROARRAY DATA

Figure 1 shows a simplified overview of the acquisition of microarray data. We begin with control and experimental tissue samples. After extracting RNA from these samples, we can label the RNA with fluorescent dye. Labeling the RNA, whether fluorescent (as shown in Fig. 1) or radio-

active, enables detection of nucleic acid sample that adheres to the complementary probes on the microarray. Modern microarrays can accommodate 10^4 to 10^6 probes/cm^2, and approximately 10^7 copies of each probe at each site on the microarray. By measuring the intensity of fluorescence or radioactivity at each site on the microarray, we obtain an estimate of relative gene expression for each of the probes.

At the risk of oversimplification, we can summarize acquisition as the process whereby a series of specimens is converted into an array of signal intensities, which in turn represent proxies for gene[a] expression. For example, the Affymetrix® HG-U133 set consists of two arrays that contain a total of almost 45,000 probe sets; thus, a series of 10 specimens each from control and experimental groups analyzed with these arrays will yield approximately 900,000 signal intensities.

Microarrays represent not only a quantum leap in the volume of data per experiment, relative to previous techniques for interrogating gene expression; microarray experiments are also yielding an exponential increase in the volume of data deposited into GenBank®,[b] as shown in Figure 2.

---

[a]We use the term "gene" to represent known genes and/or expressed sequence tags.
[b] http://www.ncbi.nlm.nih.gov/Genbank/genbankstats.html.

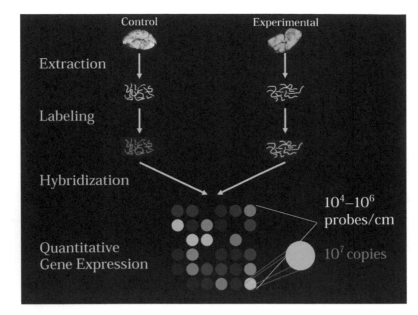

Figure 1 A simplified overview of a microarray experiment.

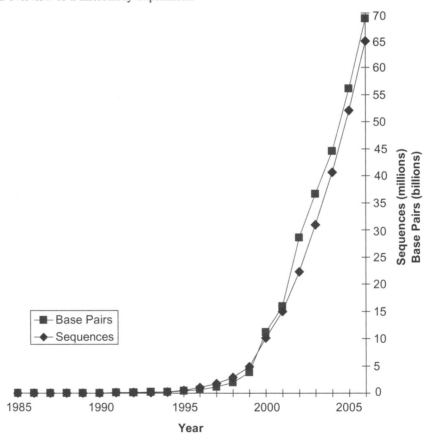

Figure 2 Numbers of base pairs and sequences entered into GenBank® (1).

ANALYTIC APPROACHES

Regardless of the purposes for having collected microarray data, the principal difficulty in analyzing these data is not the size of the data set per se, but the small number of samples relative to the number of genes interrogated. For example, a typical microarray experiment, such as that by Ross et al. (2), they interrogated 8000 genes across 60 different cancer cell lines to determine patterns of gene expression in these cell lines. From a statistician's point of view, these data are severely undersampled: one would have to analyze hundreds of thousands of cell lines to sample 8,000 genes adequately. Because so many features (e.g., gene-expression values) are measured for few samples, standard statistical techniques do not apply. For example, if these 8000 measurements were randomly distributed rather than truly associated with tissue of origin, approximately 400 false-positive associations would result from using a significance threshold of 0.05. This problem is often referred to as the "curse of dimensionality" (3,4).

Because undersampling renders infeasible standard statistical approaches to the analysis of gene-expression data, researchers have attempted to apply a wide range of data-mining and clustering techniques to determine associations among gene-expression levels and class membership (e.g., a tumor's tissue of origin), prognosis (e.g., survival), or response to therapy. These techniques range from those relatively simple to apply, such as visualization and thresholding, to simple, widely applicable clustering techniques, to more complex clustering and data-mining techniques, such as support vector machines (see Refs. 5–7 for a comprehensive review). What follows is a brief description of several representative approaches.

Thresholding is very widely employed in microarray analysis, because of its simplicity. Although there are many variations to this technique, its essence is the selection for further analysis of those genes that are expressed within a certain factor across experimental conditions, or relative to baseline. Thresholding is almost always used as a preliminary step to select a subset of candidate genes whose expression changes across experimental conditions (8).

Clustering is the most common approach to analyzing gene-expression profiles; many researchers cluster their data as an early step of microarray analysis. Most clustering algorithms consist of a similarity metric, such as a correlation coefficient or Euclidean distance, and a search algorithm. The goal of the search is to identify groups (i.e., clusters) that are homogeneous with respect to the metric (9); that is, they minimize differences within a cluster relative to differences among clusters. Among the many clustering algorithms described in the literature, three of the more commonly used include the K-means algorithm (10), self-organizing maps (11–13), and hierarchical clustering (2,14).

Clustering algorithms generally fall into one of the two broad classes: unsupervised and supervised; the former are by far more common. Unsupervised clustering is performed without labeling the samples with respect to class membership (e.g., a tumor's tissue of origin) or other information, whereas a supervised clustering algorithm incorporates this additional information. In addition, clustering may be performed with respect to genes or samples (see Ref. 2 for applications of both approaches). In gene-based clustering, genes are grouped into clusters based on similar expression patterns across samples (note that this can be performed without class-membership information); as shown in Figure 3, this process usually yields groups of functionally similar genes (14), and may thereby provide information about unknown genes. In sample-based clustering, samples that have similar gene-expression profiles are grouped together; in general, these groups share phenotypic characteristics, such as tumor cell type (15).

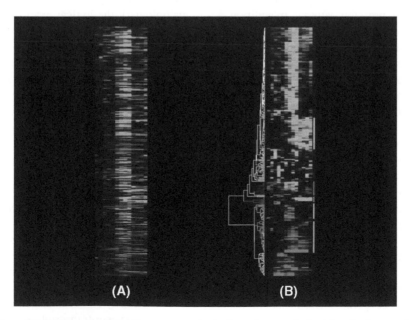

Figure 3 Microarray data (**A**) before and (**B**) after unsupervised clustering; each functional cluster of genes is colored to aid visualization. See http://rana.stanford.edu/clustering/serum.html for details (*See Color Insert*).

Unsupervised clustering is useful when the principal goal of analysis is to classify previously unknown sample types, such as tumor cells of unknown histology. Supervised analysis methods, of which only a few are based on clustering, require that each sample be labeled, for example with respect to tumor cell type (although we focus on this histological label here, other labels could be used, such as response to therapy, point in cell cycle, and so on). These algorithms take as input, a training set of labeled gene-expression profiles, and construct a classifier, which can be used to classify new samples into cell types based on their gene-expression profiles. There is a vast literature describing many examples of supervised analysis of microarray data; relatively commonly used algorithms include significance analysis of microarrays (16), support vector machines (17), k-nearest neighbors (18), and artificial neural-networks (19). Although these methods are highly sophisticated and perform fairly well in classifying new samples, they are often more difficult to implement and apply than unsupervised clustering methods, and may require the collaboration of someone with expertise in bioinformatics or biostatistics. Similarly, statistical and probabilistic methods, such as analysis of variance (6), principal components analysis (or singular-value decomposition) (20,21), decision trees (22), and Bayesian networks (23) have also been applied successfully to the analysis of microarray data, but often require experienced collaborators to guarantee that they are being used correctly.

Given the multitude of algorithms that could be applied to microarray analysis, the question of which to apply to a given data set naturally follows. Although the type of analysis will depend on the nature of the data collected and the questions being asked (24), often an unsupervised analysis, such as clustering, will be helpful to determine unexpected, novel gene-expression patterns. In addition, a permutation-based approach to analysis, in conjunction with cross-validation of classification results, will help reduce the false-discovery rate.

Microarray acquisition and analysis are susceptible to many types of errors, some of which can be subtle, many of which can lead to irreproducibility or false-positive results (25–27). However, it has been shown that meticulous attention to technique, and careful choice of analytic approach, support reproducibility across laboratories (28–32). One of the most commonly recommended techniques for ensuring reproducibility of analysis is using permutation techniques to accurately estimate the false-discovery rate (16,33). Standardization among laboratories with regard to techniques, data formats (34), data descriptors (35,36), and analytic approaches will be necessary to support interdisciplinary multi-institutional microarray research. Standardization will remain a critical factor in maturation of this field, as researchers will have to cooperate across institutions to redress the problem of low sample size, which has been shown to be a central cause of poor reproducibility in microarray experiments (37).

APPLICATIONS TO ONCOLOGY

Oncology is arguably the hallmark application of microarray technology (38–41). Indeed, many of the earliest microarray applications involved cancer cell lines or biopsy material. These experiments highlight the great promise of this technology, while underscoring the necessity for meticulous experimental design and analysis. Although most applications have focused on classification or diagnosis, researchers are also investigating potential genetic signatures of prognosis, and potential predictors of response to therapy. The major underlying assumption in the application of microarray technology to understand cancer is that gene-expression changes are an important factor in carcinogenesis, and therefore that these gene-expression changes predict prognosis and response to therapy.

Diagnosis

The publication of Golub's microarray experiments on leukemic cells was a seminal event (15); these experiments demonstrated accurate computer-based recapitulation of the well-known classification of leukemia into T-cell and B-cell subtypes, based solely on microarray-expression signatures. This publication highlighted the promise of microarray technology in basing the diagnosis of cancer on objective criteria (e.g., expression patterns), rather than subjective criteria (e.g., morphology, or mitotic activity, assessed under the microscope by a pathologist); the logical extension of this line of research will center on increasing the accuracy of prognosis and therapy selection (42,43).

Alon et al. (44) demonstrated separation of colon cancer from normal tissue based on clustering. They used an unsupervised clustering algorithm to analyze the expression of approximately 6500 genes for 40 colon-cancer and 22 normal colon samples. They found two clusters corresponding to the cancer and normal samples. Note that, when they added expression data from colon-cancer cell lines to the clustering algorithm, the cell lines formed a distinct third cluster, indicating that cell lines manifest different gene-expression signatures from tumors.

Dunican et al. analyzed approximately 18,000 genes from 6 colon-cancer cell lines to develop a 73-gene signature that distinguished between the microsatellite-instability and chromosomal-instability phenotypes (45). However, only six of nine genes validated with Northern blot and reverse-transcriptase polymerase chain reaction

(RT-PCR) could be confirmed as being differentially expressed.

Kim et al. measured the expression of approximately 7100 genes from samples of 15 normal colons, 51 colon adenocarcinomas, and 224 other normal and malignant samples (e.g., ovarian and lung cancers) (46). They found that galanin was expressed approximately 10 times higher in colon-cancer samples than in any of the other samples, thereby highlighting its promise as an early-detection marker. Galanin serum levels were found to be approximately 70% sensitive and 75% specific, which are superior to carcinoembryonic antigen, but are still inadequate for screening purposes.

Dhanasekaran et al. developed a 10,000-gene microarray to compare benign (normal, prostatic, benign hypertrophy) and malignant prostate samples (47). Clustering demonstrated clear separation of benign and malignant samples based primarily on 43 genes. They confirmed differential expression of two of these genes, HPN and PIM1, using immunohistochemistry.

Holloway et al. used thresholding and support vector machines to analyze 190 lung adenocarcinomas and 33 malignant mesotheliomas; using RT-PCR, they validated a 17-gene signature that distinguishes between these tumors (48). RT-PCR analysis of independent test samples derived from pleural effusions demonstrated 100% accuracy in distinguishing lung adenocarcinoma from malignant mesothelioma.

Wong et al. used hierarchical clustering and significance analysis of microarrays (49) to compare normal cerebellar tissue with samples obtained from 21 patients with juvenile pilocytic astrocytoma (JPA). They found 428 genes that were differentially expressed between the two groups; in particular, they found differential gene expression with respect to neurogenesis, cell adhesion, potassium-ion transport, protein dephosphorylation, and cell differentiation, among other functional groups. They also performed hierarchical cluster analysis of the normal and JPA samples, and found that, as expected normal and JPA samples formed distinct clusters. In addition, they found two potential clusters within the JPA cluster; genes related to angiogenesis, cell adhesion, cell growth, and cell motility, possibly indicating differing levels of invasiveness.

Using support vector machines, Jaeger et al. analyzed 19 primary and 22 metastatic melanoma samples using approximately 22,000 genes (50); they found that 308 genes are differentially expressed between primary tumors and metastases. In particular, they found that signatures representing cellular proliferation, cell-cycle regulation, cell adhesion, and cell-extracellular matrix interaction differentiated primary from metastatic tumor samples. The support vector machine correctly classified approximately 85% of samples using cross-validation. With respect to the two major subtypes of melanoma, they found that a 60-gene signature distinguished between superficial spreading melanoma and nodular melanoma.

To determine gene-expression taxonomy of central nervous system (CNS) embryonal tumors, Pomeroy et al. analyzed the gene-expression profiles for approximately 6800 genes from 42 patient samples [10 medulloblastomas, 5 atypical teratoid/rhabdoid tumors, 5 renal and extrarenal rhabdoid tumors, 8 supratentorial primitive neuroectodermal tumors (PNETs), 10 malignant gliomas, and 4 normal human cerebella] (18). They applied principal components analysis and hierarchical clustering; cross-validation resulted in correct classification of 35 of the samples. As expected, gliomas were readily distinguished from medulloblastomas; in addition, medulloblastomas and PNETs were readily separable, indicating different origins. The rhabdoid tumors, whether of CNS or renal origin, were readily separable from other CNS tumors, but the CNS and renal tumors could not be separated, indicating a common origin. In a sample of 34 medulloblastomas, they were further able to distinguish between classic and desmoplastic subtypes.

Godard et al. used a combination of statistical and clustering methods to distinguish among low-grade astrocytoma, secondary glioblastoma (those evolving from low-grade astrocytomas), and primary glioblastoma, based on data obtained from a 1185-gene microarray (51). They generated a classifier from clusters using a k-nearest neighbor algorithm, and tested this classifier using a 20-sample independent test set; one cluster of 9 genes related to angiogenesis correctly classified approximately 90% of test cases.

Khan et al. used principal components analysis and artificial neural networks to develop a classifier for small, round blue-cell tumors (neuroblastoma, rhabdomyosarcoma, Burkitt lymphoma, and Ewing sarcoma). Many of the genes in the resulting signatures had not been previously associated with these neoplasms. They also demonstrated high sensitivity and specificity upon applying this classifier to the samples not used in training the neural networks (52).

Ramaswamy et al. have performed one of the more ambitious experiments; they measured expression levels for approximately 16,000 genes from 308 samples, 90 of which were normal, and 218 of which were one of 14 different cancer classes, the goal being to develop a multiclass cancer diagnostic tool (53). They used support vector machines to distinguish among the 15 classes; leave-one-out cross-validation yielded 78% classification accuracy, and classification of a 54-sample independent test set also resulted in 78% accuracy. They found much lower accuracy when they applied this classifier to a set of poorly differentiated tumors, implying that these tumors may have fundamentally different gene-expression signatures.

Prognosis

In addition to diagnostic applications, many microarray experiments have been designed to determine whether differences in gene expression reflect differences in prognosis, rather than alternative genetic pathways to a similar tumor histology.

Chen et al. used decision trees to derive gene-expression signatures that predict survival in non–small cell lung cancer (22). Of note, they used microarrays followed by RT-PCR to measure gene expression, believing that RT-PCR better captures possible multivariate associations among gene-expression profiles and survival. They found a five-gene signature to be associated with survival length: patients with high-risk signatures had shorter median survival than patients with low-risk signatures.

In an effort to predict postsurgical local recurrence, Iizuka et al. examined expression values of approximately 6000 genes from 33 patients (12 with subsequent local recurrence) with hepatocellular carcinoma (HCC) (54). Using Fisher linear discriminant analysis, they developed a classifier based on 12 genes. Testing this classifier on independent samples from an additional 27 patients (8 with subsequent local recurrence) resulted in approximately 93% accuracy in predicting recurrence within one year.

Dave et al. used clustering and survival analysis to develop gene-expression signatures that predict survival in patients with follicular lymphoma (55). They used cross-validation to validate the two signatures they found. In addition, they performed flow cytometry, demonstrating that these genes were expressed by non-neoplastic immune cells infiltrating the tumor.

Because of the relatively high prevalence of breast cancer, and the difficulty in deciding which patients will benefit from adjuvant therapy, there is an extensive literature describing the prognostic factors for this disease (56). van 't Veer et al. used hierarchical clustering to analyze gene-expression profiles from 78 node-negative sporadic breast cancer patients; they derived a 70-gene classifier that correctly identified 17 of 19 additional patients with respect to metastasis within five years (57). Wang et al. performed a similar experiment (58), analyzing 115 training samples to obtain a 76-gene signature that accurately predicted metastasis within five years in an additional 171 node-negative breast cancer patients. Note, that there is only a three-gene overlap between Wang's and van 't Veer's signatures, which may be due to a combination of different microarray platforms, and inadequate sample sizes, among other factors (59).

Sørlie et al. analyzed 85 samples consisting of 78 cancers, three fibroadenomas, and four normal breast tissues, using hierarchical clustering based on 427 genes (60); they found that the cancers clustered into four groups: a basal epithelial-like group, a normal breast-like group, an ERBB2 (epidermal growth factor receptor 2; also known as HER2/neu)-overexpressing group, and a luminal epithelial/estrogen receptor–positive (ER+) group. They found that this last group, consisting of 32 tumors, could be further subdivided into at least two subgroups. They also performed significance analysis of microarrays on the cancer samples, which yielded 264 candidate genes, which they then subjected to hierarchical clustering, which resulted in 3 clusters: the luminal cluster, the basal epithelial cluster, and a proliferation cluster. They further found that these subtypes had different survival times: those patients whose tumors manifested a basal epithelial-like or ERBB2-overexpression signature having the shortest survival times.

Alizadeh et al. examined 96 samples of normal lymphocytes, diffuse large B-cell lymphoma (DLBCL), follicular lymphoma (FL), mantle cell lymphoma, and chronic lymphocytic leukemia (CLL) (61). To increase the likelihood of finding relevant gene-expression patterns, they constructed a 17,856 cDNA-clone chip, including 12,069 that they chose from a germinal-center B-cell library, and an additional 2338 cDNA clones from DLBCL, FL, and CLL libraries. They found that the relatively indolent malignancies, CLL, and FL manifested relatively low expression of a proliferation signature, relative to the more aggressive DLBCL, which itself showed variability in proliferative activity. A germinal-center B-cell signature differentiated FL from CLL. Further analysis of the DLBCL samples revealed that they were also heterogeneous with respect to a T-cell expression signature, and that varying expression of B-cell differentiation genes appears to correspond to the different stages of B-cell differentiation from which the DLBCL samples were derived. On the basis of these differentially expressed signatures, they were able to distinguish two subclasses of DLBCL: those that expressed the germinal-center B-cell signature, and those that expressed a signature suggestive of activated peripheral-blood B cells. These groups had 76% and 16% five-year survival rates on similar therapeutic regimens, respectively (see Ref. 62 for a review of the application of microarrays to the management of lymphoma patients.

Therapy

There are relatively few studies predicting response to therapy, primarily because there are often many therapeutic regimens that could be employed for a particular cancer diagnosis, thus decreasing the number of subjects available to evaluate a particular regimen. In addition, there have been reports refuting previously discovered gene-signatures that predict response to therapy (63), underscoring the difficulty of designing and analyzing these experiments.

Ayers et al. employed a variety of analytic methods on over 19,000 candidate genes measured in training samples from 24 breast cancer patients (64). They found that a 74-gene signature predicted response to paclitaxel and fluorouracil, doxorubicin, and cyclophosphamide chemotherapy in 14 of 18 test subjects (see Ref. 65 for a review of the role of microarrays in the management of breast cancer).

Sotiriou et al. analyzed fine-needle aspirate samples from 10 breast cancer patients before undergoing neo-adjuvant chemotherapy (66). Clustering of 4,803 genes yielded a 37-gene signature that they then used to construct a compound covariate predictor, which accurately distinguished responders to chemotherapy from nonresponders, as determined by cross-validation.

Based on 34 pediatric osteosarcoma samples, Man et al. constructed a support vector machine to predict which patients would respond to preoperative chemotherapy consisting of cisplatin, doxorubicin, and (in all but 3 patients) methotrexate (67). Of approximately 9200 genes on the microarray, they used approximately 3000 informative genes to construct the support vector machine; of note, 6 of the 34 samples also contributed to the test set of 14 preoperative biopsy specimens. From the 20 surgical samples, they generated a 45-gene signature that accurately predicted response to chemotherapy.

Staunton et al. examined the National Cancer Institute panel of 60 cancer cell lines (NCI-60) (68) to determine whether gene-expression signatures could predict response to any of 232 compounds (69). For 88 of the 232 compounds, they were able to predict sensitivity accurately, indicating the potential for this approach in predicting the utility of potential chemotherapeutic agents, or developing novel agents.

Similarly, Torres-Roca et al. examined a 35-sample subset of the NCI-60 cell lines to derive a gene-expression signature that would predict tumor survival fraction after radiation therapy at 2 gray (Gy) (70). To discover this four-gene signature, they measured the expression of approximately 7,100 genes from the 35 samples and analyzed these data using significance analysis of microarrays and multivariate linear regression. Cross-validation resulted in approximately 62% accuracy in predicting radiation sensitivity. Permutation testing showed this performance to be significantly better than chance ($P = 0.0002$).

As described in section "Diagnosis," Pomeroy et al. determined a gene-expression taxonomy of CNS embryonal tumors; in addition, they examined an additional group of 60 patients from whom biopsies had been obtained before the institution of therapy for medulloblastoma (18). They used self-organizing maps to group the samples into clusters; however, this approach failed to yield significant differences in response to therapy between clusters. Upon applying a k-nearest neighbors algorithm (a supervised learning method) to these data, the resulting optimal model had 8 genes, and classified 47 of 60 samples correctly by cross-validation. Those patients predicted to respond to therapy had an 80% five-year survival, compared with 17% for those predicted not to respond to therapy. Several other approaches, including support vector machines, demonstrated similar classification accuracy.

McLean et al. examined pretreatment gene-expression profiles in 66 chronic myeloid leukemia (CML) patients to determine whether they could be used to predict response to imatinib therapy (71). Comparing 53 patients with no remaining Philadelphia-chromosome–positive (Ph^+) cells remaining after treatment to 13 patients with patients who had at least 65% Ph^+ cells, they found that, of approximately 12,000 genes on the microarray, 31 genes correctly predicted response to imatinib therapy in 50 of 53 responders, and in 12 of 13 nonresponders. In addition, they found that many of the genes they identified could be related to the BCR-ABL oncogene, possibly leading to additional targets for drug discovery. Similarly, Hofmann et al. found 56 genes that predicted secondary resistance to imatinib (72), indicating potential targets for the development of novel chemotherapeutic agents.

FUTURE APPLICATIONS

Just as the combination of gene-expression profiles and sophisticated analysis software shows early indications of having profound impacts on cancer diagnosis, prognosis, and therapy, it is reasonable to expect that microarrays will also provide clues to guide the development of molecular-imaging agents. One indication of this potential is the growing body of literature describing the potential of microarray-guided drug development (69,71–79).

An early step toward microarray-guided imaging-ligand development is the work by Hundt et al., in which a murine squamous cell cancer (SCCA) model was subjected to high-intensity focused ultrasound (HIFU), and magnetic resonance (MR) examination, and microarray analysis were performed on treated and control tumor samples, in an attempt to identify gene-expression profiles characterizing successful HIFU treatment, and potentially to identify molecular-imaging agents that could be used to assess the efficacy of HIFU treatment (80). Of approximately 36,000 murine genes examined, 23 genes were found to be upregulated, and 5 genes were found to be downregulated. In treated samples, these findings predicted cell death more accurately than did MR findings (e.g., decreased enhancement reflecting devascularization). The authors speculated that these genes might serve as useful guides in the development of molecular-imaging agents for the noninvasive evaluation of HIFU efficacy.

An additional application of microarrays to molecular imaging is the assessment of the effects of molecular-imaging agents on gene expression. Ideally, the introduction of a molecular imaging agent should not alter the system being interrogated, i.e., the agent should support biochemically noninvasive imaging. In an important example of this application, Wu et al. used a microarray capable of measuring the expression of over 20,000 murine genes to characterize in detail the effects of a triple-fusion reporter gene on gene-expression profiles (81). Although the transduced and nontransduced embryonic stem cells manifested similar differentiation capabilities and viability, transduced cells manifested downregulation of 333 genes, including cell cycling, cell death, and protein and nucleic acid metabolism genes, and upregulation of 207 genes, including homeostatic and anti-apoptosis genes.

In addition, researchers have begun to ask whether findings on radiological examination are associated with gene-expression profiles. For example, Segal et al. examined computed tomography (CT) findings in 28 patients with HCC, in an attempt to determine whether these findings were associated with gene-expression profiles for these tumors (82). Of 32 CT traits that they defined for HCCs (e.g., "internal arteries") and expression values for 6732 genes, they found that most of the variation in gene-expression was manifested in 116 gene "functional modules" (e.g., cell-cycle genes), and that 28 CT findings accounted for the variation in expression for approximately 75% (5282) of the genes. Furthermore, they were able to use these 28 CT findings to successfully predict expression patterns for 74% of genes in an independent sample of 19 HCC patients.

Similarly, Bianchi et al. compared gene-expression profiles in patients whose lung cancer was detected on screening CT examination to those in patients who presented symptomatically (83). They employed a microarray containing approximately 3000 genes to analyze samples from 18 histologically proven lung cancers detected with screening CT, and compared these gene-expression values with those obtained from 19 patients who had presented with symptoms, such as cough. They were unable to construct a set of genes that distinguished between the two groups of subjects, leading them to conclude that lung cancer detected on screening CT does not differ significantly from the tumors that come to diagnosis through symptoms. Although they employed multiple-comparison correction to control the false-discovery rate, they presented no power analysis to estimate the probability of a false-negative result.

Although there are no reports in the research literature demonstrating the use of microarray analysis to guide molecular-imaging research, the combination of promising early results in cancer diagnosis, prognosis, and drug development, as well as early successes in correlating CT and MR findings with gene-expression profiles, indicate the feasibility of this endeavor.

CONCLUSION

Clearly, the promise of microarray technology to elucidate the molecular nature of cancer must be balanced against the complex logistics of carrying out such research in a reproducible manner. Multicenter trials may be necessary to ensure adequate sample sizes for producing meaningful results from severely undersampled data. In addition, collaboration among molecular biologists, oncologists, biostatisticians, and bioinformaticians will be necessary to ensure that these complex experiments are properly designed, implemented, and analyzed. As standards develop to promote collaboration, microarrays will play an increasing role in cancer diagnosis, estimating prognosis, and managing therapy. Another potential result of the increased use of gene-expression profiling for the diagnosis and management of cancer is the potential for atomization of cancer diagnosis. Although the term "cancer" currently represents a collection of hundreds of different diseases, microarray analysis may reveal many thousands of different genetic changes requiring individualized therapy. Unless the process of molecular analysis and target development for a particular neoplasm can be highly automated, the costs of cancer management could become prohibitively expensive if cancer proves to be thousands, rather than hundreds, of diseases.

REFERENCES

1. GenBank. Growth of GenBank (1982–2005). Available at: http://www.ncbi.nlm.nih.gov/Genbank/genbankstats.html. Accessed 8/1/2008.
2. Ross DT, Scherf U, Eisen MB, et al. Systematic variation in gene expression patterns in human cancer cell lines. Nat Genet 2000; 24(3):227–235.
3. Bellman R. Adaptive Control Processes: A Guided Tour. Princeton, NJ: Princeton University Press, 1961.
4. Köppen M. The curse of dimensionality. In: Proceedings of the Fifth Online World Conference on Soft Computing in Industrial Applications, 2000, WSC5.
5. Quackenbush J. Computational analysis of microarray data. Nat Rev Genet 2001; 2(6):418–427.
6. Nadon R, Shoemaker J. Statistical issues with microarrays: processing and analysis. Trends Genet 2002; 18(5):265–271.
7. Cui X, Churchill GA. Statistical tests for differential expression in cDNA microarray experiments. Genome Biol 2003; 4(4):210 [Epub March 17, 2003].
8. Perou CM, Jeffrey SS, van de Rijn M, et al. Distinctive gene expression patterns in human mammary epithelial cells and breast cancers. Proc Natl Acad Sci U S A 1999; 96(16):9212–9217.

9. Jiang D, Tang C, Zhang A. Cluster analysis for gene expression data: a survey. IEEE Trans Knowledge Data Eng 2004; 16(11):1370–1386.

10. Calza S, Hall P, Auer G, et al. Intrinsic molecular signature of breast cancer in a population-based cohort of 412 patients. Breast Cancer Res 2006; 8(4):R34.

11. Kohonen T, ed. Self-Organizing Maps. New York: Springer-Verlag, Inc.1997.

12. Tamayo P, Slonim D, Mesirov J, et al. Interpreting patterns of gene expression with self-organizing maps: methods and application to hematopoietic differentiation. Proc Natl Acad Sci U S A 1999; 96(6):2907–2912.

13. Törönen P, Kolehmainen M, Wong G, et al. Analysis of gene expression data using self-organizing maps. FEBS Lett 1999; 451(2):142–146.

14. Eisen MB, Spellman PT, Brown PO, et al. Cluster analysis and display of genome-wide expression patterns. Proc Natl Acad Sci U S A 1998; 95(25):14863–14868.

15. Golub TR, Slonim DK, Tamayo P, et al. Molecular classification of cancer: class discovery and class prediction by gene expression monitoring. Science 1999; 286(5439): 531–537.

16. Tusher VG, Tibshirani R, Chu G. Significance analysis of microarrays applied to the ionizing radiation response. Proc Natl Acad Sci U S A 2001; 98(9):5116–5121.

17. Brown MP, Grundy WN, Lin D, et al. Knowledge-based analysis of microarray gene expression data by using support vector machines. Proc Natl Acad Sci U S A 2000; 97(1):262–267.

18. Pomeroy SL, Tamayo P, Gaasenbeek M, et al. Prediction of central nervous system embryonal tumour outcome based on gene expression. Nature 2002; 415(6870):436–442.

19. O'Neill M, Song L. Neural network analysis of lymphoma microarray data: prognosis and diagnosis near-perfect. BMC Bioinformatics 2003; 4(1):13 [Epub April 10, 2003].

20. Alter O, Brown PO, Botstein D. Singular value decomposition for genome-wide expression data processing and modeling. Proc Natl Acad Sci U S A 2000; 97(18): 10101–10106.

21. Bicciato S, Luchini A, Di Bello C. PCA disjoint models for multiclass cancer analysis using gene expression data. Bioinformatics 2003; 19(5):571–578.

22. Chen H-Y, Yu S-L, Chen C-H, et al. A five-gene signature and clinical outcome in non-small-cell lung cancer. N Engl J Med 2007; 356(1):11–20.

23. Friedman N. Inferring cellular networks using probabilistic graphical models. Science 2004; 303(5659):799–805.

24. Slonim DK. From patterns to pathways: gene expression data analysis comes of age. Nat Genet 2002; 32:502–508.

25. Koren A, Tirosh I, Barkai N. Autocorrelation analysis reveals widespread spatial biases in microarray experiments. BMC Genomics 2007; 8:164.

26. Frantz S. An array of problems. Nat Rev Drug Discov 2005; 4(5):362–363.

27. Michiels S, Koscielny S, Hill C. Prediction of cancer outcome with microarrays: a multiple random validation strategy. Lancet 2005; 365(9458):488–492.

28. MAQC Consortium, Shi L, Reid LH, et al. The MicroArray Quality Control (MAQC) project shows inter- and intraplatform reproducibility of gene expression measurements. Nat Biotechnol 2006; 24(9):1151–1161.

29. Anderson K, Hess KR, Kapoor M, et al. Reproducibility of gene expression signature-based predictions in replicate experiments. Clin Cancer Res 2006; 12(6):1721–1727.

30. Fan J, Niu Y. Selection and validation of normalization methods for c-DNA microarrays using within-array replications. Bioinformatics 2007; 23(18):2391–2398.

31. Lee M-LT, Kuo FC, Whitmore GA, et al. Importance of replication in microarray gene expression studies: statistical methods and evidence from repetitive cDNA hybridizations. Proc Natl Acad Sci U S A 2000; 97(18): 9834–9839.

32. Dobbin KK, Beer DG, Meyerson M, et al. Interlaboratory comparability study of cancer gene expression analysis using oligonucleotide microarrays. Clin Cancer Res 2005; 11(2):565–572.

33. Guo X, Pan W. Using weighted permutation scores to detect differential gene expression with microarray data. J Bioinform Comput Biol 2005; 3(4):989–1006.

34. Brazma A, Hingamp P, Quackenbush J, et al. Minimum information about a microarray experiment (MIAME)-toward standards for microarray data. Nat Genet 2001; 29(4):365–371.

35. Spellman PT, Miller M, Stewart J, et al. Design and implementation of microarray gene expression markup language (MAGE-ML). Genome Biol 2002; 3(9): RESEARCH0046 [Epub August 23, 2002].

36. Whetzel PL, Parkinson H, Causton HC, et al. The MGED Ontology: a resource for semantics-based description of microarray experiments. Bioinformatics 2006; 22(7): 866–873.

37. Ein-Dor L, Zuk O, Domany E. Thousands of samples are needed to generate a robust gene list for predicting outcome in cancer. Proc Natl Acad Sci U S A 2006; 103(15): 5923–5928.

38. Macgregor PF, Squire JA. Application of microarrays to the analysis of gene expression in cancer. Clin Chem 2002; 48(8):1170–1177.

39. Ramaswamy S, Golub TR. DNA microarrays in clinical oncology. J Clin Oncol 2002; 20(7):1932–1941.

40. Bullinger L, Valk PJM. Gene expression profiling in acute myeloid leukemia. J Clin Oncol 2005; 23(26): 6296–6305.

41. Wadlow R, Ramaswamy S. DNA microarrays in clinical cancer research. Curr Mol Med 2005; 5:111–120.

42. Ebert B, Golub T. Genomic approaches to hematologic malignancies. Blood 2004; 104:923–932.

43. Chiaretti S, Ritz J, Foa R. Genomic analysis in lymphoid leukemias. Rev Clin Exp Hematol 2005; 9:E3.

44. Alon U, Barkai N, Notterman DA, et al. Broad patterns of gene expression revealed by clustering analysis of tumor and normal colon tissues probed by oligonucleotide arrays. Proc Natl Acad Sci U S A 1999; 96(12):6745–6750.

45. Dunican DS, McWilliam P, Tighe O, et al. Gene expression differences between the microsatellite instability (MIN) and chromosomal instability (CIN) phenotypes in colorectal cancer revealed by high-density cDNA array hybridization. Oncogene 2002; 21(20):3253–3257.

46. Kim KY, Kee MK, Chong SA, et al. Galanin is up-regulated in colon adenocarcinoma. Cancer Epidemiol Biomarkers Prev 2007; 16(11):2373–2378.

47. Dhanasekaran SM, Barrette TR, Ghosh D, et al. Delineation of prognostic biomarkers in prostate cancer. Nature 2001; 412(6849):822–826.

48. Holloway AJ, Diyagama DS, Opeskin K, et al. A molecular diagnostic test for distinguishing lung adenocarcinoma from malignant mesothelioma using cells collected from pleural effusions. Clin Cancer Res 2006; 12(17):5129–5135.

49. Wong K-K, Chang Y-M, Tsang YTM, et al. Expression analysis of juvenile pilocytic astrocytomas by oligonucleotide microarray reveals two potential subgroups. Cancer Res 2005; 65(1):76–84.

50. Jaeger J, Koczan D, Thiesen H-J, et al. Gene expression signatures for tumor progression, tumor subtype, and tumor thickness in laser-microdissected melanoma tissues. Clin Cancer Res 2007; 13(3):806–815.

51. Godard S, Getz G, Delorenzi M, et al. Classification of human astrocytic gliomas on the basis of gene expression: a correlated group of genes with angiogenic activity emerges as a strong predictor of subtypes. Cancer Res 2003; 63(20): 6613–6625.

52. Khan J, Wei JS, Ringner M, et al. Classification and diagnostic prediction of cancers using gene expression profiling and artificial neural networks. Nat Med 2001; 7(6):673–679.

53. Ramaswamy S, Tamayo P, Rifkin R, et al. Multiclass cancer diagnosis using tumor gene expression signatures. Proc Natl Acad Sci U S A 2001; 98(26):15149–15154.

54. Iizuka N, Oka M, Yamada-Okabe H, et al. Oligonucleotide microarray for prediction of early intrahepatic recurrence of hepatocellular carcinoma after curative resection. Lancet 2003; 361(9361):923–929.

55. Dave SS, Wright G, Tan B, et al. Prediction of survival in follicular lymphoma based on molecular features of tumor-infiltrating immune cells. N Engl J Med 2004; 351 (21):2159–2169.

56. Weigelt B, Peterse J, van 't Veer LJ. Breast cancer metastasis: markers and models. Nat Rev Cancer 2005; 5:591–602.

57. van 't Veer LJ, Dai H, van de Vijver MJ, et al. Gene expression profiling predicts clinical outcome of breast cancer. Nature 2002; 415(6871):530–536.

58. Wang Y, Klijn JG, Zhang Y, et al. Gene-expression profiles to predict distant metastasis of lymph-node-negative primary breast cancer. Lancet 2005; 365(9460):671–679.

59. Ein-Dor L, Kela I, Getz G, et al. Outcome signature genes in breast cancer: is there a unique set? Bioinformatics 2005; 21(2):171–178.

60. Sørlie T, Perou CM, Tibshirani R, et al. Gene expression patterns of breast carcinomas distinguish tumor subclasses with clinical implications. Proc Natl Acad Sci U S A 2001; 98(19):10869–10874.

61. Alizadeh AA, Eisen MB, Davis RE, et al. Distinct types of diffuse large B-cell lymphoma identified by gene expression profiling. Nature 2000; 403(6769):503–511.

62. Savage KJ, Gascoyne RD. Molecular signatures of lymphoma. Int J Hematol 2004; 80:401–409.

63. Reid JF, Lusa L, De Cecco L, et al. Limits of predictive models using microarray data for breast cancer clinical treatment outcome. J Natl Cancer Inst 2005; 97(12): 927–930.

64. Ayers M, Symmans WF, Stec J, et al. Gene expression profiles predict complete pathologic response to neoadjuvant paclitaxel and fluorouracil, doxorubicin, and cyclophosphamide chemotherapy in breast cancer. J Clin Oncol 2004; 22(12):2284–2293.

65. Chang J, Hilsenbeck S, Fuqua S. Genomic approaches in the management and treatment of breast cancer. Br J Cancer 2005; 92:618–624.

66. Sotiriou C, Powles T, Dowsett M, et al. Gene expression profiles derived from fine needle aspiration correlate with response to systemic chemotherapy in breast cancer. Breast Cancer Res 2002; 4(3):R3 [Epub March 20, 2002].

67. Man T-K, Chintagumpala M, Visvanathan J, et al. Expression profiles of osteosarcoma that can predict response to chemotherapy. Cancer Res 2005; 65(18):8142–8150.

68. Shoemaker RH. The NCI60 human tumour cell line anticancer drug screen. Nat Rev Cancer 2006; 6(10):813–823.

69. Staunton JE, Slonim DK, Coller HA, et al. Chemosensitivity prediction by transcriptional profiling. Proc Natl Acad Sci U S A 2001; 98(19):10787–10792.

70. Torres-Roca JF, Eschrich S, Zhao H, et al. Prediction of radiation sensitivity using a gene expression classifier. Cancer Res 2005; 65(16):7169–7176.

71. McLean LA, Gathmann I, Capdeville R, et al. Pharmacogenomic analysis of cytogenetic response in chronic myeloid leukemia patients treated with imatinib. Clin Cancer Res 2004; 10(1):155–165.

72. Hofmann W-K, de Vos S, Elashoff D, et al. Relation between resistance of Philadelphia-chromosome-positive acute lymphoblastic leukaemia to the tyrosine kinase inhibitor STI571 and gene-expression profiles: a gene-expression study. Lancet 2002; 359(9305):481–486.

73. Butte AJ, Tamayo P, Slonim D, et al. Discovering functional relationships between RNA expression and chemotherapeutic susceptibility using relevance networks. Proc Natl Acad Sci U S A 2000; 97(22):12182–12186.

74. Debouck C, Goodfellow PN. DNA microarrays in drug discovery and development. Nat Genet 1999; 21(1 suppl): 48–50.

75. Gunther EC, Stone DJ, Gerwien RW, et al. Prediction of clinical drug efficacy by classification of drug-induced genomic expression profiles in vitro. Proc Natl Acad Sci U S A 2003; 100(16):9608–9613.

76. Sausville EA, Holbeck SL. Transcription profiling of gene expression in drug discovery and development: the NCI experience. Eur J Cancer 2004; 40(17):2544–2549.

77. Wirth GJ, Schandelmaier K, Smith V, et al. Microarrays of 41 human tumor cell lines for the characterization of new molecular targets: expression patterns of cathepsin B and the transferrin receptor. Oncology 2006; 71(1–2):86–94.

78. Lee JK, Havaleshko DM, Cho H, et al. A strategy for predicting the chemosensitivity of human cancers and its application to drug discovery. Proc Natl Acad Sci U S A 2007; 104(32):13086–13091.

79. Chengalvala MV, Chennathukuzhi VM, Johnston DS, et al. Gene expression profiling and its practice in drug development. Curr Genomics 2007; 8(4):262–270.

80. Hundt W, Yuh EL, Bednarski MD, et al. Gene expression profiles, histologic analysis, and imaging of squamous cell carcinoma model treated with focused ultrasound beams. Am J Roentgenol 2007; 189(3):726–736.

81. Wu JC, Spin JM, Cao F, et al. Transcriptional profiling of reporter genes used for molecular imaging of embryonic stem cell transplantation. Physiol Genomics 2006; 25(1): 29–38.

82. Segal E, Sirlin CB, Ooi C, et al. Decoding global gene expression programs in liver cancer by noninvasive imaging. Nat Biotechnol 2007; 25(6):675–680.

83. Bianchi F, Hu J, Pelosi G, et al. Lung cancers detected by screening with spiral computed tomography have a malignant phenotype when analyzed by cDNA microarray. Clin Cancer Res 2004; 10(18):6023–6028

5

Molecular PET Instrumentation and Imaging Techniques

ROGER LECOMTE

Sherbrooke Molecular Imaging Center, Department of Nuclear Medicine and Radiobiology, Université de Sherbrooke, Sherbrooke, Quebec, Canada

INTRODUCTION

Positron emission tomography (PET) is a nuclear medicine imaging technique that provides a powerful and sensitive means to noninvasively investigate biological processes in vivo. After the administration of a suitably radiolabeled pharmaceutical into the subject, images of the static or dynamic distribution of the tracer can be formed that provide information on blood flow, metabolism, cellular proliferation, angiogenesis, hypoxia, receptor and enzyme concentrations, gene expression, etc. PET finds applications in the clinic for diagnosis, treatment follow-up, and therapy assessment in cardiology and oncology. In basic research, PET is used as an investigation tool for neurology and drug development, among others.

PET images are created through the observation of the annihilation radiation produced as a result of the disintegration of neutron-deficient radionuclides by positron emission. The interest of imaging with such positron-emitting radionuclides stems from three main factors. The first one is the ability to determine the direction of incidence of the radiation by electronic collimation through annihilation coincidence detection, thus avoiding the need for heavy absorptive collimators as in conventional nuclear imaging with standard gamma emitters. The resulting higher sensitivity (by two to three orders of magnitude) enables the radiotracer distribution in living subjects to be measured down to the nano- and picomolar range, levels that can be achieved by no other imaging modalities. The second related factor is the absolute quantification capability that can be achieved through accurate correction for attenuation of the annihilation radiation in the subject. The third main factor that makes PET unique among other imaging modalities is the availability of positron-emitting radionuclides that are *organic* atoms, such as ^{11}C, ^{13}N, ^{15}O, and ^{18}F, which can be substituted into molecules without modifying their biological activity (Table 1). As a result of these three unique features, PET radiotracers can, in principle, be developed to investigate virtually any biological processes without interfering with normal biochemistry. Hence, PET currently continues to hold some advantages over other molecular imaging modalities such as single photon emission computed tomography (SPECT), magnetic resonance imaging (MRI), and optical imaging due to the sensitivity, absolute quantification capability, and specificity it provides at the molecular level.

There exists an abundant literature on the topic of PET imaging. One classic on the subject is a book chapter by Hoffman and Phelps (1). An excellent introductory text can be found in Cherry et al. (2). A number of recent review papers on the instrumentation and methodology of PET imaging are also available (3–9).

Table 1 Most Popular PET Radioisotopes

Radionuclides	$T_{1/2}$ (min)	β^+ Branching ratio (%)	Production method
^{11}C	20.4	100	Cyclotron
^{13}N	9.97	100	Cyclotron
^{15}O	2.04	100	Cyclotron
^{18}F	109.7	97	Cyclotron
^{64}Cu	12.8 h	18	Cyclotron
^{68}Ga	68	89	Generator
^{82}Rb	1.25	95	Generator

HISTORICAL OVERVIEW OF POSITRON IMAGING

The idea to detect the back-to-back 511-keV radiation in coincidence for measuring internal structures of the body was first proposed independently in 1951 by Sweet (10) and Wrenn et al. (11) The first clinical positron imaging device, consisting of two coincident sodium iodide (NaI(Tl)) probes with a 2D scanning motion, was even used in 1952 to obtain images of radiotracer distribution in the brain (12). However, it was only about two decades later, with the advent of proper tomographic image reconstruction methods, researchers at the Massachusetts General Hospital, the Washington University in St. Louis, the Brookhaven National Laboratory, and later at the Montreal Neurological Institute succeeded in developing PET scanners that were eventually able to obtain true reconstructed cross-sectional images of the body. Since then, remarkable progress has been made in PET scanner design and performance through many generations of technology advancements, which have improved the spatial resolution from a coarse $\sim$2 cm to better than $\sim$2 mm and increased the sensitivity $\sim$1000-fold, but also significantly refined image quality. Some of the major technological advances that have shaped the development of PET thereafter include the discovery of bismuth germanate (BGO) and lutetium oxyorthosilicate (LSO) scintillators, the introduction of the block detector and more recently of avalanche photodiode (APD) detectors, the adjunction of CT for attenuation correction and anatomical image coregistration, the implementation of fully 3D whole-body imaging, and the recent revival of time-of-flight (TOF) PET. Such progress was boosted by the parallel development of medical cyclotrons and associated automated radiochemistry and the synthesis of a wide variety of radiopharmaceuticals, including ^{18}F-deoxyglucose (FDG), with its subsequent acceptance as a diagnostic procedure for cardiac viability and cancer. For an historical review of the timeline of significant accomplishments that have contributed to the development of PET as it is know today, see reports by Brownell (13), Lewellen (14), Nutt (15), and Muehllehner and Karp (8).

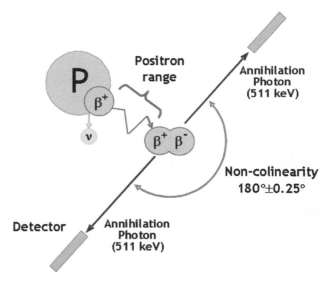

Figure 1 Positron emission and annihilation processes in PET coincidence detection.

PHYSICAL PRINCIPLES OF PET

Annihilation Coincidence Detection

PET is based on the coincidence detection of the two collinear 511-keV photons resulting from the annihilation of an electron, with the positron emitted during β^+ decay (Fig. 1). Two fundamental limits to spatial resolution result from this process: the finite distance traveled by the positron before annihilation and the small deviation from 180° of the annihilation photons due to the residual momentum of the two annihilating particles.

The effect of the positron range on resolution is radionuclide-specific and depends on the β^+ emission energy (Table 2). Its distribution profile in tissue-equivalent materials (e.g., water) has a sharply peaked shape that can be modeled as the sum of two exponentials (16,17). Although the effect on full width at half maximum (FWHM) resolution is relatively insignificant, the long exponential tails broaden the full width at tenth maximum (FWTM) resolution and will affect edge sharpness in reconstructed images. The resulting overall blurring due to positron range is better described by the root mean square (rms) effective range, which can be expressed as r = 2.35 × rms, for convenience, to be combined in quadrature with other FWHM values (18). For ^{18}F ($E_{\beta max} = 0.64$ MeV), the positron range contributes a negligible 0.1-mm FWHM and an overall 0.5-mm degradation to resolution. However, for ^{82}Rb ($E_{\beta max} = 3.4$ MeV), the FWHM contribution slightly exceeds 1 mm and the overall degradation amounts to a significant 6 mm.

The noncolinearity of annihilation photons can be described as an approximately Gaussian angular distribution

Table 2 Effect of Positron Range on Resolution in PET

Radioisotopes	β' Energy (MeV)		Resolution (mm)		
	Max	Average	FWHM	FWTM	r^a
^{11}C	0.96	0.385	0.188	1.86	0.92
^{13}N	1.20	0.491	0.282	2.53	1.35
^{15}O	1.73	0.735	0.501	4.14	2.4
^{18}F	0.64	0.242	0.102	1.03	0.54
^{64}Cu	0.65	0.278	0.104	1.05	0.55
^{68}Ga	1.90	0.836	0.58	4.83	2.8
^{82}Rb	3.36	1.52	1.27	10.5	6.1

$^a r = 2.35 \times$ rms
Abbreviations: PET, positron emission tomography; FWHM, full width at half maximum; FWTM, full width at tenth maximum.

around 180° with FWHM $\approx$ 0.5°. Its spreading effect on spatial resolution is a linear function of the distance D between coincident detectors, which can be simply expressed as $0.5D \times \tan 0.25° = 0.0022D$ for a source halfway between detectors. Therefore, for whole-body PET scanners having a diameter of $\sim$80 cm, noncolinearity entails a physical limit of about 2 mm to the achievable spatial resolution. For small-animal PET scanners having a diameter of $\sim$20 cm or less, the effect is small ($<$0.5 mm) and remains beyond other contributions to resolution. Overall, the positron emission and annihilation processes impose a physical limit of the order of 2 to 2.5 mm ($\sim$6 mm with ^{82}Rb) for clinical whole-body scanners, but of only about 0.7 mm with ^{18}F or ^{64}Cu for a small-animal scanner with a 15-cm diameter ring. This is an estimate of the overall blurring, but since the positron range distribution is sharply peaked, the FWHM resolution limit with an optimized system could be nearly 250 to 300 μm.

The spatial resolution in PET is generally dominated by the detector intrinsic resolution, which consists of a *geometric* and a *decoding* component. The geometric resolution is determined by the size of discrete detector elements or the finite pixel size of continuous detector arrays. The coincidence response function halfway between a pair of such diametrically opposed pixel detector elements in annihilation coincidence detection is simply a triangle of base equal to the pixel size d and FWHM = $d/2$ (Fig. 2A). As the source is shifted toward either detector, the response profile becomes trapezoidal and eventually square at the surface of the detectors, keeping the same base size d with a FWHM resolution varying linearly from $d/2$ to d. For coincident detectors at angle in a ring or planar arrays, the apparent width of the detectors increases the width of the tube of response because the exact depth at which annihilation photons interact in the crystal volume is unknown. This uncertainty about the depth of interaction (DOI) degrades the spatial resolution, and the magnitude of this effect depends on the length l and width d of detector elements and the source location relative to coincident detectors

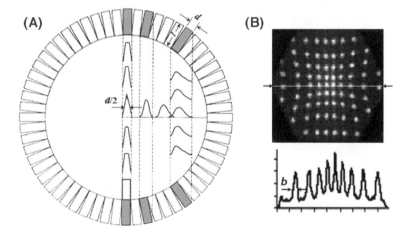

Figure 2 Illustration of the detector intrinsic resolution in PET consisting of (**A**) a geometric component determined by the size of detector element and position within the scanner FOV and (**B**) a decoding component accounting for the positioning accuracy with which crystals can be identified in coded detector arrays. *Abbreviations*: PET, positron emission tomography; FOV, field of view.

(19) (Fig. 2A). Ways to avoid this degradation include the use of a larger scanner diameter relative to the subject size to limit the incidence angle on the detectors or the measurement of DOI within the detector, for instance using multilayer crystals or depth sensitive detectors (20,21).

The decoding contribution to spatial resolution accounts for the positioning accuracy within detector arrays (Fig. 2B) and depends on the type of coupling between scintillators and photodetectors and the method used to identify the crystal of interaction. Since most detection systems cannot discriminate multiple Compton interactions in crystal arrays, the decoding resolution incorporates the effect of detector scatter (see below). The decoding resolution typically amounts to ~ 2 mm on the average for detection systems based on light-sharing or Anger-like logic and to ~ 1 mm with charge division readout schemes, but can be reduced to zero with individual pixel readout (22).

The reconstructed FWHM image resolution in PET can be described by an empirical formula combining the individual resolution components (18):

$$R = a\sqrt{g^2 + b^2 + (0.0022D)^2 + r^2},\qquad(1)$$

where a is a tomographic reconstruction degradation factor, g is the geometric resolution, b is the detector positioning accuracy, D is the distance between coincident detectors, and r is the positron range. The exact value of the factor a depends on the algorithm used to reconstruct the image ($a \approx 1.25$ for filtered backprojection (FBP) with suitable sampling, $a \approx 1.1$ with iterative reconstruction, $a = 1$ with no reconstruction).

Both annihilation photons must be detected for an event to be counted in PET. In practice, every single hit in the detectors is analyzed for energy and time, but a coincidence event is counted only when two such *singles* are validated for energy and found to occur in simultaneity. With the detectors currently used in PET, the precision with which the energy and time can be determined is limited. For instance, with scintillation detectors

achieving a rather coarse energy resolution of typically 15% to 30%, an *energy window* of ~ 350 to 650 keV must be used to accept most valid annihilation photons. Similarly, whereas the propagation time to reach detectors merely exceeds ~ 1 ns, the rather long decay time of scintillators (from ~ 20 to 300 ns) and the electronic noise in the signal processing circuitry usually require the *coincidence time window* of the scanner to be in the range of 6 to 20 ns. As a result of these uncertainties, the PET measurement is contaminated by undesirable coincident events that degrade image quality and quantitative accuracy.

Event Types in PET

The *true* events are those originating from the detection of the two singles emitted from the same positron annihilation. The *trues* count rate T is proportional to

$$T \approx A\varepsilon^2\Omega_{\text{coinc}},\qquad(2)$$

where A is the activity concentration of the source, ε is the detection efficiency of individual detectors for 511-keV photons, and Ω_{coinc} is the coincidence solid angle for detection of collinear annihilation photons, which defines a tube of response commonly referred to as a *line of response* (LOR) between opposed detectors (Fig. 3). The position of the annihilation on the LOR cannot usually be determined, although recent progress in timing resolution with fast scintillators now makes it possible to measure the TOF of the annihilation photons and restrict the position of the annihilation within less than about 10 cm along the LOR. The trues sensitivity can be enhanced by allowing all possible coincidence LORs over the source volume of interest to be measured with maximum intrinsic detection efficiency.

A consequence of the coincidence detection principle in PET is the registration of accidental or *random* events, occurring when singles originating from different annihilations are detected within the finite coincidence time

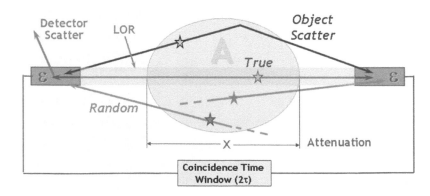

Figure 3 Various event types in PET coincidence detection.

window of the scanner (Fig. 3). The *randoms* rate R in PET is given by

$$R = 2\tau N_i N_j \approx 2\tau A^2 \Omega_s^2 \varepsilon^2, \qquad (3)$$

where 2τ is the width of the time window (conventionally so-called in reference to the width τ of the square pulses that are ANDed to perform the coincidence in electronic logic) and $N_s \approx A\,\Omega_s\varepsilon$ is the individual detector *singles* count rate, which is proportional to the activity concentration of the source A, the detection efficiency ε, and the solid angle Ω_s for direct incidence on the detectors. Since Ω_s spans a much larger fraction of the source volume, even extending to out-of-field activity, than LORs do for true coincidences (Fig. 4A), random coincidences are unavoidable and their rate may actually exceed the trues rate because it increases as the square of the activity A. Although the randoms rate can be controlled by limiting the injected activity, the shorter coincidence time window allowed by faster scintillators and the smaller singles solid angle obtained with field collimators and slice septa in 2D mode help limit the randoms-to-trues ratio. In addition to the noise contamination in images, one significant impact of a high randoms rate is the increased deadtime and pulse pileup in the front-end processing electronics that may eventually limit the sensitivity of the scanner.

Scatter events, where at least one of the photons undergoes Compton interaction before being detected, may origin from two sources in PET: from the subject and from the gantry and detection system itself, especially with small-diameter, large acceptance angle scanners dedicated to brain or small-animal imaging (23–25). Since the scatters count rate S as well as the trues count rate T are proportional to the activity concentration A, the

scatter-to-true ratio will be independent of activity for a given imaging configuration. The *detector scatter* contribution mostly affects spatial resolution in high-resolution, small-animal scanners, but can generally be neglected in clinical systems. The *object scatter* rate S is given by

$$S \approx A\varepsilon^2 \Omega_d, \qquad (4)$$

where Ω_d is the solid angle describing the field of view (FOV) for coincident scatter events. The scatters-to-trues ratio can be reduced considerably by limiting Ω_d with interslice septa in 2D PET scanners, but represents a significant background contribution that must be subtracted in fully 3D systems (Fig. 4B). However, the four- to sixfold gain in trues sensitivity in the central region of the scanner obtained by accepting all oblique coincidences (Fig. 5) generally compensate for the even larger increase in scatter and random count rates that are more uniformly spread across the entire FOV.

The trade-offs between these background contributions and sensitivity are commonly summarized into a measurement of the noise equivalent count rate (NECR), defined as

$$\text{NECR} = \frac{T \times T}{T + S + \alpha R}, \qquad (5)$$

which is the rate of true coincidences weighted by the ratio of trues-to-total events measured by the scanner. The

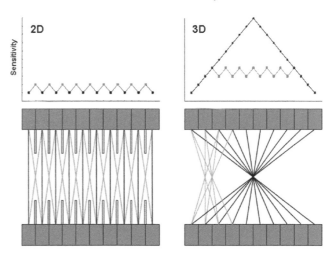

Figure 5 Comparison between 2D (*left*) and 3D (*right*) PET data acquisition modes. 2D acquisition usually involves direct (*dark lines*) and cross-plane (*gray lines*) coincidences, with cross-slices having about twice the sensitivity of direct slices. Septa removal to allow oblique coincidences between distant planes in 3D mode increases sensitivity toward the center of the FOV proportionally to the number of cross-planes ("span") allowed, as illustrated for a span of ±3 (*gray lines*) and maximum span (*dark lines*). The maximum sensitivity improvement in 3D is obtained at the center of FOV by accepting all oblique coincidence planes. Only coincidence planes for ±3 and maximum spans at selected axial positions are shown on the right for clarity. *Abbreviation*: FOV, field of view.

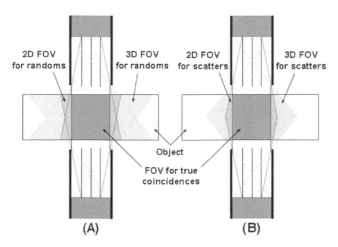

Figure 4 Schematic representation of the contributions from activity outside the useful FOV to random (**A**) and scatter coincidences (**B**) for 2D (with interslice septa) and 3D PET imaging systems. *Abbreviations*: FOV, field of view; PET, positron emission tomography.

factor α is set to 2 or 1 depending on whether randoms are measured in a delayed time window and directly subtracted or estimated from the singles count rate (Eq. 3) with reduced variance.

PET DATA RECONSTRUCTION AND CORRECTIONS

Tomographic image reconstruction has received much attention during the last three decades and several papers and textbooks exist on the subject (26,27), therefore it will not be described here. Suffice it to say that two general approaches are being used in PET: analytical reconstruction such as the FBP method (28), which has some limitations due to the discrete nature of PET data but is fast and simple to implement, and iterative reconstruction methods, such as maximum-likelihood expectation maximization (MLEM) (29) and several variants that can be more accurate by taking into account the physical and statistical characteristics of the PET data but are more difficult to implement and more computer intensive.

A number of corrections must be applied to the measured PET data in order to provide reconstructed images that faithfully reproduce the actual activity distribution in the subject being scanned. One fundamental requirement of molecular imaging is to be able to determine the absolute activity concentration of radiotracers in living subjects in units of kBq/cc (or nCi/cc) that can be converted into molar concentrations of the radiopharmaceutical being used. This is normally achieved by calibrating the measured counts per pixel (or voxel) in the PET image against a standard source of known concentration. Such absolute calibration of the PET scanners is necessary for pharmacokinetic modeling of new radiopharmaceuticals and for accurate extraction of biochemical and physiological parameters of interest. It is also important to ensure that reliable results are obtained in the same subject over time for follow-up studies and to enable comparison between different subjects.

Normalization

Variations of the coincidence detection efficiency between LORs affect image uniformity in PET. These variations may result from a number of imperfections related to physical, geometric, mechanical, and electronic properties of individual detector elements. The standard way to correct for these nonuniformities is to obtain a blank scan using a uniform plane or ring source and to compensate for deviations from the average of all LORs in the scanner. In practice, this is usually performed using a rod source extending across the entire axial FOV that is

slowly rotated at a constant speed at the periphery of the useful transaxial FOV while recording coincidence events. Ideally, the same number of counts would be recorded by all detector pairs after one complete rotation of the rod source. The deviations from the mean can thus be used to normalize the coincidence detection efficiency as

$$C_{ij} = \frac{N_{ij}}{\overline{N}}, \tag{6}$$

where the normalization coefficients C_{ij} are simply the ratio of the individual LOR counts N_{ij} to the average of all LORs $\overline{N}$. These coefficients can subsequently be used to correct counts recorded on individual LORs as

$$M_{ij}^N = \frac{M_{ij}}{C_{ij}}. \tag{7}$$

One problem with this technique is that the normalization factors extracted from a coincidence measurement are affected by significant statistical noise due to the limited number of counts per LOR. Some variance reduction must be applied to the normalization data to avoid propagation of this statistical noise in the image (30,31). Another way to improve statistical accuracy is to decouple normalization factors into its contributing components such as intrinsic detector efficiency, geometric effects, time alignment, deadtime, and crystal-specific (e.g., block profile) factors that can be characterized individually and jointly estimated (32–35). The normalization scan can also be used to identify faulty or malfunctioning detectors that should be disabled and discard corresponding LORs from contributing to the image formation. Missing data can then be interpolated to avoid artifacts in the reconstructed images (36,37).

Deadtime

Deadtime accounts for the finite time required to process and record an event during which no other events can be recorded and also accounts for pulse pileup that results in count losses. Deadtime losses occur in every single detector channel of a PET scanner and can become significant at high count rates with continuous or block detectors (38,39). Like any detection systems, PET detectors can be described by deadtime models with paralyzable, nonparalyzable, and pulse overlap components (40–42). In practice, the deadtime losses can be measured by observing the count rate as a function of activity concentration and fitted with a suitable empirical model that can be used to compensate for count losses by individually scaling up the measured LOR count rates in real time (43). Pulse processing techniques with active pileup compensation can be used to minimize deadtime losses and related mispositioning of events due to pileup (44,45).

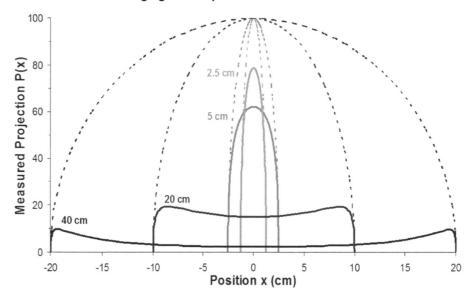

Figure 6 Effect of attenuation on measured projection in PET for water-filled cylinders with uniform concentration of a positron emitter. The dotted lines represent the actual line integral of activity along each LOR in the projection, while the full line is the measured attenuated intensity. *Abbreviations*: PET, positron emission tomography; LOR, line of response.

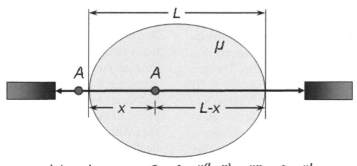

Internal source: $C = Ae^{-\mu(L-x)}\, e^{-\mu x} = Ae^{-\mu L}$

External source: $C = Ae^{-\mu(0)}\, e^{-\mu L} = Ae^{-\mu L}$

Figure 7 Attenuation in PET is dependent on the total path traveled by the two annihilation photons in tissues and is the same whether a point source of activity is inside or outside the object.

Attenuation

The most important correction in PET images is attenuation, especially for human imaging (46). Figure 6 illustrates the effect of attenuation on the measured projection for different source diameters representative of human whole-body (40 cm) and brain (20 cm) imaging, as well as for small-animal imaging with rats (5 cm) and mice (2.5 cm). For example, the attenuation factor can be as high as ~45 for a 40-cm diameter man and ~7 for the human brain, but only 1.6 for a rat and 1.25 for a mouse, which still is nonnegligible if absolute quantification of the radiotracer concentration is required. Since attenuation in PET is dependent on the path lengths l_1 and l_2 traveled by each of the two 511-keV photons through the object, it depends only on the total thickness of tissue $L = l_1 + l_2$

irrespective of the position of the source along the trajectory (Fig. 7). Hence, attenuation can be measured and corrected accurately on each LOR, enabling absolute quantification in the PET images. In many cases the shape of the body and organs can be visualized due to nonnegligible and nonspecific uptake of the radiotracer in the PET image, and the attenuation can be calculated approximately from this contour. Nevertheless, this rough anatomical estimate is often not sufficient for accurate attenuation correction due to inaccurate contour and non-uniform attenuation within different organs (e.g., bone or lung vs. soft tissue). Therefore, an independent measurement of the attenuation is usually required. Accordingly, since attenuation is not dependent on the source position along coincident LORs, this can be performed using an external source of a positron emitter such as ^{68}Ge that extends along the axial FOV and is rotated around the periphery of the FOV, first with and then without the patient in the imaging position, to acquire a transmission and a blank scan, respectively. The attenuation correction factor (ACF) on each LOR can then be derived from the ratio of the counts in these two scans as

$$\mathrm{ACF} = e^{\mu L} = \frac{C_{\mathrm{blank}}}{C_{\mathrm{trans}}}, \tag{8}$$

where C_{blank} and C_{trans} are the external source LOR counts in the blank and transmission scans, respectively. In practice, transmission scans performed using ^{68}Ge have very low counting statistics, requiring long scan times to gather enough events to ensure measurement of the ACF with good accuracy. Since only the ratio of blank to transmission LOR counts is required for attenuation correction, the measurements do not need to be registered in coincidence and a single-photon emitter such as ^{137}Cs (or ^{57}Co for small-animal imaging) can be used, provided the point source position can be accurately known (47–49). The advantage of avoiding coincidence detection is a much higher count rate and a shorter transmission scan time. In addition, ^{137}Cs (30 years) has a much longer half-life than ^{68}Ge (287 days) and does not need to be replaced periodically. The recent introduction of PET/CT scanners has enabled attenuation map to be generated using CT rather than transmission sources. A CT image is basically a 2D map of attenuation coefficients at an average X-ray effective energy of ~80 keV for clinical imaging and ~20 to 60 keV for preclinical imaging. There are several advantages of using CT for attenuation correction of the PET emission data: the transmission scan can be acquired much faster, the CT data have a much lower statistical noise, and contamination from emission photons for post-emission transmission scans is negligible because the X-ray photon flux is orders of magnitudes higher than the emission photon flux.

For attenuation correction of the PET emission data using either a single-photon source or CT, the measured ACFs must be scaled to be converted at the appropriate values for 511-keV annihilation photons (50). For transmission measurements with ^{137}Cs, the ACF can be scaled approximately linearly, since Compton interactions are the major cause of attenuation in tissues and the ratios of attenuation coefficients at 662 to 511 keV are approximately the same for any biological tissues. However, the ratios of attenuation coefficients at 122 keV (^{57}Co) or ~20 to 80 keV (CT) to 511 keV vary significantly for soft tissue, bone, and lung due to significant differences in photoelectric absorption cross sections. Thus, ACFs derived from such low energy transmission data cannot be scaled simply using a global factor. Accordingly, attenuation correction must be implemented using a combination of segmentation to delineate the soft tissue, bone,

and lung compartments, and variable scaling to account for the different attenuation coefficient ratios in these respective tissues. Each attenuation correction method involves different trade-offs, with coincidence transmission scans having the highest noise but lowest bias, whereas X-ray scans have negligible noise but the potential for increased quantitative errors (50).

Randoms

Random events reduce image contrast and distort the linear relationship between image intensity and activity concentration in the object being scanned. A common technique to estimate the rate of randoms within the coincidence time window is to measure the count rate in a delayed time window where true coincidences are impossible. Since the rate at which uncorrelated photons will be registered in the off-time and on-time windows must be the same, the former provides an estimate of the random coincidences occurring in the latter. This estimate can be used to remove the contribution due to randoms in the on-time window. This is commonly implemented in hardware as a real-time subtraction for each LOR-connecting coincident detector pairs. The disadvantage of this technique is the increased uncertainty resulting from the subtraction of estimates affected by Poisson noise ($\alpha = 2$ in Eq. 5) (51). Modern scanners acquiring data in list mode usually have the ability to histogram delayed random events, which can then be subjected to variance reduction processing prior to subtraction (52). Alternatively, the randoms rates can be computed with negligible statistical error from the singles rates using equation (3) for every coincident detector pairs. However, this approach can only be used if the singles rates are being registered as a function of time for every detector in the scanner.

Scatter

As already mentioned, scattered events in PET may origin from Compton interactions in the object or in the detectors. The detector scatter distribution has a relatively narrow extent centered on specific LORs and while it may slightly degrade spatial resolution, its inclusion into the image is generally considered useful to increase sensitivity (53). Scattered radiation from the object results in broadly diffuse background counts in reconstructed PET images, with a distribution generally concentrated toward the center but extending up to the edges of the FOV. In projections, it is well described by a broad exponential distribution centered on the source location (Fig. 8). As such, the peripheral tails presumably due exclusively to scatter after randoms subtraction can be fitted to a mathematical function in the projections or reconstructed image and then subtracted. Alternatively, scatter kernel functions determined for

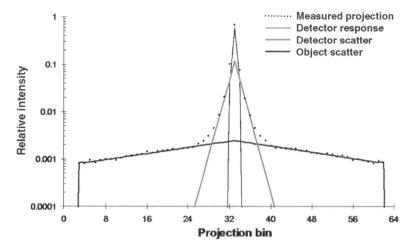

Figure 8 Projection scatter distributions from object and detectors in PET.

standard objects can be deconvolved from the measured projections to yield scatter-corrected data that can then be used for tomographic image reconstruction (54,55). The benefits of such a technique is that it can be implemented together with the filtration step of the FBP reconstruction method to both subtract object scatter and restore detector scatter (56).

Another approach to scatter correction derived from SPECT is to use dual- or multiple-energy windows in an attempt to distinguish between photoelectric and Compton scattered events (57–59). However, due to the relatively poor energy resolution of current PET detectors and because it is not possible to distinguish between scatter events in the object versus scatter events in the detector on the basis of energy, these correction schemes are far less successful than in SPECT imaging (25,60,61).

The most promising scatter compensation approaches currently use simplified Monte Carlo simulation to iteratively estimate the scatter distribution based on coarse scatter-contaminated reconstructed images and attenuation maps derived from transmission images (62,63). Although these methods are time consuming, such model-based scatter correction approaches can potentially address the problem of contamination due to activity outside the FOV in 3D PET systems (64), and some have already made their way to practical implementation in commercial PET scanners (65,66).

Partial Volume

Partial volume effect refers to two distinct phenomena resulting from the finite spatial resolution of the imaging system and the inherent sampling of discrete pixel image representation. Both phenomena contribute to reduce signal intensity by spilling out a fraction of the signal emanating from the source (67). Thus, partial volume

not only affects the apparent intensity but also the apparent size of small sources having a dimension of the order of the resolution element of the imaging system. In the absence of background, the total activity of the source can still be recovered by summing the intensities of all pixels attributable to the object. The *recovery coefficient* can be determined from the ratio of apparent intensity to the true intensity (or concentration) for known object sizes (Fig. 9). These coefficients can then be used to compensate for partial volume effect in images if the source dimension can be determined, for instance using another morphological imaging technique such as CT or MRI. However, compensation for partial volume is frequently compounded by the surrounding activity, which spills over into the structure of interest due to the same phenomena described above. Therefore, whereas several methods have been proposed to correct for partial volume, no general, widely accepted solution has yet been found. For an extensive review of the existing methods, see Soret et al. (67).

DETECTOR TECHNOLOGIES AND DESIGNS

To date all existing clinical PET scanners and the vast majority of dedicated preclinical PET systems for small-animal imaging are using scintillation detectors based on inorganic scintillators and photomultiplier tube (PMT) or APD readouts. One notable exception is the high-density avalanche chamber (HIDAC) camera (68), derived from the multiwire proportional chamber (MWPC) technology developed by Charpak (69), which uses the direct interaction of γ radiation into lead converters and the subsequent multiplication of secondary photoelectrons to detect radiation. Another promising gaseous detector technology is the resistive plate chamber (RPC), which has the potential for TOF capability and submillimeter resolution (70,71). Despite the promises for better intrinsic performance and

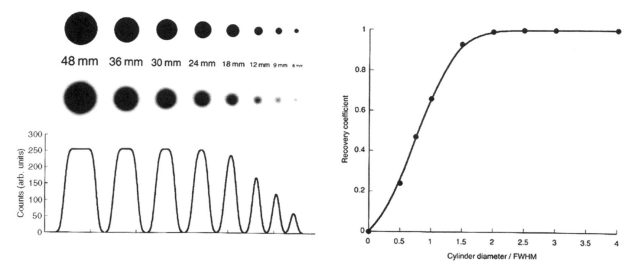

Figure 9 Illustration of partial volume effect and recovery coefficient as a function of object size. *Source*: From Ref. 234.

practicality, semiconductor detectors such as cadmium telluride (CdTe) and cadmium zinc telluride (CZT) have not yet been adopted for PET applications due to cost and technological limitations. Recent progress in basic material production and detector design may change this situation in the near future (72–76).

Scintillators

Nowadays, there is a wide variety of scintillator materials having a range of intrinsic properties that can be suitable for their use in PET imaging, although none of them combines all the characteristics of an ideal crystal. The physical properties of the most common scintillators for

PET are summarized in Table 3. With the exception of sodium iodide (NaI(Tl)) and BGO, all scintillators that are currently being used in PET scanners are materials doped with cerium in the trivalent charge state (Ce^{3+}) as the scintillation mechanism (77). While early PET systems relied on NaI(Tl), which even today remains as one of the most efficient scintillation material, BGO has been the crystal of choice in PET for more than two decades mainly due to its high effective atomic number (Z_{eff}) and high density, which results in very good stopping power (78). Indeed, while about 26 mm of NaI(Tl) is needed for 63% of 511-keV photons to interact, only 11.2 mm of BGO is required. In addition, BGO has a 2.4-fold higher photoelectric interaction probability that makes its coincidence

Table 3 Physical Properties of Common Scintillators for PET

	NaI	BGO	GSO	LSO	LYSO[a]	LGSO[b]	LuAP	YAP	LaBr$_3$
Peak emission wavelength (nm)	410	480	440	420	420	415	365	350	360
Light output (photons/MeV)	41,000	9,000	8,000	30,000	30,000	16,000	12,000	17,000	60,000
Decay time (ns)	230	300/60	60/600	40	40	65	18	30	16
I_0 @ 511 keV (photons/ns)	90	21	60	380	380	125	340	290	1900
Index of refraction	1.85	2.15	1.85	1.82	1.81	1.8	1.94	1.95	1.9
Density ρ (g/cm^3)	3.67	7.13	6.71	7.35	7.19	6.5	8.34	5.5	5.3
Effective Z (Z_{eff})	50	73	58	65	64	59	65	33	46
ρZ_{eff}^4 ($\times 10^6$)	23	202	76	131	121	79	149	7	24
$1/\mu$ at 511 keV (mm)	25.9	11.2	15.0	12.3	12.6	14.3	11.0	21.3	22.3
$\Delta E/E$ (%) @ 662 keV	6	10	8	10	10	9	15	4.5	3
PE (%)[c]	18	44	26	34	33	28	32	4.4	14
PE^2 (%)[d]	3.2	19	6.8	12	11	7.9	10	0.20	1.9

[a]5% Yttrium.
[b]80% Gadolinium.
[c]Photoelectric absorption probability, PE $= 100 \times \sigma_p/(\sigma_p + \sigma_c)$.
[d]Coincident photoelectric absorption probability.
Abbreviations: NaI, sodium iodide; BGO, bismuth germanate; GSO, gadolinium orthosilicate; LSO, lutetium oxyorthosilicate; LuAP, lutetium aluminum perovskite; YAP, yttrium aluminum perovskite; LaBr$_3$, lanthanum bromide.

detection efficiency for photoelectric events a factor of ~ 6 higher than NaI(Tl). This probability of interaction by photoelectric effect is commonly measured by the product ρZ_{eff}^4 to compare different materials (79). Because of its excellent detection efficiency, BGO allowed the design of high spatial resolution systems with small discrete crystals, in contrast to NaI(Tl)-based systems, which took advantage of the Anger positioning method to enhance detection efficiency in large continuous crystals (8). The main drawbacks of BGO are its relatively low light yield and long scintillation decay time constant (300 ns) that limit the count rate capabilities of systems using this scintillation material and increase the acceptance of unwanted random coincidences relative to true coincidences due to a broad coincidence time window. Nevertheless, a fact that is often overlooked is that BGO-based systems were able to achieve acceptable timing performance mainly due to a secondary fast emission component (60 ns), which contributes only 10% to total light output, but increases the initial emission rate I_0 that is crucial for timing performance by more than 50% (80). Another shortcoming of BGO is the mean emission wavelength of 480 nm that does not match the sensitivity of PMTs and results in a relatively poor energy resolution. However, this feature turns out to be advantageous with semiconductor photodetectors reaching quantum efficiency of more than 60% at 480 nm. Together with the small fast emission component of BGO, it enabled the first implementation of APD readout in PET (81,82).

A new breed of cerium-doped scintillators having several advantageous properties for use in PET was developed during the last 20 years. These include gadolinium orthosilicate (Gd_2SiO_5:Ce, GSO) (83–86), lutetium oxyorthosilicate (Lu_2SiO_5:Ce, LSO) (87,88), yttrium aluminum perovskite ($YAlO_3$:Ce, YAP) (89,90), lutetium aluminum perovskite ($LuAlO_3$:Ce, LuAP) (91), and a number of variants with mixed composition but similar properties, such as LGSO (92,93), LYSO (94–97), LuYAP (98,99), MLS (100,101), and LFS (102). All of these crystals have high luminosity (i.e., short scintillation decay time and/or high light yield) relative to BGO, and all except YAP have high Z_{eff} and high density that provide reasonable detection efficiency for 511 keV. An alternative approach has been proposed to increase sensitivity with YAP by selecting the whole energy spectrum instead of the photopeak only (which in this case provides an extremely low coincidence detection probability $\ll 1\%$, see Table 1), to increase the detection probability of single Compton interactions (103). In situations where scatter radiation from the object is low, as is the case with mice and rats, it was shown by Monte Carlo simulation that the fraction of misplaced events would be lower with a dense, medium-Z scintillator like YAP than with high-Z materials for ultrahigh resolution PET imaging (90,104).

One unexpected shortcoming of most of the cerium-doped scintillator crystals (GSO and YAP are noteworthy exceptions) is the relatively poor energy resolution that appears to involve systematic crystal-dependent and excess statistical contributions (96,105). The latter is commonly attributed to nonproportional photon yield as a function of energy in cerium-doped crystals (106,107), but the coexistence of two competing luminescence processes has also been postulated (108). Strangely, the energy resolution seems to improve as the lutetium content of the scintillator materials decreases, irrespective of the relative light output. Another disadvantage of the lutetium content is the presence of the naturally long-lived isotope ^{176}Lu (half-life of $\sim 4 \times 10^{10}$ years) with an estimated abundance of 2.6%, which decays by β^- emission (mean energy of 420 keV) followed by the prompt emission of γ rays (88, 202, and 307 keV). This natural radioactivity gives rise to a background count rate of 240 cps/cc in LSO (87). Although singles and trues background count rates of the order of 100,000 cps and 10,000 cps are common for LSO-based clinical scanners, the impact is generally negligible for conventional clinical scans (109). However, the singles background count rate may contaminate measurement and increase statistical uncertainty in single-photon transmission scans (e.g., with ^{137}Cs or ^{57}Co) used for attenuation correction. The effect can also be significant in small-animal PET systems commonly using lower energy thresholds, especially for research studies involving weak source distributions (110). As a result, there would be some advantage to reduce the lutetium content in the scintillators used for PET (98).

Another promising scintillator that is currently raising high interest is lanthanum bromide ($LaBr_3$:Ce), which has one of the highest light output and the best initial emission rate of all known scintillators (111,112). Not only is this new material achieving the best reported energy resolution (better than 3% at 662 keV) for a scintillator, but this crystal also appears as the most suitable to date for TOF PET, potentially achieving a time resolution of ~ 300 ps (113,114). One drawback of this material is that it is hygroscopic and, like NaI(Tl), it must be hermetically sealed to prevent discoloration and reduced light output.

Photodetectors

Even 80 years after its development, the PMT remains the photodetector of choice to convert scintillation photons into electric signals in most radiation detection applications, including PET, because of the combination of very high gain ($>10^6$), low noise, fast response, and simple signal processing. Ideally, individual coupling of discrete scintillators to PMTs as used in early PET scanners is desirable because the spatial resolution is determined by the crystal geometry and the deadtime is limited to the detector channel in which the interaction occurs. However, it is difficult to achieve one-to-one coupling with crystals smaller than the size of PMTs, which are about 10 mm in size for the smallest ones presently available, therefore limiting the achievable spatial resolution to about 5 mm at best. Position-sensitive (PS-PMT) or multichannel photomultiplier tubes (MC-PMT) with multianode readout can be used to multiplex several smaller discrete crystals into a reduced number of electronic channels (115). In these devices, the position information of the electrons ejected from the photocathode is preserved by the use of special dynode structures that maintain the focus of the electron path up to the anode. Crystals of less than 1 mm in cross section can be decoded using these devices while maintaining adequate timing and energy resolution (116–118). Whereas the position of impinging photons on the photocathode can be determined with high precision, light cross talk between adjacent crystals or through the glass envelope and photon statistics usually affect the crystal identification accuracy, resulting in some degradation of the achievable spatial resolution, as described in equation (1).

A variety of photodetecting devices and crystal-encoding strategies has been investigated to improve the resolution of PET detectors. These include photosensitive gas detectors to read out the ultraviolet (UV) scintillation light from arrays of barium fluoride (BaF_2) scintillators (119) and the use of semiconductor photodiodes. Solid-state photon detectors have several inherent advantages over PMTs: high quantum efficiency, compact and flexible shape that can be adapted to individual crystals, ruggedness, and potentially inexpensive mass production. Standard unity-gain photodiodes currently do not achieve the required signal-to-noise ratio to perform coincidence detection with scintillators in PET (120). They must be used in conjunction with another fast photodetector (121,122) or devices with an internal gain such as silicon APDs must be employed (123–125). APDs exist as small discrete devices (126,127) or as monolithic arrays (128,129), which can be used for individual or multiplexed crystal readouts (130–133). The low-noise, fast front-end electronics required for processing signals from individual APD pixels represent a serious burden to the large scale implementation of this technology in PET without suitable low-power integrated circuits (134–139). Large-area APD in small arrays and position-sensitive APDs have also been investigated to reduce the number of electronic channels and cost of APD-based detection systems for PET (140–142). One promising development in photodetecting devices for PET applications is the recent introduction of Geiger mode APDs, commonly (but not exclusively) called silicon photomultiplier (SiPM) (143).

These new devices have many attractive properties for implementing innovative detector designs in PET (144,145).

PET Detector Designs

Efforts at encoding more than one crystal per PMT naturally led to the implementation of the Anger positioning method used in γ cameras to build PET scanners based on large continuous NaI(Tl) detectors (146,147). In these detectors, the location of each scintillation event is determined by the weighted average of the signals from PMTs arranged in a close-packed hexagonal grid by analog position-encoding circuits (Fig. 10A). The high light output of NaI(Tl) allows the use of large PMTs (50-mm diameter), thus minimizing cost and complexity, and makes it possible to achieve good spatial (<4-mm FWHM) and energy resolution. However, there are two main drawbacks with these detectors, the low stopping power of NaI(Tl) and the limited count rate capability due to pulse pileup in the large area crystals. To overcome these limitations, this concept was extended to higher density, lower light output scintillators like BGO and GSO, by segmenting the crystals and by controlling the light spread to only a few PMTs with a thinner continuous or slotted light guide (Fig. 10B) (148,149). The position of interaction is still determined by a local centroid calculation involving a cluster of smaller PMTs (39-mm diameter), but the readout is limited by logic to a small number of PMTs (typically six) surrounding the one that has triggered. Because of the coarse position sampling of a large number of small cross-section crystals (typically 2 × 2 mm² to 4 × 4 mm²) with a limited number of PMTs, image is linearly distorted with gaps between PMT regions, but individual crystals are well discriminated (Fig. 10B).

A major step was the introduction of the block detector that also uses Anger positioning with a limited extent to improve spatial resolution and reduce deadtime (150). In this design, grooves are cut in a block of scintillator material (BGO or LSO), creating a matrix of typically 8 × 8 to 12 × 12 detector elements whose light output is shared by four square PMTs (Fig. 10C). The block design results in less light collection from edge crystals than from center crystals and nonuniform detection efficiency because of the larger probability of Compton scatter escapes from the edge and corner crystals (151,152). The smallest size that individual detector elements can reliably be made and uniquely identified is usually the limiting factor. A variation on the block design called quadrant sharing uses larger round PMTs, with each tube being centered over a corner of the block (Fig. 10D). The light distribution from each crystal to the PMTs is

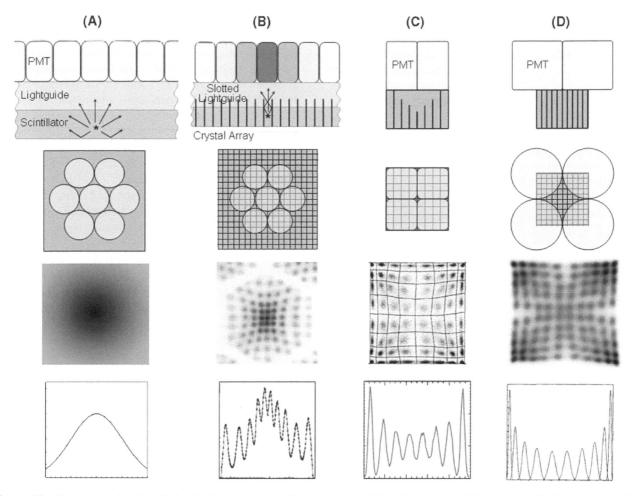

Figure 10 Illustration of various light-sharing crystal encoding schemes used in PET detectors: (**A**) Anger positioning method with a large continuous scintillator, (**B**) Anger positioning with segmented crystals, (**C**) block detector, and (**D**) quadrant-sharing block detector.

carefully controlled by surface treatment and reflector material to ensure unique identification. Thus, each tube "sees" four adjacent blocks and many blocks can be abutted to each other to form a large flat panel detector, avoiding the block edge effects. Approximately four times fewer phototubes are required and arrays of smaller cross-section crystals can be discriminated, but there are some unused crystals that cannot be discriminated on the panel edge.

Although PS-PMT and MC-PMT are available with a square shape that facilitates the assembly in larger arrays, some clever techniques must be used to avoid the gap due to the glass envelope between detectors. One way is to take advantage of light sharing across the boundary of adjacent PMTs to encode interstitial crystals (153). Another solution to maximize the packing fraction without losing positional accuracy, but at the expense of some light loss that degrades energy and timing resolution, is to use individual optical fibers or fiber bundles to pipe scintillation light to the PMT photocathode (154,155).

PRECLINICAL PET IMAGING

Although molecular imaging studies can be conducted in animals using clinical PET scanners designed for human use, they are mostly restricted to larger animals such as nonhuman primates (brain) and dogs or pigs (heart), and sometimes rabbits or cats, because of limitations in spatial resolution and sensitivity. Indeed, a 100- to 1000-fold improvement of the volumetric spatial resolution is required for imaging 250-g rats and 25-g mice with a definition similar to what is currently achieved in a 70-kg human with clinical PET scanners. Quantitatively, it means a gain from the current 5 to 10 mm ($\sim$1 cc) in the clinical PET images to $\sim$2 mm ($\sim$10 μL) for rats and $\sim$1 mm (1 μL) for mice. At the same time, the tissue radioactivity concentration would have to be increased or the scanner sensitivity improved grossly by the same volumetric factor for similar quantitative accuracy per image voxel to be achieved (156). In addition to these two stringent performance requirements, two of the major challenges of molecular imaging are to achieve the fast dynamic imaging capabilities required for pharmacokinetic modeling, with short half-life radiolabeled pharmaceuticals, and to overcome biological limitations in receptor studies with high-affinity, low specific activity radiolabeled ligands without infringing tracer kinetic principles (157–159).

Animal PET Scanners

Since the initial relatively unsuccessful attempts in the early 1990s at adapting clinical PET scanners or using clinical PET detector technologies for small-animal imaging, this field has been an extremely prolific area of research for testing novel detector technologies and original scanner concepts (160). Figure 11 displays typical images obtained with a first generation, dedicated small-animal PET prototype and with a recent commercial imager. The limitations of clinical systems have brought several groups of researchers worldwide to develop PET scanners and establish facilities designed specifically for small-animal imaging. Currently there are several small-animal PET systems based on various detector technologies that are available commercially.

The microPET Focus/Inveon systems (Siemens) are derived from the original microPET prototype developed

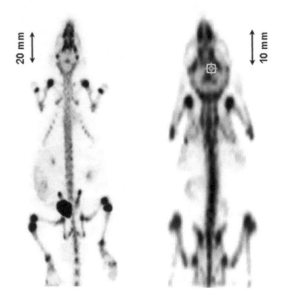

Figure 11 Whole-body Na[18]F PET images of a 250-g rat taken with the first-generation Sherbrooke APD PET scanner [2-mm resolution, 1995 (179)] (*left*) and of a 22-g mouse taken with the second-generation LabPET device [1.35-mm resolution, 2006 (235)] (*right*). The rat image (*left*) shows some residual FDG activity from a previous injection suggesting the contour of the animal's body. *Abbreviations*: APD, avalanche photodiode; PET, positron emission tomography; FDG, ^{18}F-deoxyglucose.

at University of California in Los Angeles (UCLA) (161,162). These systems use optical fiber bundles or tapered light guide in its latest version to read out large compact arrays of up to 20 × 20 small cross-section LSO crystals ($\sim 1.5 \times 1.5$ mm^2) with a PS-PMT. The coupling through light guide allows assembly of the blocks on a cylinder with minimum dead space between adjacent modules. Short crystals with a large ring diameter were selected to ensure high and relatively uniform resolution (~ 1.4-mm FWHM/2.7 μL at center) across the FOV and high sensitivity claimed to reach 7% to 10% by extending the axial length of the scanner to 12 cm. The system appears to achieve among the best NECR performance, making it well adapted to dynamic imaging of radiotracers for pharmacokinetic modeling.

The eXplore Vista (GE Medical Systems, Milwaukee, Wisconsin, U.S.) is also based on PS-PMT block detector modules implementing the phoswich detector technology initially developed at National Institutes of Health to measure DOI (163,164). It uses a dual layer of optically joined LYSO and GSO 13 × 13 scintillator arrays, which are identified by signal pulse shape analysis to reduce the aperture and increase the sensitivity using a reduced number of detectors. The useful FOV is only 6.7 cm in diameter and 4.8 cm axially, effectively limiting its application to imaging of mice. This scanner achieves a maximum sensitivity of 4% and a resolution of 1.4 mm or 2.9 μL at center that only degrades slightly when moving to the periphery of the FOV.

The ClearPET (Raytest, Germany) uses a similar detector design with LYSO/LuYAP phoswich detectors to measure DOI (165,166). Like the original microPET, the blocks are made of 8 × 8 arrays of 2 × 2 mm^2 cross-section crystals readout by a 64-channel MC-PMT, which partly avoids the inherent loss of spatial resolution resulting from light-sharing schemes. Advanced digital techniques are used to digitize and process signals at the output of each MC-PMT channel, making it possible to achieve ~ 1.3-mm spatial resolution at the FOV center (167). One interesting feature of this system is the adjustable detector diameters of 13.5 and 28.5 cm, which makes the system suitable for whole-body rodent studies as well as primate brain studies. The detectors are mounted on a rotating gantry to ensure homogeneous sampling of the image FOV.

The YAP-(S)PET scanner (ISE) is built from four planar rotating scintillator detectors, each based on a 4 × 4 cm^2 matrix made of 20 × 20 crystals of YAP, a bright but low-density scintillator (168). The arrays of 2 × 2 × 25 mm^3 crystals are coupled to 3 in. round PS-PMTs with crossed wire anodes, making the system relatively inexpensive. Interestingly, a very low energy threshold was advocated to accept the first Compton interaction events in order to compensate for the poor detection efficiency of YAP without sacrificing spatial resolution (90). This scanner is the only system providing SPECT imaging as a standard feature using the same hardware, by simply adding a lead parallel-hole collimator in front of each detector, offering an affordable multimodality imaging solution. For both PET and SPECT, the scanner has a 4-cm diameter by 4-cm axial FOV that is mostly suitable for mouse imaging. In PET mode, the scanner achieves an isotropic spatial resolution of ~1.8 mm (~6.5 μL) and a maximum sensitivity of 2.3%. Because of the incomplete ring geometry, the detectors are required to be rotated to acquire complete tomographic data sets, imposing some limitations for fast dynamic studies.

The problem of incomplete ring and gaps between detectors has been addressed in systems using quasi-continuous cylindrical configurations. The Mosaic scanner (Philips Medical Systems, Milpitas, California, U.S.), derived from the A-PET (169,170) and clinical Allegro/ Gemini PET scanners (171,172), utilizes a single annular Anger logic detector made of 16680 $2 \times 2 \times 10$ mm^3 GSO crystals coupled to the inner surface of a cylindrical, slotted light guide with 288 19-mm diameter PMTs on its outer surface. This design is less complex than most other small-animal PET scanners, leading to a compact and cost-effective configuration. The scanner was built as a 21-cm diameter cylindrical detector defining a 12.8-cm transverse FOV with an axial length of 12.8 cm. The effective axial FOV is slightly reduced to 11.6 cm because the edge crystals cannot be resolved. The GSO scintillator provides fairly good energy resolution, but relatively low detection efficiency and poor light output, which degrades the positioning accuracy with Anger logic. The intrinsic spatial resolution of the system was measured to be 2.26 mm, but reconstructed resolution was estimated to 2.7-mm transaxially and 3.4-mm axially, resulting in a volumetric resolution of ~25 μL. The system point source sensitivity with a 410- to 665-keV energy window was reported to be 1.3%, but derived to be 0.65% when measured along the lines of the NEMA (National Electrical Manufacturers Association) protocol (169,173). In spite of its moderate resolution and sensitivity values, the Mosaic has a large FOV making it suitable for whole-body imaging of medium-size rodents such as rats and rabbits. An upgraded version using LYSO scintillators was proposed to increase sensitivity to 2.5% with a default energy window of 385 to 665 keV (174).

The X-PET scanner (Gamma Medica, Northridge, California, U.S.) derived from the rodent research PET (RR-PET) (175) was designed to achieve optimum sensitivity by implementing a solid BGO ring architecture made of tapered crystals at an average detector pitch of 2.0 mm in-plane and 2.2 mm axial. An improved crystal assembly optimizing packing fraction and light output with quadrant-sharing readout (176,177) enhances crystal decoding accuracy, making it possible to achieve a spatial resolution close to 2 mm (~8 μL) and to reach a point

source efficiency exceeding 10% (250-keV lower energy threshold) at the center of a 10-cm diameter by 11.6-cm axial FOV defined by the 16.5-cm diameter solid ring (178). The high sensitivity and good NECR performance of the X-PET make it well adapted to high-throughput whole-body scanning of rats and mice.

Further improving the spatial resolution of PET scanners required to get rid of the positioning errors resulting from light- or charge-sharing decoding schemes. This can only be achieved by individually coupling discrete crystal scintillators to small photodetectors with parallel, independent signal-processing electronics. This more complex and expensive approach was originally pioneered with BGO APD–based detectors in the Sherbrooke animal PET scanner (179) and further investigated in the Munich avalanche diode PET (MADPET) prototype (180). These developments have led to the implementation of novel APD-based detector and digital electronic technologies in the MADPET-II, RatCAP, and LabPET scanners. MADPET-II consists of a ring of dual layer detector modules (71-mm inner diameter), each containing a 4×8 array of $2 \times 2 \times 6$ mm^3 (front) and $2 \times 2 \times 8$ mm^3 (back) LSO crystals that are each optically isolated and coupled one-to-one to a monolithic 4×8 APD array. Signals from each channel are individually processed using integrated analog front-end electronics and custom time and energy digitizers generate list-mode data for every single hit in detectors. The system provides an invaluable platform to investigate intercrystal scatter and random events in a small-diameter, large-aperture imaging device (24). System spatial resolution and point source sensitivity of 1.1-mm FWHM and 2.8%, respectively, are expected.

The RatCAP PET scanner is a unique design that has been developed to enable conscious rat brain imaging without the undesirable effects of anesthesia (181). This has been accomplished through the challenging miniaturization of all scanner components and direct attachment to the rat's head. The RatCAP consists of 384 $2.2 \times 2.2 \times 5$ mm^3 LSO crystals arranged in 12 blocks around an FOV of 38 mm in diameter and 18 mm axially. Each block consists of a 4×8 array of crystals coupled to a 4×8 APD array, which is read out by data acquisition hardware based on custom application specific integrated circuits (ASIC) and field programmable gate arrays (FPGA). The system measured spatial resolution is 2.1 mm and 0.7% at the FOV center. Because of its unshielded, small-diameter, large-aperture design and electronic constraints, the system has some limitations relating to out-of-field randoms and scatters contamination. Nevertheless, promising initial imaging results of awake animals with FDG and ^{11}C-raclopride were successfully obtained (182).

The LabPET scanner (AMI/Gamma-Medica) is the first commercial APD-based PET camera derived from the original Sherbrooke animal PET scanner. The system was

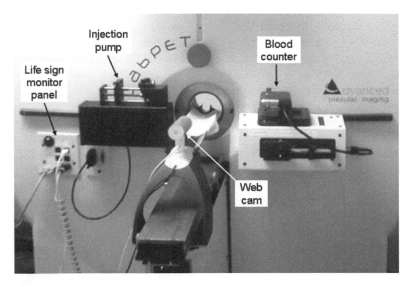

Figure 12 Animal PET scanner equipped with ancillary devices for molecular imaging procedures.

designed with several ergonomic features and ancillary devices making it an ideal platform for carrying out sophisticated molecular imaging procedures (Fig. 12). The scanner exists in two versions having a 3.75-cm and 7.5-cm axial FOV, extendable to 11.25 cm. The 16.2-cm diameter ring defines a maximum 10-cm diameter transaxial FOV. It consists of a $2 \times 2 \times 10$ to $2 \times 2 \times 12$ mm^3 LYSO and LGSO scintillators, optically coupled as a phoswich pair along one long side, read out by one single high-performance APD sitting on a $55°$ wedge. The scanner uses free-running ADCs and advanced real-time digital processing to identify the crystal of interaction and extract information for every single hit in the detectors. Data can be recorded in two modes, a research mode where single hits are saved in list mode for postprocessing and an image mode where only coincidence events sorted out in real time are written in the list-mode file. Because of undersampling resulting from gaps between hermetically packaged detector modules, the measured resolution obtained with FBP is 1.35-mm FWHM, but the effective image resolution with iterative reconstruction and full modeling of the detector response function is ~ 1.2 mm (<2 μL) at the FOV center. Sensitivity with a 250- to 650-keV energy window is 1.1% and 2.1% for the 3.75-cm and 7.5-cm axial FOV versions, respectively. The system has excellent dynamic imaging capabilities with low deadtime, making it well adapted to pharmacokinetic studies.

Another original animal PET system marketed by Oxford Positron Systems (United Kingdom) is based on the MWPC detector technology (183). Although the HIDAC detectors have some inherent drawbacks (low detection efficiency, poor coincidence time resolution, no energy resolution), large-area multilayer stacks of lead converters can be manufactured at a very low cost to compensate for the low detection efficiency. The

unique 3D detection capability of the HIDAC system provides the best spatial resolution in PET at the present time, reaching submillimeter resolution in the reconstructed image with advanced 3D iterative reconstruction techniques (184).

Several other systems with various technological advancements and innovative features are currently investigated or in development. The microPET II, a second generation LSO-based scanner with optical fiber readout of scintillator arrays achieved ~ 1-mm in-plane and 1.4-μL resolution (185). The IndyPET uses large planar detector banks made of 48×108 arrays of 0.87-mm pitch, 20-mm-long LSO crystals coupled to MC-PMT to reach high transaxial resolution (1.1 mm) and <2 μL volumetric resolution with high sensitivity (4.0%) (186). The MiCES (micro crystal element scanner) uses $0.8 \times 0.8 \times 10$ mm MLS crystal arrays coupled to PS-PMTs to achieve 1-mm reconstructed resolution (117,187). Even smaller crystals are being investigated to reach submillimeter resolution (118). The jPET scanner is using four-layer DOI-encoding detectors and smaller than usual ring diameters to obtain sensitivity with uniform spatial resolution across the useful FOV (188,189). Several other detector technologies and designs are currently being investigated for PET, making use of new scintillators and photodetecting devices, as well as semiconductor materials in nonconventional configurations. These new advancements will very likely allow the millimeter resolution barrier to be broken in the near future in molecular PET imaging.

Multimodality Imaging Systems

In spite of improved spatial resolution, a complementary noninvasive high-resolution anatomical imaging modality will sometimes be mandatory. This can be needed simply to properly define target tissues from nonspecific uptake, but sometimes to overcome one adverse feature of PET imaging deriving from its major strength, the extremely high specificity with which new molecular probes are being tailored to be directed toward one particular target, which may result in PET images lacking proper anatomical landmarks to identify and localize uptake tissues. High-resolution morphological imaging also provides the support for accurate partial volume correction in the PET emission images. Suitable methods for coregistrating and fusing images from other microimaging modalities exist, but as in clinical imaging, multimodality scanners combining X-ray computed tomography (CT), or possibly MRI in the near future, to PET is highly desirable. The relevance of collecting anatomical information in conjunction with the metabolic and functional data provided by PET has been swiftly recognized in clinical oncology. The same obviously applies for research in oncology using small-animal imaging, and researchers are actively addressing this issue.

PET/CT

A few manufacturers already offer multimodality platforms that include X-ray microCT for morphological imaging, and the combination of PET and MRI has recently become an active area of development where substantial progress is being made. Gamma Medica was the first supplier to develop the tri-modality FLEX/Triumph™ preclinical imaging system that can be configured to include any combination of PET, SPECT, and CT modalities in a single device (190). In this design, the different systems are accessible with the same bed that can be translated from one modality to the next without moving the animal. Image fusion can thus be obtained by simple 1D translation after resolution scaling (Fig. 13). A similar more flexible approach has been proposed by Siemens with its microPET Inveon system, which was designed to be abutted to a SPECT/CT system to form a multimodality platform accommodating a wide range of applications from mouse to small primate (191). Another approach first proposed by Goertzen et al. (192) and being pursued by the Ferrara group with the YAP-(S)PET small-animal scanner (193) is to use coaxial rotating scanners for simultaneous anatomical and molecular imaging of the subject, allowing direct spatiotemporal correspondence of biological processes in vivo. Enhanced capability for simultaneous dual-modality imaging was also investigated with a full-ring PET scanner using an off-centered cone beam CT geometry, which unfortunately introduces some

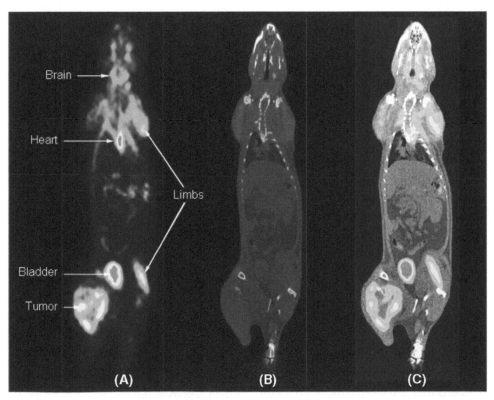

Figure 13 Multimodality imaging in a living rat showing (**A**) PET image of FDG uptake in the brain, heart, limbs, bladder, and tumor; (**B**) X-ray CT image; and (**C**) registration of the images in (**A**) and (**B**) into a fused PET/CT image. Animal PET scanner equipped with ancillary devices for molecular imaging procedures. Images obtained with the FLEX Triumph multimodality preclinical platform. *Abbreviations*: PET, positron emission tomography; FDG, ^{18}F-deoxyglucose. *Source*: Courtesy of Gamma Medica-Ideas (*See Color Insert*).

limitations for 3D tomographic reconstruction of the anatomical image (194,195).

Ideally, since both PET and CT imaging rely on radiation detection for forming images, the same detection system would be used to record both data sets. This is the challenge being undertaken by a few groups to realize true hardware fusion of the two modalities (196–201). One unique potential benefit of this achievement would be the substantial dose reduction resulting from the implementation of single photon-counting X-ray CT, contributing to solve one of the major concerns of molecular imaging for longitudinal studies where the absorbed dose by the same subject in repeated scans can be a serious issue (202–204).

PET/MRI

The alternative use of MRI would offer a high-resolution, nonionizing method and better soft tissue contrast for anatomical imaging of laboratory animals. However, MRI brings considerably more than its 3D anatomical capability, especially regarding dynamic imaging techniques, which can facilitate studies of perfusion, oxygenation, and diffusion among others. Injected contrast agents extend MRI into the domain of molecular imaging. Further, MR spectroscopy can provide images that can be related to the concentration of endogenous molecules in vivo. Therefore, in combination with PET, MRI would facilitate studies of dynamic processes such as biodistribution, pharmacokinetics, and pharmacodynamics (205,206).

The simple adjunction of a PET scanner to one end of MR magnet with the addition of a translating bed might be a workable solution, provided that relatively insensitive detectors to magnetic field can be used, but this solution has not yet been considered. One team has rather elected to introduce the PET detector ring at the center of a costly split-magnet device (207). Because of the high magnetic field, field gradients, and RF present in the MRI environment, a complete redesign of the PET detector and electronic front end is necessary. Vacuum tube–based technologies that have to be used meters away from the main magnet should obviously be avoided. APD-based detectors were demonstrated to operate normally in high magnetic field and are currently being investigated in prototype PET scanners entirely inserted within the MR tunnel (142,208,209).

METHODOLOGICAL ISSUES IN SMALL-ANIMAL PET

The logistics of molecular PET imaging with small animals is basically the same as for clinical PET. It requires similar facilities in terms of staff support, access to radiotracers, and image analysis capability. However, the limited accessibility and inadequate environment of clinical settings for animal experiments, in addition to the inappropriate human scanner performance, have prevented widespread utilization of clinical PET facilities for preclinical studies. Preclinical molecular imaging requires a distinct imaging suite to satisfy both research and regulatory issues, especially regarding animal care and housing facilities (210). Ideally, the small-animal PET imaging suite would be located adjacent to the main clinical PET facilities to share the radiotracer production/handling and image-processing resources, but also within a small distance from other preclinical imaging facilities to facilitate multimodal imaging of subjects during a single experimental procedure.

Other methodological issues must be addressed concurrently with the scanner characteristics if preclinical PET molecular imaging is to become a viable research tool in the biomedical sciences. This is mandatory to ensure the reliability and reproducibility of the PET data in challenge studies where the same subject is used as its own control, but also in longitudinal studies where the same animal must be preserved to be scanned repeatedly over days, weeks, or even months.

Still, there are a number of practical considerations that must be addressed to fully exploit the potential of PET molecular imaging for biological studies. Contrary to imaging modalities that provide information on anatomy and tissue composition, PET opens a unique window on the biochemistry, physiology, and function of living organisms at the molecular level. Not only is it necessary to immobilize the animal during the imaging procedure, the physiological conditions of the subject (depth of anesthesia, body temperature, glycemia, blood pressure and gas, ventilation, heart rate, etc.), which often will have an indirect effect on the biological parameters under investigation, must also be carefully monitored and controlled throughout the imaging session and beyond. Examples of practical issues that must also be addressed for molecular imaging of small animals relate to physiological and pharmacological constraints on radiotracer administration, the acquisition of dynamic data and the measurement of input function for kinetic modeling, physiological gating, the monitoring of the animal's vital signs and the registration of these physiological data with image data, the feasibility of intervention during imaging, and subject repositioning for serial studies, etc. These issues have been discussed in a few papers (3,7,211–214). Flexible, programmable acquisition protocols must be available to the user to satisfy the wide variety of experimental conditions encountered in biological research. It must also be realized that the PET image data is often only one component of the biological investigation that must be correlated with other physiological or biochemical data collected concurrently. In the acquisition of rapid kinetic data for blood flow studies for instance

(215–218), it is quite difficult to synchronize the image acquisition with the bolus injection of the radiotracer and with the input function obtained by drawing blood samples. Considering the shorter time scale of physiological processes in small animals, accurate estimation of the kinetic model rate constants is critically dependent on an exact timing between these three measurements. Another area of application where synchronicity is important relates to real-time follow-up of intervention. Monitoring the early effects of therapy to study the mechanisms of action of a drug or to optimize treatment delivery requires accurate timing and should avoid loss of data between change of acquisition modes.

The utility of cardiac and respiratory gating has been demonstrated for the study of left ventricular function in a few small-animal models (219–225). Both the cardiac and respiratory cycles in anesthetized and diseased animals are often subject to instabilities provoking arrhythmia and variations in the duration of heartbeat and respiration. Such irregular cycles are usually compensated for by dropping the last frame of the gated series or by rejecting bad beats on the fly until stable conditions are restored (216,226). To make the most efficient use of available data and shorten acquisition time, it is advantageous to collect all data in list mode for postacquisition processing (225,227).

Ideally, all relevant information should be recorded together with the PET image data, using the same time reference, so that external data as well as any fortuitous or provoked change of the animal's physiologic state can be related to the PET images. Available life signs monitoring devices for small animals usually offer the ability to record these data. Such capabilities also exist with list-mode data acquisition, where data from other sources can be interleaved into the PET image data stream and saved in the same data file. One key advantage of the list-mode data acquisition is the ability to resample or discard dynamic image data as desired after the measurement, thus avoiding the necessity to determine the imaging sequence beforehand and to accurately synchronize image acquisition with external intervention during the imaging session. In practice, the associated data could as well serve to monitor the physiological state of the subject during an imaging session and, if necessary, be used to discard unreliable image data a posteriori. Such real-time monitoring of the animal condition is important to ensure the validity of the acquired PET images and contributes to improve the reliability and reproducibility of molecular PET imaging investigations.

Likewise, pharmacokinetic modeling of radiotracer distribution and metabolism requires that the blood input function as well as the plasma concentration of labeled metabolites be known (228). Repeated manual blood sampling in small animals, especially mice, requires

sophisticated cannulation techniques and skillful personnel. It is hazardous due to the limited blood volume that can be drawn safely. Automated, microvolumetric blood sampling has been demonstrated using bubble segmentation in catheter tubing (229) and microfluidic devices (230). A continuous real-time microvolumetric whole-blood radioactivity counting system based on direct detection of β particles was also successfully developed (231,232). Dynamic, whole-body imaging using a large solid-angle scanner provides an alternative means to noninvasively obtain the input function from the left ventricular blood pool, large vessels, or another reference tissue (233).

REFERENCES

1. Hoffman EJ, Phelps ME. Positron emission tomography: principles and quantitation. In: Phelps ME, Mazziotta JC, Shelbert HR, eds. Positron Emission Tomography and Autoradiography: Principles and Applications for the Brain and Heart. New York, NY: Raven Press, 1986: 237–286.
2. Cherry SR, Phelps ME, Sorenson JA. Positron emission tomography. In: Physics in Nuclear Medicine. 3rd ed. Philadelphia, PA: WB Saunders, 2003:325–359.
3. Chatziioannou AF. PET scanners dedicated to molecular imaging of small animal models. Mol Imag Biol 2002; 4(1):47–63.
4. Humm JL, Rosenfeld A, Del Guerra A. From PET detectors to PET scanners. Eur J Nucl Med Mol Imaging 2003; 30(11):1574–1597.
5. Surti S, Karp JS, Kinahan PE. PET instrumentation. Radiol Clin North Am 2004; 42(6):1003–1016, vii.
6. Zanzonico P. Positron emission tomography: a review of basic principles, scanner design and performance, and current systems. Semin Nucl Med 2004; 34(2):87–111.
7. Tai YC, Laforest R. Instrumentation aspects of animal PET. Annu Rev Biomed Eng 2005; 7:255–285.
8. Muehllehner G, Karp JS. Positron emission tomography. Phys Med Biol 2006; 51(13):R117–R137.
9. Zaidi H. Recent developments and future trends in nuclear medicine instrumentation. Z Med Phys 2006; 16(1):5–17.
10. Sweet WH. The uses of nuclear disintegration in the diagnosis and treatment of brain tumor. N Engl J Med 1951; 245(23):875–878.
11. Wrenn FR Jr., Good ML, Handler P. The use of positron-emitting radioisotopes for the localization of brain tumors. Science 1951; 113(2940):525–527.
12. Brownell GL, Sweet WH. Localization of brain tumors with positron emitters. Nucleonics 1953; 11:40–45.
13. Brownell GL. A History of Positron Imaging. Available at: http://www.mit.edu/~glb/alb.html. Last updated October 15, 1999.
14. Lewellen TK. Time-of-flight PET. Semin Nucl Med 1998; 28(3):268–275.
15. Nutt R. 1999 ICP distinguished scientist award. The history of positron emission tomography. Mol Imaging Biol 2002; 4(1):11–26.

16. Levin CS, Hoffman EJ. Calculation of positron range and its effect on the fundamental limit of positron emission tomography system spatial resolution. Phys Med Biol 1999; 44(3):781–799.

17. Derenzo SE. Mathematical removal of positron range blurring in high resolution tomography. IEEE Trans. Nucl Sci 1986; 33:565–569.

18. Derenzo, SE, Moses WW, Huesman RH, et al. Critical instrumentation issues for resolution smaller than 2 mm, high sensitivity brain PET. In: Uemura K, Lassen NA, Jones T, et al., eds. Quantification of Brain Function, Tracer Kinetics and Image Analysis in Brain PET. Amsterdam: Excerpta Medica, 1993:25–40.

19. Karuta B, Lecomte R. Effect of detector weighting functions on the point spread function of high-resolution PET tomographs: a simulation study. IEEE Trans Med Imag 1992; 11(3):379–385.

20. Saoudi A, Pepin CM, Dion F, et al. Investigation of depth-of-interaction by pulse shape discrimination in multicrystal detectors read out by avalanche photodiodes. IEEE Trans Nucl Sci 1999; 46(3):462–467.

21. Moses WW, Derenzo SE, Melcher CL, et al. A room temperature LSO/PIN photodiode PET detector module that measures depth of interaction. IEEE Trans Nucl Sci 1995; 42:1085–1089.

22. Lecomte R. Technology challenges in small animal PET imaging. Nucl Instrum Meth Phys Res A 2004; 527(1–2):157–165.

23. Bentourkia M, Msaki P, Cadorette J, et al. Assessment of scatter components in high-resolution PET: correction by nonstationary convolution subtraction. J Nucl Med 1995; 36(1):121–130.

24. Rafecas, M, Boning G, Pichler BJ, et al. Inter-crystal scatter in a dual layer, high resolution LSO-APD positron emission tomograph. Phys Med Biol 2003; 48(7): 821–848.

25. Zaidi H, Koral KF. Scatter modelling and compensation in emission tomography. Eur J Nucl Med Mol Imaging 2004; 31(5):761–782.

26. Natterer F. The Mathematics of Computerized Tomography. New York: Wiley, 1986.

27. Kak AC, Slaney M. Principles of Computerized Tomographic Imaging. New York: IEEE, 1988.

28. Herman GT. Image Reconstruction from Projections. New York: Academic Press, 1980.

29. Shepp LA, Vardi Y. Maximum likelihood reconstruction for emission tomography. IEEE Trans Med Imag 1982; 1:113–122.

30. Casey ME, Hoffman EJ. Quantitation in positron emission computed tomography: 7. A technique to reduce noise in accidental coincidence measurements and coincidence efficiency calibration. J Comput Assist Tomogr 1986; 10(5):845–850.

31. Yao R, Msaki P, Lecomte R. Pre-processing variance reducing techniques in multispectral positron emission tomography. Phys Med Biol 1997; 42(11):2233–2253.

32. Defrise M, Townsend DW, Bailey D, et al. A normalization technique for 3D PET data. Phys Med Biol 1991; 36(7):939–952.

33. Oakes TR, Sossi V, Ruth TJ. Normalization for 3D PET with a low-scatter planar source and measured geometric factors. Fourth International Meeting on Fully Three-Dimensional Image Reconstruction in Radiology and Nuclear Medicine (3D97), 04. Pittsburgh, PA: IOP Publishing, 1998:961–972.

34. Badawii RD, Marsden PK. Developments in component-based normalization for 3D PET. Phys Med Biol 1999; 44(2):571–594.

35. Bai B, Li Q, Holdsworth CH, et al. Model-based normalization for iterative 3D PET image reconstruction. Sixth International Meeting on Fully Three-Dimensional Image Reconstruction in Radiology and Nuclear Medicine, 08/07. Pacific Grove, CA: IOP Publishing, 2002:2773–2784.

36. Buchert R, Bohuslavizki KH, Mester J, et al. Quality assurance in PET: evaluation of the clinical relevance of detector defects. J Nucl Med 1999; 40(10):1657–1665.

37. Baghaei H, Li H, Uribe J, et al. Compensation of missing projection data for MDAPET camera. 2000 IEEE Nuclear Science Symposium Conference Record, October 15–20, 2000. Lyon, France: IEEE, 2000:17–41.

38. Germano G, Hoffman EJ. Investigation of count rate and deadtime characteristics of a high resolution PET system. J Comput Assist Tomogr 1988; 12(5):836–846.

39. Tai YC, Chatziioannou A, Dahlbom M, et al. Investigation of deadtime characteristics for simultaneous emission-transmission data acquisition in PET. 1997 Nuclear Science Symposium. Albuquerque, NM: IEEE, 1998:2200–2204.

40. ICRU. Particle counting in radioactivity measurements. In: International Commission on Radiation Units and Measurements; Anonymous International Commission on Radiation UN: Maryland, 1994; Report 52.

41. Knoll GF. Radiation Detection and Measurement. New York: Wiley, 2000.

42. Laundy D, Collins S. Counting statistics of X-ray detectors at high counting rates. J Synchrotron Radiat 2003; 10:214–218.

43. Daube-Witherspoon ME, Carson RE. Unified deadtime correction model for PET. IEEE Trans Med Imaging 1991; 10(3):267–275.

44. Li H, Wai-Hoi Wong, Uribe J, et al. A new pileup-prevention front-end electronic design for high-resolution PET and gamma cameras. IEEE Trans Nucl Sci 2002; 49(5):2051–2056.

45. Riendeau J, Bérard P, Viscogliosi N, et al. High rate photon counting CT using parallel digital PET electronics. IEEE Trans Nucl Sci 2008; 55(1):40–47.

46. Bailey DL. Transmission scanning in emission tomography. Eur J Nucl Med 1998; 25:774–787.

47. deKemp RA, Nahmias C. Attenuation correction in PET using single photon transmission measurement. Med Phys 1994; 21:771–778.

48. Karp JS, et al. Singles transmission in volume-imaging PET with a 137Cs source. Phys Med Biol 1995; 40:929–944.

49. Lehnert W, Meikle SR, Siegel S, et al. Evaluation of transmission methodology for the microPET Focus 220 animal scanner. 2005 IEEE Nuclear Science Symposium Conference Record, October 23–29, 2005. Fajardo, Puerto Rico: IEEE; 2006:2519–2523.

50. Kinahan PE, Hasegawa BH, Beyer T. X-ray-based attenuation correction for positron emission tomography/computed tomography scanners. Semin Nucl Med 2003; 33(3):166–179.

51. Hoffman EJ, Huang SC, Phelps ME, et al. Quantitation in positron emission computed tomography: 4. Effect of accidental coincidences. J Comput Assist Tomogr 1981; 5(3):391–400.

52. Badawi RD, Miller MP, Bailey DL, et al. Randoms variance reduction in 3D PET. Phys Med Biol 1999; 44(4):941–954.

53. Bentourkia M, Msaki P, Cadorette J, et al. Nonstationary scatter subtraction-restoration in high-resolution PET. J Nucl Med 1996; 37(12):2040–2046.

54. Bailey DL, Meikle SR. A convolution-subtraction scatter correction method for 3D PET. Phys Med Biol 1994; 39(3):411–424.

55. Bentourkia M, Msaki P, Cadorette J, et al. Object and detector scatter-function dependence on energy and position in high resolution PET. IEEE Trans Nucl Sci 1995; 42(4):1162–1167.

56. Msaki P, Bentourkia M, Lecomte R. Scatter degradation and correction models for high-resolution PET. J Nucl Med 1996; 37(12):2047–2049.

57. Grootoonk S, Spinks TJ, Sashin D, et al. Correction for scatter in 3D brain PET using a dual energy window method. Phys Med Biol 1996; 41(12):2757–2774.

58. Adam LE, Karp JS, Freifelder R. Energy-based scatter correction for 3-D PET scanners using NaI(Tl) detectors. IEEE Trans Med Imaging 2000; 19(5):513–521.

59. Yao R, Bentourkia M, Lecomte R. Study of multispectral frame-by-frame convolution scatter correction in high resolution PET. IEEE Trans Nucl Sci 1997; 44(6):2489–2493.

60. Sossi V, Barney JS, Oakes TR, et al. Comparison of energy window choice and parameter implementation in dual energy window scatter correction performance in 3D PET. 1995 IEEE Nuclear Science Symposium and Medical Imaging Conference Record, October 21–28, 1995. San Francisco, CA: IEEE, 1995:1060–1063.

61. Zaidi H. Comparative evaluation of scatter correction techniques in 3D positron emission tomography. Eur J Nucl Med 2000; 27(12):1813–1826.

62. Ollinger JM. Model-based scatter correction for fully 3D PET. Phys Med Biol 1996; 41(1):153–176.

63. Wollenweber SD. Parameterization of a model-based 3-D PET scatter correction. IEEE Trans Nucl Sci 2002; 49(3):722–727.

64. Laymon CM, Harrison RL, Kohlmyer SG, et al. Characterization of single and multiple scatter from matter and activity distributions outside the FOV in 3-D PET. IEEE Trans Nucl Sci 2004; 51(1):10–15.

65. Watson CC. New, faster, image-based scatter correction for 3D PET. IEEE Trans. Nucl Sci 2000; 47(4):1587–1594.

66. Holdsworth CH, Levin CS, Farquhar TH, et al. Investigation of accelerated Monte Carlo techniques for PET simulation and 3D PET scatter correction. IEEE Trans Nucl Sci 2001; 48(1):74–81.

67. Soret M, Bacharach SL, Buvat I. Partial-volume effect in PET tumor imaging. J Nucl Med 2007; 48(6):932–945.

68. Jeavons AP, Chandler RA, Dettmar CAR. 3D HIDAC-PET camera with sub-millimetre resolution for imaging small animals. IEEE Trans Nucl Sci 1999; 46(3 II):468–473.

69. Charpak G. Applications of proportional chambers to some problems in medicine and biology. Nucl Instrum Meth 1978; 156(1–2):1–17.

70. Blanco A, Carolino N, Correia CMBA, et al. RPC-PET: a new very high resolution PET technology. IEEE Trans Nucl Sci 2006; 53(5):2489–2494.

71. Couceiro M, Blanco A, Ferreira NC, et al. RPC-PET: status and perspectives. Nucl Instrum Meth Phys Res A 2007; 580(2):915–918.

72. Vaska P, Bolotnikov A, Carini G, et al. Studies of CZT for PET applications. 2005 IEEE Nuclear Science Symposium Conference Record, Puerto Rico, October 23–29, 2005. Fajardo, Puerto Rico: IEEE, 2006:2799–2802.

73. Drezet A, Monnet O, Mathy F, et al. CdZnTe detectors for small field of view positron emission tomographic imaging. Nucl Instrum Meth Phys Res A 2007; 571(1–2): 465–470.

74. Kikuchi Y, Ishii K, Yamazaki H, et al. Feasibility of ultra high resolution better than 1 mm FWHM of small animal PET by using CdTe detector arrays. 2006 IEEE Nuclear Science Symposium Conference Record, October 29–November 4, 2006. San Diego, CA: IEEE, 2007:2454–2457.

75. Kim H, Cirignano L, Dokhale P, et al. CdTe orthogonal strip detector for small animal PET. 2006 IEEE Nuclear Science Symposium Conference Record, October 29–November 4, 2006. San Diego, CA: IEEE, 2007:3827–3830.

76. Verger L, Gros d'Aillon E, Monnet O, et al. New trends in gamma-ray imaging with CdZnTe/CdTe at CEA-Leti. Nucl Instrum Meth Phys Res A 2007; 571(1–2):33–43.

77. Melcher CL, Friedrich S, Cramer SP, et al. Cerium oxidation state in LSO:Ce scintillators. IEEE Trans Nucl Sci 2005; 52(5):1809–1812.

78. Cho ZH, Farukhi MR. Bismuth germanate as a potential scintillation detector in positron cameras. J Nucl Med 1977; 18(8):840–844.

79. van Eijk CWE. Inorganic scintillators in medical imaging. Phys Med Biol 2002; 47(8):85–106.

80. Moszynski M, Gresset C, Vacher J, et al. Timing properties of BGO scintillator. Nucl Instrum Meth Phys Res 1981; 188(2):403–409.

81. Lecomte R, Cadorette J, Jouan A, et al. High resolution positron emission tomography with a prototype camera based on solid state scintillation detectors. IEEE Trans Nucl Sci 1990; 37(2):805–811.

82. Lecomte R, Cadorette J, Richard P, et al. Design and engineering aspects of a high resolution positron tomograph for small animal imaging. IEEE Trans Nucl Sci 1994; 41(4):1446–1452.

83. Takagi K, Fukazawa T. Cerium-activated Gd_2SiO_5 single crystal scintillator. Appl Phys Lett 1983; 42(1):43–45.

84. Ishibashi H, Shimizu K, Susa K, et al. Cerium doped GSO scintillators and its application to position sensitive detectors. IEEE Trans Nucl Sci 1989; 36(1):170–172.

85. Ishii M, Kobayashi M, Ishibashi H, et al. Research and development of Ce-doped GSO scintillation crystals. In: Aprile E, ed. Gamma-Ray Detector Physics and

Applications: Proceedings of the SPIE—The International Society for Optical Engineering. San Diego, CA: SPIE Press, 1994:68–79.

86. Shimura N, Kamada M, Gunji A, et al. Zr doped GSO:Ce single crystals and their scintillation performance. IEEE Trans Nucl Sci 2006; 53(5):2519–2522.

87. Melcher CL, Schweitzer JS. Cerium-doped lutetium oxyorthosilicate: a fast, efficient new scintillator. IEEE Trans Nucl Sci 1992; 39(4):502–505.

88. Melcher CL. Scintillation crystals for PET. J Nucl Med 2000; 41(6):1051–1055.

89. Moszynski M, Kapusta M, Wolski D, et al. Properties of the YAP:Ce scintillator. Nucl Instrum Meth Phys Res A 1998; 404(1):157–165.

90. Zavattini G, Del Guerra A, Cesca N, et al. High Z and medium Z scintillators in ultra-high-resolution small animal PET. IEEE Trans Nucl Sci 2005; 52(1):222–230.

91. Lempicki A, Glodo J. Ce-doped scintillators: LSO and LuAP. Nucl Instrum Meth Phys Res A 1998; 416(2–3): 333–344.

92. Shimizu S, Kurashige K, Usui T, et al. Scintillation properties of $Lu_{0.4}Gd_{1.6}SiO_5$:Ce (LGSO) crystal. IEEE Trans Nucl Sci 2006; 53(1):14–17.

93. Usui T, Shimizu S, Shimura N, et al. 60 mm diameter $Lu_{0.4}Gd_{1.6}SiO_5$: Ce (LGSO) single crystals and their improved scintillation properties. IEEE Trans Nucl Sci 2007; 54(1):19–22.

94. Cooke DW, McClellan KJ, Bennett BL, et al. Crystal growth and optical characterization of cerium-doped $Lu_{1.8}Y_{0.2}SiO_5$. J Appl Phys 2000; 88(12):7360–7362.

95. Kimble T, Chou M, Chai BHT. Scintillation properties of LYSO crystals. 2002 IEEE Nuclear Science Symposium Conference Record, November 10–16, 2002. Norfolk, VA: IEEE, 2003:1434–1437.

96. Pepin CM, Bérard P, Perrot AL, et al. Properties of LYSO and recent LSO scintillators for phoswich PET detectors. IEEE Trans Nucl Sci 2004; 51(3):789–795.

97. Qin L, Li H, Lu S, et al. Growth and characteristics of LYSO ($Lu_{2(1-x-y)}Y_{2x}SiO_5$:Ce_y) scintillation crystals. J Cryst Growth 2005; 281(2–4):518–524.

98. Lecoq P, Korzhik M. New inorganic scintillation materials development for medical imaging. 2001 IEEE Nuclear Science Symposium Conference Record, November 4–10, 2001. San Diego, CA: IEEE, 2002:39–42.

99. Petrosyan AG, Ovanesyan KL, Shirinyan GO, et al. Growth of LuAP/LuYAP single crystals for PET applications. Rad Eff Defect Solid 2002; 157(6–12):943–949.

100. Pepin CM, Bérard P, Lecomte R. Comparison of LSO, LGSO and MLS scintillators. 2001 IEEE Nuclear Science Symposium Conference Record, November 4–10, 2001. San Diego, CA: IEEE, 2002:124–128.

101. Ramirez RA, Wong WH, Kim S, et al. A comparison of BGO, GSO, MLS, LGSO, LYSO and LSO scintillation materials for high-spatial-resolution animal PET detectors. 2005 IEEE Nuclear Science Symposium Conference Record, October 23–29, 2005. Fajardo, Puerto Rico: IEEE, 2006:2835–2839.

102. Lewellen TK, Janes M, Miyaoka RS, et al. Initial evaluation of the scintillator LFS for positron emission tomograph

applications. 2004 IEEE Nuclear Science Symposium Conference Record, October 16–22, 2004. Rome, Italy: IEEE, 2004:2915–2918.

103. Del Guerra A, Di Domenico G, Scandola M, et al. High spatial resolution small animal YAP-PET. Nucl Instrum Meth Phys Res A 1998; 409(1–3):537–541.

104. Burnham CA, Kaufman DE, Chesler DA, et al. A low-Z PET detector. IEEE Trans Nucl Sci 1990; 37(2): 832–834.

105. Lecomte R, Pepin C, Rouleau D, et al. Investigation of GSO, LSO and YSO scintillators using reverse avalanche photodiodes. IEEE Trans Nucl Sci 1998; 45(3):478–482.

106. Dorenbos P, de Haas JTM, van Eijk CWE. Nonproportionality in the scintillation response and the energy resolution obtainable with scintillation crystals. IEEE Trans Nucl Sci 1995; 42(6):2190–2202.

107. Valentine JD, Rooney BD, Li J. The light yield nonproportionality component of scintillator energy resolution. IEEE Trans Nucl Sci 1998; 45(3):512–517.

108. Saoudi A, Pepin C, Houde D, et al. Scintillation light emission studies of LSO scintillators. IEEE Trans Nucl Sci 1999; 46(6):1925–1928.

109. Yamamoto S, Horii H, Hurutani M, et al. Investigation of single, random, and true counts from natural radioactivity in LSO-based clinical PET. Ann Nucl Med 2005; 19(2): 109–114.

110. Goertzen AL, Suk JY, Thompson CJ. Imaging of weaksource distributions in LSO-based small-animal PET scanners. J Nucl Med 2007; 48(10):1692–1698.

111. van Loef EVD, Dorenbos P, van Eijk CWE, et al. High-energy-resolution scintillator: Ce^{3+} activated $LaBr_3$. Appl Phys Lett 2001; 79(10):1573–1575.

112. Shah KS, Glodo J, Klugerman M, et al. $LaBr_3$:Ce scintillators for gamma-ray spectroscopy. IEEE Trans Nucl Sci 2003; 50(6):2410–2413.

113. Kuhn A, Surti S, Karp JS, et al. Design of a lanthanum bromide detector for time-of-flight PET. IEEE Trans Nucl Sci 2004; 51(5):2550–2557.

114. Kuhn A, Surti S, Karp JS, et al. Performance assessment of pixelated $LaBr_3$ detector modules for time-of-flight PET. IEEE Trans Nucl Sci 2006; 53(3):1090–1095.

115. Shao Y, Cherry SR, Siegel S, et al. Evaluation of multichannel PMTs for readout of scintillator arrays. Nucl Instrum Meth Phys Res A 1997; 390(1–2):209–218.

116. Shao Y, Cherry SR, Chatziioannou AF. Design and development of 1 mm resolution PET detectors with position-sensitive PMTs. Nucl Instrum Meth Phys Res A 2002; 477(1–3):486–490.

117. Lee K, Miyaoka RS, Janes ML, et al. Detector characteristics of the micro crystal element scanner (MiCES). IEEE Trans Nucl Sci 2005; 52(5):1428–1433.

118. Stickel JR, Qi J, Cherry SR. Fabrication and characterization of a 0.5-mm lutetium oxyorthosilicate detector array for high-resolution PET applications. J Nucl Med 2007; 48(1):115–121.

119. Bruyndonckx P, Liu X, Tavernier S, et al. Performance study of a 3D small animal PET scanner based on BaF_2 crystals and a photo sensitive wire chamber. Nucl Instrum Meth Phys Res A 1997; 392(1–3):407–413.

120. Moses WW, Derenzo SE, Melcher CL, et al. Gamma ray spectroscopy and timing using LSO and PIN photodiodes. IEEE Trans Nucl Sci 1995; 42(4):597–600.

121. Moses WW, Derenzo SE, Nutt R, et al. Performance of a PET detector module utilizing an array of silicon photodiodes to identify the crystal of interaction. IEEE Trans Nucl Sci 1993; 40(4):1036–1040.

122. Huber JS, Moses WW, Andreaco MS, et al. An LSO scintillator array for a PET detector module with depth of interaction measurement. IEEE Trans Nucl Sci 2001; 48(3):684–688.

123. Webb PP, McIntyre RJ, Conradi J. Properties of avalanche photodiodes. RCA Rev 1974; 35(2):234–278.

124. McIntyre RJ. Recent developments in silicon avalanche photodiodes Measurement 1985; 3(4):146–152.

125. Lecomte R, Pepin C, Rouleau D, et al. Radiation detection measurements with a new "buried junction" silicon avalanche photodiode. Nucl Instrum Meth Phys Res A 1999; 423(1):92–102.

126. Lecomte R, Lightstone AW, McIntyre RJ, et al. Performance characteristics of BGO-silicon avalanche photodiode detectors for PET. IEEE Trans Nucl Sci 1985; 32(1):482–486.

127. Lecomte R, Martel C, Carrier C. Status of BGO-avalanche photodiode detectors for spectroscopic and timing measurements. Nucl Instrum Meth Phys Res A 1989; 278(2): 585–597.

128. Pichler B, Boning C, Lorenz E, et al. Studies with a prototype high resolution PET scanner based on LSO-APD modules. IEEE Trans Nucl Sci 1998; 45(3):1298–1302.

129. Pichler BJ, Bernecker F, Boning G, et al. A 4×8 APD array, consisting of two monolithic silicon wafers, coupled to a 32-channel LSO matrix for high-resolution PET. IEEE Trans Nucl Sci 2001; 48(4):1391–1396.

130. Casey ME, Dautet H, Waechter D, et al. An LSO block detector for PET using an avalanche photodiode array. 1998 IEEE Nuclear Science Symposium Conference Record, November 8–14, 1998. Toronto, Ontario, Canada: IEEE, 1998:1105–1108.

131. Lecomte R, Saoudi A, Rouleau D, et al. An APD-based quad scintillator detector module with pulse shape discrimination coding for PET. 1998 IEEE Nuclear Science Symposium Conference Record, November 8–14, 1998. Toronto, Ontario, Canada: IEEE, 1998:1445–1447.

132. Krishnamoorthy S, Vaska P, Stoll S, et al. A prototype Anger-type detector for PET using LSO and large-area APDs. 2005 IEEE Nuclear Science Symposium Conference Record, October 23–29, 2005. Fajardo, Puerto Rico: IEEE, 2006:2845–2848.

133. Maas MCm van der Laan DJ, Schaart DR, et al. Experimental characterization of monolithic-crystal small animal PET detectors read out by APD arrays. IEEE Trans Nucl Sci 2006; 53(3):1071–1077.

134. Schmitt D, Lecomte R, Lapointe M, et al. Ultra-low noise charge sensitive preamplifier for scintillation detection with avalanche photodiodes in PET applications. IEEE Trans Nucl Sci 1987; NS-34(1):91–96.

135. Binkley DM, Puckett BS, Casey ME, et al. A power-efficient, low-noise, wideband, integrated CMOS preamplifier for LSO/APD PET systems. IEEE Trans Nucl Sci 2000; 47(3):810–817.

136. Pichler BJ, Pimpl W, Buttler W, et al. Integrated low-noise low-power fast charge-sensitive preamplifier for avalanche photodiodes in JFET-CMOS technology. IEEE Trans Nucl Sci 2001; 48(6):2370–2374.

137. Pratte JF, Robert S, De Geronimo G, et al. Preamplifiers for APD-based PET scanners. IEEE Trans Nucl Sci 2004; 51(5):1979–1985.

138. Habte F, Levin CS. Study of low noise multichannel readout electronics for high sensitivity PET systems based on avalanche photodiode arrays. IEEE Trans Nucl Sci 2004; 51(3):764–769.

139. Spanoudaki VC, McElroy DP, Ziegler SI. An analog signal processing ASIC for a small animal LSO-APD PET tomograph. Nucl Instrum Meth Phys Res A 2006; 564(1):451–462.

140. Burr KC, Ivan A, LeBlanc J, et al. Evaluation of a position sensitive avalanche photodiode for PET. IEEE Trans Nucl Sci 2003; 50(4):792–796.

141. Pichler BJ, Swann BK, Rochelle J, et al. Lutetium oxyorthosilicate block detector readout by avalanche photodiode arrays for high resolution animal PET. Phys Med Biol 2004; 49(18):4305–4319.

142. Grazioso R, Zhang N, Corbeil J, et al. APD-based PET detector for simultaneous PET/MR imaging. Nucl Instrum Meth Phys Res A 2006; 569(2):301–305.

143. Renker D. Geiger-mode avalanche photodiodes, history, properties and problems. Nucl Instrum Meth Phys Res A 2006; 567(1): 48–56.

144. Miyaoka RS, Lewellen TK. Sub-millimeter intrinsic spatial resolution PET detector designs using Geiger-mode avalanche photodetectors. 2005 IEEE Nuclear Science Symposium Conference Record, October 23–29, 2005. Fajardo, Puerto Rico: IEEE, 2006:2903–2907.

145. Moehrs S, Del Guerra A, Herbert DJ, et al. A detector head design for small-animal PET with silicon photomultipliers (SiPM). Phys Med Biol 2006; 51(5): 1113–1127.

146. Muehllehner G, Colsher JG, Lewitt RM. Hexagonal bar positron camera: problems and solutions. IEEE Trans Nucl Sci 1982; NS-30(1):652–660.

147. Freifelder R, Karp JS, Geagan M, et al. Design and performance of the HEAD PENN-PET scanner. IEEE Trans Nucl Sci 1994; 41(4):1436–1440.

148. Burnham CA, Bradshaw J, Kaufman D, et al. Stationary positron emission ring tomograph using BGO detector and analog readout. IEEE Trans Nucl Sci 1983; NS-31(1): 632–636.

149. Surti S, Karp JS, Freifelder R, et al. Optimizing the performance of a PET detector using discrete GSO crystals on a continuous lightguide. IEEE Trans Nucl Sci 2000; 47(3):1030–1036.

150. Casey ME, Nutt R. A multicrystal two dimensional BGO detector system for positron emission tomography. IEEE Trans Nucl Sci 1986; NS-33(1):460–463.

151. Rogers JG, Taylor AJ, Rahimi MF, et al. An improved multicrystal 2-D BGO detector for PET. IEEE Trans Nucl Sci 1992; 39(4):1063–1068.

152. Tornai MP, Germano G, Hoffman EJ. Positioning and energy response of PET block detectors with different light sharing schemes. IEEE Trans Nucl Sci 1994; 41(4): 1458–1463.

153. Rouze NC, Schmand M, Siegel S, et al. Design of a small animal PET imaging system with 1 microliter volume resolution. IEEE Trans Nucl Sci 2004; 51(3):757–763.

154. Cherry SR, Shao Y, Siegel S, et al. Optical fiber readout of scintillator arrays using a multi-channel PMT: a high resolution PET detector for animal imaging. IEEE Trans Nucl Sci 1996; 43(3):1932–1937.

155. Chatziioannou A, Shao Y, Doshi N, et al. Evaluation of optical fiber bundles for coupling a small LSO crystal array to a multi-channel PMT. 1999 IEEE Nuclear Science Symposium and Medical Imaging Conference, October 24–30, 1999. Seattle, WA: IEEE, 1999:1483–1487.

156. Budinger TF, Derenzo SE, Greenberg WL, et al. Quantitative potentials of dynamic emission computed tomography. J Nucl Med 1978; 19(3):309–315.

157. Hume SP, Gunn RN, Jones T. Pharmacological constraints associated with positron emission tomographic scanning of small laboratory animals. Eur J Nucl Med 1998; 25(2): 173–176.

158. Meikle SR, Eberl S, Fulton RR, et al. The influence of tomograph sensitivity on kinetic parameter estimation in positron emission tomography imaging studies of the rat brain. Nucl Med Biol 2000; 27(6):617–625.

159. Jagoda EM, Vaquero JJ, Seidel J, et al. Experiment assessment of mass effects in the rat: implications for small animal PET imaging. Nucl Med Biol 2004; 31(6):771–779.

160. Chatziioannou AF. Molecular imaging of small animals with dedicated PET tomographs. Eur J Nucl Med Mol Imaging 2002; 29(1):98–114.

161. Cherry SR, Shao Y, Silverman RW, et al. MicroPET: a high resolution PET scanner for imaging small animals. IEEE Trans Nucl Sci 1997; 44(3):1161–1166.

162. Chatziioannou AF, Cherry SR, Shao Y, et al. Performance evaluation of microPET: a high-resolution lutetium oxyorthosilicate PET scanner for animal imaging. J Nucl Med 1999; 40(7):1164–1175.

163. Seidel J, Vaquero JJ, Siegel S, et al. Depth identification accuracy of a three layer phoswich PET detector module. IEEE Trans Nucl Sci 1999; 46(3):485–490.

164. Seidel J, Vaquero JJ, Green MV. Resolution uniformity and sensitivity of the NIH ATLAS small animal PET scanner: comparison to simulated LSO scanners without depth-of-interaction capability. IEEE Trans Nucl Sci 2003; 50(5):1347–1350.

165. Ziemons K, Auffray E, Barbier R, et al. The ClearPET™ project: development of a 2nd generation high-performance small animal PET scanner. Nucl Instrum Meth Phys Res A 2005; 537(1–2):307–311.

166. Mosset JB, Devroede O, Krieguer M, et al. Development of an optimized LSO/LuYAP phoswich detector head for the Lausanne ClearPET demonstrator. IEEE Trans Nucl Sci 2006; 53(1):25–29.

167. Streun M, Brandenburg G, Larue H, et al. The data acquisition system of ClearPET neuro: a small animal PET scanner. IEEE Trans Nucl Sci 2006; 53(3):700–703.

168. Del Guerra A, Bartoli A, Belcari N, et al. Performance evaluation of the fully engineered YAP-(S)PET scanner for small animal imaging. IEEE Trans Nucl Sci 2006; 53(3):1078–1083.

169. Surti S, Karp JS, Perkins AE, et al. Design evaluation of A-PET: a high sensitivity animal PET camera. IEEE Trans Nucl Sci 2003; 50(5):1357–1363.

170. Merheb C, Petegnief Y, Talbot JN. Full modelling of the MOSAIC animal PET system based on the GATE Monte Carlo simulation code. Phys Med Biol 2007; 52(3):563–576.

171. Surti S, Karp JS, Adam LE, et al. Performance measurements for the GSO-based brain PET camera (G-PET). 2001 IEEE Nuclear Science Symposium Conference Record, November 4–10, 2001. San Diego, CA: IEEE, 2002:1109–1114.

172. Surti S, Karp JS. Imaging characteristics of a 3-dimensional GSO whole-body PET camera. J Nucl Med 2004; 45(6): 1040–1049.

173. Huisman MC, Reder S, Weber AW, et al. Performance evaluation of the Philips MOSAIC small animal PET scanner. Eur J Nucl Med Mol Imaging 2007; 34(4): 532–540.

174. Surti S, Karp JS, Perkins AE, et al. Imaging performance of a-PET: a small animal PET camera. IEEE Trans Med Imaging 2005; 24(7):844–852.

175. Wong WH, Li H, Xie S, et al. Design of an inexpensive high-sensitivity rodent-research PET camera (RRPET), Conference Record, October 19–25, 2003. Portland, OR: IEEE, 2004:2058–2062.

176. Uribe J, Wong WH, Baghaei H, et al. An efficient detector production method for position-sensitive scintillation detector arrays with 98% detector packing fraction. IEEE Trans Nucl Sci 2003; 50(5):1469–1476.

177. Wong W, Xie S, Ramirez R, et al. An improved quadrant-sharing BGO detector for a low cost rodent-research PET (RRPET). 2004 IEEE Nuclear Science Symposium Conference Record, October 16–22, 2004. Rome, Italy: IEEE, 2004:3407–3411.

178. Zhang Y, Wong WH, Baghaei H, et al. Performance evaluation of the low-cost high-sensitivity rodent research PET (RRPET) camera using Monte Carlo simulations. 2005 IEEE Nuclear Science Symposium Conference Record, October 23–29, 2005. Fajardo, Puerto Rico: IEEE, 2006:2514–2518.

179. Lecomte R, Cadorette J, Rodrigue S, et al. Initial results from the Sherbrooke avalanche photodiode positron tomograph. IEEE Trans Nucl Sci 1996; 43(3):1952–1957.

180. Ziegler SI, Pichler BJ, Boening G, et al. A prototype high-resolution animal positron tomograph with avalanche photodiode arrays and LSO crystals. Eur J Nucl Med 2001; 28(2):136–143.

181. Vaska P, Woody CL, Schlyer DJ, et al. RatCAP: miniaturized head-mounted PET for conscious rodent brain imaging. IEEE Trans Nucl Sci 2004; 51(5):2718–2722.

182. Vaska P, Woody C, Schlyer D, et al. Performance enhancement of the RatCAP awake rat brain PET system. 2006 IEEE Nuclear Science Symposium Conference Record, October 29–November 4, 2006. San Diego, CA: IEEE, 2007:2443–2446.

183. Hastings DL, Reader AJ, Julyan PJ, et al. Performance characteristics of a small animal PET camera for molecular imaging. Nucl Instrum Meth Phys Res A 2007; 573(1–2):80–83.

184. Reader AJ, Ally S, Bakatselos F, et al. One-pass list-mode EM algorithm for high-resolution 3-D PET image reconstruction into large arrays. IEEE Trans Nucl Sci 2002; 49(3):693–699.

185. Tai YC, Chatziioannou AF, Yang Y, et al. MicroPET II: design, development and initial performance of an improved microPET scanner for small-animal imaging. Phys Med Biol 2003; 48(11):1519–1537.

186. Rouze NC, Soon VC, Young JW, et al. Initial evaluation of the Indiana small animal PET scanner. 2005 IEEE Nuclear Science Symposium Conference Record, October 23–29, 2005. Fajardo, Puerto Rico: IEEE, 2006: 2394–2398.

187. Lewellen TK, Janes M, Miyaoka RS, et al. System integration of the MiCES small animal PET scanner. 2004 IEEE Nuclear Science Symposium Conference Record, October 16–22, 2004. Rome, Italy: IEEE, 2004:3316–3320.

188. Yamaya T, Hagiwara N, Obi T, et al. Preliminary resolution performance of the prototype system for a 4-Layer DOI-PET scanner: jPET-D4. IEEE Trans Nucl Sci 2006; 53(3):1123–1128.

189. Nishikido F, Tsuda T, Yoshida E, et al. Spatial resolution evaluation with a pair of two four-layer DOI detectors for small animal PET scanner: jPET-RD. Nucl Instrum Meth Phys Res A 2008; 584(1):212–218.

190. Parnham K, Wagenaar DJ, Li J, et al. Second-generation, tri-modality pre-clinical imaging system. 2006 Nuclear Science Symposium Conference Record, October 29–November 4, 2006. San Diego, CA: IEEE, 2006:1802–1805.

191. Gleason SS, Austin DW, Beach RS, et al. A new highly versatile multimodality small animal imaging platform. 2006 IEEE Nuclear Science Symposium Conference Record, October 29–November 4, 2006. San Diego, CA: IEEE, 2007:3.

192. Goertzen AL, Meadors AK, Silverman RW, et al. Simultaneous molecular and anatomical imaging of the mouse in vivo. Phys Med Biol 2002; 47(24):4315–4328.

193. Cesca N, Di Domenico G, Gambaccini M, et al. A triple modality device for simultaneous small animal CT and PET-SPECT imaging. 2004 IEEE Nuclear Science Symposium Conference Record, October 16–22, 2004. Rome, Italy: IEEE, 2004:3472–3474.

194. Delpierre P, Debarbieux F, Basolo S, et al. PIXSCAN: pixel detector CT-scanner for small animal imaging. Nucl Instrum Meth Phys Res A 2007; 571(1–2 special issue):425–428.

195. Valton S, Peyrin F, Sappey-Marinier D. A FDK-based reconstruction method for off-centered circular trajectory cone beam tomography. IEEE Trans Nucl Sci 2006; 53(5): 2736–2745.

196. Saoudi A, Lecomte R. A novel APD-based detector module for multi-modality PET/SPECT/CT scanners. IEEE Trans Nucl Sci 1999; 46:479–484.

197. Fontaine R, Bélanger F, Cadorette J, et al. Architecture of a dual-modality, high-resolution, fully digital positron emission tomography/computed tomography (PET/CT) scanner for small animal imaging. IEEE Trans Nucl Sci 2005; 52(3 pt 1):691–696.

198. Bérard P, Pepin CM, Rouleau D, et al. CT acquisition using PET detectors and electronics. IEEE Trans Nucl Sci 2005; 52(3 pt 1):634–637.

199. Meyer TC, Powolny F, Anghinolfi F, et al. A time-based front end readout system for PET & CT. 2006 IEEE Nuclear Science Symposium Conference Record, October 29–November 4, 2006. San Diego, CA: IEEE, 2007:5.

200. Bérard P, Riendeau J, Pepin CM, et al. Investigation of the LabPETtm detector and electronics for photon-counting CT imaging. Nucl Instrum Meth Phys Res A 2007; 571(1–2):114–117.

201. Nassalski A, Moszynski M, Szczesniak T, et al. The road to the common PET/CT detector. IEEE Trans Nucl Sci 2007; 54(5/1):1459–1463.

202. Boone JM, Velazquez O, Cherry SR. Small-animal X-ray dose from micro-CT. Mol Imaging 2004; 3(3):149–158.

203. Goertzen AL, Janicki C, Rosa-Neto P. Dosimetry of PET tracers in mice using microPET scans as an input function. 2005 IEEE Nuclear Science Symposium Conference Record, October 23–29, 2005. Fajardo, Puerto Rico: IEEE, 2006:5.

204. Carlson SK, Classic KL, Bender CE, et al. Small animal absorbed radiation dose from serial micro-computed tomography imaging. Mol Imaging Biol 2007; 9(2):78–82.

205. Wagenaar DJ, Kapusta M, Li J, et al. Rationale for the combination of nuclear medicine with magnetic resonance for pre-clinical imaging. Technol Cancer Res Treat 2006; 5(4):343–350.

206. Zaidi H, Mawlawi O, Orton CG. Simultaneous PET/MR will replace PET/CT as the molecular multimodality imaging platform of choice. Med Phys 2007; 34(5):1525–1528.

207. Lucas AJ, Hawkes RC, Ansorge RE, et al. Development of a combined microPET-MR system. Technol Cancer Res Treat 2006; 5(4):337–341.

208. Catana C, Wu Y, Judenhofer MS, et al. Simultaneous acquisition of multislice PET and MR images: initial results with a MR-compatible PET scanner. J Nucl Med 2006; 47(12):1968–1976.

209. Pichler BJ, Judenhofer MS, Catana C, et al. Performance test of an LSO-APD detector in a 7-T MRI scanner for simultaneous PET/MRI. J Nucl Med 2006; 47(4):639–647.

210. Stout DB, Chatziioannou AF, Lawson TP, et al. Small animal imaging center design: the facility at the UCLA crump institute for molecular imaging. Mol Imaging Biol 2005; 7(6):393–402.

211. Meikle SR, Eberl S, Iida H. Instrumentation and methodology for quantitative pre-clinical imaging studies. Curr Pharm Des 2001; 7(18):1945–1966.

212. Myers R. The biological application of small animal PET imaging. Nucl Med Biol 2001; 28:585–593.

213. Myers R, Hume S. Small animal PET. Eur Neuropsychopharmacol 2002; 12(6):545–555.

214. Toyama H, Ichise M, Liow JS, et al. Evaluation of anesthesia effects on [18F]FDG uptake in mouse brain and heart using small animal PET. Nucl Med Biol 2004; 31(2):251–256.

215. Bentourkia M, Croteau É, Langlois R, et al. Cardiac studies in rats with ^{11}C-acetate and PET: a comparison with ^{13}N-ammonia. IEEE Trans Nucl Sci 2002; 49(5):2322–2327.

216. Lecomte R, Croteau É, Gauthier MÈ, et al. Cardiac PET imaging of blood flow, metabolism, and function in normal and infarcted rats. IEEE Trans Nucl Sci 2004; 51(3):696–704.

217. Kreissl MC, Wu H, Stout D, et al. Cardiovascular transit times in mice by high temporal resolution microPET. 2004 IEEE Nuclear Science Symposium Conference Record, October 16–22, 2004. Rome, Italy: IEEE, 2004:3330–3333.

218. Kreissl MC, Wu HM, Stout DB, et al. Noninvasive measurement of cardiovascular function in mice with high-temporal-resolution small-animal PET. J Nucl Med 2006; 47(6):974–980.

219. Green MV, Andrich MP, Doudet D, et al. Evaluation of cardiovascular function in small animals using a microcomputer-based scintigraphic imaging system, 91CH3116-1, September 23–26, 1991. Venice, Italy: IEEE, Computer Society Press, 1991:233–236.

220. Croteau É, Bénard F, Cadorette J, et al. Quantitative gated PET for the assessment of left ventricular function in small animals. J Nucl Med 2003; 44(10):1655–1661.

221. Kreissl MC, Stout D, Silverman RW, et al. Heart and respiratory gating of cardiac microPET[TM]/CT studies in mice. 2004 IEEE Nuclear Science Symposium Conference Record, October 16–22, 2004. Rome, Italy: IEEE, 2004:3877–3879.

222. Badea CT, Fubara B, Hedlund LW, et al. 4-D micro-CT of the mouse heart. Mol Imaging 2005; 4(2):110–116.

223. Vanhove C, Lahoutte T, Defrise M, et al. Reproducibility of left ventricular volume and ejection fraction measurements in rat using pinhole gated SPECT. Eur J Nucl Med Mol Imaging 2005; 32(2):211–220.

224. Yang Y, Rendig S, Siegel S, et al. Cardiac PET imaging in mice with simultaneous cardiac and respiratory gating. Phys Med Biol 2005; 50(13):2979–2989.

225. Woo SK, Kim KM, Cheon GJ, et al. Respiratory gating of MicroPET and clinical CT studies using list-mode acquisition. 2006 IEEE Nuclear Science Symposium Conference Record, October 29–November 4, 2006. San Diego, CA: IEEE, 2007:2761–2764.

226. Ford NL, Nikolov HN, Norley CJ, et al. Prospective respiratory-gated micro-CT of free breathing rodents. Med Phys 2005; 32(9):2888–2898.

227. Drangova M, Ford NL, Detombe SA, et al. Fast retrospectively gated quantitative four-dimensional (4D) cardiac micro computed tomography imaging of free-breathing mice. Invest Radiol 2007; 42(2):85–94.

228. Laforest R, Sharp TL, Engelbach JA, et al. Measurement of input functions in rodents: challenges and solutions. Nucl Med Biol 2005; 32(7):679–685.

229. Lapointe D, Cadorette J, Rodrigue S, et al. A microvolumetric blood counter/sampler for metabolic PET studies in small animals. IEEE Trans Nucl Sci 1998; 45(4):2195–2199.

230. Wu HM, Sui G, Lee CC, et al. In vivo quantitation of glucose metabolism in mice using small-animal PET and a microfluidic device. J Nucl Med 2007; 48(5):837–845.

231. Convert L, Morin-Brassard G, Cadorette J, et al. A new tool for molecular imaging: the microvolumetric β blood counter. J Nucl Med 2007; 48(7):1197–1206.

232. Convert L, Morin-Brassard G, Cadorette J, et al. A microvolumetric β blood counter for pharmacokinetic PET studies in small animals. IEEE Trans Nucl Sci 2007; 54(1/1):173–180.

233. Kim J, Herrero P, Sharp T, et al. Minimally invasive method of determining blood input function from PET images in rodents. J Nucl Med 2006; 47(2):330–336.

234. Cherry SR, Sorenson JA, Phelps ME. Physics in Nuclear Medicine. Philadelphia: Saunders, 2003.

235. Bergeron M, Cadorette J, Beaudoin JF, et al. Performance evaluation of the LabPET[TM] APD-based digital PET scanner. 2007 IEEE Nuclear Science Symposium Conference Record, October 26-November 3, 2007. Honolulu, Hawaii: IEEE, 2007; 6:4185–4191.

6

Molecular SPECT Imaging Instrumentation and Techniques

BENJAMIN M. W. TSUI, YUCHUAN WANG, and SENG PENG MOK
Department of Radiology, Johns Hopkins University, Baltimore, Maryland, U.S.A.

INTRODUCTION

Nuclear medicine imaging techniques traditionally involve the use of tracer amount of pharmaceuticals labeled with radionuclides or radiopharmaceuticals. By tracking the radiation, usually gamma-ray photons, emitting from distribution of the radiopharmaceutical among different tissues or organs within the human body, information about the functions of the tissues or organs can be obtained through the differential uptakes of the radiopharmaceuticals. In clinical nuclear medicine, the information leads to differentiation of normal and abnormal functions and clinical diagnosis. During the last decade, with the advances of molecular biology and radiochemistry, new agents that target tissues and organs specifically at the molecular and cellular level have been developed, which expanded the molecular imaging capabilities of nuclear medicine (1–3). At the same time, the advances of high-resolution small-animal nuclear medicine instrumentation and techniques provide unique and unprecedented tools for preclinical studies using small animals. The translational capability from small animals to human, a well-recognized major advantage of molecular imaging, is greatly facilitated by this unique imaging modality.

The conventional two-dimensional (2D) nuclear medicine images are projections of the three-dimensional (3D) distribution of radioactivity in vivo onto a 2D image plane. Emission computer tomography (ECT) is a combi-

nation of conventional 2D nuclear medicine imaging of an object from different views, or projection images, and image reconstruction methods that produce 3D images from these multiple projections. There are two categories of ECT. The first category is positron emission tomography (PET) that is designed to image radiopharmaceuticals that are labeled with radionuclides emitting positrons (4,5). An emitted positron will quickly interact with an electron and the two annihilate with each other resulting in the emission of two 511-keV photons that travel in $\sim 180°$ opposite directions. A PET system is designed to detect the pairs of 511-keV photons to form multiple projections. The advantages of PET include the desirable properties of positron-emitting radionuclides and radiopharmaceuticals and PET systems with both high photon detection efficiency and spatial resolution. The disadvantages include the difficulties involved in detecting the high-energy 511-keV photons, the need of on-site or nearby facility to produce positron-emitting radionuclides that generally have very short decay half-lives, and the high cost of PET systems. More detailed descriptions of PET in clinical and preclinical imaging are given in chapter 5.

The second category is single-photon emission computed tomography (SPECT), which utilizes radiopharmaceuticals emitting gamma-ray photons directly from the labeled radionuclide (6,7) A typical clinical SPECT system consists of a standard scintillation camera that is held by a gantry and rotated around the patient to obtain multiple projection images from different views around the patient. The formation of a projection image requires the use of a collimator that accepts only gamma-ray photons that travel to the camera at a certain direction. The spatial resolution and statistical noise of the projection images largely depend on the collimator design. Due to the use of collimator, limitation on the radiation dose that can be administered into the patient, and reasonable imaging time, clinical SPECT imaging technique suffers from much lower detection efficiency and poorer spatial resolution as compared with clinical PET. Also, available radiopharmaceuticals and molecular targets for SPECT often do not have some of the desirable biochemical properties as compared with those used in PET. However, the readily available SPECT imaging agents have relatively lower energy emitting photons for imaging, and the relatively lower system. Facility costs are the major advantages that allow SPECT to become a much widely used clinical molecular imaging technique as compared with PET. In preclinical small-animal imaging, SPECT has the advantage of being capable of achieving much higher spatial resolution than PET. Exciting advances are being made in small-animal molecular SPECT imaging that will provide ultrahigh resolution with much higher detection efficiency than that can be previously achieved.

While PET and SPECT images offer unique functional molecular information, they are often difficult to interpret due to the lack of correlation with anatomical structures or landmarks. X-ray computed tomography (CT) is an image technique that provides high-resolution 3D images that represent the distribution of X-ray attenuation property of the patient or object being imaged. Since the attenuation property largely depends on the density of the tissue, a CT image can often be used to represent the anatomical structure of the patient or object. By overlaying a PET or SPECT image with the registered CT image, one will be able to correlate the functional and molecular information with the anatomical structure. The fused image will aid in interpretation of functional and molecular information for clinical diagnosis. In preclinical small-animal imaging, the fused images provide more complete information about the biomedical process at the molecular level.

In this chapter, we will discuss the recent advances, current status, and future trend of SPECT/CT in molecular imaging. The emphasis will be in SPECT/CT instrumentation and imaging techniques for preclinical small-animal imaging studies. More detailed discussions can be found in chapter 9 on micro-CT and in chapter 5 on PET/CT.

FUNDAMENTALS OF SPECT IMAGING

Traditional SPECT for clinical applications is based on one or more standard scintillation camera mounted on a rotational gantry that places the camera at positions around the patient to acquire 2D projection images at different views (7–9). A parallel-hole collimator is normally used to form projection images of the 3D distribution of radioactivity in vivo. The quality of traditional SPECT images is largely dependent on the imaging characteristics of the parallel-hole collimator (10–12).

The two most important imaging characteristics are spatial resolution, or the ability to discern spatial details in the images, and detection efficiency, or the capability to accept gamma-ray photons from the in vivo radioactivity distribution (11,12).

High detection efficiency is desirable as an increased number of detected counts results in lower statistical fluctuations in the projection images and lower image noise. The ideal parallel-hole collimator should have the best spatial resolution and the highest detection efficiency. However, a parallel-hole collimator with improved spatial resolution will unfortunately have decreased detection efficiency. This spatial resolution and detection efficiency trade-off is the major limitation of a parallel-hole collimator. For example, a twofold improvement in spatial resolution will lead to a fourfold decrease in detection efficiency. In clinical imaging, additional considerations, including the aforementioned limitation of radiation dose to the patient, reasonable imaging time, and specific clinical application, are required in the design of parallel-hole collimators. A typical high-resolution collimator has a spatial resolution on the order of ~ 1 cm at 10 cm from the collimator face and a detection efficiency on the order of 10^{-4} to 10^{-3} (11,12).

In preclinical small-animal imaging, much higher spatial resolution than that used in clinical imaging is required. For example, the body width measured at the chest of a normal adult is about 36 cm, compared with that of about 2.5 cm for a mouse. In order to resolve similar anatomical details in a mouse, the spatial resolution of the small-animal imaging system will need to have spatial resolution that is at least 10 times better than that of a clinical system. If we were to design a parallel-hole collimator to achieve the required resolution for this application, such a parallel-hole collimator will have a detection efficiency that is 100 times lower than that used in clinical applications. In practice, other considerations, such as the intrinsic resolution of the detector, impose additional limitations on the use of parallel-hole collimator in molecular imaging of small animals.

PINHOLE SPECT IMAGING

Pinhole collimator is a simple design that has been used in clinical nuclear medicine and SPECT imaging of small organs such as the thyroid (11,13–16). By placing a small object close to the pinhole aperture, substantial increase in photon detection efficiency as compared with parallel-hole

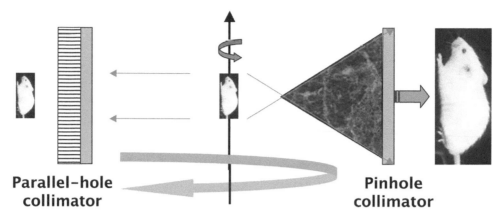

Parallel–hole collimator

Pinhole collimator

Figure 1 Comparison between the parallel-hole and pinhole SPECT imaging geometries. The parallel-hole collimation provides a 1:1 ratio between the size of the object and the acquired image while the pinhole collimation magnifies and inverts a small object placed at close distance onto the detector.

collimation can be achieved through magnification of the object onto the detector plane (16,17). Figure 1 shows the use of parallel-hole and pinhole collimator in preclinical imaging of a mouse using a standard scintillation camera. In Figure 2, we show the comparison of the spatial resolution and detection efficiency of several pinhole collimator designs, and a typical low-energy high-resolution (LEHR) parallel-hole collimator as a function of source distance from the collimator. It shows that at closer source distances, pinhole collimators can be designed to have much increased detection efficiency for the same spatial resolution as a parallel-hole collimator. However, at close source distances, the increased detection efficiency is accompanied by the concurrent decrease in the field of view (FOV). That is, the advantages of pinhole collimator over parallel-hole collimator can only be realized when imaging small objects or small animals at close distances (18–21).

In theory, the sensitivity and spatial resolution of pinhole imaging depends on the size of and the distance from the pinhole aperture (12,16,22–24). That is, a pinhole collimator with any desirable ultrahigh spatial resolution at a close distance can be designed with sufficiently small pinhole aperture. In practice, however, the realization of ultrahigh spatial resolution offered by a pinhole collimator requires the use of gamma-ray photons with low energies for minimal penetration through the pinhole aperture, careful pinhole aperture design, and radiation detector with sufficiently high intrinsic spatial resolution. Also, even though for the same resolution, pinhole collimation provide much higher detection efficiency as compared with parallel-hole collimation at close imaging distances, the detection efficiency of a pinhole collimator decreases with improved spatial resolution. Further improvement in the image quality of pinhole SPECT through increasing

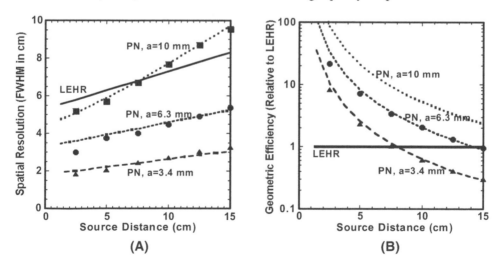

(A)

(B)

Figure 2 Comparison of (**A**) spatial resolution and (**B**) detection efficiency of a typical low-energy high-resolution (LEHR) parallel-hole collimator and several pinhole (PN) collimator designs with different aperture size as a function of source distance. The graphs show that a pinhole collimator can be designed with both better spatial resolution and higher detection efficiency than a LEHR collimator for a source at close distance.

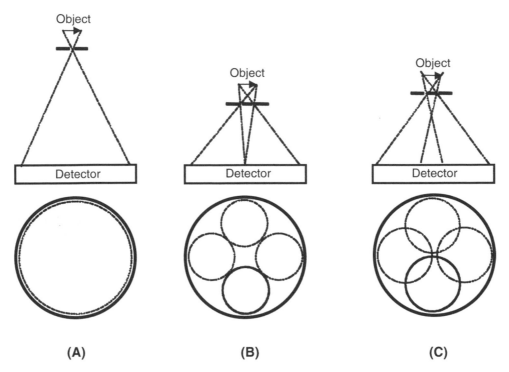

Figure 3 Pinhole and multiple pinhole collimation approaches. (**A**) Single-pinhole collimator with single detector. (**B**) Multipinhole collimator with nonoverlapping projections. (**C**) Multipinhole collimator with overlapping projections.

detection efficiency and reducing noise can be achieved by using multidetector SPECT system design and the use of multipinhole collimation (25–30).

Figure 3A shows the single-pinhole-imaging configuration where the distances from the pinhole aperture to the object and to the detector are adjusted such that the projection image of the object fits fully within the entire radiation detector area for optimal resolution–efficiency trade-off. Similar to multicamera clinical SPECT systems, a simple means to the increase detection efficiency is to place additional detectors each fitted with a single-pinhole collimator around the object to be imaged. An alternative means is the use of a multipinhole collimator that accepts multiple projection images through several pinholes apertures onto the same detector area. There are two general approaches for multiple pinhole collimator design as shown in Figure 3B, C where the projection images obtained from different pinholes are totally separated (31) or have certain degree of overlap (32,33).

Figure 3 also shows that the increase in detection efficiency offered by a multipinhole collimator is not a simple function of the number of pinhole apertures. As shown in Figure 3B, in order to fit all the projection images within the detector area, a smaller magnification than that used in single-pinhole collimator has to be used by shortening the distance between the pinhole aperture and the detector. This

results in a reduced image magnification, and consequently a worsen image resolution because the intrinsic resolution of the detector will have greater degrading effect on the total system resolution with smaller projection images. To compensate this and achieve the same image resolution, smaller pinhole apertures have to be used. The use of smaller apertures results in a reduction of detection efficiency for each pinhole as compared with the single-pinhole collimation shown in Figure 3A. A careful consideration must be given for the multipinhole collimator design by comparing the detection efficiency for the same total system resolution as the single-pinhole collimator.

Another means to further increase the detection efficiency of a multipinhole collimator is to allow some degree of overlapping of the projection images as shown in Figure 3C. The overlap will allow a larger magnification and higher detection efficiency for each pinhole. The larger magnified projection image will be less affected by the intrinsic resolution of the detector. However, while a larger degree of overlap among the multipinhole projection images provides a large increase in detection efficiency for the same spatial resolution, it may give rise to a large amount of undesirable image artifacts and distortions in the multipinhole SPECT reconstructed images. Hence, there exists an optimal number of pinholes that depends on the size and intrinsic resolution of the detector, the multipinhole image reconstruction methods, the radioactivity distribution of the object, and the diagnostic or interpretation task.

Single- and Multiple-Pinhole SPECT/CT Imaging Techniques

Image Calibration and Determination of System Misalignment Parameters

In high-resolution pinhole and multipinhole SPECT/CT imaging when the pinhole collimator detector system rotates around the object, a small system misalignment can lead to severe image degradation and reconstructed image artifacts, and distortions. Currently, it is not easy for most preclinical SPECT/CT systems to directly provide their alignment information to the users with a submillimeter mechanical accuracy, which is essential to achieve high-resolution, accurate, and artifact-free pinhole SPECT images. A careful experimental calibration method and procedures need to be performed by the users to determine the system misalignment parameters (34–40), including the exact location and orientation of the axis –of rotation (AOR) with respect to the projection image matrices as shown in Figure 4A. These experimentally determined misalignment parameters will then be used in the pinhole and multipinhole SPECT image reconstruction methods to reduce the image artifacts and distortion to achieve the best possible image quality (41). Similar calibration method is also required in micro-CT imaging. Figure 4B shows sample micro-CT and pinhole SPECT images without and with the system calibration and correction procedure.

Single-Pinhole Image Reconstruction Methods

Since the pinhole imaging geometry is similar to that of the cone-bean imaging geometry, the 3D pinhole image reconstruction problem is similar to that of the 3D cone-beam image reconstruction. For a conventional SPECT imaging acquisition using a planar circular orbit, that is, the centers of the projection images at different rotational positions lie on a plane, according to the theory of 3D image reconstruction, the only reconstructed image slice that has sufficient projection data for artifact-free image reconstruction is the one that coincides with the same central plane. For an image slice that is further away from the central plane, the data sufficiency condition becomes less satisfied resulting in increased image artifacts and distortions. For most single-pinhole SPECT applications, the main effect is degradation of spatial resolution and the occurrence of image distortions in the image slices that are further away from the central plane.

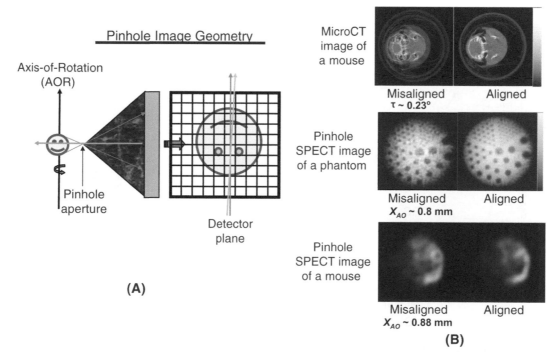

Figure 4 (**A**) The pinhole SPECT imaging geometry showing the projection of an object onto a projection image plane. The geometrical parameters that cause misalignment error include the skew angle (ρ), tilt angle (τ) of the axis of rotation (AOR), and the transverse shift of the AOR (X_{AD}). (**B**) Sample micro-CT images of a mouse, and pinhole SPECT images of a phantom and a mouse showing the reduction of the misalignment error and image artifacts before and after correction.

Pinhole SPECT image reconstruction methods can be divided into two main categories. The first is based on analytical cone-beam image reconstruction methods such as the Feldkamp reconstruction algorithm (42). The second category consists of statistical image reconstruction methods that are based on iterative algorithms (43,44). Similar to the development in clinical SPECT (45,46), 3D iterative single and multipinhole image reconstruction methods have been developed to provide improved reconstructed image quality in terms of reduction of noise amplification and streaking image artifacts found in analytically based image reconstruction methods (40,47). Furthermore, the iterative image reconstruction methods allow incorporation of the system misalignment parameter, as well as models of the imaging physics and system characteristics for substantial further improvement of the quality and quantitative accuracy of the reconstructed images (40,48). Examples include the application of iterative image reconstruction methods to compensate for the effects of photon attenuation, and scatter in the object and the blurring effect of the collimator detector system.

Figure 5A shows the schematic diagram of a typical iterative image reconstruction algorithm that incorporates models of the imaging process that is used in single and multipinhole SPECT image reconstruction. In Figure 5B, the improvement in the reconstruction is demonstrated by the improved resolution for the reconstructed line source images using an iterative ordered-subset expectation maximization (OS-EM) algorithm with model of the pinhole collimator detector response function. The improvement in image quality is demonstrated in Figure 5C where lower image noise and higher spatial resolution in the OS-EM reconstructed images of a phantom with 'hot' rods with different sizes are shown.

Fully 3D Pinhole–Imaging Methods

As described earlier, the standard single-pinhole acquisition using a circular planar orbit provides sufficient projection data for artifact-free image reconstruction only for the central image slice that lies on the same plane as the orbit. An image slice that is further from the central plane has more missing projection data, therefore does not allow accurate image reconstruction. To fully achieve 3D pinhole SPECT image reconstruction, special rotational orbits that allow acquisition of sufficient projection data are required. A typical example is the helical orbit where

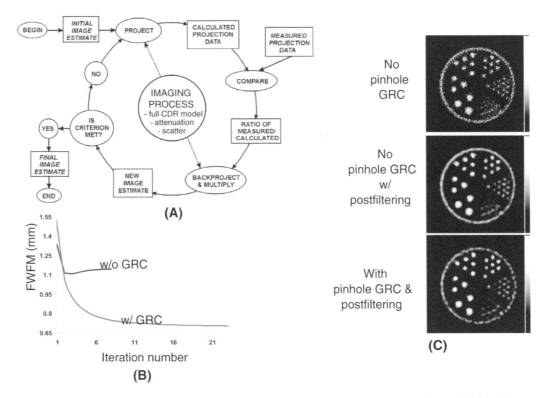

Figure 5 (**A**) Schematic diagram of a typical iterative image reconstruction algorithm with modeling of the imaging process. (**B**) The FWHM of OS-EM reconstructed images of a thin line source with (w/) and without (w/o) modeling the GRC of the pinhole collimator detector system. A pinhole collimator with a 1 mm pinhole aperture was used. (**C**) Sample results from iterative pinhole SPECT image reconstruction method without and with modeling of the pinhole GRC. *Abbreviations:* FWHM, full-width at half maximum; OS-EM, ordered-subset expectation maximization; GRC, geometric response function.

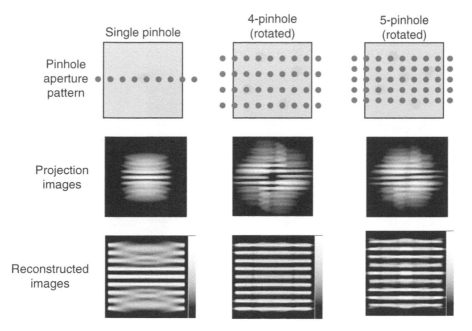

Figure 6 (*Top row*) Pinole aperture patterns of a single-, four-, and five-pinhole collimators. (*Middle row*) Sample pinhole simulated projection images from the corresponding single and multipinhole collimators. (*Bottom row*) Sample coronal SPECT images obtained using the corresponding single and multipinhole collimators and iterative single and multipinhole OS-EM image reconstruction methods. (*Left column*), (*middle column*), and (*right column*) show results from collimator with a single-pinhole, rotated four-pinhole, and five-pinhole aperture patterns.

the detector rotates around the object while moving along the rotational axis (40,49).

An alternative way to obtain projection data for fully pinhole SPECT image reconstruction is through the use of multipinhole collimator with special pinhole aperture pattern design. Figure 6A shows a single and two multipinhole aperture pattern designs. The special "rotated" pinhole patterns were designed such that the pinholes are spaced evenly along the direction of gantry AOR during acquisition of the projection data. The pinhole projection images acquired with the special "rotated" multipinhole collimator designs using a planar orbit provide more complete data for fully 3D image reconstruction over a larger reconstructed image volume than that obtained using a single-pinhole collimator with the same planar orbit. Figure 6B shows sample projection images from a simulation study using three different pinhole collimators with the pinhole aperture patterns shown in Figure 6A. In Figure 6C, sample coronal images from reconstructions of the projection datasets from the three pinhole collimators are shown. When compared with the phantom image, the coronal reconstructed images from the single-pinhole collimator show accurate and artifact-free reconstructed image only at the central image slice, and increased blurring at image slices further away from the central slice. The corresponding images from the multipinhole collimators show more accurate reconstruction with much reduced artifactual image blurring throughout the reconstruction images.

To demonstrate the limited angle and fully 3D image reconstruction in preclinical studies, a normal mouse injected with Tc-99m MDP (methylene diphosphonate) was imaged using pinhole collimators that have the single and multiple pinhole aperture pattern shown in Figure 6A. The projection data were reconstructed using the 3D iterative OS-EM single and multiple pinhole image reconstruction methods. Figure 7 shows the maximum intensity projections of the resulting 3D reconstruction images. The results from single-pinhole SPECT show increased blurring of radioactivity uptakes toward the top and bottom of the images, or further away from the central image slice. The results are consistent with those found in the phantom images shown in Figure 6.

PRECLINICAL SMALL-ANIMAL SPECT/CT INSTRUMENTATION

Accurate and high-resolution single and multipinhole SPECT have become the most popular approach employed in the preclinical SPECT/CT instrumentation and imaging techniques. Active research and development in the academia during the past decade and the industry during the past five years have propelled significant advances in this field. In the following sections, we show examples of the latest advances by selected research groups and commercial companies.

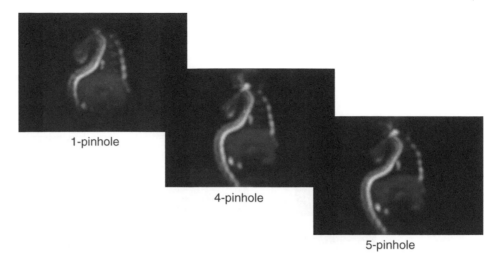

1-pinhole

4-pinhole

5-pinhole

Figure 7 Maximum intensity projection images from the 3D OS-EM (*with 20 updates*) single and multipinhole reconstructed images of a mouse injected with Tc-99m MDP for bone imaging. The single, four, and five pinholes have the aperture patterns shown in Figure 6. The 3D reconstructed images have been post-filtered with a Butterworth filter with cutoff frequency of 0.2 cycles/pixel and order 8. *Abbreviation*: OS-EM, ordered-subset expectation maximization.

Research On Small-Animal SPECT/CT Instrumentation

The application of pinhole planar and SPECT to small-animal imaging was initiated in the nineties. Most of the initial work was performed using clinical SPECT systems with standard large field of view (LFOV) scintillation cameras (28). The animal was often rotated vertically in front of the stationary camera fitted with a pinhole collimator. "The use of a conventional scintillation camera in a clinical system has several disadvantages when applied to small-animal imaging." with "While conventional scintillation camera are useful in imaging dogs, pigs, monkeys, and other larger animal models for a variety of research studies, they have several disadvantages when applied to small-animal imaging." They include the bulky size of a standard LFOV camera, the large dead space at the edge of the detector, the relatively poor intrinsic resolution that is on the order of ~3 mm (which can be reduced at the object from minification in a pinhole geometry), and the fact that a clinical system is difficult to be dedicated for small animal research. Due to these disadvantages, most of the preclinical small-animal SPECT/CT systems today have been using dedicated systems with compact modular cameras or radiation detectors (50–53). Figure 8 shows examples of the transition from the use of a standard scintillation camera to a compact modular camera in the small-animal SPECT system.

The major advance in preclinical small-animal SPECT instrumentation has been in the development of compact modular cameras with high intrinsic resolution. To overcome the limitations of a traditional scintillation camera using a continuous scintillation crystal and an array of photomultiplier tubes (PMT) for positioning information of the incident photons, pixellated scintillation crystals are used. The intrinsic resolution of the modular camera is determined by the pitch of the array elements of the pixellated crystal, that is, a smaller pitch provides better intrinsic resolution. However, the choice of the smallest pitch depends on the manufacturing process and the ability for the positioning electronics to differentiate between the neighboring pixel elements. The manufacturing technology of pixellated NaI(Tl) crystal has improved to provide the smallest pitch from about 2.5 to 1 mm today.

To resolve the intrinsic resolution offered by the pixellated crystal, an array of conventional PMT and associated positioning circuitry can be used. The current technology can resolve a pitch size of about 1.5 mm with a large dead space at the edge of the detector. An alternate is the use of multianode photomultiplier tubes (MAPMT) that allow the extension of high intrinsic resolution to the edge of the detector. A disadvantage is the cost of a MAPMT which is much higher than that of a standard PMT. Currently, the state-of-the-art MAPMT is capable of resolving a pixellated crystal with a pitch of ~1 mm. Compact modular cameras based on the pixellated scintillation crystal and MAPMT have paved the way for a rapid development of dedicated high-resolution small-animal SPECT system. Figure 8 shows a compact modular camera in a small-animal SPECT system, with a pixellated NaI(Tl) crystal and a Hamamatsu H8500 MAPMT with 16×16 anodes.

In the United States, two research groups have initiated the development of dedicated small-animal SPECT and SPECT/CT systems. The research group at the Thomas Jefferson National Accelerator Facility (TJNAF) developed several dedicated research pinhole SPECT and SPECT/CT systems consisting of single and multiple modular cameras that are based on pixellated scintillators and multi-anode

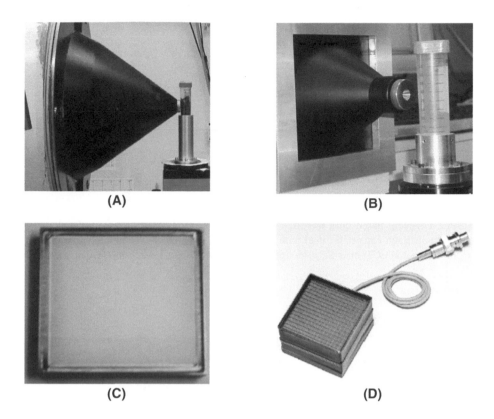

Figure 8 Transition of small-animal pinhole SPECT imaging using (**A**) a standard camera and (**B**) a compact modular camera. The animal is rotated vertically in front of the stationary camera in the early days of development. Example of (**C**) a pixellated NaI(Tl) crystal and (**D**) a Hammatsu H8500 MAPMT with 16 × 16 anodes that are often used in a compact modular camera.

photomultiplier tube (MAPMT) (51). The Center of Gamma-Ray Imaging at the University of Arizona is the largest academic research group that is dedicated to the development of small-animal SPECT and SPECT/CT systems. They have developed several innovative small-animal SPECT and SPECT/CT systems ranging from a compact dedicated SPECT/CT to a multidetector system that completely surround the animal (54–60). They have also developed 3D image reconstruction methods for high-resolution and high-sensitivity single and multipinhole small-animal SPECT imaging.

A research group at the Harvard Medical School has developed a high-resolution small-animal SPECT system based a clinical triple-head SPECT system with three standard scintillation cameras that completely surround the object (61). The large scintillation cameras are fitted with multipinhole collimators and allow high magnification and high-resolution small-animal SPECT imaging. Figure 9 shows the system configuration and sample images from of a high-resolution bone SPECT scan of a mouse. The research group has demonstrated the feasibility and high performance characteristics that can be obtained from the adaptation of a clinical SPECT system (the Trionix XLT-20) for small animal imaging research when a dedicated small animal imaging system is not available.

The research group at the Research Center, Jüilich, Germany has developed multipinhole SPECT imaging using conventional cameras. By taking advantage of the large area detection and allowing a large degree of overlap between the pinhole projections, they are able to image the entire mouse using nine pinholes and a focal area with 12 pinholes. They have shown good multipinhole reconstructed images from different SPECT imaging applications (26,32,62–64).

Innovative ultra-high resolution SPECT systems (U-SPECT-I and II) were developed by the research group at the University Medical Center Utrecht and Delft University of Technology in the Netherlands. Both systems are based on three large stationary gamma cameras (31,65). Also, different from the system developed at Harvard Medical School, the system is designed for ultra-high resolution SPECT by focusing the volume-of-interest (VOI) to a very small volume (on the order of 1.5 cm in diameter for a mouse pinhole collimator and 3 cm for a rat pinhole collimator). By using a large number of small gold pinhole apertures in a cylindrical collimator that surrounds the animal, ultra-high resolution on the order of 350 micron (65) can be achieved in mouse organs. Figure 10 shows the system configuration and a gated myocardial perfusion image of the heart of a mouse

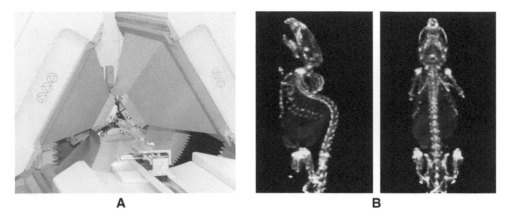

Figure 9 (**A**) The µSPECT system based on a modified Trionix XLT-20 triple-camera system developed by the research group at the Harvard Medical School. Each camera is fitted with a two-pinhole collimator with interchangeable tungsten pinhole inserts. (**B**) Sample images from a bone SPECT of a 25 g mouse injected with 710 µCi Tc-99m-MDP and 30-minute acquisition time. *Source*: From Ref. 61.

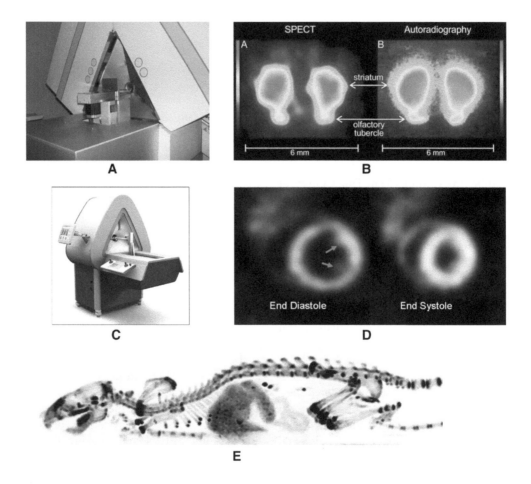

Figure 10 (**A**) U-SPECT-I system based on a clinical scanner, (**B**) mouse brain [I123]FP-CIT: U-SPECT-I image versus autoradiography (Ref. 31), (**C**) the stand alone U-SPECT-II device, (**D**) U-SPECT-II gated mouse heart perfusion image (Tetrafosmin). Arrows indicate tracer take up in papillary muscles, and (**E**) total body rat [Tc99m]HDP image acquired with U-SPECT-II. Respiratory gated version of this image can be found on www.milabs.com. (Images courtesy of Images courtesy of Beekman, van der Have and Vastenhouw (Delft University of Technology / UMC Utrecht / MILabs).

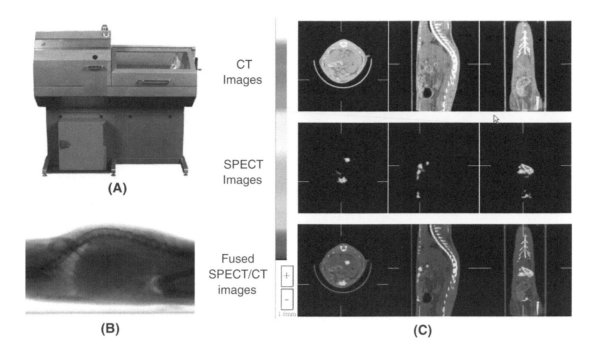

Figure 11 (**A**) Photo of a Gamma Medica-Ideas FLEX™ dual-modality SPECT/CT system. (**B**) A sample X-ray projection image from the CT subsystem and (**C**) sample transaxial, sagittal and coronal CT, SPECT, and fused SPECT/CT images of a rat with a induced shoulder wound and injected with In-111 labeled stem cells. *Source*: Courtesy of Gamma Medica-Ideas, Inc.

obtained from the system. The system allows imaging of larger objects, up to an entire rat, by automated stepping of the animal bed through the pinhole focus with an XYZ stage. 3D images of the entire animal are reconstructed by using all projections obtained from these different bed positions (66). By exploiting the full capabilities of the imaging characteristics of pinhole collimator and pinhole imaging, the unique system demonstrates the ultra-high resolution and high sensitivity capabilities of SPECT imaging for mouse organs (at sub-half–mm resolution) or entire mice (~0.5 mm resolution (66)) and total body rat imaging below 1 mm resolution. In particular, it demonstrates the ultra-high resolution capability of SPECT to be better than 0.5 mm in many cases, something that presently cannot be achieved with PET due to limitations of the high energy 511 keV photons and the physics of coincidence detection.

Commercial Small-Animal SPECT/CT Instrumentation

A multiple head commercial preclinical SPECT system was first marketed by Gamma Medica-Ideas, Inc.[a] Currently, the company offers a preclinical SPECT/CT system that allows registered multimodality SPECT/CT

imaging of small animals ranging from mice to rabbits. The SPECT subsystem was based on one or two modular cameras based on pixellated NaI(Tl) crystal and an array of PMTs. Each modular camera can be fitted with single or multiple pinhole collimator for small animals, such as mice and rats, or a parallel-hole collimator for larger animals (up to ~12 cm in size), such as small rabbits. An optional micro-CT system can be installed within the same housing into an integrated SPECT/CT system. A small animal can be imaged with the micro-CT subsystem and subsequently with the SPECT subsystem without moving the animal. Figure 11 shows the system configuration and the sampled X-ray projection, CT, SPECT, and fused SPECT/CT images. Recently, the company offers a new integrated trimodality SPECT/CT/PET system in a new gantry as shown in Figure 12. The new SPECT subsystem can be upgraded to a total of four new modular cameras that are based on solid-state cadmium zinc telluride (CZT) detector technology, which provides better energy resolution as compared with the pixellated NaI(Tl) scintillation crystal, that is, ~6% versus ~12% (67). The trimodality system provides unprecedented capability and great promises to open a new chapter in preclinical molecular imaging.

Currently, there are several other commercial companies that are also offering state-of-the-art preclinical small

---

[a] http://www.gm-ideas.com/.

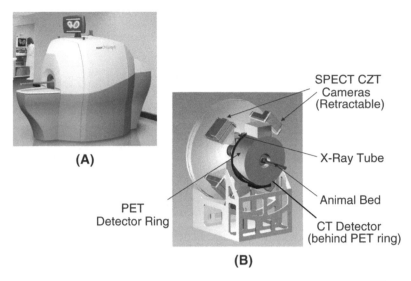

Figure 12 (**A**) Front and (**B**) inside views of the new Gamma Medica-Ideas FLEX Triumph™ tri-modality SPECT/PET/CT preclinical small-animal imaging system. The system consists of a 4-detector SPECT subsystem, an X-ray CT subsystem and a ring PET subsystem whose components can be interchanged and upgraded. *Source*: Courtesy of Gamma Medica-Ideas, Inc.

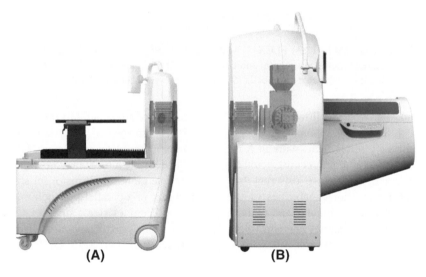

Figure 13 The Siemens InveonTM (**A**) preclinical small animal PET and (**B**) tri-modality SPECT/PET/CT imaging system. The system consists of a 4-detector SPECT subsystem, a X-ray CT subsystem, and a ring PET subsystem. *Source*: Courtesy of Siemens Medical Solutions.

animal-SPECT and SPECT/CT systems. For example, Bioscan, Inc. markets a SPECT system consists of dual or four modular cameras each is fitted with a multipinhole collimator.[b] They are working with the research group at the Research Center, Jüilich, Germany, to develop the multipinhole imaging techniques and image reconstruction for preclinical small-animal SPECT/CT applications. Based on the unique SPECT system design from the University Medical Center, Utrecht, The Netherlands described above, Molecular Imaging Laboratories in Utrecht, The Netherlands, is marketing a SPECT system with ultrahigh-resolution and sensitivity imaging of a small organ within a small animal and of a whole mouse using multisection imaging techniques. They also offer a separate CT system for CT images used in anatomical correlation. Recently, GE Healthcare revealed a small-animal SPECT system based on a ring of CZT detector and either a rotating slit or pinhole collimator.[c] The system also holds great potential to provide high-resolution and high-sensitivity preclinical small-animal SPECT imaging. Finally, Siemens Medical System is offering a new trimodality small-animal SPECT/CT/PET as shown in Figure 13 that will add to the great lineup of preclinical molecular imaging systems for small animals.[d]

[b] http://www.bioscan.com/.
[c] http://www.gehealthcare.com/usen/fun_img/pcimaging/index.html.
[d] http://www.medical.siemens.com/siemens/en_US/gg_nm_FBAs/files/multimedia/inveon/.

CONCLUSION AND FUTURE TRENDS

Rapid and significant advances have been made in the research and development in preclinical molecular SPECT/CT instrumentation and imaging techniques especially within the last five years. The major advances include new radiation detector technologies that allow high resolution imaging in a small detector area, single and multipinhole pinhole SPECT techniques for high-resolution and high-sensitivity imaging, image processing and reconstruction methods that provide quantitative accurate and artifact-free reconstructed images. These advances result in continuing improvements in the unique molecular imaging techniques in many biomedical applications, including drug development and investigations of various diseases including cancers and those related to certain organs, such as the heart and brain. Examples of the different applications of SPECT/CT are found in other chapters in this book.

In the future, we fully expect the research and development in preclinical SPECT/CT for small animals to continue in academic institutions and commercial companies around the globe. The goals will be to meet the needs of investigators in the different biomedical fields. Since there is no single instrument that meets the requirement of different applications, the trend is the ability of the instrument to adapt to the needs of different applications or dedicated instrumentation for specific applications. An example is the need to perform whole body imaging on the entire animal and another to image a specific tissue organ with a small field-of-view for better resolution. The ultrahigh-resolution SPECT system developed by the Utrecht group is a good example for a dedicated system for a small organ. Another example is the ability to perform fast dynamic SPECT acquisition to study the biodistribution and kinetics of the radiotracers. This ability is especially important in drug development studies.

An increasing number of investigators are demanding quantitative information from preclinical small-animal SPECT/CT images. Knowledge of the exact amount of radioactivity in vivo is important in many biomedical research applications. To achieve absolute quantitation from SPECT/CT images, quantitative image reconstruction methods that provide accurate compensations of different image degradation factors will be an important area of continuing research. They include accurate compensation methods for photon attenuation and scatter, the imaging characteristics of the collimator detector system, and partial volume effect to provide SPECT/CT images with high quality and quantitative accuracy.

Preclinical molecular imaging of small animals using SPECT/CT will continue to offer valuable information in the understanding of many diseases and to aid the development of a wide variety of drugs that will ultimately translate to clinical use. Also, the advance technologies developed for high-resolution and high-sensitivity SPECT/CT imaging will have great potential to directly translate to clinical imaging instrumentation and imaging techniques. For breast and brain imaging, the examples are new high-resolution detector technologies and high-resolution and high-sensitivity multipinhole SPECT imaging techniques. These exciting translational potentials of the unique molecular SPECT/CT imaging will fuel active research and development in the years to come.

ACKNOWLEDGMENTS

This work is partially supported by the Public Health Service Grants EB168, EB1558, and CA92871. The authors are grateful to several collaborators at Johns Hopkins University including Martin G. Pomper, M.D., Ph.D. and Kathleen Gabrielson, D.V.M., Ph.D. for their valuable advice.

REFERENCES

1. Blankenberg FG, Strauss HW. Nuclear medicine applications in molecular imaging. J Magn Reson Imaging 2002; 16:352–361.
2. Blankenberg FG, Strauss HW. Nuclear medicine applications in molecular imaging: 2007 update. Q J Nucl Med Mol Imaging 2007; 51:99–110.
3. Weissleder R, Mahmood U. Molecular imaging. Radiology 2001; 219:316–333.
4. Zanzonico P. Positron emission tomography: a review of basic principles, scanner design and performance, and current systems. Semin Nucl Med 2004; 34:87–111.
5. Cherry SR. Fundamentals of positron emission tomography and applications in preclinical drug development. J Clin Pharmacol 2001; 41:482–491.
6. Jaszczak RJ, Coleman RE, Lim CB. SPECT: single photon emission computed tomography. IEEE Trans Nucl Sci 1980; NS-27:1137–1153.
7. Jaszczak RJ, Tsui BMW. Single photon emission computed tomography (SPECT). In: Wagner HN, Szabo Z, Buchanan JW, eds. Principles of Nuclear Medicine. 24th ed. Philadelphia: WB Saunders, 1995:317–341.
8. Jaszczak RJ, Coleman RE. Single photon emission computed tomography (SPECT) principles and instrumentation. Invest Radiol 1985; 20:897–910.
9. Rogers WL, Ackermann RJ. SPECT Instrumentation. Am J Physiol Imaging 1992; 7(3–4):105–120.
10. Metz CE, Atkins FB, Beck RN. The geometric transfer function component for scintillation camera collimators with straight parallel holes. Phys Med Biol 1980; 25:1059–1070.
11. Tsui BMW. Collimator design, properties and characteristics. In: Simmons GH, ed. SNM The Scintillation Camera (Society of Nuclear Medicine). 1988:17–45.
12. Tsui BMW, Gunter DL, Beck RN, et al. Physics of collimator design. In: Sandler MP, Coleman RE, Wackers FJTh, et al., eds. Diagnostic Nuclear Medicine. 3rd ed. Baltimore: William and Wilkins, 1996:67–80.

13. Krausz Y, Wilk M, Saliman F, et al. Role of high-resolution pinhole tomography in the evaluation of thyroid abnormalities. Thyroid 1997; 7:847–852.

14. Wanet PM, Sand A, Abramovici J. Physical and clinical evaluation of high-resolution thyroid pinhole tomography. J Nucl Med 1996; 37:2017–2020.

15. Zaidi H. Assessment of thyroid volume with pinhole emission computed tomography. Phys Med 1996; 12:97–100.

16. Anger HO. Use of a gamma-ray pinhole camera for in vivo studies. Nature 1952; 170:200–201.

17. Anger HO. Scintillation camera. Rev Sci Instrum 1958; 29:23.

18. Weber DA, Ivanovic M. Pinhole SPECT—ultra-high-resolution imaging for small animal studies. J Nucl Med 1995; 36:2287–2289.

19. Weber DA, Ivanovic M, Franceschi D, et al. Pinhole SPECT: An approach to in vivo high resolution SPECT imaging in small laboratory animals. J Nucl Med 1994; 35(2):342–348.

20. Ishizu K, Mukai T, Yonekura Y, et al. Ultra-high resolution SPECT system using four pinhole collimators for small animal studies. J Nucl Med 1995; 36(12):2282–2287.

21. Jaszczak RJ, Li JY, Wang HL, et al. Pinhole collimation for ultra-high-resolution, small-field-of-view SPECT. Phys Med Biol 1994; 39:425–437.

22. Mortimer RK, Anger HO, Tobias CA. Visualization of the distribution of gamma emitters in vivo by means of the gamma ray pinhole camera and image amplifier. Proc Inst Radio Eng 1954; 42:612–616.

23. Mortimer RK, Anger HO, Tobias CA. The gamma ray pinhole camera with image amplifier. Conv. Rec. IRE Med Nucl Electron 1954; (pt 9):2–5.

24. Metzler SD, Bowsher JE, Smith MF, et al. Analytic determination of pinhole collimator sensitivity with penetration. IEEE Trans Med Imaging 2001; 20:730–741.

25. Vogel A, Kirch D, LeFree M, et al. A new method of multiplanar emission tomography using a seven pinhole collimator and an anger scintillation camera. J Nucl Med 1978; 19:648–654.

26. Schramm NU, Ebel G, Engeland U, et al. High-resolution SPECT using multipinhole collimation. IEEE Trans Nucl Sci 2003; 50:315–320.

27. Beekman FJ, Vastenhouw B. Design and simulation of a high-resolution stationary SPECT system for small animals. Phys Med Biol 2004; 49:4579–4592.

28. Ivanovic M, Weber DA, Loncaric S. Design of rotating multi-pinhole SPECT system for high resolution small animal imaging. J Nucl Med 1998; 39:174P.

29. Lefree MT, Vogel RA, Kirch DL, et al. 7-Pinhole tomography—a technical description. J Nucl Med 1981; 22:48–54.

30. Botsch H, Calder D, Savaser A, et al. Myocardial 7-pinhole emission tomography. Dtsch Med Wochenschr 1981; 106:1468–1471.

31. Vastenhouw, et al. Movies of dopamine transporter occupancy with ultra-high resolution focusing pinhole SPECT. Mol Psych 2007.

32. Schramm NU, Engeland U, Ebel G, et al. Multi-pinhole SPECT for small animal research. J Nucl Med 2002; 43:223P.

33. Mok G, Wang Y, Li J, et al. Development and evaluation of a novel multi-pinhole collimator system for imaging small animals with different sizes using a FLEX MicroSPECT/CT imaging system. J Nucl Med 2006; 47(suppl 1):63P.

34. Beque D, Nuyts J, Bormans G, et al. Characterization of pinhole SPECT acquisition geometry. IEEE Trans Med Imaging 2003; 22:599–612.

35. Bequé D, Nuyts J, Suetens P, et al. Optimization of geometrical calibration in pinhole SPECT. IEEE Trans Med Imaging 2004; 24:180–190.

36. Li JY, Jaszczak RJ, Wang HL, et al. Determination of both mechanical and electronic shifts in cone-beam SPECT. Phys Med Biol 1993; 38:743–754.

37. Metzler SD, Greer KL, Jaszczak RJ. Determination of mechanical and electronic shifts for pinhole SPECT using a single point source. IEEE Trans Med Imaging 2005; 24:361–370.

38. Noo F, Clackdoyle R, Mennessier C, et al. Analytic method based on identification of ellipse parameters for scanner calibration in cone-beam tomography. Phys Med Biol 2000; 45:3489–3508.

39. Rizo P, Grangeat P, Guillemaud R. Geometric calibration method for multiple-head cone-beam SPECT system. IEEE Trans Nucl Sci 1994; 41:2748–2757.

40. Wang YC, Tsui BMW. Pinhole SPECT with different data acquisition geometries: usefulness of unified projection operators in homogeneous coordinates. IEEE Trans Med Imaging 2007; 26:298–308.

41. Tsui BMW, Wang YC. High-resolution molecular imaging techniques for cardiovascular research. J Nucl Cardiol 2005; 12:261–267.

42. Feldkamp LA, Davis LC, Kress JW. Practical cone-beam algorithm. J Opt Soc Am A 1984; 1:612–619.

43. Lange K, Carson R. EM reconstruction algorithms for emission and transmission tomography. J Comput Assist Tomogr 1984; 8:306–316.

44. Shepp LA, Vardi Y. Maximum likelihood estimation for emission tomography. IEEE Trans Med Imaging 1982; MI-1:113–121.

45. Tsui BMW, Zhao XD, Frey EC, et al. Quantitative single-photon emission computed-tomography—basics and clinical considerations. Semin Nucl Med 1994; 24:38–65.

46. Tsui BMW. Quantitative SPECT. In: Henkin RE, Boles MA, Dillehay GL, et al., eds. Nuclear Medicine. 2nd ed. Philadephia: Mosby Elsevier, 2006:223–245.

47. Sohlberg A, Lensu S, Jolkkonen J, et al. Improving the quality of small animal brain pinhole SPECT imaging by Bayesian reconstruction. Eur J Nucl Med Mol Imaging 2004; 31:986–994.

48. Frey EC, Tsui BMW. Correction for collimator response function in SPECT. In: Zaidi H, ed. Quantitative Analysis in Nuclear Medicine Imaging. New York: Springer, 2005: 141–166.

49. Metzler SD, Greer KL, Jaszczak RJ. Helical pinhole SPECT for small-animal imaging: a method for addressing sampling completeness. IEEE Trans Nucl Sci 2003; 50:1575–1583.

50. McElroy DP, MacDonald LR, Beekman FJ, et al. Performance evaluation of A-SPECT: a high resolution desktop

pinhole SPECT system for imaging small animals. IEEE Trans Nucl Sci 2002; 49:2139–2147.

51. Weisenberger AG, Wojcik R, Bradley EL, et al. SPECT-CT system for small animal imaging. IEEE Trans Nucl Sci 2003; 50:74–79.

52. Qi Y, Tsui B, Yoder B, et al. Characteristics of compact detectors based on pixellated NaI(Tl) crystal arrays. In: Proceedings of the Nuclear Science Symposium and Medical Imaging Conference, Norfolk, Virginia, USA, 2002:582–588.

53. Qi Y, Tsui BMW, Wang Y, et al. Development and characterization of a high-resolution microSPECT system for small animal imaging. In: Kupinski M, Barrett H, eds. Small Animal SPECT Imaging. New York: Springer, 2005:259–266.

54. Kastis GK, Barber HB, Barrett HH, et al. High resolution SPECT imager for three-dimensional imaging of small animals. J Nucl Med 1998; 39:25.

55. Patton DD, Barrett HH, Chen JC, et al. Fastspect—a 4-dimensional brain imager. J Nucl Med 1994; 35(suppl 5): 93P.

56. Peterson TE, Kim H, Crawford MJ, et al. SemiSPECT: a small-animal imaging systems based on eight CdZnTe pixel detectors. In: Proceedings of the IEEE Nuclear Science Symposium and Medical Imaging Conference, Norfolk, Virginia, USA, 2002.

57. Kim H, Furenlid LR, Crawford MJ, et al. SemiSPECT: a small-animal single-photon emission computed tomography (SPECT) imager based on eight cadmium zinc telluride (CZT) detector arrays. Med Phys 2006; 33:465–474.

58. Liu ZL, Kastis GA, Stevenson GD, et al. Quantitative analysis of acute myocardial infarct in rat hearts with ischemia-reperfusion using a high-resolution stationary SPECT system. J Nucl Med 2002; 43:933–939.

59. Furenlid LR, Chen Y, Kim H. SPECT imager design and data acquisition systems. In: Kupinski MA, Barrett HH, eds. Small-Animal SPECT Imaging. New York: Springer Science + Business Media Inc., 2005:115–138.

60. Rowe RK, Aarsvold JN, Barrett HH, et al. A stationary hemispherical SPECT imager for 3-Dimensional brain imaging. J Nucl Med 1993; 34:474–480.

61. Moore SC, Zimmerman RE, Mellen R, et al. Modification of a triple-detector SPECT system for small-animal imaging. Paper presented at: the IEEE Nuclear Science Symposium and Medical Imaging Conference, Portland, Oregon, USA, 2003.

62. Schramm NU, Ebel G, Engeland U, et al. High-resolution SPECT using multipinhole collimation. IEEE Trans Nucl Sci 2003; 50(3):315–320.

63. Schramm NU, Behe M, Schurrat T, et al. Multi-pinhole SPECT: recent results of an animal imaging system. J Nucl Med 2003; 44:9–10.

64. Lackas C, Schramm NU, Hoppin JW, et al. T-SPECT: a novel imaging technique for small-animal research. IEEE Trans Nucl Sci 2005; 52:181–187.

65. Feekman FJ, van der Have F. The pinhole: gateway to ultra-high resolution three-dimensional radionuclide imaging. Eur J Nucl Med Mol Im 2007; 4(2):151–161.

66. Vastenhouw B, Beekman FJ. Total body murine imaging with the U-SPECT-I. J Nucl Med 2007; 48(3):487–493.

67. Takahashi T, Watanabe S. Recent progress in CdTe and CdZnTe detectors. IEEE Trans Nucl Sci 2001; 48:950–959.

7

Ultrasound Instrumentation and Techniques

PAUL A. DAYTON

Joint Department of Biomedical Engineering, University of North Carolina at Chapel Hill and North Carolina State University, Raleigh, North Carolina, U.S.A.

MARK A. BORDEN

Department of Chemical Engineering, Columbia University, New York, New York, U.S.A.

INTRODUCTION

Ultrasound is one of the most widely used imaging modalities worldwide, and it is becoming increasingly useful for molecular imaging. Ultrasound scanners are generally inexpensive and portable. For instance, laptop scanners are readily available that can serve as personal devices for physicians and technicians in the field. Beyond simple economics, ultrasound provides a facile means of fast-frame rate imaging, even deep in the body. Spatial resolution compares well with the other modalities, particularly at the high acoustic frequencies used for animal studies. Since ultrasound does not utilize radioisotopes or ionizing radiation, it is safer than CT, PET, or SPECT for both the patient and the operator over successive uses. Recently, specialized small-animal scanners and targeted microbubble formulations have been commercialized. These attributes are bringing ultrasound to the mainstream of molecular imaging.

The main limitation of ultrasound imaging is a limited field of view—ultrasound is restricted to the region accessible by the transducer rather than the whole-body imaging provided by most other imaging technologies. Additionally, although three-dimensional ultrasound is in development, ultrasound images are still typically acquired in two-dimensional format. Another limitation is that targeted contrast agents for ultrasound molecular imaging are currently too large to enter the extravascular space, and thus the accessible receptors are restricted to the vascular lumen. Finally, while ultrasound combined with targeted contrast agents appears to be safe, more work needs to be done to establish dose limits in preclinical and clinical trials.

The general concept of ultrasound molecular imaging is simple and analogous to the other modalities. First, a handheld probe, or transducer, is positioned by the sonographer and kept in place by means of a reticulating arm. Acoustic reflections from local anatomical structures help the sonographer to find the region of interest. Next, targeted contrast agents are injected intravenously in a peripheral vein. The contrast agents circulate in the blood to the tissue of interest. Ligands on the surface of the contrast agent bind specifically to the target receptors, and multiple ligand-receptor interactions act to arrest the contrast agent. The signal from the adherent contrast agent is then detected and used to assess the extent of expression and spatial distribution of the target molecule. An initial and/or follow-up bolus injection of nontargeted microbubbles helps elucidate local blood flow and nonspecific contrast. In this chapter, we review the basics of ultrasound contrast imaging and molecular imaging with ultrasound using microbubble agents.

ULTRASOUND BASICS

Sound waves are longitudinal pressure waves that travel through a medium as regions of compression and rarefaction (1). Sound waves are characterized by their amplitude, frequency (or wavelength), and phase. The wavelength λ and the frequency f of the wave are related to each other by the speed of sound as:

$$c = f\lambda. \tag{1}$$

Ultrasound refers to acoustic waves traveling at frequencies greater than 20 kHz, the detection limit of the human ear (2). Typical clinical imaging systems use a frequency range of 1 to 20 MHz. Higher frequencies are also used, particularly for intracavity or small-animal imaging. The amplitude of the acoustic pulses, also called the acoustic pressure, is usually on the order of hundreds to thousands of kilopascals (kPa). The propagation speed of the sound wave c depends on the density and compressibility of the medium as in equation (2):

$$c = \sqrt{\frac{1}{\rho\kappa}}, \tag{2}$$

where ρ is the density and κ is the compressibility of the medium. The speed of sound is approximately 1540 m/s in most tissues, with small variations depending on the local tissue density and compressibility (3). The acoustic impedance, z, of a medium is characterized by the density of the medium and the speed of sound in the medium as in equation (3):

$$z = \rho c. \tag{3}$$

When a sound wave is incident on an interface between different tissue types, some of the wave is reflected back toward the source, and some of the wave propagates through the interface. A larger mismatch in the acoustic impedance of the two tissues will result in reflection of a larger percentage of the sound energy. Typically, the impedance mismatch between different physiological tissues is less than 1%, which means that very little ultrasound is reflected, and most of the ultrasound is able to continue propagating to deeper tissues. These small differences in acoustic impedance mismatch often extend to tumor tissue as well, which makes small tumors challenging to detect with basic ultrasound. Bone has a higher acoustic impedance, approximately a factor of five greater than tissue, which is why ultrasound is largely reflected from tissue-bone interfaces. The impedance mismatch between a gas

Table 1 Values of Acoustic Impedance

Material	Acoustic impedance
Air	4.30×10^2
Blood	1.67×10^6
Bone	6.47×10^6
Fat	1.33×10^6
Kidney	1.64×10^6
Liver	1.66×10^6
Water	1.48×10^6

and a biological tissue or blood is on the order of 10,000 fold (Table 1), which means that sound waves are scattered from gas bubbles substantially more strongly than from tissue boundaries or blood components. It is for this reason that ultrasound contrast agents contain a gas (or other substance) with a substantially different acoustic impedance than tissue.

Sound waves traveling through tissue lose energy as they propagate. This loss of energy is called attenuation. Attenuation is due to a combination of effects including scattering, reflection, and absorption. Energy losses due to absorption are largely converted into heat. The attenuation of ultrasound in tissue increases as frequency increases. Hence, lower frequencies of ultrasound can propagate deeper into tissue without a reduction in amplitude. The trade-off between attenuation and resolution will be discussed later in this chapter.

IMAGING SYSTEMS

A modern clinical ultrasound transducer, or probe, consists of an array of hundreds of active elements made of a piezoelectric material. When energized with an oscillating voltage, these piezoelectric elements produce ultrasound, which can be actively focused into the tissue by tailoring the order in which the elements are excited. The elements also act as receivers, producing a voltage when they are excited by incident ultrasound. Typical ultrasound pulses are several cycles long, and clinical scanners typically transmit thousands of pulses per second to form an image.

During an ultrasound scan, the transducer probe is energized by the scanner electronics to send out pulse trains of ultrasound that enter the tissue. Ultrasound is reflected from anatomical features where there is an acoustic impedance mismatch due to differences in density and speed of sound. Echoes returned to the transducer are received, processed, and reconstructed to form a two-dimensional image of the scan plane (4). B-mode (brightness modulated) images are formed by mapping the reflected echo intensity to pixel intensity. If the anatomical feature is moving, it will shift the frequency and phase of the scattered echoes in relation to its relative velocity (Doppler shift). This shift can be represented by color overlaid on the ultrasound image, for example, to map the flow velocity within blood vessels.

The resolution of an imaging system is a function of the sound wavelength as well as the transducer design. Since the imaging frequency is inversely proportional to the wavelength, the resolution of the imaging system increases with the frequency. However, the fundamental limitation with ultrasound imaging is that as frequency increases, attenuation also increases (4). Therefore, a trade-off is made between resolution and penetration depth. For this reason, clinical imaging requiring a large depth of penetration, such as adult cardiac imaging, is performed at low frequencies, such as 1.5 to 3 MHz, whereas imaging of peripheral vasculature can be performed at higher frequencies, such as 10 to 15 MHz.

For imaging studies that do not require significant penetration depth into tissue, frequencies from 15 to 50 MHz (often referred to as high-frequency ultrasound) are often used. Transducers used for high-frequency clinical applications include intravascular, intraesophageal, and other intracavity transducers. These small transducers are typically built into the end of a thin probe (for intracavity) or a catheter (for intravascular) and used to image from within the body with high spatial resolution.

High-frequency ultrasound is also used largely in preclinical imaging, where imaging of small rodents does not require substantial penetration depth. Since a large percentage of basic research in cancer treatment is developed in animals, high-frequency ultrasound imaging is a powerful research tool in this area.

INTERACTION BETWEEN ULTRASOUND AND CONTRAST AGENTS

The use of ultrasound contrast agents significantly enhances the power of ultrasound as an imaging tool. Solid and liquid particle contrast agents scatter ultrasound due to acoustic impedance mismatch. Microbubble contrast agents, however, not only scatter ultrasound but also oscillate in an acoustic field, and therefore act as secondary ultrasound sources.

When excited by an acoustic pulse, highly compressible microbubble agents undergo cycles of expansion and compression in response to the acoustic pressure change (Fig. 1). As these microbubbles oscillate, they act as active acoustic sources and can produce echoes with harmonics of the imaging frequency as well as frequencies related to their inherent resonant frequency (5–7). Additionally, the oscillatory response of contrast agent microbubbles is nonlinear in relation to acoustic pressure, frequency, and phase. These unique qualities have pre-

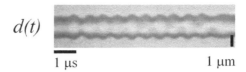

Figure 1 High-speed photography of a contrast agent microbubble oscillating in response to an acoustic pulse. The image is presented as a diameter versus time "streak" image $d(t)$. *Source*: From Ref. 8.

cipitated the development of imaging strategies, which allow the detection of small quantities of contrast agents and discrimination of echoes from contrast agents from those of biological tissue. The remainder of this chapter will focus on imaging strategies specific to microbubble contrast agents.

Microbubble Manipulations

Ultrasound is unique among the imaging modalities in that it is the only modality that can affect the location, adhesion, and clearance of contrast agents in vivo. Two important interactions between ultrasound and microbubbles, which are utilized in molecular imaging, are discussed below. The first is the ability to destroy the contrast agents with specific ultrasound pulses. The second interaction involves radiation forces, also called Bjerknes forces, which can act to displace the microbubbles in an acoustic field.

Microbubble Destruction

Microbubbles can be destroyed by inertial cavitation, which leads to disruption of the stabilizing shell and dissolution of the gas core (2). Inertial cavitation generally refers to the strong inward momentum of the surrounding fluid that collapses the gas core. Higher acoustic pressures and lower frequencies each contribute to a more substantial cavitation effect, and therefore tend to be more destructive to microbubble contrast agents (9,10).

For most medical imaging applications, the cavitation effect should be minimized to prevent bioeffects, since it is known that violently cavitating microbubbles can disrupt endothelium and cell membranes, although this mechanism may have a role in drug delivery (11–13).

Higher energy acoustic pulses are often utilized during contrast imaging to produce microbubble destruction to clear the contrast agent from the sample volume. Clearing microbubbles in this manner is often used in conjunction destruction-reperfusion imaging, where the intent is to measure the time required for contrast (and therefore blood) to flow into a tissue or organ of interest (14,15).

Additionally, microbubble destruction can be used in molecular imaging to clear a region of adherent targeted contrast agents to obtain a background signal to assess the number of bound versus free microbubbles (16,17).

Ultrasound Radiation Force

Acoustic radiation force is produced on objects in an ultrasound field, and is orders of magnitude greater on highly compressible microbubbles than surrounding tissue or blood components (18,19). This force can be maximized on contrast agents by exciting the agents near their resonant frequency and by using a low-pressure pulse with a high duty cycle. If the acoustic parameters for radiation force are optimized, microbubbles can be pushed in the direction of the ultrasound propagation at velocities on the order of hundreds of millimeters per second. The applications of radiation force to molecular imaging are discussed later in this chapter.

CONTRAST ENHANCED ULTRASOUND IMAGING

Ultrasound imaging has traditionally involved the imaging of structural and anatomical features. With the recent development of ultrasound contrast agents, ultrasound imaging has expanded into the fields of functional and molecular imaging. Contrast-enhanced ultrasound imaging can be performed in real time, and provides information about the location of the contrast agent, which can correlate with blood flow (standard contrast imaging) or with the expression of a specific molecular marker (molecular imaging).

An ultrasound contrast exam utilizes a small volume of contrast agents in solution, which is administered into the vasculature through a peripheral vein in humans and large experimental animals, or via the jugular or tail vein in small animals. In humans, a typical dose is on the order of tens of microliters of microbubble suspension per kilogram of body weight, which translates to approximately 10^8 to 10^{10} microbubbles for an 80-kg person (20). Per person, the total encapsulated gas volume injected is very small, on the order of tens of microliters. Contrast enhancement is usually apparent on the imaging system within seconds, as contrast agents are rapidly distributed by blood flow to the imaging site. Duration of contrast enhancement for most commercially available ultrasound contrast agents is on the order of several minutes. In general, this duration is dependent on the administered dose and the properties of the contrast agent. Clearance mechanisms include filtration by the reticuloendothelial system, engulfment by phagocytic cells, and entrapment in the lung and other dense capillary beds (21,22). In addition, ultrasound pulses at higher energies can destroy microbubble contrast agents (9,23).

Microbubble contrast agents exhibit rheological behavior similar to erythrocytes, and thus the most extensive uses of nontargeted microbubble contrast agents are for organ border delineation and for quantitating vascular perfusion (24–26), particularly in diagnostic cardiology (27–29). These techniques are made possible largely because microbubble agents exhibit flow characteristics similar to erythrocytes in vivo. Ultrasound contrast agents have also demonstrated diagnostic efficacy in various radiological applications, such as the evaluation of blood flow in both abdominal and peripheral vascular structures (30) and the detection of intratumoral blood vessels in liver, kidney, ovary, pancreas, prostate, and breast tumors (31).

CONTRAST-SPECIFIC IMAGING TECHNIQUES

In conventional ultrasound imaging, the imaging system transmits and receives using the same frequency band, also commonly referred to as fundamental imaging. Traditional fundamental imaging does not involve signal processing to distinguish between the scattered echoes from tissue and contrast agents. In order to specifically detect contrast agents in the blood pool, or adherent at a target site, clinical contrast imaging takes advantage of signal processing to extract the unique signatures of microbubble contrast agents.

As discussed previously, microbubble contrast agents expand and contract in an oscillatory fashion as they experience an acoustic pulse (a pressure wave). As these contrast agents oscillate, they scatter ultrasound at not only the imaging frequency that excited them but also over a range of other frequencies. Their magnitude, phase, and rate of oscillation are nonlinear with respect to the incident ultrasound wave pressure and frequency (32–37), and their responses to the acoustic pulses are uniquely different than tissue. The result is that with pulsing, detection, and signal processing strategies, the signal from contrast agents can be detected and differentiated from tissue. This allows substantially greater differentiation of contrast agents from tissue (sometimes referred to as the contrast-to-tissue ratio or CTR) than fundamental imaging can provide.

The ability to detect and differentiate small numbers of contrast agents in tissue is particularly important for imaging sensitivity in areas where only small numbers of contrast agents are present, such as in small vessels or tumors. Molecular imaging with ultrasound has produced the greatest motivation for increasing CTR, since typically only small numbers of contrast agents are adherent at the target site (often several orders of magnitude less contrast agents are adherent at a target site than are initially introduced in the contrast agent injection). For determination of the extent and degree of expression of the molecular target, it is necessary to quantify even small amounts of contrast agent adherent at the target site.

In the following sections, we review the most common contrast imaging methods. These methods are categorized based on whether a single imaging pulse (single pulse strategy) or multiple pulses (multipulse strategy) are applied per line of sight to produce one image. Single-pulse contrast imaging strategies include subharmonic imaging, second harmonic imaging, superharmonic/ultraharmonic imaging, and power imaging. Multiple pulse strategies include phase inversion imaging, power modulation, and contrast pulse sequence (CPS) imaging. Other detection methods, which are described in the literature but not reviewed here, include release burst imaging (38), frequency modulation (31,36,39), and coded excitation (40).

Single Pulse Imaging Strategies

Harmonic Imaging

Harmonic imaging relies on detecting multiples of the imaging frequency (called harmonics), which are produced by contrast agents that oscillate in response to the ultrasound pulse. Oscillating contrast agents produce a broadband response that contains energy at other integer multiples (2, 3, 4 . . .) and rational multiples (3/2, 5/2, . . .) of the fundamental frequencies. The concept of harmonic imaging methods is that oscillating microbubbles scatter energy at multiples of the imaging frequency, whereas tissue does not.

Second harmonic imaging involves signal processing where the received ultrasound echoes are filtered to retain only frequencies that are approximately twice the imaging center frequency (the second harmonic) (41–44). One

advantage to this method is that second-harmonic imaging has improved resolution because of the higher frequency produced by the microbubbles. The main limitation of this method as a contrast imaging technique is that although tissue does not produce significant harmonics at low acoustic pressures, at moderate pressures (used in most clinical imaging) tissue also produces higher harmonics, which limits the CTR.

Subharmonic imaging involves signal processing where the received ultrasound signal is filtered to retain only frequencies that are approximately half of the transmission center frequency (5,45–47). Two types of subharmonic signals are described in the literature: one where the contrast agents are excited by the imaging frequency at their natural resonant frequency, and a second where the contrast agents are excited by the imaging center frequency at their second harmonic frequency (5). In either case, the result is that the microbubbles produce echoes with frequency components at half of the imaging frequency (Fig. 2). The main advantage of this technique is that insonified tissue does not generate subharmonic echoes and scatters only frequencies that are same or higher than the transmission frequency. The result is that this imaging technique can achieve a better CTR than traditional fundamental imaging. The main drawback of subharmonic imaging is that the spatial resolution is reduced since only the lower frequencies are preferentially retained.

In addition to the second and subharmonic frequencies, oscillating contrast agents produce a broadband response that contains energy at other multiples of the fundamental frequency. By using more of this broadband response, imaging methods can provide even better CTR compared with fundamental imaging, as well as much better spatial

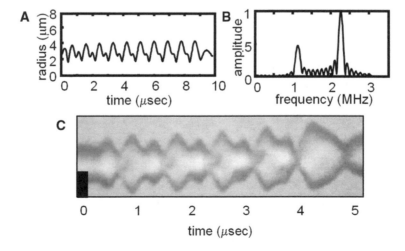

Figure 2 Example of subharmonic response of oscillating contrast agent. (**A**) Simulation of diameter versus time response for a lipid-shelled contrast agent excited at 2.25 MHz and 200 kPa. (**B**) Received echo frequency spectrum based on **A**, which illustrates both fundamental at 2.25 MHz and the subharmonic at 1.125 MHz. (**C**) High-speed photography diameter versus time image of an oscillating lipid-shelled contrast agent illustrating subharmonic response predicted in **A** (less cycles are shown in the photograph than in the simulation). *Source*: Adapted from Ref. 5.

resolution compared with subharmonic imaging (48–51). The major difficulty associated with these methods, such as ultraharmonic and transient imaging, is the extremely wide bandwidth requirement necessary, which can be beyond the limitations of current commercial ultrasound systems.

Power Imaging

Power imaging, which is also called power Doppler imaging or energy imaging, involves detecting the decorrelation of the ultrasound signal over successive pulses. This imaging method was originally designed to sensitively detect blood flow. It has also been shown to be very effective at detecting moving or breaking contrast agents (52,53). However, power imaging is most effective at higher acoustic pressures where the contrast agents are destroyed, so a constant refreshment of microbubbles in the tissue to be imaged is required. Power imaging is not a practical method for molecular imaging for this reason.

Multiple Pulse Imaging Strategies

Phase Inversion Imaging

Phase inversion or pulse inversion imaging is a technique in which two transmitted pulses of opposite phase are transmitted one after the other separated by a delay (33,54,55). This technique takes advantage of the nonlinear scattering of microbubbles. Linear scatterers such as tissue reflect the original and inverted pulses similarly, and the two opposite phase pulses will cancel when echoes from the two pulses are summed. In contrast, nonlinear scatterers, such as contrast agent microbubbles, respond differently to the different phase pulses, and the sum of the echoes from microbubbles will not be zero. This technique achieves tissue suppression in exchange for a reduction in imaging frame rate. A major limitation with this technique, as well as all multiple-pulse imaging strategies, is sensitivity to tissue or contrast motion. Additionally, the nonlinear response of tissue at higher acoustic pressures limits the ability to phase inversion imaging to fully suppress tissue.

Power Modulation Imaging

Power modulation imaging is a two pulse imaging strategy which involves transmitting pulses of different amplitude, and then multiplying by a scaling factor before subtracting received echoes (56,57). Similar to phase inversion imaging, linear components of the echo will cancel, allowing tissue suppression and enhanced contrast detection. Power modulation suffers from the same drawbacks due to tissue motion and the nonlinearity of tissue at higher acoustic pressures as phase inversion.

CPS

Cadence contrast pulse sequencing, as it is referred to by Siemens, is a multiple-pulse imaging method, which improves upon phase inversion by utilizing both the phase and amplitude response of contrast agents, as well as a correction term for the tissue signal (58). As it was originally proposed, this method involves transmission of three pulses that have the same shape but different amplitude and phase (59,60). Upon receipt, three calibrated gain factors calculated to suppress tissue echoes are applied to the received echoes, and the result is summed. This method can achieve tissue suppression greater than phase inversion imaging, but also results in reduced frame rate and more susceptibility to tissue motion.

TECHNIQUES FOR MOLECULAR IMAGING

Molecular imaging with ultrasound is still a relatively new modality, and clinical imaging scanners are not yet optimized for the detection of targeted contrast agents. Most of the ultrasonic molecular imaging described in the literature consists of a multistep process. To create an image of targeted contrast agent distribution, two images of the region of interest are acquired—one background image without targeted contrast agents and other after administration of targeted contrast agents, which have been allowed to circulate for several minutes while the agent becomes adherent to receptors at the target site (Fig. 3) (16,17). Additionally, the waiting period allows for clearance of the freely circulating (nonadherent) contrast agents,

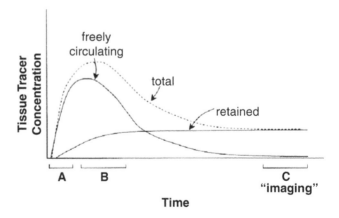

Figure 3 Imaging strategy that is commonly utilized for detection of targeted contrast agents. After a bolus administration, the total signal in an organ rises rapidly and is largely attributable to free contrast (**A**). The rate of targeted agent adhesion in diseased tissue is highest when the free contrast concentration is high (**B**). After a waiting period for clearance of freely circulating agent, remaining contrast in tissue is due to retention of targeted agents, and imaging of targeted agent is performed (**C**). *Source*: From Ref. 17.

which would otherwise interfere with the detection of the targeted agents. The original control image is subtracted from the targeted agent image to remove the signal from tissue, and the resultant image that contains the information for the distribution of targeted agents is typically color coded and may be overlaid on the tissue-only image.

NEW TECHNOLOGIES FOR MOLECULAR IMAGING

Detection Techniques

One of the major challenges of molecular imaging with ultrasound is that a very small percentage of the total injected dose of targeted contrast is retained at the diseased site. For this reason, it is challenging in some applications to isolate the signal from molecularly targeted agents from that of freely circulating agents and tissue. As described previously, most ultrasound molecular imaging studies utilize a waiting period of several minutes during which time contrast agents accumulate at the target site and at the same time freely circulating agents are cleared from the system, followed by signal subtraction with the noncontrast image. This waiting period can be problematic because adherent agents may degrade or release during this time, resulting in decreased signal intensity. Additionally, this method is cumbersome due to the time delay and the requirement for offline processing.

New molecular imaging–specific detection methods have recently been developed using custom ultrasound systems, which take advantage of trends in the scattered echoes from bound contrast agents compared with freely circulating agents. They can be used to image molecularly targeted microbubbles in near real time (51,61). However, these new detection methods rely on ultrawide band imaging and the use of ultrasound forcing to rapidly increase the adhesion rate and reduce the waiting period to a few seconds, neither of which can be implemented in currently available clinical scanners. Regardless, the ability to image targeted agents sensitively and rapidly without offline processing will be a prerequisite before ultrasonic molecular imaging becomes a practical clinical technology.

Acoustic Radiation Force–Enhanced Adhesion

Researchers have shown that radiation force, which can physically push contrast agents from the blood flow against the endothelium, can be used to enhance the retention of targeted contrast agents (62–64). The mechanisms for this adhesion enhancement include the decreased flow velocity of the contrast agents and increased ligand-receptor interaction between the bubbles and receptors when the contrast agents are pushed against the vessel wall. Additionally, radiation force has been shown to promote adhesion of buried-ligand architecture contrast agents, which exhibit reduced immunogenicity under normal conditions (65,66). In an imaging setting, radiation force would be applied by the imaging transducer during the targeted agent accumulation phase before imaging the region of interest (Fig. 4). This technique has the potential to increase targeted contrast agent retention over an order of magnitude and reduce the time required for bubble accumulation to a few seconds. However, improvements will probably be most significant in vessels larger than capillaries, where microbubble-endothelial interaction is small under normal conditions.

Hardware Improvements

A significant limitation of current clinical imaging systems with regard to molecular imaging is transducer bandwidth. High-bandwidth imaging will have the potential to improve molecular imaging with ultrasound because it will be able to take full advantage of imaging the broadband response from microbubbles (see *Harmonic Imaging*), thereby optimizing detection and differentiation of the contrast agent and tissue echoes (50). One method for enhancing transducer bandwidth is by using multifrequency arrays. Multirow, multifrequency transducers are now being developed, which have a much greater bandwidth than those currently available (67).

Additionally, recent improvements in the development of new capacitive micromachined ultrasonic transducers (CMUTs) have demonstrated that these transducers can be

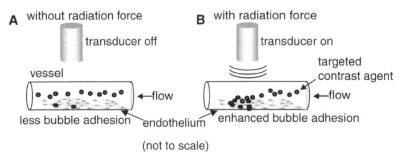

Figure 4 (**A**) Without radiation force, contrast agents accumulate slowly at a target site. (**B**) Radiation force pushes flowing targeted contrast agents into contact with endothelium, rapidly increasing adhesion. *Source*: Adapted from Ref. 62.

made with broad frequency bandwidth (130%) and high transduction efficiency (68).

The implementation of volumetric imaging for ultrasonic molecular imaging will be another substantial technology improvement. Traditional ultrasound images are two-dimensional scan planes of the region of interest, which limits the useful information about the distribution of targeted contrast agents and presents a challenge in selecting the same imaging slice during longitudinal studies. Several ultrasound manufacturers are now producing transducers, hardware, and software for three-dimensional ultrasound imaging (69–71). Volumetric contrast imaging will enable repeatable interrogation of entire tumors or other pathology.

ULTRASONIC MOLECULAR IMAGING IN APPLICATION TO ONCOLOGY

Traditional noncontrast-enhanced ultrasound imaging used to assess patients with cancer is based on structural imaging. Structural imaging entails the assessment of morphological features of tissues and organs of the body and of malignant lesions within these tissues. The structural features of lesions can be assessed over time through serial imaging. However, structural monitoring alone may not be fully indicative of the state of the lesion (72).

One challenge is that gross macroscopic changes in tissues or organs due to cancer generally lag in time following changes at the molecular, subcellular, or cellular

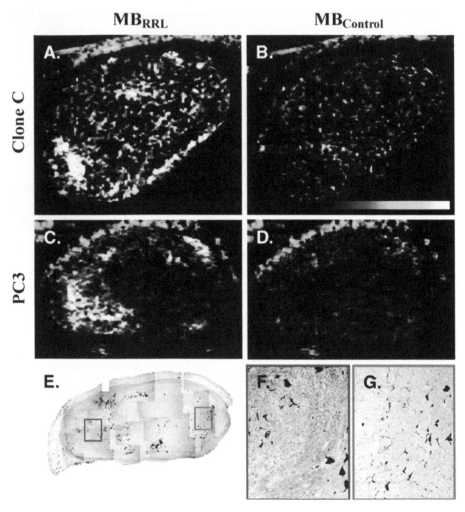

Figure 5 Ultrasonic molecular imaging of angiogenesis. (**A**) Background-subtracted, color-coded ultrasound image taken 120 seconds after injection of targeted contrast agents into a mouse bearing a clone C tumor. Within the colored areas, gradations from red to orange to yellow to white denote greater signal enhancement by contrast material. Non-color-coded portions are not background subtracted and do not influence the videointensity data. (**B**) Corresponding image for control contrast agents in the same mouse as **A**. (**C, D**) Similar ultrasound images as in **A** and **B** but from a mouse with a PC3 tumor. (**E**) Collage of high-resolution photomicrographs taken of a midline PC3 tumor section immunohistochemically stained for factor VIII, showing localization of the microvasculature predominantly to the periphery of the tumor. Cells are counterstained with hematoxylin Original magnification ×20. (**F, G**) High magnification of selected areas of image in **E**. *Source*: Adapted from Ref. 75 (*See Color Insert*).

levels. Another limitation is that structural abnormalities are often nonspecific and often seen in benign conditions (72).

Ultrasonic imaging of lesions utilizing targeted contrast agents allows noninvasive measurement of tumor molecular characteristics, which can be combined with structural imaging to maximize characterization of the tumor. One of the promising applications of ultrasonic molecular imaging in cancer medicine is measuring the response of tumors to antiangiogenic therapies. Ultrasound contrast imaging is uniquely suited to image blood flow in tissue since ultrasound contrast agents exhibit similar rheological behavior as erythrocytes, and the addition of targeted contrast allows the imaging of integrins or other molecular markers indicative of molecular changes within the tumor. Researchers have demonstrated that ultrasonic molecular imaging with contrast agents targeted to molecular markers such as integrin $\alpha_v\beta_3$ or VEGF is a promising tool for noninvasive molecular imaging of tumor angiogenesis and for monitoring vascular effects specific to antitumor therapy (Fig. 5) (76–78).

REFERENCES

1. Leighton TG. What is ultrasound? Prog Biophys Mol Biol 2007; 93(1–3):3–83.
2. Leighton TE. The Acoustic Bubble. London: Academic Press, 1994.
3. Bushberg JT, Seibert JA, Leidholdt EM, et al. The essential physics of medical imaging. Baltimore: Williams and Wilkins, 1994.
4. Szabo TL. Diagnostic Ultrasound Imaging: Inside Out. Burlington, Massachusetts: Elsevier Academic Press, 2004.
5. Chomas J, Dayton P, May D, et al. Nondestructive subharmonic imaging. IEEE Trans Ultrason Ferroelectr Freq Control 2002; 49(7):883–892.
6. de Jong N, Bouakaz A, Frinking P. Basic acoustic properties of microbubbles. Echocardiography 2002; 19(3):229–240.
7. Mayer S, Grayburn PA. Myocardial contrast agents: recent advances and future directions. Prog Cardiovasc Dis 2001; 44(1):33–44.
8. Dayton PA, Rychak JJ. Molecular ultrasound imaging using microbubble contrast agents. Front Biosci 2007; 12:5124–5142.
9. Chomas JE, Dayton P, May D, et al. Threshold of fragmentation for ultrasonic contrast agents. J Biomed Opt 2001; 6(2):141–150.
10. Bouakaz A, Versluis M, de Jong N. High-speed optical observations of contrast agent destruction. Ultrasound Med Biol 2005; 31(3):391–399.
11. Skyba DM, Price RJ, Linka AZ, et al. Direct in vivo visualization of intravascular destruction of microbubbles by ultrasound and its local effects on tissue. Circulation 1998; 98(4):290–293.
12. Stieger SM, Caskey CF, Adamson RH, et al. Enhancement of vascular permeability with low-frequency contrast-enhanced ultrasound in the chorioallantoic membrane model. Radiology 2007; 243(1):112–121.
13. Deng CX, Sieling F, Pan H, et al. Ultrasound-induced cell membrane porosity. Ultrasound Med Biol 2004; 30(4):519–526.
14. Pollard RE, Sadlowski AR, Bloch SH, et al. Contrast-assisted destruction-replenishment ultrasound for the assessment of tumor microvasculature in a rat model. Technol Cancer Res Treat 2002; 1(6):459–470.
15. Porter TR, Xie F, Kricsfeld A, et al. Noninvasive identification of acute myocardial ischemia and reperfusion with contrast ultrasound using intravenous perfluoropropane-exposed sonicated dextrose albumin. J Am Coll Cardiol 1995; 26(1):33–40.
16. Lindner JR. Microbubbles in medical imaging: current applications and future directions. Nat Rev Drug Discov 2004; 3(6):527–532.
17. Lindner JR. Molecular imaging with contrast ultrasound and targeted microbubbles. J Nucl Cardiol 2004; 11(2):215–221.
18. Dayton PA, Allen JS, Ferrara KW. The magnitude of radiation force on ultrasound contrast agents. J Acoust Soc Am 2002; 112(5 pt 1):2183–2192.
19. Dayton PA, Morgan KE, Klibanov AL, et al. Optical and acoustical observations of the effects of ultrasound on contrast agents. IEEE Trans Ultrason Ferroelectr Freq Control 1999; 46(1):220–232.
20. Becher H, Burns PN. Handbook of Contrast Echocardiography. Berlin: Springer, 2000.
21. Schneider M. Characteristics of SonoVue (TM). Echocardiogr-J Card 1999; 16(7):743–746.
22. Wei K, Jayaweera AR, Firoozan S, et al. Quantification of myocardial blood flow with ultrasound-induced destruction of microbubbles administered as a constant venous infusion. Circulation 1998; 97(5):473–483.
23. Chomas JE, Dayton P, Allen J, et al. Mechanisms of contrast agent destruction. IEEE Trans Ultrason Ferroelectr Freq Control 2001; 48(1):232–248.
24. Ismail S, Jayaweera AR, Camarano G, et al. Relation between air-filled albumin microbubble and red blood cell rheology in the human myocardium—influence of echocardiographic systems and chest wall attenuation. Circulation 1996; 94(3):445–451.
25. Lindner JR, Ismail S, Spotnitz WD, et al. Albumin microbubble persistence during myocardial contrast echocardiography is associated with microvascular endothelial glycocalyx damage. Circulation 1998; 98(20):2187–2194.
26. Lindner JR. Evolving applications for contrast ultrasound. Am J Cardiol 2002; 90(10A):72J–80J.
27. Lindner JR, Villanueva FS, Dent JM, et al. Assessment of resting perfusion with myocardial contrast echocardiography: theoretical and practical considerations. Am Heart J 2000; 139(2 pt 1):231–240.
28. Mulvagh SL, DeMaria AN, Feinstein SB, et al. Contrast echocardiography: current and future applications. J Am Soc Echocardiogr 2000; 13(4):331–342.
29. Wei K, Kaul S. Recent advances in myocardial contrast echocardiography. Curr Opin Cardiol 1997; 12(6):539–546.

30. Forsberg F, Liu JB, Merton DA, et al. Parenchymal enhancement and tumor visualization using a new sonographic contrast agent. J Ultrasound Med 1995; 14(12): 949–957.

31. Goldberg BB, Raichlen JS, Forsberg F. Ultrasound contrast agents: basic principals and clinical applications. London: Martin Dunitz, 2001.

32. Biagi E, Breschi L, Vannacci E, et al. Subharmonic emissions from microbubbles: effect of the driving pulse shape. IEEE Trans Ultrason Ferroelectr Freq Control 2006; 53(11):2174–2182.

33. Burns PN, Wilson SR, Simpson DH. Pulse inversion imaging of liver blood flow: improved method for characterizing focal masses with microbubble contrast. Invest Radiol 2000; 35(1):58–71.

34. Ganor Y, Adam D, Kimmel E. Time and pressure dependence of acoustic signals radiated from microbubbles. Ultrasound Med Biol 2005; 31(10):1367–1374.

35. Postema M, Schmitz G. Bubble dynamics involved in ultrasonic imaging. Expert Rev Mol Diagn 2006; 6(3): 493–502.

36. Sun Y, Kruse DE, Ferrara KW. Contrast imaging with chirped excitation. IEEE Trans Ultrason Ferroelectr Freq Control 2007; 54(3):520–529.

37. Wu J, Pepe J, Dewitt W. Nonlinear behaviors of contrast agents relevant to diagnostic and therapeutic applications. Ultrasound Med Biol 2003; 29(4):555–562.

38. Frinking PJ, Cespedes EI, Kirkhorn J, et al. A new ultrasound contrast imaging approach based on the combination of multiple imaging pulses and a separate release burst. IEEE Trans Ultrason Ferroelectr Freq Control 2001; 48(3): 643–651.

39. Deng CX, Lizzi FL, Kalisz A, et al. Study of ultrasonic contrast agents using a dual-frequency band technique. Ultrasound Med Biol 2000; 26(5):819–831.

40. Eckersley RJ, Tang MX, Chetty K, et al. Microbubble contrast agent detection using binary coded pulses. Ultrasound Med Biol 2007; 33(11):1787–1795.

41. Burns PN. Harmonic imaging with ultrasound contrast agents. Clin Radiol 1996; 51(1):50–55.

42. Forsberg F, Goldberg BB, Liu JB, et al. On the feasibility of real-time, in vivo harmonic imaging with proteinaceous microspheres. J Ultrasound Med 1996; 15(12):853–860; quiz 61-2.

43. Frinking PJ, Bouakaz A, Kirkhorn J, et al. Ultrasound contrast imaging: current and new potential methods. Ultrasound Med Biol 2000; 26(6):965–975.

44. Schwarz KQ, Chen X, Steinmetz S, et al. Harmonic imaging with Levovist. J Am Soc Echocardiogr 1997; 10(1):1–10.

45. Forsberg F, Shi WT, Goldberg BB. Subharmonic imaging of contrast agents. Ultrasonics 2000; 38(1–8):93–98.

46. Krishna PD, Shankar PM, Newhouse VL. Subharmonic generation from ultrasonic contrast agents. Phys Med Biol 1999; 44(3):681–694.

47. Shi WT, Forsberg F, Hall AL, et al. Subharmonic imaging with microbubble contrast agents: initial results. Ultrason Imaging 1999; 21(2):79–94.

48. Bouakaz A, Frigstad S, Ten Cate FJ, et al. Super harmonic imaging: a new imaging technique for improved contrast detection. Ultrasound Med Biol 2002; 28(1):59–68.

49. Bouakaz A, Krenning BJ, Vletter WB, et al. Contrast superharmonic imaging: a feasibility study. Ultrasound Med Biol 2003; 29(4):547–553.

50. Kruse DE, Ferrara KW. A new imaging strategy using wideband transient response of ultrasound contrast agents. IEEE Trans Ultrason Ferroelectr Freq Control 2005; 52(8): 1320–1329.

51. Zhao S, Kruse D, Ferrara K, et al. Selective imaging of adherent targeted ultrasound contrast agents. Phys Med Biol 2007; 52:2055–2072.

52. Kook SH, Kwag HJ. Value of contrast-enhanced power Doppler sonography using a microbubble echo-enhancing agent in evaluation of small breast lesions. J Clin Ultrasound 2003; 31(5):227–238.

53. Villanueva FS, Gertz EW, Csikari M, et al. Detection of coronary artery stenosis with power Doppler imaging. Circulation 2001; 103(21):2624–2630.

54. de Jong N, Frinking PJ, Bouakaz A, et al. Detection procedures of ultrasound contrast agents. Ultrasonics 2000; 38(1–8):87–92.

55. Morgan KE, Allen JS, Dayton PA, et al. Experimental and theoretical evaluation of microbubble behavior: effect of transmitted phase and bubble size. IEEE Trans Ultrason Ferroelectr Freq Control 2000; 47(6):1494–1509.

56. Eckersley RJ, Chin CT, Burns PN. Optimising phase and amplitude modulation schemes for imaging microbubble contrast agents at low acoustic power. Ultrasound Med Biol 2005; 31(2):213–219.

57. Mor-Avi V, Caiani EG, Collins KA, et al. Combined assessment of myocardial perfusion and regional left ventricular function by analysis of contrast-enhanced power modulation images. Circulation 2001; 104(3):352–357.

58. Phillips P, Gardner E. Contrast-agent detection and quantification. Eur Radiol 2004; 14(suppl 8):P4–P10.

59. Brock-Fisher GA. Inventor contrast agent imaging with suppression of nonlinear tissue response. US patent 6,361,498 B1, 2002.

60. Phillips PJ. Contrast pulse sequences (CPS): imaging nonlinear microbubbles. In: Proceedings of the 2001 IEEE Ultrasonics Symposium, 2001; 2:1739–1745.

61. Zhao S, Kruse DE, Ferrara KW, et al. Acoustic response from adherent targeted contrast agents. J Acoust Soc Am 2006; 120(6):EL63–EL69.

62. Zhao S, Borden M, Bloch SH, et al. Radiation-force assisted targeting facilitates ultrasonic molecular imaging. Mol Imaging 2004; 3(3):135–148.

63. Rychak JJ, Klibanov AL, Hossack JA. Acoustic radiation force enhances targeted delivery of ultrasound contrast microbubbles: in vitro verification. IEEE Trans Ultrason Ferroelectr Freq Control 2005; 52(3):421–433.

64. Rychak JJ, Klibanov AL, Ley KF, et al. Enhanced targeting of ultrasound contrast agents using acoustic radiation force. Ultrasound Med Biol 2007; 33(7):1132–1139. [Epub 2007 Apr 18].

65. Borden MA, Martinez GV, Ricker J, et al. Lateral phase separation in lipid-coated microbubbles. Langmuir 2006, 22(9):4291–4297.

66. Borden MA, Zhang H, Gillies RJ, et al. A stimulus-responsive contrast agent for ultrasound molecular imaging. Biomaterials 2008; 29(5):597–606.

67. Stephens DN, Ming Lu X, Proulx T, et al. Multi-frequency array development for drug delivery therapies: characterization and first use of a triple row ultrasound probe. In: Proceedings of the 2006 IEEE Ultrasonics Symposium 2006:66–69, doi:10.1109/ULTSYM.2006.30.

68. Demirci U, Ergun AS, Oralkan O, et al. Forward-viewing CMUT arrays for medical imaging. IEEE Trans Ultrason Ferroelectr Freq Control 2004; 51(7):887–895.

69. Pemberton J, Li X, Karamlou T, et al. The use of live three-dimensional Doppler echocardiography in the measurement of cardiac output: an in vivo animal study. J Am Coll Cardiol 2005; 45(3):433–438.

70. Albrecht H, Stroszczynski C, Felix R, et al. Real time 3D (4D) ultrasound-guided percutaneous biopsy of solid tumours. Ultraschall Med 2006; 27(4):324–328.

71. Voormolen MM, Krenning BJ, van Geuns RJ, et al. Efficient quantification of the left ventricular volume using 3-dimensional echocardiography: the minimal number of equiangular long-axis images for accurate quantification of the left ventricular volume. J Am Soc Echocardiogr 2007; 20(4):373–380.

72. Torigian DA, Huang SS, Houseni M, et al. Functional imaging of cancer with emphasis on molecular techniques. CA Cancer J Clin 2007; 57(4):206–224.

73. Atri M. New technologies and directed agents for applications of cancer imaging. J Clin Oncol 2006; 24(20):3299–3308.

74. Alavi A, Lakhani P, Mavi A, et al. PET: a revolution in medical imaging. Radiol Clin North Am 2004; 42(6): 983–1001, vii.

75. Weller GE, Wong MK, Modzelewski RA, et al. Ultrasonic imaging of tumor angiogenesis using contrast microbubbles targeted via the tumor-binding peptide argininearginine-leucine. Cancer Res 2005; 65(2):533–539.

76. Korpanty G, Carbon JG, Grayburn PA, et al. Monitoring response to anticancer therapy by targeting microbubbles to tumor vasculature. Clin Cancer Res 2007; 13(1): 323–330.

77. Heppner P, Lindner JR. Contrast ultrasound assessment of angiogenesis by perfusion and molecular imaging. Expert Rev Mol Diagn 2005; 5(3):447–455.

78. Leong-Poi H, Christiansen J, Klibanov AL, et al. Non-invasive assessment of angiogenesis by ultrasound and microbubbles targeted to alpha(v)-integrins. Circulation 2003; 107(3):455–460.

8

Oncological Applications of MR Spectroscopy

MARIE-FRANCE PENET, KRISTINE GLUNDE, MICHAEL A. JACOBS, NORIKO MORI, and DMITRI ARTEMOV
JHU ICMIC Program, Russell H. Morgan Department of Radiology and Radiological Science,
Johns Hopkins University School of Medicine, Baltimore, Maryland, U.S.A.

ZAVER M. BHUJWALLA
JHU ICMIC Program, Russell H. Morgan Department of Radiology and Radiological Science, and Sidney Kimmel Comprehensive Cancer Center, Johns Hopkins University School of Medicine, Baltimore, Maryland, U.S.A.

INTRODUCTION

Since the initial demonstration of the use of noninvasive magnetic resonance spectroscopy (MRS) in cancer two decades ago, MRS has found several preclinical and clinical applications in oncology. MRS is based on the detection of radiofrequency (RF) signals generated by magnetic nuclear spins precessing in an external magnetic field B0. The magnetic resonance frequency $\omega 0$ is linearly dependent on B0 and the gyromagnetic ratio of the nucleus γ as $\omega 0 = \gamma B0$. The intensity of the MR signal depends on the concentration of nuclear spins and the gyromagnetic ratio γ of the spins. In addition, the magnetization signal is characterized by two rate constants, the spin-lattice (or longitudinal relaxation time) T_1, and the spin-spin (or tranverse relaxation time) T_2. The most important aspect of MRS is its ability to distinguish a particular nucleus with respect to its environment in the molecule since the resonance frequency of a particular nucleus is dependent upon its molecular structure. MRS, therefore, provides information about the chemical environment of the nuclear spin such as number of chemical bonds, neighboring nuclei, and chemical structure. Each peak in an MR spectrum has a characteristic chemical shift defined in parts per million (ppm) that is dependent upon the chemical structure of the metabolite or compound and an area proportional to its concentration.

The incorporation of imaging with MRS has resulted in the development of spectroscopic MR imaging [chemical-shift imaging (CSI) (1)] where this chemical information is spatially encoded. Selective images of the distribution of specific chemical compounds such as metabolites, exogenous substances, or drugs can be obtained by CSI. The detection limits of proton and ^{19}F MRS are typically within the mM range, with higher concentrations required for less-sensitive nuclei such as ^{31}P and ^{13}C.

A traditional strength of MRS has always been the wealth of functional information that it provides. Some of the applications of MRS, the nuclei commonly studied, and the information that can be obtained are summarized in Table 1. From this table it is apparent that noninvasive MRS methods have wide-ranging preclinical and clinical applications in cancer. As shown in Figure 1, MRS is one of the few techniques that can be applied from bench to beside. The past decade has seen major advances in sequence design, the development of novel reporter probes, and technological advances that have significantly increased the uses of MRS in molecular-functional imaging applications in oncology. In this chapter we have reviewed some of the recent applications of ^1H, ^{13}C,

Table 1 Nuclei Commonly Studied With MRS and Some of the Applications of Multinuclear MRS

Nucleus	γ[MHz/T]	Application
^{1}H	42.58	• Total choline
		• Lactate
		• Lipid
		• Extracellular pH (pHe)
		• Treatment efficacy
		• Detection of metastasis
		• Measurement of pO_2
^{13}C	10.71	• Labeled substrate utilization to evaluate drug pharmacokinetics and metabolic pathways
^{19}F	40.08	• Drug pharmacokinetics
		• pHe
		• Measurement of pO_2
		• Enzyme activity
		• Labeled substrate utilization
^{31}P	17.25	• Energy metabolism (ATP, PCr, Pi)
		• Intracellular pH (pHi)
		• Phospholipid metabolism

^{31}P, and ^{19}F MRS in preclinical models and the current clinical uses of these spectroscopy techniques. New developments such as hyperpolarization of spins to increase the sensitivity of detection of the MR signal of ^{13}C-labeled substrates are discussed (2). The advantages and limitations of the spectroscopic techniques and challenges for the future are outlined.

^{1}H MRS

Overview, Advantages, and Disadvantages

Of all the nuclei ^{1}H MRS has the highest sensitivity and is, therefore, the most widely used in preclinical and clinical studies. Proton spectra can be obtained with high temporal as well as spatial resolution. This is advantageous because tumor blood flow is typically heterogeneous and results in a heterogeneous distribution of oxygen, pH, and metabolites. The ability to obtain spatially localized spectra can be used to acquire MRS signals from tumor tissue only, and minimize signal contribution from normal tissue. The spatial distribution of metabolites within the tumor can be obtained to better characterize different tumor regions

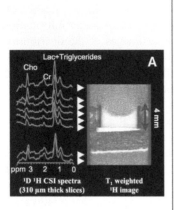
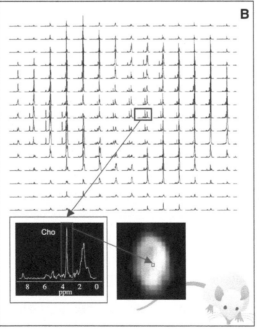
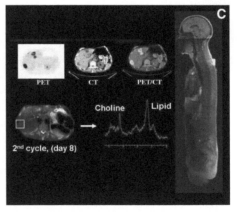

Figure 1 Scope of MRS in oncology, from studying cancer cells (**A**) to preclinical human tumor xenografts (**B**) to clinical studies (**C**). (**A**) Localized proton spectra (*left*) obtained from malignant MDA-MB-231 cells invading into a layer of matrigel (*right*). Spectra were obtained using 1D CSI and contain signal from total choline, creatine, and lactate/lipid (kindly provided by Dr. E. Ackerstaff). (**B**) Localized proton spectra (*top*) from a human prostate cancer xenograft (PC-3) in a SCID mouse, obtained with an in-plane spatial resolution of 1 mm × 1 mm and a slice thickness of 4 mm. Signal intensities of individual peaks in the spectrum obtained from each voxel can be converted into an image (*bottom*, total choline image). C. 72 year-old male with colorectal cancer and known metastatic disease in the liver detected in the PET/CT images. Single voxel MRS (TE = 270 ms) of the lesion was obtained to monitor response to treatment in conjunction with MR images.

within the tumor (Fig. 1B) as well as its response to therapy.

Unedited proton spectra are dominated by signal from water, methyl and methylene protons, and signals from metabolites are masked by these dominant signals. Water suppression methods are, therefore, required in proton spectroscopy to eliminate the signal from water during acquisition, using techniques such as VAPOR (3), CHESS (4) or band-selective refocusing (5,6). Water suppression presents some disadvantages. The water signal may be useful for absolute quantification and for correction procedures. Magnetization transfer effect may be induced by the water suppression techniques. Moreover, water suppression may affect signals from metabolites with chemical shifts close to that of water. Therefore, techniques have been developed to obtain ^{1}H MR spectra in vivo without water suppression (7). Prior to a standard localization sequence, two additional chemical shift–selective inversion pulses are either switched off or switched on to invert the metabolites' signals upfield and downfield from water. To obtain the metabolite or the water signals, the two data sets are subtracted or added, allowing the simultaneous detection of signal from water and metabolites (7).

The other dominant signal in proton spectra arises from mobile lipids and can provide useful information on apoptosis, necrosis, or lipid droplets formation (8–10). MRS-visible lipid levels have been found to accumulate with apoptosis (11), suggesting that apoptosis may be detected in vivo by ^{1}H MRS detection of cellular lipids.

Resonances from metabolites such as lactate and alanine, which resonate at frequencies close to the lipid region, are obscured by the lipid signal. These overlapping lipid resonances, therefore, also require suppression to detect signal from these metabolites. The use of longer echo times significantly reduces signal from mobile lipids, because lipid signals decay faster than metabolite signals. Localized presaturation methods are also used to suppress lipid signals when these are localized to peripheral regions (6,12). The lactate doublet may be isolated from overlapping lipid signals by using an iterative filtering process based on the continuous wavelet transform method in the time domain (13). This technique may be improved by applying a biexponential decay filter (14). Other methods for lipid suppression include gradient-filtering of lactate multiple-quantum coherences (15,16) and the application of adiabatic pulses for spectral editing (17). However, coherence selection may not be optimal, and two-dimensional experiments, difference spectra, or additional phase cycling steps may be required to obtain uncontaminated spectra. He et al. (18,19) have shown that a homonuclear gradient-coherence transfer method, combined with a frequency selective pulse, is very effective in suppressing both lipid and water in a single scan.

Preclinical Applications

Choline Metabolism

In vivo proton spectra obtained from tumors contain several resonances. At longer echo times, metabolites such as total choline [consisting of phosphocholine (PC), glycerophosphocholine (GPC), and free choline], total creatine (phosphocreatine and creatine), and lactate are detected. With shorter echo times, additional signals from mobile lipids and metabolites, such as glutamine + glutamate are also detected (20,21). [1]H MR spectra of tumors typically exhibit elevated total choline and lactate levels (22). The high levels of lactate are consistent with high glycolytic rates and poor blood flow associated with tumors (23). The high levels of total choline detected in breast, prostate, and different types of brain tumors primarily arise from increased PC levels in tumor cells, as confirmed by high-resolution ^{1}H MRS studies of cell extracts and tumors (24–27). Choline, PC, and GPC play a role in cell membrane phospholipid synthesis and breakdown (28). Molecular alterations underlying the increased PC levels observed in cancer cells include increased expression and activity of choline kinase (29–31), a higher rate of choline transport (27,32) and increased phospholipase C and D activity (33,34).

Treatment Efficacy

Proton spectroscopy has been used to investigate the effects of targeting choline kinase in preclinical studies of breast cancer (35,36). Consistent with effects observed with pharmacological inhibition (36), inhibition of choline kinase by small interfering RNA (siRNA) induced a significant reduction in PC and was associated with a reduction in proliferative rate and an increase in differentiation. As shown in Figure 2, ^{1}H MR spectra revealed a high level of PC in malignant MDA-MB-231 human mammary epithelial cells but not in nonmalignant MCF-12A human mammary epithelial cells. Transient transfection with siRNA downregulating choline kinase resulted in a significant decrease in PC levels in the malignant cells but did not alter the already low PC concentration of nonmalignant cells (35). The efficacy of pharmacological choline kinase inhibitors such as MN58b have been tested both in vivo and in vitro in human carcinoma models; MN58b resulted in a decreased total choline level in vivo. This decrease was because of a decrease in PC concentration as shown by in vitro ^{31}P MRS analysis. These data demonstrate the potential utility of using ^{1}H MRS in clinical trials to assess tumor response to choline kinase inhibition (36).

^{1}H MRS has been used to noninvasively evaluate treatment efficacy and tumor viability. An inverse correlation between the mobile lipid/total choline ratio, and the

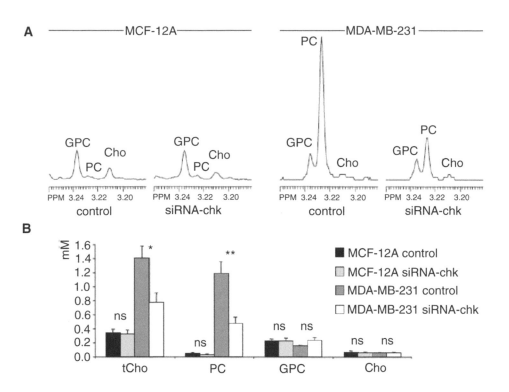

Figure 2 Choline kinase downregulation following transient transfection with choline kinase targeting siRNA. (**A**) Expanded regions of ^{1}H MR spectra from cell extracts of nonmalignant MCF-12A cells and malignant MDA-MB-231 breast cancer cells acquired at 400 MHz. Spectra are from control cells and cells obtained after 48 hours of transfection with siRNA Chk. Transfection resulted in a significant decrease of PC in the malignant MDA-MB-231 cells but not in the nonmalignant MCF-12A cells. (**B**) Quantitation of the changes induced by transfection showing a decrease of total choline resulting from the decrease in PC concentrations. *Source*: From Ref. 35.

viable tumor fraction was observed in a study using a xenograft model of human neuroblastoma treated with TNP-470 (37).

In a recent study, in vivo ^{1}H MRS was used to study metabolic pathways in tumors following induction of acute hyperglycemia in a mouse glioma model (38). The glucose signal reached a maximum one hour after injection. The data obtained suggested that there was extracellular accumulation of glucose in the tumor and that acute hyperglycemia did not change lactate concentrations (38).

High-resolution magic angle spinning (HR-MAS) spectroscopy is a technique used to characterize metabolism of intact tissues, cells, and biofluids. One- and two-dimensional ^{1}H HR-MAS has been applied to understand the effects of treatment on metabolic pathways. One such study performed following treatment of a murine melanoma and pulmonary carcinoma model with chloroethylnitrosourea revealed several metabolic alterations such as accumulation of glutamine, glutamate, and aspartate following treatment. Other metabolites such as alanine, succinate, and serine-derived compounds were also altered (39). A metabolomic characterization of tumors following therapy may allow the identification of drug

responsiveness and adaptative metabolic pathways in tumors (39).

Tumor pH and Hypoxia

Tumor pH is an important parameter that influences tumor progression and efficacy of treatment (40). Extracellular pH (pHe) is usually acidic compared to that of normal tissue (41,42). ^{1}H MRS can be used to image pHe in tumors in vivo by acquiring the signal from pH-sensitive extracellular compounds such as (imidazol-1-yl)3-ethyoxycarbonylpropionic acid (IEPA) (43). These pHe maps may be related to metabolite maps (44) or vascular volume and permeability maps (45). A recently developed probe, 2-(imidazol-1-yl)succinic acid (ISUCA), was used to demonstrate the effect of glucose infusion on both pHe and lactate concentration in a glioma model. Figure 3 demonstrates the different maps such as pHe, total choline, lactate, total creatine, and *N*-acetyl-aspartate (NAA) maps can be acquired with in vivo ^{1}H magnetic resonance spectroscopic imaging (^{1}H MRSI) (46).

Tumor hypoxia is known to result in resistance to radiation and chemotherapy (47,48). The ability to

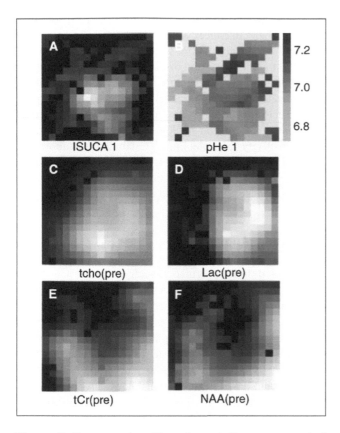

Figure 3 Representative pHe and metabolites maps acquired with ¹H MRSI of a glioma in a mouse brain. (**A**) Map of the peak areas of the ISUCA H2 resonances, (**B**) map of pHe calculated from the chemical shifts of the H2 peaks, (**C**) total choline map, (**D**) lactate map, (**E**) total creatine map, and (**F**) N-acetyl aspartate map. Metabolites maps were acquired with a echo time of 136 ms and pixel size of 0.5×0.5 mm². *Source*: From Ref. 46.

noninvasively measure tumor hypoxia would be useful for selecting an appropriate therapy. A recent exciting development is the use of ¹H MRS to perform tissue oximetry using hexamethyldisiloxane. This new pO_2 probe provides the possibility of detecting pO_2 in vivo (49).

Clinical Applications

The clinical applications of ¹H MRS in vivo and ex vivo for several cancers (breast, prostate, ovary) have recently been reviewed by Mountford et al. (50). The use of metabolic profiles and elevated choline levels to detect cancer with MRS or MRSI have been demonstrated for prostate (51–53), brain (54–56), breast (57–59), and other cancers (60). Elevated total choline was also detected in MRSI of biopsied musculoskeletal tumors (61), and a recent study showed that musculoskeletal lesions may be characterized in vivo with ¹H MRS (62). Because total choline levels are higher in malignant tissue than in benign or normal breast tissue, the detection of the total choline signal by proton MRSI, typically performed in conjunction with high-resolution anatomic MR imaging, has been shown to significantly improve the diagnosis and assessment of cancer location and aggressiveness (57). An example of the elevated total choline signal detected in breast cancer is shown in Figure 4.

Healthy and cancerous prostate tissue can be distinguished by the ratio of (choline + creatine)/citrate (63). However, a characterization of human prostate tissue performed on biopsies using ¹H MRS showed that depleted citrate and elevated choline levels alone were not accurate markers for distinguishing histologic variants of prostatic tissue. A comparison of the intensities of choline, lysine,

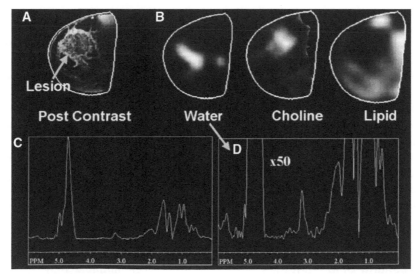

Figure 4 Proton MRI and MRSI of a 41-year-old patient with infiltrating ductal carcinoma of the breast. (**A**) Post-contrast T₁-weighted images of the breast lesion. (**B**) Spectroscopic images of water, total choline, and mobile lipids. (**C, D**) Representative spectrum of elevated total choline within the lesion. *Source*: From Ref. 57.

creatine, and lipid detected prostate carcinoma with a high degree of sensitivity and specificity (64). Metabolic profiles of human brain tumors have been established to define different classes of tumors (56). ^{1}H MRS combined with MRI has been used for noninvasive diagnostic assessment of brain tumors (65). Automated pattern recognition techniques are under development for brain tumor classification (56). The acquisition of ^{1}H MRSI at 3T with an eight-channel phased-array head coil improved sensitivity and spatial resolution to detect more subtle differences in metabolite levels (66). Metastases in lymph nodes in vivo (67) and ex vivo (68) were also detected by the elevation of total choline in vivo and by an increase of GPC + PC, choline and lactate ex vivo in ^{1}H MRS.

HR-MAS spectroscopy has been applied for quantitative analysis of metabolites in prostate biopsies. PC+GPC, total choline, alanine and lactate were higher in tumors than in control tissues, while citrate was lower (69). HR-MAS has also been applied to explore breast cancer biopsies (70,71). In a study comparing breast tumor tissues to adjacent noninvolved tissues, GPC was found to be the dominant choline signal in noninvolved tissues, whereas PC was the dominant choline signal in tumors. Signals from lactate, glycine, and taurine were also detected in tumors. HR-MAS may be a rapid and simple way to analyze healthy and cancerous tissue (70).

Pre- and post-therapy studies have demonstrated the potential of combined MRI and MRSI to provide a direct measure of the presence and spatial extent of cancer, as well as the time course and mechanism of therapeutic response (72,73). The applications of MRS in radiotherapy treatment planning for brain and prostate cancers were recently reviewed by Payne et al. (21). Meisamy et al. (74) detected the response to primary systemic therapy (PST) in breast cancer within 24 hours of treatment by monitoring the change in total tissue choline concentration. In this study, MRI and MRS were performed on a 4T research scanner prior to treatment and within 24 hours after treatment with combined doxorubicin and cyclophosphamide. A lower total choline level compared to baseline was detected within 24 hours with a further decrease after the fourth dose in patients who were objective responders. Total choline levels remained unchanged or increased in patients who were nonresponders (74). ^{1}H MRS has also been applied to monitor the effect of temozolomide on low-grade glioma; reduction in the tumor choline/water signal paralleled tumor volume decrease with treatment (75).

^{13}C MRS

Overview, Advantages, and Disadvantages

^{13}C MR spectroscopy is usually performed using a ^{13}C-labeled substrate and is uniquely suited to study glycolysis and other metabolic pathways such as choline metabolism, among others, in cancer cells and solid tumors. The flux of metabolites through various pathways can be determined through the incorporation of the label into metabolites and metabolic modeling. ^{13}C MR spectroscopy has relatively low sensitivity, but indirect detection methods (76) permit the detection of the ^{13}C label with a sensitivity approaching that of the proton nucleus and significantly increase the sensitivity of detecting ^{13}C-labeled metabolites in vivo. The use of heteronuclear cross polarization transfer to increase the sensitivity of direct ^{13}C detection has also been previously demonstrated (77).

Preclinical Applications

^{13}C-labeled lipid precursors such as [1,2-^{13}C]-choline, [3-^{13}C]-serine, [1,2-^{13}C]-ethanolamine, or [^{13}C-methyl]-methionine have been utilized for ^{13}C MRS studies to characterize the metabolism of cells and tumors (78–80). ^{13}C MRS studies investigating the metabolism of [1,2-^{13}C]-choline in a cell perfusion system demonstrated that breast cancer cells exhibited enhanced choline transport and choline kinase activity (32). This study also revealed that the rate of choline phosphorylation was much faster than the choline transport rate (32). Glunde et al. have utilized [1,2-^{13}C]-choline to follow the production of water-soluble ^{13}C-labeled choline phospholipid metabolites PC and GPC in human MDA-MB-231 breast cancer cells (81). Using a dual-phase extraction method, the lipid fraction was recovered and measured separately to assess incorporation of [1,2-^{13}C]-choline into membrane phosphatidylcholine. This study demonstrated that the elevated level of PC in cancer cells is because of increased choline kinase and phospholipase C activity (81).

Tumor glycolysis can also be investigated in vivo by using ^{13}C-labeled glucose and lactate. Glucose uptake and consumption, as well as lactate synthesis and clearance can be derived from the metabolism of these substrates (82). Glucose uptake and metabolism is very different in tumors since mitochondrial metabolism is impaired and cytosolic glycolysis is elevated (83,84). Cancer cells rapidly metabolize glucose to form lactate. Following intravenous infusion of [1-^{13}C]-labeled glucose, signals from [1-^{13}C]-glucose and [3-^{13}C]-lactate are detected in tumors by ^{13}C MRS. The conversion of [1-^{13}C]-glucose to [3-^{13}C]-lactate can, therefore, be followed in vivo. For most tumors, lactate levels are the result of an interplay between hemodynamics, substrate supply, hypoxia, venous clearance, glucose supply, extent of necrosis, and degree of inflammatory cell infiltrate (85). A clear correlation between decreasing tumor oxygenation and increasing glycolytic rate was observed in a murine mammary carcinoma model, studied by volume localized ^{13}C MRS with

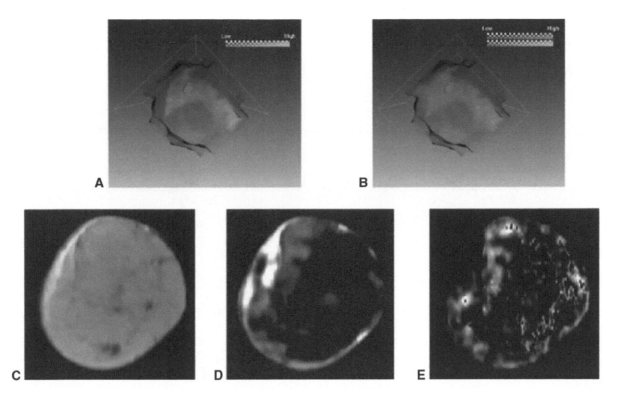

Figure 5 Biodistribution of a contrast agent and of ^{13}C-labeled TMZ (temozolomide) in MCF-7 tumor. (**A**) Gadolinium Diethylenetriaminepentaacetate (GdDTPA) uptake in the tumor. (**B**) Coregistration of GdDTPA (*green*) and ^{13}C-TMZ (*red*) in the tumor. (**C**) Precontrast image acquired before the administration of GdDTPA (**D**) Contrast map reconstructed as a difference map between pre- and postcontrast acquisitions showing the distribution of GdDTPA (**E**) Volume transfer constant (K^{trans}) map showing the vascular functions of the tumor. This map is reconstructed from a two-compartment model-based analysis. K^{trans} is generally a function of tumor blood flow and vascular permeability surface area product. These maps showed the GdDTPA uptake spatially related with the distribution of TMZ. The inhomogeneous distribution of TMZ might be because of heterogeneous tumor perfusion and vascularization. *Source*: From Ref. 95 (*See Color Insert*).

^{1}H-^{13}C cross polarization to detect the conversion of [1-^{13}C]-glucose to [3-^{13}C]-lactate (86). Rivenzon-Segal et al. have shown that in MCF-7 breast cancer xenografts, the lactate signal is visible at 10 minutes after the glucose infusion and increases for 50 minutes (82). Although [1-^{13}C]-labeled glucose is metabolized to lactate (87–90) in poorly differentiated tumors, Ronen et al. found that a well-differentiated rat hepatoma (H4IIEC3) exhibited metabolic characteristics similar to normal hepatocytes mainly utilizing alanine as a substrate and resorting to glucose only under conditions of nutrient deprivation (91). When studying perchloric acid extracts of tumors or organs from animals infused with [1-^{13}C]- or [U-^{13}C]-labeled glucose, the labeling pattern of metabolites can provide insight into metabolic compartmentalization, shuttling of metabolites between cell types or organs, and metabolic fluxes (92).

Glutathione metabolism in tumors has also been evaluated in vivo and ex vivo by infusing [2-^{13}C]-glycine in rats implanted with a fibrosarcoma. Spectroscopic imaging revealed a heterogenous distribution of glutathione within the tumor (93).

Three-dimensional maps of drug distribution can be obtained following systemic administration of ^{13}C-labeled anticancer drugs such as phenylacetate. The delivery of a low molecular weight drug was approximated by measuring the delivery of a similarly sized contrast agent (94). In another example of the detection of ^{13}C-labeled anticancer drugs by ^{13}C MRS, Kato et al. (95) imaged the intratumoral distribution of the ^{13}C-labeled anticancer agent temozolomide by ^{1}H/^{13}C MRS. This anticancer agent is used clinically to treat glioblastomas and anaplastic astrocytomas (96). This study demonstrated the heterogenous delivery of the drug by using ^{13}C MRSI as shown in Figure 5.

Treatment Response

^{13}C MRS has been used to detect the effect of treatment aimed at the selective inhibition of glycolysis in tumors (97) as well as to detect changes in glycolysis following treatments not specifically targeting glycolysis, such as tamoxifen treatment. Treatment with tamoxifen induced a reduction in glycolysis rate and lactate clearance (82).

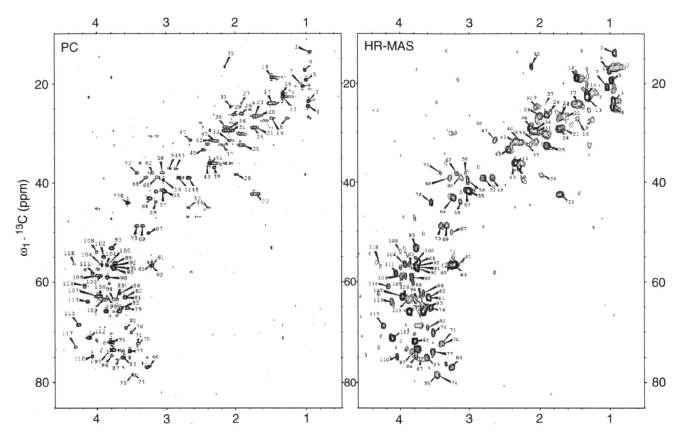

Figure 6 Representative aliphatic region of two-dimensional ^{13}C-^{1}H HSQC from perchloric acid extract on the left and from HR-MAS on the right of tumor samples acquired at 500 MHz. *Source*: From Ref. 100.

^{13}C-labeled glucose and lactate have been used to test the effect of lithium in a human neuroblastoma cell line. Treatment with lithium inhibited flux through the TCA (tricarboxylic acid) cycle (98); the conversion rate of glucose to pyruvate decreased, but lactate production was not altered. ^{13}C MRS has also been used to study the effects of imatinib treatment. Imatinib is a tyrosine kinase inhibitor used in the treatment of chronic myelogenous leukemia (99). Imatinib inhibits the ATP-binding on the BCR-ABL tyrosine kinase, which is a fused oncogene. To characterize changes in cell metabolism induced by imatinib, studies were performed on both BCR-ABL positive cells and BCR-ABL negative cells. ^{13}C MRS performed on cell extracts following an incubation of cells with [1-^{13}C]-glucose showed that imatinib induced a change in BCR-ABL positive cell metabolism by reversing the Warburg effect; cells switched from glycolytic to mitochondrial glucose metabolism (99).

Clinical Applications

HR-MAS with one- and two-dimensional ^{1}H and ^{13}C has been used to characterize metabolites in brain tumor tissue (100). Intact glioblastoma tissue was analyzed and the

results compared with those obtained after perchloric acid extraction; a good correlation between ex vivo (HR-MAS) and in vitro (perchloric acid extracts) results was observed. The resolutions of both spectra were comparable and ex vivo metabolite degradation was avoided by keeping the sample at low temperature. The data obtained demonstrate that HR-MAS spectroscopy may be a viable alternative to the classical histopathological process to classify and grade tissue samples. With this approach, 37 metabolites were identified. Representative two-dimensional spectra of extract and tissue samples are shown in Figure 6 and demonstrate the feasibility of a complete analysis of the metabolite profile of the tumor (100).

^{19}F MRS

Overview, Advantages, and Disadvantages

Poor drug delivery is a major problem in cancer chemotherapy. Like ^{13}C MRS described earlier, ^{19}F MRS can be used to determine the pharmacokinetics of ^{19}F-labeled drugs in the tumor or provide surrogate indices of drug uptake. ^{19}F MR pharmacokinetic measurements of tumors in vivo have mainly been restricted to fluorinated drugs such as 5-fluorouracil (5-FU) detected by ^{19}F MRS, since ^{19}F imaging has the advantage of a relatively high sensitivity and no background signal. For drugs lacking fluorine atoms, fluorine labeling may alter the physicochemical and pharmacological properties of the drug.

Preclinical Applications

Enzyme Activity Assay

^{19}F MRS of fluorinated markers has been used to verify transgene activity in situ by assessing endogenous and exogenous enzyme activity in vivo. In a recent study (101), ^{19}F MRS was used to report on the expression of LacZ through the hydrolysis of 2-fluoro-4-nitrophenyl β-D-galactopyranoside (OFPNPG). The cleavage of OFPNPG by LacZ induced the formation of aglycone 2-fluoro-4-nitrophenol (OFPNP). Both compounds were detected by ^{19}F MRS with a chemical shift difference of approximately 4 to 6 ppm between the two peaks (101).

^{19}F MRS was also used to measure the activity of thymidine phosphorylase in a bladder tumor model by following the formation of 5-FU (102). Capecitabine (N-pentyloxycarbonyl-5′-deoxy-5-fluorocytidine) is a pro-drug of 5-FU. Capecitabine is converted to 5′deoxy-5-fluorocytidine (5′DFCR) by hepatic carboxylesterase (102). 5′DFCR is converted to 5′deoxy-5-fluorouridine (5′DFUR) by cytidine deaminase in the liver and tumor tissue. 5′DFUR is converted to 5-FU by thymidine phosphorylase, which is active in tumor tissue. These metabolites were detected by ^{19}F MRS. This study showed that tumor thymidine phosphorylase activity correlated with the conversion rate of 5′DFUR as measured by ^{19}F MRS (102).

In another study, the activity of the enzyme histone deacetylase was monitored with ^{19}F MRS. The inhibition of this enzyme was followed in PC3 prostate cancer cells by using the fluorinated lysine derivate Bov-Lys-(Tfa)-OH (BLT) (103).

Pro-drug Therapy

^{19}F MRS has also been useful in detecting pro-drug therapy with the nonmammalian enzyme cytosine deaminase (CD) (104). CD converts the nontoxic pro-drug 5-fluorocytosine (5-FC) to 5-fluorouracil (5-FU) (104). This conversion can be followed by ^{19}F MRS in cells in culture or tumors in vivo as shown in Figure 7. The peak representing the pro-drug 5-FC decreased progressively and an increasing signal from 5-FU was observed (Fig. 7A). Other metabolites such as FUMP (fluorouridine monophosphate) were also detected (Fig. 7D). The enzyme may be either expressed by the cancer cells (104) or delivered to the tumor (105).

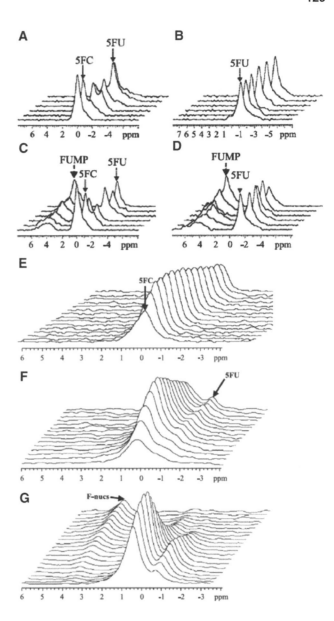

Figure 7 Visualization of the conversion of 5-FC into 5-FU and 5-FUMP in cell culture (**A–D**) and in vivo (**E–G**) by ^{19}F MRS. CD converts 5-FC into 5-FU and UPRT converts 5-FU to fluorouridine monophosphate. These metabolites are detected in the ^{19}F spectrum. (**A–D**) ^{19}F MRS plots acquired after incubation for 0, 15, 30, 45, 90, and 180 minutes with lysates containing CD (**A, B**) or CD-UPRT (**C, D**) in the presence of 2 mM of 5 FC (**A** and **C**) or 2 mM 5 FU (**B** and **D**). (**E–G**) serial spectra of (**E**) non-tumor bearing muscle, (**F**) subcutaneous tumor expressing CD, (**G**) subcutaneous tumor expressing CD-UPRT. *Source:* From Ref. 104.

pO₂ Measurements

Tumor hypoxia has been evaluated by exploiting the dependence of the T_1 relaxation of crown ethers on oxygen tension. Tumor oxygen tension was measured by injecting perfluoro-15-crown-5-ether intravenously in mice inoculated with Shionogi cells. Nonlocalized ^{19}F T_1 measurements were performed at several time points of tumor growth showing that the pO_2 values for growing androgen-dependent prostate tumors were lower than those for regressing and relapsing androgen-independent tumors (106). In another relaxometry approach, the reporter molecule hexafluorobenzene was directly injected into the tumor and the fluorocarbon relaxation maps were obtained using echo planar imaging to derive oxygen maps (FREDOM) from within the tumor (107,108).

Tumor hypoxia can also be assessed with ^{19}F MRS. Trifluoro-nitroimidazole (TF-MISO) was used as a hypoxia reporter in solid tumors as shown in a recent study (109). The uptake and retention of this probe is oxygen dependent. The spatial distribution of TF-MISO was visualized with a spectroscopic image overlaid with a T_2-weighted image (109). A phase I clinical study was performed to use SR-4554, a fluorinated 2-nitroimidazole, as a noninvasive probe of tumor hypoxia detected by ^{19}F MRS. This probe is reduced and retained within hypoxic cells. Unlocalized spectra were acquired from tumors after intravenous injection of the probe (110). The study assessed the toxicity profiles of the probe and demonstrated the feasibility of detection in human tumors. Using unlocalized ^{19}F MRS, the total SR-4554 (the sum of parent SR-4554 and retained bioreduction products) was detected but further studies optimizing timing and localization are required (110).

Clinical Applications

The pharmacokinetics of fluorine-containing drugs like 5-FU and its conversion to anabolites (fluoronuclides and nucleosides) and catabolites [α-fluoro-β-alanine FBAL, α-fluoro-β-ureidopropionic acid (FUPA), dihydrofluorouracil (DHFU)] can be detected by ^{19}F MRS. Localized ^{19}F MRS detection of capecitabine, a pro-drug of 5-FU, within the liver was performed at 3T on patients with advanced colorectal cancer (111). Absolute tissue concentrations of capecitabine and its metabolites were acquired in vivo. This study revealed heterogeneity in the spatial distribution of these compounds in the livers (111). The signal of 5-FU in human liver metastases was assessed by ^{19}F MRS to measure its uptake and conversion of the drug in order to predict therapy outcome (112).

^{31}P MRS
Overview, Advantages, and Disadvantages

Despite its low sensitivity, ^{31}P MRS has been a valuable method for evaluating tumor energy metabolism, pH, and

choline phospholipid metabolism. Metabolites detected in ^{31}P MR spectra of solid tumors are nucleoside triphosphates (NTP), phosphocreatine (PCr), inorganic phosphate (Pi), phosphodiesters (PDE), and phosphomonoesters (PME). ^{31}P MRS studies of solid tumors were amongst the first MR studies of solid tumors to be performed in vivo (113).

Preclinical Applications

^{1}H MRS studies of choline phospholipid metabolism in cancer cells and solid tumors have been complemented by an array of ^{31}P MRS investigations performed in vivo and in vitro (60,114,115). Phospholipid metabolites have been monitored in cancer, using ^{31}P MRS to determine the effects of different treatments and signaling pathways. Mutant ras-oncogene transformation (116), inhibition of hypoxia-inducible factor (HIF)-1α (117), inhibition of mitogen-activated protein kinase (MAPK) signaling, and inhibition of phosphoinositide 3-kinase (PI3K) signaling have been shown to affect choline phospholipids (118,119). The inhibition of MAPK by the drug U0126 induced a significant drop in PC levels as shown by ^{31}P spectra of cell extracts (119). The inhibition of PI3K with LY294002 induced a decrease in PC and an increase in GPC levels detected in ^{31}P spectra of cell extracts (118). Several other drugs such as microtubule inhibitors (120), indomethacin, a nonsteroidal anti-inflammatory agent (121,122), and docetaxel have resulted in a decrease of PC. These data support the use of PC as a biomarker to detect the therapeutic response to several agents. Docetaxel has been tested both in MCF-7 and MDA-MB-231 cells and tumors (123). In vivo ^{31}P spectra acquired on MCF-7 tumor before and after two days of treatment are presented in Figure 8 and demonstrated a reduction in PC levels with docetaxel treatment (123).

Many anticancer strategies are aimed at inducing apoptosis in cancer cells. Apoptosis can be induced by inhibiting NAD^+ synthesis, for example, by the novel agent FK866 (124). The action of this agent on cancer cell metabolism was explored both in vivo and in vitro by ^{31}P MRS (124). The model chosen was a mouse mammary carcinoma. Unlike the previous agents that induced a decrease of PC (a component of the PME peak), treatment with this agent induced an increase in the PME signal, and decreases in NAD^+, pH, and bioenergetic status. In vitro analysis revealed that the drug altered tumor glycolysis, guanylate synthesis, phospholipid metabolism and pyridine nucleotide pools (124).

The effect of the choline kinase inhibitor MN58b has been explored using combined ^{31}P and ^{1}H MRS. Human HT29 (colon) and MDA-MB-231 carcinoma cells were examined in culture and in xenografts by both ^{31}P and ^{1}H MRS. This study showed that detecting the decrease of

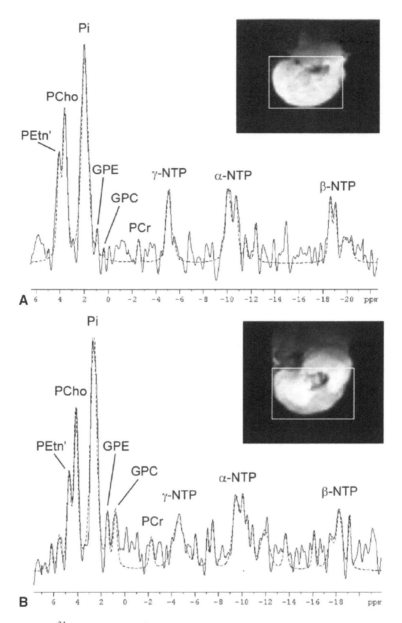

Figure 8 Typical localized in vivo ^{31}P MR spectra (**A**) pretreatment and (**B**) two days posttreatment with docetaxel from an MCF-7 tumor xenograft. The deconvolution line-fits are overlaid on the spectra (*dashed line*). MR images were used to localize the voxel to the tumor. Treatment with docetaxel induced a decrease in PC and an increase in GPC. *Source*: From Ref. 123.

PC, total choline, and PME may have potential for determining tumor response following treatment with choline kinase inhibitors (36). The effect of HIF-1α inhibition has also been studied by combined ^{31}P and ^{1}H MRS. Efficacy of treatment was assessed by in vivo ^{1}H MRS and ex vivo ^{1}H MRS and ^{31}P MRS of tumor extracts after inhibition of HIF1α with PX-478. The treatment induced a decrease in the levels of both PDE and PME (117).

^{31}P is also used to evaluate tumor pH by analyzing the chemical shift of the Pi signal or by using exogenous

^{31}P probes. The chemical shift of Pi depends on pH and mostly reports intracellular pH (125). ^{31}P MRS of tumor pH has demonstrated that intracellular tumor pH is mostly neutral to alkaline (126). Consistent with the acidic pH values reported by microelectrode measurements (23), pHe measured by an exogenous ^{31}P-detectable pH marker 3-aminopropylphosphonate (3-APP) also reported acidic pHe values (127).

Early results obtained from tumors suggested that levels of NTP, PCr, and Pi would reflect the efficiency of flow and oxygenation within a tumor (128,129). It is likely that at a given time, the levels of these metabolites in a ^{31}P spectrum from a tumor will depend on glucose and oxygen consumption rates, cell density, and nutritive blood flow. However, since both glucose and oxygen delivery are dependent on blood flow, energy metabolism should be tightly coupled to blood flow.

Clinical Applications

In a recent multi-institutional trial of characterizing ^{31}P spectral patterns and reproducibility in cancer patients, in vivo localized ^{31}P MRS was obtained at 1.5 T from non-Hodgkin's lymphomas, sarcomas of soft tissue and bone, breast carcinomas, and head and neck carcinomas. This multi-institutional trial demonstrated the utility of in vivo ^{31}P MRS to predict treatment response in the clinic (130). ^{1}H decoupled ^{31}P MRS of untreated pediatric brain tumors revealed an elevated ratio of PC/PE, PE/GPE, and PC/GPC in tumors compared to normal tissue (54). ^{31}P MRS has also been used to analyze phospholipid changes in plasma of patients with acute leukemia (131). The signals of phosphatidylcholine, lysophosphatidylcholine, sphingomyeline, phosphatidylethanolamine, and phosphatidylinositol were measured. There was no difference in phospholipid concentrations between healthy volunteers and patients on complete remission. Leukemic patients showed lower concentrations than the controls (131).

NEW ADVANCES AND CHALLENGES FOR THE FUTURE

Multinuclear MRS is increasingly being combined with MRI, and with PET and CT, in preclinical and clinical imaging, and as outlined in this review, the methods provide a wealth of information to complement the capabilities of other imaging modalities. While multinuclear MRS is being used for prognosis and detecting therapeutic response, the relatively poor sensitivity of MRS has resulted in a drive toward higher field strength magnets and strategies to increase signal-to-noise ratio. One of the most exciting developments in MRS is the use of hyperpolarized ^{13}C to increase signal-to-noise ratio. An increase of more than 10,000 times in the signal-to-noise ratio was reported in a recent study (132). Substances generated through the process of dynamic nuclear polarization (DNP) are injected, allowing real-time metabolic mapping (132–134). The DNP hyperpolarization technique allowed signal enhancement of ^{13}C-labeled substances such as pyruvate. Metabolic maps obtained from a tumor xenograft following systemic injection of hyperpolarized pyruvate (Fig. 9), show the conversion of pyruvate to lactate, alanine, and bicarbonate in vivo (135,136). This figure demonstrates the typical spectra that can be acquired from muscle, blood, and tumor after the injection of pyruvate. These tissues are characterized by different metabolite profiles, with the tumor showing the highest level of lactate and a lack of alanine.

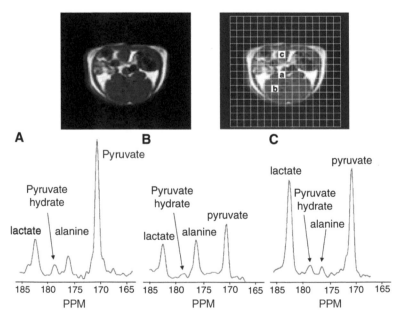

Figure 9 Metabolic patterns measured by ^{13}C MRS. The anatomical images are shown at the top. (*Bottom*) Representative spectra acquired from (**A**) the vena cava, (**B**) skeletal muscle, and (**C**) tumor tissue. The tumor is characterized by a high level of lactate and a low level of alanine. *Source*: From Ref. 136.

In conclusion, this review has summarized some of the capabilities of multinuclear MRS in preclinical and clinical applications of oncology. These capabilities together with advances in increasing sensitivity, development of novel probes, and imaging sequences should see an even greater utilization of this translational modality in oncological applications in preclinical research and the clinical management of cancer.

ACKNOWLEDGMENTS

Support from NIH P50 CA103175, R01 CA73850, and R01 CA82337 is gratefully acknowledged.

REFERENCES

1. Brown TR, Kincaid BM, Ugurbil K. NMR chemical shift imaging in three dimensions. Proc Natl Acad Sci U S A 1982; 79(11):3523–3526.
2. Golman K, Olsson LE, Axelsson O, et al. Molecular imaging using hyperpolarized 13C. Br J Radiol 2003; 76(Spec No 2):S118–S127.
3. Tkac I, Starcuk Z, Choi IY, et al. In vivo 1H NMR spectroscopy of rat brain at 1 ms echo time. Magn Reson Med 1999; 41(4):649–656.
4. Frahm J, Bruhn H, Gyngell ML, et al. Localized high-resolution proton NMR spectroscopy using stimulated echoes: initial applications to human brain in vivo. Magn Reson Med 1989; 9(1):79–93.
5. Star-Lack J, Nelson SJ, Kurhanewicz J, et al. Improved water and lipid suppression for 3D PRESS CSI using RF band selective inversion with gradient dephasing (BASING). Magn Reson Med 1997; 38(2):311–321.
6. Shungu DC, Glickson JD. Band-selective spin echoes for in vivo localized 1H NMR spectroscopy. Magn Reson Med 1994; 32(3):277–284.
7. Dreher W, Leibfritz D. New method for the simultaneous detection of metabolites and water in localized in vivo 1H nuclear magnetic resonance spectroscopy. Magn Reson Med 2005; 54(1):190–195.
8. Al-Saffar NM, Titley JC, Robertson D, et al. Apoptosis is associated with triacylglycerol accumulation in Jurkat T-cells. Br J Cancer 2002; 86(6):963–970.
9. Barba I, Cabanas ME, Arus C. The relationship between nuclear magnetic resonance-visible lipids, lipid droplets, and cell proliferation in cultured C6 cells. Cancer Res 1999; 59(8):1861–1868.
10. Callies R, Sri-Pathmanathan RM, Ferguson DY, et al. The appearance of neutral lipid signals in the 1H NMR spectra of a myeloma cell line correlates with the induced formation of cytoplasmic lipid droplets. Magn Reson Med 1993; 29(4):546–550.
11. Schmitz JE, Kettunen MI, Hu DE, et al. 1H MRS-visible lipids accumulate during apoptosis of lymphoma cells in vitro and in vivo. Magn Reson Med 2005; 54(1):43–50.
12. Bhujwalla ZM, Shungu DC, Glickson JD. Effects of blood flow modifiers on tumor metabolism observed in vivo by proton magnetic resonance spectroscopic imaging. Magn Reson Med 1996; 36(2):204–211.
13. Serrai H, Nadal-Desbarats L, Poptani H, et al. Lactate editing and lipid suppression by continuous wavelet transform analysis: application to simulated and (1)H MRS brain tumor time-domain data. Magn Reson Med 2000; 43(5):649–656.
14. Serrai H, Senhadji L, Wang G, et al. Lactate doublet quantification and lipid signal suppression using a new biexponential decay filter: application to simulated and 1H MRS brain tumor time-domain data. Magn Reson Med 2003; 50(3):623–626.
15. Sotak CH. A volume-localized, two-dimensional NMR method for the determination of lactate using zero-quantum coherence created in a stimulated echo pulse sequence. Magn Reson Med 1988; 7(3):364–370.
16. Hurd RE, Freeman D. Proton editing and imaging of lactate. NMR Biomed 1991; 4(2):73–80.
17. de Graaf RA, Luo Y, Terpstra M, et al. Spectral editing with adiabatic pulses. J Magn Reson B 1995; 109(2):184–193.
18. He Q, Bhujwalla ZM, Maxwell RJ, et al. Proton NMR observation of the antineoplastic agent Iproplatin in vivo by selective multiple quantum coherence transfer (Sel-MQC). Magn Reson Med 1995; 33(3):414–416.
19. He Q, Shungu DC, van Zijl PC, et al. Single-scan in vivo lactate editing with complete lipid and water suppression by selective multiple-quantum-coherence transfer (Sel-MQC) with application to tumors. J Magn Reson B 1995; 106(3):203–211.
20. Howe FA, Opstad KS. 1H MR spectroscopy of brain tumours and masses. NMR Biomed 2003; 16(3):123–131.
21. Payne GS, Troy H, Vaidya SJ, et al. Evaluation of 31P high-resolution magic angle spinning of intact tissue samples. NMR Biomed 2006; 19(5):593–598.
22. Howe FA, Barton SJ, Cudlip SA, et al. Metabolic profiles of human brain tumors using quantitative in vivo 1H magnetic resonance spectroscopy. Magn Reson Med 2003; 49(2):223–232.
23. Vaupel P, Okunieff P, Kluge M. Response of tumour red blood cell flux to hyperthermia and/or hyperglycaemia. Int J Hyperthermia 1989; 5(2):199–210.
24. Aboagye EO, Bhujwalla ZM. Malignant transformation alters membrane choline phospholipid metabolism of human mammary epithelial cells. Cancer Res 1999; 59(1):80–84.
25. Ackerstaff E, Pflug BR, Nelson JB, et al. Detection of increased choline compounds with proton nuclear magnetic resonance spectroscopy subsequent to malignant transformation of human prostatic epithelial cells. Cancer Res 2001; 61(9):3599–3603.
26. Bhakoo KK, Williams SR, Florian CL, et al. Immortalization and transformation are associated with specific alterations in choline metabolism. Cancer Res 1996; 56(20):4630–4635.
27. Eliyahu G, Kreizman T, Degani H. Phosphocholine as a biomarker of breast cancer: molecular and biochemical studies. Int J Cancer 2007; 120(8):1721–1730.

28. Payne GS, Leach MO. Applications of magnetic resonance spectroscopy in radiotherapy treatment planning. Br J Radiol 2006; 79(Spec No 1):S16–S26.

29. Ramirez de Molina A, Gutierrez R, Ramos MA, et al. Increased choline kinase activity in human breast carcinomas: clinical evidence for a potential novel antitumor strategy. Oncogene 2002; 21(27):4317–4322.

30. Ramirez de Molina A, Penalva V, Lucas L, et al. Regulation of choline kinase activity by Ras proteins involves Ral-GDS and PI3K. Oncogene 2002; 21(6):937–946.

31. Ramirez de Molina A, Rodriguez-Gonzalez A, Gutierrez R, et al. Overexpression of choline kinase is a frequent feature in human tumor-derived cell lines and in lung, prostate, and colorectal human cancers. Biochem Biophys Res Commun 2002; 296(3):580–583.

32. Katz-Brull R, Degani H. Kinetics of choline transport and phosphorylation in human breast cancer cells; NMR application of the zero trans method. Anticancer Res 1996; 16(3B):1375–1380.

33. Noh DY, Ahn SJ, Lee RA, et al. Overexpression of phospholipase D1 in human breast cancer tissues. Cancer Lett 2000; 161(2):207–214.

34. Iorio E, Mezzanzanica D, Alberti P, et al. Alterations of choline phospholipid metabolism in ovarian tumor progression. Cancer Res 2005;65(20):9369–9376.

35. Glunde K, Raman V, Mori N, et al. RNA interference-mediated choline kinase suppression in breast cancer cells induces differentiation and reduces proliferation. Cancer Res 2005; 65(23):11034–11043.

36. Al-Saffar NM, Troy H, Ramirez de Molina A, et al. Noninvasive magnetic resonance spectroscopic pharmacodynamic markers of the choline kinase inhibitor MN58b in human carcinoma models. Cancer Res 2006; 66(1):427–434.

37. Lindskog M, Kogner P, Ponthan F, et al. Noninvasive estimation of tumour viability in a xenograft model of human neuroblastoma with proton magnetic resonance spectroscopy (1H MRS). Br J Cancer 2003; 88(3):478–485.

38. Simoes RV, Garcia-Martin ML, Cerdan S, et al. Perturbation of mouse glioma MRS pattern by induced acute hyperglycemia. NMR Biomed 2007.

39. Morvan D, Demidem A. Metabolomics by proton nuclear magnetic resonance spectroscopy of the response to chloroethylnitrosourea reveals drug efficacy and tumor adaptive metabolic pathways. Cancer Res 2007; 67(5): 2150–2159.

40. Gillies RJ, Gatenby RA. Hypoxia and adaptive landscapes in the evolution of carcinogenesis. Cancer Metastasis Rev 2007; 26(2):311–317.

41. Cardone RA, Casavola V, Reshkin SJ. The role of disturbed pH dynamics and the Na+/H+ exchanger in metastasis. Nat Rev Cancer 2005; 5(10):786–795.

42. Gillies RJ, Raghunand N, Karczmar GS, et al. MRI of the tumor microenvironment. J Magn Reson Imaging 2002; 16(4):430–450.

43. van Sluis R, Bhujwalla ZM, Raghunand N, et al. In vivo imaging of extracellular pH using 1H MRSI. Magn Reson Med 1999; 41(4):743–750.

44. Garcia-Martin ML, Herigault G, Remy C, et al. Mapping extracellular pH in rat brain gliomas in vivo by 1H magnetic resonance spectroscopic imaging: comparison with maps of metabolites. Cancer Res 2001; 61(17):6524–6531.

45. Bhujwalla ZM, Artemov D, Ballesteros P, et al. Combined vascular and extracellular pH imaging of solid tumors. NMR Biomed 2002; 15(2):114–119.

46. Provent P, Benito M, Hiba B, et al. Serial in vivo spectroscopic nuclear magnetic resonance imaging of lactate and extracellular pH in rat gliomas shows redistribution of protons away from sites of glycolysis. Cancer Res 2007; 67(16):7638–7645.

47. Brown JM. The hypoxic cell: a target for selective cancer therapy—eighteenth Bruce F Cain Memorial Award lecture. Cancer Res 1999; 59(23):5863–5870.

48. Harada H, Kizaka-Kondoh S, Li G, et al. Significance of HIF-1-active cells in angiogenesis and radioresistance. Oncogene 2007; 26(54):7508–7516. Epub 2007 Jun.

49. Kodibagkar VD, Cui W, Merritt ME, et al. Novel 1H NMR approach to quantitative tissue oximetry using hexamethyldisiloxane. Magn Reson Med 2006; 55(4): 743–748.

50. Mountford C, Lean C, Malycha P, et al. Proton spectroscopy provides accurate pathology on biopsy and in vivo. J Magn Reson Imaging 2006; 24(3):459–477.

51. Kurhanewicz J, Vigneron DB, Nelson SJ. Three-dimensional magnetic resonance spectroscopic imaging of brain and prostate cancer. Neoplasia 2000; 2(1–2):166–189.

52. Wang L, Hricak H, Kattan MW, et al. Prediction of organ-confined prostate cancer: incremental value of MR imaging and MR spectroscopic imaging to staging nomograms. Radiology 2006; 238(2):597–603.

53. Scheenen TW, Gambarota G, Weiland E, et al. Optimal timing for in vivo 1H-MR spectroscopic imaging of the human prostate at 3T. Magn Reson Med 2005; 53(6): 1268–1274.

54. Albers MJ, Krieger MD, Gonzalez-Gomez I, et al. Proton-decoupled 31P MRS in untreated pediatric brain tumors. Magn Reson Med 2005; 53(1):22–29.

55. Li X, Lu Y, Pirzkall A, et al. Analysis of the spatial characteristics of metabolic abnormalities in newly diagnosed glioma patients. J Magn Reson Imaging 2002; 16(3):229–237.

56. Tate AR, Majos C, Moreno A, et al. Automated classification of short echo time in in vivo 1H brain tumor spectra: a multicenter study. Magn Reson Med 2003; 49(1):29–36.

57. Jacobs MA, Barker PB, Bottomley PA, et al. Proton magnetic resonance spectroscopic imaging of human breast cancer: a preliminary study. J Magn Reson Imaging 2004; 19(1):68–75.

58. Bolan PJ, Meisamy S, Baker EH, et al. In vivo quantification of choline compounds in the breast with 1H MR spectroscopy. Magn Reson Med 2003; 50(6): 1134–1143.

59. Gribbestad IS, Sitter B, Lundgren S, et al. Metabolite composition in breast tumors examined by proton nuclear magnetic resonance spectroscopy. Anticancer Res 1999; 19(3A):1737–1746.

60. Negendank W. Studies of human tumors by MRS: a review. NMR Biomed 1992; 5(5):303–324.

61. Fayad LM, Bluemke DA, McCarthy EF, et al. Musculoskeletal tumors: use of proton MR spectroscopic

imaging for characterization. J Magn Reson Imaging 2006; 23(1):23–28.

62. Fayad LM, Barker PB, Jacobs MA, et al. Characterization of musculoskeletal lesions on 3-T proton MR spectroscopy. AJR Am J Roentgenol 2007; 188(6):1513–1520.

63. Sherr DL. Advanced prostate cancer and postoperative radiotherapy. JAMA 2007; 297(9):950(author reply 1).

64. Swindle P, McCredie S, Russell P, et al. Pathologic characterization of human prostate tissue with proton MR spectroscopy. Radiology 2003; 228(1):144–151.

65. Galanaud D, Nicoli F, Chinot O, et al. Noninvasive diagnostic assessment of brain tumors using combined in vivo MR imaging and spectroscopy. Magn Reson Med 2006; 55(6):1236–1245.

66. Osorio JA, Ozturk-Isik E, Xu D, et al. 3D 1H MRSI of brain tumors at 3.0 Tesla using an eight-channel phased-array head coil. J Magn Reson Imaging 2007; 26(1):23–30.

67. Heijmink SW, Scheenen TW, Futterer JJ, et al. Prostate and lymph node proton magnetic resonance (MR) spectroscopic imaging with external array coils at 3 T to detect recurrent prostate cancer after radiation therapy. Invest Radiol 2007; 42(6):420–427.

68. Seenu V, Pavan Kumar MN, Sharma U, et al. Potential of magnetic resonance spectroscopy to detect metastasis in axillary lymph nodes in breast cancer. Magn Reson Imaging 2005; 23(10):1005–1010.

69. Swanson MG, Zektzer AS, Tabatabai ZL, et al. Quantitative analysis of prostate metabolites using 1H HR-MAS spectroscopy. Magn Reson Med 2006; 55(6): 1257–1264.

70. Sitter B, Lundgren S, Bathen TF, et al. Comparison of HR MAS MR spectroscopic profiles of breast cancer tissue with clinical parameters. NMR Biomed 2006; 19(1):30–40.

71. Sitter B, Sonnewald U, Spraul M, et al. High-resolution magic angle spinning MRS of breast cancer tissue. NMR Biomed 2002; 15(5):327–337.

72. Leach MO, Verrill M, Glaholm J, et al. Measurements of human breast cancer using magnetic resonance spectroscopy: a review of clinical measurements and a report of localized 31P measurements of response to treatment. NMR Biomed 1998; 11(7):314–340.

73. Kurhanewicz J, Vigneron DB, Males RG, et al. The prostate: MR imaging and spectroscopy. Present and future. Radiol Clin North Am 2000; 38(1):115–138, viii–ix.

74. Meisamy S, Bolan PJ, Baker EH, et al. Neoadjuvant chemotherapy of locally advanced breast cancer: predicting response with in vivo (1)H MR spectroscopy—a pilot study at 4 T. Radiology 2004; 233(2):424–431.

75. Murphy PS, Viviers L, Abson C, et al. Monitoring temozolomide treatment of low-grade glioma with proton magnetic resonance spectroscopy. Br J Cancer 2004; 90(4):781–786.

76. van Zijl PC, Chesnick AS, DesPres D, et al. In vivo proton spectroscopy and spectroscopic imaging of [1-13C]-glucose and its metabolic products. Magn Reson Med 1993; 30(5):544–551.

77. Artemov D, Bhujwalla ZM, Glickson JD. In vivo selective measurement of (1-13C)-glucose metabolism in tumors by heteronuclear cross polarization. Magn Reson Med 1995; 33(2):151–155.

78. Ronen SM, Degani H. The application of 13C NMR to the characterization of phospholipid metabolism in cells. Magn Reson Med 1992; 25(2):384–389.

79. Gillies RJ, Barry JA, Ross BD. In vitro and in vivo 13C and 31P NMR analyses of phosphocholine metabolism in rat glioma cells. Magn Reson Med 1994; 32(3):310–318.

80. Dixon RM. Phosphatidylethanolamine synthesis in the normal and lymphomatous mouse liver; a 13C NMR study. Anticancer Res 1996; 16(3B):1351–1356.

81. Glunde K, Jie C, Bhujwalla ZM. Molecular causes of the aberrant choline phospholipid metabolism in breast cancer. Cancer Res 2004; 64(12):4270–4276.

82. Rivenzon-Segal D, Margalit R, Degani H. Glycolysis as a metabolic marker in orthotopic breast cancer, monitored by in vivo (13)C MRS. Am J Physiol Endocrinol Metab 2002; 283(4):E623–E630.

83. Zhang H, Gao P, Fukuda R, et al. HIF-1 inhibits mitochondrial biogenesis and cellular respiration in VHL-deficient renal cell carcinoma by repression of C-MYC activity. Cancer Cell 2007; 11(5):407–420.

84. Dang CV, Semenza GL. Oncogenic alterations of metabolism. Trends Biochem Sci 1999; 24(2):68–72.

85. Terpstra M, High WB, Luo Y, et al. Relationships among lactate concentration, blood flow and histopathologic profiles in rat C6 glioma. NMR Biomed 1996; 9(5):185–194.

86. Nielsen FU, Daugaard P, Bentzen L, et al. Effect of changing tumor oxygenation on glycolytic metabolism in a murine C3H mammary carcinoma assessed by in vivo nuclear magnetic resonance spectroscopy. Cancer Res 2001; 61(13):5318–5325.

87. Constantinidis I, Chatham JC, Wehrle JP, et al. In vivo 13CNMR spectroscopy of glucose metabolism of RIF-1 tumors. Magn Reson Med 1991; 20(1):17–26.

88. Bhujwalla ZM, Constantinidis I, Chatham JC, et al. Energy metabolism, pH changes, and lactate production in RIF-1 tumors following intratumoral injection of glucose. Int J Radiat Oncol Biol Phys 1992; 22(1):95–101.

89. Schupp DG, Merkle H, Ellermann JM, et al. Localized detection of glioma glycolysis using edited 1H MRS. Magn Reson Med 1993; 30(1):18–27.

90. Artemov D, Bhujwalla ZM, Pilatus U, et al. Two-compartment model for determination of glycolytic rates of solid tumors by in vivo 13C NMR spectroscopy. NMR Biomed 1998; 11(8):395–404.

91. Ronen SM, Volk A, Mispelter J. Comparative NMR study of a differentiated rat hepatoma and its dedifferentiated subclone cultured as spheroids and as implanted tumors. NMR Biomed 1994; 7(6):278–286.

92. Bouzier AK, Quesson B, Valeins H, et al. [1-(13)C]glucose metabolism in the tumoral and nontumoral cerebral tissue of a glioma-bearing rat. J Neurochem 1999; 72(6): 2445–2455.

93. Thelwall PE, Yemin AY, Gillian TL, et al. Noninvasive in vivo detection of glutathione metabolism in tumors. Cancer Res 2005; 65(22):10149–10153.

94. Artemov D, Solaiyappan M, Bhujwalla ZM. Magnetic resonance pharmacoangiography to detect and predict chemotherapy delivery to solid tumors. Cancer Res 2001; 61(7):3039–3044.

95. Kato Y, Okollie B, Artemov D. Noninvasive 1H/13C magnetic resonance spectroscopic imaging of the intra-tumoral distribution of temozolomide. Magn Reson Med 2006; 55(4):755–761.

96. O'Reilly SM, Newlands ES, Glaser MG, et al. Temozo-lomide: a new oral cytotoxic chemotherapeutic agent with promising activity against primary brain tumours. Eur J Cancer 1993; 29A(7):940–942.

97. Floridi A, Paggi MG, D'Atri S, et al. Effect of lonidamine on the energy metabolism of Ehrlich ascites tumor cells. Cancer Res 1981; 41(11 pt 1):4661–4666.

98. Fonseca CP, Jones JG, Carvalho RA, et al. Tricarboxylic acid cycle inhibition by Li+ in the human neuroblastoma SH-SY5Y cell line: a 13C NMR isotopomer analysis. Neurochem Int 2005; 47(6):385–393.

99. Gottschalk S, Anderson N, Hainz C, et al. Imatinib (STI571)-mediated changes in glucose metabolism in human leukemia BCR-ABL-positive cells. Clin Cancer Res 2004; 10(19):6661–6668.

100. Martinez-Bisbal MC, Marti-Bonmati L, Piquer J, et al. 1H and 13C HR-MAS spectroscopy of intact biopsy samples ex vivo and in vivo 1H MRS study of human high grade gliomas. NMR Biomed 2004; 17(4):191–205.

101. Liu L, Kodibagkar VD, Yu JX, et al. 19F-NMR detection of lacZ gene expression via the enzymic hydrolysis of 2-fluoro-4-nitrophenyl beta-D-galactopyranoside in vivo in PC3 prostate tumor xenografts in the mouse. FASEB J 2007; 21(9):2014–2019.

102. Chung YL, Troy H, Judson IR, et al. Noninvasive meas-urements of capecitabine metabolism in bladder tumors overexpressing thymidine phosphorylase by fluorine-19 magnetic resonance spectroscopy. Clin Cancer Res 2004; 10(11):3863–3870.

103. Sankaranarayanapillai M, Tong WP, Maxwell DS, et al. Detection of histone deacetylase inhibition by noninvasive magnetic resonance spectroscopy. Mol Cancer Ther 2006; 5(5):1325–1334.

104. Hamstra DA, Lee KC, Tychewicz JM, et al. The use of 19F spectroscopy and diffusion-weighted MRI to evaluate differences in gene-dependent enzyme prodrug therapies. Mol Ther 2004; 10(5):916–928.

105. Dresselaers T, Theys J, Nuyts S, et al. Non-invasive 19F MR spectroscopy of 5-fluorocytosine to 5-fluorouracil conversion by recombinant Salmonella in tumours. Br J Cancer 2003; 89(9):1796–1801.

106. McNab JA, Yung AC, Kozlowski P. Tissue oxygen tension measurements in the Shionogi model of prostate cancer using 19F MRS and MRI. MAGMA 2004; 17(3–6):288–295.

107. Bourke VA, Zhao D, Gilio J, et al. Correlation of radiation response with tumor oxygenation in the Dunning prostate R3327-AT1 tumor. Int J Radiat Oncol Biol Phys 2007; 67(4):1179–1186.

108. Xia M, Kodibagkar V, Liu H, et al. Tumour oxygen dynamics measured simultaneously by near-infrared spec-troscopy and 19F magnetic resonance imaging in rats. Phys Med Biol 2006; 51(1):45–60.

109. Procissi D, Claus F, Burgman P, et al. In vivo 19F magnetic resonance spectroscopy and chemical shift imaging of tri-fluoro-nitroimidazole as a potential hypoxia reporter in solid tumors. Clin Cancer Res 2007; 13(12):3738–3747.

110. Seddon BM, Payne GS, Simmons L, et al. A phase I study of SR-4554 via intravenous administration for noninvasive investigation of tumor hypoxia by magnetic resonance spectroscopy in patients with malignancy. Clin Cancer Res 2003; 9(14):5101–5112.

111. Klomp D, van Laarhoven H, Scheenen T, et al. Quantita-tive 19F MR spectroscopy at 3 T to detect heterogeneous capecitabine metabolism in human liver. NMR Biomed 2007; 20(5):485–492.

112. Kamm YJ, Heerschap A, van den Bergh EJ, et al. 19F-magnetic resonance spectroscopy in patients with liver metastases of colorectal cancer treated with 5-fluorouracil. Anticancer Drugs 2004; 15(3):229–233.

113. Griffiths JR, Stevens AN, Iles RA, et al. 31P-NMR investigation of solid tumours in the living rat. Biosci Rep 1981; 1(4):319–325.

114. de Certaines JD, Larsen VA, Podo F, et al. In vivo 31P MRS of experimental tumours. NMR Biomed 1993; 6(6):345–365.

115. Podo F. Tumour phospholipid metabolism. NMR Biomed 1999; 12(7):413–439.

116. Ronen SM, Leach MO. Imaging biochemistry: applications to breast cancer. Breast Cancer Res 2001; 3(1):36–40.

117. Jordan BF, Black K, Robey IF, et al. Metabolite changes in HT-29 xenograft tumors following HIF-1alpha inhibi-tion with PX-478 as studied by MR spectroscopy in vivo and ex vivo. NMR Biomed 2005; 18(7):430–439.

118. Beloueche-Babari M, Jackson LE, Al-Saffar NM, et al. Identification of magnetic resonance detectable metabolic changes associated with inhibition of phosphoinositide 3-kinase signaling in human breast cancer cells. Mol Cancer Ther 2006; 5(1):187–196.

119. Beloueche-Babari M, Jackson LE, Al-Saffar NM, et al. Magnetic resonance spectroscopy monitoring of mitogen-activated protein kinase signaling inhibition. Cancer Res 2005; 65(8):3356–3363.

120. Sterin M, Cohen JS, Mardor Y, et al. Levels of phospho-lipid metabolites in breast cancer cells treated with anti-mitotic drugs: a 31P-magnetic resonance spectroscopy study. Cancer Res 2001; 61(20):7536–7543.

121. Natarajan K, Mori N, Artemov D, et al. Exposure of human breast cancer cells to the anti-inflammatory agent indomethacin alters choline phospholipid metabolites and Nm23 expression. Neoplasia 2002; 4(5):409–416.

122. Glunde K, Ackerstaff E, Natarajan K, et al. Real-time changes in 1H and 31P NMR spectra of malignant human mammary epithelial cells during treatment with the anti-inflammatory agent indomethacin. Magn Reson Med 2002; 48(5):819–825.

123. Morse DL, Raghunand N, Sadarangani P, et al. Response of choline metabolites to docetaxel therapy is quantified in vivo by localized (31)P MRS of human breast cancer xenografts and in vitro by high-resolution (31)P NMR spectroscopy of cell extracts. Magn Reson Med 2007; 58 (2):270–280.

124. Muruganandham M, Alfieri AA, Matei C, et al. Metabolic signatures associated with a NAD synthesis inhibitor-induced tumor apoptosis identified by 1H-decoupled-31P

magnetic resonance spectroscopy. Clin Cancer Res 2005; 11(9):3503–3513.

125. Stubbs M, Rodrigues L, Howe FA, et al. Metabolic consequences of a reversed pH gradient in rat tumors. Cancer Res 1994; 54(15):4011–4016.

126. Griffiths JR. Are cancer cells acidic? Br J Cancer 1991; 64(3):425–427.

127. Gillies RJ, Liu Z, Bhujwalla Z. 31P-MRS measurements of extracellular pH of tumors using 3-aminopropylphosphonate. Am J Physiol 1994; 267(1 pt 1):C195–C203.

128. Evanochko WT, Ng TC, Glickson JD. Application of in vivo NMR spectroscopy to cancer. Magn Reson Med 1984; 1(4):508–534.

129. Evanochko WT, Sakai TT, Ng TC, et al. NMR study of in vivo RIF-1 tumors. analysis of perchloric acid extracts and identification of 1H, 31P and 13C resonances. Biochim Biophys Acta 1984; 805(1):104–116.

130. Arias-Mendoza F, Payne GS, Zakian KL, et al. In vivo 31P MR spectral patterns and reproducibility in cancer patients studied in a multi-institutional trial. NMR Biomed 2006; 19(4):504–512.

131. Kuliszkiewicz-Janus M, Tuz MA, Baczynski S. Application of 31P MRS to the analysis of phospholipid changes in plasma of patients with acute leukemia. Biochim Biophys Acta 2005; 1737(1):11–15.

132. Ardenkjaer-Larsen JH, Fridlund B, Gram A, et al. Increase in signal-to-noise ratio of >10,000 times in liquid-state NMR. Proc Natl Acad Sci U S A 2003; 100(18): 10158–10163.

133. Golman K, Ardenkjaer-Larsen JH, Petersson JS, et al. Molecular imaging with endogenous substances. Proc Natl Acad Sci U S A 2003; 100(18):10435–10439.

134. Golman K, in 't Zandt R, Thaning M. Real-time metabolic imaging. Proc Natl Acad Sci U S A 2006; 103(30): 11270–11275.

135. Kohler SJ, Yen Y, Wolber J, et al. In vivo 13 carbon metabolic imaging at 3T with hyperpolarized 13C-1-pyruvate. Magn Reson Med 2007; 58(1):65–69.

136. Golman K, Zandt RI, Lerche M, et al. Metabolic imaging by hyperpolarized 13C magnetic resonance imaging for in vivo tumor diagnosis. Cancer Res 2006; 66(22): 10855–10860.

9

Physiological and Functional Imaging with CT: Techniques and Applications

TING-YIM LEE

Imaging Program, Lawson Health Research Institute; Imaging Research Laboratories, Robarts Research Institute; and Departments of Medical Imaging and Medical Biophysics, Schulich School of Medicine & Dentistry, The University of Western Ontario, London, Ontario, Canada

EUGENE WONG

Department of Physics, The University of Western Ontario, London, Ontario, Canada

ERROL STEWART

Department of Medical Biophysics, Schulich School of Medicine & Dentistry, The University of Western Ontario, London, Ontario, Canada

JIM XUAN

Department of Surgery, London Health Sciences Centre, London, Ontario, Canada

GLENN BAUMAN

Department of Oncology, Schulich School of Medicine & Dentistry, The University of Western Ontario, London, Ontario, Canada

PETER GABRA

Department of Medical Biophysics, Schulich School of Medicine & Dentistry, The University of Western Ontario, London, Ontario, Canada

INTRODUCTION

Rapid advances in molecular biology in the past two decades have uncovered many genetic and molecular alterations in cancer (1). Based on the newly acquired knowledge, a number of molecularly targeted cancer treatment drugs have been developed that prolong survival, induce remission of tumor, and provide better quality of life for cancer patients. Notable examples of success include the anti-HER-2/neu antibody trastuzumab for ErbB2-expressing breast cancers (2), the tyrosine kinase inhibitor imatinib for chronic myelogenous leukemia and gastrointestinal stromal tumors (3,4), the epidermal growth factor receptor (EGFR) inhibitor for non–small cell lung cancer [erlotinib (5)] and advanced colorectal cancer [cetuximab (6)], the aromatase inhibitor letrozole for unknown or hormone receptor–positive locally advanced or metastatic breast cancer in postmenopausal women (7), and the proteasome inhibitor bortezomib for multiple myeloma (8). However, evaluation of treatment responses with these molecularly targeted drugs has severely lagged behind the new advances in molecular biology and still relies heavily on conventional measurements of tumor size before and after treatment (9). The size measurement criteria were formalized in 1981 as the WHO criteria (10), and in 2000 as the response evaluation criteria in solid tumors (RECIST) criteria (11). Size measurements might not be applicable to molecularly targeted drugs since durable responses to these newer drugs might be cytostatic rather than cytotoxic and are thus not associated with tumor shrinkage. A good example of the inadequacy of size measurement in evaluating treatment response is the effects of two EGFR inhibitors, erlotinib (Tarceva) and gefitinib (Iressa) on non–small cell lung cancer. Treatment with Tarceva prolonged median overall survival of chemotherapy-refractory patients by 50%. The objective tumor response rate as measured by computerized tomography (CT) was 9% (12). In the Iressa trial, there was an identical response rate of 9% by CT; however, this CT response was *not* associated with a significant survival benefit (http://www .iressa-us.com/dr.pdf, accessed January 4, 2008). These data demonstrate that tumor size is a poor predictor of patient survival after treatment with molecularly targeted drug.

In the preclinical and clinical developments of molecularly targeted cancer drugs, it is essential to measure pharmacokinetic (PK) and pharmacodynamic (PD) end points. PK end points are concerned with whether adequate or optimal concentration of the drug is being achieved in the tissues of interest in the experimental animal or patient and whether the molecular target is being appropriately modulated, while PD end points focus on whether the desired biological effect is being achieved (13). Biomarkers of PK/PD end points can be challenging to develop because they need to be sensitive and specific and also can be difficult to implement because invasive tissue sampling is required for molecular assays. Molecular and functional imaging have emerged as new tools for PK and PD measurements in cancer drug development because of their noninvasive properties and ability to evaluate PK/PD end points in living subjects without the need for tissue samples (14). Both preclinical and clinical molecular and functional imaging have made use of positron emission tomography (PET), single-photon

emission tomography (SPECT), optical imaging, dynamic contrast-enhanced magnetic resonance imaging (DECT) and CT, magnetic resonance spectroscopy, and ultrasound (15–17). While PET is the most versatile for molecular and functional imaging because of the wide selection of physiological and molecular tracers available and high sensitivity (16), DECT has a number of advantages for functional imaging (18). First, it rivals the ability of PET for kinetics modeling of the uptake of contrast because tissue contrast concentration can be accurately and quantitatively measured. Secondly, it has the highest temporal frequency (~ 1 Hz) in dynamic studies to follow the uptake and washout of contrast without sacrificing its submillimeter spatial resolution. Thirdly, the arterial input curve can be measured from the same dynamic CT images as the tissue concentration (19) obviating the need for invasive arterial sampling or more complicated postprocessing of image data (20,21). Finally, CT is widely accessible in most hospitals and is not limited to academic or tertiary hospitals. The main disadvantage is the use of ionizing radiation. The effective dose, dependent on the application, can be as high as 15 to 30 mSv (22,23). As a result, it may not be feasible to repeat the CT functional imaging studies at regular intervals to monitor drug response.

DECT has been developed recently to investigate tumor-associated angiogenesis (24) by measuring tumor blood flow and vascular permeability (18,25,26). Tumor angiogenesis is important in neoplastic development, progression and invasion (27), and targeting angiogenesis has lead to the development of a totally new class of anticancer drugs (28–30). Inhibition of angiogenesis may also lead to normalization of blood flow in perfusion-starved tumor resulting in better oxygenation, which helps to overcome problems in drug delivery and hypoxia-induced treatment resistance (31). On the other hand, it has also been observed that resistance to EGFR inhibitor could be mediated by increased angiogenesis (32,33). In summary, to study the effects of antiangiogenic and antivascular agents as well as the newer molecularly targeted cancer drugs, such as EGFR inhibitors, methods for the evaluation of angiogenesis are required (34,35). CT functional imaging is ideally suited for measuring blood flow and vascular permeability. In this chapter we will discuss the principles involved in these measurements and describe examples of its application.

SCANNING PROTOCOL FOR A DYNAMIC CONTRAST-ENHANCED CT STUDY

In a DECT or CT perfusion (CTP) study, iodinated contrast agent is administered via a peripheral vein at a dosage of 0.5 to 1.0 mL, 1 to 2 mL, and 3 to 6 mL per

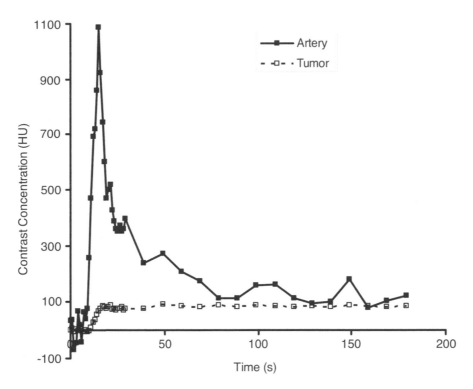

Figure 1 Arterial and tumor contrast media concentration curve in a nude rat following injection of 0.9 mL of contrast agent at a iodine concentration of 300 mg·mL^{-1} into a tail vein. *Abbreviation*: HU, Hounsfield unit.

kilogram body weight for humans, nonhuman primates (rabbits, dogs, and pigs), and rodents, respectively at an iodine concentration of 300 mg·mL^{-1}. The injection rate is 2 to 4 mL·s^{-1}, 0.5 to 1 mL·s^{-1}, and 0.03 to 0.1 mL·s^{-1} for humans, nonhuman primates (rabbits, dogs, and pigs), and rodents, respectively. A CT scanner is used to scan the tissue of interest repeatedly after the injection to measure the arterial and tissue concentration as a rate of one to two measurements per second to obtain their concentration versus time curves. In general, the higher the volume, concentration (of iodine), and injection rate of contrast agent, the higher the signal-to-noise ratio (precision) attained in the measured arterial and tissue concentration with the CT scanner. Since increase in CT number (enhancement) of an artery or tissue region is linearly related to iodine (contrast agent) concentration via the same calibration factor (36), it is the convention in CTP studies to express both arterial and tissue contrast agent concentrations in CT number or Hounsfield unit (HU).

The CT scanning protocol is divided into two phases. The first phase or vascular phase at a rate of scanning of once per second for a duration of 30 to 50 seconds is used to monitor the first circulation of the injected bolus of contrast agent through the tissue. The second phase or interstitial phase at a slower scanning rate of once every 10 to 20 seconds for a duration of 2 minutes is used to monitor the wash-in of contrast agent into the interstitial space and its subsequent washout. Most investigators have used a kVp of either 80 or 120 (37). Figure 1 shows the arterial and tumor concentration curve from a common iliac artery of a 320-g nude rate with an implanted tumor in the left flank following contrast injection into a tail vein.

TRACER KINETIC ANALYSIS

In modeling the transport and distribution of X-ray contrast agent in tissue, the following terms need to be defined first:

Blood Flow (*F*)

This is the volume flow rate of blood through the vasculature in a tissue region. It is usually expressed in units of mL·min^{-1}·(100 g)$^{-1}$. Note that blood flow measured with DECT (or CTP) includes flow in large vessels, arterioles, capillaries, venules and veins. In particular, flow in arteriovenous shunts will also be included.

Blood Volume (V_b)

This is the volume of blood within the vasculature in a tissue region that is actually "flowing." Again, as in the case of blood flow, blood volume includes blood in large vessels, arterioles, capillaries, venules, and veins. Any stagnant pool of blood will not be included in the blood volume. It is measured in units of mL·$(100 \text{ g})^{-1}$.

Mean Transit Time (T_m)

This is the average time taken by blood elements to traverse the vasculature from the arterial end to the venous end. If the perfusion pressure (or pressure head) is high, blood elements travel at a higher velocity resulting in a shorter mean transit time than when the perfusion pressure is low. In this sense, mean transit time is a surrogate measure of perfusion pressure (38). Mean transit time is measured in seconds.

Vascular Permeability–Surface Area Product (PS)

The product of permeability and blood concentration of a solute gives the unidirectional diffusional flux from blood to interstitial space per unit surface area of capillary endothelium (39). PS is the product of permeability and the total surface area of capillary endothelium in a mass of tissue (usually 100 g of tissue) and hence is the total diffusional flux across all capillaries in that mass. It is measured in units of mL·min^{-1}·$(100 \text{ g})^{-1}$, same as F. Expressed in the stated units, the unidirectional flux of solutes, PS, from blood plasma to interstitial space is equivalent to the complete transfer of all the solutes in PS mL of blood per minute to interstitial space. Note that PS applies to the experimental

setup in which a permeable membrane is separating two solvents containing a solute at different concentrations. It is equal to the diffusional flux of solute across the whole permeable membrane (capillary endothelium) when the solvent (blood) is "stationary" with respect to the membrane. For the more physiological case of blood flowing through capillaries, the unidirectional flux of blood-borne solutes through capillaries is dependent on both F and PS. This relationship will be discussed in the following with respect to equation (4).

Extraction Efficiency (Fraction) (E)

This is the fraction of solutes present in arterial inlets, with the potential to diffuse into interstitial space, which are actually transferred from blood to interstitial space during a single passage of blood from the arterial end to the venous end of the capillaries of a tissue (40).

Central Volume Principle

Blood flow, blood volume, and mean transit time are related via the Central Volume Principle (41), which states that $F = V_b/T_m$.

KINETICS MODELING

Although compartmental models have been used to describe the transport and distribution of contrast agent in tissue, they all share the drawback that F, V, T_m, and PS cannot be simultaneously and separately determined (42–45). We have pioneered the use of the Johnson and Wilson model (46) to overcome this difficulty. In this model (Fig. 2) it is assumed

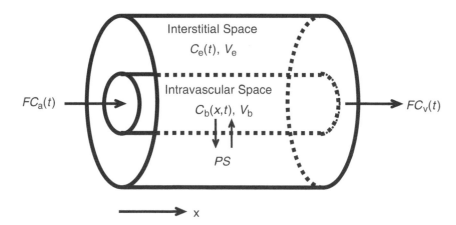

Figure 2 The Johnson and Wilson model for the distribution of blood-borne contrast media in tissue. Contrast concentration in the intravascular (blood) space, $C_b(x,t)$, is dependent on position along the capillary to reflect that it is decreasing from arterial $C_a(t)$ end to venous $C_v(t)$ end of the capillary. The interstitial space is assumed to be a compartment with no concentration gradient within it. *Abbreviations*: $C_e(t)$, interstitial concentration of solute; V_e, interstitial space of volume; F, blood flow; V_b, blood volume; x, axial position along the capillary.

that tissue consists of capillaries and interstitial tissue. All the capillaries are lumped together as a single cylinder of length L and volume V_b. The interstitial tissue is assumed to be a cylindrical annulus around the capillary. As the blood-borne contrast agent enters the capillary, it starts to diffuse across the capillary endothelium, thus the blood concentration of solute $C_b(x,t)$ is a function of both axial position x along the capillary and time t. The interstitial concentration of solute is $C_e(t)$ and depends only on time, that is, the interstitial space of volume V_e is treated as a "well-stirred" compartment. The transport and exchange of solute through the capillaries can be described by the following equation:

$$\frac{\partial C_b(x,t)}{\partial t} + \frac{FL}{V_b}\frac{\partial C_b(x,t)}{\partial x} + \frac{PS}{V_b}[C_b(x,t) - C_e(t)] = 0 \quad (1)$$

In the special case when $C_e(t)$ is a constant, say C_e, equation (1) has the solution:

$$C_b(x,t) = C_a\left(t - \frac{V_b}{FL}x\right)e^{-\frac{PS}{FL}x} + C_e$$
$$- C_e e^{-\frac{PS}{FL}x}H\left(t - \frac{V_b}{FL}x\right) \quad (2)$$

where $H(t)$ is the unit step function. As expected, at $x = 0$, $C_b(x,t) = C_a(t)$ and

$$C_v(t) = C_b(x,t)\big|_{x=L, t \geq \frac{V_b}{F}}$$
$$= C_a\left(t - \frac{V_b}{F}\right)e^{-\frac{PS}{F}} + C_e\left(1 - e^{-\frac{PS}{F}}\right)$$

Further, the arteriovenous difference can be written as

$$C_a(t - T_m) - C_v(t) = \left(1 - e^{-\frac{PS}{F}}\right) \cdot [C_a(t - T_m) - C_e]$$

where $T_m = V_b/F$ is the capillary (mean) transit time. Thus,

$$E \approx \frac{C_a(t - T_m) - C_v(t)}{C_a(t - T_m) - C_e} = 1 - e^{-\frac{PS}{F}} \quad (3)$$

or,

$$PS = -F \cdot \ln(1 - E) \quad (3a)$$

as Crone (40) and Renkin (47) had derived previously. Moreover, the Fick's Law gives the change in the interstitial concentration as

$$\frac{dC_e(t)}{dt} = F \cdot [C_a(t - T_m) - C_v(t)]$$

which, according to equation (3), can also be expressed as

$$V_e \cdot \frac{dC_e(t)}{dt} = F \cdot E \cdot [C_a(t - T_m) - C_v(t)] \quad (4)$$

Equation (4) can be interpreted as that the forward flux from the capillaries to the interstitial space is $F \cdot E \cdot C_a(t - T_m)$ and the backflux from the interstitial space to

the capillary is $F \cdot E \cdot C_e$. Thus, $F \cdot E$ is the unidirectional flux of solute per unit concentration, or transfer constant, from (flowing) blood to interstitial space or from interstitial space to (flowing) blood. There exists three regimes for the exchange of solute between blood and interstitial space: (i) when $PS \ll F$, flow extraction product (FE) approximates PS, the exchange is diffusion limited (43–45); (ii) when $PS \gg F$, so that FE approaches F, the exchange is flow limited; and (iii) when PS is of the same magnitude as F, the exchange is neither diffusion nor flow limited. The above derivation is obtained under the special case when $C_e(t)$ is held constant in time. For the general case when $C_e(t)$ is an arbitrary function of time, it has been shown that the unidirectional flux of solute per unit concentration is still $F \cdot E$ (48).

With the relationship between PS and FE clarified as above, we can now turn our attention to the solution of the Johnson and Wilson model. The governing equations of the model can be written as

$$\frac{\partial C_b(x,t)}{\partial t} + \frac{FL}{V_b} \cdot \frac{\partial C_b(x,t)}{\partial x} + \frac{PS}{V_b} \cdot [C_b(x,t) - C_e(t)]$$
$$= 0 \quad (5a)$$

$$V_e \cdot \frac{dC_e(t)}{dt} = \frac{PS}{L} \cdot \int_0^L [C_b(x,t) - C_e(t)] \cdot dx \quad (5b)$$

Equation (5a) describing the convective (blood flow) and diffusional transport of contrast agent in capillaries is the same as equation (1), while equation (5b) gives the rate of change of contrast concentration in the interstitial compartment. However, even with the simplification that the interstitial space is a compartment, the solution of the Johnson and Wilson model can only be expressed in the frequency domain with use of Laplace transform (46). This has severely limited its application until an adiabatic approximation was discovered to derive a closed-form solution of the model in the time domain (48). The motivations for the adiabatic approximation are twofold. First, the time rate of change of $C_e(t)$ is much slower than that of $C_b(x,t)$ so that $C_e(t)$ can be approximated by a staircase function consisting of discrete, finite steps provided the time interval of each step is small relative to the transit time of the tissue (capillaries). With this approximation, $C_e(t)$ is constant within each step of the staircase. Second, as discussed above in the solution of equations (1) or (5a), when $C_e(t)$ is a constant, $C_b(x,t)$ can be expressed in terms of $C_e(t)$. Thus, at each step of the staircase approximation of $C_e(t)$, equation (5a) is solved for $C_b(x,t)$ in terms of $C_e(t)$. With $C_b(x,t)$ expressed in $C_e(t)$, equation (5b) can be used to determine the increase in $C_e(t)$ at the end of the step. This procedure can be repeated for each step in the staircase approximation of $C_e(t)$, resulting in a

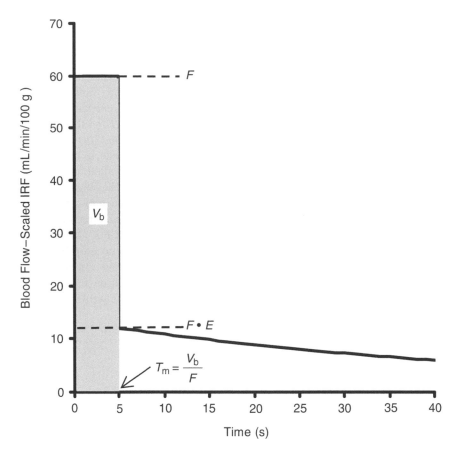

Figure 3 The blood flow–scaled impulse residue function according to the Johnson and Wilson model with the adiabatic approximation. The symbols are defined in the text. *Abbreviations*: IRF, impulse residue function; F, blood flow; V_b, blood volume; T_m, mean transit time.

time domain solution for the mass of solute per unit mass of tissue, $Q(t)$, which can be expressed as

$$Q(t) = F \cdot C_a(t) * R(t) \qquad (6a)$$

where $*$ is a convolution operator and $R(t)$, the impulse residue function (IRF), is expressed as (48)

$$R(t) = \begin{cases} 1 & 0 < t \leq \dfrac{V_b}{F} \\ E \cdot e^{-\frac{FE}{V_e} \cdot (t - \frac{V_b}{F})} \cdot H\left(t - \dfrac{V_b}{F}\right) & t > \dfrac{V_b}{F} \end{cases} \qquad (6b)$$

Figure 3 is a plot of $F \cdot R(t)$ or the blood flow–scaled IRF. It lends itself to the following interpretation: If a bolus of contrast agent is injected directly into the arterial inlet(s) of the tissue so that $C_a(t)$ is held at unity concentration for a very short while, the total mass of solute delivered to the tissue is numerically equal to F. The blood flow–scaled IRF, $F \cdot R(t)$, therefore would reach a height of F immediately and maintains this height for a duration equal to the T_m of the tissue, V_b/F. The shaded area in Figure 3 is therefore the V_b. After a time equal to

V_b/F, unextracted contrast agent starts to leave the tissue, $F \cdot R(t)$ drops to a height of $F \cdot E$, and thereafter contrast agent in the interstitial space back diffuses into the intravascular space and is washed out by blood flow. This portion of $F \cdot R(t)$ is described by a decreasing monoexponential function with a rate constant equal to $F \cdot E/V_e$. With $C_a(t)$ and $Q(t)$ measured by CT scanning as shown in Figure 1, $F \cdot R(t)$ can be determined by model deconvolution (49) according to equation (6b) and the parameters F, V_b, T_m, and E (PS) can be determined as discussed above.

APPLICATIONS

Validation of Blood Flow Measurement

For validation of blood flow measurements with the Johnson and Wilson model, we have used VX2 tumors implanted in the brain and a thigh of rabbits and compared CTP measurements against the gold-standard microsphere measurements (25,26). In each series of comparisons, the slope of the linear regression between CTP and microsphere measurement of blood flow was close to unity and the intercept was not significantly different from zero. Both studies also investigated the reproducibility of blood flow measurement with CT and determined that the coefficient of variation (CV) was about 14%. These results suggest that CTP measurement of blood flow in angiogenesis is both accurate and reproducible.

Study on the Vascular Reactivity of Tumor Neovasculature to Arterial Carbon Dioxide Tension

The structural and functional abnormalities of tumor vessels result in regions that are poorly perfused, hypoxic and high in interstitial pH (50). These characteristics of the tumor microenvironment limit the efficacy of many nonsurgical cancer treatments. For instance, poor perfusion limits the delivery of systemically administered cytotoxic agents to the tumor to achieve tissue concentrations necessary to kill tumor cells. Poor perfusion also leads to tumor hypoxia, which is a cause of resistance to cytotoxic agents (51) and in particular radiation (52). One approach to improve tumor response to therapy has been to increase the tumor oxygen and carbon dioxide levels through the inhalation of hypercarbic gases, such as carbogen (95% O_2, 5% CO_2) (53). The therapeutic

applications of carbogen have primarily focused on overcoming the resistance of hypoxic cells to radiation therapy. The rationale for using carbogen over pure oxygen is the conjecture that carbon dioxide blocks the vasoconstrictive effects of oxygen, thereby maintaining tumor blood flow to supply oxygen to the tumor (54). In practice, however, this theoretically plausible approach has shown variable results in increasing tumor blood flow (53) and tumor oxygenation (54–56) to improve the radiosensitivity of hypoxic cells (57,58).

Purdie et al. investigated the carbon dioxide reactivity of VX2 tumors implanted into a thigh of rabbits (59). Figure 4 shows a plot of the carbon dioxide reactivity of tumor blood flow as the fractional change in blood flow from normocapnia as a function of $PaCO_2$ for the eight rabbits studied. The relationship is sigmoidal ($R = 0.94$) in nature, showing a maximal decrease in blood flow of 40% at hypocapnia ($PaCO_2 < 30$ mmHg), whereas there is essentially no increase in blood flow above normocapnia ($PaCO_2 = 40$ mmHg). Figure 5 shows changes in tumor mean transit time with carbon dioxide tension in a format equivalent to Figure 4. The carbon dioxide reactivity plot of mean transit time demonstrates an exponential relationship, although the fit is poorer ($R = 0.64$). At hypocapnia there were large increases in mean transit

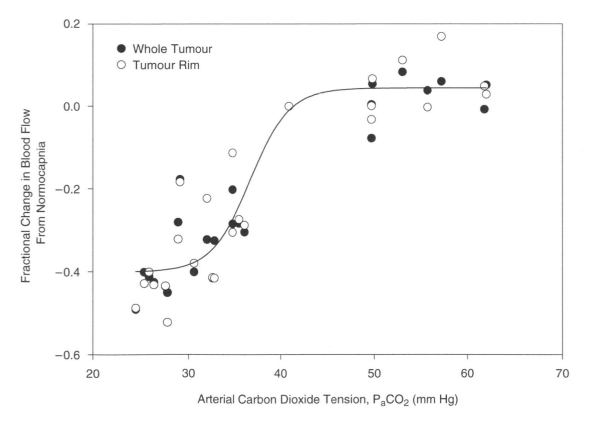

Figure 4 Carbon dioxide reactivity of blood flow of VX2 sarcoma in a rabbit thigh.

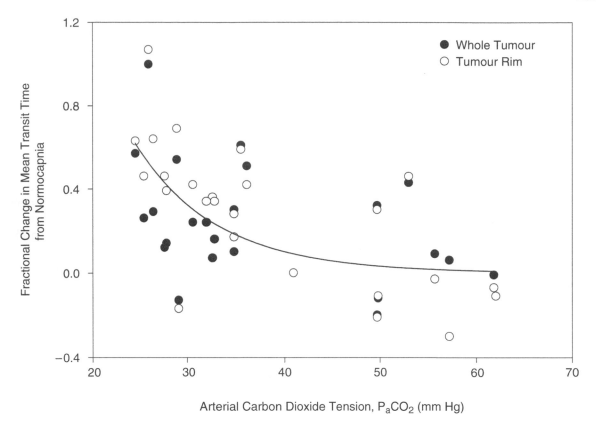

Figure 5 Carbon dioxide reactivity of mean transit time of VX2 sarcoma in a rabbit thigh.

time, that is, the time for blood elements to travel through the capillary network was longer. The effect at hypercapnia, however, was smaller and more variable with both increases and decreases in mean transit time. The carbon dioxide reactivity of tumor vascular permeability–surface area product and blood volume showed decreases in both parameters as the $PaCO_2$ was decreased below normal, and there was also a decrease above normocapnia, although to a lesser degree (data not shown). However, all these changes were not statistically significant.

These results show that lowering the $PaCO_2$ to a hypocapnic state induced decreases in tumor blood flow and increases in mean transit time, with minimal effects on the vascular permeability–surface area product and blood volume in the VX2 skeletal muscle tumor model. Hypercapnia produced insignificant effects in all parameters, presumably because of the near-maximum dilation of the tumor vessels at normocapnia. Therefore, the applicability of hypercapnia to improve tumor oxygenation and cytotoxic drug delivery appears limited. Further experiments with other tumor models are required to determine whether this finding is true in general or there exist some tumors that will respond to hypercapnia with increases in blood flow and possibly tumor oxygenation.

Study on Angiogenesis in a Murine Transgenic Model of Prostate Cancer

Since prostate secretory protein of 94 amino acids (PSP94) is one of the three most abundant proteins secreted from the human prostate, we have experimented with the promoter/enhancer region of the PSP94 gene to direct prostate targeting and expression of the SV40 Tag oncogene. The transgenic mice generated in our lab demonstrate prostatic hyperplasia as early as 10 weeks of age, with subsequent emergence of prostatic intraepithelial neoplasia (PIN) and eventually high-grade carcinoma in the prostate (60). Twelve transgenic mice were studied. Mice were screened regularly prior to CT scanning using a high-frequency small-animal ultrasound scanner (VisualSonics Vevo 770) with a 40-MHz probe to identify small tumors. CTP studies started when 1- to 2-mm diameter tumors were first detected with ultrasound (day 0) and repeated every 7 to 14 days for 9 weeks. During each session of CTP scanning, the mice were anesthetized with isoflurane and continuously scanned for 40 seconds using 80 kVp, 60 mA, an in-plane resolution of 175 μm to cover 40 × 0.9 mm thick slices with a small-animal CT scanner capable of one-second rotation speed (GE Healthcare, eXplore Locus Ultra). Two hundred

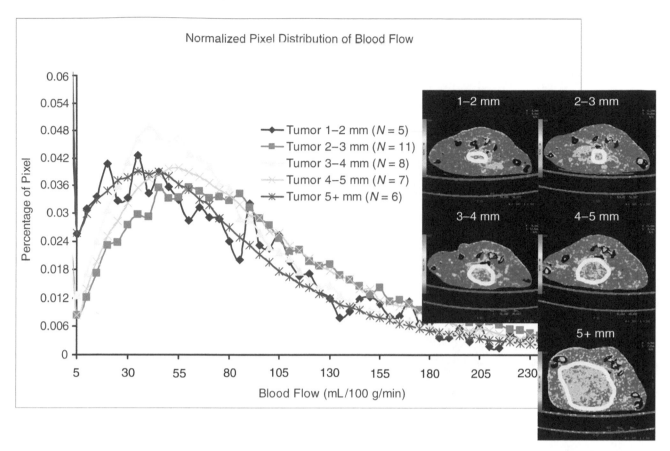

Figure 6 Blood flow maps from a transgenic mouse as the prostate tumor grew from 1 to 2 mm to over 5 mm in diameter. Also shown is the average normalized blood flow histogram for the whole tumor of the transgenic mouse studied.

microliters of an iodinated contrast agent (Hypaque 200 mgI/mL) was injected via a tail vein at an injection rate of 2.0 mL/min, five seconds after the start of CTP scanning. From the acquired series of CT images, CTP software (GE Healthcare), which implements the method discussed in the section on tracer kinetic analysis, was used to calculate functional maps of blood flow (Fig. 6) and blood volume according to equation (6) with $C_a(t)$, the arterial contrast media concentration versus time curve, measured from a common iliac artery and $Q(t)$, the tissue concentration versus time curve, from 2×2 pixel blocks in the CT images. Figure 6 shows the blood flow map of a 0.9-mm thick slice through the prostate of a transgenic mouse as the tumor grew from 1 to 2 mm to more than 5 mm in diameter. The prostate is outlined using thick white lines in the images. The normalized blood flow histogram distribution of the whole tumor, obtained by outlining the tumor in each CT slice and summing the blood flow histogram in the outlined tumor region from each slice, was also shown in Figure 6. The normalized blood flow histogram peaked at around 30 to 40 mL·min^{-1}·(100 g)$^{-1}$ at tumor diameter 1 to 2 mm before angiogenesis developed. As angiogenesis progressed and the tumor grew to 5 mm in diameter, the peak of the normalized blood

flow histogram shifted to higher blood flow around 55 to 60 mL·min^{-1}·(100 g)$^{-1}$. At tumor diameter larger than 5 mm, there was a downward shift in the peak to match that before angiogenesis developed. This also corresponded to the appearance of hypovascular regions in the blood flow map in Figure 6. The results from this study demonstrate that CTP is able to monitor angiogenesis and development of hypovascular (hypoxic) regions as the tumor grows in a preclinical transgenic murine model of prostate cancer.

Study on the Response of Brain Tumor to Radiation Treatment in Patients

CTP can also be used to monitor tumor response to radiation treatment in patients with primary brain tumor (glioblastoma multiforme). Figure 7 shows contrast-enhanced CT (CECT) scans of a patient with a right parietal and occipital enhancing mass from a glioblastoma multiforme before radiation treatment to 4000 cGy in 15 fractions. The CTP maps of blood flow, blood volume, and vascular permeability–surface area product before and one week after radiation treatment for a 5-mm CT slice through the tumor are shown in Figure 8. Both blood flow and blood volume in the tumor decreased while the *PS*

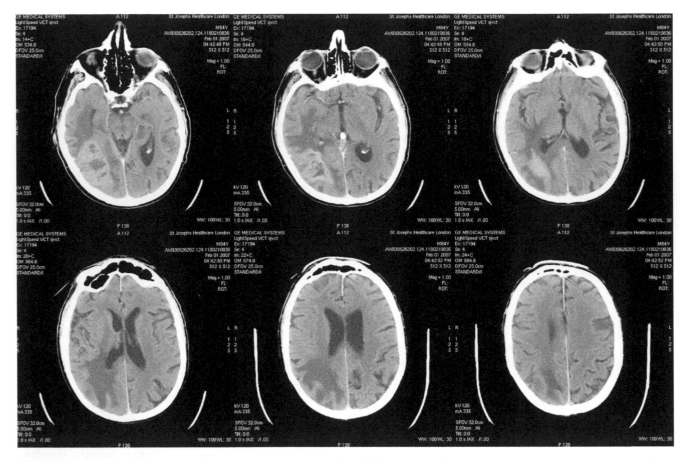

Figure 7 Contrast-enhanced computerized tomography scan of a glioblastoma multiforme patient showing the tumor in the right parietal/occipital region. There was also extensive edema surrounding the tumor.

product increased to suggest that the tumor had responded to the treatment. Figure 9 shows the CECT scans of the tumor before and three months after radiation treatment. There was extensive edema surrounding the tumor before treatment, which appeared to have resolved three months after the treatment. The conditions of the patient were also stable after the radiation treatment. These results demonstrate that CTP functional maps may give an earlier indication of response of the tumor to radiation treatment.

Study on Liver Tumor

Hepatocellular carcinoma (HCC) is the fifth most common solid tumor in the world and accounts for ~500,000 deaths each year (61). About 75% of all HCCs are associated with cirrhosis caused by Hepatitis B virus (HBV) and Hepatitis C virus (HCV) infections and alcoholic abuse (62,63). HCC develops at a rate of 1.5% to 8% per year in patients with cirrhosis caused by chronic HCV infection (64) compared to 0.03% to 0.07% among the general population in developed countries (65). The median life expectancy of untreated HCC with cirrhosis is only 6 to 13 months, with fewer than 40% of patients surviving 2 years (66,67). Small tumors

(<2 cm) have a substantially better prognosis following curative resection and/or orthotopic transplant than larger tumors (68). Current imaging modalities for early detection include ultrasonography, contrast-enhanced ultrasound, and multiphasic contrast-enhanced CT and MR (69). However, sensitivities to identify tumors less than 2 cm in diameter is uniformly low, being less than 75% on average (69–72). Therefore, there is an urgent need to develop better molecular and functional imaging biomarkers to improve detection of progression from cirrhotic/dysplastic nodules into HCC. The liver in normal human subject derives its blood flow from both the hepatic artery and the portal vein, in the ratio of ~1:3 (73). The hepatic vasculature is obliterated in cirrhosis (74) because of chronic inflammation, fibrosis, and necrosis, leading to increased intrahepatic resistance and portal hypertension. In turn, portal venous flow decreases and begins to bypass the liver parenchyma through porto-systemic venous shunts that have developed (75), but total liver blood flow is maintained by the hepatic buffer response (76). Thus, the hepatic arterial fraction (HAF) or the fraction of the total liver flow that is contributed by the hepatic artery increases. As cirrhosis evolves through regenerative nodules, dysplastic nodules to HCC, angiogenesis

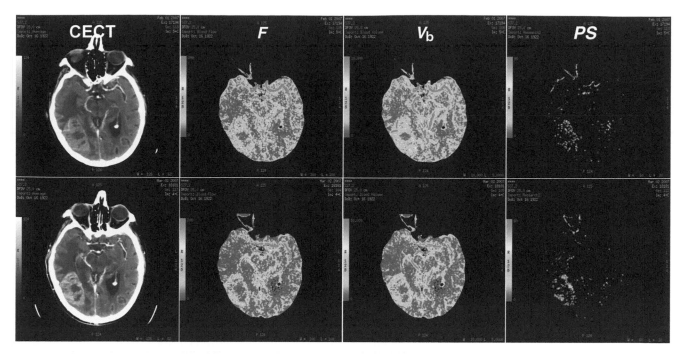

Figure 8 CECT and CT perfusion functional maps: blood flow, blood volume, and *PS* of the same glioblastoma multiforme patient as Figure 7 before (*top row*) and one week after (*bottom row*) radiation treatment. *Abbreviations*: CECT, contrast-enhanced computerized tomography; CT, computerized tomography; *F*, blood flow; V_b, blood volume (*See Color Insert*).

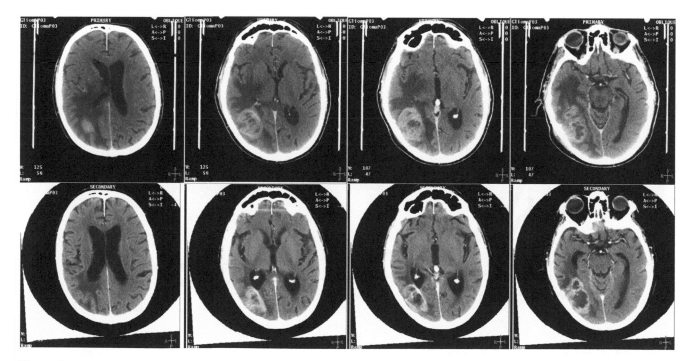

Figure 9 Contrast-enhanced computerized tomography scans of the same glioblastoma multiforme patient as Figures 7 and 8 before (*top row*) and three months after (*bottom row*) radiation treatment. The extensive edema surrounding the tumor had resolved three months after radiation treatment.

(77) also plays a major role in the remodeling of the vasculature to maximize the delivery via the hepatic artery of fully oxygenated blood to the growing lesion. Whereas regenerative nodules receive the majority of their blood supply from the portal vein like normal liver parenchyma, an increasing arterial blood supply and hence further increases in HAF accompany the evolution from a low-grade dysplastic nodule to frank HCC (78). In the progression from cirrhotic/dysplastic liver nodules to HCC, there may be a redistribution of liver blood flow to hepatic arterial rather than portal venous routes or an increase in the HAF of liver blood flow. A CT scanning method for the measurement of HAF in a rabbit model of liver tumor (implanted VX2 tumor cells) has been developed by Stewart et al. (79). VX2 carcinoma cells were implanted into the livers of eight male New Zealand white rabbits. DECT studies were performed before and every four days after implantation with a clinical multi-slice CT scanner (GE Healthcare LightSpeed). Each DECT study consists of two phases: a

30-second continuous scan with breath hold at the injection of 5 mL contrast, followed by 4-second continuous scans without breath hold every 10 seconds for 2 minutes. The scan parameters for both phases were 120 kVp, 60 mA, 1 second per rotation to cover four 5-mm thick slices. The second-phase free breathing images were registered with the first-phase breath-hold images to eliminate breathing motion. To account for the dual input of the liver, the contrast input to the liver, $I(t)$, assuming that the enhancement of the aorta can represent that of the hepatic artery input, is approximated by

$$I(t) = \alpha \cdot A(t) + (1 - \alpha) \cdot V(t) \qquad (7)$$

where $A(t)$ and $V(t)$ are the contrast concentrations (enhancements) measured in the hepatic artery (i.e., the aorta) and the portal vein, respectively and α is the fraction of liver blood flow contributed by the hepatic artery or the HAF. Figure 10 shows the aortic $A(t)$, portal vein $V(t)$, and liver enhancement $Q(t)$ curves from a rabbit study. With

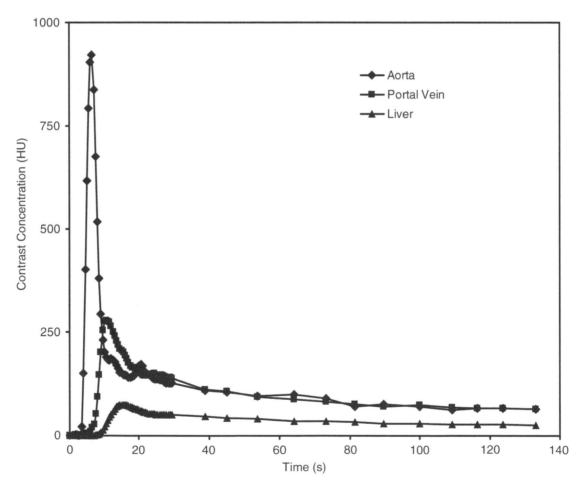

Figure 10 Contrast concentration curves from the aorta (*diamond*), the portal vein (*square*), and liver parenchyma (*triangle*) measured by a CT scanner in a rabbit following intravenous injection of contrast. The curves were measured from the co-registered first- and second-phase CT images and were deconvolved to calculate the functional parameters as described in the text. *Abbreviations*: CT, computerized tomography; HU, Hounsfield unit.

$A(t)$ and $V(t)$ measured as shown in Figure 10, the values of F, E, V_b, V_e, and α in equation (6) were changed iteratively by CTP software (GE Healthcare) in the deconvolution process to achieve an optimum fit by equation (6a) to the measured $Q(t)$. From the estimated values, PS was calculated with equation (3a) and the hepatic arterial blood flow ($H_A BF$) is equal to the product $\alpha \cdot F$, where F is the total liver

blood flow ($H_T BF$). Figure 11 shows the functional maps of a VX2 tumor in a rabbit 23 days after implantation. The tumor is visible in all of the functional maps. However, the $H_A BF$ map delineates the tumor rim from the tumor core most clearly. It also suggests that the tumor derives most of its blood flow from the hepatic artery. To investigate the change of HAF as the VX2 tumor developed, day 0

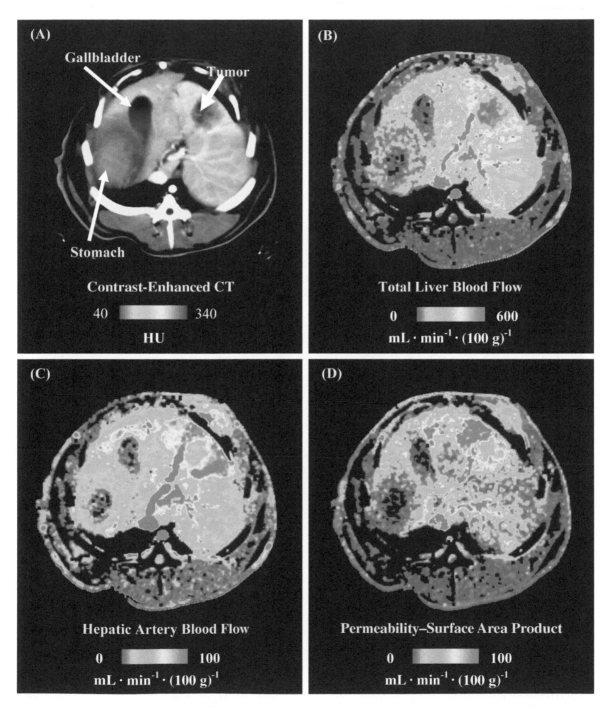

Figure 11 Functional maps of a 5 mm thick liver slice of a rabbit at 23 days post implantation of VX2 cells. (**A**) Contrast Enhanced CT. (**B**) Total liver blood Flow map. (**C**) Hepatic artery blood flow map. (**D**) Permeability-surface area map. *Abbreviations*: CT, computerized tomography; HU, Hounsfield unit (*See Color Insert*).

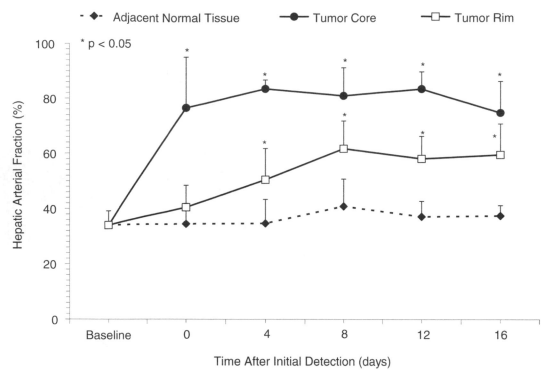

Figure 12 Measured hepatic arterial fraction (mean ± standard deviation) in the liver of eight rabbits over a period of 16 days from initial detection of the tumor developed from implanted VX2 cells.

(baseline) was set at the time when a tumor was detected by the functional maps (approximate 0.7 ± 0.1 cm diameter). HAFs measured in the tumor core and rim and adjacent normal tissue at baseline and every four days after the initial detection of the tumor were significantly different by an analysis of variance (ANOVA) (Fig. 12). Post hoc tests revealed that HAF in normal liver remained relatively constant at $36\% \pm 7\%$ throughout the study ($P > 0.05$). At the initial detection of the tumor, the HAF in the tumor core increased twofold over the baseline and adjacent normal tissue value ($P < 0.05$). Conversely, HAF in the tumor rim gradually increased and was significantly different from normal tissue starting four days after the baseline ($P < 0.05$).

To validate the CT method, $H_A BF$ measured by CTP in normal tissue, tumor rim, and core were compared with those measured by ex vivo microsphere technique (80) under normocapnia, hypercapnia, and hypocapnia conditions in seven rabbits at 16 days post tumor detection. There was a strong correlation of $H_A BF$ values from the two techniques. The average slope of the individual linear regression of $H_A BF$ measurements from a single rabbit was 0.92 ± 0.05, which was significantly different from a value of zero (the null hypothesis, $P < 0.05$), but not significantly different from the line of identity (slope = 1, $P > 0.05$). The average intercept, 4.62 ± 2.69

$mL \cdot min^{-1} \cdot (100\ g)^{-1}$, was not significantly different from zero, $P > 0.05$. The average correlation coefficient (R^2) was 0.81 ± 0.05 (range 0.64–0.96). The Bland-Altman plot (81) comparing CTP and microsphere $H_A BF$ measurements gives a mean difference of -0.13 $mL \cdot min^{-1} \cdot (100\ g)^{-1}$, which is not significantly different from zero (Fig. 13). The limits of agreement, the region in which 95% of the differences lie, are from -29.21 to $28.95\ mL \cdot min^{-1} \cdot (100\ g)^{-1}$.

The reproducibility of CTP measurements in liver tumor was investigated by scanning five rabbits with VX2 liver tumors twice at 12 and 16 days after the initial detection of liver tumor. On each study day, each rabbit was scanned twice using the protocol described above to measure $H_A BF$ under normal conditions ($PaCO_2$ of 39 ± 2 mmHg, temperature of $39.0 \pm 0.1°C$, and pH of 7.46 ± 0.01). Precision was investigated by a three-way ANOVA. The analysis was performed for each tissue type to account for the repeated scans, difference slices, and the repositioning of the animal (different scan days). Reproducibility was measured by the CV derived from the ANOVA (82). The results show that repeated measurements of $H_A BF$ with CTP on either the same day or different days are not different from each other. Further, the CVs of CTP $H_A BF$ in normal liver and tumor core and rim are 5.7%, 24.9%, and 1.4%, respectively. Parameters

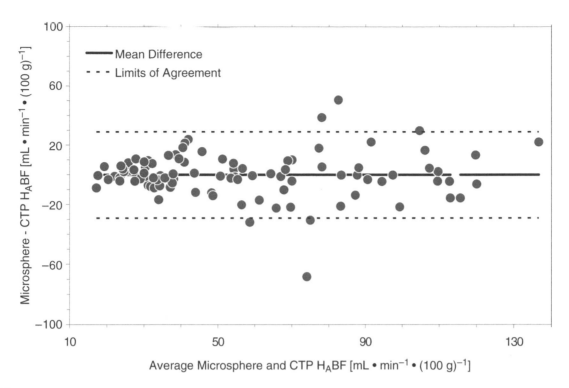

Figure 13 Bland-Altman plot comparing CTP and microsphere $H_A BF$ measurements. The mean difference (*solid line*) between the two methods is -0.13 mL·min^{-1}·(100 g)$^{-1}$. The limits of agreement (*dotted lines*), that is, the boundaries of the region in which 95% of the differences lie, are -29.21 and 28.95 mL·min^{-1}·(100 g)$^{-1}$. *Abbreviations*: CTP, computerized tomography perfusion; $H_A BF$, hepatic arterial blood flow.

Table 1 The Coefficients of Variation of Liver Functional Parameters Measured by Computerized Tomography Perfusion.

	Coefficient of variation (%)				
	$H_A BF$	α	$H_T BF$	$H_T BV$	*PS*
Tumor rim	1.4	3.5	0.5	0.5	6.7
Tumor core	24.9	14.9	41.6	16.9	42.2
Normal tissue	5.7	14.0	7.4	6.3	18.6

$H_T BV$ is equal to V_b in equation (6b) and Figure 3.
Abbreviations: $H_A BF$, hepatic arterial blood flow; $H_T BF$, total liver blood flow; $H_T BV$, total liver blood volume.

other than $H_A BF$ also showed similar results with better reproducibility in the tumor rim and normal tissue than in the tumor core (Table 1).

Table 1 shows the CV for total liver blood flow ($H_T BF$), HAF, and other functional parameters from a CTP liver scan.

CONCLUSION

With the advent of fast helical scanners and appropriate kinetics modeling method as discussed in this chapter, CT imaging of the vascular effects of angiogenesis has

become a reality both in preclinical and clinical studies. The inherent quantitative nature of CT scanning allows quantitative maps of blood flow, blood volume, mean transit time, and vascular permeability surface product to be determined simultaneously from a single study. The study can be performed with very simple procedures making it particularly suited for incorporation into the routine monitoring protocol of treatment response to angiogenesis inhibitors either in preclinical or clinical studies. The utility of imaging angiogenesis has been demonstrated in a number of experimental studies, further clinical studies will prove whether the favorable results obtained in animal models can be reproduced in clinical studies.

REFERENCES

1. Hanahan D, Weinberg RA. The hallmarks of cancer. Cell 2000; 100:57–70.
2. Albanell J, Baselga J. Trastuzumab, a humanized anti-her2 monoclonal antibody, for the treatment of breast cancer. Drugs Today (Barc) 1999; 35:931–946.
3. Nadal E, Olavarria E. Imatinib mesylate (gleevec/glivec) a molecular-targeted therapy for chronic myeloid leukaemia and other malignancies. Int J Clin Pract 2004; 58:511–516.

4. Demetri GD. Identification and treatment of chemoresistant inoperable or metastatic gist: experience with the selective tyrosine kinase inhibitor imatinib mesylate (sti571). Eur J Cancer 2002; 38(suppl 5):S52–S59.

5. Smith J. Erlotinib: small-molecule targeted therapy in the treatment of non-small-cell lung cancer. Clin Ther 2005; 27:1513–1534.

6. Wong SF. Cetuximab: an epidermal growth factor receptor monoclonal antibody for the treatment of colorectal cancer. Clin Ther 2005; 27:684–694.

7. Miller WR, Anderson TJ, Dixon JM. Anti-tumor effects of letrozole. Cancer Invest 2002; 20(suppl 2):15–21.

8. Richardson PG, Sonneveld P, Schuster MW, et al. Safety and efficacy of bortezomib in high-risk and elderly patients with relapsed multiple myeloma. Br J Haematol 2007; 137:429–435.

9. Prasad SR, Jhaveri KS, Saini S, et al. Ct tumor measurement for therapeutic response assessment: comparison of unidimensional, bidimensional, and volumetric techniques initial observations. Radiology 2002; 225:416–419.

10. Miller AB, Hoogstraten B, Staquet M, et al. Reporting results of cancer treatment. Cancer 1981; 47:207–214.

11. Therasse P, Arbuck SG, Eisenhauer EA, et al. New guidelines to evaluate the response to treatment in solid tumors. European Organization for Research and Treatment of Cancer, National Cancer Institute of the United States, National Cancer Institute of Canada. J Natl Cancer Inst 2000; 92:205–216.

12. Shepherd FA, Rodrigues Pereira J, Ciuleanu T, et al. Erlotinib in previously treated non-small-cell lung cancer. N Engl J Med 2005; 353:123–132.

13. Workman P. Challenges of pk/pd measurements in modern drug development. Eur J Cancer 2002; 38:2189–2193.

14. Sarker D, Workman P. Pharmacodynamic biomarkers for molecular cancer therapeutics. Adv Cancer Res 2007; 96:213–268.

15. Workman P, Aboagye EO, Chung YL, et al. Minimally invasive pharmacokinetic and pharmacodynamic technologies in hypothesis-testing clinical trials of innovative therapies. J Natl Cancer Inst 2006; 98:580–598.

16. Massoud TF, Gambhir SS. Molecular imaging in living subjects: seeing fundamental biological processes in a new light. Genes Dev 2003; 17:545–580.

17. Weissleder R, Mahmood U. Molecular imaging. Radiology 2001; 219:316–333.

18. Lee TY. Functional ct: physiological models. Trends Biotechnol 2002; 20:S3–S10.

19. Cenic A, Nabavi DG, Craen RA, et al. Dynamic ct measurement of cerebral blood flow: a validation study. AJNR Am J Neuroradiol 1999; 20:63–73.

20. Naganawa M, Kimura Y, Yano J, et al. Robust estimation of the arterial input function for logan plots using an intersectional searching algorithm and clustering in positron emission tomography for neuroreceptor imaging. Neuroimage 2008; 40:26–34.

21. Guo H, Renaut RA, Chen K. An input function estimation method for fdg-pet human brain studies. Nucl Med Biol 2007; 34:483–492.

22. Brenner DJ, Hall EJ. Computed tomography—an increasing source of radiation exposure. N Engl J Med 2007; 357:2277–2284.

23. Einstein AJ, Henzlova MJ, Rajagopalan S. Estimating risk of cancer associated with radiation exposure from 64-slice computed tomography coronary angiography. JAMA 2007; 298:317–323.

24. Miles KA, Charnsangavej C, Lee FT, et al. Application of ct in the investigation of angiogenesis in oncology. Acad Radiol 2000; 7:840–850.

25. Cenic A, Nabavi DG, Craen RA, et al. A CT method to measure hemodynamics in brain tumors: validation and application of cerebral blood flow maps. AJNR Am J Neuroradiol 2000; 21:462–470.

26. Purdie TG, Henderson E, Lee TY. Functional CT imaging of angiogenesis in rabbit vx2 soft-tissue tumour. Phys Med Biol 2001; 46:3161–3175.

27. Kerbel RS. Tumor angiogenesis: past, present and the near future. Carcinogenesis 2000; 21:505–515.

28. Hinnen P, Eskens FA. Vascular disrupting agents in clinical development. Br J Cancer 2007; 96:1159–1165.

29. Folkman J. Angiogenesis: an organizing principle for drug discovery? Nat Rev Drug Discov 2007; 6:273–286.

30. Kerbel R, Folkman J. Clinical translation of angiogenesis inhibitors. Nat Rev Cancer 2002; 2:727–739.

31. Jain RK. Normalizing tumor vasculature with anti-angiogenic therapy: a new paradigm for combination therapy. Nat Med 2001; 7:987–989.

32. Viloria-Petit AM, Kerbel RS. Acquired resistance to egfr inhibitors: mechanisms and prevention strategies. Int J Radiat Oncol Biol Phys 2004; 58:914–926.

33. Camp ER, Summy J, Bauer TW, et al. Molecular mechanisms of resistance to therapies targeting the epidermal growth factor receptor. Clin Cancer Res 2005; 11: 397–405.

34. Herbst RS, Mullani NA, Davis DW, et al. Development of biologic markers of response and assessment of antiangiogenic activity in a clinical trial of human recombinant endostatin. J Clin Oncol 2002; 20:3804–3814.

35. Rehman S, Jayson GC. Molecular imaging of antiangiogenic agents. Oncologist 2005; 10:92–103.

36. Lee TY, Ellis RJ, Dunscombe PB, et al. Quantitative computed tomography of the brain with xenon enhancement: a phantom study with the ge9800 scanner. Phys Med Biol 1990; 35:925–935.

37. Lee TY, Stewart E. Scientific basis and evaluation. In: Miles K, Cuenod C-A, eds. Multidetector Computed Tomography in Oncology: Ct Perfusion Imaging. London: Informa Healthcare, 2007.

38. Schumann P, Touzani O, Young AR, et al. Evaluation of the ratio of cerebral blood flow to cerebral blood volume as an index of local cerebral perfusion pressure. Brain 1998; 121(pt 7):1369–1379.

39. Rappaport S. Blood-Brain Barrier in Physiology and Medicine. New York: Raven Press, 1976.

40. Crone C. The permeability of capillaries in various organs as determined by use of the 'indicator diffusion' method. Acta Physiol Scand 1963; 58:292–305.

41. Meier P, Zierler KL. On the theory of the indicator-dilution method for measurement of blood flow and volume. J Appl Physiol 1954; 6:731–744.

42. Yeung WT, Lee TY, Del Maestro RF, et al. In vivo ct measurement of blood-brain transfer constant of iopamidol in human brain tumors. J Neurooncol 1992; 14:177–187.

43. Groothuis DR, Lapin GD, Vriesendorp FJ, et al. A method to quantitatively measure transcapillary transport of iodinated compounds in canine brain tumors with computed tomography. J Cereb Blood Flow Metab 1991; 11:939–948.

44. Patlak CS, Blasberg RG, Fenstermacher JD. Graphical evaluation of blood-to-brain transfer constants from multiple-time uptake data. J Cereb Blood Flow Metab 1983; 3:1–7.

45. Patlak CS, Blasberg RG. Graphical evaluation of blood-to-brain transfer constants from multiple-time uptake data. Generalizations. J Cereb Blood Flow Metab 1985; 5: 584–590.

46. Johnson JA, Wilson TA. A model for capillary exchange. Am J Physiol 1966; 210:1299–1303.

47. Renkin EM. Transport of potassium-42 from blood to tissue in isolated mammalian skeletal muscles. Am J Physiol 1959; 197:1205–1210.

48. St Lawrence KS, Lee TY. An adiabatic approximation to the tissue homogeneity model for water exchange in the brain: I. Theoretical derivation. J Cereb Blood Flow Metab 1998; 18:1365–1377.

49. Lawson C, Hanson R. Solving Least-Squares Problems. Englewood Cliffs, New Jersey: Prentice-Hall, Inc, 1974.

50. Jain RK. Determinants of tumor blood flow: a review. Cancer Res 1988; 48:2641–2658.

51. Teicher BA, Lazo JS, Sartorelli AC. Classification of antineoplastic agents by their selective toxicities toward oxygenated and hypoxic tumor cells. Cancer Res 1981; 41:73–81.

52. Thomlinson RH, Gray LH. The histological structure of some human lung cancers and the possible implications for radiotherapy. Br J Cancer 1955; 9:539–549.

53. Powell ME, Hill SA, Saunders MI, et al. Effect of carbogen breathing on tumour microregional blood flow in humans. Radiother Oncol 1996; 41:225–231.

54. Lanzen JL, Braun RD, Ong AL, et al. Variability in blood flow and po2 in tumors in response to carbogen breathing. Int J Radiat Oncol Biol Phys 1998; 42:855–859.

55. Martin L, Lartigau E, Weeger P, et al. Changes in the oxygenation of head and neck tumors during carbogen breathing. Radiother Oncol 1993; 27:123–130.

56. Powell ME, Collingridge DR, Saunders MI, et al. Improvement in human tumour oxygenation with carbogen of varying carbon dioxide concentrations. Radiother Oncol 1999; 50:167–171.

57. Martin LM, Thomas CD, Guichard M. Nicotinamide and carbogen: relationship between po2 and radiosensitivity in three tumour lines. Int J Radiat Biol 1994; 65:379–386.

58. Grau C, Horsman MR, Overgaard J. Improving the radiation response in a c3h mouse mammary carcinoma by normobaric oxygen or carbogen breathing. Int J Radiat Oncol Biol Phys 1992; 22:415–419.

59. Purdie TG, Lee TY. Carbon dioxide reactivity of computed tomography functional parameters in rabbit vx2 soft tissue tumour. Phys Med Biol 2003; 48:849–860.

60. Gabril MY, Onita T, Ji PG, et al. Prostate targeting: Psp94 gene promoter/enhancer region directed prostate tissue-specific expression in a transgenic mouse prostate cancer model. Gene Ther 2002; 9:1589–1599.

61. Parkin DM, Bray F, Ferlay J, et al. Estimating the world cancer burden: globocan 2000. Int J Cancer 2001; 94: 153–156.

62. Ikeda K, Saitoh S, Koida I, et al. A multivariate analysis of risk factors for hepatocellular carcinogenesis: a prospective observation of 795 patients with viral and alcoholic cirrhosis. Hepatology 1993; 18:47–53.

63. Ikeda K, Saitoh S, Suzuki Y, et al. Disease progression and hepatocellular carcinogenesis in patients with chronic viral hepatitis: a prospective observation of 2215 patients. J Hepatol 1998; 28:930–938.

64. Colombo M. Screening for cancer in viral hepatitis. Clin Liver Dis 2001; 5:109–122.

65. Di Bisceglie AM. Epidemiology and clinical presentation of hepatocellular carcinoma. J Vasc Interv Radiol 2002; 13: S169–S171.

66. Okuda K, Ohtsuki T, Obata H, et al. Natural history of hepatocellular carcinoma and prognosis in relation to treatment. Study of 850 patients. Cancer 1985; 56:918–928.

67. Llovet JM, Burroughs A, Bruix J. Hepatocellular carcinoma. Lancet 2003; 362:1907–1917.

68. Tobe T, Arii S. Improving survival after resection of hepatocellular carcinoma: characteristics and current status of surgical treatment of primary liver cancer in Japan. In: Tobe T, Kaneda H, Okudaira M, eds. Primary Liver Cancer in Japan. Tokyo: Springer, 1992.

69. Kamel IR, Bluemke DA. Imaging evaluation of hepatocellular carcinoma. J Vasc Interv Radiol 2002; 13:S173–S184.

70. Sherman M. Screening for hepatocellular carcinoma. Baillieres Best Pract Res Clin Gastroenterol 1999; 13:623–635.

71. Lencioni R, Cioni D, Della Pina C, et al. Imaging diagnosis. Semin Liver Dis 2005; 25:162–170.

72. Pandharipande PV, Krinsky GA, Rusinek H, et al. Perfusion imaging of the liver: current challenges and future goals. Radiology 2005; 234:661–673.

73. Chiandussi L, Greco F, Sardi G, et al. Estimation of hepatic arterial and portal venous blood flow by direct catheterization of the vena porta through the umbilical cord in man. Preliminary results. Acta Hepatosplenol 1968; 15:166–171.

74. Blendis L, Wong F. The hyperdynamic circulation in cirrhosis: an overview. Pharmacol Ther 2001; 89:221–231.

75. Li X, Benjamin IS, Naftalin R, et al. Location and function of intrahepatic shunts in anaesthetised rats. Gut 2003; 52:1339–1346.

76. Richter S, Mucke I, Menger MD, et al. Impact of intrinsic blood flow regulation in cirrhosis: maintenance of hepatic arterial buffer response. Am J Physiol Gastrointest Liver Physiol 2000; 279:G454–G462.

77. Folkman J. The role of angiogenesis in tumor growth. Semin Cancer Biol 1992; 3:65–71.

78. Park YN, Yang CP, Fernandez GJ, et al. Neoangiogenesis and sinusoidal "capillarization" in dysplastic nodules of the liver. Am J Surg Pathol 1998; 22:656–662.

79. Stewart EE, Chen X, Hadway J, et al. Correlation between hepatic tumor blood flow and glucose utilization in a rabbit liver tumor model. Radiology 2006; 239:740–750.

80. Heymann MA, Payne BD, Hoffman JI, et al. Blood flow measurements with radionuclide-labeled particles. Prog Cardiovasc Dis 1977; 20:55–79.

81. Bland JM, Altman DG. Statistical methods for assessing agreement between two methods of clinical measurement. Lancet 1986; 1:307–310.

82. Eliasziw M, Young SL, Woodbury MG, et al. Statistical methodology for the concurrent assessment of interrater and intrarater reliability: using goniometric measurements as an example. Phys Ther 1994; 74:777–788.

10

Multimodality Imaging Instrumentation and Techniques

DOUGLAS J. WAGENAAR and BRADLEY E. PATT

Gamma Medica-Ideas, Inc., Northridge, California, U.S.A.

INTRODUCTION

In this chapter, the topic of multimodality medical imaging will be reviewed. The context of multimodality imaging in healthcare is the subject of this introductory section. The history of multimodality imaging is then presented, followed by the most prominent current examples and promising new combinations of technology. Techniques for analysis and display of multimodality data are discussed. Only certain "winning combinations" of modalities will find clinical utility. We discuss the criteria for selecting the winning combinations and avoiding dead-ends of redundant or noncomplementary modalities.

From the earliest days of human medicine, practitioners have sought to ascertain the patient's condition and to determine the best course of action. Experience with symptoms and recorded correlations between attempted treatments and known outcomes have been handed down within human cultures over centuries. During the past century, the expansion of the knowledge base of biology, in particular the genetic nature of normal development and disease, has only amplified the responsibility of caregivers to associate symptoms and test results with the proper diagnosis of disease and stage, and to determine the most appropriate course of beneficial action.

The technology associated with assessing the patient's condition has grown in synchronization with our understanding of the underlying biology. Using only sensory inputs—visual appearance, heart and breathing sounds, olfactory and tactile clues—early physicians could categorize patients based on cultural wisdom and their personal experience. Microscopy and chemical analyses techniques have rapidly developed into the healthcare field of "diagnostic laboratory testing," which include blood, urine, sputum, and fecal analysis. In general, these tests compare an individual's measurement with a normal database. Over the decades, each test has become miniaturized, automated, and computerized such that the technician's time and the laboratory's resources are more efficiently utilized. The ultimate goal of laboratory testing that is envisioned is a "lab-on-a-chip" (1) in which multiple tests are performed on a single sample in a miniaturized biological and chemical analogue to the microchip circuitry developed in the last half of the 20th century. Multiple laboratory test results, obtained quickly, noninvasively, and at low cost, contribute to the needed accumulation of descriptive data that help direct the recommended therapeutic path in each individual's case.

The "visual inspection" aspect of clinical data gathering was greatly augmented by the invention of film radiography in the late 1890s. As mentioned above, laboratory testing, through miniaturization, can continue to become more productive and efficient, i.e., more tests can be done for the same sample volume and resource costs with no risk to the patient. X-ray and nuclear medicine tests have low levels of ionizing radiation dose associated with them, and this risk must be considered when ordering the diagnostic test. Detrimental interactions of ultrasound acoustic waves and MRI magnetic field and radio frequency (RF) energy with living tissue have not been observed. However, all imaging modalities have resource costs associated with them, beginning with the equipment itself, the imaging room, the disposable materials, such as film and contrast media, and the skilled technologists and physician interpreters. The risks and costs of imaging modalities distinguish them from laboratory tests. These issues make the use of multiple imaging studies for individual patients more complex, and the design and development of multimodality equipment a challenging proposition.

The field of medical imaging is the technological extension of the visual inspection performed by generations of physicians. For the first 70 years or so, until the introduction of tomography in about 1970, medical imaging was limited to film radiography and a far smaller but growing nuclear medicine study volume that began around 1950. When the external visual inspection, the stethoscope, and palpation failed to yield the desired answer, physicians could now have a look within the body using X-rays. The nature of radiography favors the demonstration of structural anatomy and malformations, injuries such as broken bones, swelling, and obstructive accumulations. Iodine- and barium-based contrast agents allowed the radiographic imaging of vessels, bronchi, and the digestive tract. The imaging of flow through large vessels and conduits was a step toward more "functional"

imaging as opposed to strictly anatomical or structure imaging. Nuclear medicine from the beginning was involved in functional imaging, measuring thyroid uptake with radioactive iodine, perfusion of the myocardium, lungs, kidneys, and liver, and increased regenerative metabolism in the well-known "bone-scan."

In recent years, the field of "molecular imaging" has emerged (2). What began as radiopharmaceutical research for nuclear medicine has become a broader field that encompasses optical, MRI, and even CT contrast agents that are targeted to highlight specific cellular or molecular concentrations and processes in both normal and diseased tissues. ^{18}F-labeled fluorodeoxyglucose for sugar metabolism was developed in the 1970s, ^{99m}Tc-labeled sestamibi for myocardial perfusion was developed in the 1980s, and radiolabeled antibodies (e.g., *Prostascint* by Cytogen) and peptides (e.g., *Octreoscan* by Mallinckrodt; *Neotect* by Diatide) were developed and FDA approved in the 1990s. These forerunners represent the vanguard of molecular imaging possibilities. Now hundreds of agents are under study and the National Library of Medicine and the National Institutes of Health have developed a publicly accessible database (3) to catalog these developments. In Figure 1, we schematically depict how molecular imaging is closer to the causes of, and hopefully the cures for, the diseases afflicting people today. The potential for combinations of modalities can be interpreted from this figure as well: anatomical combined with functional or molecular modalities can provide an

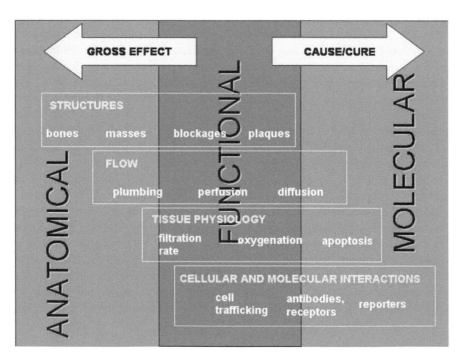

Figure 1 Medical imaging schematically represented as "anatomical" (*left*), "functional" (*center*), and "cellular and molecular" (*right*). Broad categories of applications are shown with a few examples from each category.

anatomical backdrop or context that is painted with specific information about the molecular interactions or biological functions within this context.

In the remainder of this chapter, therefore, we will continue to define the field of multimodality medical imaging and how it fits into the broader subject of healthcare. Multimodality imaging is similar to multiple, parallel analyses of blood samples. That is, more data are gathered to aid the physician's decision making. The important difference is that miniaturization, automation, and cost-reduction cannot be realized as in laboratory diagnostic testing, and therefore combinations must be carefully rationalized and justified before prototypes are built and products are clinically tested.

MULTIMODALITY IMAGING

The costs associated with bringing a new pharmaceutical to market have been estimated to be about $900 million (4). As each new candidate drug progresses from microarrays to petri dishes to microscopy slides to small-animal testing to human clinical trials, the costs exponentially increase (5). In this section, we argue that small-animal imaging is the most cost-effective and experimentally efficient way to reduce development time and costs for pharmaceutical research and development. Significantly fewer animals and less technician time must be devoted to biodistribution and pharmacokinetics studies that traditionally have required ex vivo quantitative analysis following tissue excision, isolation, and sample preparation. From the clinical side, early phase human toxicity and

pharmacodynamics studies are migrating toward in vivo animal studies. Finally, the new fields of genetic engineering, stem cell therapies, and bionanoparticle interactions can best be studied in vivo using small-animal imaging. Multimodality instrumentation extracts anatomical, functional, cellular, and molecular information for experimenters in all of these fields without the clinical needs of proving efficacy and justifying reimbursement.

Multimodality Imaging in Biomedical Research

In fields outside of preclinical and clinical medical imaging one can find multimodality imaging examples. Figure 2 shows an interesting example that combines radar topography with satellite optical imaging in representing the San Andreas Fault in southern California. Many other examples of dual- or multimodality imaging of the surface of the earth can be found in the fields of agriculture, meteorology, and of course military mapping. Other broad fields of multimodality imaging are from the very large as well as the very small: astronomy and microscopy. In astronomy, emission from various electromagnetic spectral ranges can show valuable information as multimodality overlays. In microscopy, we find the similar concepts that have grown into the subject of this chapter, namely, multimodality medical imaging.

There are many examples in the field of cellular microscopy in which the same cells can be stained for the presence of different receptors. These "hyperspectral cytometry" images are a powerful example of "multimodality" biomedical images. The labeling of cells with

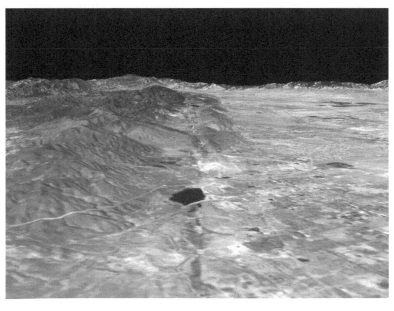

Figure 2 Dual-modality topographic image of the San Andreas fault. This is a depiction of two superimposed modalities—radar topology and optical photography in a 3D surface rendering. *Source*: From Ref. 49.

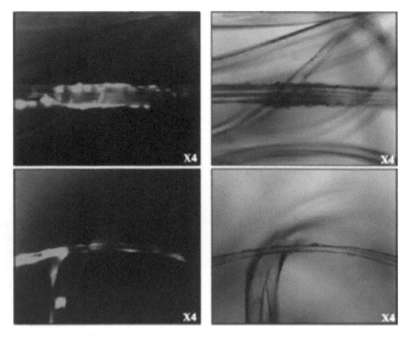

Figure 3 Fluorescent microscopy using green fluorescent protein (GFP) on the left and white light microscopy on the right. Endothelialization of the filamentous polymeric scaffold can be observed. *Source*: From Ref. 10 (with permission).

radioactive atoms of tritium (^{3}H), ^{14}C, and ^{32}P has been called the "foundation of biochemistry" (6,7). Radioactive decay of these beta emitters can, over time frames of days, expose the film placed in proximity to the sample. This is the field of autoradiography, the name resulting from the exposure being the same size of the sample (i.e., there is no lens for magnification). Film-based autoradiography is now being replaced by digital autoradiography systems (8,9). Another form of multimodality imaging is the combination of autoradiographs with optical microscopy images of the same sample.

Optical imaging of two wavelengths can be used to show newly forming cells growing within a bio-scaffold (Fig. 3) (10). As the size of the objects being imaged goes from cells to tissues, the effectiveness of high-resolution optical imaging goes down due to multiple scatters of photons. The field of nuclear microscopy is emerging for this particular application. Nuclear microscopy uses relatively low energy (5–30 keV) X-ray and gamma-ray emissions from radioactive decay to image with spatial resolution of less than 100 μm (11–13). Tissue specimens and peripheral subcutaneous lesions in animals are the subject of dual-modality nuclear microscopy and optical imaging.

Working our way up from cell samples to tissue samples, the next biological research entity to consider is the intact living specimen. The field of "preclinical imaging" has emerged from the use of separate imaging components developed at various research institutions from the 1980s until the early 2000s. Preclinical imaging is generally described as imaging of small animals such as

zebra fish, mice, rats, guinea pigs, and rabbits. Special-purpose imaging instruments, usually obsolete clinical, novel prototype, or niche-market products, are still being used for research on larger animals such as pigs, dogs, and nonhuman primates. In the following section, we concentrate on the preclinical research imaging of small animals in which a viable market for multimodality instruments has developed in the new millennium.

Preclinical Multimodality Imaging

In biomedical research involving the use of small animals, the value of the experimental results is paramount. The use of noninvasive imaging allows longitudinal study of time-course effects on a small population of animals, and this compares favorably to using many more animals with sacrifice of subpopulations, over time, to gather sufficient statistics for the experiment. The use of multiple imaging modalities in these experiments facilitates the data acquisition by minimizing preparation time and using the same physiological condition and physical orientation. The time of the laboratory technician and the integrity of the experimental results supersede duty-cycle arguments, which arise when costly clinical devices are idled by another modality (see section on Clinical Multimodality Imaging).

The first commercial SPECT/CT scanner for small-animal research was Gamma Medica-Ideas' A-SPECT™ (14,15). The CT has been used primarily to provide an anatomical backdrop. The availability of micro-focus X-ray tubes has lead to a larger market of ultrahigh

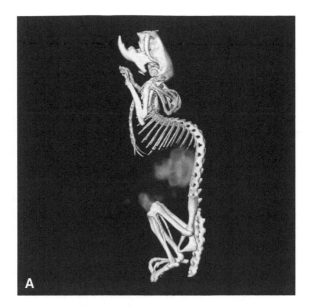
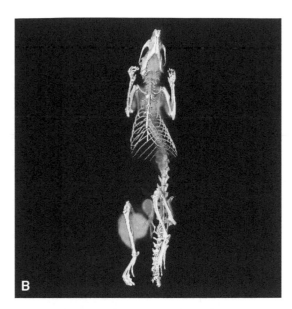

Figure 4 (**A**) SPECT/CT in use for drug development in a mouse. The tumor is growing in the shoulder of the mouse; the ^{99m}Tc-labeled folate receptor agent is present in the bowel but not in the lesion in this animal, resulting in a negative scan. (**B**) PET/CT showing positive uptake of (^{18}F) FDG in an inter-muscular tumor xenograft in the thigh muscle of a rat. **A** and **B** demonstrate the whole-body capability of combined modality instruments and the value of using CT bone windows to display anatomical context. *Source*: Images courtesy of Paul Scherrer Institute.

resolution microCT scanners capable of less than 20 μm spatial resolution. However, this CT resolution imparts a significant radiation dose to the living animal and is generally used for excised bone and joint specimens. The first trimodality SPECT/PET/CT was also introduced by Gamma Medica-Ideas, Inc. (16) and the instrument is called the Triumph™. Example images of SPECT/CT and PET/CT are shown in Figure 4.

The future of preclinical, multimodality imaging has two major branches: (*i*) optical imaging techniques combined with the above-mentioned PET/SPECT/CT instruments; and (*ii*) MRI combined with PET/SPECT/CT. Preclinical optical imagers can be multimodality within a single detector by using different wavelengths of emissions to signify different biological processes. One of the first optical/X-ray combinations is the in vivo FXPro (17). In this instrument, digital projection X-radiographs provide an anatomical context for optical fluorescence or luminescence images. Researchers from Gamma Medica-Ideas (18,19) are developing a combined SPECT/MRI imaging system for mice that is based on semiconductor cadmium zinc telluride (CZT), which has shown insensitivity to magnetic fields. This system is a stationary (to avoid eddy currents), ultrasmall (<12-cm diameter) cylinder that incorporates the RF coil and a pinhole collimator sleeve into a combined unit. Finally, researchers at the University of California, Davis led by Cherry (20) have developed a small (again, <12-cm diameter) MR-compatible mouse PET scanner based on the replacement

of photomultiplier tubes (PMTs) with position-sensitive avalanche photodiodes. The growing preclinical research market and these new combined instruments will serve as a technological proving ground for the clinical instruments of the future.

CLINICAL MULTIMODALITY IMAGING

The nuclear medicine modalities of SPECT and PET can benefit from knowledge of the attenuation properties of the tissue that is being penetrated by the detected radiation. Correction for attenuation in SPECT and PET can compensate for the "hot rim" artifact that is generated by attenuation of photons originating from substantial depths within the body. Correction for attenuation also improves the accuracy of quantitation of uptake, an improvement that is particularly necessary for SPECT imaging because of the increased attenuation of the lower energy SPECT photons.

In nuclear imaging, there are two unknown distributions: (*i*) the distribution of radioactivity in the volume of interest (the determination of which is the purpose of the nuclear scan) and (*ii*) the attenuation properties of the volume of interest (VOI) and tissues intervening between the VOI and the nuclear detector. During the 1980s and 1990s, the distribution of attenuation properties, known as the "mu map" (the Greek letter μ being the symbol for the linear attenuation coefficient), was determined by acquiring a transmission scan. The transmission scan is essentially a CT scan acquired with a known-location radioactive source that is collimated to shine a narrow beam of photons through the patient (hence transmission) and into the radiation detector. In SPECT, the 103-keV photons from a ^{153}Gd source create the projection image in the Anger camera. For PET, a ^{68}Ge source is used. Although the coarse intrinsic resolution of nuclear imagers produces poor quality CT scans, these scans have sufficient detail to provide adequate attenuation correction for nuclear tomography. Interestingly, users of attenuation-corrected nuclear scanners became the first routine practitioners of clinical multimodality imaging.

The "hot spots" being created by ^{18}F-fluorodeoxyglucose positron emission tomography (FDG PET) in the 1980s and early 1990s were often displayed in reading rooms alongside corresponding slices of the patient's CT scan, either on a digital display monitor or as film on a light box. The same can be said of hot spot uptake from early SPECT-radiolabeled antibodies and peptides such as Prostascint and Octreotide. Placing the nuclear hot spots in anatomical context was important in making the most accurate diagnostic evaluation.

Although attenuation correction and anatomical context were motivations for combining CT with nuclear scanning, the most important factor was the complementary nature of the two scans. Indeed, in attempting to document the efficacy of FDG PET in the field of oncology, it was often necessary to make comparisons with the "gold standard" modality, CT. It was found that when the data from the two modalities were acquired together there were improvements in diagnostic accuracy by up to 60%, and significant changes in patient management occurred in up to 25% of the cases (21). Publications from the initial studies of first-generation PET/CT products (22,23) provided a cogent explanation for the commercial success of a combined instrument for single-session imaging.

Historical Development

Hasegawa (24) at the University of California, San Francisco (UCSF), was the first to build a combined emission/transmission imaging system. This system used the same detector for X-ray CT as well as SPECT acquisition (see section on Multimodality Hardware). The primary rationale for this development was the need for quantitation in SPECT imaging, which requires accurate attenuation correction. The UCSF group continued development work in SPECT/CT with a linear design (25), with a commercial CT scanner adjacent to a SPECT system and a common patient bed. This "linear patient motion" from one modality to the next has become the standard for first-generation multimodality systems of SPECT/CT as well as PET/CT,

both in the clinical and preclinical instrument markets. The first commercial SPECT/CT product available for clinical use was the Hawkeye (General Electric Healthcare, Waukesha, WI) (26). Other manufacturers have introduced similar SPECT/CT products, generally combining dual-head SPECT systems with multislice CT scanners. The desire for quantitation has not yet developed into a clinically useful application of SPECT/CT. Today, the main utility of this device has been to provide an anatomical context in cases that are otherwise difficult to interpret (27). New SPECT imaging agents developed by researchers in the relatively new field of "molecular imaging" may prove to require SPECT/CT's quantitation capability. For example, in the future, physicians may need to accurately monitor changes in uptake in response to therapy.

In contrast to SPECT/CT, the development of PET/CT has recorded more evident clinical utility and rapid commercial success. In order for the PET modality to succeed at all in the commercial marketplace, researchers had to methodically compete against established CT (and to a lesser extent MRI) for the oncology imaging market. In designing and performing these comparison studies, it became evident that the data were complementary, and radiologists who were involved in these studies found both datasets provided the most accurate diagnoses and beneficial patient management decisions. The first integrated PET/CT instrument was designed and built by Townsend (28). The motivation was beyond the above-mentioned attenuation correction, anatomical context, and logistical convenience. The designers wanted to provide state-of-the-art CT and PET for the physicians to give them the best opportunity to optimally and economically manage the patient's case. The modality of PET would go from a position of competing with CT for oncology patient volume to complementing and strengthening CT—a "win-win" situation for both modalities. As of 2007, nuclear medicine market reports show virtually no market for stand-alone PET—all PET installations are now multimodality only. This success story demonstrates the need for complementary clinical information for the conception and design of future multimodality instruments.

Next Generation Clinical Multimodality

Since the unquestionable commercial success of PET/CT at the turn of the century, strategic planners and researchers have been trying to design the next clinical multimodality system. The most visible efforts have been those of the Siemens Healthcare group toward PET/MRI (29). This instrument has a stationary an MR-compatible PET ring designed for brain imaging. Applications for this system will include Alzheimer's disease using new agents targeted for plaques associated with degeneration (30).

MULTIMODALITY SOFTWARE

The "software solution" is defined as the fusion of the information from two or more modalities into one image display format. Since the early days of nuclear medicine and later ultrasound, CT, and MRI, radiologists have performed the "software solution" in their minds—imagining the data fused and determining the best estimate of the current condition of the patient under examination. Fusion software, therefore, represents a tool to enable and simplify the work of the radiologist.

There are many confounding elements that limit the accuracy of the software solution. The time between studies is probably the largest contributor to uncertainties in fused image sets. Other factors are differences in physiological condition (weight, body temperature, heart rate, respiratory rate, etc.), patient position, and position and orientation of organs relative to each other (especially in the abdomen).

The basic technique of the software solution involves first "registration" of the image data, that is, adjusting one of the image sets in scale, position, orientation, and even shape (for flexible structures) using morphing techniques to match the other image set. Once the data sets are registered, they are "fused" together in a common image display. Usually, the lower-resolution functional or molecular information is rendered in bright color such as orange or red and superimposed on the higher-resolution anatomical background. Figure 5 is perhaps the best-known example of multimodality imaging. This image shows a primary cancer and metastatic lymph node in PET superimposed on a CT background (31). This image received Society of Nuclear Medicine's "Image of the Year" honors in 2005.

The field of "quantitation" of medical images attempts to assign meaningful numerical values to the entities being visualized. Quantitation is distinguished from quantification in that the former represents absolute measures and the latter provides qualitative, comparative, or relative values. Initially, CT scans quantified the attenuation properties of tissues into Hounsfield units. Quantitation in nuclear imaging requires an accurate estimate of the attenuation properties of surrounding tissues in order to account for loss of signal through attenuation and scatter. The standardized uptake value (SUV) (32) in FDG PET imaging is the best-known quantitative measure in nuclear imaging.

Combining a high-resolution anatomical modality with a lower-resolution functional or molecular modality brings up the question of using the high-resolution information to augment the reconstruction of the low-resolution data. This is generally known as the use of "anatomical priors" (33,34) in enhancement of reconstruction and is a popular current research topic. It is anticipated that as simultaneous image acquisition techniques

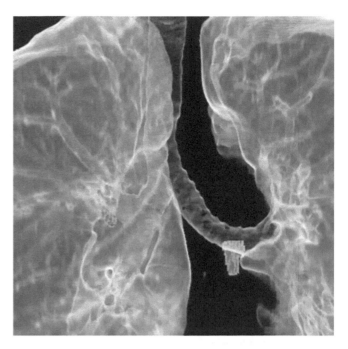

Figure 5 2005 Society of Nuclear Medicine "Image of the Year." This is a PET/CT scan showing the primary cancer lesion (*right*) and mediastinal lymph node metastasis (*left*). The backdrop of the transparently rendered CT scan of the lung makes this image especially impressive as a demonstration of the power of dual-modality imaging. *Source*: From Ref. 31 and Drs. Quon and Gambhir, Molecular Imaging Program at Stanford (with permission) (*See Color Insert*).

(see section on Multimodality Hardware below) are perfected, anatomical priors techniques will enable resolution improvements in PET and SPECT with minimal artifacts.

MULTIMODALITY HARDWARE

Cell phones, digital cameras, video viewers, and MP3 audio players are rapidly converging onto a common "multifunctional" handheld device. These are the descendents of cassette tape players that where combined with AM/FM transistor radios and first introduced in the early 1980s. In the field of medical imaging instrumentation, the combination of modalities into one system usually means that a valuable instrument with potential high duty cycle is necessarily not being used while the other modality is active. The low production cost of miniaturized handheld entertainment allows for features to be seldom or rarely used without being detriment to the user. In the field of medical imaging, the relatively high cost of each modality and the clinic space it occupies demands minimal "down time" during which any equipment is idle.

To achieve commercial and clinical success, PET/CT therefore had to surmount this significant financial barrier. CT scanners were scanning as many as 24 patients per day at some institutions, and the relatively long acquisition time of PET would limit the productivity of the CT scanner alone. Beneficial (and often less costly) changes in patient management, clinical efficacy, and improved outcomes (21) definitively counterbalanced the inefficiency of CT downtime.

There are at least three ways to combine imaging modalities. The first is the linear combination of placing one modality side by side with the other and using a common bed. This is the idea behind PET/CT, and following a few years later, SPECT/CT. The second is to use a single detection system to acquire two (or more) image sets that can be called separate "modalities" since they answer different questions. A third way to combine modalities is to integrate the acquisition methods such that there is synergistic coupling between the two modalities. The first method, the linear combination of modalities, has been reviewed in section Clinical Multimodality Imaging. We expand on the second and third methods in this section.

The use of the same detection equipment to acquire multiple image sets is best demonstrated in the field of nuclear imaging, namely, with single photon SPECT using NaI (Tl) scintillators combined with PMTs. The first PET scanners were actually NaI (Tl) crystals with special coincidence electronics (35). Since PET, SPECT, and CT all involve the detection of photons in the energy range between ~ 50 and 511 keV, the desire to expand the electronic functionality of one modality, for example, SPECT, to enable PET is natural. SPECT/PET prototypes have been built and products have been introduced to the clinical and research marketplace with little success. The first attempts involved the straightforward use of "high energy collimators" to acquire positron-annihilation photons of 511 keV in the single-photon mode. This was mainly for cardiac imaging (36). Dual-headed SPECT detectors are capable of acquiring 511-keV coincidence images simultaneously with 140-keV images from a ^{99m}Tc-labeled isotope through a low energy collimator (37). This "dual-isotope" capability of SPECT can be seen to be an elegant way of combining SPECT with PET. The SPECT camera electronics must be modified to perform *coincidence* PET, and simultaneity is possible because the low energy collimator is relatively transparent to the 511-keV photons. Several vendors offered a thicker NaI (Tl) crystal (usually 2.54 cm) and engineered a "coincidence mode" SPECT product (38,39). Both SPECT and PET quality were compromised compared with the separate, dedicated modalities, and when reimbursement of coincidence PET was withdrawn in 2002 (40), the demand for this product vanished. Another SPECT/PET device that was investigated was a high-performance phoswich combination of lutetium orthosilicate/yttrium orthosilicate (LSO/YSO) and LSO/NaI scintillators (41) that promised large axial field of view and high quality PET without

compromising SPECT quality. Because it was developed in the same timeframe as PET/CT, however, it has not generated sufficient interest to be offered in the market—likely because PET and CT together provide improved clinical efficacy, whereas PET and SPECT combined in this manner provide only flexibility in functionality.

The field of preclinical animal imaging is perhaps the best place to discover a winning combination of PET and SPECT hardware. This is because the volume of detector is much smaller than that required for human imaging, thereby limiting the cost. Full rings of PET detectors are routinely produced for preclinical imaging. Cylindrical sleeve collimator inserts with multiple pinholes provide a simple way to produce single photon images (42,43). We note that in the clinic, attempts were made to add PET functionality to existing SPECT systems. In contrast, in the preclinical application, SPECT functionality is being added to existing PET ring designs. This research is currently in progress, energy and spatial resolution of PET rings must improve for the quality of the micro-SPECT images to approach that of dedicated micro-SPECT instrumentation.

The ability of radiation detectors to discriminate photon energies provides powerful functionality. Some SPECT radionuclides, such as ^{67}Ga, emit multiple photons of different energies that can be used to improve image quality via counting statistics compared with that obtained when only one photon energy is used to form the image. When two energy windows are applied to two *different* radionuclides, the probing of separate biological processes with two different contrast-generating pharmaceuticals can be realized. This is analogous to "hyperspectral cytometry" in biomedical microscopy research as mentioned in section Multimodality Imaging. Figure 6 demonstrates the use of three radionuclides in the preclinical (mouse) imaging application in combination with a CT scan that depicts bone surfaces. The ^{99m}Tc-labeled bone agent, methylene diphosphonate, is superimposed on the CT (orange); ^{201}Tl chloride is taken up in myocardial perfusion (green); and sodium iodide (^{123}I) is taken up in the thyroid (blue). The fact that separate biological processes can be probed simultaneously with the same detection equipment, created by a simple electronic sorting by energy, makes SPECT one of the most promising multimodality technologies. It should be noted that the SPECT detectors must have high-energy resolution to ensure that there is little overlap of the detected photon spectra. Semiconductor CZT (44) operates at room temperature and has superior energy resolution to NaI (Tl) by about a factor of two. CZT will therefore be an enabling technology for the multi-isotope applications in preclinical research.

SPECT/CT and PET/CT using the same instrument is another example of second method of combining modalities. Hasegawa (24) was the first to propose and build a

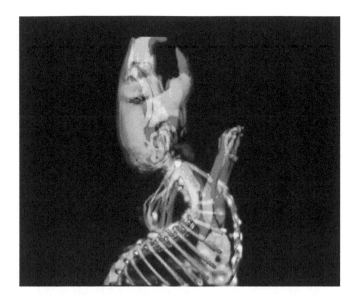

Figure 6 Tri-isotope SPECT image combined with surface-rendered CT of a mouse. The thyroid uptake of ^{123}I is shown in blue; the myocardial uptake of ^{201}Tl is shown in green; the bone uptake (superimposed with the bones depicted by CT) of ^{99m}Tc methylene diphosphonate is shown in the orange. Three biological processes can be depicted simultaneously with SPECT, with the CT providing an excellent anatomical backdrop (*See Color Insert*).

system that could acquire CT data from an X-ray source as well as SPECT data through a collimator. This approach is technologically challenging because of the vast differences in photon fluxes between nuclear and X-ray CT. Fortunately, as pixel size is diminished and electronics are miniaturized, there is a point at which "counts per pixel" (a diminishing function of pixel size) and "count rate capability" (an increasing function of electronic sophistication) are able to handle the disparate photon fluxes. This point is now being approached from two directions, that is, (*i*) PET scintillators have necessarily high count-rate capabilities (to handle singles detection), and these electronic front-ends are now being engineered to handle X-ray photons for CT imaging (45); (*ii*) the field of "color CT" or dispersive X-ray detection using ultrafast semiconductor detectors and electronic acquisition systems (46). Considering the need for a collimator to form the image in SPECT, it appears that PET and CT using the same hardware can be more easily implemented.

Synergy in Hardware

The third way to combine imaging modalities is by designing them to be integrated from the basic image formation principles. SPECT/MRI is a combination that is currently being developed (19,47,48). The use of semiconductor CZT for the SPECT detector is key to enable this combination; PMTs of conventional SPECT systems

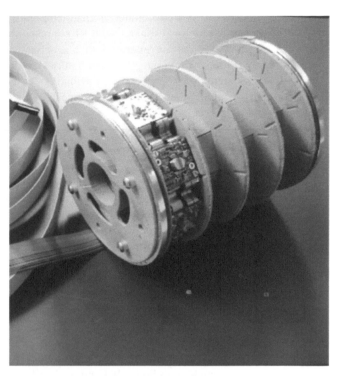

Figure 7 MR-compatible SPECT prototype based on rings of eight CZT modules arranged in an octagonal configuration around a sleeve-collimator/RF coil. When three rings are populated, 24 modules focus to provide regional tomography of a mouse of a volume of about 2.5-cm diameter. When four rings are populated, whole-body mouse imaging is enabled using 32 CZT modules. The outer diameter of this system is 12 cm. *Abbreviations*: CZT, cadmium zinc telluride; RF, radio frequency.

(and PET systems as well) cannot operate in strong magnetic fields. The small-animal imaging system being developed by Gamma Medica-Ideas (Northridge, California) for small-animal imaging is shown in Figure 7. This system is compact enough to fit into a 12-cm diameter gradient bore and is limited to mouse imaging only. In designing the collimator sleeve with pinholes for this system, our research group found that a special RF coil design is necessary to fit into the volume between the mouse and the collimator sleeve. Although special engineering measures must be taken to design the RF coil to perform similarly to when the collimator is not present, one can envision the possibility that the presence of a collimator's special materials could enhance the MRI performance. Another example is MR elastography (MRE) and single-photon nuclear imaging (SPECT) of the human breast. In this case, the compression paddles for SPECT would have acoustic drivers for MRE integrated into their design. In both modalities, the best images are obtained with the acoustic drivers and the compression paddles in contact with the skin of the patient. Another synergistic approach to SPECT/MRI would be a SPECT detector material that temporarily changes magnetic state (or resonates with RF) in response to conversion of gamma-ray energy into magnetization states. In this approach, the image formation infrastructure of the MRI system is exploited by contributing to the detection of gamma rays and the measurement of their energies and locations.

Sequential vs. Simultaneous Image Acquisitions

The linear, side-by-side designs of PET/CT and SPECT/CT enable sequential acquisition only, that is, the acquisition of one modality must necessarily precede the other. The advantages over separate instrument imaging are: misalignment is kept to a minimum; patient preparation time is reduced; and data formats and displays are provided by the same equipment vendor.

The advantages to simultaneous imaging are: duty cycles for each modality are higher and exact physiological conditions exist during acquisitions. The kinetics and dynamics of either "cocktails" (mixtures of dual-modality contrast agents) or multiply-labeled contrast agents, for example, a nanoparticle with both MRI and nuclear labels attached or within, can be analyzed best when images are acquired simultaneously because time-dependent behaviors are synchronized. In simultaneous imaging, the experimental variables are reduced, and any changes in patient stress, heartbeat, or respiratory rate are taken into account. As mentioned in the preceding section, SPECT/MRI and PET/MRI are the most promising combinations for simultaneous imaging since there are fundamental differences in their acquisition methods that minimize cross-modality interference. Since CT also uses photon detectors but has much higher photon fluxes, it is technically very challenging to simultaneously acquire in CT and nuclear modes and maintain linearity and accuracy of detector response. Many optical techniques have the advantage of being able to simultaneously acquire images from different wavelength. As we have discussed above, SPECT also has this advantage but within a higher, more penetrating photon energy range. Because different radiolabeled pharmaceuticals can probe different biological processes simultaneously, SPECT is promising as a multimodality research tool, especially in combination with an anatomical (CT) or functional (MRI) modality.

CONCLUSION

The field of radiology has progressed from the early days of X-ray film to multiple electronic and computerized modalities. Radiologists have adapted to the each new modality by broadening the scope of questions that can be answered. Multimodality medical imaging represents a physical instantiation of the abstract knowledge of radiology; the sharpest, most accurate images can be depicted clearly rather than imagined from experience. Indeed, "imagined fusion" in radiology first appeared at least 45 years ago as recalled by Wagner (6):

> As long ago as 1961 we combined the nuclear medicine images of regional chemistry and function with X-rays on which the nuclear medicine images were superimposed. Thus, even then, clinical decisions were based on the combining of anatomical and biochemical images.

In this chapter, we have shown how multimodality clinical imaging results from fundamental research efforts beginning with cellular microscopy and ascending through preclinical, small-animal imaging toward clinical human imaging. As the size of the structures and subjects being imaged increases, it becomes necessary to replace optical microscopy with more penetrating X-ray and gamma-ray imaging when probing for specific molecular and cellular interactions.

When a single patient bed moves between two modalities, such as PET and CT, advantages in removal of artifacts from time-dependent changes, and importantly, coordination of acquisition and integration of reconstruction and display software outweigh the disadvantages in reduced duty-cycle utilization. Simultaneous multimodality awaits development and is best realized when the acquisition methods are substantially different, such as with MRI and nuclear medicine imaging. Using multiple wavelengths in optical imaging or multiple photon energies in SPECT provides an elegant way for a single modality to view multiple biological processes simultaneously. In multimodality medical imaging, anatomical structure, functional environment, cellular dynamics, and molecular interactions can all be visualized and thereby understood and acted upon for the benefit of the patient.

ACKNOWLEDGMENTS

The authors wish to thank David Wilk, Samir Chowdhury, Kevin Parnham, Gunnar Maehlum, David Lapointe, Roger Lecomte, Dirk Meier, JoAnn Zhang, Koji Iwata, Koki Yoshioka, Bruce Hasegawa, and Danny Gazit for their contributions to the development and establishment of the field of multimodality preclinical imaging, as well as their individual contributions to the composition of this chapter.

REFERENCES

1. Hengerer A, Wunder A, Wagenaar DJ, et al. From genomics to clinical molecular imaging. Proc IEEE 2005; 93(4):819–828.
2. Weissleder R, Mahmood U. Molecular imaging. Radiology 2001; 219:316–333.

3. MICAD. 2007. Molecular imaging contrast agent database. NLM, NIH. Available at: http://www.ncbi.nlm.nih.gov/books/bookres.fcgi/micad/home.html.

4. DiMasi JA, Hansen RW, Grabowski HG. The price of innovation: new estimates of drug development costs. J Health Econ 2003; 22(2):151–185.

5. DiMasi JA. The value of improving the productivity of the drug development process: faster times and better decisions. In: the cost and value of new medicines in an era of change. Pharmacoeconomics 2002; 20(suppl 3):1–10.

6. Wagner H. Atoms for Peace + 50 lecture, Nuclear Energy & Science for the 21st Century, Washington DC. Available at: http://www.ifpaenergyconference.com/transcript-wagner.html. Institute for Foreign Policy Analysis energy conference, 2003.

7. Wagner HN. Principles of Nuclear Medicine. In: Wagner HN, Szabo Z, Buchanan JW, eds. Philadelphia, PA: WB Saunders, 1968:3.

8. Cabello J, Wells K, Metaxas A, et al. Digital autoradiography imaging using CMOS technology: first tritium autoradiography with a back-thinned CMOS detector and comparison of CMOS imaging performance with autoradiography film. IEEE Nucl Sci Symp/Med Imaging Conf Rec 2007; 5:3743–3746.

9. Biomolex. 2007. Available at: http://www.biomolex.com/ (Oslo, Norway).

10. Gafni Y, Zilberman Y, Ophir Z, et al. Design of a filamentous polymeric scaffold for in vivo guided angiogenesis. Tissue Eng 2006; 12(11) 3021–3034.

11. Miller BW, Barrett HH, Barber HB, et al. Gamma-ray microscopy using micro-coded apertures and Bazooka SPECT, a low-cost, high-resolution image intensifying gamma camera. J Nucl Med 2007; 48(6):47P(abstr 158, presented at SNM annual meeting, Washington DC).

12. Meng L. Adaptive apertures for microscopic SPECT imaging. J Nucl Med 2007; 48(6):458P(abstr 2116).

13. Accorsi R. A 15-micron resolution imager for soft X-ray emitters. IEEE Nucl Sci Symp/Med Imaging Conf Rec 2004; 5:2975–2979.

14. McElroy DP, MacDonald LR, Beekman FJ, et al. Evaluation of A-SPECT: a desktop pinhole SPECT system for small animal imaging. IEEE Trans Nucl Sci 2002; 49:2139–2147.

15. Iwata K, Vandehei T, Zhou H, et al. Radiotracer quantification with microSPECT-CT: phantom study. Mol Imaging 2004; 3(3):213(abstr 128).

16. Carcieri S, Kuszpit K, Iwata K, et al. Integrated imaging now: PET, SPECT, and CT imaging in small animals. Society of Nuclear Medicine Annual meeting, San Diego, California, 2006 (abstr 1517).

17. Carestream. 2007. Available at: http://www.carestreamhealth.com/en/US/en/health/s2/products/inVivoFXPro/index.jhtml.htm.

18. Wagenaar DJ, Kapusta M, Li J, et al. Rationale for the combination of nuclear medicine with magnetic resonance for pre-clinical imaging. Technol Cancer Res Treat 2006; 5(4):343–350.

19. Wagenaar DJ, Nalcioglu O, Muftuler T, et al. A multi-ring small animal CZT system for simultaneous SPECT/MRI imaging. J Nucl Med 2007; 48(suppl 2):89P–90P(abstr 302).

20. Catana C, Wu Y, Judenhofer MS, et al. Simultaneous acquisition of multislice PET and MR images: initial results with an MR-compatible PET scanner. J Nucl Med 2006; 47(12):1968–1976.

21. Watson CC, Townsend DW, Bendriem B. PET/CT Systems. In: Wernick MN, Aarsvold JN, eds. Emission Tomography. The Fundamentals of PET and SPECT. San Diego, California: Elsevier Academic Press, 2004:195–212.

22. Kluetz PG, Meltzer CC, Vellemagne VL, et al. Combined PET/CT imaging in oncology: impact on patient management. Clin Positron Imaging 2000; 3:223–230.

23. Hany TF, Steinert HC, Goerres GW, et al. PET diagnostic accuracy: improvement with in-line PET-CT system, initial results. Radiology 2002; 225:575–581.

24. Lang TF, Hasegawa BH, Liew SC, et al. Description of a prototype emission-transmission computed tomography imaging system. J Nucl Med 1992; 33(10):1881–1887.

25. Blankenspoor SC, Wu X, Kalki K, et al. Attenuation correction of SPECT using X-ray CT on an emission-transmission CT system: myocardial perfusion assessment. IEEE Trans Nucl Sci 1996; 43(4):2263–2274.

26. Patton JA, Delbeke D, Sandler MP. Image fusion using an integrated, dual-head coincidence camera with X-ray tube-based attenuation maps. J Nucl Med 2000; 41:1364–1368.

27. Even-Sapir E. Imaging of malignant bone involvement by morphologic, scintigraphic, and hybrid modalities. J Nucl Med 2005; 46(8):1356–1367.

28. Townsend DW, Beyer T, Kinahan PE, et al. The SMART scanner: a combined PET/CT tomograph for clinical oncology. IEEE Nucl Sci Symp Conf Rec 1998; 2:1170–1174.

29. Grazioso R, Zhang N, Corbeil J, et al. APD-based PET detector for simultaneous PET/MR imaging. Nucl Instrum Methods A 2006; 569(2):301–305.

30. Lockhart A, Lamb JR, Osredkar T, et al. PIB is a non-specific imaging marker of amyloid-beta (Abeta) peptide-related cerebral amyloidosis. Brain 2007; 130(10):2607–2615.

31. Quon A, Napel S, Beaulieu CF, et al. "Flying Through" and "Flying Around" a PET/CT scan: pilot study and development of 3D integrated 18F-FDG PET/CT for virtual bronchoscopy and colonoscopy. J Nucl Med 2006; 47:1081–1087.

32. Thie JA. Understanding the standardized uptake value, its methods, and implications for usage. J Nucl Med 2004; 45(9):1431–1434.

33. Somayajula S, Asma E, Leahy RM. PET image reconstruction using anatomical information through mutual information base priors. IEEE Nucl Sci Symp/Med Imaging Conf Rec 2005; 5:2722–2726.

34. Chu Y, Su M-Y, Mandelkern M, et al. Resolution improvement in positron emission tomography using anatomical magnetic resonance imaging. Technol Cancer Res Treat 2006; 5(4):311–318.

35. Wrenn FR, Good ML, Handler P. The use of positron-emitting radioisotopes for the localization of brain tumors. Science 1951; 113:525–527.

36. Chen EQ, MacIntyre WJ, Go TR, et al. Myocardial viability studies using fluorine-18-FDG SPECT: a comparison with fluorine-18-FDG PET. J Nucl Med 1997; 38(4):582–586.

37. DiBella EVR, Kadrams DJ, Christian PE. Feasibility of dual-isotope coincidence/single-photon imaging of the myocardium. J Nucl Med 2001; 42(6):944–950.

38. Patton JA, Turkington TG. Coincidence imaging with a dual-head scintillation camera. J Nucl Med 1999; 40:432–441.

39. Kunze WD, Baehre M, Richter E. PET with a dual-head coincidence camera: spatial resolution, scatter fraction, and sensitivity. J Nucl Med 2000; 41(6):1067–1074.

40. Biestendorf J. FDG PET reimbursement. J Nucl Med Tech 2004; 32(1):33–38.

41. Eriksson L, Schmand M, Eriksson M, et al. On the efficiency of NaI/LSO and YSO/LSO phoswich block detectors. IEEE Nucl Sci Symp/Med Imaging Conf Rec 2000; 2:14/65–14/69.

42. Cardi CA, Cao Z, Thakur ML, et al. Pinhole PET (pPET): a multi-pinhole collimator insert for small animal SPECT imaging on PET cameras. IEEE Nucl Sci Symp/Med Imaging Conf Rec 2005; 4:1973–1976.

43. Shao Y, Yao R, Ma T, et al. Initial studies of PET-SPECT dual-tracer imaging. IEEE Nucl Sci Symp/Med Imaging Conf Rec 2007; 6:4198–4204.

44. Wagenaar DJ. CdTe and CdZnTe semiconductor detectors for nuclear medicine imaging. In: Emission Tomography. The Fundamentals of PET and SPECT. San Diego, CA: Elsevier Academic Press, 2004:15.1–15.23.

45. Riendeau J, Berard P, Viscogliosi N, et al. High rate photon counting CT using parallel digital PET electronics. Proceedings of the 15th IEEE NPSS Real-Time Conference 2007:1–8.

46. Frey EC, Taguchi K, Kapusta M, et al. Microcomputed tomography with a photon-counting X-ray detector. Proc SPIE 2007; 6510, paper1R.

47. Després P, Izaguirre EW, Liu S, et al. Evaluation of a MR-compatible CZT detector. IEEE Nucl Sci Symp/Med Imaging Conf Rec 2007; 6:4324P–4326P (abstr M26–104).

48. Goetz C, Breton E, Choquet P, et al. SPECT low-field MRI system for small-animal imaging. J Nucl Med 2008; 49(1): 88–93.

49. NASA. 2007. Available at: http://earthobservatory.nasa.gov/Newsroom/NewImages/images.php3?img_id=3117.

11

Targeted Agents for MRI

DMITRI ARTEMOV

JHU ICMIC Program, Russell H. Morgan Department of Radiology and Radiological Science, Johns Hopkins University School of Medicine, Baltimore, Maryland, U.S.A.

INTRODUCTION

Novel approaches in molecular medicine are aimed at the development of highly specific forms of therapy that will precisely target the lesion while sparing the normal tissue from cytotoxic effects of the therapy. One highly successful example of this approach is target-specific antitumor therapy based on humanized monoclonal antibodies (mAb). The identification of a subpopulation of tumors that express therapeutic targets (such as cell surface receptors) and the monitoring of their status during treatment can help optimize the therapeutic regimen and improve cure. Magnetic resonance imaging (MRI) with highly specific targeted contrast agents (CAs) has a potential to image these targets noninvasively with high spatial and temporal resolution. On the other hand, molecular magnetic resonance imaging of cellular targets is a very challenging problem because of (*i*) inherently low sensitivity of magnetic resonance imaging and spectroscopy and (*ii*) low concentration of the target molecules in living cells. To enable reliable MR detection of these targets, efficient methods of contrast enhancement need to be developed. In this chapter we will discuss available groups of MR CAs, the general mechanisms of contrast enhancement in MRI, targeting strategies, and some applications of targeted MRI in preclinical model systems.

CLASSES OF CONTRAST AGENTS

MRI produces highest spatial resolution and strongest endogenous soft tissue contrast among all other available medical imaging modalities. There are multiple parameters that determine the amplitude of the measured MR signals such as concentration of resonating nuclei (protons), their relaxation times, diffusion parameters, flow effects, and water exchange. CAs are exogenous substances that can efficiently modify these parameters and modulate intensity of MR signals in the region where these agents accumulate, thus generating specific MR contrast. The efficiency of a CA can be measured as a ratio of the MR signal change to the concentration of the CA. Here we discuss three most important groups of MR CAs that can be used in the design of targeted MRI platforms.

Paramagnetic MR CAs

Paramagnetic MR CAs are the most important class of MR CAs that are based on the transition metal, gadolinium (Gd). Gd has nine electron coordination sites, and up to eight of them can be used to form stable biologically inert complexes with linear and cyclic chelates such as diethylenetriaminepentaacetic acid (DTPA) and tetraaza-cyclododecanetetraacetic acid (DOTA) (1). An unpaired electron that has high magnetic moment (almost 700-fold higher than magnetic moment of a proton) induces rapid T_1 and T_2 relaxation in neighboring water protons via near field (contact) interactions and far field due to the fluctuating magnetic field generated by the unpaired electron. To quantitatively measure the efficiency of a CA, relaxivity parameter R is often used. For T_1 and T_2 relaxation, R is defined as

$$R_{1,2} = \frac{(1/T_{1,2}) - (1/T_{1,2}^0)}{[C]}$$

Where $T_{1,2}^0$ and $T_{1,2}$ are corresponding relaxation times before and after addition of the CA and [C] is the concentration of the contrast. Typically, a chelator group such as DTPA or DOTA coordinates eight of the nine electrons of Gd and one remaining coordination site is used by rapidly exchanging water molecules. This results in moderate T_1 relaxivity values of low-molecular-weight GdDTPA/GdDOTA complexes that are in the range of 4 to 8 $[\text{sec} \cdot (\text{mM Gd})]^{-1}$. Interestingly, the relaxivity of the complex could be modulated by blocking the free coordination site with a cleavable chemical group as reported by Louie at al. (2). They designed a "smart" relaxation agent in which the access of water to the first coordination sphere was blocked with a β-galactosidase substrate, galactopyranose, which can be removed by enzymatic cleavage. Following the cleavage of the blocking sugar group, the paramagnetic ion can interact directly with water protons to reduce their T_1 by the inner sphere (contact) relaxation with a corresponding increase in the MR signal. A similar strategy can be implemented to design CAs with polypeptide blocking chains to probe protease activity.

Another group of paramagnetic CAs uses manganese ion (Mn^{2+}), a biological analog of calcium, to visualize calcium influx and cell activation in vivo (3) such as neuronal tract tracing (4,5). In contrast to Gd, manganese is not toxic and does not need to be sequestered in a stable complex to prevent toxicity. Up to date, no molecularly targeted CAs based on Mn^{2+} have been reported.

To estimate a minimal concentration of Gd that generates a detectable T_1 contrast in MR images, we consider a minimal required shortening of the T_1 relaxation time of the order of 10%. For a typical intrinsic T_1 value of 1 sec and CAs with the T_1 relaxivity of ~ 10 $[\text{sec} \cdot \text{mM}]^{-1}$, the required concentration of Gd-based agents should be in the range of ~ 10 μmol and above. Therefore, to detect molecular targets at micromolar biological concentrations, a single target molecule should be labeled with multiple Gd groups. One way to accomplish this is to use macromolecular carriers decorated with a large number of Gd groups. Conjugation chemistry for this type of reaction is well established and typically a free amine group is used to provide a conjugation site for derivatized Gd chelate complexes. Several imaging platforms have been explored as Gd carriers, including proteins (albumin, avidin), dendrimers, poly-L-lysine, liposomes, and nanoemulsions (6–9). Generally, larger carriers provide proportionately larger T_1 relaxivity per molecule; however, their large molecular size may present significant problems with extravasation of the molecule from blood capillaries and diffusion across tissue interstitium to access the binding site in vivo. The delivery issues will be discussed in more detail later in the chapter.

Superparamagnetic MR CAs

As was discussed above, CAs with large magnetic moments induce very efficient relaxation. Superparamagnetic iron oxide (SPIO) nanoparticles were introduced as highly efficient MR CAs. The SPIO magnetic core is typically composed from magnetite, which is an inverse spinel with formula $Fe^{2+}O \cdot Fe^{3+}_2O_3 = Fe_3O_4$. The iron oxide magnetic core is protected by various polymeric coats to ensure biocompatibility of the agent and to prevent formation of aggregates. Depending on the size, the core consists of several thousands of iron atoms and has very high magnetic moment. Because of the large molecular size of SPIO nanoparticles, they have relatively long rotational correlation time, τ_c, and they act as efficient T_1 CAs only at low magnetic fields where the condition $\omega_0 = \gamma B_0 = \tau_c^{-1}$ is fulfilled. On the other hand, strong local magnetic fields generated by SPIO make them very efficient T_2 and T_2^* CAs with typical T_2 relaxivity R_2 in the order of 50 to 100 $[\text{sec} \cdot (\text{mM Fe})]^{-1}$. A single SPIO particle consists of a large amount of iron, which results in several order of magnitude higher relaxivities per CA molecule in comparison to Gd-based agents. Several different SPIO preparations have been tested for MRI applications, including monocrystalline iron oxide nanoparticles (MION), with a core diameter of 4.6 nm and nanoparticles diameter of about 20 nm; ultrasmall SPIO (USPIO), with 3 to 4 nm core and hydrodynamic diameter <25 nm; cross-linked iron oxide (CLIO), classical SPIO such as Feridex (Berlex Laboratories, Wayne, New Jersey, U.S.) with 5- to 6-nm polycrystalline core and dextran coating and ~ 35 nm average diameter (10). Large SPIO particles with polystyrene coating and a diameter of ~ 1 μm are produced by Bangs, Inc. (Fishers, Indiana, U.S.) and are very useful as in vitro cell labeling probes (11).

As with Gd-based CA, larger SPIO particles generally provide higher relaxivity. However, in vivo, the delivery of this type of MR CAs may be not optimal for targeting tissue epitopes. Indeed, traditional use of SPIO relies on rapid internalization of the particles by macrophages in the liver, lymph nodes, and peripheral circulation. Biodistribution of CLIO particles in rats was studied by Moore et al. (12), and a relatively low biodistribution was found in tumors with presumably leaky vasculature. However, high relaxivity of the agent enabled visualization of the brain tumor from the very low background signals of a normal brain (12).

Nakahara et al. studied the delivery of mAb and fluorescent nanospheres to Lewis lung carcinoma models in mice (13). Fluorescent images of distribution of nonspecific fluorescent IgG and fluorescent 50-nm diameter nanospheres obtained six hours after IV injection are shown in Figure 1. Extravasated IgG (arrows) had a patchy distribution; on the other hand, extravasated nanospheres were closely associated with focal regions of tumor vessels. While hyperpermeable vasculature of certain tumors may support extravasation of large macromolecules (14), generally lower molecular weight imaging markers are required for molecular MRI of tissue targets, unless the target is expressed in the vasculature.

Another imaging strategy that utilizes paramagnetic properties of iron oxide is based on accumulation of endogenous iron by cells overexpressing iron-binding protein, ferritin. This method was proposed for molecular imaging of cancer cells transfected with ferritin gene, which accumulate iron and generate strong negative T_2 contrast detectable in MR images. Ferritin may be used as a universal reporter gene for successful cell transfection in vivo (15).

CEST-Based CAs

This new class of MR CA uses fast chemical exchange of protons between water molecules and an exchangeable chemical group of the agent. Selective RF irradiation on the proton frequency of this exchangeable group leads to a decrease in the amplitude of MR signal of the bulk water because of transfer of the saturated magnetization from the irradiated protons to water protons by chemical exchange. Originally proposed by Guivel-Scharen et al. (16), CEST (chemical exchange saturation transfer) contrast was demonstrated for exchangeable amide protons of proteins (17), imino and hydroxyl protons (18). A significant increase in the sensitivity of detection can be gained if a polymer with a large number of equivalent exchangeable groups is used. In experiments with polyuridine composed of 2000 uridine units, the sensitivity gain of more than 5000 per imino proton was demonstrated and the CA could be detected at concentration as low as 5 μM (18).

The efficiency of CEST contrast increases as the frequency offset, $\Delta\omega$, between the resonance frequency of the exchangeable group and water protons increases. This frequency shift can be significantly increased from several ppm to more than 20 ppm by attaching a paramagnetic shift reagent to the CEST agent. Experiments with a model poly-L-arginine/Tm(HDOTP)$^{4-}$ system lowered the detection limit to 2.8 μM in a phantom at 7-T magnetic field (19). This modification of the method was named PARACEST for paramagnetic-enhanced CEST. The major potential advantages of the CEST/PARACEST methods to generate MR contrast are (i) the ability to "turn" the contrast "on" and "off" by applying RF saturation field at the resonance frequency of the exchangeable group, (ii) high sensitivity that can be achieved by using polymer probes and/or PARACEST agents with large $\Delta\omega$ shifts and fast exchange rates, (iii) certain types of CEST agents such as poly-amino acids that can be expressed in vivo by target cells with an appropriate reporter vector (20), and (iv) the possibility to design PARACEST probes with different $\Delta\omega$ values and image them independently using RF saturation field with the appropriate frequency offset.

A similar effect can be obtained by using paramagnetic liposomes loaded with a shift reagent. Fast exchange between free water and liposomal water with shifted resonance frequency across the liposomal membrane generates strong LIPOCEST effect as reported by Terreno et al. (21).

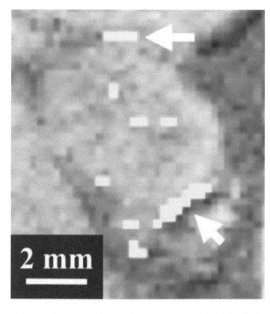

Figure 1 Enlarged section of T_1-weighted MR image showing implanted Vx-2 tumor. Bright areas indicate MRI signal enhancement 120 minutes postinjection of $\alpha_v\beta_3$-targeted nanoparticles. MRI enhancement was predominately, although not exclusively, asymmetrically distributed along the tumor periphery proximate to blood vessels and tissue fascial interfaces. *Source*: Adapted from Ref. 7.

PRECLINICAL APPLICATION OF TARGETED MR CAs

MRI of cellular molecular imaging requires (*i*) a highly efficient and specific targeting mechanism that recognizes cell surface markers and (*ii*) efficient effector molecules or MR probes that can generate strong MR contrast from very small amount of the probe targeted to the cell. Specific targeting can be achieved by mAb, mAb fragments, or specially designed minibodies, diabodies, or synthetic targeting peptides (22,23). An alternative approach is to use proteins that have high affinity binding to the cell marker of choice such as transferrin and transferrin receptor (24) or annexin V(or synaptotagmin I) that have high-affinity binding to phosphatidyl serine residues relocated to the outer surface of the plasma membrane in apoptotic cells (25). While complete antibody provides the highest binding affinity to the antigen, their large molecular size may restrict efficient delivery to the interstitium of solid tumors; on the other hand, they can provide excellent targeting properties for accessible receptors such as those expressed in the lumen of blood vessels (7,8).

Most of the MR targeting strategies are currently limited to preclinical studies due to potential toxic or immunogenic effects of the targeting molecules and/or contrast generating molecules. Nuclear imaging modalities such as SPECT or PET require tracer concentrations of imaging probes to produce an image. In contrast, low-sensitivity MRI requires high concentrations of the CAs that results in practically complete occupancy of the imaging target sites and may induce undesirable biological effect. In this section we discuss several examples of preclinical applications of MRI for targeted imaging of specific molecular epitopes in animal tumor models.

Imaging of Vascular Targets

Various mechanisms of contrast generations were explored for MRI of cell surface receptors. Several attempts to directly label mAb with Gd chelate groups did not produce satisfactory results in solid tumors primarily due to the limited number of groups that can be conjugated to the mAb without diminishing its binding affinity and limited extravasation and diffusion of the large molecular complexes in the tumor microenvironment. Vascular targets have a significant advantage for molecular imaging as (*i*) they are completely accessible to a systemically administered CA and (*ii*) large molecular size of CAs does not limit its delivery properties, although shear forces generated by blood flow may prevent specific binding of large molecules to immobile molecular targets located on the inner surface of blood capillaries (26). Several reports demonstrated successful imaging of $\alpha_v\beta_3$ integrins that are expressed in the angiogenic endothelium of tumors using nanoscale MR CAs. High accessibility of this marker enables the use of large blood-pool nanocomplexes such as paramagnetic polymerized liposomes (8) or Gd-perfluorocarbon nanoparticles (27) that can contain several thousands Gd ions per particle. To image $\alpha_v\beta_3$ receptors in rabbit Vx-2 tumor model, animals were injected with paramagnetic perfluorocarbon nanoemulsion (particle diameter of about 270 nm) containing about 94,000 Gd ions per particle. The specific targeting was provided by $\alpha_v\beta_3$ integrin peptidomimetic antagonist conjugated to the nanopartcle. T_1-weighted MRI was performed on a clinical 1.5-T clinical scanner. Typical results demonstrating a specific enhancement of the Vx-2 tumor neovasculature are shown in Figure 1.

Imaging of Cancer Cell Surface Receptors

Imaging of tumor cell receptors requires efficient extravasation and delivery of the CA from blood capillaries through the interstitium to the target cell(s). One approach that can be used to optimize molecular size of the components of a CA is multistep labeling developed by Paganelli et al. approach (28). With this approach for MRI of tissue targets, macromolecular carriers such as protein or dendrimer Gd conjugates can be administered independently from the targeting antibodies. The individual components have improved delivery properties in comparison to a single large molecular weight–targeted imaging agent. This protocol was used for in vivo imaging of HER-2/neu receptors in a preclinical model of breast cancer using biotinylated primary anti-HER-2/neu mAb and avidin(GdDTPA) conjugate (29). The combination of high receptor expression levels, relatively small molecular sizes of the components, and the amplification effect of multiple Gd ions attached to a single avidin molecule and several avidin-binding biotins per mAb resulted in detectable positive T_1 MR contrast in HER-2/neu positive tumors (29). Histological sections of HER-2/neu-expressing BT-474 tumor model (Fig. 2) demonstrated efficient and uniform labeling of the breast cancer cells with fluorescent avidin (MW = 60 kDa) and biotinylated Herceptin, 24 hours after systemic administration of this antibody, with molecular weight of 150 kDa. No specific labeling was detected in an MCF-7 tumor that expresses low number of the Her-2/neu receptors. It is likely that the use of multistep avidin-biotin labeling system in addition to the specific recognition of biotinylated mAb by avidin-based CA also induces cross-linking that results in a rapid internalization of the HER-2/neu receptors with the attached probe (30). It is also possible that the higher

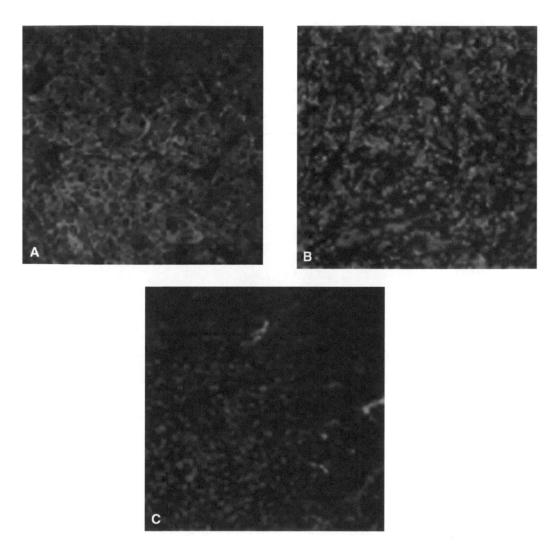

Figure 2 Cryosections of human breast cancer xenografts grown in SCID mice. (**A**) BT-474 tumor section prepared 48 hours after the mouse received biotinylated Herceptin-Alexa594. (**B**) BT-474 tumor section prepared 6 hours after the mouse received avidin, injected 48 hours after administration of biotinylated Herceptin-Alexa594. (**C**) MCF-7 tumor section prepared 48 hours after the mouse received biotinylated Herceptin-Alexa594. All slides were nuclei stained with Hoechst 33258. *Abbreviation*: SCID, severe combined immunodeficient. *Source*: Adapted from Ref. 43 (*See Color Insert*).

sensitivity of this approach resulted from efficient loading of cells with the internalized CA.

SPIO nanoparticles–based MR CAs were explored for targeted imaging of tumor cell surface receptors. One approach used a specific uptake of the SPIO via plasma membrane transporters on the target cell. Iron transport protein, transferrin, conjugated with MION was used to image 9L glioma cancer cell overexpressing engineered transferring receptor (ETR) (24). The ETR+ cancer cells internalized up to 8×10^6 of the TF-targeted CAs within an hour, and MION-loaded cancer cells generated strong negative T_2^* contrast in vivo in gradient echo MR images obtained at 1.5 T, 24 hours after IV injection of 3 mg of Tf-MION to a nude mouse.

An alternative approach relies on the use of SPIO immunoconjugates with a mAb (or other targeting molecules) specific for the molecular target. In a study by Weissleder et al., human polyclonal IgG were used to target MION to sites of inflammation (31). A similar approach was used for molecular MRI of apoptosis in EL4 solid tumor models exposed to a chemotherapy; there SPIO particles were conjugated to the C2 domain of the protein synaptotagmin that binds with high affinity to phosphatidylserine residues that translocate to the outer leaflet of the plasma membrane in apoptotic cells (25). Fluorescent CLIO particles conjugated with the targeting peptide were used to image underglycosylated MUC-1 tumor antigen (32). Combined T_2 MRI and near infrared

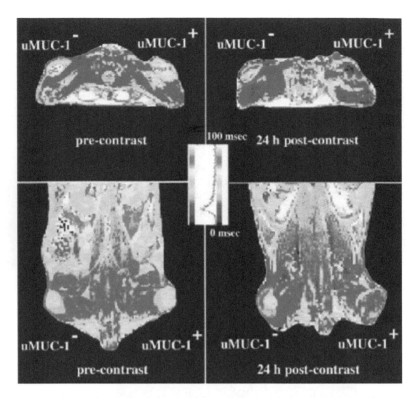

Figure 3 Representative T_2 maps of the animals bearing uMUC-1-negative (U87) and uMUC-1-positive (LS174T) tumors. Transverse (*top*) and coronal (*bottom*) images showed a significant (52%; $p < 0.0001$) decrease in signal intensity in uMUC-1-positive tumors 24 hours after administration of the CLIO-EPPT probe. *Abbreviation*: uMUC-1, underglycosylated mucin-1 antigen. *Source*: Adapted from Ref. 32 (*See Color Insert*).

fluorescence imaging demonstrated a specific accumulation of the contrast in the tumor that expressed the antigen as shown in Figure 3.

One of the potential problems of using SPIO nanoparticles for detection of cellular epitopes is their relatively poor delivery properties. The situation can be more favorable in tumors where hyperpermeable vasculature in combination with long circulation time of the agent results in an efficient extravasation and contrast enhancement. However, the question still remains regarding uniform and reliable delivery of nanosize CAs to the specific receptors expressed in tissues other than endothelial lining of blood vessels.

Functional Imaging with Targeted MR CAs

Targeted MR CAs can also be used to study physiological processes in living organisms. Here we will discuss several classes of applications where targeted MRI is feasible at least for applications in preclinical animal models.

Apoptosis

Zhao et al. demonstrated MRI of apoptosis using magnetic conjugates of SPIO nanoparticles and C2 domain of synaptotagmin I that binds to anionic phospholipids in cell membranes of apoptotic cells (25). Apoptotic cell death was detected in EL4 tumors treated with combination chemotherapy of cyclophosphamide and etoposide.

Proteolysis

An MR-activated CA was designed to detect expression of reporter gene such as β-galactosidase (2). Activated MR agents for other proteolytic enzymes including cancer proteases can be developed using similar approach based on a cleavable protective group that inhibits free water exchange with one of the coordination sites of Gd ion.

An alternative approach to detect protease activity with targeted MR CAs was developed by Zhao et al. (33). They used clustered CLIO nanoparticles with high T_2 relaxivity. Cleavage of linker molecules between SPIO (CLIO) particles results in the release of monomeric SPIOs with lower T_2 relaxivity.

Specific CEST Agents

CEST effect is inherently sensitive to the proton exchange rate between bulk water and exchangeable chemical group of the CEST agent. Therefore, different classes of CEST agents can be synthesized selectively sensitive to pH values (34), lactate concentration (19), or glucose (35). It is also possible to use CEST effect of endogenous amide protons to detect pH changes in ischemic rat brain (17).

Cell Tracking

Therapeutic stem cells or islets can be loaded with high concentration of the imaging probe such as SPIO nanoparticles or fluorinated tracers ex vivo that enables their detection and tracking in vivo in preclinical systems and also in pilot clinical studies (11,36–38). Expression of a significant number of endogenous reporter molecules such as poly-L-lysine CEST reporters (20,39) or ferritin protein (15) in the target cell is another approach to cell imaging.

MR Spectroscopy

One example of using MR spectroscopic imaging was in vivo detection of prodrug 5-fluorocytosine (5-FC) conversion to 5-fluorouracil (5-FU) chemotherapeutic compound using cytosine deaminase (CD) enzyme conjugated to antiganglioside antigen antibody. The enzymatic conversion of 5-FC substrate molecules to 5-FU resulted in an efficient multiplication of the probe and ^{19}F chemical shifts of both 5-FU and 5-FC were detected in cultured cells and in animal tumor models (40). Li et al. developed a novel imaging platform for activated drug therapy (41). It combines poly-L-lysine backbone with multiple GdDOTA relaxation groups for MR detection, fluorescent probes for optical imaging, and cytosine deaminase enzyme for 5-FC to 5-FU conversion. This platform enables detection of the delivery of active CD enzyme to the tumor site using T_1-weighted MRI, and the timing of 5-FC administration can be optimized to the point when the agent has maximal concentration in the tumor. Conversion of nontoxic 5-FC to therapeutic 5-FU can be detected by ^{19}F MR spectroscopy in vivo as described above. One potential problem of MR spectroscopy is that a limited sensitivity and a threshold concentration of the product in the range of ∼ 1 mM is required for detection.

DISCUSSION AND FUTURE

The major obstacle for successful application of MR for specific imaging of cell surface molecular targets is intrinsic low sensitivity of the method. Generally, to produce MR detectable contrast it is necessary to use highly efficient targeted CAs. The efficiency of an agent typically depends on the molecular size of the agent and larger molecular aggregates, such as SPIO nanoparticles, paramagnetic liposomes, and nanoemulsions generate the highest contrast in MR images. These highly efficient CAs can be successfully used for imaging of intravascular targets where there are practically no delivery barriers for high-molecular-weight imaging platforms to the target site. One major problem in molecular MRI of cancer cell receptors is a significantly restricted extravasation and diffusion of the large-molecular-weight targeted CAs in the solid tumor. The situation becomes even more difficult in normal tissues that are generally less permeable in comparison to tumors that are generally characterized by enhanced vascular permeability (42). In tumors relatively large molecules can escape from the leaky blood vessels as was shown for dextran-coated iron oxide nanoparticles in 9L glioma model (12). However, high permeability regions within the tumor are often present as "hot spots," while the bulk of the tumor remains inaccessible for the macromolecular probe/therapeutic agent. Indeed, a diffused distribution of IgG antibodies around blood capillaries was detected six hours after administration; however, most of 50-nm nanospheres were detected in the blood vessels within the tumor, using fluorescence microscopy of tumor histological slices (13). Our current working hypothesis is that an optimal CA for molecular imaging of solid tumors should have a molecular weight below or equal to 150 kD (as for mAb) and that it should have prolonged lifetime in plasma to ensure efficient delivery to the tumor targets. A significant advantage of molecular MRI is that MR CAs are stable substances. They can have relatively long circulation time and accumulation time for maximal tumor/blood ratio without typical concerns of the probe lifetime and radiation exposure inherent to nuclear imaging. The concept of internalization of the CA upon binding to its target on the cell plasma membrane can provide an additional amplification effect by loading the target cells with molecules of the CA.

While MRI provides excellent morphological resolution, soft tissue contrast, and functional information, its main problem is a relatively low sensitivity that requires application of efficient CAs combined with signal amplification to detect sparse molecular targets. We have reviewed several experimental approaches that may provide a framework for development of novel sophisticated MRI technique that can bring receptor imaging into the realm of radiological testing. Imaging of vascular targets appears to be the most straightforward application of molecular MRI because of accessibility of the targets to large highly efficient MR CAs.

ACKNOWLEDGMENTS

This publication was supported in part by NIH/NCI grants P50 CA103175.

REFERENCES

1. Corot C, Idee JM, Hentsch AM, et al. Structure-activity relationship of macrocyclic and linear gadolinium chelates: investigation of transmetallation effect on the zinc-dependent metallopeptidase angiotensin-converting enzyme. J Magn Reson Imaging 1998; 8:695–702.

2. Louie AY, Huber MM, Ahrens ET, et al. In vivo visualization of gene expression using magnetic resonance imaging. Nat Biotechnol 2000; 18:321–325.

3. Pautler RG, Silva AC, Koretsky AP. In vivo neuronal tract tracing using manganese-enhanced magnetic resonance imaging. Magn Reson Med 1998; 40:740–748.

4. Wadghiri YZ, Blind JA, Duan X, et al. Manganese-enhanced magnetic resonance imaging (MEMRI) of mouse brain development. NMR Biomed 2004; 17:613–619.

5. Koretsky AP, Silva AC. Manganese-enhanced magnetic resonance imaging (MEMRI). NMR Biomed 2004; 17:527–531.

6. Uzgiris EE, Cline H, Moasser B, et al. Conformation and structure of polymeric contrast agents for medical imaging. Biomacromolecules 2004; 5:54–61.

7. Winter PM, Caruthers SD, Kassner A, et al. Molecular imaging of angiogenesis in nascent Vx-2 rabbit tumors using a novel alpha(nu)beta3-targeted nanoparticle and 1.5 tesla magnetic resonance imaging. Cancer Res 2003; 63:5838–5843.

8. Sipkins DA, Cheresh DA, Kazemi MR, et al. Detection of tumor angiogenesis in vivo by alphaVbeta3-targeted magnetic resonance imaging. Nat Med 1998; 4:623–626.

9. Artemov D, Mori N, Ravi R, et al. MR molecular imaging of Her-2/Neu receptor with Gd based targeted contrast agent. In: International Society for Magnetic Resonance in Medicine, Honolulu, 2002:390.

10. Jung CW, Jacobs P. Physical and chemical properties of superparamagnetic iron oxide MR contrast agents: ferumoxides, ferumoxtran, ferumoxsil. Magn Reson Imaging 1995; 13:661–674.

11. Shapiro EM, Skrtic S, Sharer K, et al. MRI detection of single particles for cellular imaging. Proc Natl Acad Sci U S A 2004; 101:10901–10906.

12. Moore A, Marecos E, Bogdanov A Jr., et al. Tumoral distribution of long-circulating dextran-coated iron oxide nanoparticles in a rodent model. Radiology 2000; 214:568–574.

13. Nakahara T, Norberg SM, Shalinsky DR, et al. Effect of inhibition of vascular endothelial growth factor signaling on distribution of extravasated antibodies in tumors. Cancer Res 2006; 66:1434–1445.

14. Monsky WL, Fukumura D, Gohongi T, et al. Augmentation of transvascular transport of macromolecules and nanoparticles in tumors using vascular endothelial growth factor. Cancer Res 1999; 59:4129–4135.

15. Cohen B, Dafni H, Meir G, et al. Ferritin as an endogenous MRI reporter for noninvasive imaging of gene expression in C6 glioma tumors. Neoplasia 2005; 7:109–117.

16. Guivel-Scharen V, Sinnwell T, Wolff SD, et al. Detection of proton chemical exchange between metabolites and water in biological tissues. J Magn Reson 1998; 133:36–45.

17. Zhou J, Payen JF, Wilson DA, et al. Using the amide proton signals of intracellular proteins and peptides to detect pH effects in MRI. Nat Med 2003; 9:1085–1090.

18. Snoussi K, Bulte JW, Gueron M, et al. Sensitive CEST agents based on nucleic acid imino proton exchange: detection of poly(rU) and of a dendrimer-poly(rU) model for nucleic acid delivery and pharmacology. Magn Reson Med 2003; 49:998–1005.

19. Aime S, Delli Castelli D, Terreno E. Supramolecular adducts between poly-L-arginine and [TmIIIdotp]: a route to sensitivity-enhanced magnetic resonance imaging-chemical exchange saturation transfer agents. Angew Chem Int Ed Engl 2003; 42:4527–4529.

20. Gilad AA, McMahon MT, Walczak P, et al. Artificial reporter gene providing MRI contrast based on proton exchange. Nat Biotechnol 2007; 25:217–219.

21. Terreno E, Cabella C, Carrera C, et al. From spherical to osmotically shrunken paramagnetic liposomes: an improved generation of LIPOCEST MRI agents with highly shifted water protons. Angew Chem Int Ed Engl 2007; 46:966–968.

22. Li L, Yazaki PJ, Anderson AL, et al. Improved biodistribution and radioimmunoimaging with poly(ethylene glycol)-DOTA-conjugated anti-CEA diabody. Bioconjug Chem 2006; 17:68–76.

23. Olafsen T, Tan GJ, Cheung CW, et al. Characterization of engineered anti-p185HER-2 (scFv-CH3)2 antibody fragments (minibodies) for tumor targeting. Protein Eng Des Sel 2004; 17:315–323.

24. Weissleder R, Moore A, Mahmood U, et al. In vivo magnetic resonance imaging of transgene expression. Nat Med 2000; 6:351–355.

25. Zhao M, Beauregard DA, Loizou L, et al. Non-invasive detection of apoptosis using magnetic resonance imaging and a targeted contrast agent. Nat Med 2001; 7:1241–1244.

26. Ham AS, Goetz DJ, Klibanov AL, et al. Microparticle adhesive dynamics and rolling mediated by selectin-specific antibodies under flow. Biotechnol Bioeng 2007; 96:596–607.

27. Anderson SA, Rader RK, Westlin WF, et al. Magnetic resonance contrast enhancement of neovasculature with alpha(v)beta(3)-targeted nanoparticles. Magn Reson Med 2000; 44:433–439.

28. Paganelli G, Grana C, Chinol M, et al. Antibody-guided three-step therapy for high grade glioma with yttrium- 90 biotin. Eur J Nucl Med 1999; 26:348–357.

29. Artemov D, Mori N, Ravi R, et al. Magnetic resonance molecular imaging of the Her-2/neu receptor. Cancer Res 2003; 63:2723–2727.

30. Zhu W, Okollie B, Bhujwalla ZM, et al. Controlled internalization and recycling of Her-2/neu by cross-linking with an avidin/streptavidin-biotin system for MR enhancement. In: International Society for Magnetic Resonance in Medicine, Seattle, WA, 2006:1843.

31. Weissleder R, Lee AS, Fischman AJ, et al. Polyclonal human immunoglobulin G labeled with polymeric iron oxide: antibody MR imaging. Radiology 1991; 181: 245–249.

32. Moore A, Medarova Z, Potthast A, et al. In vivo targeting of underglycosylated MUC-1 tumor antigen using a multimodal imaging probe. Cancer Res 2004; 64: 1821–1827.

33. Zhao M, Josephson L, Tang Y, et al. Magnetic sensors for protease assays. Angew Chem Int Ed Engl 2003; 42: 1375–1378.

34. Aime S, Barge A, Delli Castelli D, et al. Paramagnetic lanthanide(III) complexes as pH-sensitive chemical exchange saturation transfer (CEST) contrast agents for MRI applications. Magn Reson Med 2002; 47:639–648.

35. Zhou J, Wilson DA, Sun PZ, et al. Quantitative description of proton exchange processes between water and endogenous and exogenous agents for WEX, CEST, and APT experiments. Magn Reson Med 2004; 51:945–952.

36. de Vries IJ, Lesterhuis WJ, Barentsz JO, et al. Magnetic resonance tracking of dendritic cells in melanoma patients for monitoring of cellular therapy. Nat Biotechnol 2005; 23:1407–1413.

37. Bulte JW, Bryant LH Jr., Frank JA. The challenge of genomics and proteomics to clinical practice. In: Feinendegen LE, Shreeve WW, Eckelman WC, eds. Molecular Nuclear Medicine. Springer: Birkhäuser, 2003:721–740.

38. Evgenov NV, Medarova Z, Dai G, et al. In vivo imaging of islet transplantation. Nat Med 2006;12:144–148.

39. McMahon MT, Gilad AA, Zhou J, et al. Quantifying exchange rates in chemical exchange saturation transfer agents using the saturation time and saturation power dependencies of the magnetization transfer effect on the magnetic resonance imaging signal (QUEST and QUESP): Ph calibration for poly-L-lysine and a starburst dendrimer. Magn Reson Med 2006; 55:836–847.

40. Aboagye EO, Artemov D, Senter P, et al. Intratumoral conversion of 5-fluorocytosine to 5-fluorouracil by monoclonal antibody-cytosine deaminase conjugates: noninvasive detection of prodrug activation by magnetic resonance spectroscopy and spectroscopic imaging. Cancer Res 1998; 58:4075–4078.

41. Li C, Penet MF, Winnard P Jr., et al. Image-guided enzyme/prodrug cancer therapy. Clin Cancer Res 2008; 14:515–522.

42. Jain RK. Tumor angiogenesis and accessibility: role of vascular endothelial growth factor. Semin Oncol 2002; 29:3–9.

43. Zhu W, Okollie B, Artemov D. Controlled internalization of Her-2/neu receptors by cross-linking for targeted delivery. Cancer Biol Therapy 2007; 6:1960–1966.

12

High-Throughput Screening for Probe Development

KIMBERLY A. KELLY, FRED REYNOLDS, and KELLY R. KRISTOF
Harvard Medical School, Massachusetts General Hospital, Boston, Massachusetts, U.S.A.

INTRODUCTION

Molecularly targeted affinity ligands derived from screens play an important role in furthering our understanding of human disease (1–3), in pharmaceutical discovery and development (4–6), for nanotechnology sensing applications (7), systems biology (8), and the design of molecular imaging agents (9–11). As with all potentially revolutionary ideas, the development of molecular imaging probes has faced several significant hurdles. As is the case with new cancer therapeutics, the attrition rate for new imaging agents is high. Fewer than 25% survive rigorous preclinical testing in animal models (12). This is where the similarities between therapeutics and targeted imaging agents end (Table 1). Imaging agents must display exquisite affinity (nanomolar to subnanomolar) for their molecular/biological targets, show minimal nonspecific uptake or retention (a major factor contributing to low target-to-background ratios), and have sufficiently long half-lives to be detectable but be cleared relatively quickly to allow longitudinal study (13,14). Further, the molecular imaging probe should not exert pharmacological effects. Finally, the tolerance for toxicity due to the targeted imaging agents is significantly lower than in therapeutics since the agent is used to determine putative disease burden in healthy individuals (13,14). It is one thing for a drug that will cure a disease to have unpleasant side effects, and it is another problem entirely to make someone feel sick to see if they are sick. Designing a single imaging agent with all of these features is challenging.

Although the endpoints in agent development are different, the process is similar to that of therapeutic drug discovery. Historically, drug discovery efforts depended on discrete contributions from individuals toiling to identify the active compound(s) from biological sources such as poppy (opium/morphine) or foxglove (digitalis). A large degree of serendipity and empiricism was required for success. This process has resulted in today's impressive armamentarium of drugs, including antibiotics, chemotherapeutics, anesthetics, and antihypertensives (15). Unfortunately, with today's economic and regulatory pressures, this model is no longer feasible. In addition, drug discovery done this way was time consuming, rarely or never elucidated the molecular mechanism of drug interaction, and most validation assays were performed on human subjects, a process that would be frowned upon by today's Food and Drug Administration (FDA).

High-throughput screening (HTS) has the potential to overcome the limitations of the traditional drug discovery methods since it allows the rapid screening of libraries of compounds for precise biological function. For this reason, HTS has become a successful, reliable component of the discovery process today. Technological and scientific advances (combinatorial chemistry techniques, advances in

Table 1 Design Differences of Imaging Agents and Therapeutic Agents

	Imaging agents	Therapeutic agents
Dose	Single	Multiple
Amount	Small/tracer	Large (g)
Toxicity	Minimal	Possible
Effect on target	Minimal/none	Notable
TBR requirement	Stringent	Irrelevant
Effect (timing)	Min–hr	Day–mo
Marker of success	Histology	Survival, symptoms, other
Preferred targets	1. Internalizing receptors	Many
	2. Enzymes	
	3. Matrix	
	4. Endothelium	
	5. Host response	

computing, robotics, target identification and validation through genomic sciences, and nonradioactive validation assays) have driven the development of HTS from one-by-one testing of natural products to today's industrialized automated process of assaying millions of compounds (synthetic or natural) for specific biological activity (16). HTS as a viable platform for discovery is illustrated by the growth of information generated by screening programs. In the early 1990s, typical pharmaceutical company conducted roughly 200,000 experiments (where an experiment is one compound placed on one target) whereas this number blossomed to 5 million in the mid-1990s and over 50 million today (17).

THE COMPONENTS OF HTS

The discovery of imaging agents is a complex multidisciplinary effort. It requires an infrastructure of experts from research fields as diverse as genomics, proteomics, chemical biology, engineering, image computation, and clinical trial design.

The understanding of the etiology of diseases, collections of compounds, automation, and bioinformatics are the essential core components of a successful HTS effort (16). Each core component plays a critical role: understanding the causes of diseases and identification of appropriate biomarkers drive screen design; libraries of compounds are the source of chemical diversity that will generate potential leads; robotics and automation facilitate the number of compounds that can be screened; and bioinformatics allows the data handling and complex analysis required for choosing which compounds are suitable leads.

ETIOLOGY AND TARGET SELECTION

Modern day drug discovery efforts are leading the way in exploiting molecular and biological information gathered through the sequencing of the human genome and the

flood of knowledge about aberrant pathways to develop novel targeted medicine. Advances in molecular biology and the understanding of diseases at the molecular level has allowed insight into optimal targets for drug intervention and, importantly, imaging agents. So, what makes a good target for imaging agents? The targets for imaging agents should be (*i*) readily accessible, preferably on the cell surface, since the plasma membrane presents an additional delivery barrier, (*ii*) expressed significantly different than in normal tissues, (*iii*) present in high copy numbers, and (*iv*) amplifiable to maximize target-to-background ratios (12). The latter has been accomplished through the use of activatable agents (18), where the probe is "turned on" upon binding with its substrate, or agents that facilitate receptor-mediated internalization (9,18), where the receptor is constantly being recycled back to the cell membrane, creating a very high cellular probe concentration. Appropriate target selection is critical for the successful development of probes that meet all of the criteria previously outlined.

LIBRARIES
Phage Display

Phage display employs a population of bacteriophage genetically modified to display a library on various phage coat proteins (Fig. 1). Phage display offers a number of important advantages such as rapid and economical biological expansion (rather than more time-consuming chemical resynthesis), vast peptide diversity, a rapid screening process, and the availability of many types of phage clones and libraries (19–21). Another important advantage is that bacteriophage, unlike higher organisms, have only one copy of each gene, so protein expression is not dependent on the interaction of multiple genes. Each gene leads to one protein and each protein has one gene, i.e., genotype equals phenotype. A clone isolated based on

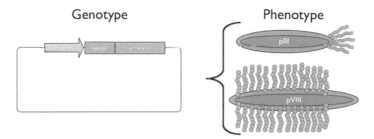

Figure 1 Schematic of typical phage display library generation. Note the link between genotype and phenotype. Sequencing the phage genome identifies the peptide that was selected for its biological activity.

phenotypic properties is easy to identify by sequencing the appropriate portion of the phage genome. The genotype equals phenotype phenomenon enables screening in a single well, thereby reducing the amount of starting material (proteins, cells, tissue, etc.) needed for the screen and also allowing the competition of displayed entities against each other.

Since it was first described by George Smith in 1985 (22), there have been over 3500 publications utilizing phage display. The most commonly used libraries are random peptide sequences, which can be found in great diversity containing linear, disulfide constrained, or various peptide lengths from 7 amino acids up to 15. In addition to the length and constraint, an important consideration when choosing a library is the number of peptides being displayed, as peptides can be displayed monovalently on pIII or multivalently on pIII or pVIII coat proteins. Whether to use monovalent or multivalent libraries is dependent on the end use of the peptide. Typically, multivalent uses generate the highest apparent affinity agents due to their avidity effects, and as such, are the main choice for the development of imaging agents. The choice of libraries is an empirical one; however, the ease and rapidity of screening facilitates the use of multiple libraries in case the screen does not yield a satisfactory outcome. Phage display peptide libraries are commercially available and represent the easiest out-of-the-box method for HTS. A close second in usage are phage libraries where the phage has been engineered to display antibody fragments from the serum of diseased patients. Less widely used, especially as lead compounds for imaging agents, are phage that display whole proteins. These libraries are complex to construct and the synthesis of the subsequent agent apart from the phage is costly, time consuming, and proteins are generally not amenable as imaging agents.

Phage display clones having the highest affinity for the target are enriched via stringent washing conditions after multiple rounds of selection. A number of modifications to traditional phage screens have been developed over the last decade. Traditional in vitro screens commonly utilize purified target proteins immobilized on plates (23).

Alternatively, screens have been performed on live cells with targets expressed in their native environments, which has allowed the development of modified screens that bias toward cell internalized phage (24,25), binding under flow conditions (9) or other biological processes. One of the most exciting recent developments has been the use of in vivo phage display to yield disease- or organ-specific phage clones (26,27). For example, a number of atherosclerosis-targeted phage have recently been developed (28) and endothelial bed–specific clones have been found in both mice and humans (2,29,30). Likewise, in vivo screening for tumor vascular targets have also produced peptides specific for tumor associated endothelial cells (31). In addition to vascular targets, researchers have extended the technology to include in vivo screening for tumor epithelial cells and have found specific peptides for cancers such as prostate (32). However, irrespective of the method employed, it is common for a given screen to yield tens to hundreds of potential phage clones that subsequently require time consuming and costly validation. In addition, once a clone is validated, developing, validating, and scaling-up an imaging agent based on lead peptides can be challenging and costly, not to mention the potential for the synthesized peptide to fail to recapitulate its selected behavior. One of the methods to ameliorate this is to use the phage as a nanoscaffold for reporter molecules. By conjugating reporter molecules to the phage coat proteins, the phage becomes a targeted imaging agent that is replenishable, cheap, and the peptides (or other displayed moieties) are in the context in which they were screened (32,33).

Aptamers

Aptamers, oligonucleotides composed of either DNA or RNA, can be selected to have a specific and high binding affinity to a target. In 1990, simultaneously and independently, three different laboratories headed by Jack W. Szostak (Massachusetts General Hospital, Boston, Massachusetts) (34), Larry Gold (University of Colorado, Boulder, Colorado) (35), and Gerald Joyce (Scripps Research Institute, La Jolla, California) (36) developed theoretically similar processes that they termed, in vitro selection, SELEX, and directed evolution, respectively. Like phage display, the developed aptamer libraries have the advantage of linking genotype to phenotype.

Both RNA and DNA can produce interesting secondary and tertiary structures, have high specificity and affinity, cause quick clearance in the bloodstream due to their small size, and as natural molecules have reduced immunogenic effects in vivo. Nonetheless, some have found RNA to be a better imaging agent because of its intramolecular forces, which allow its own bases to pair with each other to form tertiary structures that have the ability to interact with small molecules and proteins. The con of using RNA instead of DNA is that RNA is less stable and more prone to RNase activity. Modification of the 2′ position of the nucleotide [e.g., 2′-fluoro (37), a 2′-amino (38), or a 2′-methoxy substitution (39)] is a potential solution to this issue. These modifications help stabilize the molecule and decrease nuclease degradation.

The selection process is a high throughput process utilizing a random nucleic acid library composed of over 10^{15} random sequences, flanked on both ends by primer sequences and a polymerase sequence on the 5′ end (Fig. 2) (40). The base length of the random region has been varied but is usually around 40 bases in length, which facilitates tertiary structure but is still short enough to easily synthesize. As in phage display, the selection can be performed on immobilized purified protein, cells, or even, in principle, in vivo. The library is placed under selective pressure for a specific target where nonbound molecules are depleted from the library and the bound sequences are eluted and amplified. This amplified batch is used in the next round of selection and the process continues until there is a population of nucleic acids that have high affinity for the target.

Thus far, there have been aptamers isolated that bind to prostate-specific membrane antigen (PSMA) (41), a trans-membrane protein overexpressed in prostate cancer epithelial cells, tenascin-C (TN-C) (42), an extracellular matrix protein that is overexpressed during protein growth and during other tissue remodeling processes, Dazl protein (43), ancestral to human "deleted in azoospermia" protein in the Y chromosome, and many others. Another aptamer that has been extensively studied and tested and has gone to clinical trials is Macugen, also known as pegaptanib sodium, which is a 2-OMe aptamer that binds to 165 amino acid form of vascular endothelial growth factor (VEGF) with a K_D of 49 pM (37,44). This was found by affinity selection and is now used to treat neovascular macular degeneration. When Macugen binds to VEGF, VEGF cannot bind to the receptors in the eye, reducing signaling and as a result decreasing angiogenesis and vascular permeability. While these examples are not of imaging agents, it is a relatively simple modification to place a chromophore or other reporter entity on one end of the aptamer, as has been done with TN-C- (45) and elastin-binding (46) aptamers.

Taking the HTS process of SELEX one step further, Jack Szostak has developed another method known as mRNA display (47). One of the major problems with phage display is that the bacteriophage are limiting because of the bacterial transformation requirement. With mRNA display, translation is done in vitro so that the peptide or protein can be physically linked to the nucleic acid, so genotype still equals phenotype, but the process of translation has not gone through a complex biological system. The generation of the library begins with the synthesis of mRNA oligonucleotides that terminate with puromyocin, a peptidyl acceptor and a translation-terminating antibiotic. The mRNA is translated in vitro with a commercially available kit until it comes to the puromyocin, where it enters at the A site and forms a covalent bond with the nascent peptide or protein. The conjugates isolated after mRNA display were found to bind

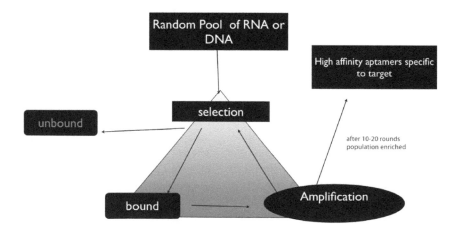

Figure 2 The selection process for mRNA-based technologies.

with an affinity in the low nanomolar range, as opposed to the micromolar affinities found after phage display. For example, 20 different aptamers were found to bind to streptavidin, a commonly screened biomarker, with an affinity between 110 nM and 2.4 nM, as opposed to "strep-tag" peptide (SNWSHPQFEK) found via phage display that has a binding affinity of about 13 μM (48).

Small Molecules and Small Molecule Conjugated Nanoparticles

The potent therapeutic effect of small molecules has been known since the caveman started brewing tea. Traditionally, small-molecule libraries have been primarily composed of natural products. However, drugs isolated from natural sources are often structurally complex, may lack selectivity, and are available in a limited supply. As such, screening with natural product based libraries fell out of favor in the early 1980s (15). To circumvent these perceived shortcomings, combinatorial chemistry was born, allowing the synthesis of thousands of molecules relatively quickly and cheaply (16,49). Today, small-molecule libraries can consist of natural products, pure synthetic compounds with known physicochemical properties, and combinatorially generated compounds (Fig. 3A). The ideal library should be large and chemically diverse. In contrast to phage display where billions of peptides can be screened at once, small-molecule libraries are generally limited to one well per compound. The pharmaceutical industry has been leading this area of research because compound collections are expensive and also the equipment and time needed to screen effective numbers of small molecules are prohibitive for most academic investigators.

Small molecules as imaging agents can present potential problems. Typically, they are excreted rapidly, which limits the bioavailability for agent binding to target, and need to be modified in order to incorporate a reporter molecule. Since non-radiation-based reporter molecules are typically the same size or larger than the small molecule, the chances of negatively impacting the affinity, specificity, or selectivity are a real risk. Radiation-based reporters are appropriate for confirmation but not general screening because of the health effects of cumulative radiation dosing. Recently, efforts have been reported that generate libraries of small-molecule-based imaging agents, where the small molecules are conjugated to nanoparticles (Fig. 3B) (50,51). These libraries have the advantage in that the pharmacokinetics may be more optimal; the nanoparticles are the reporter molecule and, as such, screening with the library results in a lead molecule that is closer to an actual imaging agent.

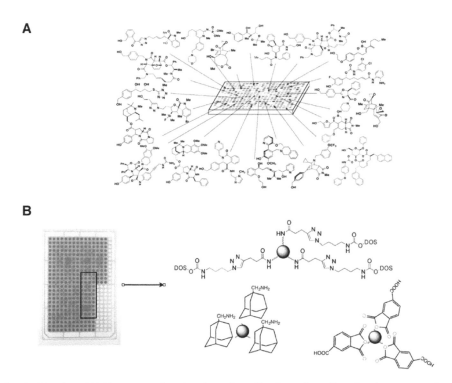

Figure 3 Small-molecule libraries. (**A**) Representative drawing of a collection of small-molecule compounds. (**B**) Library of small-molecule conjugated nanoparticles.

SCREENS FOR MOLECULAR IMAGING AGENTS

There are many factors to consider when designing a screen using libraries of compounds. The obvious ones are what target to screen and what library to use. What is the target that one would like to screen? Knowledge of the disease state allows the choice of an appropriate candidate. Here the appropriateness of phage display versus small-molecule libraries is widely divergent. With small-molecule libraries, while it is possible to find useful compounds with limited knowledge of the affliction of interest by using cells or ex vivo tissue, the odds of the hit (and the expensive validation) being poor are greatly increased. In addition, identifying the binding partner is a difficult and often Herculean task. In contrast, phage display–derived libraries and RNA techniques are more amenable to no a priori knowledge screening as the sheer number of compounds almost guarantees success and the techniques for the biochemical isolation and identification of the binding partners as well as other library techniques such as yeast two-hybrid are well established. For general imaging applications, they are often, but not always, preferred.

If the target identity is known, the screen can be performed with purified material (e.g., protein, sugars, DNA) immobilized on solid support such as immunoplates, bead, in cells that naturally have or are engineered to express the protein of interest, in ex vivo tissue sections, and in vivo.

Purified material has the advantage that the only interactions involved are between the target and the library compounds. In addition, the stringency can be better controlled by vigorous washing, addition of stronger detergents to the wash buffer, and plating less of the target material. All of these are hard to do with living cells or organisms. However, there are also several major disadvantages including (*i*) the inability to screen for receptor-mediated internalization, (*ii*) the material is not in its native environment and may produce artifacts due to its presentation on the immunoplate, and (*iii*) the density and environment is highly artificial and may not recapitulate what happens in the context of the cellular milieu.

To overcome some of these disadvantages, cells can be engineered to express the target of interest or cells can be found that naturally express the target. Screening on cells allows selection for compounds that undergo receptor-mediated internalization and also the material is closer to its native environment. Specificity can be controlled using similar techniques as described with purified material; however, the fragility of the cells greatly limits the stringency that can be achieved. Another advantage to the cell-based system is that selectivity for the target can be factored into the screen since moieties other than the target will be present on the cell surface. Like with all screens and systems, there are disadvantages to cell-based

systems. Eluting with nonspecific buffers (low pH high salt) produces the potential of compounds that can bind to other materials besides the target. To alleviate this, the compounds can be eluted with target material, but this necessitates purifying or purchasing large quantities of target, which may be prohibitively expensive.

In vitro screening has been highly successful in generating lead compounds, but recapitulation of the in vitro properties to in vivo may not occur. Further, in vitro screening does not address delivery, specificity in the background of other cell types, selectivity, and retention of the compounds; all important parameters for an imaging agent. In vivo screening has been almost solely done with phage display–derived libraries, but in principle, RNA libraries can also be utilized if the ribose sugar is properly protected from ribonucleases using fluorine or the more preferred methoxy derivatives. These libraries are preferred for in vivo screening because of the genotype equals phenotype property that allows the identification of compounds in the background of other members of the library, which is not easily done with small molecules. New synthesis schemes that combine nanoparticles with individual tags corresponding to unique small molecules have been published (51), providing a new avenue for future screening if the library can be adapted for rapid synthesis.

Screening has also been performed on cells and in vivo with no a priori knowledge of specific targets. This has the advantage with systems that are less well known biologically. In addition, genomics has outstripped proteomics in terms of target identification, and as such, proteins that become accessible through differential trafficking to the cell surface would be missed as potential targets because their mRNA is static. The advent of newer proteomics-based protocols will eliminate this discrepancy in the future.

Regardless of prior knowledge of the target, selectivity and affinity of the compounds are of paramount importance. Techniques such as negative selection or subtraction on related targets or cell lines (typically disease vs. normal cells or tissues) have been used to increase the selectivity for the target. Affinity can be increased through increasing the stringency of a screen or by optimizing lead compounds. In the case of phage display or mRNA, consensus sequences are held constant whereas the other building blocks are randomized. Small molecules may be modified using medicinal chemistry techniques and often molecular modeling to improve desired properties.

AUTOMATION

Given the large number of molecules that need to be screened, automation, i.e., robotics, electronic pipettes, etc., has become indispensable for a successful HTS effort

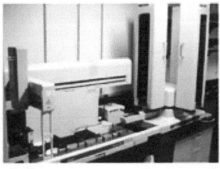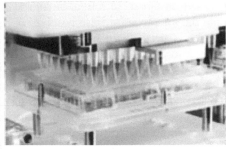

Figure 4 Biomek 2000. A multifunctional robot used for library generation, screening, and validation.

(Fig. 4). There are many places in the HTS process that is greatly simplified by automation. Indeed, without technological advances, HTS as it is performed today could not have been accomplished.

Library generation is greatly enhanced through automation. Small molecules as well as RNA and DNA for cloning into phage or direct use and peptides are synthesized by solid phase techniques and can be completely automated requiring only initial input. In addition, small molecules can be conjugated to nanoparticles through the use of liquid handlers and even the purification is automatable. Small-molecule screening itself would be almost impossible without automation and the miniaturization of assays. The advent of the 384 and 1536 well plates, the robotic equipment (plate washers, liquid handlers, and plate readers), and the highly sensitive event detection assays have enabled the rapid and economical screening of very large libraries. Miniaturization is especially important when the compounds or targets are of limited supply or are expensive. This also allows more replicates for better statistical rigor and reduction of spurious results.

Robotic systems come in various shapes, sizes, capabilities, and price ranges. In this way, there is a system for everyone from the basic plate washer and liquid handler to systems designed to screen millions of compounds at a time. Most systems, unfortunately, are not interchangeable and have limited expansion potential, with the price soaring as more sophisticated capabilities are added. Therefore, much thought and planning should go into choosing the appropriate system for the planned assays (52).

DATA MANAGEMENT AND ANALYSIS

Data flow, the quality of data generated, and distilling the large compound sets down to a few valuable "hits" with predetermined properties is another important aspect of HTS. Because of the sheer amount of data generated, data input, data management, and statistical analysis must be automated. For example, if a small-molecule library composed of 100,000 compounds is used to screen in sextuplicate 10 targets a year, the data generated would be 7 million data points not including reference compounds, blanks, and appropriate controls. All of these must be compared using statistical techniques and a list generated with the top candidates based on predetermined criteria. Manual input of this volume of data, not to mention statistical processing, is fraught with potential for errors and is prohibitively time consuming. If only 0.05% are hits (the percentage depends measurably on the screen and the target), then 500 compounds will be carried on for further validation and potential development into imaging agents, further increasing the amount of data generated. In the case of phage display or mRNA processes, the numbers are much lower. In a typical screen, 30 to 90 of the clones are sequences with a hit yield (greater than average affinity with over twofold selectivity) of $\sim 30\%$.

The key elements for a successful data management system are the ability to (i) store the data points in a usable and retrievable format, (ii) store identifying information about the compound library including source, target, location, etc., (iii) store experimental protocols relating to screen design, (iv) easily analyze the data and compare against controls, standards, other compounds, and potentially other targets, and (v) present the data in an easily understood format to facilitate choosing desired compounds. The management software should be integrated in the screening process such that the data is automatically uploaded in the correct format from the detection device to allow analysis to occur.

Bad data is costly and time consuming; therefore, it is critical to have parameters in place to quickly assess the quality of the data generated. A good data management and analysis program allows determination of the correct signal and inclusion or rejection of data based on controls. Data that do not conform to quality control standards will be rejected and provide an opportunity for the user to correct the flaw in the assay or plate.

The bioinformatics and analysis actually used in HTS is complex and varies based on target, selection, biological properties desired, and the tolerance for false-positives or false-negatives (15,53,54). One of the difficulties associated with HTS screening is to validate which clones are true hits. Analyzing all selected compounds would be costly in terms of time and resources. Conversely, if few compounds are carried through to secondary validation, the chances of obtaining a hit with the correct binding properties are diminished. A common compromise to resolve the trade-off is to conduct a rapid assay on the promising compounds to look at some of the selection criteria. An example would be a simple binding assay. After the data has been quality controlled, it is normalized using relevant criteria, usually background correction, or analyzed using multidimensional analysis based on signal from control wells. The normalized values are then sorted and ranked with hits being selected from the list generated.

VALIDATION AND DEVELOPMENT OF TARGETED IMAGING AGENTS

Once a lead is identified from the screening process, the next step is developing, validating, and scaling-up an imaging agent (Fig. 5). As mentioned previously, when setting up the screen, there is a trade-off between avoiding false-positives and collecting all the real-positives. Is the blue well in the plate a real hit, or is it just random scatter? Validation is the process of using additional experiments on the much smaller data set of hits to window the false-positives from the real compounds of interest and to determine if subsequent improvements actually generate a better probe. These compounds of interest are, by

themselves, usually not a finished imaging agent. They may have inadequate solubility in aqueous media (such as blood), poor pharmacokinetics, inadequate affinity or selectivity, or some other undesirable properties. Development is converting the initial lead from the HTS screen into a compound that can feasibly progress to human clinical trials and FDA approval. Unfortunately, space limitations and the shear breadth of material involved in these steps prevent us from giving much more than the general goals of the procedures.

The first step in validation is to investigate the parameters that were investigated in the initial screen, but in more detail. For example, if, as is often the case, the initial screen deals with affinity, the first validation experiment would be a concentration versus uptake trial to give a numeric value to the affinity. This would immediately expose the hits that are of insufficient quality to take on to development; those that hit the statistical jackpot but were not really binding or those that did bind, the binding was detected, but it was not strong enough to be usable as an imaging agent.

The next step would be to look at other parameters that may or may not have been included in the initial screen, such as specificity and selectivity. On the now much smaller set of compounds, these tests become more feasible than on the entire library.

The last and most costly step in validation is to use more complex systems to verify that the probes still work. While the last step in the validation is an FDA-approved clinical trial on the final, developed version of the compound, the steps leading up to this event will vary greatly depending on the compound (and problems associated with similar compounds in the past) and the disease state. Selection of appropriate cellular and animal models is of great importance at this stage.

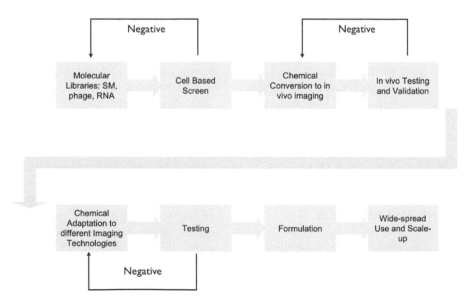

Figure 5 Work diagram depicting validation and development steps.

Development is the art of modifying an initial lead to make a compound more amenable to use as an imaging agent. The lead molecule must be functionalized with a reporter molecule in order to generate a visible agent. Common problems addressed in development are pharmacokinetics, affinity, selectivity, clearance pathways, and toxicity (both cellular and systemic). There is a constant feedback between development and validation; problems identified in validation are solved in development, and the solution tested in validation. Unfortunately, as with validation, the number of potential problems and their possible solution and the ramifications of the solutions are too large a tangle to be unknotted here.

CONCLUSION

Through a combination of various libraries, modern robotics, sensitive and miniaturized assays, and bioinformatics, HTS allows researcher to effectively conduct millions of biochemical, genetic, metabolic, pharmacological, or molecularly targeted agents in a relatively short period. The results of these experiments provide lead compounds for drug design, including the development of targeted molecular imaging agents.

HTS is an evolution of traditional methodologies done in much larger scale to produce more quickly lead compounds for further experimentation. In HTS, the time frame is hours to days not months to years. Additionally, it is an integrated process requiring multidisciplinary effort.

REFERENCES

1. Hoffman JA, Giraudo E, Singh M, et al. Progressive vascular changes in a transgenic mouse model of squamous cell carcinoma. Cancer Cell 2003; 4:383–391.
2. Joyce JA, Laakkonen P, Bernasconi M, et al. Stage-specific vascular markers revealed by phage display in a mouse model of pancreatic islet tumorigenesis. Cancer Cell 2003; 4:393–403.
3. Valadon P, Garnett JD, Testa JE, et al. Screening phage display libraries for organ-specific vascular immunotargeting in vivo. Proc Natl Acad Sci U S A 2006; 103:407–412.
4. Ladner RC, Sato AK, Gorzelany J, et al. Phage display-derived peptides as therapeutic alternatives to antibodies. Drug Discov Today 2004; 9:525–529.
5. Frank R, Hargreaves R. Clinical biomarkers in drug discovery and development. Nat Rev Drug Discov 2003; 2:566–580.
6. Rudin M, Weissleder R. Molecular imaging in drug discovery and development. Nat Rev Drug Discov 2003; 2:123–131.
7. Perez JM, Josephson L, O'Loughlin T, et al. Magnetic relaxation switches capable of sensing molecular interactions. Nat Biotechnol 2002; 20:816–820.
8. Hood L, Heath JR, Phelps ME, et al. Systems biology and new technologies enable predictive and preventative medicine. Science 2004; 306:640–643.
9. Kelly KA, Allport JR, Tsourkas A, et al. Detection of vascular adhesion molecule-1 expression using a novel multimodal nanoparticle. Circ Res 2005; 96:327–336.
10. Akerman ME, Chan WC, Laakkonen P, et al. Nanocrystal targeting in vivo. Proc Natl Acad Sci U S A 2002; 99:12617–12621.
11. Zitzmann S, Mier W, Schad A, et al. A new prostate carcinoma binding peptide (DUP-1) for tumor imaging and therapy. Clin Cancer Res 2005; 11:139–146.
12. Weissleder R. Molecular imaging in cancer. Science 2006; 312:1168–1171.
13. Gillies RJ, Hoffman JM, Lam KS, et al. Meeting report: high-throughput technologies for in vivo imaging agents. Mol Imaging 2005; 4:98–103.
14. Massoud TF, Gambhir SS. Molecular imaging in living subjects: seeing fundamental biological processes in a new light. Genes Dev 2003; 17:545–580.
15. Seethala R, Fernandes PB. Handbook of Drug Screening. New York: Marcel Dekker, 2001:xiii, 597.
16. Miertus S, Fassina G. Combinatorial chemistry and technology: principles, methods, and applications. New York: Marcel Dekker, 1999:xii, 435.
17. Drews J. Drug discovery: a historical perspective. Science 2000; 287:1960–1964.
18. Tung CH, Bredow S, Mahmood U, et al. Preparation of a cathepsin D sensitive near-infrared fluorescence probe for imaging. Bioconjug Chem 1999; 10:892–896.
19. Parmley SF, Smith GP. Filamentous fusion phage cloning vectors for the study of epitopes and design of vaccines. Adv Exp Med Biol 1989; 251:215–218.
20. Willats WG. Phage display: practicalities and prospects. Plant Mol Biol 2002; 50:837–854.
21. Smith GP, Petrenko VA. Phage display. Chem Rev 1997; 97:391–410.
22. Smith GP. Filamentous fusion phage: novel expression vectors that display cloned antigens on the virion surface. Science 1985; 228:1315–1317.
23. Koivunen E, Gay DA, Ruoslahti E. Selection of peptides binding to the alpha 5 beta 1 integrin from phage display library. J Biol Chem 1993; 268:20205–20210.
24. Hong FD, Clayman GL. Isolation of a peptide for targeted drug delivery into human head and neck solid tumors. Cancer Res 2000; 60:6551–6556.
25. Brown KC. New approaches for cell-specific targeting: identification of cell-selective peptides from combinatorial libraries. Curr Opin Chem Biol 2000; 4:16–21.
26. Rajotte D, Arap W, Hagedorn M, et al. Molecular heterogeneity of the vascular endothelium revealed by in vivo phage display. J Clin Invest 1998; 102:430–437.
27. Landon LA, Deutscher SL. Combinatorial discovery of tumor targeting peptides using phage display. J Cell Biochem 2003; 90:509–517.
28. Liu C, Bhattacharjee G, Boisvert W, et al. In vivo interrogation of the molecular display of atherosclerotic lesion surfaces. Am J Pathol 2003; 163:1859–1871.

29. Arap W, Kolonin MG, Trepel M, et al. Steps toward mapping the human vasculature by phage display. Nat Med 2002; 8:121–127.

30. Krag DN, Shukla GS, Shen GP, et al. Selection of tumor-binding ligands in cancer patients with phage display libraries. Cancer Res 2006; 66:7724–7733.

31. Bussolati B, Grange C, Tei L, et al. Targeting of human renal tumor-derived endothelial cells with peptides obtained by phage display. J Mol Med 2007; 85:897–906.

32. Newton JR, Kelly KA, Mahmood U, et al. In vivo selection of phage for the optical imaging of PC-3 human prostate carcinoma in mice. Neoplasia 2006; 8:772–780.

33. Kelly KA, Waterman P, Weissleder R. In vivo imaging of molecularly targeted phage. Neoplasia 2006; 8:1011–1018.

34. Ellington AD, Szostak JW. In vitro selection of RNA molecules that bind specific ligands. Nature 1990; 346:818–822.

35. Tuerk C, Gold L. Systematic evolution of ligands by exponential enrichment: RNA ligands to bacteriophage T4 DNA polymerase. Science 1990; 249:505–510.

36. Robertson DL, Joyce GF. Selection in vitro of an RNA enzyme that specifically cleaves single-stranded DNA. Nature 1990; 344:467–468.

37. Ruckman J, Green LS, Beeson J, et al. 2′-Fluoropyrimidine RNA-based aptamers to the 165-amino acid form of vascular endothelial growth factor (VEGF165). Inhibition of receptor binding and VEGF-induced vascular permeability through interactions requiring the exon 7-encoded domain. J Biol Chem 1998; 273:20556–20567.

38. Jellinek D, Green LS, Bell C, et al. Potent 2′-amino-2′-deoxypyrimidine RNA inhibitors of basic fibroblast growth factor. Biochemistry 1995; 34:11363–11372.

39. Burmeister PE, Lewis SD, Silva RF, et al. Direct in vitro selection of a 2′-O-methyl aptamer to VEGF. Chem Biol 2005; 12:25–33.

40. Pestourie C, Cerchia L, Gombert K, et al. Comparison of different strategies to select aptamers against a transmembrane protein target. Oligonucleotides 2006; 16:323–335.

41. Lupold SE, Hicke BJ, Lin Y, et al. Identification and characterization of nuclease-stabilized RNA molecules that bind human prostate cancer cells via the prostate-specific membrane antigen. Cancer Res 2002; 62:4029–4033.

42. Hicke BJ, Marion C, Chang YF, et al. Tenascin-C aptamers are generated using tumor cells and purified protein. J Biol Chem 2001; 276:48644–48654.

43. Venables JP, Ruggiu M, Cooke HJ. The RNA-binding specificity of the mouse Dazl protein. Nucleic Acids Res 2001; 29:2479–2483.

44. Fraunfelder FW. Pegaptanib for wet macular degeneration. Drugs Today (Barc) 2005; 41:703–709.

45. Hicke BJ, Stephens AW, Gould T, et al. Tumor targeting by an aptamer. J Nucl Med 2006; 47:668–678.

46. Charlton J, Sennello J, Smith D. In vivo imaging of inflammation using an aptamer inhibitor of human neutrophil elastase. Chem Biol 1997; 4:809–816.

47. Roberts RW, Szostak JW. RNA-peptide fusions for the in vitro selection of peptides and proteins. Proc Natl Acad Sci U S A 1997; 94:12297–12302.

48. Wilson DS, Keefe AD, Szostak JW. The use of mRNA display to select high-affinity protein-binding peptides. Proc Natl Acad Sci U S A 2001; 98:3750–3755.

49. Kubota H, Lim J, Depew KM, et al. Pathway development and pilot library realization in diversity-oriented synthesis: exploring Ferrier and Pauson-Khand reactions on a glycal template. Chem Biol 2002; 9:265–276.

50. Weissleder R, Kelly K, Sun EY, et al. Cell-specific targeting of nanoparticles by multivalent attachment of small molecules. Nat Biotechnol 2005; 23:1418–1423.

51. Lam KS, Lebl M, Krchnak V. The "one-bead-one-compound" combinatorial library method. Chem Rev 1997; 97:411–448.

52. Building a High Throughput Screening Facility in an Academic Setting. Available at: http://iccb.med.harvard.edu/screening/hts_facility.pdf.

53. Kim YK, Arai MA, Arai T, et al. Relationship of stereochemical and skeletal diversity of small molecules to cellular measurement space. J Am Chem Soc 2004; 126:14740–14745.

54. Kelly KA, Clemons PA, Yu AM, et al. High-throughput identification of phage-derived imaging agents. Mol Imaging 2006; 5:24–30.

13

Radiopharmaceuticals for SPECT

RONNIE C. MEASE

Russell H. Morgan Department of Radiology and Radiological Sciences, Johns Hopkins University School of Medicine, Baltimore, Maryland, U.S.A.

INTRODUCTION

Positron emission tomography (PET) and single photon emission computed tomography (SPECT) play important roles in the diagnosis and staging of cancer (1), as well as in the monitoring of tumor response to therapy (2). Positron and single photon-emitting radiotracers are also important tools in research including molecular imaging and gene therapy of cancer (3–6).

In this chapter we will describe the fundamental chemistry used in the preparation of small molecule SPECT radiopharmaceuticals. We will also present the elements involved in the design of SPECT tracers as well as PET tracers, which can potentially be prepared with single photon-emitting radionuclides. Antibodies (7,8) and peptides (9–13) labeled with single photon emitters will be covered in Chapter 20. Cancer-related SPECT radiopharmaceuticals, clinical and experimental, will be reviewed.

Commonly used imaging radionuclides are listed in Table 1. Compared to the PET radionuclides C-11 ($T_{1/2} =$ 20 minutes) and F-18 ($T_{1/2} =$ 110 minutes), single photon emitters have significantly longer half-lives; however, I-124, Br-76, and Cu-64 have half-lives comparable to single photon emitters. Radionuclides with longer half-lives have certain advantages. These include the ability to utilize radiopharmaceuticals that have either slow target uptake or slow background clearance, and the ability to produce the radiopharmaceuticals offsite for distribution to the clinic. In research, longer half-lives make radiopharmaceutical development more convenient. Also, multiple parameters can be studied simultaneously (small animal SPECT imaging or cut and count biodistribution) using more than one agent; each agent is labeled with a different energy single photon emitter (14).

The single photon emitters listed in Table 1 can be separated into two types, radiometals (Ga, Tl, In, and Tc) and the radiohalogens, iodine and bromine. Radiometals used in radiopharmaceuticals are either in the form of specific salts (Ga, Tl), complexes/chelates (Tc, In, Ga), or organometallic compounds (Tc) (15–20). Technetium-99m remains the workhorse radionuclide in nuclear medicine because of its low cost and widespread availability (17). It also forms many different complexes and organometallic compounds and its chemistry will be examined in more detail below.

Radioiodine is used either as its sodium/potassium salt (thyroid imaging) or is covalently bound to a pharmaceutical (21,22). Radiobromine does not localize in the thyroid and is also covalently bound to a pharmaceutical (23). The reactions used to covalently attach radioiodine and radiobromine are similar and have been reviewed (21–23) Because there are numerous chemical reactions used to covalently bind radioiodine or radiobromine to molecules, this topic will also be addressed in more detail below.

Table 1 Imaging Radionuclides

Single photon-emitting radionuclide ($T_{1/2}$)	Corresponding positron-emitting radionuclide ($T_{1/2}$)	Beta-emitting radionuclide with an imaging gamma emission
Tc-99m (6.05 hr)	Tc-94m (52 min)	
In-111 (2.8 days)		
Ga-67 (3.26 days)		
Tl-201 (3.08 days)		
I-123 (13.3 hr)	I-124 (4.2 days)	I-131 (8.05 days)
I-125[a] (60 days)		
Br-77 (2.3 days)	Br-76 (16.2 hr)	
	Br-75 (1.6 hr)	
	Cu-60 (24 min)	Cu-67 (2.6 days)
	Cu-64 (12.7 hr)	
	F-18 (110 min)	
	C-11 (20 min)	

[a]Pinhole micro SPECT only.

TECHNETIUM CHEMISTRY

For radiolabeling, ^{99m}Tc is eluted from a commercial ^{99}Mo/^{99m}Tc generator in saline as sodium pertechnetate (Na^{99m}TcO$_4$). In this form technetium is in the +7 oxidation state. With the exception of the preparation of sulfur colloids, technetium in this oxidation state is not chemically accessible for use in the preparation of radiopharmaceuticals and must be reduced to a lower oxidation state for coordination either by traditional or organometallic ligands. The actual oxidation state achieved depends on

the particular reducing agent, the specific reaction conditions (e.g., pH and temperature), and the nature and number of coordinating ligands present. Coordinating ligands L may either be multiple monodentate species or tethered together as a polydentate ligand. Specific examples of clinical radiopharmaceuticals are shown in Figure 1. Technetium-99m-sestamibi is coordinated to six individual 2-methoxy-isobutyl-3-isonitrile ligands. Technetium-99m-furifosmin (Q-12) is coordinated by two bidentate (N,O) ligands and two monodentate phosphine ligands. ^{99m}Tc-ECD and ^{99m}Tc-MAG$_3$ are all Tc mono-oxo compounds and are coordinated by a single tetradentate ligand. Technetium-99m-tetrofosmin is a Tc dioxo compound and is coordinated by two bidentate ligands.

Technetium-99m radiopharmaceuticals can be divided into two classes of compounds, "technetium essential" and "technetium tagged" (19,24). In the former, the ^{99m}Tc is an integral part of the structure of the molecule around which other components are arranged. Neither the coordinating ligands by themselves nor free ^{99m}Tc distribute in the body in the same manner as the intact ^{99m}Tc-compound. All the compounds shown in Figure 1 are technetium essential compounds. The most important technetium essential imaging agent in oncology is ^{99m}Tc-sestamibi. This agent will be discussed in more detail below. Technetium tagged compounds have ^{99m}Tc attached to a target-localizing compound in a manner and in a position that ideally does not interfere with the physiological properties of the biologically active species. Technetium tagged compounds can be further defined by the method of technetium attachment; the radiometal can either be conjugated to or integrated within the localizing

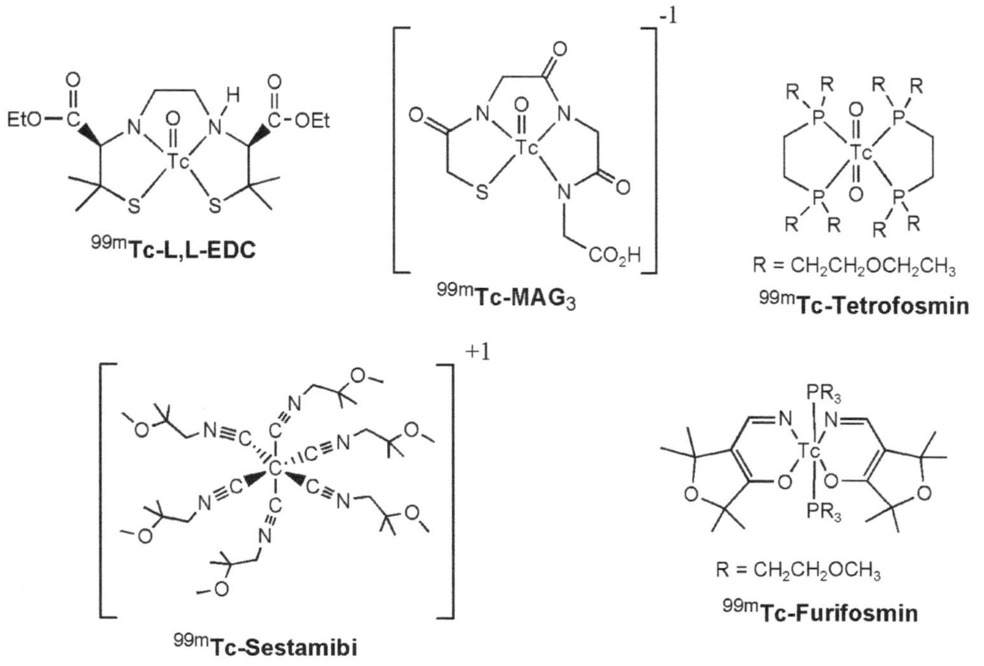

Figure 1 Technetium essential radiopharmaceuticals.

molecule. In the former method, technetium is complexed by a chelating ligand (a bifunctional chelate), which also incorporates a reactive group for attachment to the target-localizing molecule. In the integrated approach the ^{99m}Tc replaces a portion of a modified target-localizing small molecule such that there is little overall change in size, shape, charge, and structure of the resulting compound. Specific examples of each type are presented in the section on estrogen receptor (ER)–binding compounds. Many of the technetium complexes used as prototypes from which to design ^{99m}Tc-tagged pharmaceuticals incorporate a Tc oxo core coordinated by a single multi-dentate ligand. Although tethering together various coordinating atoms in a multidentate ligand improves the stability of the ^{99m}Tc coordination complex, Pietzsch found that the ligand attached to the biologically relevant molecule did not need to incorporate all requisite coordinating sites in a single polydentate ligand in order to bind technetium (25). A Tc oxo complex resulting from coordination by a tridentate ligand and a monodentate ligand is generally described as a "3+1" mixed ligand complex.

In their groundbreaking paper, Schubinger and co-workers reported the facile synthesis of the tricarbonyl complex fac-$[^{99m}Tc^I(OH_2)_3(CO)_3]^+$ via reduction of Na^{99m}TcO$_4$ with sodium borohydride in basic saline (pH 11) under a carbon monoxide atmosphere (75°C, 30 minutes) (26). The tricarbonyl-triaquo complex is stable in aqueous solution over a broad pH range, yet under the appropriate conditions undergoes facile exchange of coordinated water with a wide variety of donor ligands. It forms tricarbonyl complexes with nitrogen heterocycles (26–28), phosphines (29), multidentate dithioethers (30), O^5-cyclopentadienyl compounds (31–33), and trihydro (mercaptoazolyl)borates (34).

RADIOIODINE/RADIOBROMINE CHEMISTRY

The structure of the desired radiohalogenated compound guides the method of radioiodination/radiobromination. Radioiodine or radiobromine is usually incorporated into the molecule at or near the end of the synthesis. Because an sp^2 carbon (vinylic or aromatic)-iodine bond is stronger (268–297 kJ/mole) than an sp^3 aliphatic carbon-iodide bond (222 kJ/mole), radioiodine is usually attached to an unsaturated carbon. Furthermore, unsaturated carbon-iodine bonds are less prone to in vivo deiodination than saturated carbon-iodine bonds. Methods to covalently attach radioiodine or radiobromine directly to a molecule are as follows: (*i*) Direct electrophilic addition to an activated position of an aromatic ring (method used in radioiodination of peptides and proteins via tyrosine); (*ii*) Nucleophilic exchange of radioiodine for either bromine or iodine on the molecule; (*iii*) Electrophilic addition of a specie of general structure I-Y to a conjugated double

bond followed by elimination of H-Y to reform the conjugated system; (*iv*) Electrophilic addition, i.e., deme-tallation using either trialkylstananne, trialkylsilane, boronic acid, organomercury, or organothalium precursors. Examples of each are shown in Figure 2. Direct electrophilic addition of radioiodine to alpha-methyl tyrosine to yield 3-[^{125}I]iodo-alpha-methyl tyrosine (35) is shown in Reaction 1 (Fig. 2). Nucleophilic exchange of the bromine in bromophenylalanine for ^{123}I$^-$ to give p-[^{123}I]iodo-phenylalanine (36) is shown in Reaction 2. Cu(I)-assisted nucleophilic isotopic exchange of nonradioactive iodine in meta-iodobenzylguanidine (MIBG) with ^{123}I$^-$ to yield [^{123}I]MIBG (37,38) is shown in Reaction 3. Radioiodinated FIAU can be prepared either by electrophilic addition-elimination via FAU (39) (Reaction 4) or from the trimethylstannane FTAU via electrophilic addition-destannylation (40) (Reaction 5). Nucleophilic isotopic exchange reactions yield lower specific activity product than the other methods because the labeled product and starting material are chemically equivalent and cannot be separated.

Radioiodinated and radiobrominated compounds can also be prepared by the attachment of either radiohalogenated prosthetic groups or prosthetic groups that contain radiohalogenation precursor moieties like trialkylstannanes to the desired compound. These prosthetic groups can be functionalized small aromatic (41) or vinylic (42,43) compounds. The preparation and use of amine, thiol, and carbohydrate reactive prosthetic groups for protein radioiodination has been reviewed (41). Where appropriate, these methods can be used for tagging small molecules.

CLINICAL SPECT AGENTS

With the exception of technetium-99m colloids, all the clinical SPECT agents have a localizing mechanism, which has been utilized in the design of the radiotracer. The localizing mechanism can be as simple as the similarity of gallium to iron or as complex as the need for a specific amino acid transporter for localization.

Technetium-99m Colloids

Technetium-99m colloids were among the very first technetium radiopharmaceuticals (44). In breast cancer these radiolabeled particles have been used to follow lymphatic drainage after interstitial injection and identify lymph nodes, which are likely to contain metastatic disease. Detection can be performed either by imaging or with an intraoperative gamma-probe during surgery. It is believed that a particle size between 100 and 200 nm gives the best combination of fast lymphatic drainage and retention in the sentinel lymph node. The technetium-99m colloids in

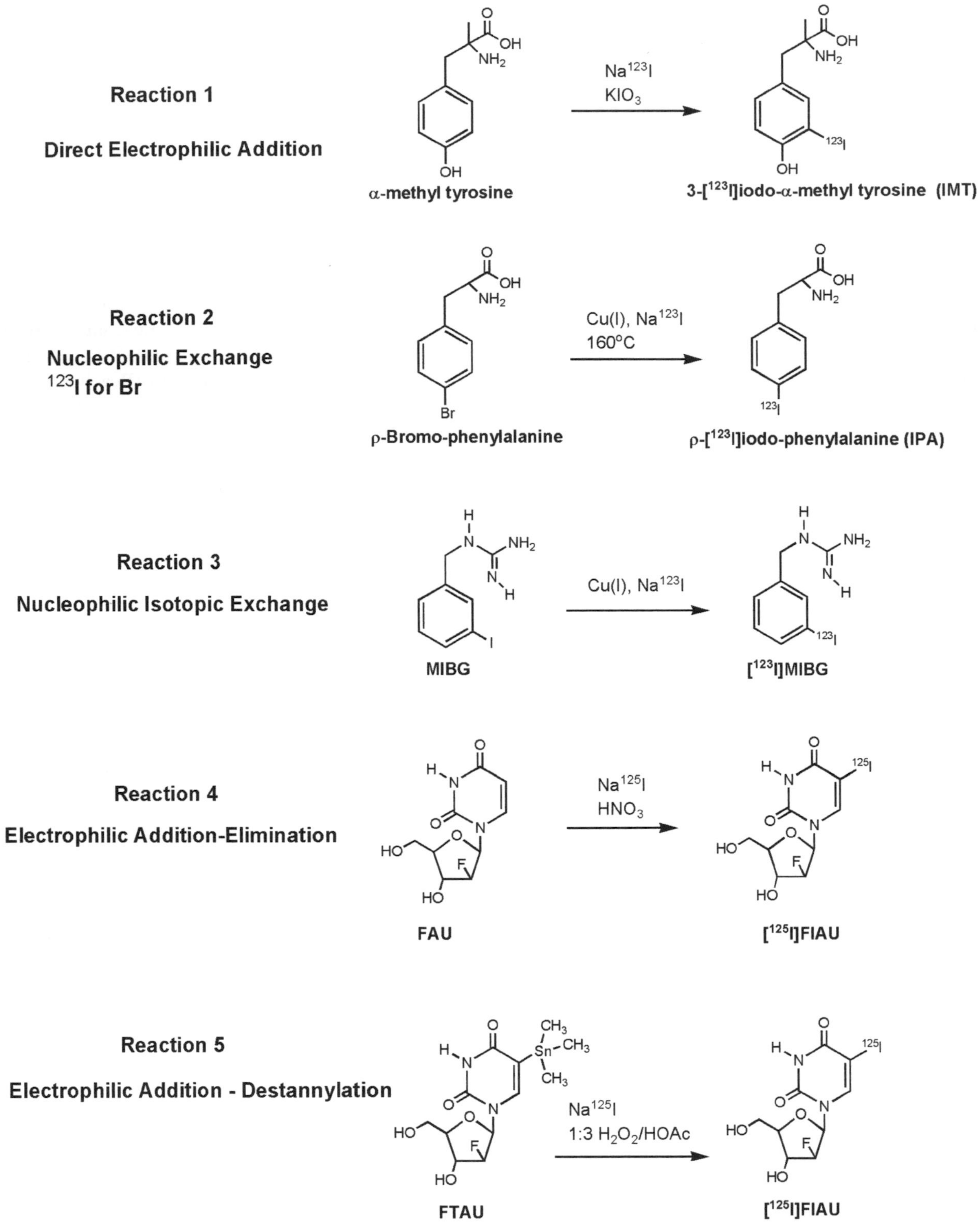

Figure 2 Radioiodination reactions.

clinical use include ^{99m}Tc-sulfur colloid, which has particles ranging in size from 15 to 5000 nm and ^{99m}Tc-nanocolloid human serum albumin (HSA), which has particles ranging in size from 4 to 100 nm (45).

Gallium-67 Citrate

Gallium-67 localizes in sites of lymphoma including non-Hodgkin's lymphoma and Hodgkin's Disease (46). Since

[67]Ga uptake occurs in viable lymphomas but not in necrotic or fibrotic tissue, it is primarily used for monitoring the response to therapy (47). The exact mechanism of tumor localization of ^{67}Ga is not fully understood. Gallium is a transition metal, acts like ferric ion, and can bind to transferrin in the blood. Although a direct correlation between the number of transferrin receptors on tumor cells and ^{67}Ga uptake has been demonstrated (48,49), there is also evidence for transferrin-independent mechanisms for non-Hodgkin's lymphoma and Hodgkin's Disease (50,51). Therefore, tumor localization of ^{67}Ga is probably the result of a combination of mechanisms including nonspecific uptake via the increased permeability of tumors and a transferrin-dependent mechanism. PET imaging with F-18 fluoro-2-deoxyglucose (FDG) has recently been shown to be superior to ^{67}Ga imaging for detecting non-Hodgkin's lymphoma and Hodgkin's Disease (52,53). Therefore, FDG-PET imaging, where available, is replacing ^{67}Ga-SPECT imaging as the preferred imaging procedure for these tumors.

Technetium-99m Bone Agents

The first technetium bone agents were inorganic polyphosphonates containing P–O–P bonds; however, they were rapidly hydrolyzed in vivo and were replaced by the more stable organophosphonates, which contained P–C–P bonds (54). Technetium diphosphonates accumulate in tissues as a function of their calcium content with bone tissue having the highest uptake (55). Technetium diphosphonates act as chelating agents, which coordinate tissue calcium, thereby localizing the technetium diphosphonate in the mineral phase of the bone. The calcium-phosphate molar ratio, crystalline surface area, and presence of other metals are also important factors in the uptake of diphosphonates (56). In general, growing bones and hyperactive metabolic bone tissue including bone lesions have higher concentrations of amorphous calcium phosphate than mature or normal bone tissue, which results in higher adsorption of technetium diphosphonate in the lesion (56). Bone uptake is also a function of local blood flow and osteoblast activity (57). As a result technetium-99m diphosphonates are used for imaging a variety of skeletal conditions including osteomyelitis, Paget's disease, occult fracture, primary bone sarcomas, osteoid osteoma, early aseptic necrosis, osteomalacia, migratory osteoporosis, and metastatic carcinoma.

The technetium-99m diphosphonates currently in clinical use include methylene diphosphonate (MDP, Osteolite/Osteoscan), hydroxymethylene diphosphonate (HMDP, Technescan), and 1-hydroxyethylidiene diphosphonate (HEDP). These Tc-diphosphonate complexes exist as a mixture of oligomers and polymers. Recently, ^{99m}Tc complexes of the tetraphosphonate ligand trans-1,2-cyclohexyldinitrilo tetramethylene phosphonic acid (CDTMP) have shown high in vitro stability and bone-lesion uptake comparable to ^{99m}Tc-MDP (58). Unlike the diphosphonates above, this polydentate ligand built on a semirigid cyclohexane backbone favors the formation of a single 1:1 ligand to metal complex.

Meta-iodobenzylguanidine

MIBG is a catecholamine analog that accumulates in tumors arising from the adrenal medulla. It is structurally similar to norepinephrine (noradrenaline) and the noradrenaline and adrenergic neuron blockers bretylium and guanethidine (Fig. 3). Ninety percent of neuroblastomas show a positive uptake of radioiodinated MIBG (I-123 or I-131 labeled) (59). Radioiodinated MIBG is more sensitive for adrenomedullary tumors than the somatostatin analog In-111 pentetreotide; however, in certain neuroendocrine tumors they can be complementary since each agent had different localization foci in the same patient (60).

MIBG enters cells by two mechanisms (i) nonspecific passive diffusion that is energy independent and unsaturable and (ii) a specific, energy dependent, saturable uptake via the noradrenaline transporter (NAT) (61). The uptake of MIBG is proportional to NAT expression (62,63). There is also a correlation between human norepinephrine transporter (hNET) expression and MIBG uptake in human neuroblastoma cell lines (62,64). Numerous ring and side chain–substituted MIBG analogs have been synthesized and tested but none have produced any significant improvements over MIBG (65,66). It was hoped that polar analogs of MIBG would be eliminated more rapidly thereby producing higher tumor to background ratios. Analogs containing polar substituents on carbon 5 did not bind in vitro. Analogs containing substituents on carbon 4 were active in vitro with the 4-chloro analog being more potent than MIBG. However, it was more lipophilic than MIBG and suffered extensive deiodination in vivo (65,66).

Metabolism Tracers

Amino Acids

Metabolically active tumors have a greater need for amino acids than normal tissue. Cells acquire aminoacids either from outside the cell or from intracellular protein recycling. For this reason many tumors overexpress amino acid transporters in order to increase their intake of amino acids. For imaging brain tumors, radiolabeled amino acids should be superior to [^{18}F]FDG because of low amino acid uptake in normal brain tissue. Also, unlike FDG, amino acid uptake should not be affected by inflammation. Many radiolabeled amino acids have been investigated as

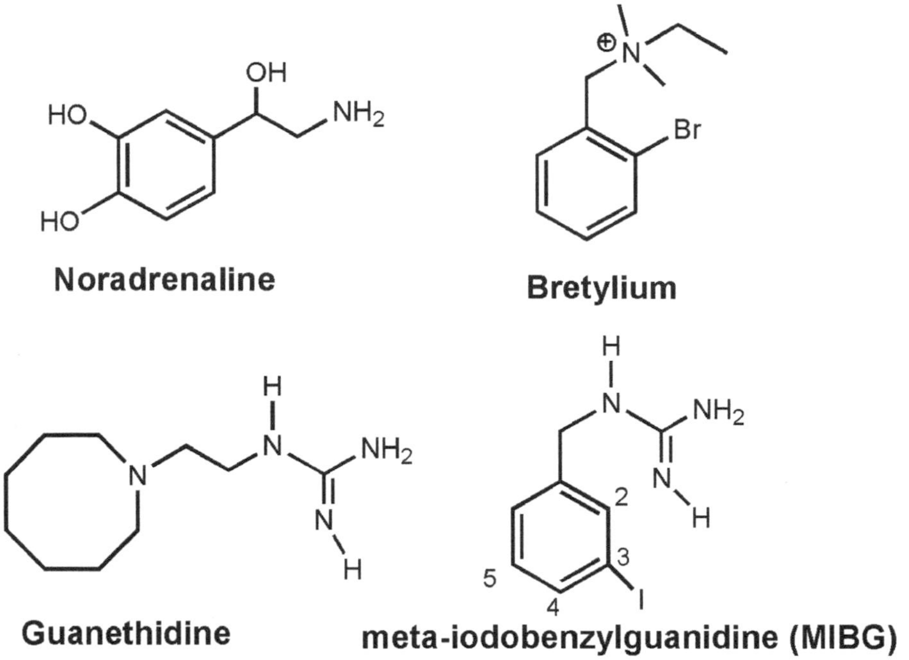

Figure 3 Adrenergic compounds.

imaging agents (67). Most have been labeled with the positron emitters C-11 and F-18 since these atoms cause little or no change in the size and properties of the molecule compared to labeling with bromine or iodine. The artificial amino acid 3-[^{123}I]iodo-α-methyl-L-tyrosine (IMT, Fig. 2) has shown promising results in imaging brain tumors in the clinic using SPECT (68–72). PET tracers [methyl-^{11}C]-L-methionine (MET) and O-(2-[^{18}F]fluoroethyl)-L-tyrosine (FET) are also effective imaging agents. IMT, MET, and FET are all transported into cells via the sodium-independent L transporter system (68,70,73). The L-type transporter consists of LAT1 and LAT2 subtypes. IMT is transported by LAT1 (74). Soft tissue tumors can also be visualized with IMT but there is no clear advantage over [^{18}F]FDG when both agents are available (67). Another tyrosine analog, 2-[^{123}I]iodo-tyrosine (2-IT), is also transported by LAT1. In rats, it had tumor uptake comparable to IMT with sixfold lower kidney retention (75,76).

Two other radioiodinated amino acid analogs p-[^{123}I]iodo-1-phenylalanine (IPA, Fig. 2) and L-8-[^{123}I]iodo-1,2,3,4-tetrahydro-7-hydroxyisoquinoline (ITIC) have been used to image orthotopic pancreatic (77) and prostate (78,79) tumor xenografts, respectively.

^{99m}Tc-methoxyisobutylisonitrile (Sestamibi)

The ^{99m}Tc-labeled lipophilic cation ^{99m}Tc-methoxyisobu-tylisonitrile (sestamibi) as well as ^{99m}Tc-tetrofosmin, and ^{99m}Tc-furifosmin (Fig. 1) were originally developed as myocardial perfusion agents. These agents localize in

cardiac cells because of both the greater number of mitochondria in these cells and the higher negative membrane potential of the mitochondrial membrane (80). They accumulate in malignant cells by similar mechanisms (81) and have been used to image breast, lung, and brain tumors (73,82,83). Although other modalities such as mammography or radiopharmaceuticals such as [^{18}F] FDG remain the frontline imaging choices for breast cancer, SPECT or pinhole SPECT using ^{99m}Tc-sestamibi may provide valuable information on tumor biology and response to treatment. For example, anti-apoptotic protein Bcl-2 is overexpressed in many cancers including breast cancer and correlates with resistance to chemotherapy and radiation therapy. Bcl-2 is found in the outer mitochondrial membrane. It inhibits the permeability of mitochondrial membranes and disrupts mitochondrial membrane potentials. This can prevent or reduce the uptake of ^{99m}Tc-sestamibi. The early uptake of ^{99m}Tc-sestamibi may reflect the mitochondrial status of breast cancer cells such that the reduced or lack of uptake of ^{99m}Tc-sestamibi at early time points may represent an elevation of Bcl-2 and predict a poor response to therapy (84,85). On the other hand ^{99m}Tc-sestamibi uptake in sarcomas does not appear to be able to predict the response to therapy (86).

Drug Efflux Substrates

^{99m}Tc-Sestamibi

Lipophilic cations are also substrates for P-glycoprotein (Pgp), which is an energy-dependent drug efflux pump

(87,88). Several clinical studies have shown that the rapid clearance of ^{99m}Tc-sestamibi from breast cancer generally corresponds with a lack of response to chemotherapy (89–92), although a direct correlation with Pgp expression has not been demonstrated. However, imaging with ^{99m}Tc-sestamibi may become a useful tool in evaluating new Pgp modulators and inhibitors (93).

Radiolabeled Chemotherapeutics

Chemotherapeutics and their analogs radiolabeled with PET and SPECT radionuclides have been prepared to directly measure the drug efflux status of tumors prior to and during chemotherapy. Radioiodinated analogs include daunorubicin (94), doxorubicin (94), and paclitaxel (95,96). Daunorubicin, doxorubicin, and their radioiodinated analogs are shown in Figure 4. Compounds *1* and *2* were prepared by reacting the chemotherapeutic with the appropriate stannane containing active ester followed by radioiodination-destannylation. Compounds *3*

and *4* were prepared by direct radioiodination of an *N*-benzylphenol derivative. Paclitaxel, its stannane radioiodination precursor *5* and radioiodinated analog *6* are shown in Figure 5. Radiolabeling at this position was performed because it has been demonstrated that paclitaxel analogs with a halogen on this position were as biologically active as paclitaxel (97).

Research Imaging Agents

Hypoxia Imaging Agents

Tumor hypoxia has long been recognized as a contributing factor in tumor resistance to radiation therapy. Oxygen is needed for radiation-induced DNA damage. Hypoxic tumor cells can more readily survive radiotherapy and live to repopulate the tumor during reoxygenation. Hypoxia can also induce proteomic and genetic changes such as increasing heat shock proteins and mutations in p53, which increases radioresistance and reduces apoptosis,

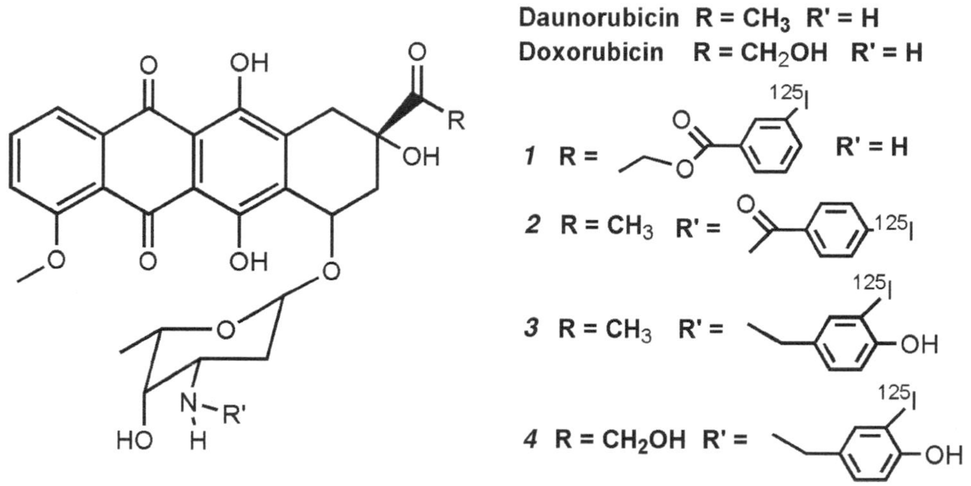

Figure 4 Radioiodinated daunorubicin and doxorubicin.

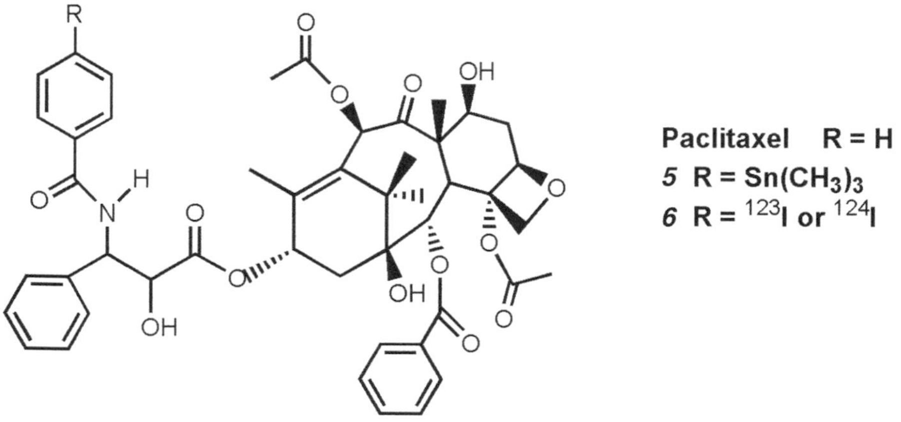

Figure 5 Radioiodinated paclitaxel.

respectively. During hypoxia, the hypoxia-inducible factor 1 (HIF1α) accumulates in cells and induces genetic and metabolic events that increase the cellular uptake of glucose thereby promoting the survival of hypoxic cells. Because many chemotherapeutics are more effective on rapidly dividing cells and hypoxic cells are less metabolically active, hypoxia may affect chemotherapy. Hypoxia alters the pH of tumors so this may affect chemotherapy as well. For these reasons, the ability to measure tumor hypoxia is important in tumor treatment planning. Oxygen concentrations in tumors can be measured directly using polarographic microelectrodes. Although this method is considered the "gold standard," it suffers from sampling errors and is an invasive procedure. On the other hand, radionuclide imaging using hypoxia localizing agents may provide noninvasive methods of assessing tumor hypoxia. Reviews on image-guided treatment planning as well as the recommendations of a recent NCI Workshop on Hypoxia have been published (98–103).

The design of hypoxia localizing compounds has been reviewed by Wardman (104). In general, hypoxia localizing compounds must possess redox properties, which can be activated by reductase enzymes or react to the presence or absence of oxygen. Such compounds include nitro-

arenes, quinones, and aromatic N-oxides (104). The development of hypoxia localizing imaging agents has been an active area of research for the last twenty years. The progress in this field has been reviewed (105–107). Radiolabeled hypoxia imaging agents prepared thus far fall into two categories: (i) Nitroimidazoles and (ii) metal complexes that are selectively reduced and trapped in hypoxic cells.

2-Nitroimidazoles

All the first and second generations of radiolabeled hypoxia imaging agents contain the 2-nitroimidazole moiety. The mechanism of localization of nitroimidazoles in hypoxic cells is shown in Scheme 1. Nitroimidazoles freely diffuse into all cells. Once inside viable cells, the nitroimidazole undergoes a one-electron reduction to a nitro-radical anion. In normal oxygenated cells, the anion rapidly reacts with oxygen to produce an oxygen radical anion and regenerate the original nitro imidazole, which is free to diffuse out of the cell. However, in hypoxic cells the nitroimidazole radical anion undergoes a series of further one-electron reductions to yield nitroso , hydroxylamine, and amine analogs. The nitroso and hydroxylamine

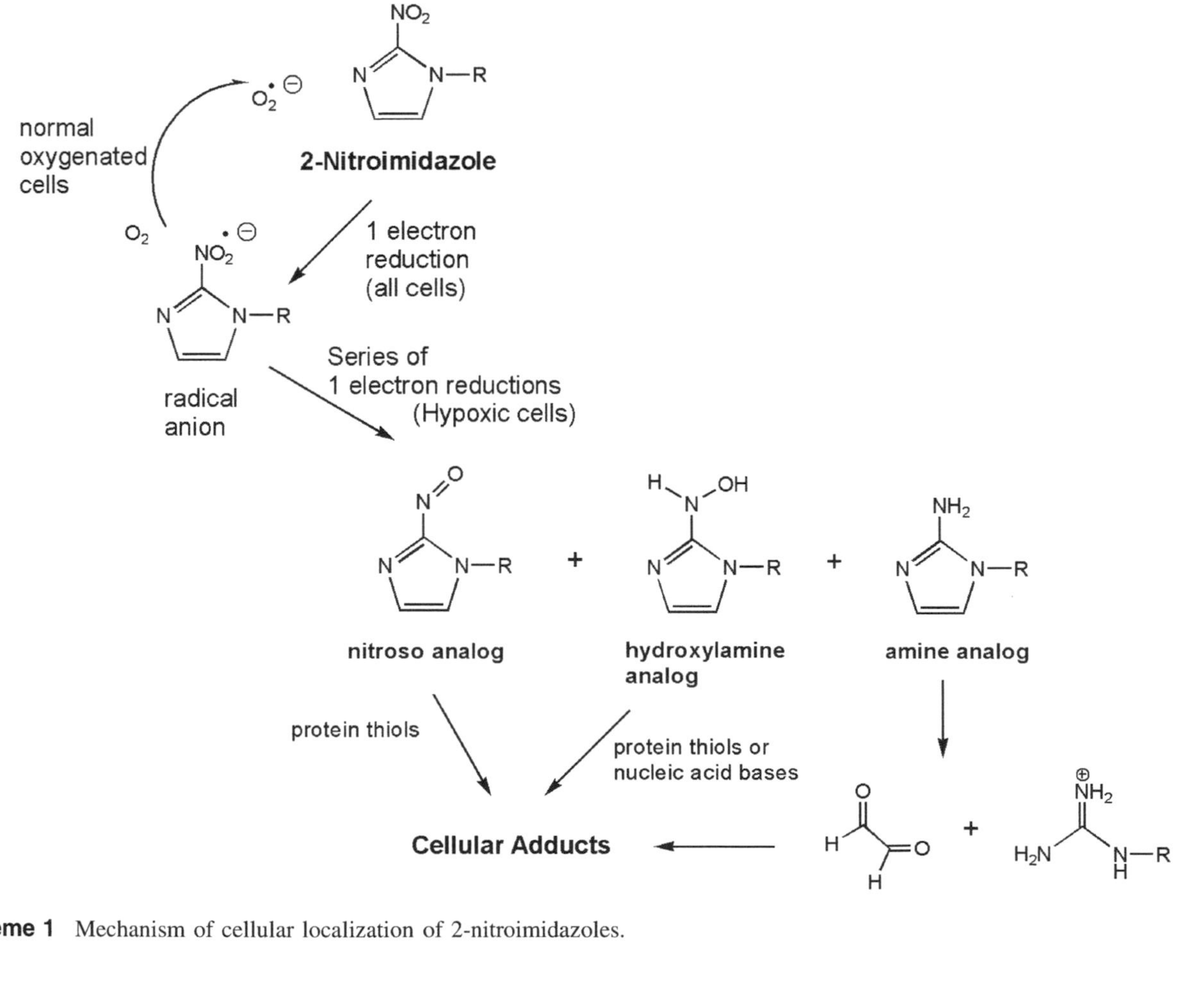

Scheme 1   Mechanism of cellular localization of 2-nitroimidazoles.

analogs are both reactive with protein thiols like gluta-thione, while the hydroxylamine can also react with nucleic acid bases. The amine analog fragments to form glyoxal and a guanidino fragment; the former can also react with cellular components. These reactions trap the 2-nitroimidazole in hypoxic cells (104,108).

The first generation radiolabeled hypoxia localizing compounds were halogenated analogs of the hypoxia cell radiosensitizer, misonidazole (Fig. 6). One of the first compounds 4-[^{82}Br]BrMISO was more lipophilic than the parent compound misonidazole, which resulted in high retention in nontargeted organs (109). Substitution of the methoxy group of misonidazole by a vinyl iodide to give [^{131}I]IMV did not significantly decrease the lipophilicity compared to 4-[^{82}Br]BrMISO (110,111). Analogs incorporating the smaller halogen, fluorine, produced compounds with lipophilicity similar to misonida-zole. [^{18}F]FMISO where the methoxy group of misonidazole is substituted with a fluorine has been used in the clinic to evaluate tumor hypoxia (112,113).

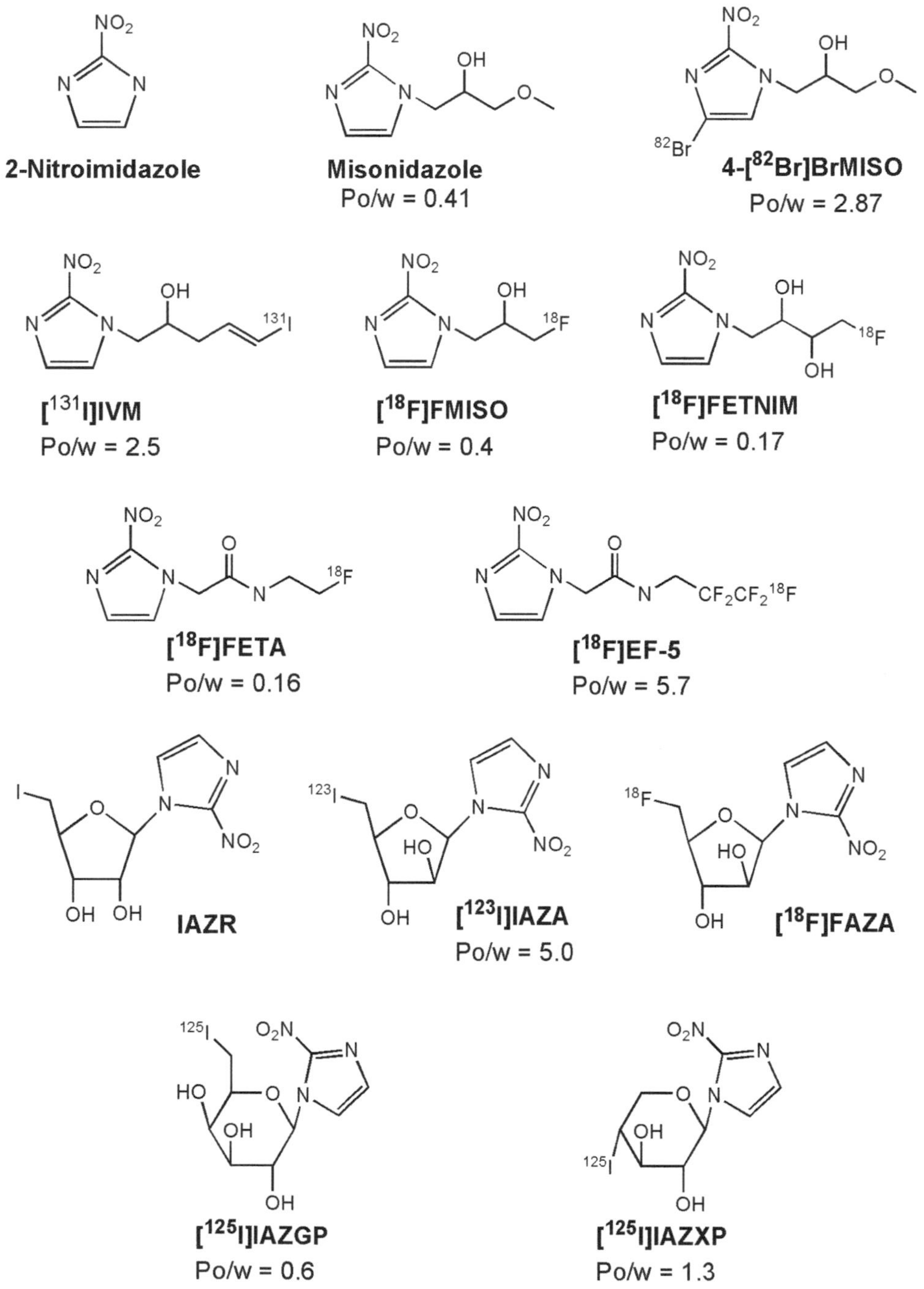

Figure 6 Radiohalogenated nitroimidazoles.

When combined with FDG imaging, it could predict radiation therapy outcomes in head and neck cancer (114). However, [^{18}F]FMISO still suffers from low relative hypoxic tumor uptake, slow blood clearance, and high background levels (98). As a result, more fluorinated analogs have been prepared and tested including [^{18}F]FETNIM, [^{18}F]FETA, and the poly fluorinated [^{18}F]EF5 (115–119). In rodent studies, [^{18}F]FETA retention in hypoxic tumors was related to the oxygen concentration of the tumor (116). Although [^{18}F]EF5 is more lipophilic than [^{18}F]FMISO it was eliminated via urine and gave tumor to organ ratios that increased with time (119).

The attachment of a sugar moiety to a radiopharmaceutical to increase nontarget organ clearance or increase renal excretion is a common strategy in radiopharmaceutical development. IAZR, one of the first misonidazole analogs to contain a sugar nucleoside, was a better radiosensitizer than miconidazole but when radiolabeled, suffered significant deiodination in vivo (120). Arabinosyl sugar nucleosides such as [^{123}I]IAZA are more promising. Although [^{123}I]IAZA is still more lipophilic than [^{18}F]FMISO, it cleared faster from the blood than [^{18}F]FMISO (121). Preliminary human imaging studies using [^{123}I]IAZA demonstrated good tumor to normal ratios when imaged at later time points (122,123). The synthesis of the F-18 analog [^{18}F]FAZA followed (124,125). FAZA has been shown by a reverse phase HPLC method to be less lipophilic than either F-MISO or IAZA (126). In rodent tumor models [^{18}F]FAZA had a lower absolute tumor update than [^{18}F]FMISO but [^{18}F]FAZA cleared more quickly from the blood and normal organs resulting in higher tumor to normal organ ratios (124,125). Schneider et al. continued this theme by preparing analogs containing 6-carbon sugars including IAZGP and IAZXP. In mice [^{123}I]IAZGP and [^{123}I]IAZXP had rapid blood clearance resulting in high tumor to blood ratios (127). A comparison of [^{18}F]FMISO and [^{124}I]IAZGP in mice showed higher tumor to normal organ rations for [^{124}I]IAZGP at 24 hours postinjection compared to [^{18}F]FMISO at 3 hours postinjection (128).

The second generation of 2-nitroimidazole based hypoxia imaging agents involved replacing the radiohalogen with chelated technetium-99m. The first promising compound was BMS181321 (129) (Fig. 7). This compound utilized a propylene aminooxime (PnAO) chelating group, which is structurally related to ^{99m}Tc-HMPAO. ^{99m}Tc-HMPAO is used clinically for measuring cerebral blood flow and as a leukocyte-labeling agent. BMS181321 is very lipophilic and exhibited slow clearance from the blood in mice, resulting in very low tumor to blood and tumor to organ ratios (130). A substitution of oxygen on carbon 5 of the PnAO backbone as well as moving the 2-nitroimidazole group to carbon 6 produced the more hydrophilic compound BRU59-21 (131). In mice BRU59-21 had lower absolute tumor uptake than BMS181321 but it cleared faster from the blood, which resulted in higher tumor to organ ratios. In a phase 1 study in head and neck cancers, BRU59-21 detected hypoxic tumors and the tumor to normal organ ratio correlated with hypoxia measured by histopathology of tumor biopsies (132). However, both of these technetium agents suffer instability and in-vivo metabolism (105,132). This should not be surprising since the cellular trapping mechanism of the related compound ^{99m}Tc-HMPAO involves the conversion of the neutral lipophilic ^{99m}Tc-HMPAO complex to a polar compound. Cyclams form complexes with various metals including technetium and copper. Engelhardt et al. prepared a series of cyclam-2-nitroimidazole derivatives where the number of 2-nitroimidazole groups and their substitution pattern on the cyclam were varied (133). Two of the most promising compounds were Cu-64 and Tc-99m-labeled FC-327 and FC-334. In rats, the absolute uptake of the labeled cyclams was low but blood clearance was rapid enough to give good tumor to blood and tumor to muscle ratios. The absolute uptake of the ^{64}Cu-cyclams was tenfold higher than the corresponding ^{99m}Tc-cyclams (133). All the Tc-99m-labeled hypoxia agents described thus far had four metal-coordinating groups contained in a single ligand. Recently Chu described the hypoxia localizing ability of a ^{99m}Tc complex prepared with the ligand N2IPA (134). No structure of the actual ^{99m}Tc complex has been reported but it is likely that two molecules of the N2IPA ligand (each with a single coordinating amine and oxime group) are required to fulfill the coordination requirements of technetium. In mice, the absolute tumor uptake was low but blood clearance was fast enough to produce good tumor to blood and tumor to muscle ratios by four hours post injection.

Bioreductive Complexes

Copper(II)bis(thiosemicarbazone) complexes possess redox potentials in a range where they can be reduced by intracellular components. Radiolabeled $^{60/62/64}$Cu PTSM (Fig. 8) is a nonspecific selective blood-perfusion PET Tracer (Mathias, 1990) whereas $^{60/62/64}$Cu ATSM is a PET tracer for hypoxia imaging (135). The differing biological properties of these very similar complexes (ASTM has an additional methyl group on the diimine backbone) has been explained as follows: Cu(II)PTSM, with a reduction potential of −0.53 V, diffuses into all cells where it is reduced to Cu(I)PTSM, which then dissociates and the free copper binds to cellular components. Cu(II)ATSM with a lower reduction potential of −0.59 V is also reduced in all cells but in the presence of oxygen is rapidly reoxidized where it can now diffuse out of the cell. In hypoxic cells, the lack of oxygen decreases reoxidation and permits complex dissociation with subsequent intracellular trapping of copper. Structure-activity studies (136) have shown that electron-donating

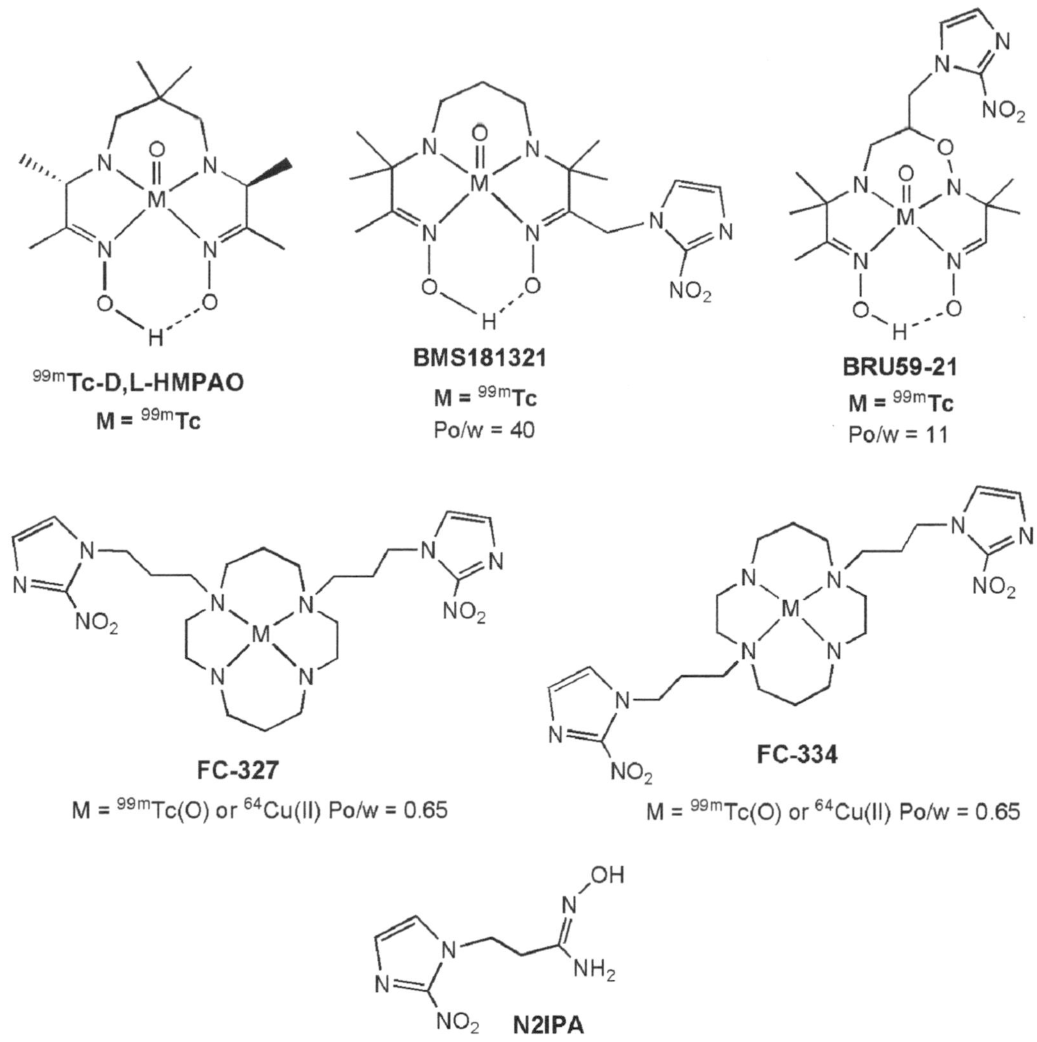

Figure 7 Technetium-99m or Copper-64-labeled nitroimidazoles.

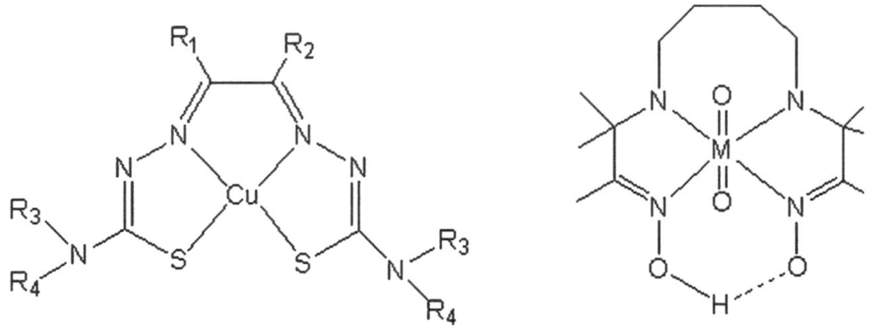

	R$_1$	R$_2$	R$_3$	R$_4$	Log P	Electrochemical Potentials
Cu(II)PSTM	CH$_3$	H	CH$_3$	H	1.45	-0.53v
Cu(II)ATS	CH$_3$	CH$_3$	H	H	0.65	-0.59v
Cu(II)ATSM	CH$_3$	CH$_3$	CH$_3$	H	1.48	-0.59v
Cu(II)DTS	C$_2$H$_5$	C$_2$H$_5$	H	H	1.69	-0.59v
Cu(II)DTSM	C$_2$H$_5$	C$_2$H$_5$	CH$_3$	H	2.34	-0.58v

Figure 8 Bioreductive complexes.

substituents on both carbons of the diimine backbone are required to decrease the reduction potential (Fig. 8). All copper complexes, with this substitution pattern, showed uptake in hypoxic cells in vitro but at different rates. The uptake of Cu(II)DTS and Cu(II)DTSM were actually higher than Cu(II)ASTM at 5 to 20 minutes where as Cu(II)ASTM was highest at 1 hour (136). Cu(II)ASTM has recently been shown to be selective for certain types of hypoxic tumors (137). A limited clinical study of [60]Cu (II)ASTM in cervical cancer demonstrated that tumor to muscle ratios of greater than 3.5 were predictive of disease recurrence (138).

The non-nitroimidazole technetium-oxime complex ^{99m}Tc-BnAO (HL-91) where the propyldiamine backbone of PnAO has been extended by one carbon to a butyldiamine has demonstrated uptake in hypoxic cells and tumors (139). HL-91 may exist as an equilibrium between mono and dioxo forms (140). The mechanism of localization in hypoxic cells is unknown but it may be related to the redox properties of the mono-dioxo technetium core (139). In mice, the absolute uptake of HL-91 in tumors is low and comparable to BMS181321; however, it clears faster from the blood and has renal clearance (139). In clinical imaging studies, HL-91 localized in squamous cell carcinomas, head and neck cancers, and non–small cell

ling cancer (3). In non–small cell lung cancer patients, the tumor to normal ratio was predictive for tumor response and patient survival (141). However, Hl-91 requires lower oxygen concentrations for uptake into hypoxic cells than the 2-nitroimidazole compounds IAZA, IAZGP, MISO, and FMISO (107). Because oxygen requirements for cellular retention of the 2-nitroimidizoles are similar to that needed for radioresistance, HL-91 may miss low and moderately hypoxic tumors (107).

Which agent is best? The recent NCI Workshop on Hypoxia concluded that there is still no clear "gold standard" of hypoxia measurements because the field of hypoxia measurement is still new, the biology of hypoxia is still poorly understood, and the best factor by which to assess hypoxia is still unclear. However, they did identify [^{18}F]FMISO, [^{18}F]FAZA, [^{18}F]EF5, [^{123}I] and [[124]I] IAZGP, [^{64}Cu]ASTM, and possibly [[67]Cu]ASTM as promising agents (103).

Metabolism Tracers

PET imaging of metabolically active tumors using 2-[^{18}F] fluoro-deoxyglucose [^{18}F]FDG (Fig. 9) is an important tool in the detection and diagnosis of cancer. [^{18}F]FDG enters tumors through the Glut1 glucose transport protein.

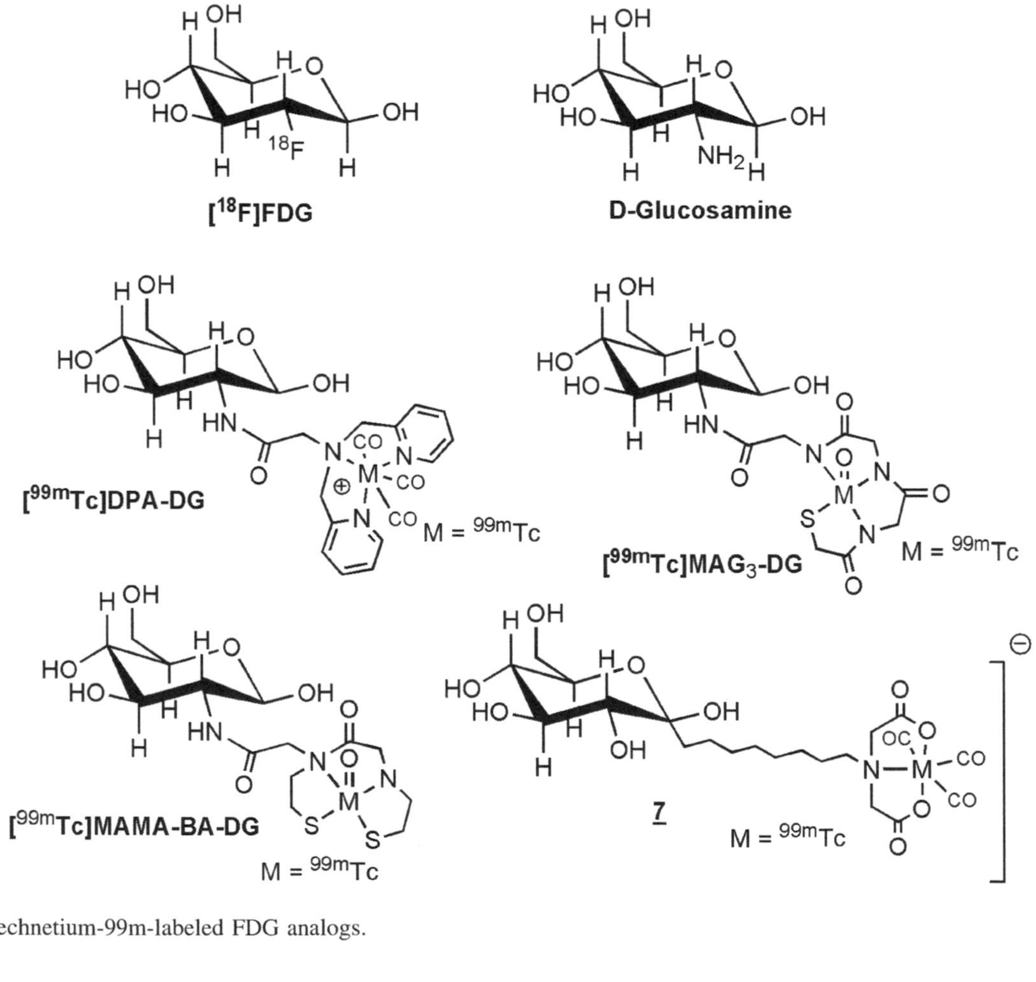

Figure 9 Technetium-99m-labeled FDG analogs.

Phosphorylation of [^{18}F]FDG to [^{18}F]-2-fluoro-deoxyglucose-6-phosphate (FDG-6-P) is catalyzed by hexokinase to trap FDG-6-P inside the cell. Because of the low cost and longer half-life of Tc-99m as compared to F-18, there has been a considerable amount of effort toward the development of a "^{99m}Tc-FDG." The amine group on C-2 of glucosamine (Fig. 9) has been conjugated with several Tc/Re chelating agents resulting in [^{99m}Tc]DPA-DG (142), [^{99m}Tc]MAG$_3$-DG (143), and [^{99m}Tc]MAMA-BA-DG (143). In addition, [^{99m}Tc]EC-DG, a glucosamine dimer containing an internal ethylenedicysteine group for coordination of ^{99m}Tc, has been prepared (144). Although these compounds have exhibited uptake in lung tumor (144) and breast tumor xenografts (143), they lack the characteristic [^{18}F]FDG localization in brain, heart, and muscle suggesting that tumor localization may be occurring by a nonspecific mechanism. Furthermore, Schibli et al. have prepared a series of substituted glucose analogs where various ^{99m}Tc/Re complexes were attached at either C-1, C-2, C-3, or C-6 via a spacer chain of varying lengths (145). Only ^{99m}Tc/Re complexes attached to C-2 with a long alkyl chain such as compound 7 (Fig. 9) successfully competed with glucose for hexokinase; however, none of these analogs were transported via Glut1. Therefore, a ^{99m}Tc-FDG has not yet been realized (75,76).

Proliferation Agents

Cells incorporate thymidine into their DNA during cell division. Therefore, radiolabeled thymidine analogs have been investigated as agents for imaging proliferation in rapidly dividing cancer cells. Radioiodinated 5-iodo-2'-deoxyuridine (IUdR) (Fig. 10) has long been used to measure proliferation in vitro. However, IUdR undergoes extensive deiodination in vivo (146). The brominated analog, BUdR has been radiolabeled with ^{77}Br, ^{76}Br, ^{82}Br, and ^{80m}Br. Although radiobrominated BUdR also suffers from in vivo debromination, it has been shown to be a marker for proliferation by its incorporation into DNA of rodents (147,148). However, PET imaging of tumor proliferation

was unsuccessful because of prolonged retention of metabolites (149). Diuretics have been utilized to increase the elimination of metabolites (150).

In order to prepare IUdr/BUdr analogs with greater in vivo stability, a fluorine was placed in the 2 position in the sugar. It is thought that the fluorine would be small enough to permit biological activity but also lock the sugar base into the anti-conformation to provide resistance to glycosidic bond cleavage (151). Mercer et al. demonstrated that FIRU and FBRU, which have the 2-fluorine in the "down" position were more stable than the corresponding IUdR or BUdR but did not show proliferation associated uptake in vivo (152). Changing the stereochemistry by having the 2-fluorine in the "up" position to give FIAU and FBAU retained the stability and produced compounds that were incorporated into DNA (152–154). However, FBAU and FIAU are also phosphorylated and trapped by cells expressing Herpes simplex virus type-1 thymidine kinase (HSV1-*tk*) (155–158). This may complicate interpreting results in gene therapy studies where HSV1-*tk* is present.

Toyohara et al. reported an alternate approach to preparing a more stable IUdR. They replaced the 4' oxygen in IUdR with a 4' thio group giving [^{125}I]ITdU (159). This compound suffered less deiodination than [^{125}I]IUdR, was incorporated into the DNA of proliferating tissues (160), and gave higher proliferating tissue to background ratios than [^{125}I]IUdR and [^{125}I]FIAU (161).

Estrogen Receptor–Binding Compounds

Knowledge of the ER status is important in the treatment of breast cancer because only ER+ cancers respond to antiestrogen therapy (162). Furthermore, ER negative cancers are more aggressive and patients have a poorer chance of survival (163,164). Tumor biopsies can provide ER status but this method suffers from sampling errors and often cannot be applied to metastatic disease. Metastases can have ER status different from the primary tumor (165). Therefore, imaging using radiolabeled ER-binding

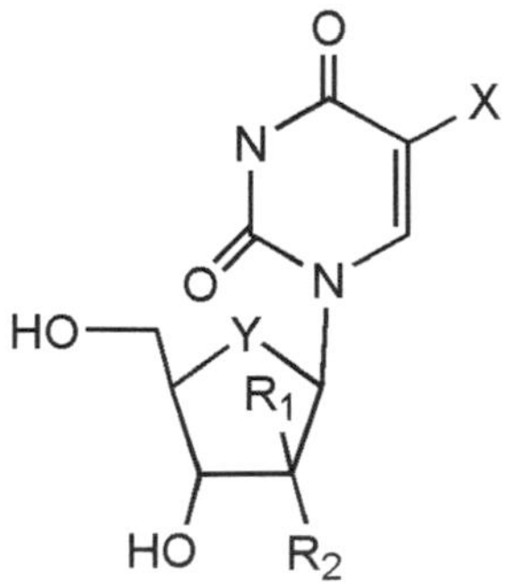

Thymidine: X = CH$_3$, R$_1$ = H, R$_2$ = H, Y = O
IUdR: X = I, R$_1$ = H, R$_2$ = H, Y = O
BUdR: X = Br, R$_1$ = H, R$_2$ = H, Y = O
FIRU: X = I, R$_1$ = H, R$_2$ = F, Y = O
FBRU: X = Br, R$_1$ = H, R$_2$ = F, Y = O
FIAU: X = I, R$_1$ = F, R$_2$ = H, Y = O
FBAU: X = Br, R$_1$ = F, R$_2$ = H, Y = O
ITdU: X = I, R$_1$ = H, R$_2$ = H, Y = S

Figure 10 Radiohalogenated thymidine analogs.

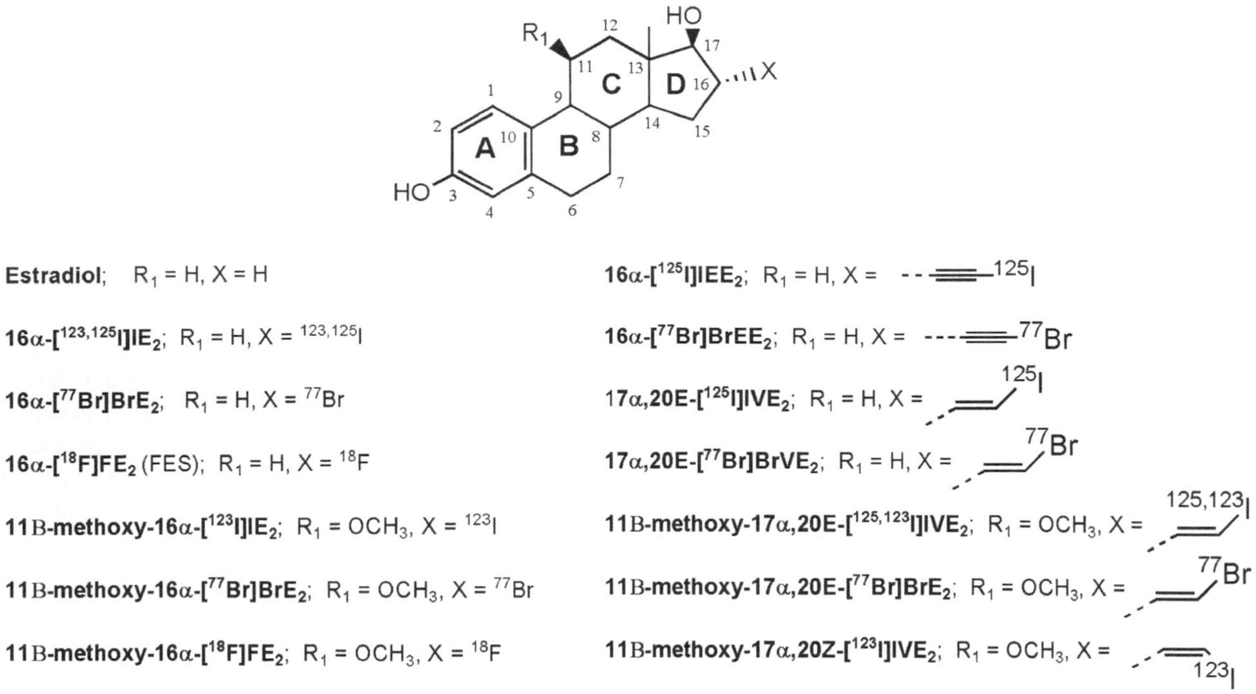

Figure 11 Radiohalogenated estradiol analogs.

compounds has been investigated as a means to provide a noninvasive measurement of ER status in primary and metastatic breast cancer. Many steroidal and nonsteroidal estrogens as well as antiestrogens have been synthesized and tested for contraception and hormonal therapy. Structure-activity relationships of ER-binding compounds have been reviewed (166,167). Many ER-binding compound are analogs of estradiol (E$_2$) (Fig. 11). Structural components on the steroid molecule necessary for ER binding and the positions that will tolerate substituents have been identified (167). The OH moiety in the 3 position of the A ring is required for binding. Loss of the OH in the 17β position reduces ER binding. The 17α position tolerates substituents but is dependant on size and polarity. The 11β and 7α positions tolerate large nonpolar substituents. These well-characterized structure-activity relationships have guided the design of this class of radiotracers.

The first high-affinity radioiodinated ligand for the ER, 16α[^{125}I]IE$_2$ (Fig. 11), was reported by Hochberg in 1979 (168). Successful imaging of ER+-rich tissues and tumors in rabbits using 16α[^{125}I]IE$_2$ has been demonstrated (169). The preparation of the bromine analog, 16α[^{77}Br]BrE$_2$, soon followed the synthesis of 16α[^{125}I]IE$_2$ (170,171). In rats, 16α[^{77}Br]BrE$_2$ behaved similarly to 16α[^{125}I]IE$_2$ (172) and showed uptake in rat mammary tumors (171). Breast cancer tumors in patients were also imaged with this agent (173). The F-18 analog 16α[^{18}F]FE$_2$ (FES) has been prepared for PET imaging (174). In clinical studies FES-detected breast cancer tumors and the uptake correlated with ER status was determined by in vitro assay of

tumor biopsies (175). From ongoing clinical PET studies, it has been determined that FES has acceptable radiation dosimetry (176) and is the ER-binding agent that is the closest to widespread clinical use. The 11β-methoxy analogs of the 16α-halo estradiols were also synthesized and in general these compounds had lower nontarget uptake (170,177–179).

Ethynyl or vinyl groups in the 17α position have higher binding affinities than estradiol. Therefore, a series of 17α-substituted radiohalogenated alkynes and alkenes have been prepared and tested. The earliest, 17α-[^{125}I] IEE$_2$ was reported a year after 16α[^{125}I]IE$_2$ (180). Unfortunately, this compound deiodinated in the presence of proteins. However, the radiobrominated analog 17α-[^{77}Br]BrEE$_2$ was stable (181). The 17α vinyl halo analogs 17α,20E-[^{125}I]IVE$_2$, 17α,20E-[^{77}Br]BrVE$_2$, 11β-methoxy-17α,20E-[^{125}I]IVE$_2$, and 11β-methoxy-17α,20E-[^{77}Br]BrVE$_2$ were synthesized from either vinyl stannanes (182–185) or vinyl boronic acid precursors (186). As seen with the 16α-halo-E$_2$ compounds, the 11β-methoxy-17α,20E–Br/IVE$_2$ compounds gave higher target to nontarget ratios in rats than 17α,20E–Br/IVE$_2$ (184–186). Ali et al. prepared the 20Z isomers of 17α-[^{125}I]IVE$_2$ and 11β-methoxy-17α-[^{125}I]IVE$_2$ and demonstrated that the 20Z isomers had higher ER binding in vitro and higher uptake in ER-rich tissues (IV injection) than the corresponding 20E isomers (187,188). Hughes et al. confirmed the higher binding of the 20Z isomers in vitro but found no difference in ER-rich tissues uptake when the estrogens were injected intraperitoneally (189).

8; R_1 = H, R_2 = CH_2CH_3, R_3 = ^{131}I, R_4 = $N(CH_3)_2$

9; R_1 = ^{125}I, R_2 CH_2CH_3, R_3 = H, R_4 = $N(CH_3)_2$

123ITX; R_1 = H, R_2 = $CH_2CH_2CH_2{}^{123}I$, R_3 = H, R_4 = $N(CH_2CH_3)_2$

10; R_1 = H, R_2 = $(CH_2)_3NH(CH_2CH_2)$-C_6H_4-NH-DTPA, R_3 = H, R_4 = $N(CH_2CH_3)_2$

[^{125}I]I-TAM-AZ; R_1 = H, R_2 = ^{125}I, R_3 = H, R_4 = N⊲

[^{80m,77}Br]Br-BHPE; R_1 = OH, R_2 = OH, R_3 = H, X = ^{80m,77}Br

[^{123,125}I]I-BHPE; R_1 = OH, R_2 = OH, R_3 = H, X = ^{123,125}I

[^{125}I]I-THPE; R_1 = OH, R_2 = OH, R_3 = OH, X = ^{125}I

Figure 12 Triphenylethylene compounds.

Furthermore, these investigators demonstrated that the 20Z isomer was converted into the 20E isomer in vivo (189). In clinical studies 11β-methoxy-(17α, 20Z) [^{123}I] IVE$_2$ successfully detected breast cancer lesions and the tumor uptake correlated with ER status (190–192).

The antiestrogen tamoxifen has also been a substrate for radiolabeling. The first two radiolabeled analogs 8 and 9 (Fig. 12) were radioiodinated on the aromatic rings (193,194). Compound 9 exhibited low uptake in ER-rich tissue. The aliphatic portion of tamoxifen has been radioiodinated to give 123-ITX (195). Although aliphatic radiohalogens usually suffer from extensive deiodination in vivo, 123-ITX was tested in the clinic. In patients, this compound did not appear to be very promising; only 4 of 9 patients with ER+ tumors had their tumors visualized (196). Delpassand et al. attached diethylenetriamine-pentaacetic acid (DTPA) to the aliphatic portion of tamoxifen to give 10. The absolute uptake of the In-111-labeled compound in ER+ tumor xenografts was low; however, the tumors were clearly visualized (197). The ability of an ER-binding compound to contain such a large substituent may be surprising but this position likely corresponds to substituents on the 7α position of estradiol. Salituro et al. prepared a novel tamoxifen analog [^{125}I]I-TAM-Az. This compound was a mixture of cis/trans isomers, had a vinyl radiohalogen, and the dimethylaminogroup was replaced with an aziridine moiety. This compound binds irreversibly to the ER via the aziridine group (198). In order to eliminate the possibility of cis/trans isomerization, the nonsteroidal

vinyl-halo estrogens bis-hydroxy-triphenylethylenes [^{80m,77}Br]Br-BHPE and [^{125,123}I]I-BHPE (Fig. 12) were prepared (185,199,200). In rats, the specific uptake in ER target tissues by [^{77}Br]Br-BHPE and [^{123}I]I-BHPE were comparable to 11β-methoxy-(17α,20E)-[^{77}Br]BrVE$_2$ and -[^{125}I]IVE$_2$ (185,201). In rats, [^{125}I]I-THPE, which has a third phenol moiety unexpectedly showed prolonged retention (up to three days) in ER target tissue and very high uterus to blood and ovary to blood ratios (202).

The second generation of ER-binding compounds contains a coordinated rhenium or technetium metal. Because of their size, the coordinated metal must reside either as a pendant of one of the positions of the steroid that can accommodate bulky substituents or the metal must be incorporated within the steroid-like structure.

The first pendant compound with high ER-binding, compound 11 (Fig. 13), had a cyclopentadienyl rhenium tricarbonyl group attached to the 17α ethynyl group (203). Replacing the cyclopentadienyl-coordinating group with a hydrazine moiety to give 12 increased the binding affinity (204). Compound 13, where the hydrazine now contributes three coordinating groups also had high-binding affinity (205). When 3 + 1 Re/^{99m}Tc oxo complexes were prepared at this position, a carbon linker between the ethynyl group and the complex was needed for high binding. Compound 14 had the highest binding affinity of a series of compounds where the complex and chain length were varied (206). Re/Tc complexes attached to the 7α positions have also been investigated (207–209).

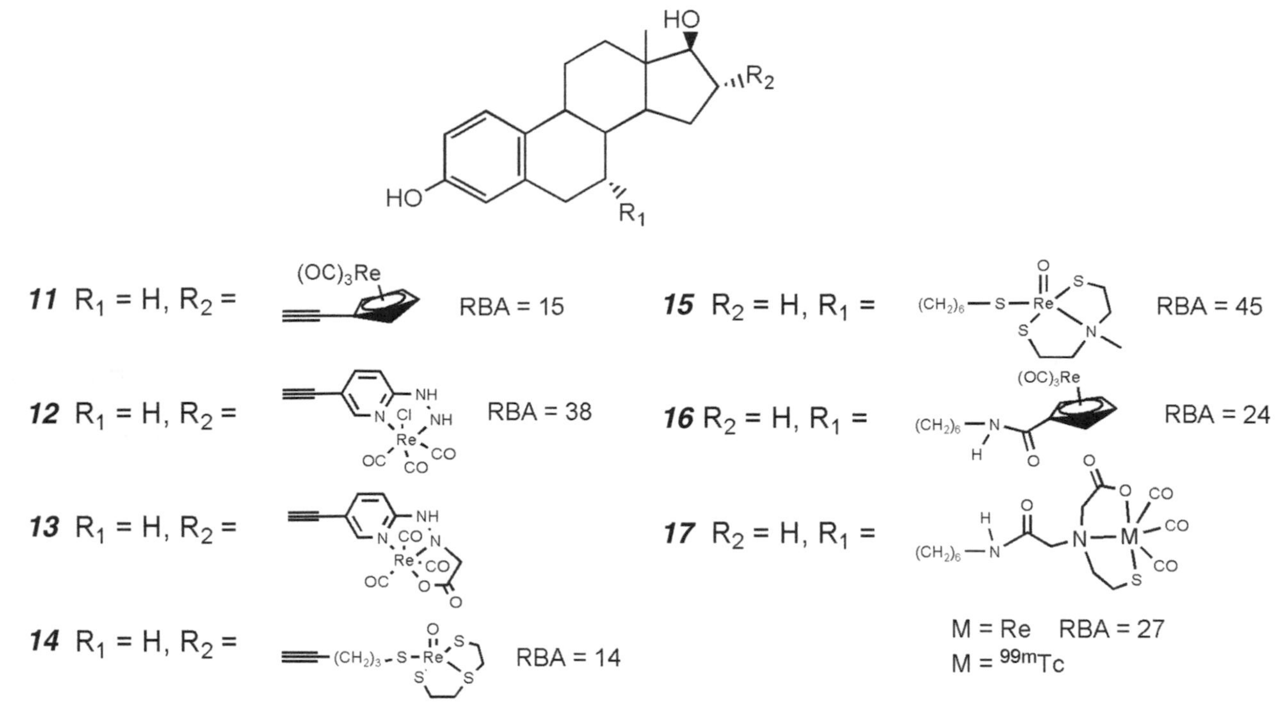

Figure 13 Pendant rhenium/technetium-99m estradiols.

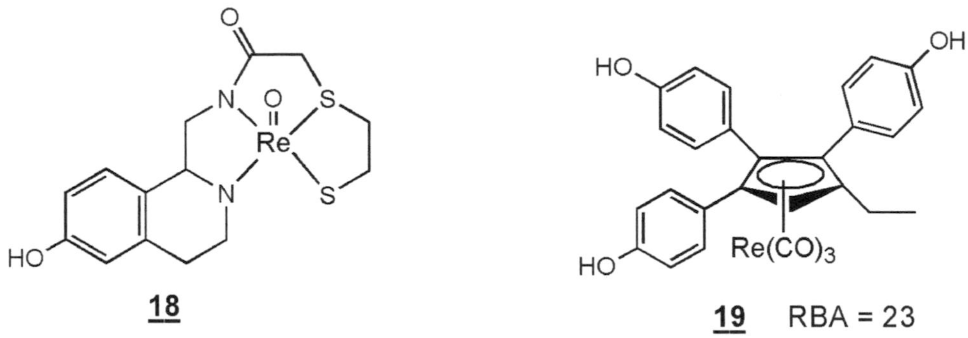

Figure 14 Steroid and triphenylethylene-like inclusion compounds.

Potent compounds included *15*, *16*, and *17*; however, the ^{99m}Tc version of *17* failed to show specific uptake in ER-rich tissues (209).

The first inclusion complex was compound *18* (Fig. 14). In this molecule the coordination of Re assembled the pseudo C and D rings of a steroid. Although this retains the overall size and shape of the estrogen, it exhibited low binding to ER (210). Mull et al. reported the synthesis of a very novel triphenylethylene like estrogen, compound *19*. In *19*, three phenols and one ethyl group are substituents on the cyclopentadienyl moiety. Rhenium tricarbonyl is coordinated to the cyclopentadienyl moiety (211). This molecule takes advantage of extra space within the ER-binding cavity and bears a striking resemblance to I-THPE.

Sigma Receptor Ligands

Sigma receptors are membrane-bound proteins and are expressed on many human cancer cells including breast tumors, lung tumors, melanomas, glioblastomas, neuroblastomas, and prostate tumors (212). There are two types of sigma receptors, sigma-1 and sigma-2. Sigma-2 receptors appear to be a biomarker of tumor-cell proliferation (213). The radioiodinated sigma receptor ligand BZA (Fig. 15) was first prepared by Michelot et al. (214) by a Cu^{+2}-assisted isotopic iodide exchange and used to image malignant melanomas in patients (215). An alternate synthesis utilizing a tributyl stannane precursor for radioiodination, which yielded higher specific activity product, was later reported by John et al. (216). Extensive

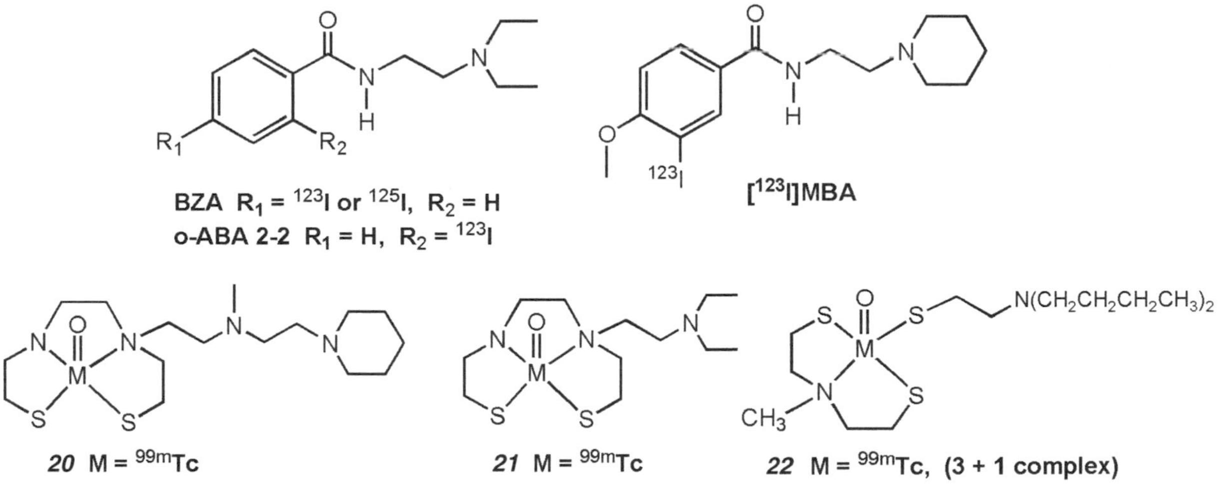

Figure 15 Sigma receptor–binding compounds.

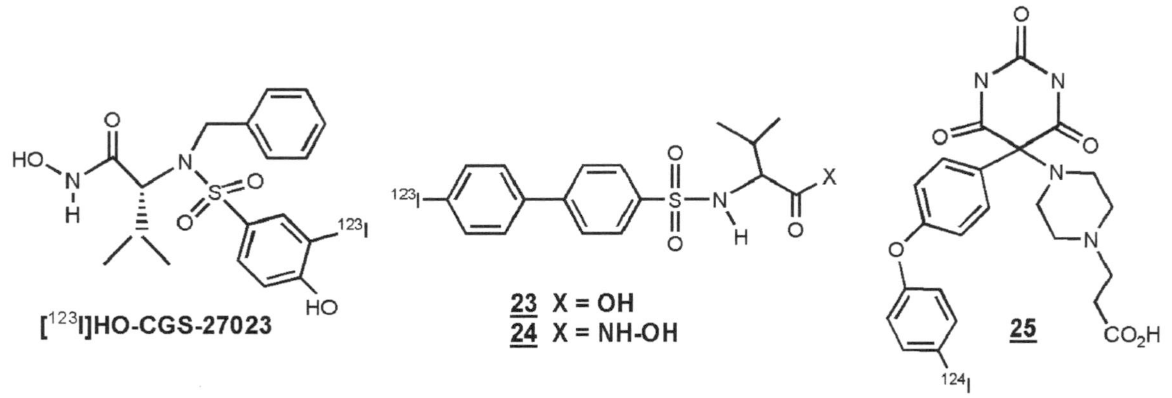

Figure 16 Matrix metalloproteinase inhibitors.

structure-activity studies in this system have been carried out by several investigators (217–222). From these studies two additional compounds have been evaluated in patients. Breast cancer tumors were visualized using [^{123}I]MBA (223) (Fig. 15) and melanoma was imaged in a single patient using [^{123}I]o-ABA 2-2 (218). Sigma receptors can accommodate some changes in ligand structure. For example, the iodobenzamide moiety in the compounds discussed above can be substituted with ^{99m}Tc oxo complexes such as in compounds 20 (224) and 21 (225) and the 3 + 1 mixed ligand 22 (226). These ^{99m}Tc analogs retained their ability to bind sigma receptors in vitro and bound to sigma receptor–rich tissues and murine melanomas in vivo.

Matrix Metalloproteinase Inhibitors

Matrix metalloproteinases (MMPs) are a family of zinc-dependent endopeptidases that cleave components of the extracellular matrix and basement membrane of the epithelium. MMPs are involved in cancer cell growth, migration,

invasion, and tumor angiogenesis (227–229). The synthesis of MMP inhibitors as therapeutic and/or imaging agents has been an active area of research and has been reviewed recently (230). Synthetic MMP inhibitors include peptidometic and nonpeptidometic compounds. Many have been radiolabeled with either PET or SPECT radionuclides. Promising nonpeptidometic radioiodinated agents include [^{123}I]HO-CGS-27023A (231) (Fig. 16), the valine-based compounds 23 and 24 (232), and the trione 25 (233). A common component of these inhibitors is the presence of a Zn-coordinating carboxylic or hydroxamic acid group.

Folic Acid Conjugates

Higher amounts of folic acid are needed by rapidly dividing malignant cells than normal cells. Folic acid enters cells by endocytosis via the folate receptor (FR), which is a high-affinity membrane protein. Many cancers including ovarian, endometrial, breast, lung, renal, and colorectal express high levels of FR making it an attractive target for imaging and therapeutic agents (234). The structure of

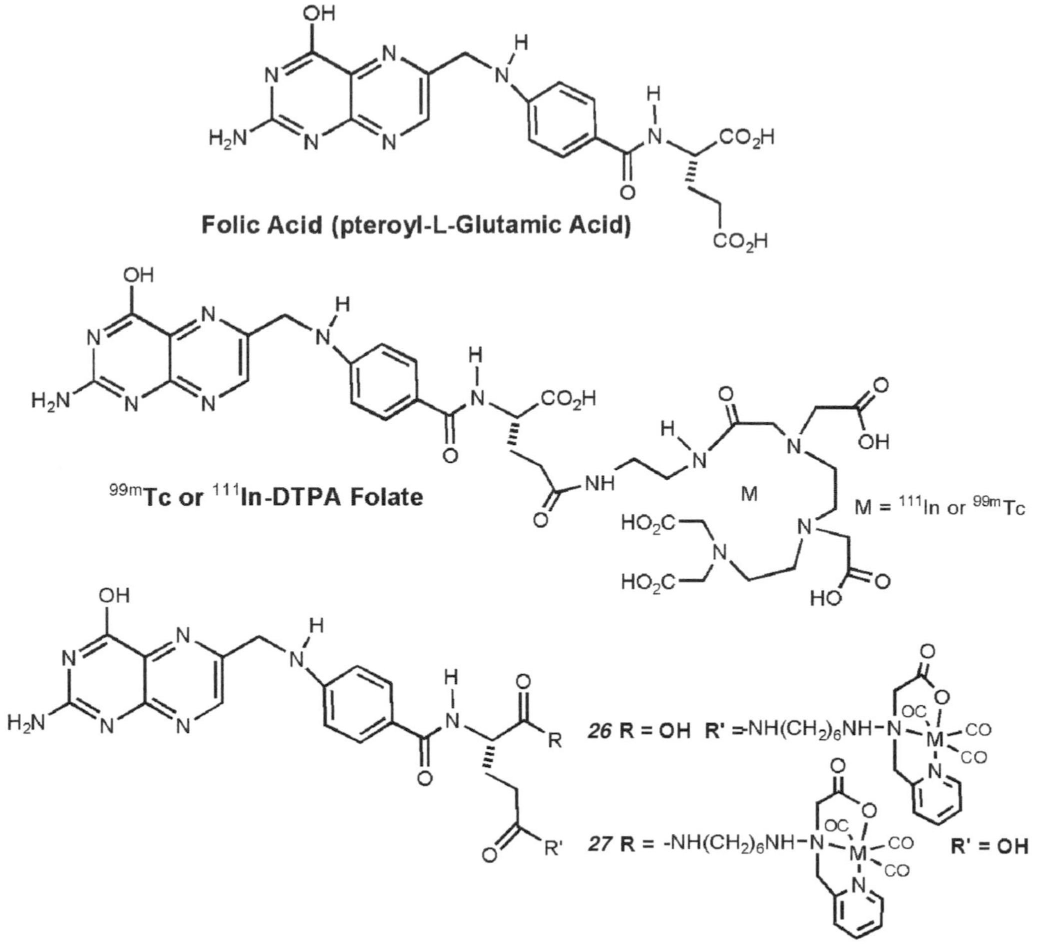

Figure 17 Folic acid conjugates.

folic acid is shown is Fig. 17. The FR is relatively insensitive to groups conjugated to the glutamate portion such that folic acid conjugates containing such large groups as radiometal chelates, MRI contrast agents, and drugs still enter cancer cells (234). Several of the many examples of FR-binding SPECT tracers are shown in Fig. 17 and include [111]In- or ^{99m}Tc-DTPA-folate (235,236) and compounds 26 and 27 where a neutral [99m]Tc(CO)$_3$ complex is conjugated to either the gamma or alpha carboxylate (237). In initial clinical studies SPECT imaging with ^{111}In-DTPA-folate successfully differentiated between new malignant and benign ovarian masses (100% sensitivity); however, detection of recurrent malignant masses required concurrent CT imaging (238).

Prostate-Specific Membrane Antigen Inhibitors

Prostate-specific membrane antigen (PSMA) is an integral membrane protein with an enzymatic active site in an extracellular domain. PSMA is upregulated in prostate cancer, particularly in advanced, hormone-independent and metastatic disease (239). It is also expressed in the neovasculature of nearly all solid tumors (240). Adding further to the attractiveness of PSMA as an imaging target is its limited pattern of expression, primarily within prostate, small bowel, proximal renal tubule and brain (241). Within the brain PSMA is known as glutamate carboxypeptidase II (GCPII, also known as NAAG peptidase), where it catalyzes the hydrolysis of NAAG to glutamate and N-acetylaspartate (242). PSMA/GCPII is an active target for the development of imaging agents and has recently been reviewed (243). One class of PSMA inhibitors has been designed by replacing the glutamide moiety of a PSMA substrate-like NAAG with a urea. Two urea based PSMA inhibitors DCIT and compound 28 labeled with single photon emitters that have shown high specific uptake in PSMA + mouse tumor xenografts are shown in Figure 18 (244,245).

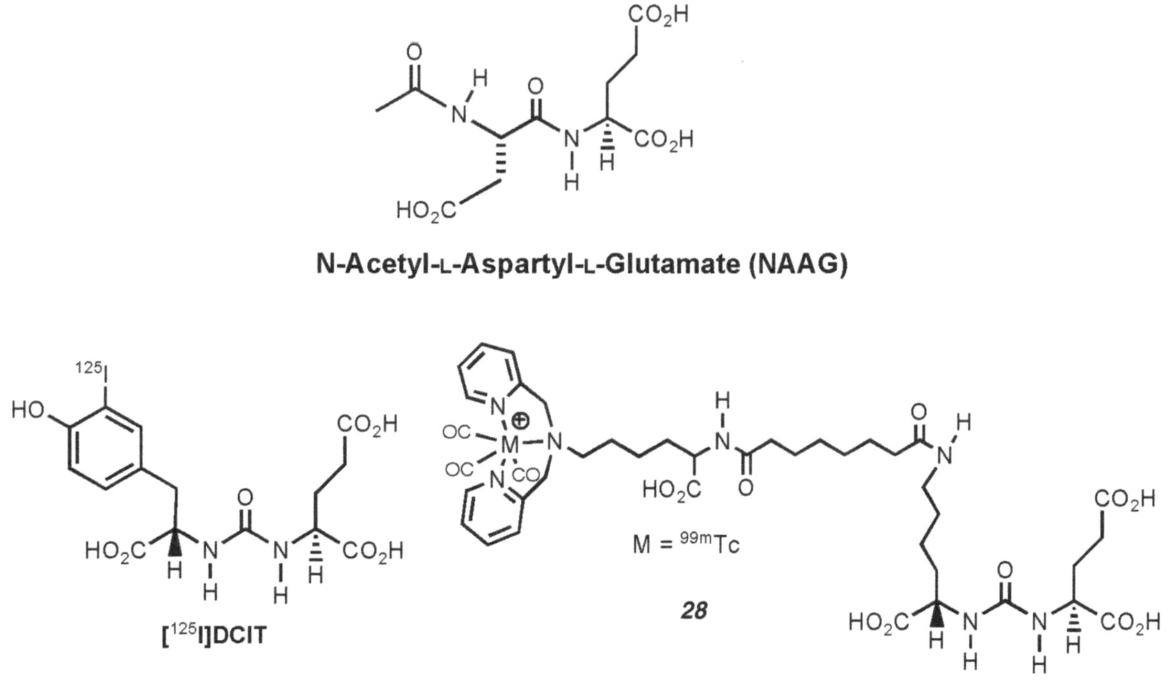

N-Acetyl-L-Aspartyl-L-Glutamate (NAAG)

[125I]DCIT

28

M = 99mTc

Figure 18 Prostate-specific membrane antigen substrates and inhibitors.

CONCLUSIONS

Single photon-emitting imaging agents have played important roles in the diagnosis and study of cancer. New technetium chemistry and the application of existing radiometal and radiohalogen chemistry to new biologically relevant small molecules will continue to produce new SPECT agents to detect and study cancer.

REFERENCES

1. Barentsz J, Takahashi S, Oyen W, et al. Commonly used imaging techniques for diagnosis and staging. J Clin Oncol 2006; 24(20):3234–3244.
2. Giannopoulou C. The role of SPET and PET in monitoring tumour response to therapy. Eur J Nucl Med Mol Imaging 2003; 30(8):1173–1200.
3. Cook GJ. Oncological molecular imaging: nuclear medicine techniques. Br J Radiol 2003; 76(Spec No 2): S152–S158.
4. Shah K, Jacobs A, Breakefield XO, et al. Molecular imaging of gene therapy for cancer. Gene Ther 2004; 11(15):1175–1187.
5. Sharma V, Luker GD, Piwnica-Worms D. Molecular imaging of gene expression and protein function in vivo with PET and SPECT. J Magn Reson Imaging 2002; 16(4):336–351.
6. Imam SK. Molecular nuclear imaging: the radiopharmaceuticals (review). Cancer Biother Radiopharm 2005; 20(2):163–172.
7. Griffiths GL, Goldenberg DM, Jones AL, et al. Radiolabeling of monoclonal antibodies and fragments with technetium and rhenium. Bioconjug Chem 1992; 3(2):91–99.
8. Moffat FL Jr., Gulec SA, Serafini AN, et al. A thousand points of light or just dim bulbs? radiolabeled antibodies and colorectal cancer imaging. Cancer Invest 1999; 17(5): 322–334.
9. Liu S, Edwards DS, Barrett JA. 99mTc labeling of highly potent small peptides. Bioconjug Chem 1997; 8(5): 621–636.
10. Liu SE, Edwards DS. 99mTc-labelled small peptide as diagnostic radiopharmaceuticals. Chem Rev 1999; 99:2235–2268.
11. Lister-James J, Moyer BR, Dean T. Small peptides radiolabeled with 99mTc. Q J Nucl Med 1996; 40(3):221–233.
12. Gotthardt M, Boermann OC, Behr TM, et al. Development and clinical application of peptide-based radiopharmaceuticals. Curr Pharm Des 2004; 10(24):2951–2963.
13. Aloj L, Morelli G. Design, synthesis and preclinical evaluation of radiolabeled peptides for diagnosis and therapy. Curr Pharm Des 2004; 10(24):3009–3031.
14. Meikle SR, Kench P, Kassiou M, et al. Small animal SPECT and its place in the matrix of molecular imaging technologies. Phys Med Biol 2005; 50(22):R45–R61.
15. Anderson CJ, Welch MJ. Radiometal-labeled agents (nontechnetium) for diagnostic imaging. Chem Rev 1999; 99:2219–2234.
16. Storr T, Thompson KH, Orvig C. Design of targeting ligands in medicinal inorganic chemistry. Chem Soc Rev 2006; 35:534–544.

17. Schwochau K. Technetium radiopharmaceuticals—fundamentals, synthesis, structure, and development. Angew Chem Int Ed Engl 1994; 33:2258–2267.

18. Schibli R, Schubiger PA. Current use and future potential of organometallic radiopharmaceuticals. Eur J Nucl Med Mol Imaging 2002; 29(11):1529–1542.

19. Jurisson S, Lydon JD. Potential technetium small molecule radiopharmaceuticals. Chem Rev 1999; 99:2205–2218.

20. Banerjee SR, Maresca KP, Francesconi L, et al. New directions in the coordination chemistry of 99mTc: a reflection on technetium core structures and a strategy for new chelate design. Nucl Med Biol 2005; 32(1):1–20.

21. Baldwin RM. Chemistry of Radioiodine. Appl Radiat Isot 1986; 37:817–821.

22. Seevers RH, Counsell RE. Radioiodination techniques for small organic molecules. Chem Rev 1982; 82:575–590.

23. Maziere B, Loc'h C. Radiopharmaceuticals labelled with bromine isotopes. Int J Rad Appl Instrum [A] 1986; 37(8): 703–713.

24. Abrams MJ, Juweid M, tenKate CI, et al. Technetium-99m-human polyclonal IgG radiolabeled via the hydrazino nicotinamide derivative for imaging focal sites of infection in rats. J Nucl Med 1990; 31(12):2022–2028.

25. Pietzsch HJ, Spies H, Hoffman S. Lipophilic Tc complexes. VI. neutral oxotechnetium(V) complexes with monothiol/tridentate coordination. Inorg Chim Acta 1989; 165:163–166.

26. Alberto R, Schibli R, Egli A, et al. A novel organometallic aqua complex of technetium for the labeling of biomolecules.: synthesis of $[^{99m}Tc)OH_2)_3(CO)_3]^+$ from $[^{99m}TcO_4^-]$ in aqueous solution and its reaction with a bifunctional ligand. J Am Chem Soc 1998; 120:7987–7988.

27. Schibli R, La Bella R, Alberto R, et al. Influence of the denticity of ligand systems on the in vitro and in vivo behavior of (99m)Tc(I)-tricarbonyl complexes: a hint for the future functionalization of biomolecules. Bioconjug Chem 2000; 11(3):345–351.

28. Alberto R, Schibli R, Schubiger PA, et al. First application of fac-$[^{99m}Tc(OH_2)_3(CO)_3]^+$ in bioorganometallic chemistry: design, structure, and in vitro affinity of a 5-HT$_{1A}$ receptor ligand labeled with ^{99m}Tc. J Am Chem Soc 1999; 121:6076–6077.

29. Schibli R, Katti KV, Higginbotham C, et al. In vitro and in vivo evaluation of bidentate, water-soluble phosphine ligands as anchor groups for the organometallic fac-[99mTc(CO)3]+-core. Nucl Med Biol 1999; 26(6): 711–716.

30. Pietzsch HJ, Gupta A, Reisgys M, et al. Chemical and biological characterization of technetium(I) and rhenium(I) tricarbonyl complexes with dithioether ligands serving as linkers for coupling the Tc(CO)(3) and Re(CO)(3) moieties to biologically active molecules. Bioconjug Chem 2000; 11 (3):414–424.

31. Minutolo F, Katzenellenbogen JA. Three component synthesis of substituted h5-cyclopentadienyl tricarbonylrhenium complexes: scope, limitations, and mechanistic interpretations. Organometallics 1998; 18:2519–2530.

32. Minutolo F, Katzenellenbogen JA. Boronic acids in the three-component synthesis of carbon-substituted cyclpen-

tadienyl tricarbonyl rhenium complexes. J Am Chem Soc 1998; 120:13264–13265.

33. Minutolo F, Katzenellenbogen JA. A convenient three-component synthesis of substituted cyclopentadienyl tricarbonyl rhenium complexes. J Am Chem Soc 1998; 120:4515–4515.

34. Maria L, Paulo A, Santos IC, et al. Very small and soft scorpionates: water stable technetium tricarbonyl complexes combining a bis-agnostic (k$_3$-H, H, S) binding motif with pendant and integrated bioactive molecules. J Am Chem Soc 2006; 128:14590–14598.

35. 'Langen KJ, Ziemons K, Kiwit JC, et al. 3-[123I]iodo-alpha-methyltyrosine and [methyl-11C]-L-methionine uptake in cerebral gliomas: a comparative study using SPECT and PET. J Nucl Med 1997; 38(4):517–522.

36. Samnick S, Schaefer A, Siebert S, et al. Preparation and investigation of tumor affinity, uptake kinetic and transport mechanism of iodine-123-labelled amino acid derivatives in human pancreatic carcinoma and glioblastoma cells. Nucl Med Biol 2001; 28(1):13–23.

37. Prabhakar G, Mehra KS, Ramamoorthy N, et al. Evaluation of radioiodination of meta-iodobenzylguanidine (MIBG) catalysed by in situ generated Cu(I) and directly added Cu(II). Appl Radiat Isot 1999; 50(6):1011–1014.

38. Eersels JLH, Travis J, Herscheid JDM. Manufacturing I-123 -labelled radiopharmaceuticals. pitfalls and solutions. J Label Comp Radiopharm 2005; 48:241–257.

39. Misra HK, Knaus EE, Weibe LI, et al. Synthesis of ^{131}I, ^{125}I, ^{123}I, and ^{82}Br labelled 5-halo-1-(2-deoxy-2-fluoro-B-D-arabino-furanosyl)uracils. Int J Rad Appl Instrum [A] 1986; 37:901–905.

40. Vaidyanathan G, Zalutsky MR. Preparation of 5-[131I] iodo- and 5-[211At]astato-1-(2-deoxy-2-fluoro-beta-D-arabinofuranosyl) uracil by a halodestannylation reaction. Nucl Med Biol 1998; 25(5):487–496.

41. Wilbur DS. Radiohalogenation of proteins: an overview of radionuclides, labeling methods, and reagents for conjugate labeling. Bioconjug Chem 1992; 3(6):433–470.

42. Lambert C, Mease RC, Avren L, et al. Radioiodinated (aminostyryl)pyridinium (ASP) dyes: new cell membrane probes for labeling mixed leukocytes and lymphocytes for diagnostic imaging. Nucl Med Biol 1996; 23(4): 417–427.

43. Musachio JL, Lever JR. Vinylstannylated alkylating agents as prosthetic groups for radioiodination of small molecules: design, synthesis, and application to iodoallyl analogues of spiperone and diprenorphine. Bioconjug Chem 1992; 3(2):167–175.

44. Harper PV, Beck R, Charleston D, et al. Optimization of scanning method using Tc-99m. Nucleonics 1964; 22:50.

45. Mariani G, Erba P, Villa G, et al. Lymphoscintigraphic and intraoperative detection of the sentinel lymph node in breast cancer patients: the nuclear medicine perspective. J Surg Oncol 2004; 85(3):112–122.

46. Edwards CL, Hayes RL. Tumor scanning with 67Ga citrate. J Nucl Med 1969; 10(2):103–105.

47. Even-Sapir E, Israel O. Gallium-67 scintigraphy: a cornerstone in functional imaging of lymphoma. Eur J Nucl Med Mol Imaging 2003; 30(suppl 1):S65–S81.

48. Nejmeddine F, Caillat-Vigneron N, Escaig F, et al. Mechanism involved in gallium-67 (Ga-67) uptake by human lymphoid cell lines. Cell Mol Biol (Noisy-le-grand) 1998; 44(8):1215–1220.

49. Feremans W, Bujan W, Neve P, et al. CD71 phenotype and the value of gallium imaging in lymphomas. Am J Hematol 1991; 36(3):215–216.

50. Sohn MH, Jones BJ, Whiting JH Jr., et al. Distribution of gallium-67 in normal and hypotransferrinemic tumor-bearing mice. J Nucl Med 1993; 34(12):2135–2143.

51. Chen DC, Newman B, Turkall RM, et al. Transferrin receptors and gallium-67 uptake in vitro. Eur J Nucl Med 1982; 7(12):536–540.

52. Shen YY, Kao A, Yen RF. Comparison of 18F-fluoro-2-deoxyglucose positron emission tomography and gallium-67 citrate scintigraphy for detecting malignant lymphoma. Oncol Rep 2002; 9(2):321–325.

53. Wirth A, Seymour JF, Hicks RJ, et al. Fluorine-18 fluorodeoxyglucose positron emission tomography, gallium-67 scintigraphy, and conventional staging for Hodgkin's disease and non-Hodgkin's lymphoma. Am J Med 2002; 112(4):262–268.

54. Subramanian G, McAfee JG. A new complex for ^{99m}Tc for skeleton imaging. Radiology 1971; 99:192–196.

55. Silberstein EB, Francis MD, Tofe AJ, et al. Distribution of ^{99m}Tc-Sn diphosphonate and free ^{99m}Tc-pertechnetate in selected soft and hard tissues. J Nucl Med 1975; 16:58–61.

56. Francis MD, Ferguson DL, Tofe AJ, et al. Comparative evaluation of three diphosphonates: in vitro adsorption (C- 14 labeled) and in vivo osteogenic uptake (Tc-99m complexed). J Nucl Med 1980; 21(12):1185–1189.

57. Malhotra P, Berman CG. Evaluation of bone metastases in lung cancer. Cancer Control 2002; 9(254):259–260.

58. Panwar P, Chuttani K, Mishra P, et al. Synthesis of trans-1,2-cyclohexyldinitrilo tetramethylene phosphonic acid and its radiolabelling with 99mTc for the detection of skeletal metastases. Nucl Med Commun 2006; 27(8):619–626.

59. Ilias I, Pacak K. Diagnosis and management of tumors of the adrenal medulla. Horm Metab Res 2005; 37(12): 717–721.

60. Kaltsas G, Korbonits M, Heintz E, et al. Comparison of somatostatin analog and meta-iodobenzylguanidine radionuclides in the diagnosis and localization of advanced neuroendocrine tumors. J Clin Endocrinol Metab 2001; 86(2):895–902.

61. Mairs RJ, Gaze MN, Barrett A. The uptake and retention of metaiodobenzyl guanidine by the neuroblastoma cell line NB1-G. Br J Cancer 1991; 64(2):293–295.

62. Mairs RJ, Livingstone A, Gaze MN, et al. Prediction of accumulation of 131I-labelled meta-iodobenzylguanidine in neuroblastoma cell lines by means of reverse transcription and polymerase chain reaction. Br J Cancer 1994; 70(1):97–101.

63. Glowniak JV, Kilty JE, Amara SG, et al. Evaluation of metaiodobenzylguanidine uptake by the norepinephrine, dopamine and serotonin transporters. J Nucl Med 1993; 34(7):1140–1146.

64. Lode HN, Bruchelt G, Seitz G, et al. Reverse transcriptase-polymerase chain reaction (RT-PCR) analysis of monoamine transporters in neuroblastoma cell lines: correlations to meta-iodobenzylguanidine (MIBG) uptake and tyrosine hydroxylase gene expression. Eur J Cancer 1995; 31A(4):586–590.

65. Vaidyanathan G, Shankar S, Affleck DJ, et al. Biological evaluation of ring- and side-chain-substituted m-iodobenzylguanidine analogues. Bioconjug Chem 2001; 12(5): 798–806.

66. Vaidyanathan G, Shankar S, Zalutsky MR. Synthesis of ring- and side-chain-substituted m-iodobenzylguanidine analogues. Bioconjug Chem 2001; 12(5):786–797.

67. Jager PL, Vaalburg W, Pruim J, et al. Radiolabeled amino acids: basic aspects and clinical applications in oncology. J Nucl Med 2001; 42(3):432–445.

68. Vander Borght T, Asenbaum S, Bartenstein P, et al. EANM procedure guidelines for brain tumour imaging using labelled amino acid analogues. Eur J Nucl Med Mol Imaging 2006; 33(11):1374–1380.

69. Langen KJ, Roosen N, Coenen HH, et al. Brain and brain tumor uptake of L-3-[123I]iodo-alpha-methyl tyrosine: competition with natural L-amino acids. J Nucl Med 1991; 32(6):1225–1229.

70. Langen KJ, Pauleit D, Coenen HH. 3-[(123)I]Iodo-alpha-methyl-L-tyrosine: uptake mechanisms and clinical applications. Nucl Med Biol 2002; 29(6):625–631.

71. Woesler B, Kuwert T, Morgenroth C, et al. Non-invasive grading of primary brain tumours: results of a comparative study between SPET with 123I-alpha-methyl tyrosine and PET with 18F-deoxyglucose. Eur J Nucl Med 1997; 24(4): 428–434.

72. Weber W, Bartenstein P, Gross MW, et al. Fluorine-18-FDG PET and iodine-123-IMT SPECT in the evaluation of brain tumors. J Nucl Med 1997; 38(5):802–808.

73. Del Vecchio S, Salvatore M. ^{99m}Tc-MIBI in the evaluation of breast cancer biology. Eur J Nucl Med Mol Imaging 2004; 31(suppl 1):S88–S96.

74. Shikano N, Kanai Y, Kawai K, et al. Isoform selectivity of 3-125I-iodo-alpha-methyl-L-tyrosine membrane transport in human L-type amino acid transporters. J Nucl Med 2003; 44(2):244–246.

75. Lahoutte T, Mertens J, Caveliers V, et al. Comparative biodistribution of iodinated amino acids in rats: selection of the optimal analog for oncologic imaging outside the brain. J Nucl Med 2003; 44(9):1489–1494.

76. Lahoutte T, Caveliers V, Camargo SM, et al. SPECT and PET amino acid tracer influx via system L (h4F2hc-hLAT1) and its transstimulation. J Nucl Med 2004; 45(9): 1591–1596.

77. Hellwig D, Menges M, Schneider G, et al. Radioiodinated phenylalanine derivatives to image pancreatic cancer: a comparative study with [18F]fluoro-2-deoxy-D-glucose in human pancreatic carcinoma xenografts and in inflammation models. Nucl Med Biol 2005; 32(2):137–145.

78. Fozing C, Wagner M, Menger MD, et al. Preparation, in-vitro and in-vivo evaluation of 8-(^{123}I)iodo-L-1,2,3, 4-tetrahydro-7-hydroxyisoquinoline-3-carboxylic acid as an imaging agent for prostate cancer. 17th International Symposium on Radiopharmaceutical Sciences, Aachen, Germany, 2007, April 30–May 4 (abstr S69).

79. Samnick S, Fozing T, Kirsch CM. Preparation and tumor affinity testing of the radioiodinated tetrahydroisoquinoline derivative [123I]TIC(OH) for targeting prostate cancer. Appl Radiat Isot 2006; 64(5):563–569.

80. Piwnica-Worms D, Kronauge JF, Chiu ML. Uptake and retention of hexakis (2-methoxyisobutyl isonitrile) technetium(I) in cultured chick myocardial cells. mitochondrial and plasma membrane potential dependence. Circulation 1990; 82(5):1826–1838.

81. Delmon-Moingeon LI, Piwnica-Worms D, Van den Abbeele AD, et al. Uptake of the cation hexakis(2-methoxyisobutylisonitrile)-technetium-99m by human carcinoma cell lines in vitro. Cancer Res 1990; 50(7): 2198–2202.

82. Schillaci O, Spanu A, Madeddu G. [99mTc]sestamibi and [99mTc]tetrofosmin in oncology: SPET and fusion imaging in lung cancer, malignant lymphomas and brain tumors. Q J Nucl Med Mol Imaging 2005; 49(2):133–144.

83. Spanu A, Schillaci O, Madeddu G. 99mTc labelled cationic lipophilic complexes in malignant and benign tumors: the role of SPET and pinhole-SPET in breast cancer, differentiated thyroid carcinoma and hyperparathyroidism. Q J Nucl Med Mol Imaging 2005; 49(2): 145–169.

84. Kapucu LO, Akyuz C, Vural G, et al. Evaluation of therapy response in children with untreated malignant lymphomas using technetium-99m-sestamibi. J Nucl Med 1997; 38(2):243–247.

85. Yuksel M, Cermik TF, Doganay L, et al. 99mTc-MIBI SPET in non-small cell lung cancer in relationship with Pgp and prognosis. Eur J Nucl Med Mol Imaging 2002; 29(7):876–881.

86. Van de Wiele C, Rottey S, Goethals I, et al. 99mTc sestamibi and 99mTc tetrofosmin scintigraphy for predicting resistance to chemotherapy: a critical review of clinical data. Nucl Med Commun 2003; 24(9):945–950.

87. Piwnica-Worms D, Chiu ML, et al. Functional imaging of multidrug-resistant P-glycoprotein with an organotechnetium complex. Cancer Res 1993; 53(5):977–984.

88. Piwnica-Worms, D, Rao VV, Kronauge JF, et al. Characterization of multidrug resistance P-glycoprotein transport function with an organotechnetium cation. Biochemistry 1995; 34(38):12210–12220.

89. Takamura Y, Miyoshi Y, Taguchi T, et al. Prediction of chemotherapeutic response by Technetium 99m-MIBI scintigraphy in breast carcinoma patients. Cancer 2001; 92(2):232–239.

90. Sciuto R, Pasqualoni R, Bergomi S, et al. Prognostic value of (99m)Tc-sestamibi washout in predicting response of locally advanced breast cancer to neoadjuvant chemotherapy. J Nucl Med 2002; 43(6):745–751.

91. Fujii H, Nakamura K, Kubo A, et al. Preoperative evaluation of the chemosensitivity of breast cancer by means of double phase 99mTc-MIBI scintimammography. Ann Nucl Med 1998; 12(6):307–312.

92. Ciarmiello A, Del Vecchio S, Silvestro P, et al. Tumor clearance of technetium 99m-sestamibi as a predictor of response to neoadjuvant chemotherapy for locally advanced breast cancer. J Clin Oncol 1998; 16(5): 1677–1683.

93. Pusztai L, Wagner P, Ibrahim N, et al. Phase II study of tariquidar, a selective P-glycoprotein inhibitor, in patients with chemotherapy-resistant, advanced breast carcinoma. Cancer 2005; 104(4):682–691.

94. Ghirmai S, Mume E, Tolmachev V, et al. Synthesis and radioiodination of some daunorubicin and doxorubicin derivatives. Carbohydr Res 2005; 340(1):15–24.

95. Kiesewetter DO, Jagoda EM, Kao CH, et al. Fluoro-, bromo-, and iodopaclitaxel derivatives: synthesis and biological evaluation. Nucl Med Biol 2003; 30(1):11–24.

96. Roh EJ, Park YH, Song CE, et al. Radiolabeling of paclitaxel with electrophilic 123I. Bioorg Med Chem 2000; 8(1):65–68.

97. Georg GI, Cheruvallath ZS, Harriman GCB, et al. Topliss approach to the synthesis of biologically active substituted N-benzoyl taxol analogues. Bioorg Med Chem Lett 1994; 4:1825–1830.

98. Apisarnthanarax S, Chao KS. Current imaging paradigms in radiation oncology. Radiat Res 2005; 163(1):1–25.

99. Serganova I, Humm J, Ling C, et al. Tumor hypoxia imaging. Clin Cancer Res 2006; 12(18):5260–5264.

100. Padhani AR, Krohn KA, Lewis JS, et al. Imaging oxygenation of human tumours. Eur Radiol 2007; 17(4): 861–872.

101. Davda S, Bezabeh T. Advances in methods for assessing tumor hypoxia in vivo: implications for treatment planning. Cancer Metastasis Rev 2006; 25(3):469–480.

102. Rajendran JG, Hendrickson KR, Spence AM, et al. Hypoxia imaging-directed radiation treatment planning. Eur J Nucl Med Mol Imaging 2006; 33(suppl 1):44–53.

103. Tatum JL, Kelloff GJ, Gillies RJ, et al. Hypoxia: importance in tumor biology, noninvasive measurement by imaging, and value of its measurement in the management of cancer therapy. Int J Radiat Biol 2006; 82(10): 699–757.

104. Wardman P. Electron transfer and oxidative stress as key factors in the design of drugs selectively active in hypoxia. Curr Med Chem 2001; 8(7):739–761.

105. Ballinger JR. Imaging hypoxia in tumors. Semin Nucl Med 2001; 31(4):321–329.

106. Chapman JD, Engelhardt EL, Stobbe CC, et al. Measuring hypoxia and predicting tumor radioresistance with nuclear medicine assays. Radiother Oncol 1998; 46(3):229–237.

107. Chapman JD, Schneider RF, Urbain JL, et al. Single-photon emission computed tomography and positron-emission tomography assays for tissue oxygenation. Semin Radiat Oncol 2001; 11(1):47–57.

108. Hodgkiss RJ. Use of 2-nitroimidazoles as bioreductive markers for tumour hypoxia. Anticancer Drug Des 1998; 13(6):687–702.

109. Grunbaum Z, Freauff SJ, Krohn KA, et al. Synthesis and characterization of congeners of misonidazole for imaging hypoxia. J Nucl Med 1987; 28(1):68–75.

110. Biskupiak JE, Grierson JR, Rasey JS, et al. Synthesis of an (iodovinyl) misonidazole derivative for hypoxia imaging. J Med Chem 1991; 34(7):2165–2168.

111. Martin GV, Biskupiak JE, Caldwell JH, et al. Characterization of iodovinylmisonidazole as a marker for myocardial hypoxia. J Nucl Med 1993; 34(6):918–924.

112. Rasey JS, Koh WJ, Evans ML, et al. Quantifying regional hypoxia in human tumors with positron emission tomography of [18F]fluoromisonidazole: a pretherapy study of 37 patients. Int J Radiat Oncol Biol Phys 1996; 36(2): 417–428.

113. Bruehlmeier M, Roelcke U, Schubiger PA, et al. Assessment of hypoxia and perfusion in human brain tumors using PET with 18F-fluoromisonidazole and 15O-H2O. J Nucl Med 2004; 45(11):1851–1859.

114. Thorwarth D, Eschmann SM, Holzner F, et al. Combined uptake of [18F]FDG and [18F]FMISO correlates with radiation therapy outcome in head-and-neck cancer patients. Radiother Oncol 2006; 80(2):151–156.

115. Yang DJ, Wallace S, Cherif A, et al. Development of F-18-labeled fluoroerythronitroimidazole as a PET agent for imaging tumor hypoxia. Radiology 1995; 194(3):795–800.

116. Barthel H, Wilson H, Collingridge DR, et al. In vivo evaluation of [18F] fluoroetanidazole as a new marker for imaging tumour hypoxia with positron emission tomography. Br J Cancer 2004; 90(11):2232–2242.

117. Dolbier WR Jr., Li AR, Koch CJ, et al. [18F]-EF5, a marker for PET detection of hypoxia: synthesis of precursor and a new fluorination procedure. Appl Radiat Isot 2001; 54(1):73–80.

118. Lehtio K, Oikonen V, Gronroos T, et al. Imaging of blood flow and hypoxia in head and neck cancer: initial evaluation with [(15)O]H(2)O and [(18)F] fluoroerythronitroimidazole PET. J Nucl Med 2001; 42(11):1643–1652.

119. Ziemer LS, Evans SM, Kachur AV, et al. Noninvasive imaging of tumor hypoxia in rats using the 2-nitroimidazole 18F-EF5. Eur J Nucl Med Mol Imaging 2003; 30(2):259–266.

120. Jette DC, Wiebe LI, Flanagan RJ, et al. Iodoazomycin riboside (1-(5′-iodo-5′-deoxyribofuranosyl)-2-nitroimidazole), a hypoxic cell marker. I. Synthesis and in vitro characterization. Radiat Res 1986; 105(2):169–179.

121. Mannan RH, Somayaji VV, Lee J, et al. Radioiodinated 1-(5-iodo-5-deoxy-beta-D-arabinofuranosyl)-2-nitroimidazole (iodoazomycin arabinoside: IAZA): a novel marker of tissue hypoxia. J Nucl Med 1991; 32(9):1764–1770.

122. Groshar D, McEwan AJ, Parliament MB, et al. Imaging tumor hypoxia and tumor perfusion. J Nucl Med 1993; 34(6):885–888.

123. Parliament MB, Chapman JD, Urtasun RC, et al. Noninvasive assessment of human tumour hypoxia with 123I-iodoazomycin arabinoside: preliminary report of a clinical study. Br J Cancer 1992; 65(1):90–95.

124. Piert M, Machulla HJ, Picchio M, et al. Hypoxia-specific tumor imaging with 18F-fluoroazomycin arabinoside. J Nucl Med 2005; 46(1):106–113.

125. Sorger D, Patt M, Kumar P, et al. [18F]Fluoroazomycinarabinofuranoside (18FAZA) and [18F]Fluoromisonidazole (18FMISO): a comparative study of their selective uptake in hypoxic cells and PET imaging in experimental rat tumors. Nucl Med Biol 2003; 30(3):317–326.

126. Kumar P, Stypinski D, Xia H, et al. Fluoroazomycin arabinoside (FAZA): synthesis, ^{3}H and ^{3}H-labelling and preliminary biological evaluation of a novel 2-nitroimidazole marker of hypoxia. J Label Comp Radiopharm 1999; 42:3–16.

127. Schneider RF, Engelhardt EL, Stobbe CC, et al. The synthesis and radiolabeling of novel markers of tissue hypoxia of the iodinated azomycin nucleoside class. J Label Comp Radiopharm 1997; 39(7):541–557.

128. Zanzonico P, O'Donoghue J, Chapman JD, et al. Iodine-124-labeled iodo-azomycin-galactoside imaging of tumor hypoxia in mice with serial microPET scanning. Eur J Nucl Med Mol Imaging 2004; 31(1):117–128.

129. Linder KE, Chan YW, Cyr JE, et al. TcO(PnA.O-1-(2-nitroimidazole)) [BMS-181321], a new technetium-containing nitroimidazole complex for imaging hypoxia: synthesis, characterization, and xanthine oxidase-catalyzed reduction. J Med Chem 1994; 37(1):9–17.

130. Ballinger JR, Kee JW, Rauth AM. In vitro and in vivo evaluation of a technetium-99m-labeled 2-nitroimidazole (BMS181321) as a marker of tumor hypoxia. J Nucl Med 1996; 37(6):1023–1031.

131. Melo T, Duncan J, Ballinger JR, et al. BRU59-21, a second-generation 99mTc-labeled 2-nitroimidazole for imaging hypoxia in tumors. J Nucl Med 2000; 41(1): 169–176.

132. Hoebers FJ, Janssen HL, Olmos AV, et al. Phase 1 study to identify tumour hypoxia in patients with head and neck cancer using technetium-99m BRU 59-21. Eur J Nucl Med Mol Imaging 2002; 29(9):1206–1211.

133. Engelhardt EL, Schneider RF, Seeholzer SH, et al. The synthesis and radiolabeling of 2-nitroimidazole derivatives of cyclam and their preclinical evaluation as positive markers of tumor hypoxia. J Nucl Med 2002; 43(6): 837–850.

134. Chu T, Li R, Hu S, et al. Preparation and biodistribution of technetium-99m-labeled 1-2(nitroimidazole-1-yl)-propanhydroxyiminoamide (N2IPA) as a tumor hypoxia marker. Nucl med Biol 2004; 31:199–203.

135. Fujibayashi Y, Taniuchi H, Yonekura Y, et al. Copper-62-ATSM: a new hypoxia imaging agent with high membrane permeability and low redox potential. J Nucl Med 1997; 38(7):1155–1160.

136. Dearling JL, Lewis JS, Mullen GE, et al. Copper bis (thiosemicarbazone) complexes as hypoxia imaging agents: structure-activity relationships. J Biol Inorg Chem 2002; 7(3):249–259.

137. Burgman P, O'Donoghue JA, Lewis JS, et al. Cell line-dependent differences in uptake and retention of the hypoxia-selective nuclear imaging agent Cu-ATSM. Nucl Med Biol 2005; 32(6):623–630.

138. Dehdashti F, Grigsby PW, Mintun MA, et al. Assessing tumor hypoxia in cervical cancer by positron emission tomography with 60Cu-ATSM: relationship to therapeutic response-a preliminary report. Int J Radiat Oncol Biol Phys 2003; 55(5):1233–1238.

139. Zhang X, Melo T, Ballinger JR, et al. Studies of 99mTc-BnAO (HL-91): a non-nitroaromatic compound for

hypoxic cell detection. Int J Radiat Oncol Biol Phys 1998; 42(4):737–740.

140. Brauers G, Archer CM, Burke JF. The chemical characterization of the tumor imaging agent 99mTc-HL91. Eur J Nucl Med Mol Imaging 1997; 24:943.

141. Li L, Yu J, Xing L, et al. Serial hypoxia imaging with 99mTc-HL91 SPECT to predict radiotherapy response in nonsmall cell lung cancer. Am J Clin Oncol 2006; 29(6):628–633.

142. Storr T, Fisher CL, Mikata Y, et al. A glucosamine-dipicolylamine conjugate of 99mTc(I) and 186Re(I) for use in imaging and therapy. Dalton Trans 2005; (4):654–655.

143. Chen X, Li L, Liu F, et al. Synthesis and biological evaluation of technetium-99m-labeled deoxyglucose derivatives as imaging agents for tumor. Bioorg Med Chem Lett 2006; 16(21):5503–5506.

144. Yang DJ, Kim CG, Schechter NR, et al. Imaging with 99mTc ECDG targeted at the multifunctional glucose transport system: feasibility study with rodents. Radiology 2003; 226(2):465–473.

145. Schibli R, Dumas C, Petrig J, et al. Synthesis and in vitro characterization of organometallic rhenium and technetium glucose complexes against Glut 1 and hexokinase. Bioconjug Chem 2005; 16(1):105–112.

146. Kriss JP, Maruyama Y, Tung LA, et al. The fate of 5-bromodeoxyuridine, 5-bromodeoxycytidine, and 5-iododeoxycytidine in man. Cancer Res 1963; 23:260–268.

147. Ryser JE, Blauenstein P, Remy N, et al. [76Br]-Bromodeoxyuridine, a potential tracer for the measurement of cell proliferation by positron emission tomography, in vitro and in vivo studies in mice. Nucl Med Biol 1999; 26(6):673–679.

148. Bergstrom M, Lu L, Fasth KJ, et al. In vitro and animal validation of bromine-76-bromodeoxyuridine as a proliferation marker. J Nucl Med 1998; 39(7):1273–1279.

149. Gardelle O, Roelcke U, Vontobel P, et al. [76Br]Bromodeoxyuridine PET in tumor-bearing animals. Nucl Med Biol 2001; 28(1):51–57.

150. Lu L, Bergstrom M, Fasth KJ, et al. Elimination of nonspecific radioactivity from [76Br]bromide in PET study with [76Br]bromodeoxyuridine. Nucl Med Biol 1999; 26(7):795–802.

151. Conti PS, Alauddin MM, Fissekis JR, et al. Synthesis of 2'-fluoro-5-[11C]-methyl-1-beta-D-arabinofuranosyluracil ([11C]-FMAU): a potential nucleoside analog for in vivo study of cellular proliferation with PET. Nucl Med Biol 1995; 22(6):783–789.

152. Mercer JR, Xu LH, Knaus EE, et al. Synthesis and tumor uptake of 5-82Br- and 5-131I-labeled 5-halo-1-(2-fluoro-2-deoxy-beta-D-ribofuranosyl) uracils. J Med Chem 1989; 32(6):1289–1294.

153. Lu L, Bergstrom M, Fasth KJ, et al. Synthesis of [76Br] bromofluorodeoxyuridine and its validation with regard to uptake, DNA incorporation, and excretion modulation in rats. J Nucl Med 2000; 41(10):1746–1752.

154. Lu L, Samuelsson L, Bergstrom M, et al. Rat studies comparing 11C-FMAU, 18F-FLT, and 76Br-BFU as proliferation markers. J Nucl Med 2002; 43(12):1688–1698.

155. Cho SY, Ravasi L, Szajek LP, et al. Evaluation of (76)Br-FBAU as a PET reporter probe for HSV1-tk gene expression imaging using mouse models of human glioma. J Nucl Med 2005; 46(11):1923–1930.

156. Alauddin MM, Shahinian A, Park R, et al. Synthesis of 2'-deoxy-2'-[18F]fluoro-5-bromo-1-beta-D-arabinofuranosyluracil ([18F]-FBAU) and 2'-deoxy-2'-[18F]fluoro-5-chloro-1-beta-D-arabinofuranosyluracil ([18F]-FCAU), and their biological evaluation as markers for gene expression. Nucl Med Biol 2004; 31(4):399–405.

157. Morin KW, Duan W, Xu L, et al. Cytotoxicity and cellular uptake of pyrimidine nucleosides for imaging herpes simplex type-1 thymidine kinase (HSV-1 TK) expression in mammalian cells. Nucl Med Biol 2004; 31(5):623–630.

158. Tjuvajev JG, Doubrovin M, Akhurst T, et al. Comparison of radiolabeled nucleoside probes (FIAU, FHBG, and FHPG) for PET imaging of HSV1-tk gene expression. J Nucl Med 2002; 43(8):1072–1083.

159. Toyohara J, Hayashi A, Sato M, et al. Rationale of 5-(125)I-iodo-4'-thio-2'-deoxyuridine as a potential iodinated proliferation marker. J Nucl Med 2002; 43(9):1218–1226.

160. Toyohara J, Gogami A, Hayashi A, et al. Pharmacokinetics and metabolism of 5-125I-iodo-4'-thio-2'-deoxyuridine in rodents. J Nucl Med 2003; 44(10):1671–1676.

161. Toyohara J, Hayashi A, Sato M, et al. Development of radioiodinated nucleoside analogs for imaging tissue proliferation: comparisons of six 5-iodonucleosides. Nucl Med Biol 2003; 30(7):687–696.

162. Rose C, Thorpe SM, Anderson KW, et al. Beneficial effect of adjuvant tamoxifen therapy in primary breast cancer patients with high oestrogen receptor values. Lancet 1985; 1(8419):16–19.

163. Clark GM, Sledge GW Jr., Osborne CK, et al. Survival from first recurrence: relative importance of prognostic factors in 1,015 breast cancer patients. J Clin Oncol 1987; 5(1):55–61.

164. Vollenweider-Zerargui L, Barrelet L, Wong Y, et al. The predictive value of estrogen and progesterone receptors' concentrations on the clinical behavior of breast cancer in women. clinical correlation on 547 patients. Cancer 1986; 57(6):1171–1180.

165. Holdaway IM, Bowditch JV. Variation in receptor status between primary and metastatic breast cancer. Cancer 1983; 52(3):479–485.

166. Gao H, Katzenellenbogen JA, Garg R, et al. Comparative QSAR analysis of estrogen receptor ligands. Chem Rev 1999; 99(3):723–744.

167. Anstead GM, Carlson KE, Katzenellenbogen JA. The estradiol pharmacophore: ligand structure-estrogen receptor binding affinity relationships and a model for the receptor binding site. Steroids 1997; 62(3):268–303.

168. Hochberg RB. Iodine-125–labeled estradiol: a gamma-emitting analog of estradiol that binds to the estrogen receptor. Science 1979; 205(4411):1138–1140.

169. Pavlik EJ, Nelson K, Gallion HH, et al. Characterization of high specific activity [16 alpha-123I] iodo-17 beta-estradiol as an estrogen receptor-specific radioligand

capable of imaging estrogen receptor-positive tumors. Cancer Res 1990; 50(24):7799–7805

170. Senderoff SG, McElvany KD, Carlson KE, et al. Methodology for the synthesis and specific activity determination of 16 alpha-[77Br]-bromoestradiol-17 beta and 16 alpha-[77Br]-11 beta-methoxyestradiol-17 beta, two estrogen receptor-binding radiopharmaceuticals. Int J Appl Radiat Isot 1982; 33(7):545–551.

171. Katzenellenbogen JA, Senderoff SG, McElvany KD, et al. 16 alpha-[77Br] bromoestradiol-17 beta: a high specific-activity, gamma-emitting tracer with uptake in rat uterus and uterus and induced mammary tumors. J Nucl Med 1981; 22(1):42–47.

172. McElvany KD, Carlson KE, Welch MJ, et al. In vivo comparison of 16 alpha[77Br]bromoestradiol-17 beta and 16 alpha-[125I]iodoestradiol-17 beta. J Nucl Med 1982; 23(5):420–424.

173. McElvany KD, Katzenellenbogen JA, Shafer KE, et al. 16 alpha-[77Br]bromoestradiol: dosimetry and preliminary clinical studies. J Nucl Med 1982; 23(5):425–430.

174. Kiesewetter DO, Kilbourn MR, Landvatter SW, et al. Preparation of four fluorine- 18-labeled estrogens and their selective uptakes in target tissues of immature rats. J Nucl Med 1984; 25(11):1212–1221.

175. Dehdashti F, Mortimer JE, Siegel BA, et al. Positron tomographic assessment of estrogen receptors in breast cancer: comparison with FDG-PET and in vitro receptor assays. J Nucl Med 1995; 36(10):1766–1774.

176. Mankoff DA, Peterson LM, Tewson TJ, et al. [18F] fluoroestradiol radiation dosimetry in human PET studies. J Nucl Med 2001; 42(4):679–684.

177. Katzenellenbogen JA, McElvany KD, Senderoff SG, et al. 16 alpha-[77Br]bromo-11 beta-methoxyestradiol-17 beta: a gamma-emitting estrogen imaging agent with high uptake and retention by target organs. J Nucl Med 1982; 23(5):411–419.

178. Zielinski JE, Larner JM, Hoffer PB, et al. The synthesis of 11 beta-methoxy-[16 alpha-123I] iodoestradiol and its interaction with the estrogen receptor in vivo and in vitro. J Nucl Med 1989; 30(2):209–215.

179. Pomper MG, VanBrocklin H, Thieme AM, et al. 11 beta-methoxy-, 11 beta-ethyl- and 17 alpha-ethynyl-substituted 16 alpha-fluoroestradiols: receptor-based imaging agents with enhanced uptake efficiency and selectivity. J Med Chem 1990; 33(12):3143–3155.

180. Mazaitis JK, Gibson RE, Komai T, et al. Radioiodinated estrogen derivatives. J Nucl Med 1980; 21(2):142–146.

181. Gibson RE, Eckelman WC, Francis B, et al. [77Br]-17-alpha-Bromoethynylestradiol: in vivo and in vitro characterization of an estrogen receptor radiotracer. Int J Nucl Med Biol 1982; 9(4):245–250.

182. Hanson RN, Seitz DE, Botarro JC. E-17 alpha[125I] iodovinylestradiol: an estrogen-receptor-seeking radiopharmaceutical. J Nucl Med 1982; 23(5):431–436.

183. Hanson RN, Seitz DE, Bottaro JC. Radiohalodestannylation: synthesis of 125I-labeled 17 alpha-E-iodovinylestradiol. Int J Appl Radiat Isot 1984; 35(8):810–812.

184. Hanson RN, Franke LA. Preparation and evaluation of 17 alpha-[125I] iodovinyl-11 beta-methoxyestradiol as a highly selective radioligand for tissues containing estrogen receptors: concise communication. J Nucl Med 1984; 25(9):998–1002.

185. DeSombre ER, Hughes A, Mease RC, et al. Comparison of the distribution of bromine-77-bromovinyl steroidal and triphenylethylene estrogens in the immature rat. J Nucl Med 1990; 31(9):1534–1542.

186. Nakatsuka I, Ferreira NL, Eckelman WC, et al. Synthesis and evaluation of (17 alpha, 20E)-21-[125I]iodo-19-norpregna-1,3,5(10), 20-tetraene-3,17 -diol and (17 alpha,20E)-21-[125I]iodo-11 beta-methoxy-19-norpregna-1,3,5(10), 20-tetraene-3,17-diol (17 alpha-(iodovinyl)estradiol derivatives) as high specific activity potential radiopharmaceuticals. J Med Chem 1984; 27(10):1287–1291.

187. Ali H, Rousseau J, Ghaffari MA, et al. Synthesis, receptor binding, and tissue distribution of (17 alpha, 20E)- and (17 alpha, 20Z)-21-[125I]iodo-19-norpregna-1,3,5(10), 20-tetraene-3,17-diol. J Med Chem 1988; 31(10):1946–1950.

188. Ali H, Rousseau J, Ghaffari MA, et al. Synthesis, receptor binding, and tissue distribution of 7 alpha- and 11 beta-substituted (17 alpha, 20E)- and (17 alpha, 20Z)-21-[125I] iodo-19-norpregna-1,3,5(10),20-tetraene-3,17-diols. J Med Chem 1991;34(2):854–860.

189. Hughes A, Larson SM, Hanson RN, et al. Uptake and interconversion of the Z and E isomers of 17 alpha-iodovinyl-11 beta-methoxyestradiol in the immature female rat. Steroids 1997; 62(2):244–252.

190. Rijks LJ, Bakker PJ, van Tienhoven G, et al. Imaging of estrogen receptors in primary and metastatic breast cancer patients with iodine-123-labeled Z-MIVE. J Clin Oncol 1997; 15(7):2536–2545.

191. Nachar O, Rousseau JA, Lefebvre B, et al. Biodistribution, dosimetry and metabolism of 11beta-methoxy-(17alpha,20E/Z)-[123I]iodovinylestradiol in healthy women and breast cancer patients. J Nucl Med 1999; 40(10):1728–1736.

192. Nachar O, Rousseau JA, Ouellet R, et al. Scintimammography with 11beta-methoxy-(17alpha,20Z)-[123I]iodovinylestradiol: a complementary role to 99mTc-methoxyisobutyl isonitrile in the characterization of breast tumors. J Nucl Med 2000; 41(8):1324–1331.

193. Hanson RN, Seitz DE. Tissue distribution of the radio-labeled antiestrogen [125I]iodotamoxifen. Int J Nucl Med Biol 1982; 9(2):105–107.

194. Hunter DH, Strickland LA. An iodine-131 iodotamoxifen: no carrier added iodination via diazonium salt. Appl Radiat Isot 1986; 37(8):889–891.

195. Van de Wiele C, De Vos F, De Sutter J, et al. Biodistribution and dosimetry of (iodine-123)-iodomethyl-N, N-diethyltamoxifen, an (anti)oestrogen receptor radioligand. Eur J Nucl Med 1999; 26(10):1259–1264.

196. Van de Wiele C, Cocquyt V, VandenBroecke R, et al. Iodine-labeled tamoxifen uptake in primary human breast carcinoma. J Nucl Med 2001; 42(12):1818–1820.

197. Delpassand ES, Yang DJ, Wallace S, et al. Synthesis, biodistribution, and estrogen receptor scintigraphy of indium-111-diethylenetriaminepentaacetic acid-tamoxifen analogue. J Pharm Sci 1996; 85(6):553–559.

198. Salituro FG, Carlson KE, Elliston JF, et al. [125I]iododesethyl tamoxifen aziridine: synthesis and covalent labeling of the estrogen receptor with an iodine-labeled affinity label. Steroids 1986; 48(5–6):287–313.

199. DeSombre ER, Mease RC, Hughes A, et al. Bromine-80m-labeled estrogens: auger electron-emitting, estrogen receptor-directed ligands with potential for therapy of estrogen receptor-positive cancers. Cancer Res 1988; 48(4):899–906.

200. Gatley SJ, Desombre ER, Mease RC, et al. Synthesis, purification and stability of no carrier added radioiodinated 1,1-bis(4-hydroxyphenyl)-2-iodo-2-phenylethylene (IBHPE), a prototype triphenylethylene estrogen-receptor binding radiopharmaceutical. Int J Rad Appl Instrum B 1991; 18(7):769–775.

201. Hughes A, Gatley SJ, DeSombre ER. Comparison of the distribution of radioiodinated-E-17 alpha-iodovinyl-11 beta-methoxyestradiol and 2-iodo-1,1-bis(4-hydroxyphenyl)-phenylethylene estrogens in the immature female rat. J Nucl Med 1993; 34(2):272–280.

202. Desombre ER, Pribish J, Hughes A. Comparison of the distribution of radioiodinated di- and tri-hydroxyphenylethylene estrogens in the immature female rat. Nucl Med Biol 1995; 22(5):679–687.

203. Top S, El Hafa H, Vessieres A, et al. Rhenium carbonyl complexes of B-estradiol derivatives with high selectivity for the estradiol receptor: an approach to selective organometallic radiopharmaceuticals. J Am Chem Soc 1995; 117:8372–8380.

204. Arterburn JB, Corona C, Rao KV, et al. Synthesis of 17-alpha-substituted estradiol-pyridin-2-yl hydrazine conjugates as effective ligands for labeling with Alberto's complex fac-[Re(OH2)3(CO)3]+ in water. J Org Chem 2003; 68(18):7063–7070.

205. Ramesh C, Bryant B, Nayak T, et al. Linkage effects on binding affinity and activation of GPR30 and estrogen receptors ERalpha/beta with tridentate pyridin-2-yl hydrazine tricarbonyl-Re/(99m)Tc(I) chelates. J Am Chem Soc 2006; 128(45):14476–14477.

206. Wust F, Carlson KE, Katzenellenbogen JA, et al. Synthesis and binding affinities of new 17 alpha-substituted estradiol-rhenium "n + 1" mixed-ligand and thioethercarbonyl complexes. Steroids 1998; 63(12):665–671.

207. Skaddan MB, Wust FR, Katzenellenbogen JA. Synthesis and binding affinities of novel re-containing 7alpha-substituted estradiol complexes: models for breast cancer imaging agents. J Org Chem 1999; 64(22):8108–8121.

208. Skaddan MB, Wust FR, Jonson S, et al. Radiochemical synthesis and tissue distribution of Tc-99m-labeled 7alpha-substituted estradiol complexes. Nucl Med Biol 2000; 27(3):269–278.

209. Luyt LG, Bigott HM, Welch MJ, et al. 7alpha- and 17alpha-substituted estrogens containing tridentate tricarbonyl rhenium/technetium complexes: synthesis of estrogen receptor imaging agents and evaluation using microPET with technetium-94m. Bioorg Med Chem 2003; 11 (23):4977–4989.

210. Hom RK, Katzenellenbogen JA. Synthesis of a tetradentate oxorhenium(V) complex mimic of a steroidal estrogen. J Org Chem 1997; 62:6290–6297.

211. Mull ES, Sattigeri VJ, Rodriguez AL, et al. Aryl cyclopentadienyl tricarbonyl rhenium complexes: novel ligands for the estrogen receptor with potential use as estrogen radiopharmaceuticals. Bioorg Med Chem 2002; 10(5): 1381–1398.

212. Vilner BJ, John CS, Bowen WD. Sigma-1 and sigma-2 receptors are expressed in a wide variety of human and rodent tumor cell lines. Cancer Res 1995; 55(2):408–413.

213. Mach RH, Smith CR, al-Nabulsi I, et al. Sigma 2 receptors as potential biomarkers of proliferation in breast cancer. Cancer Res 1997; 57(1):156–161.

214. Michelot JM, Moreau MF, Labarre PG, et al. Synthesis and evaluation of new iodine-125 radiopharmaceuticals as potential tracers for malignant melanoma. J Nucl Med 1991; 32(8):1573–1580.

215. Michelot JM, Moreau MF, Veyre AJ, et al. Phase II scintigraphic clinical trial of malignant melanoma and metastases with iodine-123-N-(2-diethylaminoethyl 4-iodobenzamide). J Nucl Med 1993; 34(8):1260–1266.

216. John CS, Saga T, Kinuya S, et al. An improved synthesis of [125I]N-(diethylaminoethyl)-4-iodobenzamide: a potential ligand for imaging malignant melanoma. Nucl Med Biol 1993; 20(1):75–79.

217. Mohammed A, Nicholl C, Titsch U, et al. Radioiodinated N-(alkylaminoalkyl)-substituted 4-methoxy-, 4-hydroxy-, and 4-aminobenzamides: biological investigations for the improvement of melanoma-imaging agents. Nucl Med Biol 1997; 24(5):373–380.

218. Brandau W, Niehoff T, Pulawski P, et al. Structure distribution relationship of iodine-123-iodobenzamides as tracers for the detection of melanotic melanoma. J Nucl Med 1996; 37(11):1865–1871.

219. John CS, Vilner BJ, Gulden ME, et al. Synthesis and pharmacological characterization of 4-[125I]-N-(N-benzylpiperidin-4-yl)-4-iodobenzamide: a high affinity sigma receptor ligand for potential imaging of breast cancer. Cancer Res 1995; 55(14):3022–3027.

220. John CS, Gulden ME, Li J, et al. Synthesis, in vitro binding, and tissue distribution of radioiodinated 2-[125I]N-(N-benzylpiperidin-4-yl)-2-iodo benzamide, 2-[125I]BP: a potential sigma receptor marker for human prostate tumors. Nucl Med Biol 1998; 25(3):189–194.

221. John CS, Bowen WD, Fisher SJ, et al. Synthesis, in vitro pharmacologic characterization, and preclinical evaluation of N-[2-(1'-piperidinyl)ethyl]-3-[125I]iodo-4-methoxybenzamide (P[125I]MBA) for imaging breast cancer. Nucl Med Biol 1999; 26(4):377–382.

222. John CS, Bowen WD, Saga T, et al. A malignant melanoma imaging agent: synthesis, characterization, in vitro binding and biodistribution of iodine-125-(2-piperidinylaminoethyl)4-iodobenzamide. J Nucl Med 1993; 34(12):2169–2175.

223. Caveliers V, Everaert H, John CS, et al. Sigma receptor scintigraphy with N-[2-(1'-piperidinyl)ethyl]-3-(123) I-iodo-4-methoxybenzamide of patients with suspected primary breast cancer: first clinical results. J Nucl Med 2002; 43(12):1647–1649.

224. John CS, Lim BB, Geyer BC, et al. 99mTc-labeled sigma-receptor-binding complex: synthesis, characterization, and

specific binding to human ductal breast carcinoma (T47D) cells. Bioconjug Chem 1997; 8(3):304–309.

225. Friebe M, Mahmood A, Bolzati C, et al. [99mTc]oxotechnetium(V) complexes amine-amide-dithiol chelates with dialkylaminoalkyl substituents as potential diagnostic probes for malignant melanoma. J Med Chem 2001; 44(19):3132–3140.

226. Friebe M, Mahmood A, Spies H, et al. '3 + 1' mixed-ligand oxotechnetium(V) complexes with affinity for melanoma: synthesis and evaluation in vitro and in vivo. J Med Chem 2000; 43(14):2745–2752.

227. Egeblad M, Werb Z. New functions for the matrix metalloproteinases in cancer progression. Nat Rev Cancer 2002; 2(3):161–174.

228. Coussens LM, Werb Z. Matrix metalloproteinases and the development of cancer. Chem Biol 1996; 3(11):895–904.

229. Vihinen P, Kahari VM. Matrix metalloproteinases in cancer: prognostic markers and therapeutic targets. Int J Cancer 2002; 99(2):157–166.

230. Van de Wiele C, Oltenfreiter R. Imaging probes targeting matrix metalloproteinases. Cancer Biother Radiopharm 2006; 21(5):409–417.

231. Kopka K, Breyholz HJ, Wagner S, et al. Synthesis and preliminary biological evaluation of new radioiodinated MMP inhibitors for imaging MMP activity in vivo. Nucl Med Biol 2004; 31(2):257–267.

232. Oltenfreiter R, Staelens L, Kersemans V, et al. Valine-based biphenylsulphonamide matrix metalloproteinase inhibitors as tumor imaging agents. Appl Radiat Isot 2006; 64(6):677–685.

233. Kopka K, Breyholz HJ, Wagner S, et al. Radioiodinated pyrimidine-2,4,6-triones as model probes for the in-vivo molecular imaging of activated MMPs. 17th International Symposium on Radiopharmaceutical Sciences, Aachen, Germany, 2007, April 30–May 4 (abstr P310).

234. Ke CY, Mathias CJ, Green MA. The folate receptor as a molecular target for tumor-selective radionuclide delivery. Nucl Med Biol 2003; 30(8):811–817.

235. Mathias CJ, Wang S, Waters DJ, et al. Indium-111-DTPA-folate as a potential folate-receptor-targeted radiopharmaceutical. J Nucl Med 1998; 39(9):1579–1585.

236. Mathias CJ, Hubers D, Low PS, et al. Synthesis of [(99m)Tc] DTPA-folate and its evaluation as a folate-receptor-targeted radiopharmaceutical. Bioconjug Chem 2000; 11(2):253–257.

237. Muller C, Hohn A, Schubiger PA, et al. Preclinical evaluation of novel organometallic 99mTc-folate and 99mTc-pteroate radiotracers for folate receptor-positive tumour targeting. Eur J Nucl Med Mol Imaging 2006; 33(9): 1007–1016.

238. Siegel BA, Dehdashti F, Mutch DG, et al. Evaluation of 111In-DTPA-folate as a receptor-targeted diagnostic agent for ovarian cancer: initial clinical results. J Nucl Med 2003; 44(5):700–707.

239. Schulke N, Varlamova OA, Donovan GP, et al. The homodimer of prostate-specific membrane antigen is a functional target for cancer therapy. Proc Natl Acad Sci U S A 2003; 100(22):12590–12595.

240. Kinoshita Y, Kuratsukuri K, Landas S, et al. Expression of prostate-specific membrane antigen in normal and malignant human tissues. World J Surg 2006; 30(4): 628–636.

241. Silver DA, Pellicer I, Fair WR, et al. Prostate-specific membrane antigen expression in normal and malignant human tissues. Clin Cancer Res 1997; 3(1):81–85.

242. Slusher BS, Tsai G, Yoo G, et al. Immunocytochemical localization of the N-acetyl-aspartyl-glutamate (NAAG) hydrolyzing enzyme N-acetylated alpha-linked acidic dipeptidase (NAALADase). J Comp Neurol 1992; 315(2):217–229.

243. Zhou J, Neale JH, Pomper MG, et al. NAAG peptidase inhibitors and their potential for diagnosis and therapy. Nat Rev Drug Discov 2005; 4(12):1015–1026.

244. Foss CA, Mease RC, Fan H, et al. Radiolabeled small-molecule ligands for prostate-specific membrane antigen: in vivo imaging in experimental models of prostate cancer. Clin Cancer Res 2005; 11(11):4022–4028.

245. Ray S, Foss C, Mease R, et al. Synthesis and biodistribution of Re/99mTc-labeled PSMA inhibitors. 17th International Symposium on Radiopharmaceutical Sciences, Aachen, Germany, 2007, April 30–May 4 (abstr).

14

Radionuclides for Therapy

GEORGE SGOUROS

Russell H. Morgan Department of Radiology and Radiological Science, Johns Hopkins University School of Medicine, Baltimore, Maryland, U.S.A.

INTRODUCTION

Advances in our understanding of the molecular biology of cancer and other diseases have helped identify targets for radionuclide therapy, making it possible to target radiation at the cellular and molecular level. Molecular radiotherapy (MRT) is a systemically administered targeted radionuclide therapy. In contrast to chemotherapy, wherein all proliferating cells are affected, MRT delivers radiation to only those cells that express cancer markers. Table 1 lists radionuclides that have been used, investigated, or considered for therapy.

RADIOIODINE THERAPY OF THYROID CANCER

The prototypical example of radionuclide therapy is radioidine treatment of thyroid cancer. Differentiated (papillary and follicular) thyroid carcinoma cells have the ability to concentrate iodine as part of the molecular machinery for making thyroid hormone. This feature of the disease has made it possible to deliver very high radiation doses (in excess of 30–60 Gy) to thyroid carcinoma cells and cell clusters using radioactive iodine, typically [131]I (8-day half-life). To insure treatment with the largest safe amount of administered activity, treatment planning, involving a pretreatment trace-level administration of ^{131}I, to collect biodistribution for dosimetry, was described early in the development of this treatment approach (1–3). Highly sophisticated, present-day treatment of this disease can include a series of [124]I PET scans for detailed dosimetry and treatment planning and an FDG PET scan to identify pockets of anaplastic (undifferentiated) disease that no longer concentrates iodine (4,5). In the latter case, the patient is referred to alternate treatment modalities.

RADIOLABELED ANTIBODY THERAPY OF NON-HODGKIN'S LYMPHOMA: BEXXAR AND ZEVALIN

Medullary thyroid cancer treatment with radioiodine illustrates targeting of the radionuclide without the need for a carrier that recognizes tumor cells. The majority of targeted radionuclide therapy has been performed with radiolabeled antibodies. There are two FDA-approved antibody-based molecular radiotherapeutics, Bexxar and Zevalin, for Non-Hodgkin's Lymphoma (NHL). Both ^{131}I-tositumomab (Bexxar) and ^{90}Y-ibritumomab tiuxetan (Zevalin) are radiolabeled antibodies; they target different regions (epitopes) on the B-cell-associated CD20 antigen. Experience with these two agents over the past 15 years illustrates a number of important principles regarding MRT.

1. These agents are more effective, by a substantial margin, than any other single agent examined in late-stage patients that have failed multiple courses and different types of chemotherapy; effective treatment (high and durable rates of CR) is achieved with a single course of treatment lasting a total of 1.5 to 2 weeks (this includes the dosimetry/imaging phase of the treatment).

2. Aside from their greater effectiveness and short treatment time, these agents are considerably less toxic compared with chemotherapy with toxicity limited largely to hematologic suppression.

3. Comparisons of the unlabeled antibody with the corresponding radiolabeled antibody have been made, and the results show far greater efficacy of the radiolabeled construct. Evidence for this is provided by the demonstrated efficacy in patients that have become refractory to rituximab [the unlabeled analog of ^{90}Y-ibritumomab tiuxetan (Zevalin)] and also by a direct comparison of unlabeled versus ^{131}I-labeled tositumomab (6,7).

4. There is increasing evidence that these agents provide a substantial advantage as first line therapy.

5. In combination with chemotherapy, which may be used to reduce tumor burden in marrow and also reduce the size of existing lesions, these agents may show even greater effectiveness (8). How exactly these agents will fit into NHL treatment is still being established. Newer MRTs against NHL are also being developed (9,10).

Table 1 Summary List of Radionuclides Considered for Therapy

Radionuclide	Decay mode	Half-life	References
Ac-225	α	10 day	33–36
As-77	β⁻	38.83 hr	37,38)
Ag-111	β⁻	7.45 day	37–39
Au-199	β⁻	3.14 day	37,38
At-211	α, ε	7.2 hr	38,40–43
Bi-212	β⁻, α	60.55 min	41,44–47
Bi-213	β⁻, α	45.6 min	38,41,47
Br-77	ε, β⁺	57.0 hr	38,40
Br-80m/Br-80	IT/ε, β⁻	17.7 min/4.4 hr	38,48)
Br-82	β⁻	35.3 hr	40,48
Ce-134/La-134	ε/ε+β⁺	3.16 day/6.45 min	38,49
Co-58m	IT	9.04 h	38,50
Cr-51	ε	27.7 day	38
Cs-129	ε	32.06 hr	38,51
Cu-64	ε+β⁺, β⁻	12.7 hr	38,39,52
Cu-67	β⁻	61.83 hr	37–41,50,53
Er-165	ε	10.36 hr	38,54
Fm-255	α	20.07 hr	38,55
Ga-67	ε	3.26 day	38,39,41,50,56
Ge-71	ε	11.43 day	38,57
Gd-159	β⁻	18.48 hr	37,58
Hg-197	ε	64.14 hr	38,59
Ho-161	ε	2.48 hr	38,50
Ho-166	β⁻	26.8 hr	37–39,53,60–62
I-123	ε	13.22 hr	38,41,63,64
I-124	ε+β⁺	4.17 day	38,63–65)
I-125	ε	59.4 day	38,41,66,67
I-131	β⁻	8.02 day	37,39,41,50,68,69
Ir-194	β⁻	19.28 hr	37,38,58)
In-111	ε	2.80 day	37,39,40,50
In-114m	IT, ε	49.5 day	38,70
In-115m	IT, β⁻	4.49 hr	38,71
Lu-177	β⁻	6.65 day	(38,39,41,50,53,72,73
Os-189m	IT	5.81 hr	38,50
P-32	β⁻	14.26 day	15,37–39,53
P-33	β⁻	25.34 day	37,38,53,74
Pb-212	β⁻	10.64 hr	38,41,75
Pd-109	β⁻	13.70 hr	37,38,58,76,77

Table 1 Summary List of Radionuclides Considered for Therapy (*Continued*)

Radionuclide	Decay mode	Half-life	References
Pm-149	β^-	53.08 hr	37–39,58,78,79
Pr-142	β^-, ε	19.12 hr	37,58,80
Pr-143	β^-	13.57 day	37,58)
Pt-193m	IT	4.33 day	38,71,81,82
Pt-195m	IT	4.01 day	38,41,81,83s
Ra-223	α	11.43 day	38,84–90
Ra-224	α	3.66 day	91–93)
Re-186	ε, β^-	3.72 day	37–41,53,94–101
Re-188	β^-	17.00 hr	37–39,41,50,102,103
Rh-105	β^-	35.36 hr	37–39,58,104,105
Rh-103m	IT	56.1 min	38,50,72
Ru-97	ε	2.9 day	38,106,107
Sb-119	ε	38.2 hr	38,50
Sc-47	β^-	3.35 day	37–39,58,108
Se-73	$\varepsilon+\beta^+$	7.15 hr	38,55)
Sm-153	β^-	46.5 hr	37–39,41,109–112
Sn-117m	IT	13.6 day	15,39,113–115
Sn-121	β^-	27.03 hr	37,38,58
Sr-89	β^-	50.53 day	15,38,39,53,116
Ta-177	ε	56.56 hr	38
Tb-149	ε, α	4.12 hr	38,117–119
Tb-161	β^-	6.91 day	38,50,120
Tc-94	$\varepsilon+\beta^+$	293 min	38,55
Tm-167	ε	9.25 day	38,55
Y-90	β^-	64.0 hr	37,39,40,50,72

α, Alpha decay; β^-, Beta decay; ε, Electron capture; IT, internal transition; β^+, Positron decay.

RADIOPEPTIDES

The Bexxar and Zevalin therapeutic regimens are based on intact antibodies. A lower molecular weight class of molecular radiotherapeutics, radiolabeled peptides (peptides are typically made up of less than 50 amino acids), has been the focus of European investigators. These peptides can achieve binding affinities in the low nanomolar range and have been found to be nonimmunogenic. One of the first of these, ^{111}In-DTPA-octreotide (Octreoscan) was approved by the FDA in 1994 for imaging/detection of neuroendocrine tumors with somatostatin receptors based on trials conducted exclusively outside the United States (in Europe). It was subsequently investigated as a radiotherapeutic, based on the expectation that the Auger and conversion electron emissions of ^{111}In would by cytotoxic once the peptide internalizes. Since these initial efforts, new agents that target a wider range of somatostatin and other receptor types with a higher affinity and using beta-particle emitters such as ^{90}Y, ^{188}Re, and ^{177}Lu have been investigated (11). Beta particles have been favored because they have a substantially longer range than Auger and conversion electrons and can provide a cross-fire component to tumor targeting by irradiating both the targeted cell and neighboring, possibly receptor-negative cells.

MIBG

Metaiodobenzylguanidine (MIBG) is an aralkylguanidine analog of catecholamine precursors, structurally similar to norepinephrine, which concentrates within secretory granules of catecholamine producing cells. It has been labeled with ^{123}I for diagnostic imaging and with ^{131}I for therapy of neuroblastoma, pheochromocytoma and, to a lesser extent, other neuroendocrine tumors (12). Neuroblastoma constitutes approximately 8% to 10% of pediatric cancers at an annual incidence of 8 to 10 cases per million children. Approximately 600 new cases are seen in the United States each year. Once metastasized, the five-year survival rate is only 30% to 40%. In these trials, ^{131}I-MIBG has demonstrated highly specific uptake and prolonged intracellular retention in tumor and not in normal organs. ^{131}I-MIBG has also been investigated in pheochromocytoma in adults (13). In neuroblastoma treatment, ^{131}I-MIBG has been investigated in progressive or recurrent neuroblastoma after conventional therapy or in combination with myeloablative therapy; it has also been applied prior to surgery in inoperable stage III and IV disease. In a very difficult patient population, a 40% to 60% rate of objective responses has been observed, including some complete responses. These responses are typically observed at doses that lead to high-grade hematologic toxicity.

MRTs AGAINST BONE METASTASES

Perhaps the greatest impact of MRTs on patient care will be in the targeting of bone metastases. A number of radionuclide constructs, including ^{153}Sm-EDTMP (Lexidronam), ^{89}SrCl$_2$ (Metastron), which have been FDA approved for pain palliation, are currently being investigated as potential therapeutics against bone metastases (14,15). Skeletal metastases are a major cause of morbidity and mortality in advanced breast, lung, colon, and prostate cancer patients. In many cases, the skeleton is the first (and sometimes the only) site of metastatic disease. Each year, 200,000 new cases of painful bone metastases are diagnosed and require palliative care; 73% of these are attributable to breast, prostate, and lung cancers. Radionuclide therapy for bone pain has been shown to be more effective and is accompanied by fewer side effects than opiate and external beam–based approaches; dose-limiting toxicity has been limited to the bone marrow in almost all cases. Pain palliation is typically seen 1 week to 10 days after administration. In the majority of cases, the pain relief is longer lasting and more cost-effective. Studies have also suggested that up-front use of these agents can reduce the incidence of metastatic progression and the subsequent need for pain palliation. Like the anti-NHL agents, however, these radiopharmaceuticals have not been incorporated, to the extent merited by their demonstrated clinical success, in the management of patients that have or are susceptible to bone metastases. New agents in this class of MRTs that are currently under investigation/development include ^{186}Re and ^{188}Re etidronates and ^{117m}Sn-DTPA. The latter, due to the short range of its emissions and demonstrated efficacy in an early clinical trial, holds the potential of high efficacy with substantially reduced hematologic toxicity. Unfortunately, development of this agent has come to a near halt, in part, because of issues related to U.S. supply of the radionuclide and lack of commercial support for its further development.

RADIOLABELED ANTIBODY THERAPY

As noted above, the greatest effort in targeted radionuclide therapy has been with radiolabeled antibodies (radioimmunotherapy). The radionuclide properties required for radioimmunotherapy should generally be matched with the disease architecture and stage of disease being targeted. For example, beta-particle emitters such as ^{131}I and ^{90}Y are preferred for bulky tumor targeting. The rationale for this is that the range of beta particles (0.8–2 mm) in tissue is sufficient to irradiate tumor cells that are not specifically targeted by the antibody. If the distribution is uniform and the radionuclide is internalized then shorter ranged conversion or Auger electron–emitting radionuclides would be appropriate. Beyond the emission type, internalization also impacts upon radionuclide selection in terms of the chemistry of the radionuclide. Unless residualized, by incorporating sugar molecules (16,17), halogens such as I-131 or I-125 clear rapidly from tumor cells and are excreted via the kidneys. Radiometals such as Y-90 or ^{111}In are retained within tumor cells and thereby provide a longer residence time in tumor cells.

Radionuclides that emit alpha particles have been gaining considerable attention for therapy; the first two trials were initiated in the past two years and are still ongoing. Alpha-particle emitters are seen as particularly promising because alpha particles are several thousand-fold more efficient at tumor cell killing than beta or electron emitters.

Linear Energy Transfer

An important aspect in characterizing the biological effects of different emission types (beta vs. Auger vs. alpha) is the amount of energy transferred to the cell as the particle traverses the cell. This is characterized by the linear energy transfer (LET), which is the energy transferred per unit distance traveled by the particle. LET will influence the likely biological effect for a given amount of energy deposition to a cell. For example, high LET emissions (e.g., alpha particles, low-energy Auger electrons) yield a very dense track of ionization-induced damage that is capable of causing irreparable double-strand DNA damage (18–20). The same amount of total energy deposition by low-LET emissions (beta particles) have a very low probability of yielding irreparable double-stranded DNA damage since the track is much less dense and double-stranded DNA breaks are infrequent. In cell culture experiments, the absorbed dose (energy per unit mass) required to achieve a particular level of cell kill is approximately five to eight times greater for low-LET emissions relative to that required for high LET emissions.

Dosimetry

The energy deposited per unit mass of tissue is defined as the absorbed dose. The absorbed dose is a measure of potential therapeutic efficacy and toxicity, in this sense it is analogous to "dose" as applied to chemotherapy. Absorbed dose is calculated as the total number of radionuclide transformations (also referred to as decays or disintegrations) occurring in a particular tissue (i.e., the source), multiplied by the energy emitted per transformation, and by a factor that represents the fraction of energy emitted by the source that is absorbed by a target tissue. The total energy absorbed by a target tissue from all source tissues is then divided by the mass of the target tissue to give the absorbed dose (21). Although all radioactivity-containing tissues will contribute dose to a particular target, the dominant contribution arises from the self-dose, that is, the fraction of energy emitted by the target (assuming it has taken up radioactivity) that is absorbed within the target. Mathematically, this may be represented by:

$$D = \frac{\tilde{A} \cdot \Delta \cdot \varphi}{M}$$

where $\tilde{A}, \cdot \Delta$, and φ are the total number of transformations, the energy emitted per transformation, and the fraction of the energy that is absorbed in the tissue, respectively; M is the mass of the target tissue and D is the target tissue self-dose. The energy emitted per transformation, Δ, and fraction absorbed, φ, are listed by radionuclide and source-target organ combination in compilations provided by the Medical Internal Radionuclide Dose Committee (22–27). The mass must generally be determined by CT or other imaging modality. The number of transformations, $\tilde{A}$, are generally obtained by imaging or sampling at different times after injection of the radiolabeled antibody (28).

Beta emitters

Table 2 lists beta emitters that have been used in radiolabeled antibody therapy. Beta particles may be thought of as electrons that originate from the nucleus. Unlike orbital shell electron emissions, they do not have a single value for the initial energy, rather the emitted energy is selected from a range of possible initial energies according to a probability function that provides the likelihood that a particle with a chosen energy will be emitted in a given decay. Tabulated values of the energy or range of beta particle emissions, therefore, typically list the most likely (mean) energy emitted or the maximum possible (end-point) energy. Since the range of a particle depends upon its initial energy, the range of beta particle emissions is correspondingly represented by a probability distribution of possible ranges with the mean or maximum ranges typically provided in tabulations. The two most popular radionuclides for radioimmunotherapy, ^{131}I and ^{90}Y, are beta emitters. ^{131}I was used almost exclusively in initial trials of radioimmunotherapy because the behavior of I-131 (as a free radionuclide) in humans had been well established in the treatment of thyroid cancer and also because of the ease with which antibodies may be labeled with this radionuclide. Yttrium-90 has gained in popularity recently because it provides the following advantages over ^{131}I: (*i*) No gamma-particle (photon) emissions, thereby eliminating the need to keep patients in radiation isolation. (*ii*) Longer range of beta particle emissions, an advantage in overcoming a non-uniform distribution of antibody within tumors. (*iii*) It is a metal that is retained within the cytosol of cells following internalization of the radiolabeled antibody. A drawback related to the second advantage of this radionuclide is that it is not possible to obtain imaging-based biodistribution information directly from ^{90}Y since it does not emit photons. This problem has been overcome by using ^{111}In as a surrogate for its biodistribution. The long range of the beta emission can be a drawback due to the potential for normal organ irradiation and increased toxicity (29).

Positron emitters

Table 3 lists positron emitters that have either been used or are being considered for use with antibodies (primarily for diagnosis). The description provided above for beta emitters also applies to positron emitters with the exception that positrons are the antimatter of electrons and are, therefore, positively charged. When positrons encounter electrons, the two particles annihilate each other leading to the release of energy in the form of high-energy

Table 2 Beta-Electron Emitters

Radionuclide	Half-life (hr)	Mean energy (keV)
I-131	193	182
Y-90	64	934
Re-188	17	765
Re-186	91	323
Cu-67	62	142
Lu-177	161	133

Table 3 Positron (β^+) Emitters

Radionuclide	Half-life (hr)	Mean energy (keV) (%β^+)
I-124	100	188 (25)
Y-86	15	219 (34)
Br-76	16	642 (57)
Ga-66	10	986 (57)

Table 4 Auger or Conversion Electron Emitters

Radionuclide	Half-life (hr)	Mean energy (keV)
I-125	1440	18
In-111	67	34
I-123	13	28

Table 5 Alpha Particle Emitters

Radionuclide	Half-life	%[a]	Emissions	
Daughters			Particle	Energy[b]
Bi-213	45.6 min	2	α	6 MeV
		98	β⁻	444 keV
		17	γ	440 keV
Po-213	4.2 μsec	98	α	8 MeV
Tl-209	2.2 min	2	β⁻	659 keV
Pb-209	3.25 hr	100	β⁻	198 keV
Bi-209	Stable			
Bi-212	1.0 hr	36	α	6 MeV
		64	β⁻	492 keV
Po-212	298 nsec	64	α	9 MeV
Tl-208	3.05 min	36	β⁻	560 keV
		8	γ	510 keV
		31	γ	580 keV
		36	γ	2.6 MeV
Pb-208	Stable			
At-211	7.21 hr	42	α	6 MeV
		19	γ	80 keV
Po-211	516 msec	58	α	7.5 MeV
Bi-207	32 yr	24	γ	70 keV
		41	γ	570 keV
		31	γ	1 MeV
Pb-207	Stable			
Ac-225	10 day	100	α	6 MeV
Fr-221	4.9 min	100	α	6 MeV
		10	γ	218 keV
At-217	32.3 msec	100	α	7 MeV
Bi-213	See Bi-123			
Ra-223	11.4 day	100	α	6 MeV
		40	γ	80 keV
		14	γ	270 keV
Rn-219	4 sec	100	α	7 MeV
		10	γ	270 keV
Po-215	1.8 msec	100	α	7 MeV
Pb-211	36.1 min	100	β⁻	447 keV
Bi-211	2.1 min	16	α	6 MeV
		84	α	7 MeV
		13	γ	350 keV
Tl-207	4.8 min	100	β⁻	493 keV
Pb-207	Stable			

[a]Percent emitted per decay of parent radionuclide.
[b]Mean β⁻ energy and approximate α and γ energies are listed.

photons. The high-energy photons are emitted in opposite direction, and this aspect of positron emitters is used for imaging with positron emission tomography (PET).

Auger emitters

In contrast to beta particles, Auger electrons are emitted from the orbital shells of atoms. They are characterized by a single energy (they are monoenergetic) and, therefore, by a single range. Table 4 lists Auger emitters that have been used or considered for use in targeted radionuclide therapy, the best studied of these is ^{125}I. The range of Auger electrons is from a few nanometers to several micrometers. Emissions in the nanometer range are therapeutically effective only if the radionuclide is incorporated into the DNA, but micrometer-ranged emissions, if of sufficient abundance, may be effective in tumor cell killing even if the radiolabeled antibody remains on the surface. In general, however, radionuclides with such emissions demonstrate enhanced cell killing if the radionuclide-carrier complex is internalized and remains within the cell and in proximity to the cell nucleus (30).

Alpha-Particle Emitters

Table 5 lists alpha-particle emitters that have been used or considered for use in therapy. The range of alpha particles in tissues is on the order of 40 to 90 μm; the LET is 100 to 1000-fold greater than that of beta particles. In most cases, one to three alpha particle traversals through the cell nucleus are sufficient to sterilize the cell. This is in contrast to the thousands to tens of thousands required of beta particles. The first two alpha-particle emitters used clinically (31,32), ^{211}At and ^{213}Bi, have relatively short half-lives and are, therefore, best suited for locoregional injection or in targeting rapidly accessible disease such as micrometastases. A clinical trial using a longer-lived alpha-particle emitter, ^{225}Ac, with a 10-day half-life has recently been initiated.

The compilation of radionuclides listed in Table 1 reflects the large number of radionuclides that have been considered for possible therapy. Only a small fraction of these have been investigated clinically or even preclinically.

An even smaller number have been approved by the FDA and are commercially available for therapeutic use in humans. As issues of supply, conjugation chemistry and the economics of targeted radionuclide therapy are resolved; many more radionuclides remain to be investigated.

REFERENCES

1. Benua RS, Leeper RD. A method and rationale for treatment of thyroid carcinoma with the largest, safe dose of 131-I. In: Meideros-Neto GA, Gaitan E, eds. Frontiers in Thyroidology. Vol 2. New York: Plenum Medical, 1986:1317–1321.

2. Benua RS, Rawson RW, Sonenberg M, et al. Relation of radioiodine dosimetry to results and complications in treatment of metastatic thyroid cancer. Am J Roentgenol Radium Ther Nucl Med 1962; 87(1):171–182.

3. Rall JE, Alpers JB, Lewallen CG, et al. Radiation pneumonitis and fibrosis—complication of radioiodine treatment of pulmonary metastases from cancer of the thyroid. J Clin Endocrinol Metab 1957; 17(11):1263–1276.

4. Wang WP, Larson SM, Fazzari M, et al. Prognostic value of [F-18]fluorodeoxyglucose positron emission tomographic scanning in patients with thyroid cancer. J Clin Endocrinol Metab 2000; 85(3):1107–1113.

5. Sgouros G, Kolbert KS, Sheikh A, et al. Patient-specific dosimetry for 131I thyroid cancer therapy using 124I PET and 3-dimensional-internal dosimetry (3D-ID) software. J Nucl Med 2004; 45(8):1366–1372.

6. Davis TA, Kaminski MS, Leonard JP, et al. Results of a randomized study of Bexxar (TM) (tositumomab and iodine I 131 tositumomab) vs. unlabeled tositumomab in patients with relapsed or refractory low-grade or transformed non-Hodgkin's lymphoma (NHL). Blood 2001; 98(11):843A.

7. Davis TA, Kaminski MS, Leonard JP, et al. The radioisotope contributes significantly to the activity of radioimmunotherapy. Clin Cancer Res 2004; 10(23):7792–7798.

8. Dreyling M, Trumper L, von Schilling C, et al. Results of a national consensus workshop: therapeutic algorithm in patients with follicular lymphoma—role of radioimmunotherapy. Ann Hematol 2007; 86(2):81–87.

9. Chatal JF, Harousseau JL, Griesinger F, et al. Radioimmunotherapy in non-Hodgkin's lymphoma (NHL) using a fractionated schedule of DOTA-conjugated, Y-90-radiolabeled, humanized anti-CD22 monoclonal antibody, epratuzumab. J Clin Oncol 2004; 22(14):174S.

10. Leahy MF, Seymour JF, Hicks RJ, et al. Multicenter phase II clinical study of iodine-131-rituximab radioimmunotherapy in relapsed or refractory indolent non-Hodgkin's lymphoma. J Clin Oncol 2006; 24(27):4418–4425.

11. Weiner RE, Thakur ML. Radiolabeled peptides in oncology—role in diagnosis and treatment. Biodrugs 2005; 19(3):145–163.

12. Pasieka JL, McEwan AJB, Rorstad O. The palliative role of I-131-MIBG and In-111-octreotide therapy in patients with metastatic progressive neuroendocrine neoplasms. Surgery 2004; 136(6):1218–1226.

13. Pashankar FD, O'Dorisio MS, Menda Y. MIBG and somatostatin receptor analogs in children: current concepts on diagnostic and therapeutic use. J Nucl Med 2005; 46:55S–61S.

14. Damerla V, Packianathan S, Boerner PS, et al. Recent developments in nuclear medicine in the management of bone metastases—a review and perspective. Am J Clin Oncol 2005; 28(5):513–520.

15. Pandit-Taskar N, Batraki M, Divgi CR. Radiopharmaceutical therapy for palliation of bone pain from osseous metastases. J Nucl Med 2004; 45(8):1358–1365.

16. Maxwell JL, Baynes JW, Thorpe SR. Inulin-125I-tyramine, an improved residualizing label for studies on sites of catabolism of circulating proteins. J Biol Chem 5 1988; 263(28):14122–14127.

17. Patel S, Stein R, Ong GL, et al. Enhancement of tumor-to-nontumor localization ratios by hepatocyte-directed blood clearance of antibodies labeled with certain residualizing radiolabels. J Nucl Med 1999; 40(8):1392–1401.

18. Zirkle RE. Some effects of alpha radiation upon plant cells. J Cell Comp Physiol 1932; 2(3):251–274.

19. Zirkle RE, Marchbank DF, Kuck KD. Exponential and sigmoid survival curves resulting from alpha and X-irradiation of Aspergillus spores. J Cell Comp Physiol 1952; 39(3):A75–A85.

20. Barendsen GW. Impairment of the proliferative capacity of human cells in culture by alpha-particles with differing linear-energy transfer. Int J Radiat Biol Relat Stud Phys Chem Med 1964; 8(5):453–466.

21. Loevinger R, Budinger TF, Watson EE. MIRD Primer for Absorbed Dose Calculations, revised edition. New York, NY: The Society of Nuclear Medicine, Inc., 1991.

22. Eckerman KF, Endo A. MIRD Radionuclide Data and Decay Scheme, 2nd edition. Reston VA:SNM press, 2008.

23. Weber DA, Eckerman KF, Dillman LT, et al. MIRD: Radionuclide Data and Decay Schemes. New York: The Society of Nuclear Medicine, 1989.

24. Bolch WE, Bouchet LG, Robertson JS, et al. MIRD pamphlet No. 17: the dosimetry of nonuniform activity distributions—radionuclide S values at the voxel level. J Nucl Med 1999; 40(1):11S–36S.

25. Bouchet LG, Bolch WE, Blanco HP, et al. MIRD Pamphlet No 19: absorbed fractions and radionuclide S values for six age-dependent multiregion models of the kidney. J Nucl Med 2003; 44(7):1113–1147.

26. Bouchet LG, Bolch WE, Howell RW, et al. S values for radionuclides localized within the skeleton. J Nucl Med 2000; 41(1):189–212.

27. Bouchet LG, Bolch WE, Weber DA, et al. MIRD Pamphlet No. 15: radionuclide S values in a revised dosimetric model of the adult head and brain. Medical Internal Radiation Dose. J Nucl Med 1999; 40(3):62S–101S.

28. Siegel JA, Thomas SR, Stubbs JB, et al. MIRD pamphlet no. 16: techniques for quantitative radiopharmaceutical biodistribution data acquisition and analysis for use in human radiation dose estimates. J Nucl Med 1999; 40(2):37S–61S.

29. Song H, Du Y, Sgouros G, et al. Therapeutic potential of 90Y- and 131I-labeled anti-CD20 monoclonal antibody in treating non-Hodgkin's lymphoma with pulmonary involvement: a Monte Carlo-based dosimetric analysis. J Nucl Med 2007; 48(1):150–157.

30. Kassis AI. The amazing world of auger electrons. Int J Radiat Biol 2004; 80(11–12):789–803.

31. Jurcic JG, Larson SM, Sgouros G, et al. Targeted alpha-particle immunotherapy for myeloid leukemia. Blood 2002; 100(4):1233–1239.

32. Zalutsky MR, Reardon DA, Akabani G, et al. Clinical experience with {alpha}-Particle emitting 211At: treatment of recurrent brain tumor patients with 211At-labeled chimeric antitenascin monoclonal antibody 81C6. J Nucl Med 2008; 49(1):30–38.

33. Geerlings MW. Radionuclides for radioimmunotherapy: criteria for selection. Int J Biol Markers 1993; 8(3):180–186.

34. Geerlings MW, Kaspersen FM, Apostolidis C, et al. The feasibility of 225Ac as a source of alpha-particles in radioimmunotherapy. Nucl Med Commun 1993; 14(2): 121–125.

35. McDevitt MR, Ma D, Simon J, et al. Design and synthesis of 225Ac radioimmunopharmaceuticals. Appl Radiat Isot 2002; 57(6):841–847.

36. McDevitt MR, Ma D, Lai LT, et al. Tumor therapy with targeted atomic nanogenerators. Science 2001; 294(5546): 1537–1540.

37. O'Donoghue JA, Bardies M, Wheldon TE. Relationships between tumor size and curability for uniformly targeted therapy with beta-emitting radionuclides. J Nucl Med 1995; 36(10):1902–1909.

38. Uusijarvi H, Bernhardt P, Ericsson T, et al. Dosimetric characterization of radionuclides for systemic tumor therapy: influence of particle range, photon emission, and subcellular distribution. Med Phys 2006; 33(9): 3260–3269.

39. Volkert WA, Hoffman TJ. Therapeutic radiopharmaceuticals. Chem Rev 1999; 99(9):2269–2292.

40. Wessels BW, Rogus RD. Radionuclide selection and model absorbed dose calculations for radiolabeled tumor associated antibodies. Med Phys 1984; 11(5):638–645.

41. Milenic DE, Brady ED, Brechbiel MW. Antibody-targeted radiation cancer therapy. Nat Rev Drug Discov 2004; 3(6): 488–499.

42. Bloomer WD, McLaughlin WH, Lambrecht RM, et al. 211At radiocolloid therapy: further observations and comparison with radiocolloids of 32P, 165Dy, and 90Y. Int J Radiat Oncol Biol Phys 1984; 10(3):341–348.

43. Zalutsky MR, Vaidyanathan G. Astatine-211-labeled radiotherapeutics: an emerging approach to targeted alpha-particle radiotherapy. Curr Pharm Des 2000; 6(14):1433–1455.

44. Atcher RW, Friedman AM, Hines JJ. An improved generator for the production of Pb-212 and Bi-212 from Ra-224. Appl Radiat Isot 1988; 39(4):283–286.

45. Macklis RM, Kaplan WD, Ferrara JL, et al. Alpha particle radio-immunotherapy: animal models and clinical prospects. Int J Radiat Oncol Biol Phys 1989; 16(6):1377–1387.

46. Macklis RM, Kinsey BM, Kassis AI, et al. Radioimmunotherapy with alpha-particle emitting immunoconjugates. Science 1988; 240(4855):1024–1026.

47. McDevitt MR, Sgouros G, Finn RD, et al. Radioimmunotherapy with alpha-emitting nuclides. Eur J Nucl Med 1998; 25(9):1341–1351.

48. Wong S, Ache HJ. On the preparation of 80Br- or 82Br-biomolecules via excitation labelling methods. Int J Appl Radiat Isot 1976; 27(1):19–25.

49. Lubberink M, Lundqvist H, Tolmachev V. Production, PET performance and dosimetric considerations of 134Ce/134La, an Auger electron and positron-emitting generator for radionuclide therapy. Phys Med Biol 2002; 47(4): 615–629.

50. Bernhardt P, Forssell-Aronsson E, Jacobsson L, et al. Low-energy electron emitters for targeted radiotherapy of small tumours. Acta Oncol 2001; 40(5):602–608.

51. Scholz KL, Sodd VJ, Blue JW. Spallation production of 127Cs-129Cs mixtures for medical use. Int J Appl Radiat Isot 1974; 25(5):203–208.

52. DeNardo SJ. Radioimmunodetection and therapy of breast cancer. Semin Nucl Med. 2005; 35(2):143–151.

53. Kassis AI, Adelstein SJ. Radiobiologic principles in radionuclide therapy. J Nucl Med 2005; 46:4S–12S.

54. Rao DV, Hallee GJ, Ottlinger ME, et al. Radiations emitted in the decay of 165Er: a promising medical radionuclide. Med Phys 1977; 4(3):177–186.

55. Stepanek J, Larsson B, Weinreich R. Auger-electron spectra of radionuclides for therapy and diagnostics. Acta Oncol 1996; 35(7):863–868.

56. Govindan SV, Goldenberg DM, Elsamra SE, et al. Radionuclides linked to a CD74 antibody as therapeutic agents for B-cell lymphoma: comparison of Auger electron emitters with beta-particle emitters. J Nucl Med 2000; 41(12):2089–2097.

57. von Neumann-Cosel P. Electron capture radioactive sources for intravascular brachytherapy: a feasibility study. Phys Med Biol 2003; 48(12):1855–1862.

58. Bardies M, Chatal JF. Absorbed doses for internal radiotherapy from 22 beta-emitting radionuclides: beta dosimetry of small spheres. Phys Med Biol 1994; 39:961–981.

59. Larsson I, Lindstedt E, Ohlin P, et al. A scintillation camera technique for quantitative estimation of separate kidney function and its use before nephrectomy. Scand J Clin Lab Invest 1975; 35(6):517–524.

60. Marques F, Paulo A, Campello MP, et al. Radiopharmaceuticals for targeted radiotherapy. Radiat Prot Dosimetry 2005; 116(1–4 pt 2):601–604.

61. Breitz H, Wendt R, Stabin M, et al. Dosimetry of high dose skeletal targeted radiotherapy (STR) with (166)Ho-DOTMP. Cancer Biother Radiopharm 2003; 18(2): 225–230.

62. Giralt S, Bensinger W, Goodman M, et al. Ho-166-DOTMP plus melphalan followed by peripheral blood stem cell transplantation in patients with multiple myeloma: results of two phase 1/2 trials. Blood 2003; 102(7): 2684–2691.

63. O'Donoghue JA, Wheldon TE. Targeted radiotherapy using Auger electron emitters. Phys Med Biol 1996; 41(10):1973–1992.

64. Kassis AI, Adelstein SJ, Mariani G. Radiolabeled nucleoside analogs in cancer diagnosis and therapy. Q J Nucl Med. 1996; 40(3):301–319.

65. Veach DR, Namavari M, Beresten T, et al. Synthesis and in vitro examination of [124I]-, [125I]- and [131I]-2-(4-iodophenylamino) pyrido[2,3-d]pyrimidin-7-one radiolabeled Abl kinase inhibitors. Nucl Med Biol 2005; 32(4): 313–321.

66. Scott AM, Lee FT, Jones R, et al. A phase I trial of humanized monoclonal antibody A33 in patients with colorectal carcinoma: biodistribution, pharmacokinetics, and quantitative tumor uptake. Clin Cancer Res Jul 1 2005; 11(13):4810–4817.

67. Panyutin IG, Sedelnikova OA, Karamychev VN, et al. Antigene radiotherapy: targeted radiodamage with 125i-labeled triplex-forming oligonucleotides. Ann N Y Acad Sci 2003; 1002:134–140.

68. Hamilton JG, Soley MH. Studies in iodine metabolism of the thyroid gland in situ by the use of radio-iodine in normal subjects and in patients with various types of goiter. Am J Physiol 1940; 131(1):0135–0143.

69. Soley MH, Foreman N. Radioiodine therapy in Graves' disease: a review. J Clin Invest 1949; 28(6, pt. 1):1367–1374.

70. Li M, Meares CF. Synthesis, metal chelate stability studies, and enzyme digestion of a peptide-linked DOTA derivative and its corresponding radiolabeled immunoconjugates. Bioconjug Chem 1993; 4(4):275–283.

71. Howell RW. Radiation spectra for Auger-electron emitting radionuclides: report No. 2 of AAPM Nuclear Medicine Task Group No. 6. Med Phys 1992; 19(6): 1371–1383.

72. Bernhardt P, Ahlman H, Forssell-Aronsson E. Model of metastatic growth valuable for radionuclide therapy. Med Phys 2003; 30(12):3227–3232.

73. Pandit-Taskar N, Hamlin PA, Reyes S, et al. New strategies in radioimmunotherapy for lymphoma. Curr Oncol Rep 2003; 5(5):364–371.

74. Goddu SM, Bishayee A, Bouchet LG, et al. Marrow toxicity of 33P-versus 32P-orthophosphate: implications for therapy of bone pain and bone metastases. J Nucl Med 2000; 41(5):941–951.

75. Ruble G, Wu C, Squire RA, et al. The use of 212Pb-labeled monoclonal antibody in the treatment of murine erythroleukemia. Int J Radiat Oncol Biol Phys 1996; 34(3):609–616.

76. Silberstein EB. Radionuclide therapy of hematologic disorders. Semin Nucl Med 1979; 9(2):100–107.

77. Chakraborty S, Das T, Banerjee S, et al. Preparation and preliminary biological evaluation of a novel 109Pd labeled porphyrin derivative for possible use in targeted tumor therapy. Q J Nucl Med Mol Imaging 2007; 51(1): 16–23.

78. Hu F, Cutler CS, Hoffman T, et al. Pm-149 DOTA bombesin analogs for potential radiotherapy. In vivo comparison with Sm-153 and Lu-177 labeled DO3A-amide-betaAla-BBN(7-14)NH(2). Nucl Med Biol 2002; 29(4): 423–430.

79. Mohsin H, Jia F, Sivaguru G, et al. Radiolanthanide-labeled monoclonal antibody CC49 for radioimmunotherapy of cancer: biological comparison of DOTA conjugates and 149Pm, 166Ho, and 177Lu. Bioconjug Chem 2006; 17(2):485–492.

80. Lee SW, Reece WD. Dose calculation of 142Pr microspheres as a potential treatment for arteriovenous malformations. Phys Med Biol 2005; 50(1):151–166.

81. Areberg J, Norrgren K, Mattsson S. Absorbed doses to patients from 191Pt-, 193mPt- and 195mPt-cisplatin. Appl Radiat Isot 1999; 51(5):581–586.

82. Howell RW, Rao DV, Sastry KS. Macroscopic dosimetry for radioimmunotherapy: nonuniform activity distributions in solid tumors. Med Phys 1989; 16(1):66–74.

83. Willins JD, Sgouros G. Modeling analysis of platinum-195M for targeting individual blood-borne cells in adjuvant radioimmunotherapy. J Nucl Med 1995; 36(2): 315–319.

84. Bruland OS, Nilsson S, Fisher DR, et al. High-linear energy transfer irradiation targeted to skeletal metastases by the alpha-emitter Ra-223: adjuvant or alternative to conventional modalities? Clin Cancer Res 2006; 12(20): 6250S–6257S.

85. Durbin PW, Asling CW, Jeung N, et al. The Metabolism and Toxicity of Radium-223 in rats. Berkely, CA: University of California Radiation Laboratory, 1958. UCRL-8189.

86. Fisher DR, Sgouros G. Dosimetry of radium-223 and progeny. In: Proceedings of the Sixth International Radiopharmaceutical Dosimetry Symposium. Paper presented at: Sixth International Radiopharmaceutical Dosimetry Symposium; 1999, 1996; Gatlinburg, TN.

87. Henriksen G, Fisher DR, Roeske JC, et al. Targeting of osseous sites with alpha-emitting Ra-223: comparison with the beta-emitter Sr-89 in mice. J Nucl Med 2003; 44(2):252–259.

88. Howell RW, Goddu SM, Narra VR, et al. Radiotoxicity of gadolinium-148 and radium-223 in mouse testes: relative biological effectiveness of alpha-particle emitters in vivo. Radiat Res 1997; 147(3):342–348.

89. Jonasdottir TJ, Fisher DR, Borrebk J, et al. First in vivo evaluation of liposome-encapsulated 223Ra as a potential alpha-particle-emitting cancer therapeutic agent. Anticancer Res 2006; 26(4 B):2841–2848.

90. Nilsson S, Larsen RH, Fossa SD, et al. First clinical experience with alpha-emitting radium-223 in the treatment of skeletal metastases. Clin Cancer Res 2005; 11(12):4451–4459.

91. Muller WA, Gossner W, Hug O, et al. Late effects after incorporation of the short-lived alpha-emitters 224Ra and 227Th in mice. Health Phys 1978; 35(1):33–55.

92. Lassmann M, Nosske D, Reiners C. Therapy of ankylosing spondylitis with Ra-224-radium chloride: dosimetry and risk considerations. Radiat Environ Biophys 2002; 41(3):173–178.

93. Tiepolt C, Gruning T, Franke WG. Renaissance of 224 Ra for the treatment of ankylosing spondylitis: clinical experiences. Nucl Med Commun 2002; 23(1):61–66.

94. Breitz HB, Durham JS, Fisher DR, et al. Radiation-absorbed dose estimates to normal organs following intraperitoneal 186Re-labeled monoclonal antibody: methods and results. Cancer Res 1995; 55(23 suppl): 5817s–5822s.

95. Breitz HB, Durham JS, Fisher DR, et al. Pharmacokinetics and normal organ dosimetry following intraperitoneal rhenium-186-labeled monoclonal antibody. J Nucl Med 1995; 36(5):754–761.

96. Breitz HB, Fisher DR, Weiden PL, et al. Dosimetry of rhenium-186-labeled monoclonal antibodies: methods, prediction from technetium-99m-labeled antibodies and results of phase I trials. J Nucl Med 1993; 34(6):908–917.

97. Breitz HB, Fisher DR, Wessels BW. Marrow toxicity and radiation absorbed dose estimates from rhenium-186-labeled monoclonal antibody. J Nucl Med 1998; 39(10):1746–1751.

98. Breitz HB, Fisher DR, Wessels BW. Marrow toxicity and radiation absorbed dose estimates from rhenium-186-labeled monoclonal antibody. J Nucl Med 1998; 39(10):1746–1751.

99. Breitz HB, Weiden PL, Vanderheyden JL, et al. Clinical experience with rhenium-186-labeled monoclonal antibodies for radioimmunotherapy: results of phase I trials. J Nucl Med 1992; 33(6):1099–1109.

100. Weiden PL, Breitz HB. Pretargeted radioimmunotherapy (PRIT) for treatment of non-Hodgkin's lymphoma (NHL). Crit Rev Oncol Hematol 2001; 40(1):37–51.

101. Weiden PL, Breitz HB, Seiler CA, et al. Rhenium-186-labeled chimeric antibody NR-LU-13: pharmacokinetics, biodistribution and immunogenicity relative to murine analog NR-LU-10. J Nucl Med 1993; 34(12):2111–2119.

102. Kotzerke J, Bunjes D, Scheinberg DA. Radioimmunoconjugates in acute leukemia treatment: the future is radiant. Bone Marrow Transplant 2005; 36(12):1021–1026.

103. Miao Y, Owen NK, Fisher DR, et al. Therapeutic efficacy of a 188Re-labeled alpha-melanocyte-stimulating hormone peptide analog in murine and human melanoma-bearing mouse models. J Nucl Med 2005; 46(1):121–129.

104. Brooks RC, Carnochan P, Vollano JF, et al. Metal complexes of bleomycin: evaluation of [Rh-105]-bleomycin for use in targeted radiotherapy. Nucl Med Biol 1999; 26(4):421–430.

105. Yorke ED, Beaumier PL, Wessels BW, et al. Optimal antibody-radionuclide combinations for clinical radioimmunotherapy: a predictive model based on mouse pharmacokinetics. Int J Rad Appl Instrum B. 1991; 18(8):827–835.

106. Tanabe M, Yamamoto G. Tissue distributions of 97Ru and 103Ru in subcutaneous tumor of rodents. Acta Med Okayama 1975; 29(6):431–436.

107. Lagunas-Solar MC, Avila MJ, Johnson PC. Targetry and radiochemical methods for the simultaneous cyclotron production of no-carrier-added radiopharmaceutical-quality 100Pd, 97Ru and 101mRh. Int J Rad Appl Instrum [A]. 1987; 38(2):151–157.

108. Kolsky KL, Joshi V, Mausner LF, et al. Radiochemical purification of no-carrier-added scandium-47 for radioimmunotherapy. Appl Radiat Isot 1998; 49(12):1541–1549.

109. Anderson P, Nunez R. Samarium lexidronam (153Sm-EDTMP): skeletal radiation for osteoblastic bone metas-

tases and osteosarcoma. Expert Rev Anticancer Ther 2007; 7(11):1517–1527.

110. Liepe K, Kotzerke J. A comparative study of 188Re-HEDP, 186Re-HEDP, 153Sm-EDTMP and 89Sr in the treatment of painful skeletal metastases. Nucl Med Commun 2007; 28(8):623–630.

111. Ricci S, Boni G, Pastina I, et al. Clinical benefit of bone-targeted radiometabolic therapy with 153Sm-EDTMP combined with chemotherapy in patients with metastatic hormone-refractory prostate cancer. Eur J Nucl Med Mol Imaging 2007; 34(7):1023–1030.

112. Strigari L, Sciuto R, D'Andrea M, et al. Radiopharmaceutical therapy of bone metastases with 89SrCl2, 186Re-HEDP and 153Sm-EDTMP: a dosimetric study using Monte Carlo simulation. Eur J Nucl Med Mol Imaging 2007; 34(7):1031–1038.

113. Kvinnsland Y, Skretting A, Bruland OS. Radionuclide therapy with bone-seeking compounds: Monte Carlo calculations of dose-volume histograms for bone marrow in trabecular bone. Phys Med Biol 2001; 46(4):1149–1161.

114. Bishayee A, Rao DV, Srivastava SC, et al. Marrow-sparing effects of 117mSn(4+)diethylenetriaminepentaacetic acid for radionuclide therapy of bone cancer. J Nucl Med 2000; 41(12):2043–2050.

115. Krishnamurthy GT, Swailem FM, Srivastava SC, et al. Tin-117m(4+)DTPA: pharmacokinetics and imaging characteristics in patients with metastatic bone pain. J Nucl Med 1997; 38(2):230–237.

116. Finlay OG, Mason MD, Shelley M. Radioisotopes for the palliation of metastatic bone cancer: a systematic review. Lancet Oncol 2005; 6(6):392–400.

117. Charlton DE, Utteridge TD, Allen BJ. Theoretical treatment of human haemopoietic stem cell survival following irradiation by alpha particles. Int J Radiat Biol 1998; 74(1):111–118.

118. Abbas Rizvi SM, Henniker AJ, Goozee G, et al. In vitro testing of the leukaemia monoclonal antibody WM-53 labeled with alpha and beta emitting radioisotopes. Leuk Res 2002; 26(1):37–43.

119. Beyer GJ, Miederer M, Vranjes-Duric S, et al. Targeted alpha therapy in vivo: direct evidence for single cancer cell kill using 149Tb-rituximab. Eur J Nucl Med Mol Imaging 2004; 31(4):547–554.

120. de Jong M, Breeman WA, Bernard BF, et al. Evaluation in vitro and in rats of 161Tb-DTPA-octreotide, a somatostatin analogue with potential for intraoperative scanning and radiotherapy. Eur J Nucl Med Jul 1995; 22(7):608–616.

15

CEST Contrast Agents

JASON M. ZHAO,[1] ASSAF A. GILAD,[2] MICHAEL T. McMAHON,[1] JEFF W. M. BULTE,[2] and PETER C. M. VAN ZIJL[1]

[1]Russell H. Morgan Department of Radiology and Radiological Science, Division of MR Research, Johns Hopkins University School of Medicine, Baltimore, Maryland, U.S.A. and F.M. Kirby Research Center for Functional Brain Imaging, Kennedy Krieger Institute, Baltimore, Maryland, U.S.A.

[2]Russell H. Morgan Department of Radiology and Radiological Science, Division of MR Research, and Cellular Imaging Section, Institute for Cell Engineering, Johns Hopkins University School of Medicine, Baltimore, Maryland, U.S.A.

INTRODUCTION

Cancer development involves deleterious genetic (1) and epigenetic (2) alternations that are augmented by external carcinogenic influences such as smoking and diet (3). Genetic studies in mice have identified two classes of genes called oncogenes and tumor-suppressor genes (4). Oncogenes are dominant genes whose mutation can manifest as cancer cell phenotypes, while tumor-suppressor genes control cellular growth and differentiation. The occurrence of an oncogenic mutation or the loss of a tumor-suppressor gene function can cause normal cells to become cancerous and proliferate rapidly, establishing their survival advantage by releasing cytokines into the host tissue environment, thereby creating a unique local "microenvironment" (5). Cytokines such as vascular endothelial growth factor (VEGF) promote angiogenesis. In addition, the high metabolic rate of cancer cells increases the glucose-to-lactate conversion and acid release, creating a low-pH condition in the extracellular space. Cancer cells thrive under this microenvironment owing to their high genomic instability, high proliferation rates, and a natural-selection pressure that favors those

mutations most adaptive to hypoxia and acidosis. The intricate relationship between cancer cells and their microenvironment is responsible for the morphological and physiological characteristics of solid tumors, accelerating their potential to invade healthy tissues and metastasize into other parts of the body. Thus, understanding this relationship is essential not only for new ways to characterize and stage tumors but also for treatment planning and efficacy evaluation of the existing and new drugs.

Magnetic resonance (MR) imaging and spectroscopy have shown great promise in the multiparametric characterization of the tumor microenvironment (5,6). More recently, a new area of research, called "molecular imaging," has begun to take shape (7–9). The task force of the Molecular Imaging Center of Excellence of the Society of Nuclear Medicine defines molecular imaging as "the visualization, characterization, and measurement of biological processes at the molecular and cellular levels in humans and other living systems." A marker of interest can be imaged by a contrast agent modified with a targeting moiety or by introducing an artificial reporter gene into the genome of host cell whose expression is downstream of this marker. One important potential application of molecular imaging is the early detection of cancer. Long before morphological changes take place, cancer cells release biochemical signaling molecules such as VEGF to prepare for proliferation and to establish their unique microenvironment. If molecular imaging could catch these molecular footprints, treatments could start early and the chance of managing the cancer would be significantly improved. Another advantage would lie in monitoring the therapeutic response of a treatment. For example, monitoring the VEGF density in the tumor would be a more accurate and reliable way of assessing the effectiveness of an antiangiogenic drug than monitoring either the vascular density or perfusion.

A central challenge in developing MR molecular imaging is the inherent low sensitivity of the MR modality. Compared with nuclear medicine and fluorescence, which can detect relatively few radionuclides or fluorophores, MR usually requires millimolar to micromolar concentrations of contrast agents. Common approaches to improve MR sensitivity involve designing chelates with optimal exchange and relaxation properties or carriers with a high payload of contrast agents (10,11). For example, gadolinium (Gd) chelates with more than one inner sphere–coordinated water are desirable because their Gd center is accessible to multiple inner-sphere water molecules, and these water molecules can efficiently exchange with the bulk water molecules. Another example is to attach the Gd chelate to a larger macromolecule to decrease the tumbling rate and enhance the relaxation process. Macromolecular carriers such as linear polymers (12) and dendrimers (13,14) can have hundreds or even thousands of Gd chelates covalently linked together, further enhancing the relaxation effects of these contrast agents on a per-Gd basis. Nanoparticle carriers have also been shown to enhance sensitivity. Tilcock et al. encapsulated ∼ 100 mM of Gd-DTPA in liposomes to image hepatic metastasis in rats (15,16); Winter et al. used Gd-containing lipid emulsions with thousands of Gd-carriers to image $\alpha_v\beta_3$ integrins in a rabbit tumor model (17,18). One important consideration of nanoparticle carriers is their size and ability to extravasate into the tumor interstitium. The requirement is less strict under conditions where the vascular membrane integrity is compromised such as tumor or stroke. For example, liposomal nanoparticles with sizes 90 to 110 nm can achieve high levels of localization inside tumors via the enhanced permeability and retention (EPR) effect with or without targeting antibodies (19).

Chemical exchange saturation transfer (CEST) is a novel approach to increase MR sensitivity (20–22). In contrast to the common gadolinium- or iron oxide–based contrast agents that affect the relaxation properties of nearby water, the CEST mechanism involves the physical transfer of saturated protons from a contrast agent to the surrounding water, resulting in a reduction of the water signal. If this transfer rate is high or if there are many saturated protons on the contrast agent, CEST can efficiently reduce the water signal in a matter of seconds and detect the presence of micromolar concentrations of the contrast agent (23,24). Moreover, when the proton transfer rate is optimized and carriers such as liposomes are used, micromolar or even picomolar carrier concentrations can be detected using the CEST mechanism (25). CEST as a signal amplification scheme comes at a crucial time in the development of MR molecular imaging techniques. The usage of CEST agents and imaging may become more prevalent in future diagnostics, treatment, and management of cancer and other diseases.

The development of CEST agents has involved an interdisciplinary effort of MR imaging scientists, chemists, and biologists. The rapid progress in this area has produced a new class of agents that are not only sensitive and biocompatible but also sophisticated and responsive to local changes in pH, temperature, and metabolites, and can differentiate various cancer cell types after labeling. This review highlights some of these recent developments and their biomedical applications with a focus on cancer research. Interested readers are referred to other reviews for further reading (10,26–28).

CEST CONTRAST MECHANISM

CEST involves the exchange between solute protons and bulk water protons (Fig. 1A). When the chemical exchange between these two proton populations is slow on the NMR time scale, the proton NMR spectrum of the system shows two distinct peaks (Fig. 1B). Under this condition, the solute proton peak can be selectively irradiated by a radiofrequency (RF) presaturation pulse. The solute protons can exchange with the bulk water protons in the process, reducing the MR signal intensity of the bulk water (Fig. 1B). Hence, CEST agents constitute a new class of negative contrast agents that create local hypointensity on an MR image.

A complete theoretical treatment of the CEST effect is quite involved and is beyond the scope of this review; thus interested readers are referred to the Refs. 29 to 35. Here we present a brief qualitative description and quote only the main results from other theoretical papers. The modified Bloch equations describe the time evolution of spins in two chemical environments in the presence of an external magnetic field. Their solution can be simplified under two assumptions: (i) a frequency match between the RF irradiation pulse and the solute protons and (ii) a large spectral separation between the solute and water proton frequencies (33). Let "s" and "w" denote the solute and the bulk water protons, respectively. Let ω be the frequency of the presaturation RF pulse; ω_{0s}, ω_{0w} the resonance frequencies of

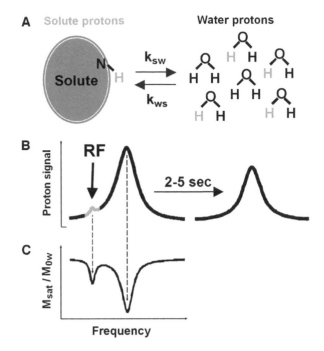

Figure 1 CEST involves chemical exchange between solute protons (e.g., amide protons on a protein) and bulk water protons. (A) A cartoon representation of the proton exchange from solute to water (k_{sw}) and vice versa (k_{ws}). (B) High-resolution proton spectrum of the system depicted in (a) showing two distinct peaks corresponding to the solute and water protons. Upon RF irradiation of the solute proton peak for two to five seconds, the saturated solute protons exchange with water protons to reduce the signal intensity of water. (C) The z-spectrum measures the saturated water signal, M_{sat}/M_{0w}, as a function of the RF irradiation frequencies.

solute and bulk water; k_{sw}, k_{ws} the solute to water exchange and vice versa; R_{1s}, R_{1w} the longitudinal relaxation rates of solute and bulk water; R_{2s}, R_{2w} the transverse relaxation rates of solute and bulk water; and $r_{1w} = R_{1w} + k_{ws}$, $r_{2w} = R_{2w} + k_{ws}$, $r_{1s} = R_{1s} + k_{sw}$, $r_{2s} = R_{1s} + k_{sw}$ the effective relaxation rates. Furthermore, M_{0w} is the total magnetization of bulk water without RF presaturation and M_{sat} with RF presaturation. In these notations, the assumption (*i*) for frequency matching means $\omega = \omega_{0s}$, and the assumption (*ii*) for large spectral separation means $|\omega - \omega_{0w}| \gg 0$. The efficiency of the proton transfer process for a CEST agent is commonly expressed as the so-called proton transfer ratio (PTR). Under these two assumptions, the time-dependent PTR following a RF pulse duration of T_{sat} is

$$\mathrm{PTR}(T_{sat}) = 1 - \frac{M_{sat}(T_{sat})}{M_{0w}}$$
$$= \frac{x_s k_{sw} \alpha}{r_{1w}}[1 - \exp(-r_{1w} \cdot T_{sat})] \qquad (1)$$

where x_s is the molar fraction of the solute protons compared to the water protons, and the saturation

efficiency α is determined by the power of the RF pulse and the exchange and relaxation rates of the solute protons. The dynamics of PTR is dictated by the effective relaxation rate r_{1w}: the larger the r_{1w}, the shorter is the RF pulse needed for the PTR to reach its steady-state value. Since $r_{1w} = R_{1w} + k_{ws}$ and $k_{ws} = x_s + k_{sw}$, this dynamical rate is determined by the proton exchange rate k_{sw} and x_s. In other words, equation (1) can be used to measure the proton exchange rate k_{sw} based on the dynamics of PTR.

The reason why PTR is important in CEST applications is that it is a direct measure of the expected CEST imaging contrast; in other words, maximizing CEST contrast is equivalent to maximizing PTR. Equation (1) shows that PTR can be maximized by either increasing the number of solute protons that are saturable (x_s), the proton exchange rate k_{sw}, the saturation efficiency α, or decreasing the effective water relaxation rate r_{1w} (note that has k_{ws} in it). The saturation efficiency α can be maximized by increasing presaturation pulse power, but this may not be practical in vivo because of specific absorption rate (SAR) limitations on human scanners. The five most common ways to achieve optimal CEST contrast are: (*i*) increase the exchange rate of the exchangeable proton group, for example, by modulating accessibility or the chemical environment catalyzing transfer, (*ii*) maximize the number of exchangeable protons per molecular weight of the agent, (*iii*) work at the highest possible agent concentrations within toxicity tolerance, (*iv*) use high presaturation pulse powers to ensure a high saturation efficiency within the SAR limit, and (*v*) work at high fields where R_{1w} is small, more importantly, where the frequency separation between water and the exchangeable protons is increased.

CEST is a MR signal amplification scheme that enhances MR sensitivity. Typical proton MR sensitivity is determined by proton density of water and the slight population asymmetry of the two spin states because of the presence of an external magnetic field. CEST, on the other hand, relies on the magnetization transfer (MT) from the continuously saturated solute protons to the bulk water protons. Since the solute proton population is usually in the millimolar concentration range compared to the molar range of the water proton population, a small signal decrease because of the solute saturation would normally not be detectable. However, it is amplified into a large signal decrease in the water signal because of the continuous exchange process between the saturated solute protons and the unsaturated water protons.

Sensitivity and sensitivity enhancement are often used to quantify and compare the sensitivities of contrast agents (CA). Sensitivity is defined as the minimum concentration required to produce an observable contrast. In the case of CEST, a common definition of sensitivity is the minimum concentration of a CEST agent that can produce 5% reduction in the bulk water signal. CEST agent sensitivities

Table 1 Proton Transfer Ratio [PTR, Eq. (1)] and Proton Transfer Efficiency [PTE, Eq. (2)] of Selected CEST Contrast Agents at the Specified Concentrations [CA]

Type	Contrast agent	[CA] (mM)	PTR	PTE ($\times 10^3$)	References
DIACEST	NH$_4$Cl	63	0.50	0.88	21
	L-lysine	125	0.66	0.59	22
	Poly-L-lysine	0.1	0.43	480	23
	Poly(rU)	0.005	0.49	10900	24
PARACEST	Eu-DOTA-4AmCE	250	0.60	0.27	95
	Yb-DOTAM-Gly	30	0.80	3	63
LipoCEST	Liposomes	9×10^{-8}	0.05	6×10^7	25
HyperCEST	Hyperpolarized Xe	0.26	0.30	130	66

are usually in the mM to μM range (Table 1). The sensitivity enhancement is quantified by the proton transfer enhancement (PTE) as follows:

$$PTE = \frac{PTR \cdot 111M}{[CA]}$$
$$= \frac{N_{CA}M_{CA}k_{sw}\alpha}{r_{1w}}[1 - \exp(-r_{1w} \cdot T_{sat})] \quad (2)$$

where 111 M is the proton concentration of water, N_{CA} the number of exchangeable saturable protons per molecular weight unit of the agent and M_{CA} its molecular weight. Table 1 lists the PTR and PTE of common CEST agents that will be discussed in more details below. To calculate the PTE of poly-L-lysine (PLL), for example, the measured PTR of 43% is multiplied by 111 M and divided by the agent concentration of 0.1 mM to yield a PTE of 480,000. Comparing equations (1) and (2), we see that the optimum PTE can be achieved by increasing the proton exchange rate k_{sw}, the saturation efficiency α, or decreasing the effective water relaxation rate r_{1w}.

Equations (1) and (2) assume a RF presaturation pulse of a single frequency ω. In practice, each RF pulse has a bandwidth positively correlated with its power, so the system is actually saturated by a range of RF frequencies. Sometimes, "direct saturation" can happen when the RF bandwidth is broad enough to overlap with the bulk water frequency. To take into account the direct saturation effect as much as possible, we define the MTR$_{asy}$ (Magnetization Transfer Ratio asymmetry) as

$$MTR_{asy} = \frac{M_{sat}(-\Delta\omega) - M_{sat}(+\Delta\omega)}{M_{0w}} \quad (3a)$$

MTR$_{asy}$ is a quantity commonly used in MT experiments and is the difference between saturated water magnetization at the positive and negative RF pulse frequencies symmetric about the water frequency, which is normally set to zero. It is an effective way to remove the bulk of the direct saturation effect from the measured M_{sat}. Another common way to express MTR$_{asy}$ is by normalizing

the saturated water magnetization to the opposite side ($-\Delta\omega$) of the water frequency, thereby excluding the dependence on the power of irradiation as long as the magnitude of saturation is not too large

$$MTR_{asy} = \frac{M_{sat}(-\Delta\omega) - M_{sat}(+\Delta\omega)}{M_{sat}(-\Delta\omega)} \quad (3b)$$

When M_{sat}/M_{0w} and MTR$_{asy}$ are plotted against the RF presaturation pulse frequencies, the graphs are called z-spectrum (Fig. 1C) and MTR$_{asy}$-spectrum, respectively.

Finally, when applying RF saturation in vivo, conventional semisolid-based MT effects will occur, which also interfere with CEST detection. These effects are also slightly asymmetric with respect to the water frequency (36–39). This MT asymmetry can be taken into account by taking a larger offset (i.e., just outside the frequency range of exchangeable protons), where such effects are approximately constant, to correct the total effects close to water for this contribution (37).

CEST CONTRAST AGENTS

CEST contrast agents can be broadly divided into two categories: diamagnetic (DIACEST) and paramagnetic (PARACEST). Alternatively, some CEST agents are named after their special composition or function, such as lipoCEST (liposome-based CEST agents) or glycoCEST (glycogen-based CEST agents). Below we will discuss each category in more details.

DIACEST Contrast Agents

Small Molecules

Early CEST experiments involved small diamagnetic molecules with −NH or −OH groups. In the early 1960s, Forsen and Hoffman pioneered the saturation transfer experiments in the presence of chemical exchange by studying the proton exchange of hydroxyl groups in a mixture of two compounds (20). Later Wolff and Balaban performed a CEST experiment using a dilute solution of ammonium chloride (21). The proton spectrum of a 63 mM NH$_4$Cl solution did not show any NH$_4$$^+$ resonance; however, when applying a presaturation pulse at the frequency offset of 2.5 ppm, a 50% decrease in the bulk water signal was observed, corresponding to a 880-fold sensitivity enhancement (Table 1). Further CEST imaging experiments of a partitioned phantom revealed hypointensity in the NH$_4$Cl partition and normal intensity in the water partition.

Ward et al. subsequently performed a systematic study on CEST effects of common small molecules of biological interest (22). They found that sugars gave a PTR of 7% to 21% at 250 mM when irradiating at the −OH group frequency in the chemical shift range of 1.0–1.5 ppm above water. When studying the −NH$_2$ group in amino acids, larger PTRs were found. In particular, L-Ala, L-Arg, and L-Lys, resonating at a chemical shift difference of about 3 ppm showed a PTR of 66% to 67% at 125 mM (Table 1). The compound 5,6-dihydrouracil, a pyramidine product in DNA repair, exchanging through two −NH groups with chemical shifts of 2.7 and 5 ppm, showed a PTR of 22% at 62.5 mM. All measurements here were done in 20 mM phosphate buffered saline at 37°C at 7 T. The pH was 7 for sugar molecules and 2–3 for amino acids. Since PTR in general depends on concentration, the presence of catalyzing agents, pH, and temperature, it is imperative to report the experimental conditions under which the CEST experiment was performed in order to be able to properly compare experimental results from different research groups and to evaluate the contrast agent for in vivo applications, where pH, temperature, and toxicity must be within the acceptable ranges.

There are a few technical challenges when CEST imaging of exchangeable protons in small mobile molecules is carried out in tissue. One is simultaneous saturation transfer of the bound protons because of the conventional MT effect of solid-like cell constituents (40–42). This problem can be partially alleviated by the fact that the bound proton resonance is broad (a few hundred Hz) and approximately symmetric about the bulk water resonance, so a MTR$_{asy}$ analysis such as equation (3) could be used to subtract out the MT contribution to CEST. However, recent work shows that even the conventional MT effect is slightly asymmetric (36–39). Another challenge is the fast transverse relaxation of water in the tissue and the resulting broad water resonance. Direct saturation of water can occur when the CEST presaturation pulse bandwidth overlaps with that of the water resonance (43,44), which reduces the total water signal and the sensitivity of the CEST technique. One solution to this problem is to use low-power pulses

with narrow bandwidth. Additionally, shimming and spectral centering are also challenging in tissues with high heterogeneity.

Guivel-Scharen et al. carefully addressed these challenges and were able to obtain MTR$_{asy}$ spectra of various rabbit tissues ex vivo (45). In particular, they found a large 10% MTR$_{asy}$ for rabbit kidney medulla between a chemical shift of 1.0 and 2.6 ppm. This effect could be attributed to small nitrogen-containing molecules in urine such as urea and ammonia. As a final proof of principle, the authors imaged whole rabbit kidney ex vivo with a presaturation pulse at 1.74 ppm at 11.7 T and observed hypointensity in the medulla region in the difference image with and without the presaturation pulse.

Macromolecules

Macromolecular DIACEST agents are mainly polymers of amino acids, nucleotides, and sugars. Cationic polymers recently attracted attention because of their potential as nonviral gene-delivery vehicles for gene therapy (46). Goffeney et al. (23) evaluated five types of such polymers: PLL, poly-L-glutamate (PLE), polyethylenimine (PEI), polyallylamine (PAA), and a generation-5 starburst PAMAM dendrimer (SPD-5) (Fig. 2A, Table 1). All the polymers studied have exchangeable protons; while PLL, PLE, and SPD-5 have amide protons and displayed a CEST effect, PEI and PAA did not. PTRs calculated using the theory agreed reasonably well with the measured values for PLL and SPD-5, the small differences being attributed to possible back exchange and insufficient saturation efficiency.

A subsequent study (24) focused on a 2000-unit polymer of uradine, poly(rU), consisting of two exchangeable protons groups: imino and hydroxyl protons resonating at 10.8 and 6.3 ppm (Fig. 2B). Although the imino protons have a large exchange rate of 5880 sec^{-1} at pH = 7.3 and 37°C, CEST experiments were possible because the experiments were performed at 11.7 T with a sufficiently large chemical shift difference from water to satisfy the slow exchange condition for CEST. At a concentration of 5 µM, poly(rU) showed a PTR = 0.49 at the imino proton resonance of 10.8 ppm, representing a factor of 20 improvement in sensitivity compared to PLL (Table 1), making it one of the most sensitive DIACEST agent studied so far. When complexed with dendrimers, the proton transfer efficiency [PTE, Eq. (2)] dropped by about 50% at 10 µM poly(rU) and 100 µM dendrimer concentrations. The authors noted that a tripling in concentration of poly(rU) only resulted in a 30% increase in PTR, implying that the agent concentration was much higher than the linear response regime of PTR and the back exchange became a limiting factor in the CEST enhancement scheme.

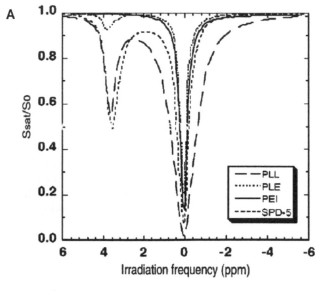

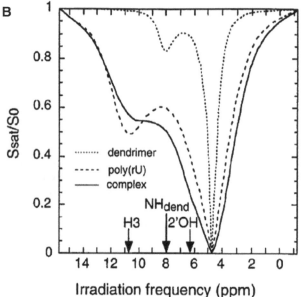

Figure 2 (**A**) Z-spectra of poly-L-lysine (PLL, 100 μM), poly-L-glutamate (PLE, 500 μM), polyethylenimine (PEI, 150 μM), and a generation-5 starburst PAMAM dendrimer (SPD-5, 1 mM). The number of exchangeable protons/kD of PLL, PLE, and SPD-5 (1 mM) are 4.58, 6.62, and 8.74, giving rise to PTR of 0.43, 0.07, and 0.51 at 3.5 ppm and PTE of 6×10^5, 1.6×10^4, and 4×10^4, respectively at pH = 7.3, 37°C, and 11.7 T. (**B**) Z-spectra of 100 μM dendrimer, 5 μM poly (rU), and a complex of 10 μM poly(rU) and 100 μM dendrimer. Poly(rU) alone has PTR = 0.49 at 10.8 ppm and PTE = 10^7, and the poly(rU)-dendrimer complex has PTR = 0.49 at 10.8 ppm and PTE = 4.6×10^6, under the same experimental conditions as (**A**). *Source*: (**A**) and (**B**) adapted from Refs. 23 and 24, respectively.

In a more recent study, McMahon et al. extended these studies by investigating different poly-amino acid sequences that can be tuned to different RF frequencies (47). They found that PLL resonates at around 8.4 ppm, poly-L-arginine at 6.5 ppm, and poly-L-threonine at 8.4 and 5.3 ppm. Thus the amino acid sequences can be tuned to distinct resonance frequencies, which could allow labeling and separation of different cell populations for cell tracking and imaging applications. Such approach is akin to "multicolor" imaging commonly used in optical imaging applications.

Another notable example of novel CEST agents involves the use of glycogen hydroxyl group for liver imaging (glycoCEST) (48). Here van Zijl et al. demonstrated a decrease in water signal (M_{sat}/M_{0w}) to 35% at 9.4 T and 50% at 4.7 T upon the saturation of −OH group on glycogen at 1.2 ppm and 37°C. Concentration studies showed an increase of 0.66% MTR_{asy}/mM glycogen in the range of 0–50 mM. Perfused mouse liver study showed a 50% larger increase in M_{sat}/M_{0w} at +1 ppm than at −1 ppm. Authors attributed the increase at +1ppm to depletion of glycogen because of the addition of glucagon.

PARACEST Contrast Agents

In the last 15 years, the majority of inorganometallic chemistry research on lanthanides (Ln) has focused on the Gd(III) ion because of its fast inner-sphere water exchange rate and superb longitudinal relaxation properties (49). Since Gd(III) has seven unpaired electrons, Gd(III) chelates, such as Gd-DTPA (diethylenetriamine penta-acetic acid) and Gd-DOTA (1,4,7,10-tetraazacyclo-dodecane-1,4,7,10-tetraacetic acid), can be designed that occupy six of the coordination sites with the remaining site occupied by an inner-sphere water. The large library of Gd(III) chelates available today offers not only reduced toxicity compared to bare Gd(III) ions, but also a tunable range of pharmacokinetics. They are routinely used as MR contrast agents to highlight brain lesions where the blood-brain barrier has been compromised as in stoke or tumors (10). Gd(III) chelates are relaxation agents, not shift agents, in that they are effective in shortening the relaxation time but do not change the chemical shift of water. Other members of the lanthanide family are effective as shift agents, so they are commonly used in spectroscopy studies to resolve overlapping resonances of nuclei in biological systems (50–52).

The invention of CEST spectroscopy and imaging have spurred a rapid development in the design and synthesis of novel lanthanide compounds for medical imaging. One important advantage of using the lanthanide family of metal ions lies in their similarity in coordination chemistry (53). Ligand conjugation protocols used for one lanthanide ion can be readily generalized to other ions, yielding a family of complexes with a range of tunable RF excitation frequencies. This dynamic range of excitation frequencies demonstrates the versatility of paramagnetic lanthanide complexes, and mimics the range of emission frequencies of fluorescent proteins commonly used for fluorescence microscopy, making them attractive candidates for "multi-frequency" imaging using MR (47,54).

The saturated water signal intensity and the proton transfer ratio depends on the exchange rate k_{sw} in equation (1). Optimizing the CEST efficiency requires rational design of compounds that maximize k_{sw}. There are several factors that influence the $k_{sw} = (1/\tau_M$, bound-water life-time) of a lanthanide compound (27). First, common chelates such as DOTA exist in two isomeric forms in solution that differ by a rotation of the acetate side chain: M isomer (or square antiprism) and m isomer (or twisted square antiprism). The m isomers usually exhibit a faster bound-water exchange rate than the M isomers. For example, the m isomer of Eu-DOTMA (1,4,7,10-tetraaza-cyclododecane-tetrakis(methylacetamide)) has an exchange rate of 5×10^5 sec^{-1} while the M isomer has a rate of 8×10^3 sec^{-1} (55,56).

Second, the exchange rate depends on the charge and polarity of the side chains (27). Coordinating a more polar side chain such as a simple amide can increase the exchange rate because of the increase in accessible surface area of the bound-water molecule, since the polar side chain creates a more favorable surface for the bulk water to access (57). For example, by coordinating side chains with increasing polarity, phosphonate ester < carboxylate ester < alkyl groups < simple amides, Aime et al. showed that the bound-water exchange rate in Eu-DOTA-tetraamide complexes can be increased by a factor of 6. Conversely, coordinating a less-polar side chain can decrease the exchange rate. For example, Zhang et al. (58) designed Gd(III) chelates with mono-, bis-, and tetra-phosphonate-amides and found that the exchange rates decreased with increasing number of phosphonate amide side chains: Gd-DOTA-1AmP (monoamide phosphonate) > Gd-DOTA-2AmP > Gd-DOTA-4AmP. The decrease in exchange rates coincides with the fact that phosphonate esters are the least polar of common side chains.

Third, the lanthanide ion sizes also influence the exchange rates (27). Figure 3A shows the ^{1}H chemical shifts ($\Delta\omega$) of Ln-DOTA-4AmCE (tetraamide CH2COOEt) for 10 lanthanide ions (59). Among all the ions, Tm(III) and Dy(III) complexes have the most positive (+500 ppm) and the most negative (−720 ppm) chemical shifts, respectively. Figure 3B shows the bound-water lifetime (τ_M) and the product, $\Delta\omega \cdot \tau_M$, calculated from the data in Fig. 3A at 11.7 T, with increasing atomic numbers (thus decreasing ionic sizes) on the abscissa (59). First, we note that the lifetimes exhibit biphasic behavior:

they first increase with decreasing ionic sizes until Eu, then decrease with decreasing ionic sizes (60). This biphasic behavior suggests different mechanisms for exchange: the exchange is likely prototropic for larger ions, but involves whole water exchange for smaller ions (61,62). Second, it can be noted that $\Delta\omega \cdot \tau_M > 1$ for all the Ln-DOTA-4AmCE at 11.7 T, implying that all the compounds are suitable CEST agents at this field strength. At lower fields, say at the clinical field strength of 1.5 T, only the four ions (Eu, Tb, Dy, and Ho) with the highest $\Delta\omega \cdot \tau_M$ are eligible CEST agents, illustrating again the advantage of working at high fields for CEST applications. These three factors affecting exchange rates discussed above should be evaluated together with those affecting chemical shifts for the design of optimal CEST agents.

Besides tetraamide derivatives of DOTA, a related class of lanthanide ligands are tetraglycineamide derivatives of DOTA (Ln-DOTAM-Gly) (63). In these compounds, the exchange between the lanthanide-bound and the bulk water are too fast to be observed on the ^{1}H spectrum. However, the protons from −NH groups show a well-separated peak away from the bulk water, implying slow exchange on the NMR time scale. Opposite to the DOTA-4Am chelates, the Tm(III) chelate of DOTAM-Gly now have the most negative (−51 ppm) and Dy(III) chelate the most positive (+77 ppm) chemical shifts. Taking into account the exchange rates, Yb-DOTAM-Gly was found to have the best transfer efficiency of 80% when irradiated at the resonance frequency of −16 ppm. Since amide proton exchange is pH dependent, the CEST effect of these compounds is also pH dependent. For example, the transfer efficiency of Yb-DOTAM-Gly changes by 22% for every unit change in pH at 30mM concentration at 312 K and 7 T (Table 1). The pH effects of paramagnetic and amide-proton CEST agents are discussed below.

Other CEST Contrast Agents

As equation (2) shows, to increase the sensitivity of CEST detection, we have to either increase the number of exchangeable protons or the exchange rate. Large macro-molecular CEST agents such as PLL and poly(rU) typically have 10^3 to 10^4 exchangeable protons per macro-molecule. Aime and coworkers recently developed a nanoparticle CEST system (LIPOCEST) that contained ~10^8 exchangeable protons inside a nanoparticle of about 200 nm (25). This 4–5 orders of magnitude increase in the number of exchangeable protons resulted in a 4–5 orders of magnitude increase in sensitivity, extending the detectable range of contrast agents from micromolar down to sub-nanomolar range (Table 1). They encapsulated 100 mM Tm-DOTMA ($\alpha,\alpha',\alpha'',\alpha'''$-tetramethyl-1,4,7,10-tetraacetic acid) inside liposomes composed of POPC:DPPG:

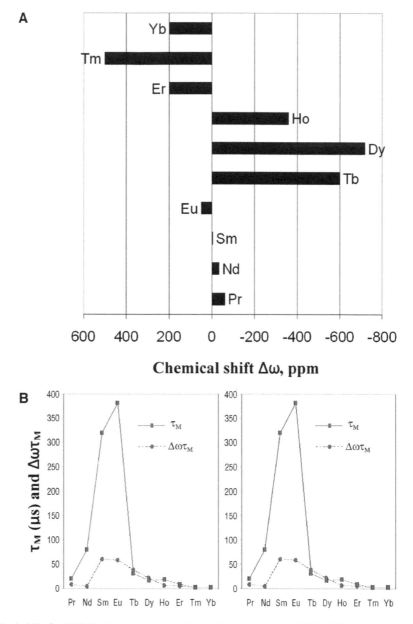

Figure 3 Proton chemical shift $\Delta\omega$ (**A**) lifetimes τ_M and their product $\Delta\omega\cdot\tau_M$ at 11.7 T, (**B**) of the bound water in the Ln-DOTA-4AmCE complexes for 10 lanthanide (Ln) ions. *Source*: Adapted from Ref. 59.

chol = 55:5:40 (POPC, palmitoyl-oleoyl-phosphatidyl-choline; DPPG, dipalmitoyl-phosphatidylglycerol; chol, cholesterol) with a mean diameter of 270 nm. The liposome concentration was 2.8 nM, yielding an effective Tm-DOTMA solution concentration of 1.3 mM. At 7T and 39°C, the high-resolution ^{1}H spectrum showed a small peak 3.1 ppm downfield of the bulk water peak, representing the shifted intraliposomal water. To test the sensitivity of the LIPOCEST technique, the authors prepared samples with liposome concentrations ranging from 90 pM to 2.88 nM. Difference images acquired with a presaturation pulse at ±3.1 ppm showed contrast for all the samples.

The same researchers also realized that the bulk magnetic susceptibility can be enhanced by making liposomes nonspherical and by aligning them along the direction of the magnetic field (64). Toward this end, they constructed two types of nonspherical shrunken liposomes. The first type encapsulates a shift agent, while the second type both encapsulates a shift agent and incorporates a lanthanide lipid in the membrane. The first type achieved an intra-liposomal water shift of 10 ppm (cf. 4 ppm of spherical liposomes) at an osmolarity of 0.05 osm for Ln(hpdo3a), Ln = Tm or Dy, after the liposomes were prepared in a hypotonic solution and dialyzed against an isotonic solution. [hpdo3a = 10-(2-hydroxypropyl)-1,4,7,10-tetraaza-cyclododecane-1,4,7-triacetic acid.] The second type shifted the intraliposomal water even more to −45 ppm upfield for liposomes encapsulating Dy(hpdo3a) and incorporating Dy-lipid in the membrane, and +18 ppm downfield for liposomes with the corresponding Tm agents. The additional enhancement in the second type was because of the alignment of the liposomes along the external magnetic field when the lanthanide lipid was incorporated into the membrane.

To explore the possibility of generating different types of MR contrast, Aime et al. encapsulated a T_1 contrast agent, Gd(hpdo3a), inside osmotically shrunken liposomes (65). The nonspherical shape of the liposomes gave rise to a bulk magnetic susceptibility effect, which shifted the intraliposomal water downfield by +7 ppm. As a result, these agents not only displayed T_1 contrast because of the encapsulated Gd(III) chelate, but the trans-membrane water exchange was slow enough that they also displayed CEST contrast. Additionally, the authors tested their susceptibility induced T_2 relaxivity and found that the agents also displayed good T_2 relaxivity ($\sim 5 \text{ sec}^{-1}$ mM^{-1}). This is the first report of an MR contrast agent that functions as a T_1, T_2, and CEST agent, all in one.

Another interesting example of novel CEST agents involves a hyperpolarized xenon biosensor for molecular imaging (hyperCEST) (66). Schroder et al. presented a signal amplification scheme based on a combination of hyperpolarized xenon and CEST. The chemical shift of free Xe = 193.6 ppm, while that of the bound Xe = 65.4 ppm inside a molecular cage coupled to a biotin side chain for targeted imaging of avidin. The authors tested the hyper-CEST xenon biosensor in a perfused avidin bead medium with a sensor concentration of 50 μM and a free Xe concentration of 260 μM (natural abundance of 25% ^{129}Xe hyperpolarized to 3%). Chemical shift imaging showed a decrease of around 30% in the free xenon signal when an on-resonance saturation pulse is applied at the xenon sensor frequency (Table 1).

Undoubtedly, the use of CEST agents will expand in the coming years. New chelating agents for lanthanide ions or lipid- and polymer-based nanoparticles will be synthesized that will exhibit superior chemical exchange properties and have a higher number of exchangeable protons. CEST agents will become a platform with which other functional chemical groups can be added for molecular targeting, cellular internalization, or conjugation to other agents for multimodality imaging (67). These unlimited possibilities could make CEST agents key players in the molecular imaging of cancer.

APPLICATIONS

pH Responsive Contrast Agents

pH is a fundamental physiological parameter that affects basic biochemical reactions for cellular function and metabolism. In the context of cancer, the tumor micro-environment often exhibits hypoxia, nutrient deprivation, and low extracellular pH, which promotes angiogenesis and activates the overexpression of a host of cytokines and proteolytic enzymes (5). The absolute pH can be quantified with either phosphorus or proton MR spectroscopy. Although the intracellular pH is neutral-to-alkaline, the extracellular pH is consistently measured acidic in majority of cancer cell lines, ranging from 6.23 in CaNT adenocarcinoma cells to 6.99 in MCF-7 breast cancer cells (5). The acidic extracellular pH in the tumor environment is partly because of the overproduction of lactic acid under anaerobic conditions. pH is a crucial parameter that characterizes the tumor microenvironment, and the local detection of pH in vivo can aid our understanding of the environmental contributions to tumor progression and metastasis. Since CEST relies on the chemical exchange between the solute and the water protons, it is an intrinsically pH-sensitive technique, and pH imaging has been a main application from the beginning. The early pH responsive agents were small DIACEST molecules whose proton chemical shifts are sensitive to changes in pH (22,68).

Using the macromolecular DIACEST agents, PLL and a generation-5 polyamidoamine dendrimer, McMahon et al. (35) demonstrated that the proton exchange rates k_{sw} of the amide protons (+3.6 ppm downfield from the bulk water, Fig. 4A) were pH dependent: increasing from 50 to 1250 Hz in the pH range from 6.0 to 7.9 in PLL, and from 40 to 540 Hz in the pH range from 5.6 to 8.1 in the dendrimer. The resulting MTR_{asy} increased from 5% to 60% between pH = 6.0 and 7.9 in PLL, and from 15% to 60% between pH = 5.6 and 8.1 in the dendrimer. Using relatively low concentrations (in the 50 μM range) of PLL and dendrimers, small changes in pH were detectable, making them sensitive agents for CEST-based pH imaging.

For in vivo imaging applications, the absolute concentrations of the administered contrast agents are often difficult to determine. Ward and Balaban devised a ratiometric pH technique that only requires the knowledge of the relative concentrations (68). At high saturation efficiencies ($\alpha \rightarrow 1$), it is not difficult to show from the expression of PTR (Eq. 1) that the quantity ($M_{0w}/M_{sat} - 1$) is proportional to the absolute concentration of exchangeable protons. Thus if two magnetically distinct proton sites are available on either one or two different agents, the ratio $(M_{0w}/M_{sat} - 1)^{site1}/(M_{0w}/M_{sat} - 1)^{site2}$ only depends on

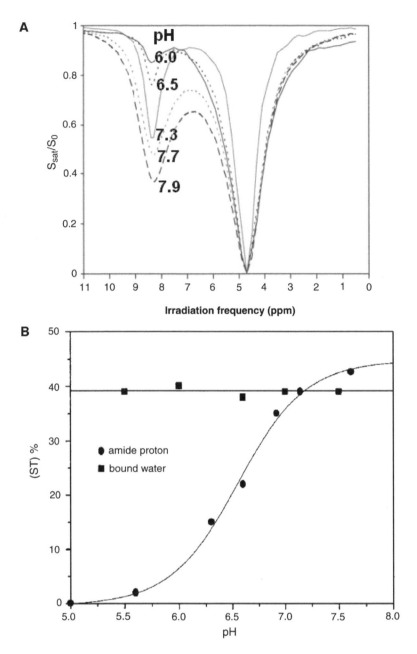

Figure 4 pH responses of a DIACEST agent, poly-L-lysine (PLL) (**A**) and a PARACEST agent, Pr-DOTAM-Gly (**B**). The concentration of the 706 kD PLL was 50 μM or less in phosphate-buffered saline and the saturated water signals was measured at 37°C and 11.7 T. Pr-DOTAM-Gly has two exchangeable proton groups: amide protons on glycine and protons of the bound-water molecule. Experiments were performed with 30 mM of Pr-DOTAM-Gly at 39°C and 7 T. *Source*: Adapted from Refs. 35 and 70.

the relative proton molar ratio of the two sites. Aime et al. applied this ratiometric technique and two PARACEST agents, Yb-DOTAM-Gly and Eu-DOTAM-Gly, to quantify the pH changes in the range of 7.0 to 8.0 (63). Since mainly Eu-DOTAM-Gly is responsive to the pH changes in this range, Yb-DOTAM-Gly was used effectively as a concentration marker in the pH quantification. In another example, Aime and colleagues (69,70) applied the

ratiometric technique to the bound-water protons and the amide protons on the PARACEST agent, Pr-DOTAM-Gly (Fig. 4B). They found that the amide protons showed their usual pH responsiveness between pH = 6.0 and 7.5, while the water protons remained essentially independent of pH changes. After taking the ratio of $(M_{0w}/M_{sat} - 1)$ between the two sites, Pr-DOTAM-Gly showed a response curve most sensitive in the pH range of 6.0 to 7.5.

Temperature Responsive Contrast Agents

Temperature is another important physiological parameter that reflects cell function and metabolism. Monitoring tissue temperature is not only a valuable diagnostic tool to locate cancerous or inflamed tissues, but also useful for MR-guided, local thermal ablation during cancer therapy (71). The linewidth of the proton signal of an exchangeable chemical group may broaden as the temperature increases, resulting in a decrease in the signal intensity on the NMR spectrum. For a narrow frequency-selective presaturation pulse, the lower proton density implies that a smaller number of protons are available for saturation and a smaller CEST effect. However, the proton exchange rate on a per-proton basis increases as a function of temperature, so the overall CEST either increases or decreases depending on which of the two competing effects dominate. Terreno et al. examined the temperature response of the PARACEST agent, Pr-DOTAM-Gly (70). They found that the PTR decreases linearly as a function of temperature for the Pr-bound water, while the amide protons remain essentially constant in the temperature range of 25–55°C. A ratiometric technique, similar to the one used for pH imaging, can then produce a concentration-independent calibration of temperature as a function of the measurable PTR of Pr-DOTAM-Gly. The temperature sensitivity is about 0.4°C for a 1% change in PTR near the physiological temperature of 37°C.

An alternative approach to measure temperature is to use the temperature-dependent chemical shift of the lanthanide-bound water. As an improvement of the traditional MR thermometry where the hyperfine shift of a nucleus is measured against a temperature change, Zhang et al. used two PARACEST agents, Dy-4Am-CH2COOH and Eu-4Am-CH2COOH, and measured their lanthanide-bound water chemical shifts (72). Since the CEST technique was used for detection of the bulk water signal, they were able to detect the shifts with higher sensitivity and at a higher spatial resolution. For example, testing on a phantom of 10 mM Eu-4Am-CH2COOH heated by temperature-controlled air flow, they measured sample temperatures ranging 25–40°C with an in-plane spatial resolution of 0.15×0.15 mm^2. This improved sensitivity and resolution can be useful for applications that require the monitoring of the local tissue temperatures.

Metabolite/Enzyme Responsive Contrast Agents

Several "smart" CEST agents have been developed to detect metabolites (73,74), caspase-3 (75), poly-L-arginine (76), and zinc (77). Lactate is an important metabolite active in anaerobic glycolysis and is involved in a wide range of physiological and pathological conditions such as stroke and brain tumors. CEST-based metabolite imaging was first demonstrated in lactate phantoms using a heptadentate ligand of Yb, Yb-MBDO3AM (73). The free Yb-MBDO3AM has six amide protons, giving rise to a broad peak at −28.5 ppm on the ^{1}H spectrum. Upon lactate binding to the amides, two narrower peaks appear centered at −20 and −14 ppm. Using a 30 mM solution of Yb-MBDO3AM, the authors showed that the MTR$_{asy}$ of the free Yb-MBDO3AM decreased by ∼6% for every 1 mM increase in the lactate concentration, while the MTR$_{asy}$ of the lactate-bound Yb-MBDO3AM increased by ∼1% for the same increase in the lactate concentration. Although this technique lacked good sensitivity to lactate concentrations and required the knowledge of the contrast agent concentration a priori to determine the lactate concentration, it represented the first successful attempt to image a metabolite using CEST agents.

A second study focused on imaging glucose, which is involved in cellular energy metabolism through glycolysis and the subsequent ATP production during Krebs cycle. Zhang et al. (74) designed and synthesized a DOTA-tetraamide ligand of Eu modified by two phenyl boronate groups (Eu-DOTA-4AmBoron). When glucose is added, the exchange between the Eu-bound water and the bulk water is slowed down because of the binding of glucose to the boronate group, resulting in a peak at 50 ppm in the ^{1}H spectrum. In a phantom of 10 mM Eu-DOTA-4AmBoron, the investigators added 0–90 mM of glucose and found that the z-spectrum lineshape became narrower around 50 ppm with increasing glucose concentrations, possibly because of slower exchange rates and a sharper bound-water linewidth. They used the CEST ratio, M$_{sat}$(30 ppm)/M$_{sat}$(50 ppm), as a benchmark for the influence of glucose on the exchange rate. This CEST ratio increased in a single-exponential fashion with the added glucose concentration with an association constant of 383 M^{-1}, in agreement with the circular dichroism spectroscopy results. CEST difference images, representing (M_{sat}(30 ppm) − M_{sat}(50 ppm)) at four different glucose concentrations, showed a higher contrast at higher glucose concentrations.

In a study that used CEST to detect the activity of the enzyme caspase-3, which is important in triggering cellular apoptosis, Yoo and Pagel synthesized a complex of Tm-DOTA and a short peptide, Asp-Glu-Val-Asp (DEVD) (75). Without the presence of caspase-3, the z-spectrum of the complex showed a dip at −51 ppm corresponding to an amide group in proximity to the Tm center. After reaction, the z-spectrum showed a much-reduced dip at −51 ppm with an additional asymmetry about the water peak. An asymmetry analysis similar to equation (3) yielded a broad peak centered around +8 ppm, indicating the cleavage of the DEVD peptide and conversion of the amide to an amine group. A 14.5%

reduction in water signal is observed at the presaturation frequency of −51 ppm before the reaction, while no significant change was seen after the reaction. Calculations also concluded a 5–50 nM caspase-3 detection sensitivity at 5.2 mM concentration of the DEVD-Tm-DOTA complex.

Labeling and Imaging of Cells

Iron oxide is the most commonly used MR contrast agent for cell labeling and tracking (78). Common methods to label cells magnetically involves incubation, electroporation (79), modifying the iron oxide with transfection agents such as dendrimers (80), cationic polymers (81,82) or peptides (83,84). One disadvantage of these labeling approaches is that administered contrast agents become diluted in each cell division, which may limit its applicability for tracking of asymmetrically dividing cells with rapid turnover (85). An alternative approach is to infect the cells with a ferritin transgene that labels the cells magnetically as ferritins are expressed and begin to sequester the endogenous iron (86,87). Since a copy of the ferritin gene is duplicated in each cell division, the constant intracellular ferritin expression ensures a stable concentration of iron oxide inside each cell. Both the direct and reporter gene approaches have now been applied for cell labeling using CEST agents in vitro (54) and in vivo (47).

Aime and colleagues explored the use of PARACEST agents as potential cell labeling agents (54). They chose Eu-DOTAM-Gly and Tb-DOTAM-Gly for their similarities in chemical synthesis and cytotoxicity and their large difference in resonance frequencies: the bound water of Eu-DOTAM-Gly resonates at +50 ppm while that of Tb-DOTAM-Gly at −600 ppm. CEST imaging with frequency-selective excitation can distinguish phantoms of 1 mM Eu-DOTAM-Gly from 1 mM Tb-DOTAM-Gly. To demonstrate frequency-selective imaging of cells labeled with the two PARACEST agents, the authors incubated 10^6 rat hepatoma cells (HTC) with 40 mM of each type of agents for six hours. After washing, the cell pellets were imaged at 7 T and 12% and 11.2% reduction in water signal intensity because of CEST were observed selectively at 50 ppm for Eu-DOTAM-Gly and −600 ppm for Tb-DOTAM-Gly. These results illustrate the potential of PARACEST agents for simultaneously labeling different cell types for cell tracking studies in vivo.

More recently, Gilad et al. (47) developed an artificial CEST reporter gene (Fig. 5). The reporter, named lysine-rich protein (LRP), was generated by cloning synthetic eight oligonucleotides in tandem encodes to protein with high lysine content (200 lysine residues per protein) into a vector that also expresses enhanced green fluorescent protein (EGFP). A control vector consisted of EGFP only. These vectors were transfected into a 9L rat glioma cell line. The transfected cells showed no cytotoxicity with respect to metabolic mitochondrial rate, as based on measurement of the release of glucose 6-phosphate dehydrogenase from dead cells, and the hydrolysis of calcein-AM by intracellular esterases in living cells. In vitro MR imaging of four separate LRP clones and one pooled clone show a statistically significant increase in MTR_{asy} compared to control cells that only expressed EGFP. The authors also tested their CEST reporter gene approach in vivo by inoculating the LRP-expressing (pooled clone) and control EGFP-expressing cells into contralateral hemispheres of mouse brains. The LRP-expressing tumor showed a 8.2% increase in signal relative to brain baseline, which is statistically significant compared to the 3.5% increase in the control tumor (Fig. 5B). This new technology could potentially be useful to track dividing cells in vivo and to image multiple cell populations with MRI.

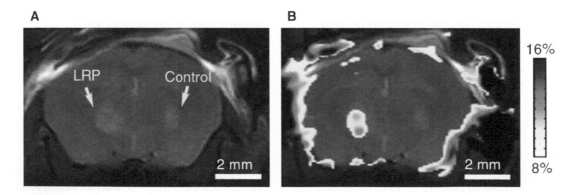

Figure 5 In vivo CEST experiments in a brain tumor mouse model. (**A**) MR anatomical image of a mouse brain inoculated by a 9L glioma tumor expressing lysine-rich protein (LRP) versus a control xenograft on the contralateral hemisphere. (**B**) Map of CEST signal changes relative to the brain baseline overlaid on top of (**A**), demonstrating that the LRP-expressing tumor can be distinguished from the control tumor. *Source*: Adapted from Ref. 47 (*See Color Insert*).

Cytotoxicity of CEST contrast agents is an important issue for their future clinical translation. Gd-based MR contrast agents recently caught public attention because nearly all reported nephrogenic systemic fibrosis (NSF) cases have been associated with their administration (88). Since lanthanide chelates share similar coordination chemistry and pharmacokinetics, other lanthanide-based CEST agents may also have deleterious effects in the body. Neither intracellular concentration nor cytotoxicity of exogenous CEST agents has been carefully studied except a few examples (89,90). Risk assessment of newly developed CEST agents should become an integral part of the research and development effort in order to expedite their clinical translation and application.

ENDOGENOUS CEST EFFECTS

In contrast to using artificially synthesized lanthanide-based PARACEST or macromolecular DIACEST agents, there are endogenous compounds in tissue that exhibit CEST effects. These are generally based on diamagnetic molecules with exchangeable amide, amine, or OH groups. Amide proton transfer (APT) imaging is a special type of CEST imaging that relies on detecting the endogenous amide protons on mobile proteins and peptides in tissue and has the advantage of not requiring the administration of any contrast agents. The MR signature of these amide protons at +3.5 ppm were first observed in ^{1}H spectra of perfused cells when the pH-sensitive amide proton exchange rates were used to quantify cellular and tissue pH (91).

Zhou et al. demonstrated the effect of ischemia on the amide proton exchange with water in rat brains (37). In tissue, the conventional MT that involves the exchange between the immobile, tissue-bound protons and the bulk water dominates the proton exchange process in the tissue water signal, for example, resulting in a 50% signal reduction at +5 ppm away from the water resonance. On top of the MT-driven proton exchange, however, close examination of the z-spectrum revealed an additional water saturation because of the amide proton exchange at a saturation frequency of +3.5 ppm. Under cardiac arrest, the MTR$_{asy}$ at 3.5 ppm changed by 2%, which is called ΔPTR (26). The authors hypothesized that the measured ΔPTR was because of the pH changing from 7.11 to 6.66 within the first two hours of postmortem, which was confirmed by ^{31}P spectroscopy. This sensitive dependence of ΔPTR on pH formed the basis for APT pH imaging in rat models with middle cerebral artery occlusion (MCAO). Figure 6A shows a MTR$_{asy}$ image with the ischemic region being hypointense. The ΔPTR contribution to MTR$_{asy}$ can be calibrated with respect to pH to construct an absolute pH map of the same ischemic rat brain (Fig. 6B). The ischemic regions captured by these images were confirmed by histology, suggesting the feasibility of the APT technique for in vivo pH imaging. This was recently confirmed in a systematic stroke model study (92).

APT imaging was also applied to brain tumors in both animals and humans. In a rat brain tumor study, Zhou et al. showed that the MT-saturated water signal is larger in the tumor than within the peritumoral edema and contralateral region (93). When ΔPTR was calculated, the tumor showed an enhanced ΔPTR $\approx$ 3% in the frequency range from 2 to 3.5 ppm, while the effect in the contralateral region was close to 0%. This increased amide proton exchange was attributed to increased protein and peptide content, although the authors did not exclude possible contributions from larger water content and longer water T_1 inside tumors.

More recently, Jones et al. reported APT imaging of human brain tumors on a 3T clinical scanner, making

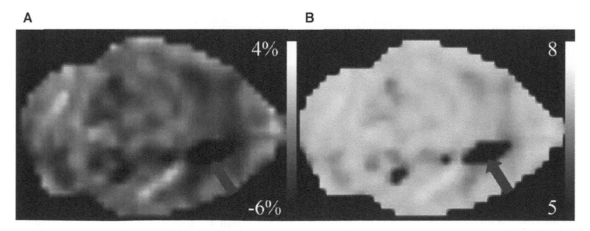

Figure 6 In vivo CEST experiments in a stroke mouse model. Demonstration of amide proton transfer (APT) imaging of endogenous proteins and peptides in terms of MTR$_{asy}$ (**A**) and absolute pH (**B**) during focal ischemia of a rat model. The histological section (not shown) validated the ischemic, low-pH region on the APT image (*arrow* in **B**). *Source*: Adapted from Ref. 37.

CEST-based MR imaging a clinical reality for the first time (94). Ten brain tumor patients with different grades of glioma were scanned and their tumor APT levels were quantified. In eight out of ten cases, APT images showed areas with elevated intensities consistent with those outlined by conventional MR sequences including T_1-weighted, T_2-weighted, Gd T_1-weighted, fluid-attenuated inversion recovery (FLAIR), and apparent diffusion constant (ADC). In six out of ten patients, statistically significant differences in APT were observed with $P < 0.001$ in high-APT regions versus contralateral normal-appearing white matter regions. More importantly, in contrast to conventional MRI, APT could distinguish the tumor from edema, thus offering a potential tool to delineate the tumor boundary for surgical intervention.

CONCLUSIONS

The application of CEST imaging has expanded from the first demonstration of an effect in small molecules to the use of a range of macromolecules, lanthanide chelates, liposomal nanoparticles, and a reporter gene. The overall pace of the developments in this field is impressive. Its sensitivity has improved dramatically from the order of a millimolar range in small molecules to a micromolar range in large macromolecules, and to a pico- to nanomolar range in LIPOCEST agents. At the same time, in vivo experiments showed that endogenous proteins and peptides with exchangeable proton concentration of ~ 70 mM in brain and brain tumors and glycogen of $\sim 200–400$ mM (glucose concentration) in livers can be detected via proton exchange with water in the surrounding tissue. The first CEST reporter gene experiment mentioned above shows great promise to track cells noninvasively in vivo for a period of time without losing signal intensity because of cell divisions and may also be exploited to report on cell survival and cellular differentiation.

There are several challenges for in vivo CEST imaging using exogenous agents, which offer plenty of research opportunities in the field of CEST agent development in the coming years. First, the agent should be water soluble and exhibit low cellular toxicity. As such, DIACEST agents involving sugar, peptides, and oligonucleotides, may be better tolerated by biological systems. Biodegradable nanocapsules such as liposomes could prove to be highly useful for encapsulating and delivering more toxic CEST agents to their targets, in particular when the goal is to target cancer cells and kill them with these substances. Second, the agent should have a long circulation time and be able to cross biological barriers to reach its target. In this regard, conjugation chemistry approaches that have been used for Gd(III) chelate-based imaging applications may be applied to new CEST agents to improve their

ability to reach the desired target. Finally, CEST agents whose resonance frequencies are close to water require additional effort in pulse sequence optimization and data analysis. The optimum presaturation pulse power and duration should be determined experimentally to ensure high saturation efficiency of the agent and low direct saturation of the bulk water. Also, shimming and centering of the bulk water frequency are crucial for the MTR_{asy} analysis to work properly [see Eq. (3)]. However, it is likely that many of these challenges can be met and that CEST imaging will develop into an important field of both exogenous and endogenous contrast for MRI.

ACKNOWLEDGMENTS

We thank Kristine Glunde and Jinyuan Zhou for critical reading of the manuscript. This work is supported by R21EB005252 (J.W.M.B.), P41RR015241 (P.C.M.v.Z.) and K01EB006394 (M.T.M).

REFERENCES

1. Vogelstein B, Kinzler KW. Cancer genes and the pathways they control. Nat Med 2004; 10(8):789–799.
2. Feinberg AP, Ohlsson R, Henikoff S. The epigenetic progenitor origin of human cancer. Nat Rev Genet 2006; 7:21–33.
3. Colditz GA, Sellers TA, Trapido E. Epidemiology—identifying the causes and preventability of cancer? Nat Rev Cancer 2006; 6:75–83.
4. Pickeral OK, Li JZ, Barrow I, et al. Classical oncogenes and tumor suppressor genes: a comparative genomics perspective. Neoplasia 2000; 2:280–286.
5. Gillies RJ, Raghunand N, Karczmar GS, et al. MRI of the tumor microenvironment. J Magn Reson Imaging 2002; 16:430–450.
6. Pathak AP, Gimi B, Glunde K, et al. Molecular and functional imaging of cancer: advances in MRI and MRS. Methods Enzymol 2004; 386:3–60.
7. Weissleder R, Mahmood U. Molecular imaging. Radiology 2001; 291:316–333.
8. Sosnovik DE, Weissleder R. Emerging concepts in molecular MRI. Curr Opin Biotechnol 2007; 18:4–10.
9. Glunde K, Pathak AP, Bhujwalla ZM. Molecular-functional imaging of cancer: to image and imagine. Trends Mol Med 2007; 13:287–297.
10. Aime S, Crich SG, Gianolio E, et al. High sensitivity lanthanide(III) based probes for MR-medical imaging. Coord Chem Rev 2006; 250:1562–1579.
11. Caravan P. Strategies for increasing the sensitivity of gadolinium based MRI contrast agents. Chem Soc Rev 2006; 35:512–523.
12. Casali C, Janier M, Canet E, et al. Evaluation of Gd-DOTA-labeled dextran polymer as an intravascular MR contrast agent for myocardial perfusion. Acad Radiol 1998; 5:S214–S218.

13. Bryant LH, Brechbiel MW, Wu C, et al. Synthesis and relaxometry of high-generation (G = 5, 7, 9, and 10) PAMAM dendrimer-DOTA-gadolinium chelates. J Magn Reson Imaging 1999; 9:348–352.

14. Kobayashi H, Brechbiel MW. Nano-sized MRI contrast agents with dendrimer cores Adv Drug Deliv Rev 2005; 57:2271–2286.

15. Tilcock C, Unger E, Cullis P, et al. Liposomal Gd-DTPA: preparation and characterization of relaxivity. Radiology 1989; 171:77–80.

16. Unger E, Winokur T, MacDougall P, et al. Hepatic metastases: liposomal Gd-DTPA-enhanced MR imaging. Radiology 1989; 171:81–85.

17. Winter PM, Caruthers SD, Kassner A, et al. Molecular imaging of angiogenesis in nascent Vx-2 rabbit tumors using a novel alpha(nu)beta3-targeted nanoparticle and 1.5 tesla magnetic resonance imaging. Cancer Res 2003; 63:5838–5843.

18. Lim EH, Danthi N, Bednarski M, et al. A review: integrin alphav-beta3-targeted molecular imaging and therapy in angiogenesis. Nanomedicine 2005; 1:110–114.

19. Kirpotin DB, Drummond DC, Shao Y, et al. Antibody targeting of long-circulating lipidic nanoparticles does not increase tumor localization but does increase internalization in animal models. Cancer Res 2006; 66:6732–6740.

20. Forsen S, Hoffman RA. Study of moderately rapid chemical exchange reactions by means of nuclear magnetic double resonance. J Chem Phys 1963; 39:2892–2901.

21. Wolff SD, Balaban RS. NMR imaging of labile proton exchange. J Magn Reson 1990; 86:164–169.

22. Ward KM, Aletras AH, Balaban RS. A new class of contrast agents for MRI based on proton chemical exchange dependent saturation transfer (CEST). J Magn Reson 2000; 143:79–87.

23. Goffeney N, Bulte JWM, Duyn J, et al. Sensitive NMR detection of cationic-polymer-based gene delivery systems using saturation transfer via proton exchange. J Am Chem Soc 2001; 123:8628–8629.

24. Snoussi K, Bulte JWM, Gueron M, et al. Sensitive CEST agents based on nucleic acid imino proton exchange: detection of poly(rU) and of a dendrimer-poly(rU) model for nucleic acid delivery and pharmacology. Magn Reson Med 2003; 49:998–1005.

25. Aime S, Delli Castelli D, Terreno E. Highly sensitive MRI chemical exchange saturation transfer agents using liposomes. Angew Chem Int Ed 2005; 44:5513–5515.

26. Zhou J, van Zijl PCM. Chemical exchange saturation transfer imaging and spectroscopy. Prog Nucl Magn Reson Spectrosc 2006; 48:109–136.

27. Zhang S, Merritt M, Woessner DE, et al. PARACEST agents: modulating MRI contrast via water proton exchange. Acc Chem Res 2003; 36:783–790.

28. Modo MMJ, Bulte JWM, eds. Molecular and Cellular MR Imaging. Part I. Contrast agents for molecular and cellular imaging. Boca Raton: CRC Press, 2007.

29. McConnell HM. Reaction rates by nuclear magnetic resonance. J Chem Phys 1958; 28:430–431.

30. Mulkern RV, Williams ML. The general solution to the Bloch equation with constant rf and relaxation terms: application to saturation and slice selection. Med Phys 1993; 20(1):5–13.

31. Kingsley PB, Monahan WG. Effects of off-resonance irradiation, cross-relaxation, and chemical exchange on steady-state magnetization and effective spin-lattice relaxation times. J Magn Reson 2000; 143:360–375.

32. Kingsley PB, Monahan WG. Correction for off-resonance effects and incomplete saturation in conventional (two-site) saturation-transfer kinetic measurements. Magn Reson Med 2000; 43:810–819.

33. Zhou J, Wilson DA, Sun PZ, et al. Quantitative description of proton exchange processes between water and endogenous and exogenous agents for WEX, CEST, and APT experiments. Magn Reson Med 2004; 51:945–952.

34. Woessner DE, Zhang S, Merritt M, et al. Numerical solution of the Bloch equations provides insights into the optimum design of PARACEST agents for MRI. Magn Reson Med 2005; 53:790–799.

35. McMahon MT, Gilad AA, Zhou J, et al. Quantifying exchange rates in chemical exchange saturation transfer agents using the saturation time and saturation power dependencies of the magnetization transfer effect on the magnetic resonance imaging signal (QUEST and QUESP): pH calibration for poly-L-lysine and a starburst dendrimer. Magn Reson Med 2006; 55:836–847.

36. Pekar J, Jezzard P, Roberts DA, et al. Perfusion imaging with compensation for asymmetric magnetization transfer effects. Magn Reson Med 1996; 35:70–79.

37. Zhou J, Payen J, Wilson DA, et al. Using the amide proton signals of intracellular proteins and peptides to detect pH effects in MRI. Nat Med 2003; 9:1085–1090.

38. Swanson SD, Pang Y. MT is Symmetric but Shifted With Respect to Water. International Society for Magnetic Resonance Imaging in Medicine 11th Scientific Meeting. Toronto, 2003:660. Available at: http://www.ismrm.org/meetings/index.htm

39. Hua J, Jones CK, Blakeley J, et al. Quantitative description of the asymmetry in magnetization transfer effects around the water resonance in the human brain. Magn Reson Med 2007; 58(4):786–793.

40. Henkelman RM, Stanisz GJ, Graham SJ. Magnetization transfer in MRI: a review. NMR Biomed 2001; 14:57–64.

41. Wolff SD, Balaban RS. Magnetization transfer contrast (MTC) and tissue water proton relaxation in vivo. Magn Reson Med 1989; 10:135–144.

42. Balaban RS, Ceckler TL. Magnetization transfer contrast in magnetic resonance imaging. Magn Reson Q 1992; 8:116–137.

43. Spencer RGS, Horska A, Ferretti JA, et al. Spillover and incomplete saturation in kinetic measurements. J Magn Reson B 1993; 101:294–296.

44. Baguet E, Roby C. Off-resonance irradiation effect in steady-state NMR saturation transfer. J Magn Reson 1997; 128:149–160.

45. Guivel-Scharen V, Sinnwell T, Wolff SD, et al. Detection of proton chemical exchange between metabolites and water in biological tissues. J Magn Reson 1998; 133:36–45.

46. Park TG, Jeong JH, Kim SW. Current status of polymeric gene delivery systems. Adv Drug Deliv Rev 2006; 58:467–486.

47. Gilad AA, McMahon MT, Walczak P, et al. Artificial reporter gene providing MRI contrast based on proton exchange. Nat Biotech 2007; 25:217–219.

48. van Zijl PCM, Jones CK, Ren J, et al. MRI detection of glycogen in vivo by using chemical exchange saturation transfer imaging (glycoCEST). Proc Natl Acad Sci U S A 2007; 104:4359–4364.

49. Caravan P, Ellison JJ, McmMurray TJ, et al. Gadolinium (III) chelates as MRI contrast agents: structure, dynamics, and applications. Chem Rev 1999; 99:2293–2352.

50. Peters JA, Huskens J, Raber DJ. Lanthanide induced shifts and relaxation rate enhancements. Prog Nucl Magn Reson Spec 1996; 28:283–350.

51. Winter PM, Bansal N. TmDOTP(5-) as a (23)Na shift reagent for the subcutaneously implanted 9L gliosarcoma in rats. Magn Reson Med 2001; 45(3):436–442.

52. Aime S, Botta M, Mainero V, et al. Separation of intra- and extracellular lactate NMR signals using a lanthanide shift reagent. Magn Reson Med 2002; 47(1):10–13.

53. Woods M, Woessner DE, Sherry AD. Paramagnetic lanthanide complexes as PARACEST agents for medical imaging. Chem Soc Rev 2006; 35:500–511.

54. Aime S, Carrera C, Delli Castelli D, Geninatti Crich S, Terreno E. Tunable imaging of cells labelled with MRI-PARACEST agents. Angew Chem Int Ed 2005; 44: 1813–1815.

55. Aime S, Barge A, Botta M, et al. Direct MMR spectroscopic observation of a lanthanide-coordinated water molecule whose exchange rate is dependent on the conformation of the complexes. Angew Chem Int Ed 1998; 37:2673–2675.

56. Aime S, Barge A, Bruce JI, et al. NMR, relaxometric, and structural studies of the hydration and exchange dynamics of cationic lanthanide complexes of macrocylic tetraamide ligands. J Am Chem Soc 1999; 121:5762–5771.

57. Aime S, Barge A, Batsanov AS, et al. Controlling the variation of axial water exchange rates in macrocyclic lanthanide (III) complexes. Chem Commun 2002(10):1120–1121.

58. Zhang S, Kovacs Z, Burgess S, et al. DOTA-bis(amide) lanthanide complexes: NMR evidence for differences in water-molecule exchange rates for coordination isomers. Chemistry 2001; 7:288–296.

59. Zhang S, Sherry AD. Physical characteristics of lanthanide complexes that act as magnetization transfer (MT) contrast agents. J Solid State Chem 2003; 171:38–43.

60. Zhang S, Wu K, Sherry AD. Unusually sharp dependence of water exchange rate versus lanthanide ionic radii for a series of tetra-amide complexes. J Am Chem Soc 2002; 124:4226–4227.

61. Cubans D, Gonzalez G, Powell DH, et al. Unexpectedly large change of water exchange rate and mechanism on [Ln (DTPA-BMA)(H2O)] complexes along the lanthanide(III) series. Inure Chem 1995; 34:4767–4768.

62. Aime S, Botta M, Fusion M, et al. Prosodic and water exchange processes in aqueous solutions of Gd(III) chelates. Acc Chem Res 1999; 32:941–949.

63. Aime S, Barge A, Castelli DD, et al. Paramagnetic lanthanide(III) complexes as pH-sensitive chemical exchange saturation transfer (CEST) contrast agents for MRI applications. Magn Reson Med 2002; 47:639–648.

64. Terreno E, Cabala C, Carrera C, et al. From spherical to osmotically shrunken paramagnetic liposomes: an improved generation of LIPOCEST MRI agents with highly shifted water protons. Angew Chem Int Ed 2006; 45:1–4.

65. Aime S, Castelli DD, Lawson D, et al. Gd-loaded liposomes as T1, susceptibility, and CEST agents, all in one. J Am Chem Soc 2007; 129(9):2430–2431.

66. Schrader L, Lowery TJ, Hilt C, et al. Molecular imaging using a targeted magnetic resonance hyperpolarized biosensor. Science 2006; 314:446–449.

67. Adair C, Woods M, Zhao P, et al. Spectral properties of a bifunctional PARACEST europium chelate: an intermediate for targeted imaging applications. Contrast Media Mol Imaging 2007; 2(1):55–58.

68. Ward KM, Balaban RS. Determination of pH using water protons and chemical exchange dependent saturation transfer (CEST). Magn Reson Med 2000; 44:799–802.

69. Aime S, Delli Castelli D, Terreno E. Novel pH-reporter MRI contrast agents. Angew Chem Int Ed 2002; 41: 4334–4336.

70. Terreno E, Castelli DD, Cravotto G, et al. Ln(III)-DOTAMGly complexes: a versatile series to assess the determinants of the efficacy of paramagnetic chemical exchange saturation transfer agents for magnetic resonance imaging applications. Invest Radiol 2004; 39(4):235–243.

71. Nour SG, Lewin JS. Radiofrequency thermal ablation: the role of MR imaging in guiding and monitoring tumor therapy. Magn Reson Imag Clin N Am 2005; 13:561–581.

72. Zhang S, Malloy CR, Sherry AD. MRI thermometry based on PARACEST agents. J Am Chem Soc 2005; 127:17572–17573.

73. Aime S, Delli Castelli D, Fedeli F, Terreno E. A paramagnetic MRI-CEST agent responsive to lactate concentration. J Am Chem Soc 2002; 124:9364–9365.

74. Zhang S, Trokowski R, Sherry AD. A paramagnetic CEST agent for imaging glucose by MRI. J Am Chem Soc 2003; 125:15288–15289.

75. Yoo B, Pagel MD. A PARACEST MRI contrast agent to detect enzyme activity. J Am Chem Soc 2006; 128:14032–114033.

76. Aime S, Castelli DD, Terreno E. Supramolecular adducts between poly-L-arginine and [Tm III dotp]: a route to sensitivity-enhanced magnetic resonance imaging-chemical exchange saturation transfer agents. Angew Chem Int Ed 2003; 42:4527–4529.

77. Trokowski R, Ren J, Kalman FK, et al. Selective sensing of zinc ions with a PARACEST contrast agent. Angew Chem Int Ed 2005; 44:6920–6923.

78. Bulte JWM, Kraitchman DL. Iron oxide MR contrast agents for molecular and cellular imaging. NMR Biomed 2004; 17(7):484–499.

79. Walczak P, Kedziorek DA, Gilad AA, et al. Instant MR labeling of stem cells using magnetoelectroporation. Magn Reson Med 2005; 54:769–774.

80. Bulte JWM, Douglas T, Witwer B, et al. Magnetodendrimers allow endosomal magnetic labeling and in vivo tracking of stem cells. Nat Biotech 2001; 19:1141–1147.

81. Arbab AS, Bashaw LA, Miller BR, et al. Characterization of biophysical and metabolic properties of cells labeled

with superparamagnetic iron oxide nanoparticles and transfection agent for cellular MR imaging. Radiology 2003; 229:838–846.

82. Frank JA, Miller BR, Arbab AS, et al. Clinically applicable labeling of mammalian and stem cells by combining superparamagnetic iron oxides and transfection agents. Radiology 2003; 228:480–487.

83. Josephson L, Tung CH, Moore A, et al. High-efficiency intracellular magnetic labeling with novel superparamagnetic-Tat peptide conjugates. Bioconjug Chem 1999; 10: 186–191.

84. Montet-Abou K, Montet X, Weissleder R, et al. Cell internalization of magnetic nanoparticles using transfection agents. Mol Imaging 2007; 6:1–9.

85. Walczak P, Kedziorek DA, Gilad AA, et al. Applicability and limitations of MR tracking of neural stem cells with asymmetric cell division and rapid turnover: the case of the Shiverer dysmyelinated mouse brain. Magn Reson Med 2007; 58:261–269.

86. Cohen B, Dafni H, Meir G, et al. Ferritin as an endogenous MRI reporter for noninvasive imaging of gene expression in C6 glioma tumors. Neoplasia 2005; 7:109–117.

87. Genove G, DeMarco U, Xu H, et al. A new transgene reporter for in vivo magnetic resonance imaging. Nat Med 2005; 11:450–454.

88. Peak AS, Sheller A. Risk factors for developing gadolinium-induced nephrogenic systemic fibrosis. Ann Pharmacother 2007; 41:1481–1485.

89. Heinrich MC, Kuhlmann MK, Kohlbacher S, et al. Cytotoxicity of iodinated and gadolinium-based contrast agents in renal tubular cells at angiographic concentrations: in vitro study. Radiology 2007; 242:425–434.

90. Oliver M, Ahmad A, Kamaly N, et al. MAGfect: a novel liposome formulation for MRI labelling and visualization of cells. Org Biomol Chem 2006; 4:3489–3497.

91. Mori S, Eleff SM, Pilatus U, et al. Proton NMR spectroscopy of solvent-saturable resonance: a new approach to study pH effects *in situ*. Magn Reson Med 1998; 40:36–42.

92. Sun PZ, Zhou J, Sun W, et al. Detection of the ischemic penumbra using pH-weighted MRI. J Cereb Blood Flow Metab 2007; 27:1129–1136.

93. Zhou J, Lal B, Wilson DA, et al. Amide proton transfer (APT) contrast for imaging of brain tumors. Magn Reson Med 2003; 50:1120–1126.

94. Jones CK, Schlosser MJ, van Zijl PC, et al. Amide proton transfer imaging of human brain tumors at 3T. Magn Reson Med 2006:585–592.

95. Zhang S, Winter P, Wu K, et al. A novel europium(III)-based MRI contrast agent. J Am Chem Soc 2001; 123(7): 1517–1578.

16

Optical Imaging Probes

ALEXEI A. BOGDANOV JR.

Departments of Radiology and Cell Biology, University of Massachusetts Medical School, Worcester, Massachusetts, U.S.A.

INTRODUCTION

In recent years, optical imaging has gained popularity in cancer research as an option for in vivo imaging of animal models of cancer. Optical imaging is sometimes viewed as an alternative to more traditional imaging modalities (such as MRI, CT, and radionuclide-based methods). The reason of such optimistic view is in lower operation costs and relative ease of use, which enables rapid screening of imaging and therapeutic drug candidates in cancer models and assists in preliminary testing of imaging concepts (1). The initial feasibility experiments in molecular optical imaging resulted in a spurt of development of multi-modality imaging markers that potentially allow seamless transition from optical screening to more sophisticated imaging experiments. These studies ultimately provide higher resolution images and/or easily quantifiable data (2–4). The development of alternative, probe-free fluorescence imaging methods for detecting early cancers accelerated relevant instrumentation development (5). However, the issues associated with complexity of light propagation in living tissues and the need in endogenous expression or exogenous delivery of optical imaging markers and probes strongly indicate that optical imaging in animals should not be trivialized and should be viewed as a multidisciplinary area of research. This chapter will focus on properties, characterization, and design of optical imaging probes for oncological applications.

BIOPHOTONIC IMAGING

In vivo optical (biophotonic) imaging is based on gathering and processing information encoded in signals that are generated as a result of interaction of light photons with cellular components that make up the live tissue.

Biophotonic applications use a wide range of light frequencies—from the long-range ultraviolet to near-infrared (approximate quantum energy span, 1.55–4.13 eV). Since the energy of these photons corresponds to wavelengths in the range of 300 to 800 nm, photons interact with individual molecules of the tissue. This interaction can potentially result in photonic energy transformation into the following types of energy: light, chemical, motion, and heat. The light emitted by an electromagnetic field source (i.e., illumination source) can either pass through (transmit), be reflected, refracted, scattered, or absorbed by these components. Ultraviolet light is usually absorbed by thin surface layers of tissue as a result of electronic transitions of molecules interacting with the photons. Ultraviolet light can readily cause photoionization (and molecular damage), especially at shorter wavelengths. Photons in the visible light range are usually very strongly absorbed since there are many available electronic states in molecules interacting with these photons, while near-infrared light causes less electronic transitions, thus having a higher probability of tissue transmission. By detecting transmitted (ballistic and near-ballistic) photons, using special ultrasensitive photon detection devices (streak cameras), or by detecting scattered photons using monitoring of the resultant waveform or phase changes, one can obtain information about the sources of light energy absorption and transformation even if these sources are located in turbid media. Deciphering of this information theoretically enables one to predict, with a high degree of certainty, the position of light-interacting object in a 3D space and concentration of the light-interacting compound in the given object. This information is much more amenable to interpretation if the nature of light-absorbing or transforming molecules (e.g., via fluorescence or phosphorescence effects) is known a priori. This is why in biophotonic imaging applications light with well-defined spectral characteristics is usually used and the energy of this light is matched to the spectral characteristics of optical imaging probes. These probes are either endogenously present in the tissue (e.g., pigments, cofactors, or fluorescent proteins) or need to be administered exogenously, e.g., into the systemic circulation (exogenous probes) (Fig. 1).

ENDOGENOUS OPTICAL IMAGING PROBES

Light-Absorbing, Nonemitting Optical Imaging Probes

Most of the colored (light-absorbing) compounds in living organisms carry chromophores, i.e., conjugated π-systems (including alternating single and double bonds) and metal complexes in which electrons absorb light photons with resultant higher energy transition. This is typical for π-systems, metal orbital electron excitation, and charge-transfer effects in metal-ligand systems (6). Deoxyhemoglobin, hemoglobin, and melanin are the most efficient pigments of mammalian tissues that are responsible for the majority of absorbed visible light photons. The most important is oxygen carrying hemoglobin—a tetrameric protein that has a porphyrin-bound iron (2+) serving as a classic metal chromophore in optical imaging. If detected in a tumor, hemoglobin presence could indicate either perfusion with blood (i.e., angiogenesis in tumors) or hemorrhage as a result of vessel integrity loss, which could also be a case of irregular blood supply and angiogenesis. Near-infrared spectroscopy (NIRS) approach, which detects oxyhemoglobin and deoxyhemoglobin was found useful for monitoring oxygenation of blood in the fetal brain and striated muscle for intrapartum

monitoring. In functional brain imaging, both frequency domain and continuous wave NIRS utilize the fact that with the increase of local blood flow, the relative concentrations of oxy- and deoxyhemoglobin change. In the spectral range between 760 and 830 nm, blood volume change causes strong changes in absorption of light almost exclusively due to hemoglobin in the blood (7). NIRS allows the evaluation of the regional increase of cerebral blood flow with good temporal resolution, but low spatial resolution (8).

Detection of chromophores in tissues is facilitated by recent progress in developing photoacoustic methods (9), which are capable of providing imaging of light absorption at several wavelengths (10). Photoacoustic imaging is based on detecting wideband ultrasonic waves that are emitted due to local optical energy deposition (10). Ultrasonic waves are less scattered than light and this allows to image strongly absorbing compounds at the depth of several millimeters. Photoacoustic microscopy can utilize imaging at 584 nm at which both forms of hemoglobin have the same molar extinction. This enables to detect angiogenesis and melanin in experimental peripheral tumors at microscopic resolutions at the depth of up to 3 mm. The above approach appears to have a potential for obtaining tomographic reconstructions for imaging tumors in vivo. For example, spectral differences between deoxy- and oxyhemoglobin allowed noninvasive assessment of hypoxia in a model of breast cancer metastasis to the brain (11).

Melanins (eumelanin, pheomelanin) are complex oligomeric pigments with no defined structure that are synthesized in normal melanocytes and in the majority of melanoma cells. Imaging of melanin formation was proposed for imaging gene expression using production of melanins by tyrosinase. However, imaging of these pigments alone does not provide sensitivity necessary for melanoma detection, unless this is done in spectroscopic mode using photoacoustic monitoring of near-infrared light interaction with melanins (10). Unlike hemoglobin, melanin absorbs near-infrared light thereby allowing sufficient contrast for subcutaneous melanoma tumor cell imaging.

Endogenous Fluorescent Probes

Cell metabolism requires the presence of certain molecules, which exhibit fluorescent light emission upon irradiation with the light of suitable wavelength (12). Endogenous fluorochromes result in so-called autofluorescence, which appear to be associated mainly with tryptophans (13) and intracellular organelles (primarily with cofactors of mitochondrial enzymes, such as nicotinamide adenine dinucleotide phosphate (NADPH) and flavin

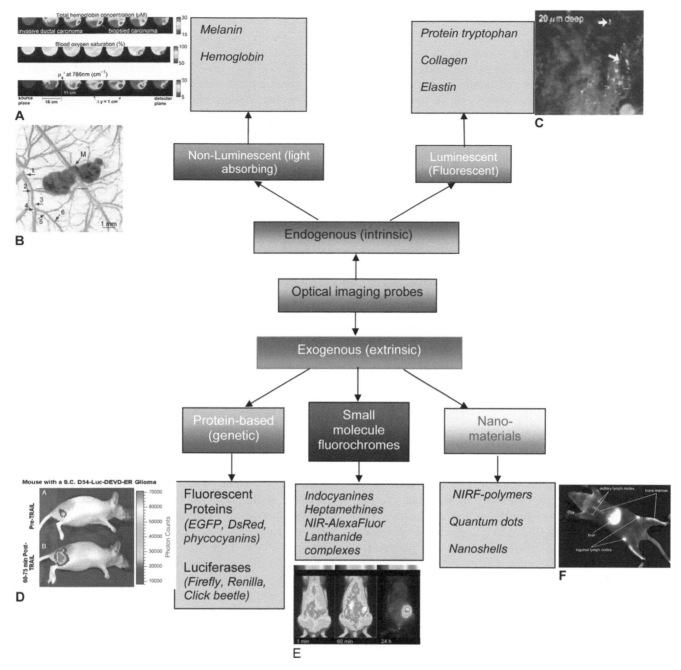

Figure 1 (**A**) Macroscopic optical imaging of hemoglobin in breast cancer (123). (**B**) Microscopic pseudocolored maximum photoacoustic amplitude projection image. Microscopic blood vessels are imaged at 584 nm and the melanoma is imaged using 764-nm image. Numbers indicate order of vessel branching (10). (**C**) Collagen (*purple*) and elastin (*white*) imaging in mouse skin, 20-μm deep, using a two-photon microscope (124); (**D**) luciferase imaging as a marker of apoptosis induced by TRAIL; (**E**) imaging using tricarbocyanine diglucamide (125); (**F**) quantum dot distribution in vivo (126). *Source*: (**D**) from ref. 51 (*See Color Insert*).

adenine dinucleotide (FAD). Tryptophan autofluorescence was reportedly stronger in normal cells than in cancer cell lines (13). Autofluorescence was also attributed to cross-linked elastins and collagens of extracellular matrix, partially due to glycation and oxidation (14,15). These natural products of protein modification in tissues have relatively high quantum yields. Autofluorescence analysis can be performed in real time in peripheral layers of tissue, primarily epithelial layers. This analysis can be useful in assessing changes during the early onset of cancer (carcinoma in situ) that results in various changes of the amount and distribution of endogenous fluorochromes.

EXOGENOUS OPTICAL IMAGING PROBES

Exogenous optical imaging probes are not intrinsically present in cancer cells and have to be delivered to tumors. In the case of fluorescent and luminescent proteins, this can be achieved by using expression vectors encoding protein cDNA sequences. The latter can also be introduced into blastocysts to generate reporter-expressing transgenic animals (16,17). Most of the exogenous optical probes are luminescent. Luminescence is usually defined as light emission from electronically excited states that involves any substance, thus fluorescence is merely a case of luminescence. However, in practice, it is convenient to differentiate between fluorescence (that does require excitation light as a source of energy) and chemiluminescence that requires energy of chemical reaction as a source of electronic excitation. If chemiluminescent processes take place in live organisms they are defined as "bioluminescent." It should be noted that the use of luminescent proteins has applications exclusively in basic and preclinical oncology research. The immunogenicity of these proteins combined with the need to deliver them encoded in expression vectors make their clinical use as diagnostic tools unlikely.

Fluorescent Proteins

The use of recombinant fluorescent protein expression as stable or inducible transgenes in live cells and tissues created a revolution in cell and developmental biology. For the first time, the monitoring of live and intact cells in their natural or semiartificial environments became feasible by using genetic labeling that did not require any additional cell manipulation. The evolvement of fluorescent proteins into a laboratory tool created a convenient alternative to prelabeling of cells with fluorochromes, which usually provide a short-term solution for cell tracking.

Fluorescent proteins found in cnidarians (jellyfishes, anemones, and corals) function as acceptors of blue bioluminescence produced by aquaporins and luciferases. In other words, fluorescent proteins are essential components of bioluminescence resonance energy transfer (BRET) systems that are found in nature. In BRET, photons emitted by luciferases are absorbed by fluorescent proteins and excite the fluorophore, as a result a red-shifted (lower energy) photon can be emitted. Fluorophore of natural fluorescent proteins is spontaneously generated upon oxidation of folding-dependent proximal side groups of amino acids. Exogenous substrates and cofactors are not required for fluorescence of these proteins; however, the amino acid oxidation requires the presence of oxygen. Most of the fluorescent proteins are multimeric, for example, enhanced green fluorescent protein (EGFP) forms weak dimers while most of the red fluorescent proteins are tetramers. The most commonly used fluorescent protein in oncology is EGFP. This engineered fluorescent protein is a product of several stages of mutagenesis and codon usage design: Phe64→Leu mutation improved maturation at higher temperatures (37°C), 190 silent base changes for improving expression in mammals; Ser65→ Thr mutation to shift excitation peak to convenient 488 nm wavelength. The resultant protein is approximately twice as bright as the wild-type protein. Expression of fluorescent proteins can be used to monitor gene expression and protein localization in living organisms. The reason for this is the ability of EGFP to fold into a fluorescent product thereby forming an independent domain of many fusion proteins with little interference with the function of the fusion partner (18,19). Unfortunately, due to multimerization of red fluorescent proteins [e.g., sea anemone *Discosoma striata* red protein, DsRed (20)], the above fusion approach is not always successful because of the tendency of red fluorescence fusion proteins to aggregate and their slow maturation (i.e., appearance of a fluorescent product), which can take several hours and interfere with double fluorescent protein labeling experiments. These potential problems can be dealt by using mutagenesis (21): the removal of several positively charged N-terminal amino acids in DsRed2 mutant decreases the stability of multimers, and the introduction of several silent mutations yielded DsRed-Express, which matures within an hour after transfection of cells with cDNA. It has been reported that cervical carcinomas stably transfected with DsRed2 are easier to detect in vivo than EGFP-expressing tumors (22) (Fig. 2).

In addition, EGFP can be expressed as a marker of gene transfer in tumor cells. EGFP messenger RNA (mRNA) is transcribed in parallel to the transgene mRNA using bidirectional promoters. Alternatively, a viral internal ribosome entry site (IRES) can be used in the case of a single transcribed mRNA. This approach is widely used for constructing viral expression vectors since the expression of a fluorescent protein marker is a convenient approach for selecting transduced cells in vitro or imaging these cells in vivo.

Fluorescent proteins can be expressed in experimental tumors to image tumor cell invasion and track metastasis, and specifically label tumor compartments. For example, human pancreatic tumor cell variants (BxPC-3 and MiaPaCa-2) expressing high levels of EGFP resulted in formation of metastases in the spleen, bowel, portal lymph nodes, and other sites (23). It is technically possible to detect fluorescent metastasis of PC-3 prostate cancer cells in the bone (24). Using a xenon wide-spectrum lamp or a mercury lamp as an excitation source and thermoelectrically cooled color charge-coupled device (CCD) camera

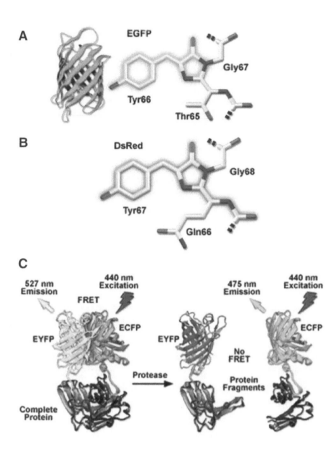

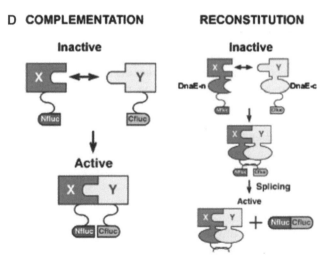

Figure 2 (**A**) An 11-strand β-sheet barrel structure of green fluorescence protein (127) and the chromophore formed as a result of spontaneous oxidation and cyclization of Tyr66 residue and neighboring glycine and serine residues. (128); (**B**) chromophore of the red fluorescence protein; (**C**) fluorescent protease sensor based on resonance energy transfer between cyan and yellow fluorescent proteins (129); (**D**) schematic diagram of complementation-mediated and reconstitution (intein-mediated) restoration of luciferase activity (130).

as a photon detection device, one can detect the presence of small tumors in intact animals. It has been reported that a 60-μm diameter tumor experimentally grown from B16-GFP cells in immunocompetent mice was detectable at a depth of 0.5 mm (25). To detect tumors at the depth of 2 mm, tumors had to be 30 times larger. Since the ratio of the volumes of two tumors is the third power of the ratio of their radii, a 27,000 larger volume of tumor cells would be needed to provide detectability of GFP at this depth. This experiment proves that the fluorescence signal recorded with CCD using a planar ("surface weighted") mode exhibits a prominent nonlinear decrease as a function of depth. Recently, a variant of fluorescence molecular tomography (FMT) imaging (termed FPT, fluorescent protein tomography) was used to image two spectrally distinct protein markers (EGFP and YFP, yellow fluorescent protein). These proteins were expressed in deeper layers of tissue in mice using spectral deconvolution approach and forward model of photon propagation in tissues at visible spectral range (26). This approach allowed imaging tumors at 6-mm depth at 0.4-mm resolution, using fluorescent proteins (26). GFP can also be utilized as specific marker of certain cell types (e.g., endothelial cells, if EGFP is expressed under endothelial Tie-2 promoter) or, conversely, as "negative" contrast to differentiate tumor cells from infiltrating cells and vascular space to image angiogenesis (27). This is feasible because nonfluorescent blood vessels are visible on the background of fluorescent tumor cells (28,29).

Recent mutagenesis experiments resulted in relatively stable true far-red fluorescent proteins (mPlum 590/649 and AQ143 590/655 from *Actinia equina*) that can be expressed in live cells (30,31). These proteins have more favorable light scattering/absorption profiles for in vivo imaging. Recently engineered monomeric Keima red fluorescent protein (32) with a large Stokes shift is useful in designing fusion reporters based on cross-correlation fluorescence spectroscopy, which is extremely sensitive to protein-protein interactions. However, the excitation band of 450 nm is less useful for in vivo applications. The disadvantage of these far-red proteins, including engineered monomeric fluorescent proteins is low quantum yield (brightness), which is 10% or even lower than that of EGFP. One member of phycocyanin protein family (allophycocyanin, a 100-kDa protein with six bilin fluorochromes per protein molecule) has maximum emission of 660 nm and extremely high photostability. However, in vivo use of phycocyanins is limited by their cost, potential high immunogenicity, and high molecular mass. As in the case of any other protein-based exogenous probe, the investigators should be aware of immune response to fluorescent proteins that can significantly alter the progression, therapeutic response, and regrowth of experimental tumors expressing fluorescent proteins (33).

Luminescent Proteins in Optical Imaging

Measuring emitted bioluminescence photons using photon counting devices or CCDs provides one of the most sensitive means of detecting the exogenous marker protein expression enabling the detection of single transfected cells in vitro (34). Likewise, because of the extremely low levels of background bioluminescence in mammals one can detect a very low number of luciferase-positive cells in vivo. This is very useful if the evidence of tumor proliferation or firefly (*Photinus pyralis* beetle) luciferase marker protein expression in HeLa cells enabled the detection of only about 1000 cells injected in peritoneal cavity of rats (35). Firefly luciferase (61 kDa) and *Renilla* (sea pansy) luciferase (36 kDa) are both monomeric proteins that do not require posttranslational processing for enzymatic activity. Unlike fluorescent proteins, luciferases do not require a maturation period and newly translated products are already catalytically active. Firefly luciferase chemiluminescence has a range of approximately 550 to 570 nm, whereas click beetle (*Pyrophorus* sp.) red-shifted luciferase emits photons with a spectral maximum of 635 nm. The latter enables spectral separation of luminescence peaks and dual reporter detection, which is usually performed by using click beetle luciferase mutants. However, dual detection of *Renilla* and firefly luciferases more convenient since the enzymes utilize chemically distinct substrate systems. Beetle luciferase photon emission results from the oxidation of beetle luciferin to oxyluciferin in the presence of ATP, Mg^{2+}, and oxygen, which occurs via luciferyl-AMP intermediate and results in a very rapidly decaying intense release of light. Firefly luminescence in vivo can have more favorable kinetics, which depend on coenzyme A concentration. Wild-type *Renilla* luciferase (RLuc) as well as its improved mutant forms catalyze oxidation of coelenterazine into coelenteramide, proceeds in the absence of ATP, and results in a release of blue light (480-nm maximum). Because of the high level of light output, mutant RLuc is indispensable as a source of excitation of EGFP in emerging in vivo BRET assays (36). The mainstay of luciferase use as tumor marker is the noninvasive imaging of tumor cell numbers (37), which shows excellent correlation with tumor volumes determined by using high-resolution magnetic resonance imaging (38,39). Recently, luciferase imaging found applications for determining kinetics of cell proliferation using transgenic models (40) as well as for performing promoter analysis in vivo (41). These applications are feasible due to the fact that luciferases mature rapidly and have a relatively short intracellular life (about 3 hours in mammals, spanning from translation to degradation) (42).

The fact that there are spectral differences between various luciferases and the application of spectrochromatic imaging to detection of luciferases holds promise in detecting the depth of luminescence sources in vivo, which otherwise is complicated by challenges of reconstructing propagation of visible photons in turbid media (43).

Sensors Based on Protein-Based Optical Imaging Probes

The detection of altered signal transduction pathways in vivo would likely involve imaging of protein phosphorylation. This is an extremely challenging task considering the number, the rate, and the diversity of phosphorylation/dephosphorylation events in live cells. Fluorescent protein pairs and split reporters are connected with a peptide linker that on phosphorylation by insulin receptor kinase (44) undergoes conformational changes. These changes are translated into the efficacy of resonance energy transfer or fluorescence intensity changes, respectively (44,45). Unfortunately, in both scenarios fluorescence changes are at the level of 5% to 10% of the equilibrium intensity, which is likely to be insufficient for reliable in vivo sensing.

Reconstitution or complementation (i.e., the reconstitution of functional activity rather than the integrity of protein) of a split-reporter protein (firefly and RLucs) were previously used for constructing more robust protein sensors. These fragmented reporters could be used for imaging nuclear receptor translocation into the nucleus or protein-protein interactions in the cell. Initially this was achieved by using intein-driven approach (46,47). Intein (DnaE) is a catalytic subunit of DNA polymerase III. To utilize intein-driven protein splicing, the full length of the nuclear receptor [e.g., androgen receptor (48)], split RLuc, and split DnaE (a protein splicing element) were used. The obtained reporting construct consisted of (*i*) cytoplasmic receptor–containing fusion protein with C-terminal fragments of DnaE and luciferase and (*ii*) nucleus-localized fusion counterpart containing N-terminal halves of DnaE and RLuc. These two fusion proteins exhibit no luciferase activity. Upon ligand (dihydrotestosterone) stimulation, the receptor is translocated into the cellular nucleus (46,48) where protein splicing occurs as a consequence of interaction between the splicing junctions of each DnaE fusion fragment. Later it was shown that alternative approaches could be used for RLuc complementation. Rapamycin was shown to drive interaction between FK506-binding protein (FKBP12) mTOR rapamycin-binding domain (FRB) and FKBP12, which if fused to split-RLuc fragments cause the latter to regain some of its catalytic activity (49,50). A similar strategy based on split EGFP protein was also tested for in vivo imaging of subcutaneously injected cells (50).

Split reporter approach has also been successfully applied for imaging chemotherapy-induced apoptosis in vivo (51). This was achieved by fusing luciferase sequence with two estrogen receptor regulatory domains via caspase-3 cleavable linkers (amino acid sequence DEVD) between the luciferase and regulatory domains. Caspase-3 cleavage and restoration of catalytically active luciferase activity results in several folds of luminescence increase.

Probes for Biosynthesis of Fluorescent Molecules

The most commonly used exogenously administered precursor, which is involved in biosynthesis of tetrapyrroles, is 5-aminolevulinic acid (ALA). Eight molecules of ALA are involved in the formation of each molecule of protoporphyrin IX. To increase the protoporphyrin content in cancer cells, ALA or its hexyl ester can be either administered orally or topically (52). Fluorescence of protoporphyrin IX can be excited at 405 nm (blue light). Protoporphyrin has photosensitizing properties, thus biosynthesis of this tetrapyrrole can be used to visualize and to eradicate malignant cells. Several clinical applications of ALA in cancer treatment are currently at the stage of clinical trials (53,54).

Extrinsic Optical Probes

Exogenous organic dyes in optical imaging of cancer are used mostly for in vitro microscopy because most of the cellular components are optically transparent or nonfluorescent. The use of fluorochromes allows to use longer wavelengths for excitation and emission and to achieve good spectral separation between characteristic emissions of various labeled cellular components. However, in vivo imaging requires fluorochromes with special characteristics: they need to be excitable in a convenient range of wavelengths with corresponding photon energies allowing propagation in the tissues and emitting fluorescence in the range that has minimal absorption and scattering in the body. Recently, nanoparticles and polymers with such fluorescence characteristics were designed and added to armamentarium of in vivo optical imaging. These and other exciting developments are reviewed below.

Low Molecular Weight Fluorochromes in Optical Imaging

In vivo imaging is frequently attempted in conjunction with long-wavelength emitters because of lower absorption and scattering of near-infrared range photons in live tissues. There are many chemically distinct dyes, which exhibit light emission in this range. They include very high quantum yield boron-containing BODIPY dye (BODIPY-Texas Red, emission maximum at 675 nm), Alexa Fluor 700 dye, thiasole orange, as well as cyanine

(Cy) dyes. The latter family of fluorochromes includes dyes excitable at 780 nm and fluorescent at wavelengths beyond 800 nm [IR-125 and heptamethine Cy dyes (55)]. Cy dyes have much higher extinction coefficients than BODIPY but lower quantum yields.

Currently, the only clinically approved near-infrared fluorochrome is indocyanine green. This dye is used for detecting sentinel lymph nodes, which assists in resection in breast cancer and colon cancer patients. Visualization of primary lesions is also possible (56) and correlates with MRI findings in breast cancer. However, indocyanine green is still mostly used in ophthalmology as angiographic agent and its use in surgical oncology could potentially find a wider use with the development of more sophisticated interoperation room viewing equipment, which would allow fluorescence detection off the surface of tissues in real time. Several other alternative near-infrared dyes were tested for breast cancer imaging as permeability markers (57).

The major impact on fluorescence imaging in live animals and beyond was made as a result of introduction of carbocyanine dye derivatives that could be covalently linked to amino groups of proteins and other macromolecules. Initially, isothiocyanate and iodoacetamide derivatives of several Cy dyes were shown to form covalent bonds with amino- and sulfhydryl groups of proteins and other macromolecules (58). These derivatives had insufficient hydrophilicity and were replaced by improved hydroxysuccinimide esters carboxylated dyes (59) and eventually were significantly improved by adding sulfate group substitutions in aromatic rings to increase solubility (60). The family of sulfated dyes included Cy5, which could be excited with the 633-nm HeNe laser and laser diodes emitting near 650 nm that are excellent excitation sources for Cy5 and related Cy5.5 dyes. The major application for some of these "early" Cy dye derivatives was found in labeling of oligonucleotides for genomic hybridization assays that allowed multiplexing because Cy3 and Cy5 dye fluorescence could be easily spectrally resolved.

A substantial effort was directed recently at further improvement of Cy dyes (61), including further increase of hydrophilicity by using N-alkylation with dicarboxylic (alkyl-N,N'-bis-carboxymethylamine) groups for cyanine nitrogen modification (62). The search for far-infrared dyes with improved photostability resulted in several heptamethine (i.e., having five conjugated methine double bonds) Cy dyes that could be relatively easily converted into highly reactive compounds because of a moderately reactive chlorine substitution in cyclohexene ring that can undergo attack by various nucleophiles (55,63). The obtained fluorochromes were successfully used for antibody labeling for the purpose of intravital imaging of mouse blood vessels (64). Some novel heptamethine dyes have unusually large Stokes shifts (65,66). Unlike most of the cyanine fluorochromes, which have Stokes shifts less than 30 nm, two reported heptamethines had Stokes shifts >100 nm because of the effect of charge transfer in excited state, which could potentially enable better filtering of excitation light. On the downside, some blue-shifting of fluorescence is also characteristic of these compounds. It should be noted that the charge transfer state is sensitive to many quenching compounds, including disulfides, and the results need to be treated with caution. Tetrasulfonated heptamethine dyes find applications mainly as covalently attached to proteins and nanoparticles, for example, as sentinel lymph node imaging agents for intraoperative mapping agents (67).

Targeted Fluorescent Imaging Agents

The initial experience accumulated in human experimental optical imaging with fluorescein-conjugated antibodies directed against carcinoembrionic antigen (CEA) in colon cancer patients during the surgery (68) suggested that imaging could be performed in intact living animals if the scattering and absorption parameters of emitted light could be improved. By tagging antibodies specific for squamous cell carcinoma with Cy5 dye (two molecules/antibody molecules), the same research group demonstrated the feasibility of tumor imaging in intact mice by using a powerful medical laser for excitation of fluorescence at 640 nm and by using photographic fluorescence detection (69). Optical imaging in the far-red range showed that (*i*) fluorescent antibody had a biodistribution similar to that of radioiodinated antibody, (*ii*) the peak of tumor signal is achieved approximately at 24 hours after injection, (*iii*) there was nonspecific accumulation of fluorescent antibody in the skin, and (*iv*) free dye did not accumulate in the tumor. This study ("infrared photodetection") was supported by other similar findings (70–72) performed by using monoclonal antibodies and recombinant diabodies labeled with Cy5.5 and Cy7 dyes using improved CCD-enabled fluorescence detection. The use of longer wavelength emitting dyes resulted in further improvement of imaging quality and tumor signal detection (73). However, both tumor/skin contrast signal stability over time were improved only marginally. In part, this resulted from nonspecific accumulation of antibodies and their degradation products in the skin and also because of poor photostability of cyanine fluorochromes.

Small molecules (receptor ligands and ligand mimetics) can also be labeled with fluorochromes with the preservation of receptor-binding properties. For example, indotricarbocyanine-octreotate was synthesized by conjugating carboxylated indodicarbo- and an indotricarbocyanine dye with the N-terminal amino group of octreotide and was shown to internalize specifically by human neuroendocrine cells (74). This probe was shown to accumulate progressively in tumor tissue for 24 hours after intravenous administration in vivo. Tumor fluorescence rapidly increased and was more than threefold higher than that of normal tissue from 3 to 24 hours after application (75). Other examples of tumor-targeted imaging agents include near-infrared analogs of cell adhesion molecule $\alpha_v\beta_3$ integrin ligands [c(RGDyK) cyclic peptide labeled with Cy5.5 or other NIR dyes] (76–78). Imaging experiments in human glioma xenografts suggested that the dose of 0.5 nmol of peptide/mouse is optimal and can be used for noninvasive imaging of integrin expression and monitoring anti-integrin treatment efficacy. The development of multimeric RGD agents (79) can potentially further improve the detection of integrin expression (Fig. 3A).

Near-infrared-labeled apoptosis-imaging agents were developed by using human recombinant annexin V (80). The latter has high affinity to phosphatidylserine, a lipid that normally resides on cytoplasmic leaflet of plasma membrane, and binds to cells exposing this lipid on the surface. The experiments involving annexin modification with amino-reactive Cy5.5 succinimide ester demonstrated that only low Cy5.5/annexin ratios result in active conjugate. The increase of these ratios during protein modification resulted in inactive protein, supposedly, because of the loss of binding to phosphatidylserine (81). Using multichannel in vivo fluorescence imaging in GFP- or DsRed2-expressing tumors, the effect of cyclophosphamide was confirmed by both TUNEL assay (that detects DNA strand breaks in apoptotic cells) and near-infrared imaging (82). Tumor NIR fluorescence (NIRF) signal increased two to three times after the treatment, 75 minutes after active Cy-annexin injection, and was detectable for a period of 20 hours after the administration (80). Annexin labeled with NIR800 dye also showed an early optimal signal-to-background ratio evolution after intravenous injection (83).

Quenched Probes Based on Near-Infrared Fluorochromes

The ability of Cy dyes to form aggregates in solutions with a resultant loss of fluorescence was recognized earlier as a significant drawback. The problem was partially solved by using indolyl group modifications by introducing various hydrophilic charged moieties in the ring. However, better understanding of quenching mechanisms in the case of Cy dyes allowed using this Cy-Cy quenching effect to the advantage of molecular sensor design.

It is well known that Cy can undergo either self-quenching (fluorochrome-fluorochrome, F-F interactions) or engage in interaction with nonfluorescent quenching molecules. The self-quenching (F-F) effect is more typical

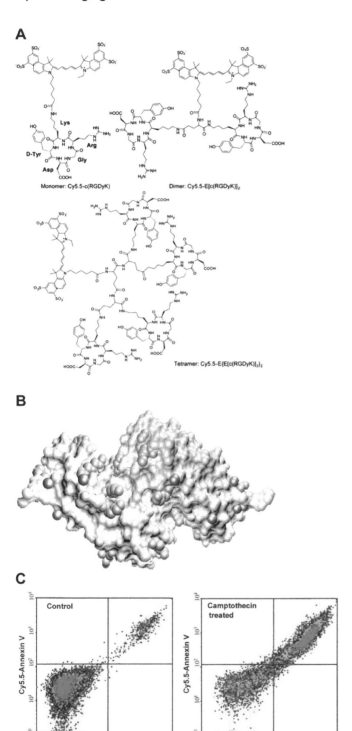

A

Monomer: Cy5.5-c(RGDyK)

Dimer: Cy5.5-E[c(RGDyK)]₂

Tetramer: Cy5.5-E{E[c(RGDyK)]₂}₂

B

C

Figure 3 Targeted optical imaging agents. (**A**) Structure of RGD cyclic peptides labeled with near-infrared Cy5.5 (131). (**B**) Amino-phospholipid binding surface of annexin V. Lysine residues are shown in blue. Biological activity of active near-infrared Cy5.5–annexin V conjugate (81). (**C**) Apoptotic cells bind Cy5.5 and fluorescein isothiocyanate (FITC)-labeled annexin V equally well, suggesting minimal interference with the binding site as a result of Cy5.5 covalent linking (81) (*See Color Insert*).

for dyes fluorescent in far-red (Cy5 and Cy5.5) (84,85). The pairs of (F-Q) dye-quenchers are widely used for designing molecular beacons (86). The chemical structure differences between various pairs of F and Q molecules in their ability to interact with each other allow fine tuning of quenching effects essential for for molecular target identification. If fluorescence of F is spectrally close to absorption range of Q, a dynamic quenching of F occurs (Forster mechanism). Forster quenching occurs because the energy of excited state of one molecule is transferred to a nearby molecule without emission. This effect takes place if the energy of electron transition in F molecule is close to the energy of a corresponding transition in Q. The probability of Forster quenching depends greatly on the distance between F and Q since the probability of fluorescence quenching $W(r) = [1+(r/R_0)^6]^{-1}$, where R_0 is Forster radius corresponding to $W(r) = 0.5$, or critical energy transfer distance. Forster quenching takes place if the distance between F and Q does not exceed 0.6 nm. If both Q and F are so close spatially that their electron orbitals start to overlap, another dynamic quenching mode dominates (Dexter exchange mechanism) (87). In both cases of dynamic fluorescence quenching, both Q and F preserve their individual spectral properties. Closely positioned Q and F can form a complex with static quenching properties, i.e., when light absorbance of two molecules no longer resemble a sum of two individual molecules, but comprise entirely different heterodimer with unique spectral properties because of coupling of excited state energy levels (88). One-dimentional aggregate of a quencher and a dye can form either H- (blue-shifted) or J- (red-shifted) aggregate (88,89). Blue-shifted aggregates are low fluorescent or completely quenched, which makes them useful in various imaging applications, because low or absent fluorescence in a gound-state complex results in an extremely low background signal of the intact fluorochrome-labeled molecule (e.g., molecular beacon). Common quenchers (DABCYL and BHQ) quench fluorescence of Cy5.5 with static quenching being much more efficient than dynamic. The efficacy of quenching reaches about 97%. Currently, more efficient quenching reagents for near-infrared dyes are available, which push quenching efficiencies close to 100%.

Ideally, optimized fluorescent imaging probe should result in specific on-target emission of photons. In most cases it is impossible to control the removal of optical signal from non-target tissues (see previous section) in live animals, and the decreased nonspecific optical signal is highly desirable for achieving high signal-to-background ratios. Unlike the most of the known imaging techniques, because of the quenching-dequenching effect, fluorescence optical imaging enables signal "caging." The effect of fluorescence release after degradation of imaging probe in tumors was initially demonstrated by using a long-circulating

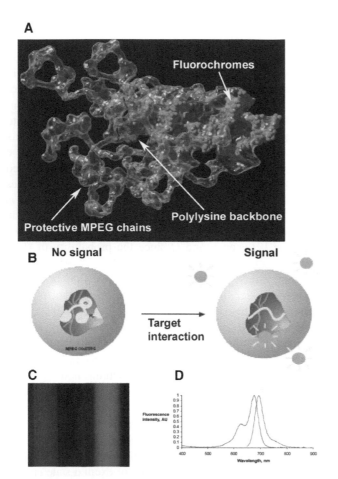

Figure 4 (**A**) Hypothetical structure of self-quenched Cy5.5-PGC imaging probe fragment based on interaction of fluorochromes linked to the central poly amino acid backbone and surrounded by poly(ethylene glycol) linked to the same backbone. (**B**) Schematic diagram of PGC probe activation. The initial proximity of the fluorochrome molecules to each other results in signal quenching (91); (**C**) NIRF image of nonactivated (*left*) and protease-activated Cy5.5-PGC (*right*). (91); (**D**) absorbance and fluorescence spectra of Prosense 680 (VisEn Medical, Inc., Woburn, Massachusetts, U.S.) probe based on copolymer similar to shown in (**A**). *Abbreviations*: PGC, polyethylene glycol; NIRF, near-infrared fluorescence. *Source*: Fig. 4A courtesy of CMIR and Fig. 4D courtesy of VisEn Medical, Inc.

graft copolymer of polylysine and polyethylene glycol (PGC) (90) as a carrier of covalently linked self-quenched Cy5.5 fluorochrome (91, 92) (Fig. 4). The dye was linked to poly-L-lysine backbone, which allowed the release of near-infrared fluorescence after the cleavage of poly-L-lysine, by several cathepsins in vivo. In the observed tumor-specific effect, several independent synergistically acting factors contributed to the high fluorescent signal: (*i*) the polymer was accumulating in the tumors via the leakage through highly permeable tumor blood vessels, (*ii*) the cathepsins are expressed at high levels in cells populating

the tumors, (*iii*) the degradation of the polymer proceeds predominantly in lysosomes, and fluorescent degradation products are thus retained at the tumor site, and (*iv*) the combination of peripheral tumor implantation site and near-infrared fluorescence enabled differentiating between nontumor and tumor tissues using a relatively simple CCD camera detection system. The specificity of this initial probe to any particular cathepsin appears low, and based on enzyme inhibition assays, several cathepsins appear to be involved in the cleavage (cathepsins B, H, and L) of the long-circulating NIRF probe, but referred to as "cathepsin B" probe in the literature. Further studies involving in vivo transcutaneous fluorescence microscopy and fluorescence-activated cell sorting (FACS) analysis showed that the proteolytic activity expressed in stromal, rather in cancer cells is mostly responsible for the cleavage of the long-circulating polymer and overall tumor fluorescence synergistic effects contributed to the tumor fluorescence (93). By using cathepsin B probe, overexpression of cathepsin B enzyme was imaged in dysplastic intestinal adenomas (94), suggesting a potential method of early dysplatic phase of cancer imaging. The uncovered correlation between tumor aggressiveness and the level of near-infrared fluorescence observed in orthotopic breast cancer xenografts was explained by the fact that highly aggressive tumors exhibit elevated levels of cathepsin B (95). It usually required 24-hour period for the probe activation. It was apparent that PGC polymer can serve as a platform for a variety of hydrolases, including metalloproteases, serine, and cysteine proteases. The useful examples of long-circulating self-quenched probes include cathepsin D–sensitive probe (96,97), metalloproteinase-2 and -7 (98,99), matrix metalloproteinase 2 (MMP-2) (100), urokinase (101,102), and caspase-1 (103) sensitive probes. The difference between the initial PGC-based cathepsin B probe and the others was in the design of self-quenched enzyme-specific linkers. Instead of covalent linking of Cy5.5 (or Cy7) dyes to the backbone, the dyes were linked to the peptides that were conjugated to PGC via sulfhydryl group of cysteine. Toward this, PGC was modified with iodoacetic acid anhydride to enable such modification. Alternatively, the fluorochromes could be introduced in peptides during the solid-phase synthesis. The peptide-encoded protease specificity requires conjugating Cy dyes via linkers, which may affect the efficacy of self-quenching. Despite spatial separation from each other, the latter approach showed feasibility of F-F dequenching in the case of relatively long "stalks" cleavable by cathepsin D (104). There are two potential problems associated with this design. First, relatively small fragments of dye-containing peptides are released from PGC carrier, which may result in lower tissue contrast than in the case of cathepsin B probe. Second, nonspecific cell uptake of the probe can result in a nonspecific cleavage of the backbone by cathepsin B and a nonspecific signal. However, the feasibility imaging studies performed with MMP-2 inhibitor prinomastat showed that the administration of MMP-2 inhibitor in animals bearing fibrosarcoma tumors resulted in a markedly lower fluorescence after the injection of the probe, suggesting that MMP-2 probe could be used as a sensor of MMP-2 or other metalloproteinases in tumors.

The feasibility of pretargeting of activatable optical imaging probes has been demonstrated using avidin-biotin system in vivo (105,106). The above scenario requires administration of biotinylated cell-surface-specific antibody followed by a waiting period. After the clearance of the antibody, self-quenched streptavidin is injected. Cell-surface-bound biotinylated antibody-streptavidin complex accumulates in lysosomes of target cells where it undergoes degradation. Proteolysis results in dequenching of fluorescence and the resultant optical signal amplification effect. The direct injection of labeled avidin into the peritoneal cavity allowed visualization of small ovarian cancer deposits because of binding of avidin to cell-surface lectins (106).

Nanoparticles as Optical Imaging Agents

A variety of nanosized materials can be used in optical imaging as contrast agents (107). Imaging of cancer-specific molecules is usually achieved with either fluorochrome-labeled nanopaticles or nanosized semiconductor monocrystals (quantum dots, QDs) (Fig. 5). Because of the fact that tumor blood vessels are usually highly permeable to macromolecules and nanoparticles, the latter can diffuse out of circulation either due to the defects in endothelial lining or because of activated transcytosis and accumulate in the tumor interstitium. Most of the large particles accumulate at the basal membrane, whereas the smaller ones apparently are capable of more extensive permeation into the tumor. In the interstitium, a fraction of nanomaterials get retained due to specific binding (targeting effect) or nonspecific accumulation in stromal and tumor cells, and the rest leave the interstitium against the concentration gradient. When targeting effect is not required, demarcation of tumor using nanoparticles does not usually present challenges, especially if permeability of nearby normal blood vessels is low (specifically, in the case of normal tight junctions in blood brain barrier). This case was explored by using cross-linked superparamagnetic nanoparticles (CLIO) labeled with NIR fluorochrome for imaging of glioma margins (108,109) The advantage of such particles is in that they have low toxicity and can be imaged before surgery to localize tumor margins using MRI. Subsequently, an intraoperative fluorochrome detection system can be used to identify the tumor margin and assist in a more complete surgical removal of the tumor. It was further demonstrated that Cy5.5-CLIO particles can be endowed with molecular specificities by covalent linking

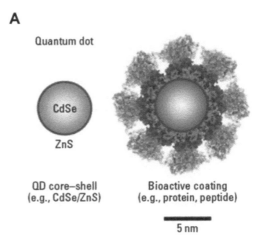

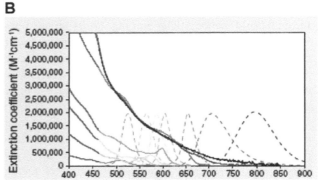

Figure 5 (**A**) QDs consist of a metalloid core and a cap/shell that shields the core and renders the QD bioavailable. The further addition of biocompatible coatings or functional groups can give the QD a desired bioactivity. (**B**) Spectral properties of QDs: excitation of QD fluorescence in the range of 500 to 800 nm is possible using a single wavelength. *Abbreviation*: QDs, quantum dots. *Source*: (**A**) Adapted from Ref. 121.

of annexin V (110) or E-selectin-specific peptide CDSDSDITWDQLWDLMK (111). The latter results in efficient binding and rapid uptake of the particles by IL-1 activated human endothelial cells and some additional affinity toward Lewis lung carcinoma (LLC) cells (111). The E-selectin targeted particles also showed higher accumulation in LLC tumors in vivo than particles carrying a scrambled peptide.

Luminescent semiconducting nanoparticles (QDs) (112) were originally developed for applications unrelated to cancer imaging. However, in addition to many various fields of use, QDs can be successfully applied for cancer imaging as a platform for labeling of antibodies due to their stable and intense luminescence (113–115). A typical QD is a monodisperse population of particles with 2- to 12-nm diameter (can be controlled during the synthesis) consisting of a CdSe core coated with ZnS layer and stabilized with mercaptoacetic acid and additional polymers (e.g., polyethylene glycols) to improve stability in water (73). Three important recent findings could potentially expand the use of QDs in optical imaging: (*i*) the development of water-based synthetic route for preparation of QDs (116), (*ii*) successful demonstration of targetability (117), (*iii*) the use of luminescence energy transfer phenomena that includes QD absorption of blue-light photons emitted due to luciferase-mediated catalysis into red-shifted photons emitted by QDs (118). The latter effect is potentially important for designing beacons because red-shifted fluorescence has better in vivo imaging characteristics. Another important feature of such light energy transfer is in elimination of excitation source and associated problems with excitation light filtering. The recent demonstration of QD use in detecting apoptotic cells via annexin V interaction (119) and the use of proteolysis-sensitive quenching of QD fluorescence through gold nanoparticle binding (120) suggest that QDs could potentially replace small organic fluorochromes as tools for designing optical "sensing" beacons. There are two problems associated with a more widespread application of QDs for in vivo imaging: the use of metals as a core building block and the size. The first suggest potential toxicity due to the presence of cadmium, selenium (or tellurium) core (121); the second limits penetration into the tissues. Larger QDs usually give red-shifted fluorescence because the energy of emitted light is inversely proportional to the square of QD diameter; hence, coincidentally, they are also less toxic than smaller "blue" luminescent QDs (121). The toxicity of such dots is usually revealed only after a prolonged coincubation of QDs with cells. Short-term incubation usually produces no toxic effects. The main advantage of QDs over organic fluorescent molecules is in high quantum yields and the potential use of multiphoton imaging (122) through excitation of luminescence at a single wavelength, eliminating the need in many excitation sources. It is apparent that QD technology will be rapidly evolving enabling new applications for targeted optical imaging in cancer models.

SUMMARY

Optically active imaging probes can be coarsely classified into two groups: endogenous and exogenous. Both types of probes are rapidly becoming essential tools of experimental oncology. Genetically encoded luminescent proteins, organic fluorochromes and QDs are currently the mainstay in noninvasive imaging in small animals. The application of these platforms for detecting various molecular species in living cells and animals will continue in parallel since the platforms complement each other, depending on the focus of a particular imaging task. The most exciting future lies ahead for sensing agents, which will be used more widely for investigating tumor responses to therapy and probing tumor microenvironment.

REFERENCES

1. Choy G, Choyke P, Libutti SK. Current advances in molecular imaging: noninvasive in vivo bioluminescent and fluorescent optical imaging in cancer research. Mol Imaging 2003; 2:303–312.
2. De A, Lewis XZ, Gambhir SS. Noninvasive imaging of lentiviral-mediated reporter gene expression in living mice. Mol Ther 2003; 7:681–691.
3. Ray P, De A, Min JJ, et al. Imaging tri-fusion multimodality reporter gene expression in living subjects. Cancer Res 2004; 64:1323–1330.
4. Doubrovin M, Ponomarev V, Serganova I, et al. Development of a new reporter gene system—dsred/xanthine phosphoriboyltransferase-xanthine for molecular imaging of processes behind the intact blood-brain barrier. Mol Imaging 2003; 2:93–112.
5. Mycek MA, Schomacker KT, Nishioka NS. Colonic polyp differentiation using time-resolved autofluorescence spectroscopy. Gastrointest Endosc 1998; 48:390–394.
6. Lakowicz J. Principles of Fluorescence Spectroscopy. 2nd ed. New York, NY: Plenum Press, 1999.
7. Cope M, Delpy D, Reynolds E, et al. Methods of quantitating cerebral near infrared spectroscopy data. Adv Exp Med Biol 1988; 222:183–189.
8. Kleinschmidt A, Obrig H, Requardt M, et al. Simultaneous recording of cerebral blood oxygenation changes during human brain activation by magnetic resonance imaging and near-infrared spectroscopy. J Cereb Blood Flow Metab 1996; 16:817–826.
9. Rosencwaig A. Potential clinical applications of photoacoustics. Clin Chem 1982; 28:1878–1881.
10. Zhang HF, Maslov K, Stoica G, et al. Functional photoacoustic microscopy for high-resolution and noninvasive in vivo imaging. Nat Biotechnol 2006; 23(7):879–884; 24:848–851.
11. Lungu GF, Li ML, Xie X, et al. In vivo imaging and characterization of hypoxia-induced neovascularization and tumor invasion. Int J Oncol 2007; 30:45–54.
12. Monici M. Cell and tissue autofluorescence research and diagnostic applications. Biotechnol Annu Rev 2005; 11:227–256.
13. Palmer GM, Keely PJ, Breslin TM, et al. Autofluorescence spectroscopy of normal and malignant human breast cell lines. Photochem Photobiol 2003; 78:462–469.
14. Fujimori E. Cross-linking and fluorescence changes of collagen by glycation and oxidation. Biochim Biophys Acta 1989; 998:105–110.
15. Izuishi K, Tajiri H, Fujii T, et al. The histological basis of detection of adenoma and cancer in the colon by autofluorescence endoscopic imaging. Endoscopy 1999; 31(7):511–516.
16. Hoffman RM. In vivo cell biology of cancer cells visualized with fluorescent proteins. Curr Top Dev Biol 2005; 70:121–144.
17. Hsieh CL, Xie Z, Liu ZY, et al. A luciferase transgenic mouse model: visualization of prostate development and its androgen responsiveness in live animals. J Mol Endocrinol 2005; 35:293–304.

18. Miyawaki A, Tsien RY. Monitoring protein conformations and interactions by fluorescence resonance energy transfer between mutants of green fluorescent protein. Methods Enzymol 2000; 327:472–500.

19. Tsien RY. The green fluorescent protein. Annu Rev Biochem 1998; 67:509–544.

20. Matz MV, Fradkov AF, Labas YA, et al. Fluorescent proteins from nonbioluminescent anthozoa species. Nat Biotechnol 1999; 17:969–973.

21. Campbell RE, Tour O, Palmer AE, et al. A monomeric red fluorescent protein. Proc Natl Acad Sci U S A 2002; 99:7877–7882.

22. Cairns RA, Hill RP. A fluorescent orthotopic model of metastatic cervical carcinoma. Clin Exp Metastasis 2004; 22(8):674–684; 21:275–281.

23. Bouvet M, Wang J, Nardin SR, et al. Real-time optical imaging of primary tumor growth and multiple metastatic events in a pancreatic cancer orthotopic model. Cancer Res 2002; 62:1534–1540.

24. Burton DW, Geller J, Yang M, et al. Monitoring of skeletal progression of prostate cancer by GFP imaging, X-ray, and serum opg and pthrp. Prostate 2005; 62(3): 253–259, 62:275–281.

25. Yang M, Baranov E, Jiang P, et al. Whole-body optical imaging of green fluorescent protein-expressing tumors and metastases. Proc Natl Acad Sci U S A 2000; 97:1206–1211.

26. Zacharakis G, Kambara H, Shih H, et al. Volumetric tomography of fluorescent proteins through small animals in vivo. Proc Natl Acad Sci U S A 2005; 102:18252–18257.

27. Hoffman RM. Imaging tumor angiogenesis with fluorescent proteins. APMIS 2004; 112:441–449.

28. Moore A, Marecos E, Simonova M, et al. Novel gliosarcoma cell line expressing green fluorescent protein: a model for quantitative assessment of angiogenesis. Microvasc Res 1998; 56:145–153.

29. Yang M, Baranov E, Li XM, et al. Whole-body and intravital optical imaging of angiogenesis in orthotopically implanted tumors. Proc Natl Acad Sci U S A 2001; 98:2616–2621.

30. Lukyanov KA, Chudakov DM, Fradkov AF, et al. Discovery and properties of GFP-like proteins from nonbioluminescent anthozoa. Methods Biochem Anal 2006; 47:121–138.

31. Matz MV, Lukyanov KA, Lukyanov SA. Family of the green fluorescent protein: journey to the end of the rainbow. BioEssays 2002; 24:953–959.

32. Kogure T, Karasawa S, Araki T, et al. A fluorescent variant of a protein from the stony coral montipora facilitates dual-color single-laser fluorescence cross-correlation spectroscopy. Nat Biotechnol 2006; 24:577–581.

33. Castano AP, Liu Q, Hamblin MR. A green fluorescent protein-expressing murine tumour but not its wild-type counterpart is cured by photodynamic therapy. Br J Cancer 2006; 94:391–397.

34. Hooper CE, Ansorge RE, Browne HM, et al. Ccd imaging of luciferase gene expression in single mammalian cells. J Biolumin Chemilumin 1990; 5:123–130.

35. Edinger M, Sweeney TJ, Tucker AA, et al. Noninvasive assessment of tumor cell proliferation in animal models. Neoplasia 1999; 1:303–310.

36. De A, Gambhir SS. Noninvasive imaging of protein-protein interactions from live cells and living subjects using bioluminescence resonance energy transfer. FASEB J 2005; 19:2017–2019.

37. Contag CH, Jenkins D, Contag PR, et al. Use of reporter genes for optical measurements of neoplastic disease in vivo. Neoplasia 2000; 2:41–52.

38. Contag CH, Bachmann MH. Advances in in vivo bioluminescence imaging of gene expression. Annu Rev Biomed Eng 2002; 4:235–260.

39. Szentirmai O, Baker CH, Lin N, et al. Noninvasive bioluminescence imaging of luciferase expressing intracranial u87 xenografts: correlation with magnetic resonance imaging determined tumor volume and longitudinal use in assessing tumor growth and antiangiogenic treatment effect. Neurosurgery 2006; 58:365–372.

40. Momota H, Holland EC. Bioluminescence technology for imaging cell proliferation. Curr Opin Biotechnol 2005; 8:449–454; 16:681–686.

41. Gueven N, Fukao T, Luff J, et al. Regulation of the Atm promoter in vivo. Genes Chromosomes Cancer 2006; 45:61–71.

42. Carey M, Smale S. Transcriptional regulation in eukaryotes: concepts, strategies, and techniques. Cold Spring Harbor, NY: CHSL Press, 2001.

43. Chaudhari AJ, Darvas F, Bading JR, et al. Hyperspectral and multispectral bioluminescence optical tomography for small animal imaging. Phys Med Biol 2005; 46(8): 2239–2253, 50:5421–5441.

44. Sato M, Ozawa T, Inukai K, et al. Fluorescent indicators for imaging protein phosphorylation in single living cells. Nat Biotechnol 2002; 20:287–294.

45. Kawai Y, Sato M, Umezawa Y. Single color fluorescent indicators of protein phosphorylation for multicolor imaging of intracellular signal flow dynamics. Anal Chem 2004; 77:6588–6593.

46. Ozawa T, Kaihara A, Sato M, et al. Split luciferase as an optical probe for detecting protein-protein interactions in mammalian cells based on protein splicing. Anal Chem 2001; 77:6588–6593.

47. Paulmurugan R, Umezawa Y, Gambhir SS. Noninvasive imaging of protein-protein interactions in living subjects by using reporter protein complementation and reconstitution strategies. Proc Natl Acad Sci U S A 2002; 99:15608–15613.

48. Kim SB, Ozawa T, Watanabe S, et al. High-throughput sensing and noninvasive imaging of protein nuclear transport by using reconstitution of split renilla luciferase. Proc Natl Acad Sci U S A 2004; 101:11542–11547.

49. Paulmurugan R, Massoud TF, Huang J, et al. Molecular imaging of drug-modulated protein-protein interactions in living subjects. Cancer Res 2004; 64:2113–2119.

50. Paulmurugan R, Gambhir SS. Novel fusion protein approach for efficient high-throughput screening of small molecule-mediating protein-protein interactions in cells and living animals. Cancer Res 2005; 65:7413–7420.

51. Laxman B, Hall DE, Bhojani MS, et al. Noninvasive real-time imaging of apoptosis. Proc Natl Acad Sci U S A 2002; 99:16551–16555.

52. Campo MA, Lange N. Fluorescence diagnosis using enzyme-related metabolic abnormalities of neoplasia. J Environ Pathol Toxicol Oncol 2006; 25:341–372.

53. Olivo M, Wilson BC. Mapping ALA-induced PPIX fluorescence in normal brain and brain tumour using confocal fluorescence microscopy. Int J Oncol 2004; 25:37–45.

54. Jocham D, Witjes F, Wagner S, et al. Improved detection and treatment of bladder cancer using hexaminolevulinate imaging: a prospective, phase iii multicenter study. J Urol 2005; 174:862–866.

55. Zaheer A, Wheat TE, Frangioni JV. Irdye78 conjugates for near-infrared fluorescence imaging. Mol Imaging 2002; 1:354–364.

56. Ntziachristos V, Yodh AG, Schnall M, et al. Concurrent MRI and diffuse optical tomography of breast after indocyanine green enhancement. Proc Natl Acad Sci USA 2000; 97:2767–2772.

57. Licha K, Riefke B, Ntziachristos V, et al. Hydrophilic cyanine dyes as contrast agents for near-infrared tumor imaging: synthesis, photophysical properties and spectroscopic in vivo characterization. Photochem Photobiol 2000; 72:392–398.

58. Ernst L, Gupta R, Mujumdar R, et al. Cyanine dye labeling reagents for sulfhydryl groups. Cytometry 1989; 46:271–280.

59. Southwick PL, Ernst LA, Tauriello EW, et al. Cyanine dye labeling reagents—carboxymethylindocyanine succinimidyl esters. Cytometry 1990; 46:271–280.

60. Mujumdar RB, Ernst LA, Mujumdar SR, et al. Cyanine dye labeling reagents: sulfoindocyanine succinimidyl esters. Bioconjug Chem 1993; 4:105–111.

61. Lin Y, Weissleder R, Tung CH. Novel near-infrared cyanine fluorochromes: synthesis, properties, bioconjugation. Bioconjug Chem 2002; 13:605–610.

62. Achilefu S. Lighting up tumors with receptor-specific optical molecular probes. Technol Cancer Res Treat 2004; 3:393–409.

63. Hilderbrand SA, Kelly KA, Weissleder R, et al. Monofunctional near-infrared fluorochromes for imaging applications. Bioconjug Chem 2005; 16:1275–1281.

64. Runnels JM, Zamiri P, Spencer JA, et al. Imaging molecular expression on vascular endothelial cells by in vivo immunofluorescence microscopy. Mol Imaging 2006; 5:31–40.

65. Bertolino C, Caputo G, Barolo C, et al. Novel heptamethine cyanine dyes with large Stokes' shift for biological applications in the near infrared. J Fluorescence 2006; 16:221–225.

66. Peng X, Song F, Lu E, et al. Heptamethine cyanine dyes with a large stokes shift and strong fluorescence: a paradigm for excited-state intramolecular charge transfer. J Am Chem Soc 2005; 127:4170–4171.

67. Ohnishi S, Lomnes SJ, Laurence RG, et al. Organic alternatives to quantum dots for intraoperative near-infrared fluorescent sentinel lymph node mapping. Mol Imaging 2005; 4:172–181.

68. Folli S, Wegnires G, Pelegrin A, et al. Immunophotodiagnosis of colon carcinomas in patients injected with fluoresceinated chimeric antibodies against carcinoembryonic antigen. Proc Natl Acad Sci U S A 1992; 89:7973–7977.

69. Foilli S, Westermann P, Braichotte D, et al. Antibody-indocyanin conjugates for immunophotodetection of human squamous cell carcinoma in nude mice. Cancer Res 1994; 54:2643–2649.

70. Ballou B, Fisher GW, Deng JS, et al. Cyanine fluorochrome-labeled antibodies in vivo: assessment of tumor imaging using cy3, cy5, cy5.5, and cy7. Cancer Detect Prev 1998; 22:251–257.

71. Neri D, Carnemolla B, Nissim A, et al. Targeting by affinity-matured recombinant antibody fragments of an angiogenesis associated fibronectin isoform. Nat Biotechnol 1997; 23:879–884.

72. Fitz Gerald K, Holliger P, Winter G. Improved tumor targeting by disulphide stabilized diabodies expressed in Pichia pastoris. Protein Eng 1997; 10:1221–1225.

73. Ballou B. Quantum dot surfaces for use in vivo and in vitro. Curr Top Dev Biol 2005; 70:103–120.

74. Licha K, Hessenius C, Becker A, et al. Synthesis, characterization, and biological properties of cyanine-labeled somatostatin analogues as receptor-targeted fluorescent probes. Bioconjug Chem 2001; 12:44–50.

75. Becker A, Hessenius C, Licha K, et al. Receptor-targeted optical imaging of tumors with near-infrared fluorescent ligands. Nature Biotechnol 2001; 19:327–331.

76. Chen X, Conti PS, Moats RA. In vivo near-infrared fluorescence imaging of integrin alphavbeta3 in brain tumor xenografts. Cancer Res 2004; 64:8009–8014.

77. Wang W, Ke S, Wu Q, et al. Near-infrared optical imaging of integrin alphavbeta3 in human tumor xenografts. Mol Imaging 2004; 3:343–351.

78. Gurfinkel M, Ke S, Wang W, et al. Quantifying molecular specificity of alphavbeta3 integrin-targeted optical contrast agents with dynamic optical imaging. J Biomed Opt 2005; 10:034019.

79. Ye Y, Bloch S, Xu B, et al. Design, synthesis, and evaluation of near infrared fluorescent multimeric RGD peptides for targeting tumors. J Med Chem 2006; 49:2268–2275.

80. Petrovsky A, Schellenberger E, Josephson L, et al. Near-infrared fluorescent imaging of tumor apoptosis. Cancer Res 2003; 63:1936–1942.

81. Schellenberger EA, Bogdanov A Jr., Petrovsky A, et al. Optical imaging of apoptosis as a biomarker of tumor response to chemotherapy. Neoplasia 2003; 5:187–192.

82. Ntziachristos V, Schellenberger E, Ripoll J, et al. Visualization of antitumor treatment by means of fluorescence molecular tomography with an annexin v-cy5.5 conjugate. Proc Natl Acad Sci USA 2004; 101:12294–12299.

83. Ohnishi S, Vanderheyden JL, Tanaka E, et al. Intraoperative detection of cell injury and cell death with an 800 nm near-infrared fluorescent annexin V derivative. Am J Transplant 2006; 6:2321–2331.

84. t Hoen PA, de Kort F, van Ommen GJ, et al. Fluorescent labelling of cRNA for microarray applications. Nucleic Acids Res 2003; 34:322–333.

85. Metelev V, Weissleder R, Bogdanov A Jr. Synthesis and properties of fluorescent nf-kappa b-recognizing hairpin oligodeoxyribonucleotide decoys. Bioconjug Chem 2004; 15:1481–1487.

86. Marras SA, Kramer FR, Tyagi S. Efficiencies of fluorescence resonance energy transfer and contact-mediated quenching in oligonucleotide probes. Nucleic Acids Res 2002; 34:322–333.

87. Hungerford G, Donald F, Birch DJ, et al. Influence of secondary structure on the decay kinetics of fluorescent donor-acceptor labelled peptides. Biosens Bioelectron 1997; 12:1183–1190.

88. Johansson MK, Cook RM. Intramolecular dimers: a new design strategy for fluorescence-quenched probes. Chemistry 2003; 9:3466–3471.

89. Johansson M, Fidder H, Dick D, et al. Intramolecular dimers: a new strategy to fluorescence quenching in dual-labeled oligonucleotide probes. J Am Chem Soc 2002; 124:6950–6956.

90. Bogdanov AA, Weissleder R, Frank HW, et al. A new macromolecule as a contrast agent for mr angiography: preparation, properties, and animal studies. Radiology 1993; 187:701–706.

91. Weissleder R, Tung CH, Mahmood U, et al. In vivo imaging of tumors with protease-activated near-infrared fluorescent probes. Nat Biotechnol 1999; 17:375–378.

92. Mahmood U, Tung CH, Bogdanov A Jr., et al. Near-infrared optical imaging of protease activity for tumor detection. Radiology 1999; 213:866–870.

93. Bogdanov AJ, Lin C, Simonova M, et al. Cellular activation of the self-quenched fluorescent reporter probe in tumor microenvironment. Neoplasia 2002; 4:228–236.

94. Marten K, Bremer C, Khazaie K, et al. Detection of dysplastic intestinal adenomas using enzyme-sensing molecular beacons in mice. Gastroenterology 2002; 122 (2):406–414.

95. Bremer C, Tung CH, Bogdanov A Jr., et al. Imaging of differential protease expression in breast cancers for detection of aggressive tumor phenotypes. Radiology 2002; 222:814–818.

96. Tung CH, Bredow S, Mahmood U, et al. Preparation of a cathepsin d sensitive near-infrared fluorescence probe for imaging. Bioconjug Chem 1999; 10:892–896.

97. Tung CH, Mahmood U, Bredow S, et al. In vivo imaging of proteolytic enzyme activity using a novel molecular reporter. Cancer Res 2000; 60:4953–4958.

98. Lamfers ML, Gianni D, Tung CH, et al. Tissue inhibitor of metalloproteinase-3 expression from an oncolytic adenovirus inhibits matrix metalloproteinase activity in vivo without affecting antitumor efficacy in malignant glioma. Cancer Res 2005; 65:9398–9405.

99. Pham W, Choi Y, Weissleder R, et al. Developing a peptide-based near-infrared molecular probe for protease sensing. Bioconjug Chem 2004; 15:1403–1407.

100. Bremer C, Tung CH, Weissleder R. In vivo molecular target assessment of matrix metalloproteinase inhibition. Nat Med 2001; 7:743–748.

101. Law B, Curino A, Bugge TH, et al. Design, synthesis, and characterization of urokinase plasminogen-activator-sensitive near-infrared reporter. Chem Biol 2004; 11:99–106.

102. Hsiao JK, Law B, Weissleder R, et al. In-vivo imaging of tumor associated urokinase-type plasminogen activator activity. J Biomed Opt 2006; 10:41205.

103. Messerli SM, Prabhakar S, Tang Y, et al. A novel method for imaging apoptosis using a caspase-1 near-infrared fluorescent probe. Neoplasia 2004; 6:95–105.

104. Tung C, Mahmood U, Bredow S, et al. A cathepsin d sensitive near infrared fluorescence probe for in vivo imaging of enzyme activity. Bioconjug Chem 1999; 10:892–896.

105. Hama Y, Urano Y, Koyama Y, et al. Activatable fluorescent molecular imaging of peritoneal metastases following pretargeting with a biotinylated monoclonal antibody. Cancer Res 2007; 67:3809–3817.

106. Hama Y, Urano Y, Koyama Y, et al. A target cell-specific activatable fluorescence probe for in vivo molecular imaging of cancer based on a self-quenched avidin-rhodamine conjugate. Cancer Res 2007; 67:2791–2799.

107. West JL, Halas NJ. Engineered nanomaterials for biophotonics applications: improving sensing, imaging, and therapeutics. Annu Rev Biomed Eng 2003; 5:285–292.

108. Kircher MF, Mahmood U, King RS, et al. A multimodal nanoparticle for preoperative magnetic resonance imaging and intraoperative optical brain tumor delineation. Cancer Res 2003; 63:8122–8125.

109. Trehin R, Figueiredo JL, Pittet MJ, et al. Fluorescent nanoparticle uptake for brain tumor visualization. Neoplasia 2006; 8:302–311.

110. Schellenberger EA, Sosnovik D, Weissleder R, et al. Magneto/optical annexin v, a multimodal protein. Bioconjug Chem 2004; 15:1062–1067.

111. Funovics M, Montet X, Reynolds F, et al. Nanoparticles for the optical imaging of tumor e-selectin. Neoplasia 2005; 7:904–911.

112. Murray C, Norris D, Bawendi M. Synthesis and characterization of nearly monodisperse cde (e = S, Se, Te) semiconductor nanocrystallites. J Am Chem Soc 1993; 115:8706–8715.

113. Ben-Ari ET. Nanoscale quantum dots hold promise for cancer applications. J Natl Cancer Inst 2003; 95:502–504.

114. Wu X, Liu H, Liu J, et al. Immunofluorescent labeling of cancer marker her2 and other cellular targets with semiconductor quantum dots. Nat Biotechnol 2003; 21:41–46.

115. Michalet X, Pinaud FF, Bentolila LA, et al. Quantum dots for live cells, in vivo imaging, and diagnostics. Science 2005; 307:538–544.

116. Li Z, Wang K, Tan W, et al. Immunofluorescent labeling of cancer cells with quantum dots synthesized in aqueous solution. Anal Biochem 2006; 354:169–174.

117. Cai W, Shin DW, Chen K, et al. Peptide-labeled near-infrared quantum dots for imaging tumor vasculature in living subjects. Nano Lett 2006; 6:669–676.

118. So MK, Xu C, Loening AM, et al. Self-illuminating quantum dot conjugates for in vivo imaging. Nat Biotechnol 2006; 24:339–343.

119. van Tilborg GA, Mulder WJ, Chin PT, et al. Annexin a5-conjugated quantum dots with a paramagnetic lipidic coating for the multimodal detection of apoptotic cells. Bioconjug Chem 2006; 17:865–868.

120. Chang E, Miller JS, Sun J, et al. Protease-activated quantum dot probes. Biochem Biophys Res Commun 2005; 334:1317–1321.

121. Hardman R. A toxicologic review of quantum dots: toxicity depends on physicochemical and environmental factors. Environ Health Perspect 2006; 114:116–172.

122. Larson DR, Zipfel WR, Williams RM, et al. Water-soluble quantum dots for multiphoton fluorescence imaging in vivo. Science 2003; 300:1434–1436.

123. Yodh A. UPENN. Available at: http://www.physics.upenn.edu/yodhlab/research_BO.html.

124. Palero JA, de Bruijn HS, van der Ploeg van den Heuvel A, et al. Spectrally resolved multiphoton imaging of in vivo and excised mouse skin tissues. Biophys J 2007; 93:992–1007.

125. Becker A, Riefke B, Ebert B, et al. Macromolecular contrast agents for optical imaging of tumors: comparison of indotricarbocyanine-labeled human serum albumin and transferrin. Photochem Photobiol 2000; 72:234–241.

126. Ballou B, Lagerholm B, Ernst L, et al. Noninvasive imaging of quantum dots in mice. Bioconjug Chem 2004; 15:79–86.

127. Ormo M, Cubitt AB, Kallio K, et al. Crystal structure of the aequorea victoria green fluorescent protein. Science 1996; 273:1392–1395.

128. Yang F, Moss LG, Phillips GN Jr. The molecular structure of green fluorescent protein. Nat Biotechnol 1996; 14:1246–1251.

129. Vanderklish PW, Krushel LA, Holst BH, et al. Marking synaptic activity in dendritic spines with a calpain substrate exhibiting fluorescence resonance energy transfer. Proc Natl Acad Sci U S A 2000; 97:2253–2258.

130. Massoud T, Gambhir S. Molecular imaging in living subjects: seeing fundamental biological processes in a new light. Genes Dev 2003; 17:545–580.

131. Cheng Z, Wu Y, Xiong Z, et al. Near-infrared fluorescent rgd peptides for optical imaging of integrin alphavbeta3 expression in living mice. Bioconjug Chem 2005; 16:1433–1441.

17

Nanoparticle-Based Molecular Imaging in Living Subjects

BRYAN RONAIN SMITH and SANJIV SAM GAMBHIR

Molecular Imaging Program at Stanford, Department of Radiology, Stanford School of Medicine, Stanford, California, U.S.A.

INTRODUCTION

Drawing from many of the latest discoveries in the basic sciences of chemistry, physics, and biology, the field of nanotechnology is growing into a broad, application-oriented transdiscipline described by as many definitions as applications it generates. For the purposes of this chapter, we adopt the National Cancer Institute's definition of nanotechnology as "the field of research that deals with the engineering and creation of things from materials that are less than 100 nanometers in size, especially single atoms or molecules." Nanoparticles are therefore particles that fall within this metric. This definition notably excludes purely biological molecules; however, pure biomolecules are important when combined with nanoparticles for functionalization, biocompatibility, and clinically relevant nanodevices. Other definitions of nanotechnology apply less stringent restrictions on size, focusing instead on functionality in addressing unmet needs (1). This is especially true in definitions attempting to address the intersection between nanotechnology, biology, and medicine—often called nanobiotechnology (2,3). For space constraints, we confine ourselves to the above size restriction in at least one dimension, though in principle, the precise definition of nanotechnology need not include a similarly precise specification of size.

Many facets of nanotechnology are emerging in scientific inquiry with a plethora of potential applications in various stages of development. However, this chapter will focus on highly engineered, multifunctional nanoparticles that have been tested in living subjects to characterize their imaging and/or therapeutic capabilities. The frequently modular nature of these multifunctional particles often allows them to be useful across a spectrum of diseases. However, we will concentrate on those nanostructures that have a direct effect on oncological applications. Readers interested in nanoparticles in the molecular imaging of atherosclerosis and other diseases are directed to excellent reviews, which have recently been published (4–6). Moreover, we restrict ourselves to more contemporary nanoparticulate platforms, even though innovations continue to flourish in the domains of liposomal (7–9), micellar (10,11), and pure polymeric (12–15) nanoparticle formulations (16–18). Further, we refer readers to other references for nanoparticulate formulations without strong ties to molecular imaging, even in cases where recent work suggests that molecular imaging may be viable; gold nanoparticles and iodinated nanoparticles, for example, are relative newcomers as molecular contrast in computed tomography (CT) and optical coherence tomography (OCT) (19,20). Studies on cell trafficking and tracking in living subjects have also been performed using molecular imaging techniques, which are not addressed here (e.g., stem cell tracking of migration, division, and viability) (21–23).

With our focus now on multifunctional nanoparticles for clinical/preclinical applications defined, we list some of the many ways biomedical nanoparticles can be classified

1. Materials composition
2. Modalities with which they can be imaged (e.g., diagnostic nanoparticles)
3. The disease(s) for which they seek to provide therapy and/or images
4. Their common terminology
5. By size, shape, charge, surface coating, or other physical characteristic.

These features are all critical for nanoparticles to perform their intended function in vivo. However, by their very definition multifunctional nanoparticles often fall into multiple subcategories, making organization of these nanoparticle types akin to a labyrinthine Venn diagram. This is because the nanoparticles may comprise multiple materials (e.g., hybrid nanoparticles), treat/image multiple diseases, and/or be imageable with multiple modalities.

Therefore, in this chapter we adopt a classification system that differentiates nanoparticles by their most prominent (i.e., most relevant to imaging/therapy) materials compositions and structures and associate them with a common terminology. Examples include carbon nanotubes, nanoshells, dendrimers, magnetically active nanomaterials [e.g., iron oxide, iron cobalt (FeCo), etc.], and quantum dots (qdots) (as well as hybrids thereof). The underlying chemistries of construction for each nanoparticulate type comprise the subject of a separate section within the chapter (Fig. 1).

Nanoparticles in oncological molecular imaging are not valuable solely because of their minute dimensions, but their size regime does enable them to interact uniquely with biomolecules. In particular, this property allows for direct interaction between nanoparticles and the biomolecules implicated in the genesis, progression, and viability of various cancers at their own scale. This capability is of intense interest to biologists and clinicians because it allows very fine, specific detection and even control

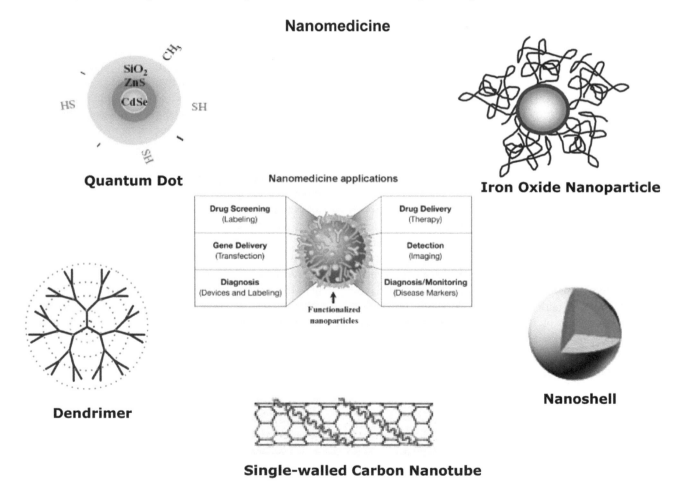

Figure 1 Nanomedicine. The center of the image displays applications and research targets of nanomedicine with an idealized, multifunctionals nanoparticle construct. Nanoparticles have been designed with chemically modifiable surfaces onto which various ligands attach, which can turn these nanomaterials into biosensors, molecular-scale fluorescent tags, imaging agents, targeted molecular delivery vehicles, and other useful biological tools. Surrounding the center image are the nanoparticle varieties we focus on in this review, from top left, counterclockwise: quantum dots, dendrimers, single-walled carbon nanotubes, nanoshells, and iron oxide nanoparticles.

over physiological parameters. On the other hand, physicists, engineers, and chemists find many size-based and other emergent physicochemical properties of nanoparticles to be intrinsically intriguing without regard to application. Yet, physical science advances in the field of nanotechnology have rapidly turned into biological utility as a consequence of the recent emphasis on interdisciplinary collaborations. The field of carbon nanotubes, where materials scientists and chemists often work closely with biologists, is representative of this trend. Collaborations between physical and biological scientists thus have the capacity to effect direct, significant, and exciting preclinical and presumably clinical advances as technical breakthroughs are achieved.

Many of the explicitly designed interactions between nanoparticles and an organism's biochemistry are mediated by specifically chosen biomolecules (e.g., DNA, proteins, and other biopolymers) that are linked to the nanoparticle. This configuration almost invariably restricts targeting of nanoparticles to cell surface molecules, rather than to the likewise rich constellations of biomarkers flowing through blood and those localized within subcellular compartments. Note that the burgeoning field of cell-penetrating peptides seeks to revolutionize this approach by providing access to intracellular compartments, though the initial burst of optimism may be somewhat unfounded (24). Nevertheless, when targeting nanoparticles to cell surface molecules, one or both of the reporter and therapeutic functions are often the responsibility of the nanoparticle construct itself. This makes control and understanding of the nanoparticle conjugate's construction and chemistry vital for exploring its biological applications. Nanoparticle chemistry is also important in helping to understand and manipulate nanoparticle circulation times. Circulation time is a critical element in targeting as parenteral nanoparticles must circulate for a sufficient time to localize at a desired site. To improve circulation times, decoration of nanoparticles by biomolecules can often become essential. Thus biomolecules not only serve to help mediate specific interactions with cells and molecules, but may also facilitate a "Trojan Horse" approach so that nanoparticles are not rapidly identified by the immune system nor taken up by the reticuloendothelial system (RES). RES cells, such as the spleen and the Kupffer cells of the liver, comprise part of the immune system. These cells serve to protect an organism as a sort of biological particle filter, filtering foreign bodies from the bloodstream. An organism generally considers injectable nanoparticle technologies as foreign bodies. Thus the utility of such nanoparticles in living subjects is critically dependent on evading the RES for sufficient time to enable desired efficacy. Various methods are used to evade the RES, from decreasing nanoparticle size to that of a small protein to optimizing the surface charge to attaching certain biomolecules to the surface (1,25–29).

Nanoparticles developed for clinical biomedicine are designed with significant consideration of materials toxicity, structure, size, geometry, and dispersity. Each factor contributes greatly to whether a nanoparticle will be able to perform the function for which it was devised and its likelihood for regulatory approval in humans. Moreover, each of these factors can be modulated by the incredibly diverse array of nanoparticle fabrication approaches available, which make extensive use of chemical, physical, and even biological (generally self-assembly related) methods (30). The construction of nanotechnological devices is often partitioned into two main nanofabrication approaches: top-down and bottom-up. Top-down techniques generally employ microfabrication or similar processes to create nano-sized assemblies via removal or modification of adjacent materials, while bottom-up methods often adopt chemical and assembly approaches to construct nanoparticles from constitutive elements. Some recent methods seek to hybridize these two main construction approaches (31–33). No matter which fabrication method is chosen, we seek here to elucidate the principal chemical methods in current, state-of-the-art nanoparticle construction and reveal their significance in the capability of a nanoparticle to function as a well-designed molecular imaging nanoagent in living subjects.

DENDRIMERS

Dendrimers, which are dendritric molecules reminiscent of trees (and termed such accordingly), generally remain without a precise, consistent definition in the literature. At their most basic, they are repeatedly branching structures comprising monomeric units of any chemical structure—they are thus by definition a form of polymer. However, dendrimers are considered here outside the purview of linear or block (co)polymer nanostructures because of their multifunctional status and intricate potential geometries. These features are conducive to therapeutic delivery and imaging as molecule carriers; indeed, dendrimers' biocompatibility, versatility, and size make them ideal nanostructures in many ways. The precision with which dendrimers can be assembled at the nanoscale with respect to size, shape, surface chemistry, solubility, and amenability to decoration with desired imaging and therapeutic molecules make these innately modular nanoparticles clinically attractive (34). It is clear that the key physical and medical properties of dendrimers are intimately related to their structure, which is a function of the chemical methods and components used in their construction. Properties such as the specific utility, encapsulation parameters, and performance of dendrimers have been reviewed well elsewhere (34–36).

In whichever form they take, dendrimers are polymers containing central cores in which concentric layers form

Dendrimers

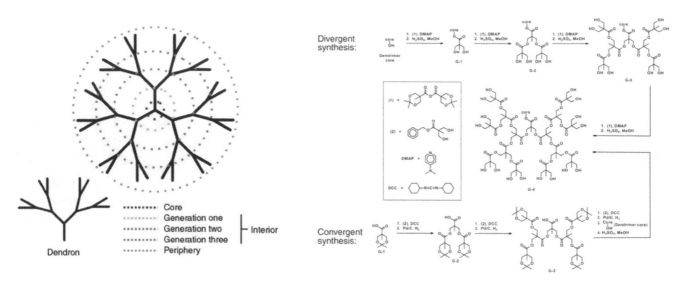

Figure 2 Dendimers. (*Left*) Anatomy of a dendrimer. A dendrimer and dendron are represented with solid lines. The broken lines identify the various key regions of the dendrimer. (*Right*) Synthesis of a polyester dendron. An example of a typical dendrimer synthesis via divergent (*top*) and convergent (*bottom*) approaches from G1 through G4. Note that in the convergent approach, dendrons are grown separately and attached to the dendrimer core in the final steps; in the divergent approach, dendrons are grown outward starting from the dendrimer core. Dendrimer synthesis is stepwise and results in a product with a defined structure, unlike typical polymerization reactions.

the bulk of the nanoparticle (Fig. 2). Each layer is termed a "generation" (G-1, G-2, etc. extending radially outward). Dendrimer biocompatibility tends to be inversely proportional to G; however, as G increases, so does the number of surface functional groups available for functional utility via chemical modification, which can be calculated according to published formulae (34) (depending on shape). The properties of dendrimers are often dominated by the surface groups' chemistries, as the outer branches tend to shield the inner core. This shielding effect can facilitate delivery of hydrophobic or other otherwise biologically difficult-to-deliver materials (such as drugs or immunogenic molecules) exposing the in vivo milieu only to a desired surface. Furthermore, the shielding effect is sometimes absolutely necessary, as the core may be toxic.

In dendrimer chemistry, each separate, identical "branch" is generally termed a dendron. Dendrimers are assembled in stepwise fashion by one of the two general methods: divergent or convergent synthesis (Fig. 2) (34,35). Though stepwise schemes can involve many steps and much time, the exquisite control over size, uniformity, and shape in bulk solutions makes such methods nevertheless quite valuable from the imaging and therapeutic perspective. In divergent synthetic methods, dendrimers are grown from their cores radially outward, exhibiting nearly exponential growth (37). Alternatively, convergent synthesis involves growing each dendron independently and linking to a core in the final production step.

This approach is generally limited to low-generation dendrimers because of steric issues in the construction (36).

The flexibility of dendrimer applications is partially derived from their ability to be constructed by nearly any type of chemistry for a wide variety of polymers (35). More than 100 dendrimer varieties exist, including polyester, poly(lysine), and poly(propyleneimine), which can provide greater than 1000 different chemical surface modifications (36,37). Polyamidoamine (PAMAM) dendrimers are the most common variety, which are produced by Michael addition of methyl acrylate to an amine-based core; however, simplifications to the chemistry have been achieved via "click" and "lego" chemistries (36) that beneficially impact reaction reliability and environmental safety of byproducts. Perhaps most importantly, these chemistries should aid in the commercial viability of dendrimers via scalable manufacturing. Lego chemistry exploits highly functionalized cores with branched dendrons to create phosphorus dendrimers, while click chemistry makes use of the extraordinary consistency of Cu(I)-catalyzed synthesis of 1,2,3-triazoles to form azides to alkynes (36). We next discuss two types of multifunctional PAMAM dendrimers that have been tested in animal models to demonstrate their versatility and encapsulate the basis for the use of dendrimers in nanomedicine (38,39).

In the first instance, multimodality imaging is achieved by linking both magnetic resonance imaging (MRI) and optically active molecules to dendrimers (39). G-6 PAMAM dendrimers (5.5 nm in hydrodynamic radius) were selected as carrier nanoparticles. Thiourea linkages were formed to covalently bind DTPA chelators to reactive functional groups on the dendrimer surface in non-saturating quantities. Remaining surface amines were then bound via amide bonds to Cy5.5 dye. Understanding of steric hindrance and (non)saturating conditions are critical parameters to such chemistries. This is because reactions can unintentionally either saturate or be far from saturation sans careful calculations and consideration of the size, shape, and hydrophobicity of the molecules involved, as well as solvents and other factors. Alternatively, titrations can be performed to obtain desired saturations. It is particularly important for saturation conditions to be carefully considered in this manner when surface functional groups are all identical. Conversely, if different surface functional groups are presented, chemistries can be designed to be specific to each type of functional group. For the G-6 PAMAM magneto-optical dendrimer, after Cy5.5 is appended, the chemistry is completed by adding an MR-active metal complex based on gadolinium (Gd(III)) to the dendrimer solution for direct chelation to DTPA.

In another study, G-5 PAMAM dendrimers were used to target Her-2/neu receptors for fluorescence imaging (38). A fraction of the amine functional groups on the dendrimer surface were first modified by acetylation. They were subsequently bound to a heterobifunctional cross-linker. A fluorophore was then linked via NHS ester chemistry to un-reacted amines. To prepare Her-2/neu antibodies for linkage to the nanoparticle, a thiol-reactive maleimide was generated on each antibody. The disulfide bonds on the heterobifunctional cross-linker, already attached to the nanoparticle, were then reduced. Reaction between the Her-2/neu antibody and dendrimer occurred readily, thereby producing the Her-2/neu-targeted optically responsive dendrimer.

The two multimodal dendrimers discussed above were tested in animals with good results: Magneto-optical dendrimers displayed high spatial resolution in MRI and high sensitivity in their optical capacity, while Her-2/neu receptors were successfully targeted and imaged by dendrimers carrying fluorescent molecules. The chemistry of nanoparticle construction was critical to maintain particle monodispersity and conjugation chemistries were developed to yield specific quantities of targeting and/or imaging agents per particle. The chemical standardization of these features allowed nanoparticles all to behave similarly to one another in living subjects to obtain a predictable and repeatable effect. Furthermore, recent data suggests that prudent modulation of dendrimer chemistry by design into certain asymmetric shapes may facilitate glomerular (i.e., kidney) filtration at unusually large sizes (35,40), as larger nanoparticles are otherwise taken up by the RES rather than renally.

Clinical applications drive the creation and use of dendrimeric agents, as is the case for multimodal nanoscale imaging agents in general. In particular, several simultaneous imaging modalities could be facilitated by dendrimers for patient use; for example, MRI and optical visualization in particular are appealing because (*i*) these imaging modalities can provide co-registration, (*ii*) combining high spatial resolution, 3-dimensional MR information with high-sensitivity optical data blends the best features of each modality, which could be useful in practice in circumstances such as (*iii*) MR-guided surgical planning with subsequent fluorescence-aided surgical intervention, assisting the surgeon with disease localization during the procedure (39). Nevertheless, despite their potential advantages, much work remains to be explored on dendrimers' biological properties and toxicity in living subjects to facilitate their viability as imaging reagents (37). Still, it appears promising for multifunctional dendrimers capable of targeting, imaging, and therapeutic delivery to become a standard in the field. The work of Shukla et al. is emblematic of the paradigm, in which antibodies to a well-characterized cancer growth receptor were bound to the nanoparticle surface in addition to functionalization with an optical dye (38). The dye could be substituted by a number of other imaging or therapeutic moieties. Assembling dendrimeric nanostructures with three or more different targeting, imaging, and/or therapeutic molecules may require more sophisticated chemistries or synthetic designs, or potentially simplifications to existing approaches (36). Despite these hurdles, the promise of dendrimers appears to be nearing fulfillment in preclinical models (34), and perhaps in the clinic in the not-so-distant future.

QUANTUM DOTS AND SEMICONDUCTOR NANOPARTICLES

The typical qdot is a colloidal semiconductor nanostructure in which one material is enclosed within another that has a higher band gap, yielding a band-gap mismatch. The core-shell configuration is most commonly used (Fig. 3). Qdots generally comprise 2 to 10 nm crystals of cadmium selenide (CdSe) or indium arsenide (InAs) [and other materials (22)] cores with thin shells of materials such as zinc sulfide, as in Figure 3. Qdots behave in some ways like a single atom despite the fact that they comprise hundreds to thousands of atoms, the effect from which they derive their name. The desirable aspect of qdots is their superior, reproducible ability to be excited by, and emit, light. The mechanism of photon emission entails absorption of an incident photon by an electron at a certain energy level in the qdot, moving it to a higher energy level (creating an electron-hole pair). The electron then rapidly drops into its original energy level (or band), emitting a

Quantum Dots

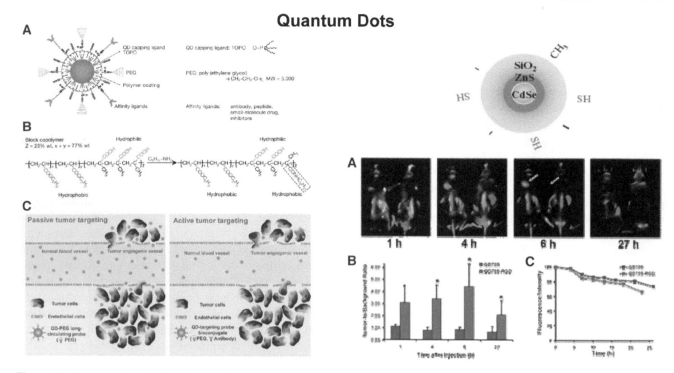

Figure 3 Quantum dots. (*Left*) Schematic illustration of biconjugated qdots for in vivo cancer targeting and imaging. (**A**) Structure of a multifunctional qdot probe, showing the capping ligand TOPO, an encapsulating copolymer layer, tumor-targeting ligands (such as peptides, antibodies or small-molecule inhibitors) and polyethylene glycol (PEG). (**B**) Chemical modification of a triblock copolymer with an 8-carbon side chain. This hydrophobic side chain is directly attached to the hydrophilic acrylic acid segment and interacts strongly with the hydrophobic tails of TOPO. Dynamic light scattering shows a compact qdot-polymer structure, indicating that qdots are tightly wrapped by the hydrophobic segments and hydrocarbon side chains. (**C**) Permeation and retention of qdot probes via leaky tumor vasculatures (passive targeting) and high affinity binding of qdot-antibody conjugates to tumor antigens (active targeting). (*Right, top*) A silanized CdSe/ZnS nanocrystal is depicted. The CdSe/ZnS core is embedded in a glass-like shell. The surface of the shell exposes thiol (−SH) groups, negatively charged phosphonate groups (−), and methyl (−CH3) groups that originate from the chlorotrimethylsilane, which is used to stop the cross-linking process. Alternatively, nanocrystals with positively charged ammonium groups (+) or neutral polyethylene groups can be synthesized (not shown). Images of mice using targeted RGD-qdot constructs. (*Bottom*) (**A**) In vivo NIR fluorescence imaging of U87MG tumor-bearing mice (left shoulder, pointed by *white arrows*) injected with 200 pmol of qdot705-RGD (*left*: 705 nm is the emission wavelength) and QD705 (*right*), respectively. All images were acquired under the same instrumental conditions. The mice autofluorescence is color coded green while the unmixed QD signal is color coded red. Prominent uptake in the liver, bone marrow, and lymph nodes was also visible. (**B**) Tumor-to-background ratios of mice injected with QD705 or QD705-RGD. The data were represented as mean ± standard deviation (SD). Using one-tailed paired Student's *t* test ($n = 3$), "*" denotes where $p < 0.05$ as compared to the mice injected with QD705. (**C**) Serum stability of QD705 and QD705-RGD in complete mouse serum over the course of 24 hours (*See Color Insert*).

photon with an energy exactly that of the band gap between higher and lower energy levels. The diameter of semiconductor qdots of specified composition determines the energy, and thus color, of the photon emitted. Smaller qdots emit shorter wavelength photons and vice versa. The utility of qdots in living subjects is critically dependent on the wavelength of emission because of the variable absorption properties of different wavelengths through tissue (41). Indeed, qdots and their derivatives (quantum rods, etc.) have become highly pursued in materials and engineering, as well as in biological and medical applications from colorful cellular and subcellular microscopy "tags" to tiny probes capable of mining the answers to biological research questions in living subjects.

Though qdots are highly valuable research tools in small living subjects such as mice, their clinical utility is also of increasing interest. Many qdot properties lend themselves to eventual clinical use: photostability, lack of phototoxicity, brightness, broad-absorption/narrow-emission spectra, potential for multifunctional delivery vehicles/platforms of multiple imaging or therapeutic agents, targeting capacity, and potential for multimodal detection through both customized emission color and bioconjugation to enable detection of multiple target molecules using a single excitation wavelength. However, toxicity concerns and the fact that qdot-generated light will not traverse significant distances in human tissues are critical hurdles. Qdot toxicity is variable, depending in part on the materials comprising the core and coatings, and is reviewed extensively elsewhere (42,43). Obstacles in tissue light absorption can be circumvented by intelligent choice of applications, such as highlighting the outline of tumor boundaries during surgery, sentinel lymph node mapping, surface lesions, or breast imaging (44–48). There is currently a drive toward the use of qdots emitting in the near-infrared (NIR) spectrum (~ 700–900 nm) to maximize their utility in living subjects, including humans, by increasing tissue penetration to emitted light. In As-based qdots are better suited to infrared applications than CdSe and are smaller (for comparable emission wavelengths), which imparts advantages in living subjects. Smaller-sized particles may prove crucial for qdots to be clinically useful because nanoparticles beneath a threshold diameter of $< \sim 5$ nm can lead to predominant renal uptake and safe excretion via urine of unbound nanoparticles, depending on qdot charge and coating material (49). This is particularly important in cases where long-term materials toxicity is a major concern.

Qdots are generally fabricated via epitaxy, lithography, pyrolytic, or colloidal methods. Batch synthesis using colloidal techniques is most economically viable, can be performed using a bench-top environment, and is considered the least toxic. Control over nucleation and growth of the nanocrystals by regulation of duration, temperature, and ligands used in the synthetic method governs the resultant qdot size (22). These parameters then determine many critical physical (e.g., emission wavelength) and in vivo (e.g., clearance parameters) properties. Further influencing in vivo behavior (e.g., such as toxicity, uptake, and immune response) are the methods and molecules by which qdots are solubilized and functionalized. Since qdots are commonly solubilized in organic solvents, hydrophobic surface ligands must be replaced with amphiphilic ones to facilitate transfer to aqueous phase, further derivatization with biomolecules, and use in living subjects. Functionalization methods used to date to replace hydrophobic ligands include ligand exchange with thiol-containing molecules, encapsulation by a layer of amphiphilic multi-block copolymers, combinations of layers of different molecules, which impart colloidal stability to the qdots, and even aqueous synthetic methods (22).

Applications for qdots in living subjects rely on the nanoparticles accumulating at the desired site via either passive (e.g., because of size, charge, shape, or some combination) or active targeting (generally ligand mediated). While passive targeting methods such as the enhanced permeability and retention (EPR) effect have been used to coax qdots to target tumors because of their size, most methods exploit surface-conjugated antibody-ligand and similar biomolecular interactions (50) (Fig. 3). The EPR effect can occur in tumors and is because of rapid angiogenesis and thus leaky blood vessels with pores

(space between endothelial cells) wide enough to allow drug or nanoparticles through. However, poor lymphatic drainage and other parameters can lead to high interstitial pressures, which may negate the impact of the EPR effect. Nevertheless, most passive targeting strategies result in low yield to the target site, unless the target site happens to be the organ(s) which naturally take up qdots. For example, since the RES takes up most qdots, RES organs such as liver and spleen display high uptake naturally. Targeting biomolecules, for example, aptamers, peptides, or proteins targeted to cell surface proteins, may be required to enable high yields of qdots to collect in non-RES tissues (and non-excretory organs, if small qdots are used) such as tumors and other lesions by attaching the biomolecules to qdot surfaces. Biomolecules can be covalently linked to surface ligands such as carboxyl or amine groups in relatively high concentrations because of the ~ 10 to 100 surface groups per qdot available for conjugation. Alternatively, biomolecules can be non-covalently bound by simply solubilizing the qdots in a solution of the desired biomolecule (22). Representative of this strategy, peptide coating via hydrophobic interactions allows rapid surfactant exchange to create qdots that are protected from photo-physical and materials degradation, solubilization in aqueous solutions, qdots to remain small in diameter, provide a labile biological interface for flexibility, control over peptide density on qdot surface, have customizable surface chemistries [for anything from targeting reagents to releasable drugs to other nanoparticles (51)], and may even be useful as a targeting reagent in itself if so designed. Given the advantages of peptide coating strategies, the marriage of peptides with qdots will surely continue synergistically as developments in these fields converge (22,52).

In living subjects, antibodies are too large for practical qdot targeting strategies since circulation time, extravasation capability, etc. are intimately related to the size of the overall qdot bioconjugate. Therefore qdot chemistries are geared toward small molecule–targeting moieties, which include peptides, aptamers, ligands, and derivations of antibodies such as minibodies, diabodies, etc. (22,28, 29,53). RGD peptides were conjugated to qdots via a maleimide-presenting heterobifunctional cross-linker, which was linked to RGD's lysine ε-amino group in order to target integrin $\alpha_v\beta_3$ (53). Because this integrin is overexpressed in new blood vessels (and some cancer cells themselves), angiogenic cancer vessels were thus targeted and imaged in mice using NIR-emitting qdots using whole animal optical scanners (Fig. 3). In other work in small living subjects, qdots were targeted via chemical linkage of a prostate cancer–binding antibody and homing peptides by carbodiimide chemistry and thiol exchange, respectively (29,50). In the case of the antibody-qdot conjugates, the EPR effect allowed the nanostructures to passively target tumors, after which the extravasated particles bound to tumor cells via surface protein interactions.

Innovations for solving some of the more critical problems plaguing qdots include the development of organic qdots to decrease toxicity concerns (54), increasing the tissue penetration depth while simultaneously decreasing tissue autofluorescence (55), and developments toward multiplexing [using multiple colors of qdots within living subjects in order to simultaneously converge on a single diagnosis using a constellation of biomarkers (56)]. A great advantage for qdot multiplexing is the inherent broad qdot absorption spectrum—that is, qdots with a range of emission spectra can all be simultaneously excited by a single wavelength (below their emission wavelengths). For multiplexing, note that although NIR light is in the optimal range for tissue penetration, much scattering and absorption still occurs for both incident and emitted photons. Thus standard qdot formulations cannot be used for deep tissue imaging (except in surgical or endoscopical procedures where a tissue surface is exposed directly to imaging equipment). Therefore, a recent qdot advance has used chemistry and bioluminescence to develop a system wherein photons must only traverse tissue in their emission, cutting in half the amount of scattering/absorption and more than doubling the depth limit for tissue imaging (55). The strategy involved linking a mutant renilla luciferase enzyme to qdots in close proximity so that BRET (bioluminescence resonance energy transfer) occurred between the enzyme and the qdot on exposure to the enzyme's substrate (coelenterazine). BRET is a non-radiative energy-transfer mechanism (57) that has been exploited here so that no external illumination source is required to excite qdots, yielding no autofluorescence and excellent tissue penetration properties.

In addition to semiconductor qdots, silicon-based nanoparticles comprise a potentially interesting area for clinical development. Nanoporous silicon, constructed either via electrochemical anodization or chemical (stain) etching, has been shown to be biocompatible, nontoxic, and degradable (58). Indeed, the nanostructured porosity of the silicon facilitates decomposition of the material into biologically innocuous silicic acid in physiological solutions. Clinical studies have been performed with larger porous silicon structures, indicating its safety (58,59). The porous structure has utility beyond the fact that it allows the silicon material to degrade. These structures can be designed to photoluminesce, or generate light upon illumination. Furthermore, the pores can be functionalized to facilitate uptake of hydrophilic or hydrophobic entities—porous silicon may thus be configured to take up molecules ranging from therapeutics and imaging agents to magnetic materials and dyes (58,60,61).

Qdots have a number of advantages over conventional fluorophores. Fluorophores are plagued by considerable photobleaching, low photostability and chemical stability, have narrow excitation and relatively broad emissions, low quantum yield, and display an inability to easily tune emission wavelength. Each of these issues is often a critical impediment for applications in living subjects for many reasons beyond the scope of this section. This is the reason for the excitement about qdots in the scientific community—nanoscale qdot beacons solve these problems. Further, the prospect of using a single laser to simultaneously excite an array of qdot colors, each targeted to a different cell surface or intracellular disease marker, to monitor the complex cellular changes because of disease is potentially revolutionary. Nevertheless, autofluorescence and sensitivity remain problems for qdots. Solutions to these may exist in the form of a novel in vivo imaging modality—Raman imaging in living subjects (see sections "Nanoshells" and "Carbon Nanotubes"), which has shown subcutaneous sensitivity down to 8.175 pM (62–64).

CARBON NANOTUBES

Carbon nanotubes have captured the imaginations of biomedical and materials scientists alike because of the smorgasbord of exceptional and unique properties they offer. We focus here exclusively on single-walled nanotubes (SWNTs), though many applications also exist for their multiwalled cousins (65). SWNTs are chemically stable, hollow cylinders of hexagonal arrays of carbon atoms (Fig. 4). They resemble rolled up (high strength, sp^2 bonded) graphene sheets that are often capped by half a fullerene on each end. SWNTs may exhibit assorted helical structures (e.g., armchair, zig-zag, chiral), electrical character (metallic or semiconductor), and a range of diameters that is dependent on which of several available methods is chosen to synthesize them (and the specific conditions used therein). While nanotubes are often selected for materials and electronic applications on the basis of their extraordinary electrical, mechanical, and physical properties (e.g., to strengthen materials, as sensitive biomedical sensors, or consistent field emitters for screens) (66), their in vivo clinical utility is more strongly a function of their intriguing optical properties (e.g., infrared fluorescence, Raman, and photonic conversion to heat), loading capacity (e.g., of imaging molecules, drugs, or targeting reagents), nanoscale character, and aspect ratio to allow them to reach sites other nanoparticles may be unable to achieve (67). Though there remains some controversy on SWNT biocompatibility (68), recent in vivo studies indicate a potentially promising future for SWNTs in medicine (69–71). Because of the variety of things SWNTs do well, they may be used in

Single-walled Carbon Nanotubes

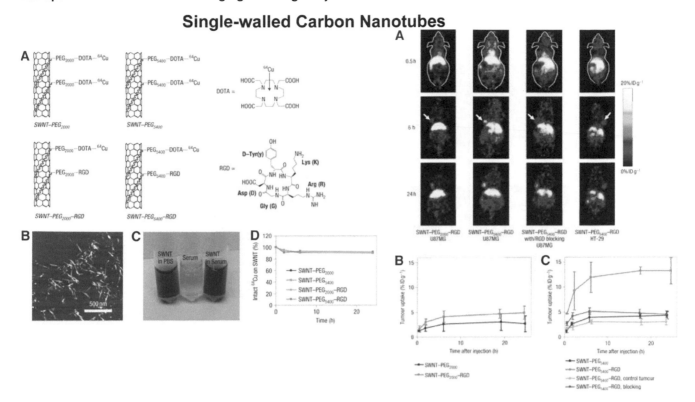

Figure 4 Single-walled carbon nanotubes. (Left, **A**) Schematic drawings of noncovalently functionalized SWNT–PEG$_{2000}$, SWNT–PEG$_{5400}$, SWNT–PEG$_{2000}$–RGD, SWNT–PEG$_{5400}$–RGD with DOTA–^{64}Cu. The hydrophobic carbon chains (*blue segments*) of the phospholipids strongly bind to the sidewalls of the SWNTs, and the PEG chains render water solubility to the SWNTs. The DOTA molecules on the SWNTs are used to chelate ^{64}Cu for radio labeling. (**B**) An atomic force microscope AFM image of SWNT–PEG$_{5400}$ deposited on a silicon substrate. (**C**) A photograph of stable SWNT–PEG$_{2000}$ suspensions in PBS and full fetal bovine serum. (**D**) Serum stability test showing that ^{64}Cu remains intact on carbon nanotubes over 24-hour incubation in full mouse serum. The slight reduction during the early two time points was due to the removal of residual-free ^{64}Cu radio labels in the nanotube solution by filtration. (*Right*) Tumor targeting of RGD-SWNTs in mice. (**A**) MicroPET images of mice. The arrows point to the tumors. High tumor uptake (15% ID g-1) of SWNT–PEG$_{5400}$–RGD is observed in the U87MG tumor (*second column*), in contrast to the low tumor uptake (*first column*) of SWNT–PEG$_{2000}$–RGD. The third column is a control experiment showing blocking of SWNT–PEG$_{5400}$–RGD tumor uptake by co-injection of free c(RGDyK). The fourth column is a control experiment showing low uptake of SWNT–PEG$_{5400}$–RGD in an integrin v 3-negative HT-29 tumor. U87MG tumor uptake curves for mice injected with SWNT–PEG$_{2000}$ (**B**) and SWNT–PEG$_{5400}$ (**C**), with and without RGD. All data shown represent three mice per group (*See Color Insert*).

conjunction with many different in vivo imaging modalities, such as in Raman microscopy, photoacoustic imaging (Fig. 5 for SWNTs targeted to tumor and imaged via photoacoustics), optical microscopy, MRI via hyperpolarization, etc. For molecular imaging applications, understanding how to exploit the potential utility of SWNTs must begin with their construction. The major methods used to synthesize SWNTs include carbon arc-discharge, laser ablation, and chemical vapor deposition (CVD). After these techniques are described, the chemical functionalization of the resulting structures will be discussed because derivatization chemistries allow SWNTs to be tolerable and practical for in vivo applications.

The carbon arc-discharge method is characterized by moving a positive carbon electrode closer to a negative carbon electrode in a vacuum chamber under an inert gas environment. The resulting electric arc heats the electrodes, causing plasma formation and nanotube deposition on the negative electrode. The presence of a catalyst (e.g., Co or Ni-Y) is necessary for SWNT growth. Unfortunately, the SWNTs that accumulate are generally highly entangled, making subsequent purification difficult. Still, high quality/purity and a high degree of control over nanotube diameters are possible using this technique (72). On the other hand, instead of an electric arc, the laser-ablation technique relies on laser energy to produce the heat necessary for nanotube formation. A laser focused on a carbon target (e.g., a graphite block) in the presence of catalyst leads to formation of SWNTs. However, as in the arc-discharge method, disorganized, tangled masses of nanotubes are formed. Though laser ablation has a high (~70%) yield, produces mainly SWNTs (as opposed to multiwalled nanotubes), and allows fine control over nanotube diameter, it is the most expensive of the three methods.

Photoacoustics

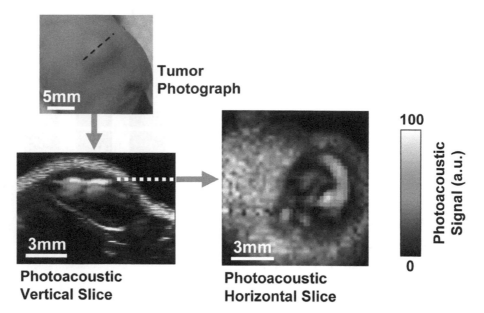

Figure 5 Photoacoustic imaging with SWNTs. A tumor-bearing mouse was injected with a photoacoustic molecular imaging agent: single-walled carbon nanotubes conjugated to cyclic Arg-Gly-Asp peptides (RGD). After injection, 3D ultrasound and photoacoustic images of the tumor were acquired. The ultrasound and photoacoustic images were overlaid and vertical and horizontal slices of the 3D images (see dotted lines) are shown. Note that while the ultrasound image shows the skin and tumor boundaries, the photoacoustic image shows the exact location of the imaging agents with high spatial resolution through several millimeters of tissue depth.

CVD offers a more precise, scalable technique for nanotube formation. In this method, gaseous hydrocarbons such as methane or ethylene are heated so that the molecular bonds are broken and the component-reactive radical species are free to diffuse to metal catalysts on the substrate. Nanotubes form at sites of these catalysts, which are most commonly iron nanoparticles or layers of Co or Ni. The diameter of the nanotubes formed is dependent on the dimensions of the catalysts and can thus be controlled. Furthermore, excellent control of growth rate is feasible. The advantages of CVD over other techniques include its potential for large-scale synthesis, and most significantly for electronics/sensor applications, the precise placement, alignment, and ordered arrays of nanotubes. While CVD suffers from significantly lower yields than the other techniques, purification is considerably easier as nanotubes are not tangled. Many different purification methods are in common use to prepare SWNTs for their intended applications (72). The purification method should be chosen prudently according to the application. Purification can modify nanotubes' electrical and mechanical properties, which may affect their use as ex vivo sensors, but most in vivo utility does not depend on such properties. However, purification alters nanotubes' surface structural features. Since the surface is the portion exposed to the in vivo environment when injected, especially in the case of nanotubes where

the surface area-to-volume ratio is enormous, it is imperative that the purification method be chosen to optimize the resultant nanotube biological tolerability and ease of subsequent bio-functionalization.

Derivatization chemistries for carbon nanotubes are not trivial and have thus consumed a great deal of effort for a projected payoff in both clinical and sensor applications. One major obstacle on the path to biological utility is that naked nanotubes are insoluble in all types of solvents (73,74). Thus, these chemistries are critical and are used to produce solubilizable nanotubes with chemical and/or biological functionality (75). Methods for circumventing the need for covalent derivatization include using biomolecules for direct, spontaneous nonspecific adsorption to SWNT surfaces (76). Similarly, nonspecific adsorption of phospholipid molecules (such as polyethylene glycol, or PEG) to SWNT surfaces facilitates solubility and subsequent functionalization with proteins or other desired biomolecules (75). However, while such non-covalent methods have implicit advantages in simplicity and cost, they may not hold long-term promise for use in living subjects. Covalent derivatization chemistries linking biomolecules directly and robustly to the surface of SWNTs are ideal, but the processes involved can be difficult, time-consuming, and can cause SWNT properties (electrical, mechanical, and optical) to be significantly altered (77). This is because the properties of SWNTs are dependent on the integrity of the structure. Thus, when the original configuration must be broken in order to free a carbon atom for bonding with another molecule rather than its typical 4-carbon partners, the physical properties change. Current methods to functionalize SWNTs include hydrogenation and hydrocarbonation/etching (78), dipolar cycloaddition of azomethine ylides (73), diazonium salts (79,80), use of oleum (80,81), nitrene and carbine chemistries, as well as many others (80). Tasis et al. provide an excellent review of SWNT functionalization chemistries (79).

The azomethine cycloaddition reaction, for instance, provides great flexibility for solubilization and subsequent linkage to amino acids. The reaction is accomplished by suspending SWNTs in dimethylformamide and adding a glycine derivative and an aldehyde (73). The resulting intermediates can then be characterized separately or further modified by linking to proteins and other biomolecules via amine end groups on the chemically functionalized SWNTs (73).

Most of the relevant [i.e., intravenously (IV) and intraperitoneally (IP) administered] SWNT studies in living subjects to date have involved biodistribution, pharmacokinetic, and toxicity studies (69,71,82,83). For clinical applications, IV administration is generally most relevant. Note, however, that IP-administered ^{125}I-radiolabeled, hydroxylated SWNTs intriguingly displayed uptake in bone (83), which was not observed with IV administered SWNTs chelated with radioactive [111]In (69). These studies suggest there may be significant clinical applications for both IV and IP administration modes. However, the range of options found in the literature in SWNT functionalization, length, and even diameter illustrates the need to standardize the studies being performed so that the properties of SWNTs can be properly evaluated across studies.

Systematic studies observing the blood half-life, toxicity, and behavior of SWNTs in living subjects are critical to their in vivo future use. As a relative newcomer to the molecular imaging arena, these initial studies form the backbone for SWNT clinical applications. For instance, experiments indicating that the blood half-life of SWNTs is longer than a relatively robust three hours with major renal excretion are exciting for clinical applicability (69). Long blood half-lives allow more time for nanoparticles to cluster at their desired target, therefore enabling smaller doses, lower costs, decreased toxicity, and better efficacy. Furthermore, a recent study provocatively indicated that nitrogen-doped nanotubes (in which pyridine-N or substitutional-N replaces a C in the carbon framework) could be significantly more biocompatible and less toxic than pure carbon nanotubes in living mice (84). Even at very high doses, such as ∼5 mg/kg, at which SWNTs were previously shown to be toxic or even lethal, N-doped nanotubes were demonstrated to be safe (84–86). Another study illustrated the significance of surface functionalization

by showing that purified, nonfunctionalized open SWNTs were found to activate blood platelets and accelerate the rate of vascular thrombosis when injected into living rats (87). It will be important to study the effects of surface functionalization on nanotubes' interaction with blood cells and proteins in order to minimize such adverse effects. Yet surface chemistry is not the only critical factor for nanotubes to be safely administered into living subjects—nanotube length, for instance, may also significantly factor into responses such as inflammation (88).

Proof-of-principle experiments involving SWNTs have been performed to demonstrate methods by which SWNTs may be targeted and used for therapeutic and imaging purposes (67,70,71,73,89) (Fig. 4). These provide a glimpse into the promise and potential approaches for using SWNTs to better human health. Therapeutic applications of SWNTs include delivery of strands of RNA for siRNA (small interfering RNA) therapeutics (67), vaccination (73), and targeting with the potential for specific heating and killing of cancer cells (71,89–91). There is much potential for therapeutic applications of SWNTs, as there is for the molecular imaging of cancer using intrinsic SWNT reporter properties such as their infrared emission and unique Raman spectra (70,71). Further, because of the extreme high surface area and space in the center of the nanotube, various molecular imaging reporter agents may be attached or trapped (71,92–94). Current methods have imaged and localized carbon nanotubes in living subjects by radiolabeling them and using nuclear imaging modalities such as PET and SPECT, or by attaching fluorescent molecules and imaging via optical means. The Dai group used SWNTs non-covalently functionalized with various lengths of PEG molecules and conjugated DOTA (for chelation to ^{64}Cu) and RGD. Sulfo-NHS and EDC was used to attach DOTA, while RGD was linked via sulfo-SMCC and thiolated RGD peptides. [64]Cu was used to identify the SWNT biodistribution by PET imaging, while the RGD allowed targeting to specific tumor sites in mice. Molecular imaging of integrin $\alpha_v\beta_3$ using SWNTs was verified by PET. Moreover, the organs/tissues shown to take up SWNTs (the tumor, liver, and kidney) displayed the distinct SWNT Raman signature when examined ex vivo (71). Similarly, the Weisman group injected SWNTs into rabbits and studied their localization by fluorescent microscopic detection of the SWNTs' infrared signal ex vivo. Studies have thus begun to optimize use of SWNTs as molecularly targeted agents capable of both intrinsic reporter and therapeutic (e.g., heat) functions such as infrared fluorescence and Raman signatures. The utility of SWNTs for oncological applications would be greatly enhanced if these reporter functions could be more fully exploited in living subjects. Proofs-of-principle utilizing many of the extraordinary properties of SWNTs are in progress and will hopefully move beyond the research stage with improvements and studies on long-term toxicity and biocompatibility.

NANOSHELLS

Nanoshells, like qdots, are optically responsive nanoparticles that can be tuned from the near-ultraviolet to infrared wavelengths (Fig. 6). However, nanoshells differ in a number of fundamental ways. Most prominent is the mechanism by which they produce light—because metal nanoshells comprise a spherical dielectric core surrounded by a very thin metallic coating (often silica and gold, respectively), they are able to produce optical resonance of surface plasmons in the metal as a response to incident photons. The thicknesses and materials compositions of the dielectric core and metal coating, which can be very finely controlled, govern nanoshell optical tunability. They are thus unlike qdots, in which core size dictates emission properties, and because of the differing synthetic protocols, nanoshells are often considerably larger—generally 10 to 500 nm in diameter, and greater than 50 nm for the typical silica-gold construct (95,96). This is

disadvantageous for nanoshells because biodistribution characteristics depend strongly on size; however, nanoshells lack heavy metals and therefore do not suffer from possible heavy metal toxicity like qdots. As contrast agents, nanoshells are potentially useful as optical, photoacoustic, and Raman nanoparticles in living subjects. As therapeutic agents, nanoshells can be tethered to drugs or can be tuned to heat up on exposure to a specific wavelength of light (96–99). Highly monodisperse silica nanospheres (50–500 nm) can be nucleated and grown by reducing TEOS (tetraethylorthosilicate) in ethanol. Amine groups are then introduced onto the silica sphere surface via treatment with APTES (aminopropyltriethoxysilane) so that 1 to 2 nm gold nanoparticles can subsequently be adsorbed at aminated sites (Fig. 6). The colloidal gold provides nucleation locations for controlled growth of gold via Au reduction in a $HAuCl_4$ solution. This confers the desired gold shell thickness (~ 5–30 nm) to help control the ratio of core diameter to gold shell thickness for precise optical tuning (96), especially in the NIR for biomedical applications. For purely optical imaging, nanoshells can be tuned to scatter rather than absorb incident photons. The NIR range allows for deep

Nanoshells

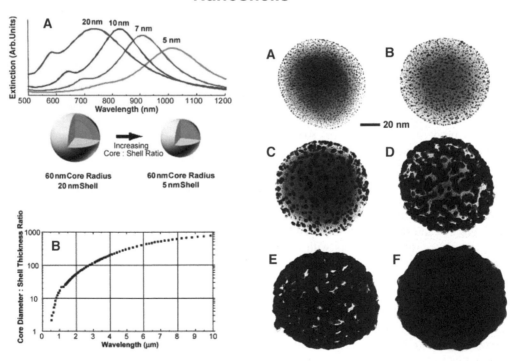

Figure 6 Nanoshells. (*Left, top*) Optical tunability is demonstrated for nanoshells with a 60-nm silica core radius and gold shells 5, 7, 10, and 20 nm thick calculated theoretically. Observe that the plasmon resonance (extinction) of the particles with decreasing thickness of the gold shell (or an increasing core:shell ratio). Nanoshells are easily fabricated with resonance in the NIR. Greater tunability can be achieved by also altering the core size, changing the composition of the core and shell, and forming multilayered structures. (*Bottom*) Calculation of optical resonance wavelength versus core diameter/shell thickness ratio for metal nanoshells (silica core, gold shell). (*Right*) TEM images of nanoshell growth on 120-nm diameter silica dielectric nanoparticle. (**A**) Initial gold colloid-decorated silica nanoparticle. (**B–E**) Gradual growth and coalescence of gold colloid on silica nanoparticle surface. (**F**) Completed growth of metallic nanoshell.

imaging in living subjects using optical technologies such as OCT, diffuse optical tomography, confocal imaging, and spectroscopic methods (96). These imaging modalities are conducive to molecularly targeted nanoshell contrast. Alternatively, nanoshells can be used as excellent photon absorbing materials, which rapidly heat up for imaging (as well as therapeutic) objectives. Photoacoustic tomography involves shining light onto a target, which rapidly heats up target molecules. These molecules thus expand, producing ultrasonic waves detectable by traditional transducers. Nanoshells are interesting materials for photoacoustic contrast because of their ability to be tuned for optimal absorption and subsequent energy dissipation as localized heat generators. Advances in photoacoustic tomography for nanoshells parallel those in optical imaging, and are clinically relevant as photoacoustics offers significantly increased spatial resolution and imaging depth compared with standard ultrasound and optical imaging, respectively (100–102). Also note that the photoacoustic strategy of nanoshells (or nanotubes, Fig. 5) chemically designed and tuned to absorb light could instead be configured for rapid heating and ablation of cancer cells to which they are molecularly targeted (97–99). Another alternative is Raman imaging, a method founded on Raman scattering. This is based on the inelastic scattering of incident photons on vibrational, rotational, and electronical molecular modes. The acquired spectra result in specific molecular signatures that can be used to identify and localize Raman-active molecules such as nanoshells. Because nanoshells are SERS (surface-enhanced Raman scattering) nanoparticles, they have been used in spectroscopic detection of intracellular molecules in vitro. Their robust signal is also useful for diagnostic imaging of living subjects using a Raman-enabled system (62–64).

The gold nanoshell surface serves as an excellent substrate replete with functional groups from which to link biological molecules. Moreover, as a noble metal, the gold surface is considered a non-toxic, corrosion-resistant, and biocompatible interface to the in vivo milieu (96). Potential chemistries are broad and flexible, from non-covalent spontaneous chemisorption to self-assembly employing strong sulfur-gold interactions to covalent bonding of biomolecules such as antibodies (96,103). Using covalent sulfhydryl chemistries, nanoshells can be decorated with hydrophobic or hydrophilic molecules that help target to molecular markers of disease, to stabilize, to reduce opsonization, or to evade immune responses. Chemical modifications of nanoshells allow targeting of cancer cells, which may then be detected by means of optical, photoacoustic, or Raman systems (96,97,100–103).

Highly engineered nanoshells have been shown to scatter light at a certain intensity (optical imaging) and absorb light at increased intensities (therapeutics/photoacoustics) so that both functionalities are integrated within the same

multifunctional nanoparticle for detection using optical methods (97). Thus this entity is capable of enabling both diagnosis and treatment without any external modification—addition of targeting capacity, feedback, and/or other "smart" systems might easily be incorporated to help fulfill this nanoparticle's utility and multifunctionality. Photoacoustic teams have likewise engineered nanoshells to image tumors via the EPR effect (100–102,104). These photoacoustic nanoshells also seamlessly integrate diagnostics and therapeutics, as the heat generated is simply a matter of the degree of incident photon intensity. Because the heating effect is in fact the mechanism of photoacoustic imaging, it would be feasible to image nanoshells as they destroy tumor cells. Present optical and photoacoustic nanoshell iterations simply employ the EPR effect to accumulate in tumors (97,100–102,104), but in vitro testing of nanoshell targeting capabilities (103,105,106) indicates a bright future for diagnostic and therapeutic oncology with all the advantages that molecular targeting offers. These advantages, which can be generalized for most targeted nanoparticles with diagnostic/therapeutic capabilities, include a very high percent of injected dose accumulating at target site. This is critical for earlier detection (because of increased signal) and for avoiding collateral damage to healthy tissue when nanoparticles are not predominantly attached to tumor, as well as decreased toxicity from reduction in dose.

MAGNETIC NANOMATERIALS

Magnetic nanoparticles, especially those with superparamagnetic properties, are principally useful for imaging in applications associated with improving contrast in MRI and spectroscopy. Superparamagnetism indicates that the material retains no magnetism on removal of magnetic field and the entire 1 to 10 nm nanocrystal tends to align with the applied magnetic field. Iron oxide nanoparticles were developed as early as the late 1980s (107) to provide MRI contrast because of their very high magnetic susceptibility, even higher than the often-used metal gadolinium. As their FDA approval for clinical use in humans suggests, iron oxides and gadolinium remain the most commonly used magnetic materials. Nevertheless, a wealth of other magnetically active nanoparticles have been created and tested in vitro and in living animals. For brevity, we primarily focus in this section on the prevalent ultrasmall superparamagnetic iron oxide (USPIO) family (Fig. 7). It is nonetheless important to mention the fascinating advances that are being achieved and optimized in the materials synthesis of various magnetic nanoparticles. For example, nanoparticles comprising FeCo, gold copper (Au_3Cu_1), iron hydroxide (FeOOH), and other materials have been constructed with superior magnetic properties that increase MR signal and have the potential to help

Ultra-small Iron Oxide Nanoparticles

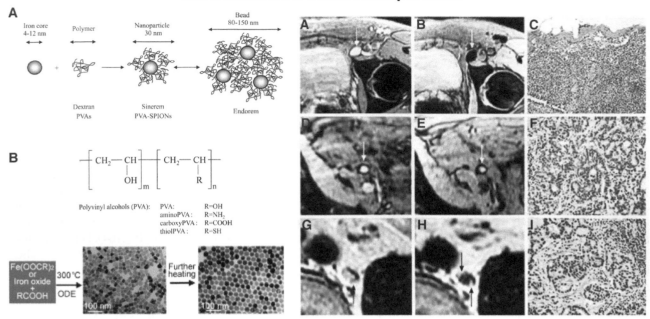

Figure 7 Iron oxide nanoparticles. (*Left*) The top shows various structures of superparamagnetic iron oxide nanoparticles with dextran and polyvinyl alcohol coatings. The bottom displays one method of iron oxide formation—the formation of Fe_3O_4 nanocrystals. The middle and right panels are TEM images of the As-synthesized nanocrystals taken at different reaction times. (*Right*, human MRI) MRI nodal abnormalities in three patients with prostate cancer. As compared with conventional MRI (*Panel A*), MRI obtained 24 hours after the administration of lymphotropic superparamagnetic nanoparticles (*Panel B*) shows a homogeneous decrease in signal intensity due to the accumulation of lymphotropic superparamagnetic nanoparticles in a normal lymph node in the left iliac region (*arrow*). (Panel C) The corresponding histologic findings (hematoxylin and eosin, 125×). Conventional MRI shows a high signal intensity in an unenlarged iliac lymph node completely replaced by tumor (*arrow in Panel D*). Nodal signal intensity remains high (*arrow in Panel E*). Panel F shows the corresponding histologic findings (hematoxylin and eosin, 200×). Conventional MRI shows high signal intensity in a retroperitoneal node with micrometastases (*arrow in Panel G*). MRI with lymphotropic superparamagnetic nanoparticles demonstrates two hyperintense foci (*arrows in Panel H*) within the node, corresponding to 2-mm metastases. Corresponding histologic analysis confirms the presence of adenocarcinoma within the node (*Panel I*, hematoxylin and eosin, 200×).

revolutionize the field of MR-based diagnoses (108–111). FeCo nanoparticles were scalably synthesized using CVD, coated with a thin graphitic shell, and have been demonstrated to yield a long-lasting MRI signal in living subjects (108). Furthermore, similar to nanoshells, these FeCo nanoparticles are capable of simultaneous diagnosis/therapy with the potential for simultaneous imaging (MRI) and therapy (photothermal ablation via NIR light absorption). FeOOH nanoparticles, which were prepared electrostatically, displayed significant accumulation in a solid tumor of a murine tumor model (110). All three of the FeCo, Au_3Cu, and FeOOH nanoparticles have excellent magnetic properties and preliminarily display overall biocompatibility and low toxicity (108–110). The promise and expectations for these nanomaterials remain lofty, and with time, the targeting and molecular imaging studies performed with USPIOs that are described below are presumably achievable and surpassable with the aforementioned novel nanomaterials. While much research is underway on the creation of novel magnetic nanomaterials,

others focus on unique combinations of nanomaterials, such as magnetic dendrimers (39,112). Both varieties will likely be attractive candidates for molecular imaging. However, as is the case for nanoparticles in human imaging in general, the major obstacle for all these nanoparticles' clinical diagnostic utility remains regulatory approval and reimbursement.

The relatively lengthy existence of nanoparticulate iron oxides in science and imaging has generated a corresponding degree of breadth and depth in the literature. A great deal of work has thus gone into detailed characterization and optimized synthesis for USPIOs, leading to a variety of compositions and phases. These include the pure metal (i.e., Fe), Fe_3O_4, γ-Fe_2O_3, higher alloys of $MgFe_2O_4$, $MnFe_2O_4$, and $CoFe_2O_4$, among others (111). The advantages of using USPIOs in living subjects are critical to their ongoing successes: USPIOs offer high MR signal change per unit of metal, afford excellent biocompatibility via their ability to degrade into safe constituents under physiological conditions, provide flexible functional groups for facile linkage to biomolecules for targeting and therapeutics, they are detectable by a wide range of modalities—from MRI to optical and electron microscopies, bridging the macroscopic-to-nanoscopic gaps, they can be purified and manipulated magnetically for high ease-of-use in bioconjugations and other protocols, their size and properties allow them to remain in circulation from tens of minutes to hours without being cleared by the RES, and their magnetic properties, shape, size, stability, and monodispersity can be intelligently modulated by well-characterized synthetic chemistries (111,113,114). Because even the breadth of USPIO synthetic protocols far exceeds the scope of this chapter, we simply list some of the most prevalent protocols and briefly expand on one of the most-used methods as it impacts oncological nanotechnology. Co-precipitation, thermal decomposition and/or reduction, hydrothermal synthesis, micelle synthesis, and laser hydrolysis comprise the most commonly used techniques to construct iron oxide nanoparticles (Fig. 7). In particular, thermal decomposition requires a relatively intricate synthetic chemistry under inert conditions, but delivers very tight monodispersity, excellent shape control, and scalable chemistries for manufacturing (111), which are all very desirable for use in living subjects.

USPIOs can be synthesized via the thermal decomposition of organometallic materials in organic solvents by using stabilizing surfactants (111). Strict modulation of the ratio of starting reagents (organometallic compound, solvent, and surfactant), reaction temperature, reaction time, and the aging period confers very fine control of the size and shape of the resultant magnetic nanoparticles. The choice of USPIO physical attributes such as size, shape, and magnetization should be directed by the user's specific application (i.e., imaging modality such as MRI, desired localization parameters, circulation time, etc.) and should thus be synthesized accordingly.

In cancer applications, because of the direct relationship between nanoparticle size/shape/circulation time and the tumor extravasation parameters, USPIO synthetic parameters should be carefully chosen to correlate with the physical characteristics that optimize the USPIOs' use in vivo. For example, decomposition of iron pentacarbonyl in octyl ether and oleic acid leads to monodisperse γ-Fe_2O_3 nanoparticles of 13 nm; alternatively, water-soluble, monodisperse Fe_3O_4 nanoparticles can be formed by mixing $FeCl_3 \cdot 6H_2O$ and 2-pyrrolidone and they can be controllably sized at 4, 12, or 60 nm by refluxing for 1, 10, or 24 hours, respectively. To induce, for instance, extravasation of nanoparticles across the blood-brain barrier, optimization of attributes such as size, charge, and partition coefficients must be emphasized. On the other hand, some tumor vasculatures are very leaky, and nanoparticles hundreds of nanometers in diameter will extravasate (115). In this case, other parameters may be more important, such

as focusing on the ability of the nanoparticle to provide maximal contrast change. Indeed, for use as MR contrast agents in living subjects, not only are the biological parameters of USPIOs such as circulation time important to consider, but the nanoscale material's physical characteristics such as magnetic anisotropy, relaxivity, magnetic susceptibility, and coercivity are implicated in, and have a significant impact on, effective contrast enhancement. Thus, choosing the appropriate nanoparticle for an application is undeniably a complex activity, and in an ideal environment this selection process would clearly be individualized, i.e., personalized (diagnostic) medicine.

The chemistry of USPIOs is ultimately driven by the resultant nanoparticles' magnetic properties. These properties are characterized by a wide range of techniques, including SQUID (Superconducting Quantum Interference Device) and vibrating sample magnetometry (111). Chemicals, coatings, and surface effects can all affect a nanoparticle's magnetization. For instance, a magnetic coating on a magnetic nanomaterial often has a tremendous effect on its magnetic properties, and must thus be chosen and characterized very carefully (111). Hence this area has the potential to effect great advances in magnetic nanomaterials as new insights evolve into novel nanotechnologies. However, for clinical applications it is critical that colloidal stability, protection of the nanoparticles in solution, and biocompatibility in physiological environments are maintained. Many methods are used for stability, including both organic techniques (e.g., via surfactants and polymers) and inorganic techniques (e.g., coating with oxides, silica, carbon, or other metals). Most clinically directed USPIOs utilize various polymers which are chemically linked or physically adsorbed to the nanoparticle surface to provide some protection and steric repulsion, leading to a stable (low aggregation) colloidal suspension (111). Moreover, the polymers can be selected specifically to have certain functional groups that can be exploited for binding to biomolecules to extend their usage to molecular targeting and imaging.

MRI-based molecular imaging has been considered challenging, perhaps because of the relatively low sensitivity of MRI [e.g., for detection of atherosclerosis (116)]. Nevertheless, because of the high resolution and soft tissue contrast provided by MRI, developing MR-based nanoparticle molecular imaging reagents became a major objective in the field; numerous groups have shown proof-of-feasibility (109,117–120). Despite the fact that USPIOs generally yield negative contrast (i.e., signal hypointensity) in MRI, a feature most radiologists prefer to avoid, they remain among the most highly investigated molecular imaging nanoparticles. This may in part be because the basic iron oxide nanoparticle is already approved, in multiple forms, by regulatory agencies around the world. However, increasing the efficacy and specificity and lowering the necessary iron dose remain major objectives. Thus, optimization and testing of bioconjugation chemistries stands as the chief hurdle to realizing MR-based molecular imaging with USPIOs in humans.

The chemistries that link targeting biomolecules to the polymer coating of USPIOs are in some ways similar to the chemistries of other nanoparticles mentioned above. They vary widely because they depend on the functional groups presented on the chosen polymer coating, rather than direct conjugation to the iron oxide lattice. We therefore focus on recent applications of polymer-coated USPIOs rather than the specific chemistries that link targeting molecules to polymer coatings.

Recent reviews and studies highlight the use of dextran-coated USPIOs for clinical MR imaging in humans (121–124) [see Fig. 7 for an example of human MR imaging with USPIOs (125)]. While nonspecific contrast enhancement certainly boosts the utility of MRI, promising studies in animal models lead to the conviction that MR-rooted molecular imaging in the clinic would lead to critical improvements in detecting early stage cancers and other diseases as well as monitoring of therapeutic response. It is thus somewhat surprising that the molecular targeting of USPIOs to specific tumor antigens has been reported for nearly 20 years in animal models (126,127). Clearly, much optimization has been required to move toward clinical trials. The body of work leading to the current state of MR molecular imaging in animals is massive in breadth and depth. This work displays astonishing improvements over nonmolecular approaches including reduction of dose, increased yields to disease sites, and improved images through a combination of enhanced USPIO bioconjugate formulations and MRI hardware and sequence advances. Lee et al. provide an excellent example of this development (128). They first optimized the magnetic, crystallinity, and monodispersity of iron oxide nanocrystals, then chose the optimal dopant by screening a variety of metal-doped (Mn, Co, Fe, or Ni) Fe_2O_4 nanoparticles. Thus $MnFe_2O_4$ was selected as the optimal material for mass magnetization, magnetic susceptibility, and relaxation values (128). By conjugating Her-2/neu antibodies to 12 nm crystals of this material via standard chemistries, they demonstrated detection of cancers with a mass of 50 mg in living subjects, which is smaller than that detectable in a comparable radiotracer study (128,129). Indeed, studies on oncological targeting of antibody-conjugated USPIOs in living subjects have become increasingly common and display promising results, such as in hepatocellular carcinomas and lymphomas (120,130). Nevertheless, the size of antibodies can dominate the properties of injected USPIOs. Therefore, smaller molecules such as smaller proteins [e.g., Annexin V for apoptosis-targeted USPIOs (117)], peptides, or aptamers are increasingly popular choices.

In attempts to preserve the pharmacokinetic properties of bare USPIOs, to facilitate their entry into otherwise inaccessible regions, and potentially to increase the polyvalent effect, smaller molecules such as peptides and aptamers are frequently employed as the targeting domain. The polyvalent effect refers to the increase in the probability of nanoparticle binding and remaining bound to a surface via greater than one binding event by the synergistic increase in affinity. Since peptides are small, the USPIO can maintain its approximate size, a higher density of targeting molecules can be appended (resulting in increased targeting molecules per nanoparticle), and surface charge distributions can be better controlled. For instance, RGD peptides (see qdot section) and the synaptotagmin domain have been shown, using MRI on living subjects, to target USPIOs to angiogenic tumor vasculature and apoptotic tumor cells, respectively (131,132).

A recent study displayed the ability to image gene transcripts via MRI for cerebral ischemia in the central nervous system using oligodeoxynucleotide-conjugated USPIOs (linked by neutravidin-biotin association) (133). The work showed the feasibility of monitoring mRNA alterations in mouse models. Also, an area gaining increasing interest involves USPIO labeling and MR tracking of exogenously administered cells, such as stem cells (134–136). In this work, cells are exogenously labeled with USPIOs and tracked to confirm localized cellular delivery, cell-based repair, replacement, and treatment, and to monitor their short-term migration/trafficking into adjacent tissues.

Recent studies by Medarova et al. display many of the features that epitomize the vast potential held by the targeted USPIO field (137,138). Multimodal nanoparticles were constructed (i) solely for imaging purposes (138) and (ii) for a combination of therapeutics/diagnostics, or theranostics (137). USPIOs were demonstrated not only to target an orthotopic human pancreatic adenocarcinoma mouse model, but also addressed the critical field of monitoring of therapeutic response via MRI. To achieve this, aminated USPIOs were first conjugated to Cy 5.5 dye. These Cy 5.5-USPIOs were then conjugated via thioether linkage to EPPT peptide, which targets underglycosylated muc-1 antigen (umuc-1). This antigen is an early tumorigenic marker that is overexpressed on most human epithelial cell adenocarcinomas. Furthermore, the EPPT peptide is labeled with FITC (fluorescein isothiocyanate, a green dye). Thus the Cy 5.5-USPIO-EPPT bioconjugate is a targeted magneto-optical nanoparticle capable of detection by magnetic resonance and by optical colocalization of two spectrally separated dyes. Studies in mice revealed up to a 46.5% MR signal decrease in umuc-1 positive tumors. In accordance with these findings, optical analyses showed a nearly twofold signal increase in tumor over background. Furthermore, when given the chemotherapeutic agent 5-FU, use of the multimodal USPIOs–enabled tracking of the tumor response. Good correlation between MRI signal and tumor shrinkage was shown, indicating that the molecular imaging approach generated an accurate oncologic representation. While this multimodal USPIO was successful in proving its potential for diagnostic imaging in the preclinical model using both MRI and optical means (138), the second study established a USPIO-based therapeutic delivery and monitoring approach using siRNA (single interfering RNA) and MRI (137).

CONCLUSIONS

The extensive variety of nanoparticle types, materials, geometries, surface functionalizations, etc. makes the precise engineering of nanoparticles for very specific applications (e.g., the monitoring of a certain disease, such as the metastases of prostate cancer, with a specific molecule overexpressed) not only feasible, but eminently practical and likely critical to medicine's future. In molecular imaging, nanoparticles are employed because they display many advantages over their small molecule relatives. For example, nanoparticles may be designed as multifunctional, integrated platforms (139), unlike small molecules. These nanoparticles can embody one or more of the following: imaging, targeting, therapeutic, and feedback for real-time monitoring or therapeutic capabilities. This platform capability is ideal for theranostic applications—i.e., the tasks involved in diagnosing, treating, and monitoring may be most efficiently accomplished via an "all-in-one" platform in which the theranostic process is all performed by the same agent. Furthermore, the abundant surface area on nanoparticles allows many targeting moieties to be attached on each nanoparticle. This allows nanoparticles to harness superior avidity capabilities via multivalent and synergistic binding. Also, because of their size, nanoparticles can deliver large "payloads" of whatever material is desired (e.g., high quantity of contrast material for molecular imaging or therapeutic molecule for treatment) compared to small molecule agents. Nanoparticles also have major advantages for drug delivery applications, for example, aptly designed nanoparticle formulations can enhance the bioavailability of the associated therapeutic (and even imaging agent in some cases) as well as improve timed/controlled release profiles (140). For approaches requiring entry into cells, nanoparticles may be ideal as the most efficient vehicle to penetrate cell membranes and deliver cargo, for example, for gene delivery and/or therapy. This is because gene delivery is dependent on the process of insertion of a gene vector into a cell and subsequently into the nucleus (all while being protected from the severe environment of the cytoplasm)

(141). Also, delivery of injected agents from the vasculature to the disease site is often passive, via leaky vasculature (the EPR effect). Nanoparticles are the appropriate size to exploit the power of this effect as they are typically $\sim$10 to 200 nm, the range in which many tumor vasculatures are leaky [endothelial pores may even go up to $\sim$1 μm (115)]. While small molecules will also extravasate in these vessels, unlike nanoparticles they are also prone to extravasate in normal blood vessels because of their size. From an industry standpoint, nanoparticle formulations provide added value by enabling pharmaceutical companies to extend intellectual property holdings on their drug and imaging agents via new patent filings. They may also provide new niche markets and sales (141). Perhaps the most important advantage of nanoparticles over small molecules lies in their as yet predominantly untapped wealth of potential as the most efficient, efficacious vehicle to target effectively and simultaneously deliver imaging and therapeutic materials because of the ability of nanotechnologists to specifically engineer and modulate the desired effect, i.e., the potential of personalized medicine.

The main disadvantages of nanoparticles compared to small molecules involve dissemination of the agent and toxicity issues. In some diseases, small molecules may be able to extravasate in areas in which nanoparticles cannot. More importantly, once extravasated, small molecules diffuse to surrounding areas considerably more easily than the more bulky nanoparticles. For therapy, this effect is often very important, as therapeutic effects dominate only near the blood vessels and are thus often not sufficient to destroy the entire lesion. Furthermore, nanoparticles introduce the potential for materials toxicity (e.g., heavy metals with qdots), while small molecules do not. Furthermore, more studies must be performed on the potential environmental toxicity of nanoparticles and the feasibility of their inhalation and size-based lung toxicity to determine the level of concern necessary. Higher masses of materials are also generally introduced in vivo with nanoparticle formulations. Toxicity concerns must thus be thoroughly addressed prior to use in humans.

After toxicity issues are mitigated, the pharmacokinetics of nanoparticles remain a critical obstacle. The difficulties arise from the fact that nanoparticle pharmacokinetics vary as broadly as the combination of nanoparticle types, materials, shapes, surface coatings, and sizes. Thus each individual nanoparticle formulation must be independently studied. For instance, a certain type of iron oxide nanoparticle was engineered to exhibit a plasma half-life of greater than 10 hours; however, when peptides were attached, the plasma half-life diminished to less than 1 hour (142). Relatively small changes to the nanoparticles often result in great differences in nanoparticle pharmacokinetics. Biodistribution and other pharmacokinetic studies are critical to perform to ensure the ability of the nanoparticle to perform its intended funtion in living subjects. Biodistribution is often performed by radiolabeling the nanoparticle and following the nano-particle distribution via PET or SPECT in living subjects at set time points. Qdots and SWNTs, for example, have been systematically studied in this manner (28,71). This data will help direct researchers toward which indications are most appropriate for these nanoparticles based on their biodistribution/pharmacokinetic parameters, and are criti-cal toward potential regulatory approval.

Most nanoparticles suffer uptake by RES organs (such as liver and spleen) and thus shortened circulation times because blood proteins and opsonins adsorb to the nano-particle surface. These proteins signal RES macrophages to clear the nanoparticles. Thus, the serum stability of the nanoparticles (a parameter that is particularly dependent on nanoparticle aggregation properties in whole blood, which in turn is mainly a function of nanoparticle surface characteristics) helps determine RES clearance. Surface modifications, such as use of PEG, help to increase circu-lation times by helping to deter blood protein binding. While myriad pharmacokinetic profiles have been observed, the ideal pharmacokinetic profile in most cases of targeted nanoparticles would display circulation through the vasculature for a number of hours prior to renal clearance. This would provide sufficient time for nanoparticles to reach their disease target site, while concurrently exposing the patient only to the precise amount of nanoparticles used to image/treat the disease.

While most issues in nanoparticle-based molecular imaging are specific to the nanoparticle system investigated, a few problems are common to the field at large. First, RES uptake/clearance must be addressed more completely than current solutions, presumably by evading opsonization. Second, the overall safety of particulates in the nanoscale must be adequately analyzed. As mentioned, environmental safety and lung toxicity of these nanoparticles are of grave concern to the community (143,144). Individual patient safety is also a concern for those injected with nanoparticles. In particular, oxidative stress, free radical effects, and hydrophobic interactions may adversely affect patients as a function of nanoparticle size. This is because these effects are surface-modulated, and the smaller a nanoparticle is, the greater the overall surface area-to-volume ratio. The increased relative surface area (proportional to the square of the radius for spherical nanoparticles) for smaller nanpo-particles can in some cases thus become detrimental.

While the potential for nanoparticles in molecular imaging oncology is immense, very few have yet reached Phase I clinical trials. This is partially because many of the basic medical questions underlying nanoparticles in medicine are still not well understood (e.g., RES uptake); nevertheless, the scientific foundation for studying both the medical and the nanotechnological parameters has

been established. For new nanoparticles to achieve human utility, it will be important to study the nano-particles that have already been approved. Most nanoparticle formulations reaching the clinic to date are drug/protein-based or polymer solutions, in addition to well-studied USPIOs, for example, Feridex and Abraxane (145–148). They are well-tolerated and highly efficacious and the lessons from their paths to human use will be instructive. These nanoparticles have passed through clin-ical trials and been approved by regulatory agencies, portending success in the clinical trials of future, more sophisticated platform nanoparticle systems if the issues raised above can be satisfactorily addressed. Indeed, with continued systematic toxicity/pharmacokinetic studies and appropriate redesign, many types of highly efficacious nanoparticles are anticipated to infiltrate the clinics in the form of trials over the next 5 to 10 years.

REFERENCES

1. Ferrari M. Cancer nanotechnology: opportunities and challenges. Nat Rev 2005; 5(3):161–171.
2. LaVan DA, McGuire T, Langer R. Small-scale systems for in vivo drug delivery. Nat Biotechnol 2003; 21(10): 1184–1191.
3. Whitesides GM. The 'right' size in nanobiotechnology. Nat Biotechnol 2003; 21(10):1161–1165.
4. Leary SP, Liu CY, Apuzzo ML. Toward the emergence of nanoneurosurgery. Part II—Nanomedicine: diagnostics and imaging at the nanoscale level. Neurosurgery 2006; 58(5):805–823; discussion 23.
5. Pison U, Welte T, Giersig M, et al. Nanomedicine for respiratory diseases. Eur J Pharmacol 2006; 533(1–3): 341–350.
6. Wickline SA, Neubauer AM, Winter PM, et al. Molecular imaging and therapy of atherosclerosis with targeted nanoparticles. J Magn Reson Imaging 2007; 25(4): 667–680.
7. Bhattacharya S, Bajaj A. Recent advances in lipid molec-ular design. Curr Opin Chem Biol 2005; 9(6):647–655.
8. Douglas SJ, Davis SS, Illum L. Nanoparticles in drug delivery. Crit Rev Ther Drug Carrier Syst 1987; 3(3): 233–261.
9. Minko T, Pakunlu RI, Wang Y, et al. New generation of liposomal drugs for cancer. Anticancer Agents Med Chem 2006; 6(6):537–552.
10. Liu J, Lee H, Allen C. Formulation of drugs in block copolymer micelles: drug loading and release. Curr Pharm Des 2006; 12(36):4685–4701.
11. Torchilin VP. Micellar nanocarriers: pharmaceutical perspectives. Pharm Res 2007; 24(1):1–16.
12. Duncan R. Designing polymer conjugates as lysosomo-tropic nanomedicines. Biochem Soc Trans 2007; 35(pt 1): 56–60.
13. Lee LJ. Polymer nano-engineering for biomedical appli-cations. Ann Biomed Eng 2006; 34(1):75–88.

14. van Vlerken LE, Amiji MM. Multi-functional polymeric nanoparticles for tumour-targeted drug delivery. Expert Opin Drug Deliv 2006; 3(2):205–216.

15. Moghimi SM. Recent developments in polymeric nanoparticle engineering and their applications in experimental and clinical oncology. Anticancer Agents Med Chem 2006; 6(6):553–561.

16. Mitra A, Nan A, Line BR, et al. Nanocarriers for nuclear imaging and radiotherapy of cancer. Curr Pharm Des 2006; 12(36):4729–4749.

17. Letchford K, Burt H. A review of the formation and classification of amphiphilic block copolymer nanoparticulate structures: micelles, nanospheres, nanocapsules and polymersomes. Eur J Pharm Biopharm 2006; 65(3):259–269.

18. Torchilin VP. Multifunctional nanocarriers. Adv Drug Deliv Rev 2006; 58(14):1532–1555.

19. Kah JCY, Sheppard CJR, Lee CGL, et al. Application of antibody-conjugated gold nanoparticles for optical molecular imaging of epithelial carcinoma cells. In: Nanobiophotonics and Biomedical Applications III. San Jose, CA: SPIE, 2006:609503–609506.

20. Hyafil F, Cornily JC, Feig JE, et al. Noninvasive detection of macrophages using a nanoparticulate contrast agent for computed tomography. Nat Med 2007; 13(5):636–641.

21. Cambi A, Lidke DS, Arndt-Jovin DJ, et al. Ligand-conjugated quantum dots monitor antigen uptake and processing by dendritic cells. Nano Lett 2007; 7(4):970–977.

22. Michalet X, Pinaud FF, Bentolila LA, et al. Quantum dots for live cells, in vivo imaging, and diagnostics. Science 2005; 307(5709):538–544.

23. Sykova E, Jendelova P. Migration, fate, and in vivo imaging of adult stem cells in the CNS. Cell Death Differ 2007; 14(7):1336–1342.

24. Herbig ME, Weller KM, Merkle HP. Reviewing biophysical and cell biological methodologies in cell-penetrating peptide (CPP) research. Crit Rev Ther Drug Carrier Syst 2007; 24(3):203–255.

25. Fischer H, Liu L, Pang K, et al. Pharmacokinetics of nanoscale quantum dots: in vivo distribution, sequestration, and clearance in the rat. Adv Funct Mater 2006; 16:1299–1305.

26. Klibanov AL, Maruyama K, Beckerleg AM, et al. Activity of amphipathic poly(ethylene glycol) 5000 to prolong the circulation time of liposomes depends on the liposome size and is unfavorable for immunoliposome binding to target. Biochimica et biophysica acta 1991; 1062(2):142–148.

27. Lockman PR, Mumper RJ, Khan MA, et al. Nanoparticle technology for drug delivery across the blood-brain barrier. Drug Dev Ind Pharm 2002; 28(1):1–13.

28. Schipper ML, Cheng Z, Lee SW, et al. MicroPET-based biodistribution of quantum dots in living mice. J Nucl Med 2007; 48(9):1511–1518.

29. Akerman ME, Chan WC, Laakkonen P, et al. Nanocrystal targeting in vivo. Proc Natl Acad Sci U S A 2002; 99(20): 12617–12621.

30. Simberg D, Duza T, Park JH, et al. Biomimetic amplification of nanoparticle homing to tumors. Proc Natl Acad Sci U S A 2007; 104(3):932–936.

31. Hess H, Bachand GD, Vogel V. Powering nanodevices with biomolecular motors. Chemistry (Weinheim an der Bergstrasse, Germany) 2004; 10(9):2110–2116.

32. Soong RK, Bachand GD, Neves HP, et al. Powering an inorganic nanodevice with a biomolecular motor. Science 2000; 290(5496):1555–1558.

33. Teo B, Sun X. From top-down to bottom-up to hybrid nanotechnologies: road to nanodevices. J Cluster Sci 2006; 17(4):529–540.

34. Tomalia DA, Reyna LA, Svenson S. Dendrimers as multipurpose nanodevices for oncology drug delivery and diagnostic imaging. Biochem Soc Trans 2007; 35(pt 1):61–67.

35. Lee CC, MacKay JA, Frechet JM, et al. Designing dendrimers for biological applications. Nat Biotechnol 2005; 23(12):1517–1526.

36. Svenson S, Tomalia DA. Dendrimers in biomedical applications—reflections on the field. Adv Drug Deliv Rev 2005; 57(15):2106–2129.

37. Portney NG, Ozkan M. Nano-oncology: drug delivery, imaging, and sensing. Anal Bioanal Chem 2006; 384(3): 620–630.

38. Shukla R, Thomas TP, Peters JL, et al. HER2 specific tumor targeting with dendrimer conjugated anti-HER2 mAb. Bioconjug Chem 2006; 17(5):1109–1115.

39. Talanov VS, Regino CA, Kobayashi H, et al. Dendrimer-based nanoprobe for dual modality magnetic resonance and fluorescence imaging. Nano Lett 2006; 6(7):1459–1463.

40. Lee CC, Gillies ER, Fox ME, et al. A single dose of doxorubicin-functionalized bow-tie dendrimer cures mice bearing C-26 colon carcinomas. Proc Natl Acad Sci U S A 2006; 103(45):16649–16654.

41. Massoud TF, Gambhir SS. Molecular imaging in living subjects: seeing fundamental biological processes in a new light. Genes Dev 2003; 17(5):545–580.

42. Tsay JM, Michalet X. New light on quantum dot cytotoxicity. Chem Biol 2005; 12(11):1159–1161.

43. Hardman R. A toxicologic review of quantum dots: toxicity depends on physicochemical and environmental factors. Environ Health Perspect 2006; 114(2):165–172.

44. Kim S, Lim YT, Soltesz EG, et al. Near-infrared fluorescent type II quantum dots for sentinel lymph node mapping. Nat Biotechnol 2004; 22(1):93–97.

45. Hama Y, Koyama Y, Urano Y, et al. Simultaneous two-color spectral fluorescence lymphangiography with near infrared quantum dots to map two lymphatic flows from the breast and the upper extremity. Breast Cancer Res Treat 2007; 103(1):23–28.

46. Ballou B, Ernst LA, Andreko S, et al. Sentinel lymph node imaging using quantum dots in mouse tumor models. Bioconjug Chem 2007; 18(2):389–396.

47. Popescu MA, Toms SA. In vivo optical imaging using quantum dots for the management of brain tumors. Expert Rev Mol Diagn 2006; 6(6):879–890.

48. Frangioni JV, Kim SW, Ohnishi S, et al. Sentinel lymph node mapping with type-II quantum dots. Methods Mol Biol 2007; 374:147–160.

49. Soo Choi H, Liu W, Misra P, et al. Renal clearance of quantum dots. Nat Biotechnol 2007; 25(10):1165–1170.

50. Gao X, Cui Y, Levenson RM, et al. In vivo cancer targeting and imaging with semiconductor quantum dots. Nat Biotechnol 2004; 22(8):969–976.

51. Iyer G, Pinaud F, Tsay J, et al. Peptide coated quantum dots for biological applications. IEEE Trans Nanobioscience 2006; 5(4):231–238.

52. Zhou M, Ghosh I. Quantum dots and peptides: a bright future together. Biopolymers 2007; 88(3):325–339.

53. Cai W, Shin DW, Chen K, et al. Peptide-labeled near-infrared quantum dots for imaging tumor vasculature in living subjects. Nano Lett 2006; 6(4):669–676.

54. Ohnishi S, Lomnes SJ, Laurence RG, et al. Organic alternatives to quantum dots for intraoperative near-infrared fluorescent sentinel lymph node mapping. Mol Imaging 2005; 4(3):172–181.

55. So MK, Xu C, Loening AM, et al. Self-illuminating quantum dot conjugates for in vivo imaging. Nat Biotechnol 2006; 24(3):339–343.

56. Fountaine TJ, Wincovitch SM, Geho DH, et al. Multi-spectral imaging of clinically relevant cellular targets in tonsil and lymphoid tissue using semiconductor quantum dots. Mod Pathol 2006; 19(9):1181–1191.

57. De A, Loening AM, Gambhir SS. An improved bioluminescence resonance energy transfer strategy for imaging intracellular events in single cells and living subjects. Cancer Res 2007; 67(15):7175–7183.

58. Smith BR, Nijdam AJ, Cheng MC, et al. A biological perspective of particulate nanoporous silicon. Mater Technol 2004; 19(1):16–20.

59. Zhang K, Loong SL, Connor S, et al. Complete tumor response following intratumoral 32P BioSilicon on human hepatocellular and pancreatic carcinoma xenografts in nude mice. Clin Cancer Res 2005; 11(20):7532–7537.

60. Dorvee JR, Derfus AM, Bhatia SN, et al. Manipulation of liquid droplets using amphiphilic, magnetic one-dimensional photonic crystal chaperones. Nat Mater 2004; 3(12):896–899.

61. Park JH, Derfus AM, Segal E, et al. Local heating of discrete droplets using magnetic porous silicon-based photonic crystals. J Am Chem Soc 2006; 128(24):7938–7946.

62. Qian X, Peng XH, Ansari DO, et al. In vivo tumor targeting and spectroscopic detection with surface-enhanced Raman nanoparticle tags. Nat Biotechnol 2008; 26(1):83–90; [Epub 2007, Dec 23].

63. Keren S, Zavaleta C, Cheng Z, et al. Noninvasive Molecular Imaging of Small Living Subjects Using Raman Spectroscopy and Raman Nanoparticles. In: Joint AMI/SMI Molecular Imaging Conference. Providence, RI: 2007.

64. Zavaleta C, Keren S, Cheng Z, et al. Use of Non-invasive Raman Spectroscopy Imaging in Living Mice for Evaluation of Tumor Targeting with Carbon Nanotubes. In: Joint AMI/SMI Molecular Imaging Conference; 2007 September 8–11, 2007; Providence, RI: 2007.

65. Rojas-Chapana JA, Giersig M. Multi-walled carbon nanotubes and metallic nanoparticles and their application in biomedicine. J Nanosci Nanotechnol 2006; 6(2):316–321.

66. Dai H. Carbon nanotubes: synthesis, integration, and properties. Acc Chem Res 2002; 35(12):1035–1044.

67. Yang R, Yang X, Zhang Z, et al. Single-walled carbon nanotubes-mediated in vivo and in vitro delivery of siRNA into antigen-presenting cells. Gene Ther 2006; 13(24):1714–1723.

68. Worle-Knirsch JM, Pulskamp K, Krug HF. Oops they did it again! Carbon nanotubes hoax scientists in viability assays. Nano Lett 2006; 6(6):1261–1268.

69. Singh R, Pantarotto D, Lacerda L, et al. Tissue biodistribution and blood clearance rates of intravenously administered carbon nanotube radiotracers. Proc Natl Acad Sci U S A 2006; 103(9):3357–3362.

70. Cherukuri P, Gannon CJ, Leeuw TK, et al. Mammalian pharmacokinetics of carbon nanotubes using intrinsic near-infrared fluorescence. Proc Natl Acad Sci U S A 2006; 103(50):18882–18886.

71. Liu Y, Cai W, He L, et al. In vivo biodistribution and highly efficient tumour targeting of carbon nanotubes in mice. Nat Nanotechnol 2007; 2(1):47–52.

72. Sinha N, Yeow JT. Carbon nanotubes for biomedical applications. IEEE Trans Nanobioscience 2005; 4(2): 180–195.

73. Bianco A, Kostarelos K, Partidos CD, et al. Biomedical applications of functionalised carbon nanotubes. Chem Commun (Camb) 2005; (5):571–577.

74. Chen J, Hamon MA, Hu H, et al. Solution properties of single-walled carbon nanotubes. Science 1998; 282(5386): 95–98.

75. Kam NW, Liu Z, Dai H. Functionalization of carbon nanotubes via cleavable disulfide bonds for efficient intra-cellular delivery of siRNA and potent gene silencing. J Am Chem Soc 2005; 127(36):12492–12493.

76. Kam NW, Dai H. Carbon nanotubes as intracellular protein transporters: generality and biological functionality. J Am Chem Soc 2005; 127(16):6021–6026.

77. Kamaras K, Itkis ME, Hu H, et al. Covalent bond formation to a carbon nanotube metal. Science 2003; 301(5639): 1501.

78. Zhang G, Qi P, Wang X, et al. Hydrogenation and hydrocarbonation and etching of single-walled carbon nanotubes. J Am Chem Soc 2006; 128(18):6026–6027.

79. Tasis D, Tagmatarchis N, Bianco A, et al. Chemistry of carbon nanotubes. Chem Rev 2006; 106(3):1105–1136.

80. Dyke CA, Tour JM. Covalent functionalization of single-walled carbon nanotubes for materials applications. J Phys Chem A 2004; 108(51):11151–11159.

81. Sayes CM, Liang F, Hudson JL, et al. Functionalization density dependence of single-walled carbon nanotubes cytotoxicity in vitro. Toxicol Lett 2006; 161(2):135–142.

82. Lacerda L, Bianco A, Prato M, et al. Carbon nanotubes as nanomedicines: from toxicology to pharmacology. Adv Drug Deliv Rev 2006; 58(14):1460–1470.

83. Wang H, Wang J, Deng X, et al. Biodistribution of carbon single-wall carbon nanotubes in mice. J Nanosci Nanotechnol 2004; 4(8):1019–1024.

84. Carrero-Sanchez JC, Elias AL, Mancilla R, et al. Biocompatibility and toxicological studies of carbon nanotubes doped with nitrogen. Nano Lett 2006; 6(8):1609–1616.

85. Lam C-W, James JT, McCluskey R, et al. Pulmonary toxicity of single-wall carbon nanotubes in mice 7 and

90 days after intratracheal instillation. Toxicol Sci 2004; 77(1):126–134; [Epub 2003, Sep 26].

86. Warheit DB, Laurence BR, Reed KL, et al. Comparative pulmonary toxicity assessment of single-wall carbon nanotubes in Rats. Toxicol Sci 2004; 77(1):117–125; [Epub 2003, Sep 26].

87. Radomski A, Jurasz P, Alonso-Escolano D, et al. Nanoparticle-induced platelet aggregation and vascular thrombosis. Br J Pharmacol 2005; 146(6):882–893.

88. Sato Y, Yokoyama A, Shibata K, et al. Influence of length on cytotoxicity of multi-walled carbon nanotubes against human acute monocytic leukemia cell line THP-1 in vitro and subcutaneous tissue of rats in vivo. Mol Biosyst 2005; 1(2):176–182.

89. Liu Y, Wang H. Nanomedicine: nanotechnology tackles tumours. Nat Nanotechnol 2007; 2(1):20–21.

90. Kam NW, O'Connell M, Wisdom JA, et al. Carbon nanotubes as multifunctional biological transporters and near-infrared agents for selective cancer cell destruction. Proc Natl Acad Sci U S A 2005; 102(33):11600–11605.

91. Gannon CJ, Cherukuri P, Yakobson BI, et al. Carbon nanotube-enhanced thermal destruction of cancer cells in a noninvasive radiofrequency field. Cancer 2007; 110(12): 2654–2665.

92. McDevitt MR, Chattopadhyay D, Jaggi JS, et al. PET imaging of soluble yttrium-86-labeled carbon nanotubes in mice. PLoS ONE 2007; 2(9):e907.

93. Sitharaman B, Kissell KR, Hartman KB, et al. Superparamagnetic gadonanotubes are high-performance MRI contrast agents. Chem Commun (Camb) 2005; (31): 3915–3917.

94. Sitharaman B, Wilson LJ. Gadonanotubes as new high-performance MRI contrast agents. Int J Nanomedicine 2006; 1(3):291–295.

95. Cuenca AG, Jiang H, Hochwald SN, et al. Emerging implications of nanotechnology on cancer diagnostics and therapeutics. Cancer 2006; 107(3):459–466.

96. Hirsch LR, Gobin AM, Lowery AR, et al. Metal nanoshells. Ann Biomed Eng 2006; 34(1):15–22.

97. Gobin AM, Lee MH, Halas NJ, et al. Near-infrared resonant nanoshells for combined optical imaging and photothermal cancer therapy. Nano Lett 2007; 7(7):1929–1934.

98. Hirsch LR, Stafford RJ, Bankson JA, et al. Nanoshell-mediated near-infrared thermal therapy of tumors under magnetic resonance guidance. Proc Natl Acad Sci U S A 2003; 100(23):13549–13554.

99. O'Neal DP, Hirsch LR, Halas NJ, et al. Photo-thermal tumor ablation in mice using near infrared-absorbing nanoparticles. Cancer Lett 2004; 209(2):171–176.

100. Wang X, Ku G, Wegiel MA, et al. Noninvasive photoacoustic angiography of animal brains in vivo with near-infrared light and an optical contrast agent. Opt Lett 2004; 29(7):730–732.

101. Wang Y, Xie X, Wang X, et al. Photoacoustic tomography of a nanoshell contrast agent in the in vivo Rat Brain. Nano Lett 2004; 4(9):1689–1692.

102. Xiang L, Da X, Gu H, et al. Gold Nanoshell-Based Photoacoustic Imaging Application in Biomedicine: Biophotonics, Nanophotonics and Metamaterials. Meta-

materials 2006. An International Symposium, Hangzhou, China, October 16–19, 2006. New York: IEEE; 2006: 76–79.

103. Loo C, Lin A, Hirsch L, et al. Nanoshell-enabled photonics-based imaging and therapy of cancer. Technol Cancer Res Treat 2004; 3(1):33–40.

104. Li Meng-Lin, Schwartz JA, Wang J, et al. In-vivo imaging of nanoshell extravasation from solid tumor vasculature by photoacoustic microscopy. In: Oraevsky AA, Wang LV, eds. Photons Plus Ultrasound: Imaging and Sensing 2007: The Eighth Conference on Biomedical Thermoacoustics, Optoacoustics, and Acousto-optics. Proceedings of the SPIE. Vol 6437, Bellingham, WA: SPIE; 2007:64370B.

105. Bernardi RJ, Lowery AR, Thompson PA, et al. Immunonanoshells for targeted photothermal ablation in medulloblastoma and glioma: an in vitro evaluation using human cell lines. J Neurooncol 2008; 86(2):165–172.

106. Stern JM, Stanfield J, Lotan Y, et al. Efficacy of laser-activated gold nanoshells in ablating prostate cancer cells in vitro. J Endourol 2007; 21(8):939–943.

107. Stark DD, Weissleder R, Elizondo G, et al. Superparamagnetic iron oxide: clinical application as a contrast agent for MR imaging of the liver. Radiology 1988; 168(2): 297–301.

108. Seo WS, Lee JH, Sun X, et al. FeCo/graphitic-shell nanocrystals as advanced magnetic-resonance-imaging and near-infrared agents. Nat Mater 2006; 5(12):971–976.

109. Su CH, Sheu HS, Lin CY, et al. Nanoshell magnetic resonance imaging contrast agents. J Am Chem Soc 2007; 129(7):2139–2146.

110. Kumagai M, Imai Y, Nakamura T, et al. Iron hydroxide nanoparticles coated with poly(ethylene glycol)-poly (aspartic acid) block copolymer as novel magnetic resonance contrast agents for in vivo cancer imaging. Colloids Surf, B 2007.

111. Lu AH, Salabas EL, Schuth F. Magnetic nanoparticles: synthesis, protection, functionalization, and application. Angew Chem Int Ed Engl 2007; 46(8):1222–1244.

112. Koyama Y, Talanov VS, Bernardo M, et al. A dendrimer-based nanosized contrast agent dual-labeled for magnetic resonance and optical fluorescence imaging to localize the sentinel lymph node in mice. J Magn Reson Imaging 2007; 25(4):866–871.

113. Liu Y, Miyoshi H, Nakamura M. Nanomedicine for drug delivery and imaging: a promising avenue for cancer therapy and diagnosis using targeted functional nanoparticles. Int J Cancer 2007; 120(12):2527–2537.

114. Thrall JH. Nanotechnology and medicine. Radiology 2004; 230(2):315–318.

115. Yuan F, Dellian M, Fukumura D, et al. Vascular permeability in a human tumor xenograft: molecular size dependence and cutoff size. Cancer Res 1995; 55(17):3752–3756.

116. Qin G, Zhang Y, Cao W, et al. Molecular imaging of atherosclerotic plaques with technetium-99m-labelled antisense oligonucleotides. Eur J Nucl Med Mol Imaging 2005; 32(1):6–14.

117. Smith BR, Heverhagen J, Knopp M, et al. Localization to atherosclerotic plaque and biodistribution of biochemically

derivatized superparamagnetic iron oxide nanoparticles (SPIONs) contrast particles for magnetic resonance imaging (MRI). Biomed Microdevices 2007; 9(5):719–727.

118. Sosnovik DE, Weissleder R. Emerging concepts in molecular MRI. Curr Opin Biotechnol 2007; 18(1):4–10.

119. Hu G, Lijowski M, Zhang H, et al. Imaging of Vx-2 rabbit tumors with alpha(nu)beta(3)-integrin-targeted (111)In nanoparticles. Int J Cancer 2007; 120(9):1951–1957.

120. Baio G, Fabbi M, de Totero D, et al. Magnetic resonance imaging at 1.5 T with immunospecific contrast agent in vitro and in vivo in a xenotransplant model. MAGMA 2006; 19(6):313–320.

121. Jander S, Schroeter M, Saleh A. Imaging inflammation in acute brain ischemia. Stroke 2007; 38(2 suppl):642–645.

122. Saksena MA, Saokar A, Harisinghani MG. Lymphotropic nanoparticle enhanced MR imaging (LNMRI) technique for lymph node imaging. Eur J Radiol 2006; 58(3):367–374.

123. Heesakkers RA, Futterer JJ, Hovels AM, et al. Prostate cancer evaluated with ferumoxtran-10-enhanced T2*-weighted MR Imaging at 1.5 and 3.0 T: early experience. Radiology 2006; 239(2):481–487.

124. Aguirre DA, Behling CA, Alpert E, et al. Liver fibrosis: noninvasive diagnosis with double contrast material-enhanced MR imaging. Radiology 2006; 239(2):425–437.

125. Harisinghani MG, Barentsz J, Hahn PF, et al. Noninvasive detection of clinically occult lymph-node metastases in prostate cancer. N Engl J Med 2003; 348(25):2491–2499.

126. Cerdan S, Lotscher HR, Kunnecke B, et al. Monoclonal antibody-coated magnetite particles as contrast agents in magnetic resonance imaging of tumors. Magn Reson Med 1989; 12(2):151–163.

127. Reimer P, Weissleder R, Lee AS, et al. Receptor imaging: application to MR imaging of liver cancer. Radiology 1990; 177(3):729–734.

128. Lee JH, Huh YM, Jun YW, et al. Artificially engineered magnetic nanoparticles for ultra-sensitive molecular imaging. Nat Med 2007; 13(1):95–99.

129. Sharkey RM, Cardillo TM, Rossi EA, et al. Signal amplification in molecular imaging by pretargeting a multivalent, bispecific antibody. Nat Med 2005; 11(11):1250–1255.

130. Towner RA, Smith N, Tesiram YA, et al. In vivo detection of c-MET expression in a rat hepatocarcinogenesis model using molecularly targeted magnetic resonance imaging. Mol Imaging 2007; 6(1):18–29.

131. Zhang C, Jugold M, Woenne EC, et al. Specific targeting of tumor angiogenesis by RGD-conjugated ultrasmall superparamagnetic iron oxide particles using a clinical 1.5-T magnetic resonance scanner. Cancer Res 2007; 67(4):1555–1562.

132. Zhao M, Beauregard DA, Loizou L, et al. Non-invasive detection of apoptosis using magnetic resonance imaging and a targeted contrast agent. Nat Med 2001; 7(11):1241–1244.

133. Liu CH, Huang S, Cui J, et al. MR contrast probes that trace gene transcripts for cerebral ischemia in live animals. Faseb J 2007; 21(11):3004–3015; [Epub 2007, May 3].

134. Verdijk P, Scheenen TW, Lesterhuis WJ, et al. Sensitivity of magnetic resonance imaging of dendritic cells for in vivo tracking of cellular cancer vaccines. Int J Cancer 2007; 120(5):978–984.

135. Daldrup-Link HE, Meier R, Rudelius M, et al. In vivo tracking of genetically engineered, anti-HER2/neu directed natural killer cells to HER2/neu positive mammary tumors with magnetic resonance imaging. Eur Radiol 2005; 15(1):4–13.

136. Frank JA, Anderson SA, Kalsih H, et al. Methods for magnetically labeling stem and other cells for detection by in vivo magnetic resonance imaging. Cytotherapy 2004; 6(6):621–625.

137. Medarova Z, Pham W, Farrar C, et al. In vivo imaging of siRNA delivery and silencing in tumors. Nat Med 2007; 13(3):372–377.

138. Medarova Z, Pham W, Kim Y, et al. In vivo imaging of tumor response to therapy using a dual-modality imaging strategy. Int J Cancer 2006; 118(11):2796–2802.

139. Goldin DS, Dahl CA, Olsen KL, et al. Biomedicine. The NASA-NCI collaboration on biomolecular sensors. Science 2001; 292(5516):443–444.

140. Galindo-Rodriguez SA, Allemann E, Fessi H, et al. Polymeric nanoparticles for oral delivery of drugs and vaccines: a critical evaluation of in vivo studies. Crit Rev Ther Drug Carrier Syst 2005; 22(5):419–464.

141. Emerich DF, Thanos CG. The pinpoint promise of nanoparticle-based drug delivery and molecular diagnosis. Biomol Eng 2006; 23(4):171–184.

142. Wunderbaldinger P, Josephson L, Weissleder R. Tat peptide directs enhanced clearance and hepatic permeability of magnetic nanoparticles. Bioconjug Chem 2002; 13(2):264–268.

143. Medina C, Santos-Martinez MJ, Radomski A, et al. Nanoparticles: pharmacological and toxicological significance. Br J Pharmacol 2007; 150(5):552–558.

144. Nel A, Xia T, Madler L, et al. Toxic potential of materials at the nanolevel. Science 2006; 311(5761):622–627.

145. Socinski M. Update on nanoparticle albumin-bound paclitaxel. Clin Adv Hematol Oncol 2006; 4(10):745–746.

146. Stinchcombe TE, Socinski MA, Walko CM, et al. Phase I and pharmacokinetic trial of carboplatin and albumin-bound paclitaxel, ABI-007 (Abraxane) on three treatment schedules in patients with solid tumors. Cancer Chemother Pharmacol 2007; 60(5):759–766.

147. Choi JY, Kim MJ, Kim JH, et al. Detection of hepatic metastasis: manganese- and ferucarbotran-enhanced MR imaging. Eur J Radiol 2006; 60(1):84–90.

148. Savranoglu P, Obuz F, Karasu S, et al. The role of SPIO-enhanced MRI in the detection of malignant liver lesions. Clin Imaging 2006; 30(6):377–381.

18

Long Lived and Unconventional PET Radionuclides

JASON S. LEWIS

Department of Radiology, Memorial-Sloan Kettering Cancer Center, New York, New York, U.S.A.

RAJENDRA K. SINGH and MICHAEL J. WELCH

Department of Radiology, Washington University School of Medicine, St. Louis, Missouri, U.S.A.

INTRODUCTION

Positron emission tomography (PET) is a fundamental component in the field of molecular imaging. The inherent quantitative nature of PET combined with the high sensitivity of the instrumentation makes this imaging modality ideal for many clinical applications. PET, in general, relies on the radionuclides ^{11}C, ^{13}N, ^{15}O, and ^{18}F for labeling to targeting molecules. These nuclides are often considered the more "traditional" PET nuclides but are limited by their short radioactive half-lives, often requiring in-house production. In 2003, a comprehensive review of the chemistry and production methods for these radionuclides was published as part of *The Handbook of Radiopharmaceuticals*, which contains chapters describing the chemistry of ^{13}N, ^{15}O, and ^{18}F as well as extensive chapters on the synthesis of radiolabeled compounds of ^{11}C and ^{18}F (1). Another book *PET Chemistry: the Driving Force in Molecular Imaging* also contains extensive discussion on ^{18}F production, chemistry, and radiopharmaceuticals as well as chapters on ^{11}C, ^{68}Ga, and nonstandard nuclide production (2). The focus of this chapter will be on the "nonstandard" PET radionuclides (Table 1). Most of the nuclides being discussed have radioactive half-lives > 2 hours, and have <90% positron emission.

They can all be produced on small cyclotrons (Fig. 1) (3), and their improved dissemination is generating increased interest within the medical imaging research community. Although not every PET imaging site has accessibility to an in-house cyclotron, with the half-lives of most of the nuclides under discussion being relatively long (>2 h), networks of production sites could be setup (Fig. 1A) and could be the foundation for a reliable and convenient network supplying these PET nuclides to clinical PET centers.

The selection of the appropriate PET nuclide for an agent is essential to achieve adequate contrast between target tissue and normal tissue activity levels. This must be achieved in a time frame compatible with the physical half-life of the radionuclide. The half-life of the radionuclide, the energy of the radioactive emissions, and the cost and the general availability of the nuclide must all be considered prior to application. In many instances, biomolecules require longer circulation times than small molecules, and therefore longer-lived PET nuclides are required to achieve the highest target to background ratios. This chapter will discuss, in brief, a series of nonstandard PET nuclides with a range of half-lives and nuclear properties that had been receiving wider attention by the PET community in the last few years (4). This chapter is by no means an exhaustive review of the nonstandard nuclide literature, but it will

Table 1 Decay Characteristics of the Nonstandard Positron-Emitting Nuclides

Isotope	$T_{1/2}$	Decay mode (branching ratio percentage)	β_{max} (MeV)	β_{mean} (MeV)	Main γ (abundance percentage)
^{60}Cu	23.7 min	β^+ (93) EC (7)	3.92	0.98	0.511 (185.2) 0.826 (21.7) 1.333 (88.0) 1.791 (45.4)
^{61}Cu	3.33 hr	β^+ (60) EC (40)	1.22	0.50	0.283 (12.2) 0.511 (122.9) 0.656 (10.8)
^{64}Cu	12.7 hr	β^+ (19) β^- (38) EC (43)	0.66 0.57	0.28 0.19	0.511 (34.8) 1.346 (0.47)
^{66}Ga	9.49 hr	β^+ (57) EC (43)	4.15	1.74	0.511 (112.0) 1.039 (36.9) 2.752 (23.3)
^{71}As	65.3 hr	β^+ (30) EC (70)	0.81	0.35	0.175 (90.0) 0.511 (60.0)
^{72}As	26.0 hr	β^+ (88) EC (12)	3.34	1.17	0.511 (150.0) 0.835 (78.0)
^{74}As	17.8 days	β^+ (29) β^- (32) EC (39)	1.36	0.44	0.511 (59.0) 0.596 (61.0) 0.635 (14.0)
^{76}Br	16.2 hr	β^+ (67) EC (33)	3.60	1.18	0.511 (109.5) 0.559 (74.0) 0.657 (15.9) 1.854 (14.7)
^{86}Y	14.7 hr	β^+ (26) EC (74)	3.15	0.66	0.443 (16.9) 0.511 (63.9) 0.627 (32.6) 0.777 (22.4) 1.077 (82.5) 1.115 (30.5) 1.921 (20.8)
^{89}Zr	78.4 hr	β^+ (22) EC (78)	0.90		0.511 (44.0) 0.91 (99.0)
^{94m}Tc	52.0 min	β^+ (72) EC (28)	2.47	1.07	0.511 (140.4) 0.871 (94.2)
^{124}I	4.18 days	β^+ (26) EC (74)	2.14	0.82	0.511 (45.9) 0.603 (62.9) 0.723 (10.4)

Source: From Ref. 92.

focus on the most common methods of *production and purification* with an overall focus on the practical aspects of their eventual use in clinical applications. The reader is directed to other reviews that discuss the *application* of these nuclides in greater detail (1,3–7).

COPPER-60, COPPER-61, AND COPPER-64

The copper PET nuclides (^{60}Cu, ^{61}Cu, ^{62}Cu, and ^{64}Cu) have been extensively studied because of their range of decay schemes allowing for versatile and selective use of the

copper nuclide depending on the application (1,5). Among all the copper PET nuclides, ^{64}Cu, with a half-life of 12.7 hours, is ideally suited for PET studies that can be conducted over 2 to 3 days. Copper-64 decays 19% by positron emission and has a β^+ maximum energy of 0.66 MeV with an average energy of 0.28 MeV. It also decays by electron capture (38%) and β^- (43%) and has therefore been studied as both a diagnostic and a therapeutic radionuclide (5). Since ^{64}Cu has a β^+ maximum energy of 0.66 MeV, which is almost identical in energy to the most widely used PET nuclide ^{18}F, which has a β^+ maximum energy of 0.63 MeV, the resulting PET images are of very good quality (Fig. 2)

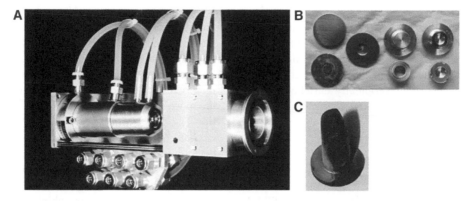

Figure 1 (**A**) Target holder designed for use on the Cyclotron Corporation CS-15 cyclotron at Washington University School of Medicine. This technology can be adapted to fit to multiple types of small cyclotrons and can be used for the production of all of the nonstandard radionuclides. (**B**) Targets that can be prepared for irradiation, a target on which the target material has been electroplated (left), and targets where the material is in a powder or foil form. (**C**) A high-powered slanted target designed for the production of ^{76}Br and ^{124}I.

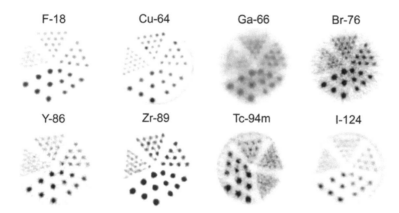

Figure 2 A mini Derenzo phantom filled with various radionuclides imaged on a microPET focus scanner (Siemens Medical Systems). This phantom consists of radioactive rods of specified diameter (1.0, 1.25, 1.5, 2.0, and 2.5 mm) separated by a distance four times the diameter. These images were reconstructed utilizing the filtered back projection. It is seen that the nuclides with higher-energy positrons and prompt gamma rays produce images that are degraded compared to those with a single low-energy positron (for example, ^{64}Cu and ^{18}F) (23). It is important to note that although this degradation is noted with small-animal PET scanners with high resolution (1–2 mm), it is often not seen with clinical scanners with 4- to 5-mm resolution. New reconstruction algorithms can also be used to enhance image quality (81). *Abbreviation*: PET, positron emission tomography.

(8). The use of ^{64}Cu has dramatically increased in the past decade and its production has now been reported by academic sources in the United States (9,10), Europe (11,12), and Japan (13). A number of commercial sources are also producing and supplying ^{64}Cu in North America (e.g., MDS Nordion and Trace Radiochemical Life Sciences) and Europe (e.g., ACOM, Italy).

The most common production method for ^{64}Cu utilizes the ^{64}Ni$(p,n)^{64}$Cu reaction (9,11,13–15). The irradiation of the target material normally involves bombardment of enriched ^{64}Ni, which has been electroplated on a gold (9,10,13,14,16) or rhodium platform (12). Yields of ^{64}Cu on small cyclotrons have varied, for example, McCarthy et al. reported production runs using 19 to 55 mg of 95% enriched Ni-64, which have yielded 150 to 600 mCi of

^{64}Cu (2.3–5.0 mCi/μAh) in high specific activity (9). This same methodology can be used to produce ^{61}Cu and ^{60}Cu from the corresponding enriched nickel targets (16). Obata et al. reported yields of 0.6 to >3.0 mCi/μAh, averaging 1.983 mCi/μAh with a radionuclidic purity of over 99% using a 12-MeV cyclotron (13). Using a tangential target on the National Institutes of Health (NIH) CS-30 cyclotron, Szajek et al. reported yields of 10.5 ± 3 mCi/μAh when bombarded with a 12.5-MeV proton beam, which was comparable to the theoretical yield and over three hours produced >1 Ci of radioactivity (10).

Multiple methods are available for the separation of radiocopper from enriched nickel. These include precipitation, solvent extraction, and electroplating. However, ion chromatography is the most effective method of isolating high-purity no-carrier-added radionuclide. Anion exchange chromatography has been the most widely used method of ion exchange separation (9,11,14–16) resulting in high specific activity ^{64}Cu, but the use of cation exchange methods has been reported (17). Separation of the ^{64}Cu from the expensive isotopically enriched nickel results in the ability to recycle the target material, which in turn dramatically reduces costs.

GALLIUM-66

Gallium-66 [$t_{1/2}$ = 9.49 hr; β^+ (57%), electron capture (EC) (43%)] can be used as a substitute for the photon emitter ^{67}Ga commonly used in single photon emission computed tomography (SPECT) imaging. Gallium-66 does, however, emit high-energy positrons (up to 4.15 MeV) and prompt high-energy gamma rays (up to 4 MeV), which can degrade the quality of the PET image (Fig. 2), but it still produces higher image quality than is available with ^{67}Ga-SPECT (18,19). Gallium-66 can be used for the labeling proteins, peptides, and small molecules allowing gallium radiopharmaceuticals intermediate to long biological half-lives to be used for PET imaging (19–21). For example, Goethals et al. have labeled an antimyosin monoclonal antibody with ^{66}Ga (19), and Jalilian et al. have labeled bleomycin (22), circumventing the PET imaging limitations of ^{68}Ga, which has a 68-minute half-life. A publication by Ugur et al. has also shown the feasibility of ^{66}Ga for both PET imaging and radiotherapy (20) since the ^{66}Ga decay process results in both β^+ emission and electron capture, suggesting a potential application in the targeted radiotherapy of cancer.

Gallium-66 production can be achieved by the proton irradiation of zinc targets on small cyclotrons. Yields of ^{66}Ga from both natural and enriched ^{66}Zn targets [^{nat}Zn(p,n)^{66}Ga and ^{66}Zn(p,n)^{66}Ga] were compared with theoretical values, and radionuclidic purity was determined for ^{66}Ga produced on ^{nat}Zn versus ^{66}Zn (23). Gallium-66 was produced by the irradiation of natural Zn (27.8% ^{66}Zn, 48.9% ^{64}Zn, 4.1% ^{67}Zn, 18.6% ^{68}Zn, 0.6% ^{70}Zn) and enriched ^{66}Zn (98.92% ^{66}Zn, 0.66% ^{64}Zn, 0.19% ^{67}Zn, 0.23% ^{68}Zn, <0.03% ^{70}Zn) foils, using a Cyclotron Corporation CS-15 cyclotron. These foils provided a highly uniform target of known thickness with which to compare measured yields of ^{66}Ga with theoretical predictions (23). Agreement between predicted and observed yields was excellent at an incident proton energy of 14.5 MeV. The observed rate of production of ^{66}Ga on the enriched ^{66}Zn foil was 13.8 mCi/µAh, a value that was within 5% of the predicted yield. Using the natural zinc foil, the observed ^{66}Ga production rate was 3.7 mCi/µAh. When extrapolated to 100% target enrichment, the measured yield of

^{66}Ga on ^{nat}Zn was within 1% of the predicted value. These values are similar to those obtained by Jalilian et al., where bombardment of ^{66}Zn with 15-MeV protons at 180 µA resulted in a yield of 11.2 mCi/µAh (22).

The quality of ^{66}Ga obtained by the cation exchange method (23) was compared with that of ^{66}Ga processed by the more conventional method of diisopropyl ether extraction (24,25). Cumulative processing time for the cation exchange method is approximately three hours, and decay-corrected recovery of ^{66}Ga ranged from 33% to 90%. However, it was shown that the contaminants, namely iron and zinc, were an order of magnitude higher following cation exchange, which subsequently resulted in higher labeled yields with the ^{66}Ga purified by the diisopropyl ether extraction method (23).

ARSENIC-71, ARSENIC-72, AND ARSENIC-74

There are a myriad of arsenic nuclides of which some are attractive positron-emitting nuclides, namely, ^{71}As, ^{72}As, and ^{74}As. Arsenic-71 has a half-life of 2.7 days (EC 70%, β^+ 30%, $E_{\beta^+ mean}$ = 350 keV), arsenic-72 has a half-life of 1.1 days (EC 12%, β^+ 88%, $E_{\beta^+ mean}$ = 1.17 MeV), and arsenic-74 has a half-life of 17.8 days (EC 32%, β^+ 29%, $E_{\beta^+ mean}$ = 440 keV). With the low positron energy of ^{74}As, PET images with a resolution similar to ^{18}F are achievable, whereas ^{72}As with the higher energy is likely to degrade the image quality to levels similar to ^{124}I (26). Although a limited amount of work has been undertaken with the arsenic PET nuclides to date, interest lies in their clinical application, not only in their use as long-lived nuclides for labeling biomolecules, but also in the fact that arsenic compounds are used as chemotherapeutic agents, for example, arsenic trioxide for the treatment of promyelocytic leukemia (27).

Arsenic-72 and ^{74}As, because of their decay properties, are the most likely arsenic nuclides to be utilized in clinical PET imaging. Arsenic-72 is available from a generator reaction ^{70}Ge($\alpha,2n$)^{72}Se→^{72}As (28,29) and can also be produced directly in high yields via the ^{72}Ge(p,n)^{72}As reaction on small biomedical cyclotrons (30). The most convenient method of production of ^{74}As utilizes either ^{74}Ge(p,n)^{74}As or ^{73}Ge(d,n)^{74}As nuclear reaction on small cyclotrons (30). The work by Jennewein et al. describes the most convenient method of arsenic nuclide production by the irradiation of enriched germanium oxide followed by dissolving the target in concentrated hydrofluoric acid and using a polystyrene-based solid-phase extraction method to isolate [*GeF$_6$]$^{2-}$ for recycling. The remaining solution can then be converted to the reactive As synthon *As[AsI$_3$] by adding potassium iodide (26).

BROMINE-76 AND IODINE-124

The applications of positron-emitting halogen nuclides in PET oncology have significantly increased over the last decade, and an exhaustive review on this subject was published in 2003 (1,7). ^{76}Br has been reported as a nuclide for the labeling of small molecules targeted toward σ_2 receptors (31) and PPARγ antagonists (32) and in the form of ^{76}Br-FBAU for imaging gene expression and proliferation (33–35). The half-life of ^{76}Br is 16.2 hours and it decays via positron emission 55% of the time. Bromine-76 does have some high-energy emitted positrons, however, only a minor increase in spatial resolution has been noted on comparison with ^{18}F (36). The ^{76}Se$(p,n)^{76}$Br is the nuclear reaction that is often used to produce ^{76}Br on small cyclotrons. This same reaction can be used to produce the therapeutic bromine nuclide ^{77}Br from enriched ^{77}Se. In general, the target material Cu$_2$Se is used, which is enriched in both copper (^{63}Cu) and selenium (^{76}Se). The synthesis of this target material requires stoichiometric quantities of Cu and Se (2:1) to be mixed in a quartz ampoule. The quartz is then sealed under vacuum and taken through a series of heating steps. This method was developed by Tolmachev et al., who exploited the ^{76}Se$(p,n)^{76}$Br reaction and on a 180 mg/cm^3 target with 16→8 MeV protons produced ^{76}Br in a yield of 1.75 to 1.89 mCi/μAh (37). Szajek et al. exploited a different reaction, namely, As(^{3}He,2n) on the NIH CS-30 cyclotron and a 19.8-MeV ^{3}He beam at 20 μA for six hours on high-purity naturally abundant arsenic targets. This method of production produced 32 ± 7 mCi at end of bombardment in 50 preparations of the nuclide. The ^{76}Br, in the form of [^{76}Br]NH$_4$Br, was usable for the synthesis of bromine radiopharmaceuticals, including [^{76}Br]FBAU, in high specific activity (33,34,38). In 2000 Forngren et al. reported a straightforward liquid chromatography-mass spectroscopy method for determining the specific activity of ^{86}Br-labeled agents, which is particularly important in the design and eventual application of brominated agents targeted at receptor-based systems (39).

Iodine-124 has a half-life of 4.18 days and decays by 26% positron emission and has already found a niche in oncological PET imaging (7,40,41). The positron emissions of ^{124}I are of relatively high energy (Table 1) and are accompanied by many high-energy gamma rays, however, it has been shown that quantitative PET imaging is possible with clinical PET scanners (40). Iodine-124 is conveniently produced by the cyclotron bombardment of ^{124}Te$(p,n)^{124}$I (42), where the target material is enriched [^{124}Te]TeO$_2$ (6,43–45). For example, using these methods Glaser et al. reported thick target yields of 0.24 mCi/μAh with over 90% recovery efficiencies from a [^{124}Te]TeO$_2$ target (6). Nye et al. produced ^{124}I on an 11-MeV cyclotron, using a glassy [^{124}Te]TeO$_2$ target that had been

doped with 6% Al$_2$O$_3$. The same group improved on these results with an Al$_2$Te$_3$ binary alloy, which showed good yields (0.23 mCi/μAh) and led to over 95% recovery of the ^{124}I from the target substrate (46). Qaim et al. also used a [^{124}Te]TeO$_2$ target that had been doped with 5% Al$_2$O$_3$. Sixteen-MeV proton beam intensities of 10 μA for eight hours yielded an average of 12.7 mCi of ^{124}I (0.16 mCi/μAh) (44).

There is often an inherently low production rate for some of the linear type of targets described above, so an alternative inclined target design has been employed to allow higher beam currents (Fig. 1C). This concept has been applied to ^{76}Br production using a ^{76}Se target (47) and ^{124}I production from TeO$_2$ (45,48,49). Since the target is slanted, the beam is spread over a greater surface area leading to a greater dissipation of heat. In addition, with a thinner layer of material, heat may be better dissipated into the tungsten, while the same effective target thickness is achieved. At the same time, these features allow for higher beam currents. This inclined target method has been tested up to 20 μA without degradation of the target (49).

Separation of the halogens from the target matrix has been performed by dry distillation using either a conventional oven (37,44,48,49) or an induction furnace (50). A review of the distillation methods and a report of an improved system was described by Glaser et al. in 2004 (6). The dry distillation method allows for multiple irradiations before the target needs replenishing with more Cu$_2$Se or Cu$_2$Te. The induction furnace apparatus consists of an upright bell-shaped quartz tube that is placed over the target, sealed and flushed with argon gas. A coil encircles the quartz tube and generates an radio frequency signal that is picked up by the tungsten disk. An electrical current is induced in the target, and the electrical resistance leads to the heating of the target. For the Cu$_2$Se target, typically high-frequency 115 VAC is applied to the coil. The approximate temperature of the target material is determined with an infrared detector. As stated above, Szajek et al. have reported the production of ^{76}Br by utilizing As(^{3}He,2n)^{76}Br reaction, and the isolation of the ^{76}Br in this study was done by chromic acid oxidation followed by distillation of hydrogen bromide using a semi-remote apparatus (34).

YTTRIUM-86

Yttrium-90 has been used extensively in nuclear medicine as a therapeutic isotope. In order to assess the biodistribution and absorbed dose for ^{90}Y, the positron-emitting isotope ^{86}Y can be used as a surrogate or the basis for yttrium-based imaging agents (51–60). It has a relatively long half-life, 14.7 hours, compared to the standard PET nuclides and has considerable positron intensity at 26%. The maximum energy of the positron is quite high, 3.15 MeV, which leads to degradation in image resolution (Fig. 1). The mean energy of the positrons is however much lower at 0.66 MeV resulting in less image degradation than what one would expect after knowing the maximum energy.

Yttrium-86 can be produced on small biomedical cyclotrons via the $^{86}Sr(p,n)^{86}Y$ reaction (61) using an enriched $^{86}SrCO_3$ (57,62–67) or ^{86}SrO target (58). It was shown that a ^{86}SrO target can withstand at least 6 μA of beam current, a significant improvement over a maximum of 2 μA on the traditional $^{86}SrCO_3$ target (58). The use of ^{86}SrO has several advantages over $^{86}SrCO_3$ as the target material: (i) It has a much higher thermal stability (mp 2430°C) than $^{86}SrCO_3$, which clearly decomposes at temperatures reached during irradiation; and (ii) ^{86}SrO has a strontium content per unit mass of 85%, while that of $^{86}SrCO_3$ is just 59%. Therefore, the same mass of target material gives a 40% higher theoretical yield of ^{86}Y for ^{86}SrO than for $^{86}SrCO_3$ (6.34 vs. 3.83 mCi/μAh). Using this target substrate, average yields of 4.5 mCi/μAh were achieved with ^{86}SrO, which represent 71% of the theoretical yield, compared to 2.3 mCi/μAh with $SrCO_3$ (58).

Yttrium-86 has been previously separated from target solutions by cation exchange chromatography followed by co-precipitation of ^{86}Y with La(III) (57) or Fe(III) (63). However, these methods are often multistep separations and require the addition of carrier, and so more efficient no-carrier-added ion exchange methods using a Sr/Y-selective resin have been reported (64,65). In 2002, Reischl et al. reported that simple electrolysis can provide high-purity ^{86}Y in a short time (62).

ZIRCONIUM-89

The radionuclide ^{89}Zr is an attractive target for further research for use in PET imaging because of its long half-life of 78.4 hours, which makes it ideal for the radiolabeling of slowly localizing antibodies (68). It has also been suggested as a surrogate for monitoring ^{90}Y- and ^{111}In-antibody distribution (69,70). It decays to ^{89}Y via positron emission (22% with a maximum energy of 0.90 MeV) and an accompanying 0.91 MeV γ emission (99.9% abundance) (71). The nuclide has been produced on biomedical cyclotrons from ^{89}Y (100% natural abundance) via the (p,n) reaction (72,73) or a $(d,2n)$ reaction (74). The reaction cross section has a maximum of 720 ± 79 mb at a bombardment energy of 12 MeV. Meijs et al. have reported that a 14-MeV proton bombardment at 100 μA for one hour produces 130 mCi of ^{89}Zr using a solid target of ^{89}Y sputtered onto a solid copper support (75). Yttrium foil has also been found to be a suitable target material (72,73).

In the past, the main difficulty has been in obtaining the ^{89}Zr in high enough chemical purity for efficient labeling of biomolecules. Link et al. dissolved the target foils in HCl and extracted the Zr(IV) into 4,4,4-trifluoro-1-(2-thienyl)-1,3-butanedione (TTA) in xylene followed by anion exchange chromatography, resulting in only a 25% recovery of the zirconium produced (73). Dejesus and Nickles utilized a similar isolation procedure, extracting the zirconium from a HCl solution with di-n-butyl phosphate in di-n-butyl ether, followed by anion exchange chromatography, with an overall recovery of zirconium of 87% (72). An improved isolation procedure was developed by Meijs et al., where the target was dissolved in HCl and the zirconium was isolated via an elution from a hydroxamate column, giving a 98% recovery of the zirconium (75).

As previously described, ^{89}Zr emits a positron with a maximum energy of 0.897 MeV; this is higher than the positron maximum of 0.64 MeV for ^{18}F but is significantly lower than that of equally long-lived positron emitter ^{124}I (positron maximum of 2.15 MeV) (Fig. 1). Data from a CTI HRRT PET scanner shows that ^{89}Zr behaves close to ^{18}F in terms of resolution (71).

TECHNETIUM-94m

^{99m}Tc is the most widely used SPECT radionuclide in nuclear medicine; ^{94m}Tc, with a half-life of 52 minutes, is a cyclotron-produced nuclide that can be used as an alternative to ^{99m}Tc but can also be used in quantitative PET imaging (72,76–79). The nuclear processes $^{94}Mo(p,n)$, $^{93}Nb(3He,2n)$, $^{92}Mo(\alpha,pn)$, and $^{92}Mo(\alpha,2n)^{94}Ru \rightarrow$ ^{94m}Tc can be used to produce ^{94m}Tc, but detailed cross section and yield measurements showed that the $^{94}Mo(p,n)$ reaction over the energy range Ep = 13 → 7 MeV is the most convenient method (80). The production of ^{94m}Tc from natural molybdenum on an 11-MeV cyclotron, with isolation using an electrochemical etching technique has been reported, but the use of natural molybdenum resulted in multiple Tc products (79). This report was the first to confirm the potential of ^{94m}Tc PET for quantitatively studying the pharmacokinetics of old and new Tc agents in humans. ^{94m}Tc has a positron branching ratio of 72% with a $E_{\beta^+ max}$ of 2.47 MeV. As such, the image quality (spatial resolution) of ^{94m}Tc on high-resolution animal scanners can degrade (Fig. 2), but this can be improved with new reconstruction techniques (81). This degradation is not significant on standard human PET cameras. The presence of other Tc nuclides, produced from the irradiation of both natural and enriched targets, can be corrected for, allowing for the routine use of ^{94m}Tc in quantitative PET (82,83).

Utilizing the $^{94}Mo(p,n)^{94m}Tc$ reaction Qaim reported a high yield of nuclide (54 mCi/μAh) (80) that was isolated in high purity when a convenient thermochromatographical separation of ^{94m}Tc from the enriched molybdenum was used (57). A wet chemistry separation procedure using a semi-automated apparatus has also been reported

Table 2 Reported Specific Activities of Nonstandard Nuclides Produced on Small Cyclotrons and Selected Radiopharmaceuticals.[a]

Radionuclide (theoretical specific activity)[b]	Radiochemical	Specific activity (Ci/μmol)	References
^{60}Cu	^{60}CuCl$_2$	4.8–18	16
^{61}Cu	^{61}CuCl$_2$	1.22–4.94	16
^{64}Cu (235.0 Ci/μmol)	^{64}CuCl$_2$	6.01–19.84	9
	^{64}CuCl$_2$	1.52–5.02	13
	^{64}CuCl$_2$	8.98 ± 3.20	10
	^{64}Cu-ATSM	0.001	10
	^{64}Cu-TETA-octreotide	1.75	8
	^{64}Cu-DOTA-ReCCMSH(Arg^{11})	0.6	55
	^{64}Cu-CBTE2A-ReCCMSH(Arg^{11})	0.6–5.0	93
^{66}Ga (314.5 Ci/μmol)	^{66}Ga-DOTA-Tyr-octreotide	0.13	23
	^{66}Ga-DOTA-biotin	0.08	23
^{76}Br (184.3 Ci/μmol)	^{76}Br, N-[(3-aminomethyl)benzyl]-4-bromobenzamide	0.97	39
	2-^{76}Br-5-nitro-N-phenylbenzamide	1.16	32
	^{76}Br σ$_2$-receptor ligands	2.42	31
	^{76}Br-FBAU 3′5′-dibenzoate	0.59	38
	^{76}Br-FBAU	10.98 ± 4.20	33
	^{76}Br-FBAU	0.05	35
^{124}I (29.9 Ci/μmol)	^{124}I	>30	45
	^{124}I	12.2	48
	1-[^{124}I]iodo-2-naphtol	0.75	6
^{86}Y (202.5 Ci/μmol)	^{86}Y(OAc)$_3$	0.08	58
	^{86}Y-DOTA-ReCCMSH(Arg^{11})	0.60	55
	^{86}Y-DTPA-(D)-phe^1-octreotide	0.46	60
	^{86}Y-Herceptin	<0.003	64

[a]The data presented in Table 2 should be reviewed with caution. The values presented in the literature are specific activities quoted at different times during radiopharmaceutical production (e.g., end of bombardment vs. end of synthesis) using different chemical synthetic routes (e.g., direct reaction or via a precursor) and have also been calculated using different analytical methodologies.
[b]Theoretical specific activity of ^{18}F = 1628 Ci/μmol.

(84). Additional advances were made in the production of ^{94m}Tc by Bigott et al., where following irradiation of an enriched ^{94}Mo and separation of the ^{94m}Tc by thermal distillation, the ^{94m}TcO$_4^-$ was isolated in either organic or aqueous solvents (81). These methods quickly yielded a highly concentrated solution of pure ^{94m}Tc in organic solvent ready for subsequent organic synthesis and eliminated a time-consuming evaporation step.

SPECIFIC ACTIVITY OF THE NONSTANDARD PET NUCLIDES

In many of the production schemes presented above, the nuclear transformations are often just a metal (or halogen) or two away from the product. The target purification step is fundamental in isolating the PET nuclide in high specific activity since many of the tracers being labeled with the nuclide are targeted to receptors and antigens. The concepts of specific activity, radioactive concentration, isotopic and non-isotopic carriers, and carrier-free and no-carrier-added have been defined and clarified in a review by Bonardi et al. (85). Ultimately, quantitative PET imaging is based on the tracer principle (86,87), and the

tracer principle requires high effective specific activity of the radiopharmaceutical produced. Not achieving this may lead to problems in the preclinical study of a new PET radiopharmaceutical and the ultimate clinical application of a new agent (88–91). Table 2 presents examples of the specific activity of the nuclide following production as well as examples of the specific activities of the final labeled products. The data presented in Table 2 should be reviewed with caution. The values presented in the literature are specific activities quoted at different times during radiopharmaceutical production (e.g., end of bombardment vs. end of synthesis) using different chemical synthetic routes (e.g., direct reaction or via a precursor) and have also been calculated using different analytical methodologies (85).

SUMMARY

This review discusses the production and separation of a number of nonstandard PET radionuclides, which will not replace the conventional PET nuclides, but instead, offer the opportunity of alternative applications. They all have diverse chemistry allowing for the labeling of different systems, but more importantly, their extended half-lives generate the possibility of imaging biomolecules and small molecules that require longer circulation times to achieve optimal target accumulation.

Since the half-lives of these nuclides allow for their distribution from a central production site to remote PET centers, they can be used by researchers who do not have in-house access to a cyclotron. These nuclides ^{64}Cu, ^{66}Ga, ^{71,72,74}As, ^{76}Br, ^{124}I, ^{86}Y, and ^{89}Zr offer new and exciting opportunities for the development of novel radiopharmaceuticals that can play an integral part in the rapidly expanding field of molecular imaging with PET.

ACKNOWLEDGMENTS

We are grateful to Dr. Richard Laforest, Washington University School of Medicine, for the images demonstrating nuclide image quality on a small-animal PET system. We also acknowledge the National Cancer Institute at the National Institutes of Health (R24 CA86307) and the Department of Energy (DE-FG02-84ER60218 and DE-FG02-87ER60512) for their support in the production of the nonstandard PET nuclides at Washington University School of Medicine.

REFERENCES

1. Welch MJ, Redvanly CS, eds. Handbook of Radiopharmaceuticals. Chichester, West Sussex: John Wiley & Sons, 2003.
2. Schubiger PA, Lehmann L, Friebe M, eds. PET Chemistry: The Driving Force of Molecular Imaging. Ernst Schering Research Foundation Workshop. Vol. 62. Berlin: Springer, 2007.
3. McQuade P, Rowland DJ, Lewis JS, et al. Positron-emitting isotopes produced on biomedical cyclotrons. Curr Med Chem 2005; 12:807–818.
4. Lucignani G. Non-standard PET radionuclides: time to get ready for new clinical PET strategies. Eur J Nucl Med Mol Imaging 2007; 34:294–300.
5. Blower PJ, Lewis JS, Zweit J. Copper radionuclides and radiopharmaceuticals in nuclear medicine. Nucl Med Biol 1996; 23:957–980.
6. Glaser M, Mackay DB, Ranicar ASO, et al. Improved targetry and production of iodine-124 for PET studies. Radiochim Acta 2004; 92:951–956.
7. Glaser M, Luthra SK, Brady F. Applications of positron-emitting halogens in PET oncology. Int J Oncol 2003; 22:253–268.
8. Anderson CJ, Dehdashti F, Cutler PD, et al. Cu-64-TETA-Octreotide as a PET imaging agent for patients with neuroendocrine tumors. J Nucl Med 2001; 42:213–221.
9. McCarthy DW, Shefer RE, Klinkowstein RE, et al. Efficient production of high specific activity ^{64}Cu using a biomedical cyclotron. Nucl Med Biol 1997; 24:35–43.
10. Szajek LP, Meyer W, Plascjak P, et al. Semi-remote production of [^{64}Cu]CuCl$_2$ and preparation of high specific

11. Hou X, Jacobsen U, Jorgensen JC. Separation of no-carrier added ^{64}Cu from a proton irradiated enriched nickel target. Appl Radiat Isot 2002; 57:773–777.
12. Zeisler SK, Pavan RA, Orzechowski J, et al. Production of ^{64}Cu on the Sherbrooke TR-PET cyclotron. J Radioanal Nucl Chem 2003; 257:175–177.
13. Obata A, Kasamatsu S, McCarthy DW, et al. Production of therapeutic quantities of ^{64}Cu using a 12 MeV cyclotron. Nucl Med Biol 2003; 30:535–539.
14. Szelecsényi F, Blessing G, Qaim SM. Excitation functions of proton induced nuclear reaction on enriched ^{61}Ni and ^{64}Ni: possibility of production of no-carrier added ^{61}Cu and ^{64}Cu at a small cyclotron. Appl Radiat Isot 1993; 44:575–580.
15. Zweit J, Smith AM, Downey S, et al. Excitation functions for deuteron induced reactions in natural nickel: production of no-carrier added ^{64}Cu from enriched ^{64}Ni target for positron emission tomography. Appl Radiat Isot 1991; 42:193–197.
16. McCarthy DW, Bass LA, Cutler PD, et al. High purity production and potential applications of copper-60 and copper-61. Nucl Med Biol 1999; 26:351–358.
17. Fan X, Parker DJ, Smith MD, et al. A simple and selective method for the separation of Cu radioisotopes from nickel. Nucl Med Biol 2006; 33:939–944.
18. Graham MC, Pentlow KS, Mawlawi O, et al. An investigation of the physical characteristics of ^{66}Ga as an isotope for PET imaging and quantification. Med Phys 1997; 24:317–326.
19. Goethals P, Coene M, Slegers G, et al. Production of carrier-free ^{66}Ga and labeling of antimyosin antibody for positron imaging of acute myocardial infarction. Eur J Nucl Med 1990; 16:237–240.
20. Ugur O, Kothari PJ, Finn RD, et al. Ga-66 labeled somatostatin analogue DOTA-DPhe1-Tyr3-octreotide as a potential agent for positron emission tomography imaging and receptor mediated internal radiotherapy of somatostatin receptor positive tumors. Nucl Med Biol 2002; 29: 147–157.
21. Mathias CJ, Lewis MR, Reichert DE, et al. Preparation of ^{66}Ga and ^{68}Ga-labeled Ga(III)-deferoxamine-folate as potential folate-receptor-targeted PET radiopharmaceuticals. Nucl Med Biol 2003; 30:725–731.
22. Jalilian AR, Rowshanfarzad P, Sabet M, et al. Preparation of [^{66}Ga]bleomycin complex as a possible PET radiopharmaceutical. J Radioanal Nucl Chem 2005; 264:617–621.
23. Lewis MR, Reichert DE, Laforest R, et al. Production and purification of gallium-66 for preparation of tumor-targeting radiopharmaceuticals. Nucl Med Biol 2002; 29:701–706.
24. Brown LC. Chemical processing of cyclotron-produced ^{67}Ga. Appl Radiat Isot 1971; 22:710–713.
25. Brown LC, Callahan AP, Skidmore MR, et al. High-yield zinc-68 cyclotron targets for carrier-free gallium-67 production. Appl Radiat Isot 1973; 24:651–655.
26. Jennewein M, Qaim SM, Hermanne A, et al. A new method for radiochemical separation of arsenic from irradiated germanium oxide. Appl Radiat Isot 2005; 63:343–351.
27. Di Noto R, Boccuin P, Costanti S, et al. In vitro exposure of acute promyelocytic leukemia cells to arsenic trioxide (As$_2$O$_3$) induces the solitary expression of CD66c

activity [^{64}Cu]Cu-ATSM for PET studies. Radiochim Acta 2005; 93:239–244.

(NCA-50/90), a member of the CEA family. Tissue Antigens 1999; 54:597–602.

28. Phillips DR, Hamilton VT, Taylor WA, et al. Generator-produced arsenic-72 positron emission tomography. Radioact Radiochem 1991; 3:53–58.

29. Jennewein M, Schmidt A, Novgorodov AF, et al. A no-carrier added ^{72}Se/^{72}As radionuclide generator based on distillation. Radiochim Acta 2004; 92:245–249.

30. Basile D, Birattari C, Bonardi M, et al. Excitation functions and production of arsenic radioisotopes for environmental toxicology and biomedical purposes. Int J Appl Radiat Isot 1994; 32:403–410.

31. Rowland DJ, Tu Z, Xu J, et al. Synthesis and in vivo evaluation of 2 high-affinity ^{76}Br-labeled σ_2-receptor ligands. J Nucl Med 2006; 47:1041–1048.

32. Lee H, Finck BN, Jones LA, et al. Synthesis and evaluation of a bromine-76-labeled PPARγ antagonist 2-bromo-5-nitro-N-phenylbenzamide. Nucl Med Biol 2006; 33: 847–854.

33. Cho SY, Ravasi L, Szajek LP, et al. Evaluation of ^{76}Br-FBAU as a PET reporter probe for HSV1-tk gene expression imaging using mouse models of human glioma. J Nucl Med 2005; 46:1923–1930.

34. Szajek LP, Kao C-HK, Kiesewetter DO, et al. Semi-remote production of Br-76 and preparation of high specific activity radiobrominated pharmaceuticals for PET studies. Radiochim Acta 2004; 92:291–295.

35. Bergström M, Lu L, Fasth KJ, et al. In vitro and animal validation of bromine-76-bromodeoxyuridine as a proliferation marker. J Nucl Med 1998; 39:1273–1279.

36. Lövqvist A, Sundin A, Ahlströ H, et al. Pharmacokinetics and experimental PET imaging of a bromine-75-labeled monoclonal anti-CEA antibody. J Nucl Med 1997; 38: 395–401.

37. Tolmachev V, Lovqvist A, Einarsson L, et al. Production of ^{76}Br by a low-energy cyclotron. Appl Radiat Isot 1998; 49:1537–1540.

38. Kao C-HK, Waki A, Sassaman MB, et al. Evaluation of [^{76}Br]FBAU 3′5′-dibenzoate as a lipophilic prodrug for brain imaging. Nucl Med Biol 2002; 29:527–535.

39. Forngren BH, Yngve U, Forngren T, et al. Determination of specific radioactivity for ^{76}Br-labeled compounds measuring the ratio between ^{76}Br and ^{79}Br using packed capillary liquid chromatography mass spectrometry. Nucl Med Biol 2000; 27:851–853.

40. Pentlow KS, Graham MC, Lambrecht RM, et al. Quantitative imaging of iodine-124 with PET. J Nucl Med 1996; 37:1557–1562.

41. Williams H, Julyan P, Ranson M, et al. Does ^{124}Iodo-deoxyuridine measure cell proliferation in NSCLC? Initial investigations with PET imaging and radio-metabolite analysis. Eur J Nucl Med Mol Imaging 2007; 34:301–303.

42. Bastian T, Coenen HH, Qaim SM. Excitation functions of ^{124}Te(d,xn)^{124,125}I reactions from threshold up to 14 MeV: comparative evaluation of nuclear routes for the production of ^{124}I. Appl Radiat Isot 2001; 55:303–308.

43. Scholten B, Kovacs Z, Tarkanyi F, et al. Excitation function of ^{124}Te(p,xn)^{123,124}I reaction from 6 to 31 MeV with special reference to the production of ^{124}I at a small cyclotron. Appl Radiat Isot 1995; 46:255–259.

44. Qaim SM, Hohn A, Bastian T, et al. Some optimisation studies relevant to the production of high-purity ^{124}I and ^{120g}I at a small-sized cyclotron. Appl Radiat Isot 2003; 58:69–78.

45. Sheh Y, Koziorowski J, Balatoni J, et al. Low energy cyclotron production and chemical separation of "no carrier added" iodine-124 from a reusable, enriched tellurium-124 dioxide/aluminum oxide solid solution target. Radiochim Acta 2000; 88:169–173.

46. Nye JA, Nickels RJ. Strategies in choosing binary alloys for the production of I-124: proof of principle studies using Al$_2$Te$_3$. Fifth International Symposium on Radiohalogens. Canada: Whistler, BC, 2004.

47. Kovacs Z, Blessing G, Qaim SM, et al. Production of bromine-75 via the ^{76}Se($p,2n$)^{75}Br reaction at a compact cyclotron. Int J Appl Radiat Isot 1985; 36:635–42.

48. Knust EJ, Dutschka K, Weinreich R. Preparation of ^{124}I solutions after thermodistillation of irradiated ^{124}TeO$_2$ targets. Appl Radiat Isot 2000; 52:181–184.

49. Nye JA, Avila-Rodriguez MA, Nickels RJ. Production of [^{124}I]-iodine on an 11 MeV cyclotron. Radiochim Acta 2006; 94:213–216.

50. Michael H, Rosezin H, Apelt H, et al. Some technical improvements in the production of iodine-123 via the ^{124}Te ($p,2n$)^{123}I reaction at a compact cyclotron. Int J Appl Radiat Isot 1981; 32:581–587.

51. Parry R, Schneider D, Hudson D, et al. Identification of a novel prostate tumor target, mindin/RG-1, for antibody-based radiotherapy of prostate cancer. Cancer Res 2005; 65:8397–8405.

52. Buchholz HG, Herzog H, Forster GJ, et al. PET imaging with yttrium-86: comparison of phantom measurements acquired with different PET scanners before and after applying background subtraction. Eur J Nucl Med Mol Imaging 2003; 30:716–720.

53. Jamar F, Barone R, Mathieu I, et al. ^{86}Y-DOTA-D-Phe^1-Tyr^3-octreotide (SMT487)–a phase 1 clinical study: pharmacokinetics, biodistribution and renal protective effect of different regimens of amino acid co-infusion. Eur J Nucl Med Mol Imaging 2003; 30:510–518.

54. Lövqvist A, Humm JL, Sheikh A, et al. PET imaging of ^{86}Y-labeled anti-Lewis Y monoclonal antibodies in a nude mouse model: comparison between ^{86}Y and ^{111}In radiolabels. J Nucl Med 2001; 42:1281–1287.

55. McQuade P, Miao Y, Yoo J, et al. Imaging of melanoma using ^{64}Cu and ^{86}Y-DOTA-ReCCSMH(Arg^{11}), a cyclized peptide analog of α-MSH. J Med Chem 2005; 48: 2985–2992.

56. Pentlow KS, Finn RD, Larson SM, et al. Quantitative imaging of yttrium-86 with PET. The occurrence and correction of anomalous apparent activity in high density regions. Clin Positron Imaging 2000; 3:85–90.

57. Roesch F, Qaim SM, Stoecklin G. Production of the positron emitting radioisotope yttrium-86 for nuclear medical application. Appl Radiat Isot 1993; 44:677–681.

58. Yoo J, Tang L, Perkins TA, et al. Preparation of high specific activity ^{86}Y using a small biomedical cyclotron. Nucl Med Biol 2005; 32:891–897.

59. Clifford T, Boswell CA, Biddlecombe GB, et al. Validation of a novel CHX-A″ derivative suitable for peptide

conjugation: small animal PET/CT imaging using yttrium-86-CHX-A''-octreotide. J Med Chem 2006; 49:4297–4304.

60. Wester HJ, Brockmann J, Rosch F, et al. PET-pharmacokinetics of ^{18}F-octreotide: a comparison with ^{67}Ga-DFO- and ^{86}Y-DTPA-octreotide. Nucl Med Biol 1997; 24:275–286.

61. Rösch F, Qaim SM, Stöcklin G. Nuclear data relevant to the production of the positron emitting radioisotope ^{86}Y via the ^{86}Sr(p,n)- and ^{nat}Rb(^{3}He,xn)-processes. Radiochim Acta 1993; 61:1–8.

62. Reischl G, Rosch F, Machulla HJ. Electrochemical separation and purification of yttrium-86. Radiochim Acta 2002; 90:225–228.

63. Finn RD, McDevitt M, Ma D, et al. Low energy cyclotron production and separation of Yttrium-86 for evaluation of monoclonal antibody pharmacokinetics and dosimetry. In: Application of Accelerators in Research and Industry AIP Conference Proceedings. vol. 475. New York, NY: American Institute of Physics, 1999:991–993.

64. Garmestani K, Milenic DE, Plascjak PS, et al. A new and convenient method for purification of ^{86}Y using a Sr(II) selective resin and comparison of biodistribution of ^{86}Y and ^{111}In labeled Herceptin. Nucl Med Biol 2002; 29:599–606.

65. Park LS, Szajek LP, Wong KJ, et al. Semi-automated ^{86}Y purification using a three-column system. Nucl Med Biol 2004; 31:297–301.

66. Kettern K, Linse KH, Spellerberg S, et al. Radiochemical studies relevant to the production of ^{86}Y and ^{88}Y at a small-sized cyclotron. Radiochim Acta 2002; 90:845–849.

67. Rösch F, Qaim SM, Stöcklin G. Production of the positron emitting radioisotope ^{86}Y for nuclear medical application. Appl Radiat Isot 1993; 44:677–681.

68. Verel I, Visser GWM, Boellaard R, et al. ^{89}Zr immuno-PET: Comprehensive procedures for the production of ^{89}Zr-labeled monoclonal antibodies. J Nucl Med 2003; 44:1271–1281.

69. Perk LR, Visser OJ, Stigter-van Walsum M, et al. Preparation and evaluation of ^{89}Zr-Zevalin for monitoring of ^{90}Y-zevalin biodistribution with positron emission tomography. Eur J Nucl Med Mol Imaging 2006; 33:1337–1345.

70. Perk LR, Visser GWM, Vosjan MJWD, et al. ^{89}Zr as a PET surrogate radioisotope for scouting biodistribution of the therapeutic radiometals ^{90}Y and ^{177}Lu in tumor-bearing nude mice after coupling to the internalizing antibody cetuximab. J Nucl Med 2005; 46:1898–1906.

71. Verel I, Visser GW, Boellaard R, et al. Quantitative ^{89}Zr immuno-PET for in vivo scouting of ^{90}Y-labeled monoclonal antibodies in xenograft-bearing nude mice. J Nucl Med 2003; 44:1663–70.

72. Dejesus OT, Nickles RJ. Production and purification of zirconium-89, a potential PET antibody label. Appl Radiat Isot 1990; 41:789–90.

73. Link JM, Krohn KA, Eary JF. ^{89}Zr for antibody labeling and positron emission tomography. J Labelled Compd Radiopharm 1986; 23:1297–1298.

74. Zweit J, Downey S, Sharma HL. Production of no-carrier-added zirconium-89 for positron emission tomography. Appl Radiat Isot 1991; 42:199–201.

75. Meijs WE, Herscheid JDM, Haisma HJ, et al. Production of highly pure no-carrier added ^{89}Zr for the labeling of anti-bodies with a positron emitter. Appl Radiat Isot 1994; 45:1143–7.

76. Griffiths GL, Goldenberg DM, Roesch F, et al. Radiolabeling of an anti-carcinoembryonic antibody Fab' fragment (CEA-Scan) with positron-emitting radionuclide Tc-94m. Clin Cancer Res 1999; 5:3001s–3003s.

77. Bigott HM, Parent E, Luyt LG, et al. Design and synthesis of functionalized cyclopentadienyl tricarbonylmetal complexes for technetium-94m PET imaging of estrogen receptors. Bioconjug Chem 2005; 16:255–264.

78. Bigott HM, Prior JL, Piwnica-Worms DR, et al. Imaging multidrug resistance P-glycoprotein transport function using microPET with Technetium-94m-sestamibi. Mol Imaging 2005; 4:30–39.

79. Nickels RJ, Nunn AD, Stone CK, et al. Technetium-94m-teboroxime: synthesis, dosimetry and initial PET imaging studies. J Nucl Med 1993; 31:1058–1066.

80. Qaim SM. Production of high purity ^{94m}Tc for positron emission tomography studies. Nucl Med Biol 2000; 27:323–328.

81. Bigott HM, Laforest R, Liu X, et al. Advances in the production, processing and microPET image quality of technetium-94m. Nucl Med Biol 2006; 33:923–933.

82. Smith MF, Daube-Witherspoon ME, Plascjak PS, et al. Device-dependent activity estimation and decay correction of radionuclide mixtures with application to Tc-94m PET studies. Med Phys 2001; 28:36–45.

83. Barker WC, Szajek LP, Green SL, et al. Improved quantification for Tc-94m PET imaging. IEEE Trans Nucl Sci 2001; 48:739–742.

84. Szajek LP, Der M, Divel J, et al. Production and radioassay of Tc-94m for PET studies. Radiochim Acta 2003; 91:613–616.

85. Bonardi ML, Goeij JJM. How do we ascertain specific activities in no-carrier-added radionuclide preparations? J Radioanal Nucl Chem 2005; 263:87–92.

86. de Hevesy GV. The absorption and translocation of lead (ThB) by plants [ThB = ^{212}Pb]. Biochem J 1923; 17:439–435.

87. Chievitz O, Bohr N, de Hevesy G. Radioactive indicators in the study of phosphorous metabolism in rats. Nature 1935; 136:754.

88. Eckelman WC, Kilbourn MR, Mathis CA. Discussion of targeting proteins in vivo: in vitro guidelines. Nucl Med Biol 2006; 33:449–451.

89. Eckelman WC, Mathis CA. Targeting proteins in vivo: in vitro guidelines. Nucl Med Biol 2006; 33:161–164.

90. Kung MP, Kung HF. Mass effect of injected dose in small rodent imaging by SPECT and PET. Nucl Med Biol 2005; 32(7):673–678.

91. Eckelman WC. Receptor Binding Radiotracers. Vols 1 and 2. Boca Raton, FL: CRC Press, 1982:1–80; 1–230.

92. Lederer CM, Hollander JM, Perlman I. Table of Isotopes. Sixth ed. New York: John Wiley & Sons, 1967.

93. Wei L, Butcher C, Miao Y, et al. Synthesis and biologic evaluation of ^{64}Cu-labeled rhenium-cyclized α-MSH peptide analog using a cross-bridged cyclam chelator. J Nucl Med 2007; 48:64–72.

19

Design of New Imaging Agents Using Positron-Emitting Radionuclides as the Reporter

WILLIAM C. ECKELMAN
Molecular Tracer LLC, Bethesda, Maryland, U.S.A.

INTRODUCTION

This review will address the use of short-lived, positron-emitting [positron emission tomography, PET] radionuclides as reporters for external imaging of physiology associated with cancer. The uses of PET radionuclides to determine anatomical definition have been mostly supplanted by other imaging techniques with higher resolution. Therefore, this chapter will concentrate on the discussion of targeted radiotracers at the expense of non-targeted radiotracers.

COMPARING IMAGING TECHNIQUES

There are now a number of imaging techniques that can be used for external detection of either anatomical or physiological changes in animals and humans (Table 1). The anatomical techniques are important for determining the size, shape, and position of abnormalities with high resolution and the measurement of the longest dimension of the tumor by X-ray is still the gold standard for tumor regression (RECIST) (1). The nontargeted agents, those distributed or excreted through high-capacity systems (e.g., blood pool, kidney, liver, and bone), have been used to better define either blood flow (BF) or permeability or the excretory processes. The targeted radiotracers

are generally considered as those radioligands binding to receptors, enzymes, and other protein sites (2). The separation between targeted and nontargeted radioligands is arbitrary given the range of target densities. In general, receptors are present in the lowest density, followed by enzymes. But there are receptors in the liver, asialoglycoprotein receptors, which are present in high enough density (~ 500 nM) to permit the use of magnetic resonance imaging (MRI) contrast agents (3,4). These generalities apply mainly to mechanisms where cellular metabolic trapping is not a major component of the biochemical localization and where cellular internalization is not a predominant mechanism during the time of measurement. In these cases, more mass can be localized in the target, but care must be taken to avoid pharmacological effects. Two examples will illustrate the point. Fluorine-19 can be detected externally using MRI. The glucose analog, 2-[^{18}F]fluoro-2-deoxyglucose (FDG), is commonly used to measure a parameter related to glucose metabolism at human doses of 10 to 20 mCi (370–740 MBq) and specific activities from the original 1 Ci/mmol (37 GBq/mmol) to the present 5000 Ci/mmol (185 TBq/mmol) at end of synthesis (EOS). If 2-[^{19}F]fluoro-2-deoxyglucose is used with MRI, the amount of glucose analog needed to give an external image causes severe pharmacological effects (5). Another example, which is one of the first proofs of principle for targeted MRI,

Table 1 The Imaging Uses for the Various Imaging Techniques

	Anatomy	Excretion	Perfusion/permeability	High-capacity proteins	Low-capacity proteins
CT					
MRI					
SPECT					
PET					
Ultrasound					
Fluorescence					

investigated the detection of the transferrin receptors by external imaging using the T2 agent, iron oxide, linked to transferrin. In order to obtain an external image of mouse tumors, the transferrin receptor was genetically upregulated and receptor downregulation in the presence of excess iron was blocked. Nevertheless, in vivo imaging in a mouse bearing a transferrin receptor–containing tumor was visualized and the control tumor was not (6).

Also, the experience with the allometric effect on percentage injected dose per gram of tissue (% ID/g) going from rodents to man with radiolabeled antibodies suggests that the concentration requirements for a targeted MRI contrast agent will be more difficult to achieve in humans than in rodents (7).

LABELING SMALL MOLECULES, PEPTIDES, PROTEINS, AND NANOPARTICLES

Positron emission tomography (PET) was developed using the short-lived radionuclides of oxygen, nitrogen, carbon, and fluorine. Their advantage in radiolabeling small molecules was readily recognized because these radionuclides represent the smallest perturbation of the chemical structure, whereas single-photon computed tomography (SPECT) radiotracers, MRI contrast agents, and fluorescent reporter probes create larger perturbations, in general. Readily available SPECT radionuclides include one halogen (^{123}I) and several metallic radionuclides, such as ^{99m}Tc and ^{111}In. The single-photon-emitting radionuclides, for

example, ^{111}In and ^{99m}Tc and MRI active metals, for example, Gd require a chelating agent to form a stable bond and this represents a major perturbation limiting them to tracing peptides, proteins, and nanoparticles. This perturbation is only important for tracing small molecules that have a well-defined biochemical mechanism (MW < 300 Da). Iodine has been used to label small molecules but the additional lipophilicity (+1 Log P unit) must be addressed. There are, nevertheless, several small molecules labeled with radioiodine that track biochemical pathways in vivo (8). Recently, SEVERAL small molecules labeled with 99mTc have been added to the long-standing first example, TRODAT-1 (9,10).

THE ROLE FOR SHORT-LIVED ($T_{1/2}$ < 110 MINUTES) PET RADIONUCLIDES

There are six major PET radionuclides with a half-life of less than 110 minutes, two of which are available from generator systems (Table 2). An advantage of these radionuclides is the near quantitative emission of positrons (>90%) from the nucleus. As a result, the majority of the emitted photons (511 keV) contribute to the image. The alternate decay pathway is predominately electron capture and those radionuclides that have a lower fraction of positron emission, in general, emitted more gamma rays that do not contribute to the image, but represent shielding challenges and dosimetry limitations. These radionuclides also have higher positron energies (11). The advantage is

Table 2 Production and Decay Characteristics of PET Radionuclides

	Production	Half-life (min)	% β^+ emission	Maximum energy (MeV)	Maximum range (mm)[a]
O-15	^{14}N (d,n)	2.03	99+	1.723	8
N-13	^{16}O (p,α)	9.97	99+	1.190	4.5
C-11	^{14}N (p,α)	20.4	99+	0.961	3.5
F-18	^{18}O (p,n)	109.7	96.9	0.635	2 (0.35)
Rb-82	Sr-82 generator	1.25	96	3.35	14
Ga-68	Ga-68 generator	68.3	90	1.88	

[a]Calculated range in water with the average value in parentheses.

the longer half-lives. The use of these longer-lived PET radionuclides with a lower fraction of positron emission is discussed by Lewis et al. (this volume).

The ideal situation for monitoring the entire biochemical pathway is achieved when ^{11}C is substituted for a stable ^{12}C in the native molecule; then there is no detectable chemical perturbation in the small molecule behavior in vivo. Of the short-lived PET radionuclides, [^{18}F]fluorine represents a solution to the short half-life of ^{11}C (20 minutes), yet is isosteric with a methyl group such that it does not represent a perturbation in size, but its increased electronegativity must be taken into consideration.

In addition, these short-lived PET radionuclides are produced by a nuclear transformation so, by the nature of the production method, these radionuclides are at high specific activity (radioactivity/mass). As a result, any small molecule radiolabeled with a PET radionuclide will require the injection of a very small amount of material to obtain sufficient annihilation photons to obtain a satisfactory external image. A practical dose for ^{18}F compounds is 10 mCi (370 MBq) and the specific activity is more than 1000 Ci/mmol (37 TBq/mmol) at the time of injection. This represents the injection of less than 10 nmol, which is orders of magnitude smaller than what must be injected to obtain MR images using a Gd chelate and fits the definition of the tracer principle developed by Hevesy and Paneth (12).

The concept of specific activity as it applies to radio-pharmaceuticals has evolved from the classical definition of the ratio of the number of radioactive atoms to the total number of atoms of a given element. Since the specific activity of the final product is the important factor in radiopharmaceuticals, other definitions have been described for particular situations when analyzing the final radioactive product. Kilbourn defined apparent specific activity where the denominator is the total mass eluted at the same time as the radioactive product. These may be different chemical species or the same chemical specie containing the nonradioactive element that was present in the reagents or materials in contact with the solution. One further definition is that of effective specific activity. The effective specific activity is defined as the specific activity determined by a biological or biochemical assay. The bioassay is carried out on the purified final product so that the apparent specific activity would come into play, but would be affected by the binding constants for the impurity (13). One example of the source of bromine in the production and isolation of ^{76}Br by a wet chemistry method describes the sources of bromine from those in the target to those in the reagents used in the process (14). A recent example of a different chemical species that is eluted with the intended product, thereby lowering the effective specific activity, is a side reaction

that occurred when converting from a multiple-reaction paradigm to a one-pot synthesis (15).

The combination of the advantages of the tracer principle (12) and the concept of a magic bullet developed by Ehrlich (16) for PET and SPECT dictate that the emphasis is on radiolabeling small molecules that follow a specific, low-density biochemical pathway. Most PET studies in oncology (and neurology) do, in fact, represent targeting of low-density sites, such as receptors, transporters, and enzymes.

PET SENSITIVITY AND RESOLUTION IN HUMANS AND ANIMALS

This review will address the use of short-lived PET radionuclides, ^{15}O, ^{13}N, ^{11}C, ^{68}Ga, and ^{18}F. The current resolution of PET capable of imaging human subjects is ~ 5 mm, and the current resolution of PET dedicated to imaging small animals is 1.2 to 1.5 mm with ordered subset-expectation maximum (OSEM) reconstruction software (17). This relatively low resolution is compensated for by combining the PET imaging device with a CT unit with higher resolution. This results in superior anatomical definition of the biochemical event. The sensitivity of these devices for small animal imaging is between 5% and 10%. On the other hand, for the ex vivo technique of autoradiography using X-ray film or a phosphorimager, ^{14}C autoradiographic resolution is approximately 25 μm full width, half maximum (FWHM) (18). It is important to note that if small animal imaging studies in rodents are to have the same "quality" as human PET studies, the same number of coincidence events must be detected from a typical rodent imaging "voxel" as from the human imaging voxel. To achieve this using the same specific activity preparation, we show that roughly the same total amount of radiopharmaceutical must be given to a rodent as to a human subject (19). If the specific activity is not high enough to still follow the tracer principle, pharmacological effects can occur and mathematical analysis can be more complex.

USE OF PET FOR NONTARGETED RADIOTRACERS

PET has been to measure blood volume (BV) using [^{11}CO]-labeled red blood cells, BF using [^{15}O]-labeled water, and permeability (P) of tumors in oncology. The most recent use of radiotracers to measure these parameters has come from the recognition that angiogenesis plays a major role in cancer development and that a measure of changes in BV and BF may be useful imaging tools. Kurdziel et al. found that the percent change in prostate specific antigen (PSA) in androgen independent prostate cancer patients undergoing treatment with thalidomide correlated with the FDG percent change in standard uptake value (SUV) mean and percentage change in metabolic tumor volume, but less well with the change in percent BV. Percent change in BF values showed an inverse correlation with percent changes in PSA (20).

Permeability studies have been carried out in experimental tumors using ^{18}F-labeled human serum albumin, although this was not used in a treatment paradigm (21). It was used as a control for specific binding studies. Although transferrin receptors were present in high concentration in mouse tumor xenografts, ^{18}F-labeled human serum albumin had high tumor uptake because of its higher permeability compared with that of the targeted ^{18}F-labeled transferrin. For the ^{18}F transferrin, the rate-determining step appeared to be permeability rather than receptor binding.

In both cases, the resolution of PET imaging with respect to the heterogeneity of tumors needs to be considered (22). It may be that MRI or CT may be more sensitive to change in the angiogenesis process if these two approaches can produce quantitative evaluations of BF or BV for smaller resolution–voxel sizes (23).

USE OF PET IN METABOLIC TRAPPING OR HIGH-CAPACITY TARGETS

The major emphasis of PET in oncology is to monitor glucose metabolism, cellular proliferation, hypoxia, apoptosis, protein synthesis, lipid metabolism, neuroendocrine dependencies, and receptors found to be upregulated in tumors.

Glucose Metabolism: 2-[18F]fluoro-2-deoxyglucose Indications

The clinical indications of characterization, staging, and restaging for solitary pulmonary nodules was the first approval followed by approvals for similar clinical indications in esophageal cancer, colorectal cancer, lymphoma, melanoma, breast cancer, head and neck cancers, and thyroid cancer. Other studies are reimbursed in the United States if they are accompanied by an evidence-development program, that is, an FDG PET clinical study that is designed to collect additional information at the time of the scan to assist in patient management. PET is not reimbursed as a screening test (i.e., testing patients without specific signs and symptoms of disease). Hoh has recently defined a paradigm by which FDG-PET is the imaging agent of choice in staging recurrent cancer. Three clinical questions were applied to the various clinical applications of FDG to understand this difference: (*i*) Are there competing tests? (*ii*) Is there a cost-effective role in the clinical management? (*iii*) Is the

interpretation of the imaging study easy? Melanoma recurrence seems to be the cancer in which FDG is used most often as a first-line diagnostic (24).

What is unique about the probe design for FDG? This bears on the question of what is being measured when gamma rays are being detected, rather than chemical composition. Magnetic resonance spectroscopy is capable of measuring chemical structure, but other imaging modalities only measure the emitted electromagnetic radiation. Therefore, if there is extensive metabolism, the analysis is increasingly difficult. The beauty of monitoring a limited number of biochemical steps is exemplified by the properties of 2-deoxy-[14C]glucose (DG), which were elucidated by Sokoloff and colleagues (25). DG and FDG are transported and phosphorylated, but proceed no further because neither one is a substrate for the next enzyme in the many step process of glucose metabolism. In addition, the 6-phosphatase that removes the phosphate and regenerates DG or FDG is usually not present in tumors (26). The relative properties of FDG and DG in the normal brain were determined for the glucose transporter (GLUT) and hexokinase, and this led to the development of a lumped constant–relating FDG to glucose biochemical processing (25). This relationship is less certain in tumors and therefore attributing glucose metabolism to the distribution of FDG in tumors has to be made with caution. Krohn et al. have written about the relationship between a fluorinated compound and the parent compound radiolabeled with [11]C. The advantage of FDG is that it is metabolically trapped as the 6-phosphate and after a certain length of time, only the 6-phosphate is present in the target so a complicated model is not needed to account for free FDG or metabolites in the target tissue. On the other hand, FDG is not glucose and in disease states, the ratio of rate constants for FDG and glucose for GLUT and hexokinase may not remain a constant. Therefore, statements about glucose metabolism must be made with the understanding of what is involved in using an analog. PET has developed over the years to produce quantitative renderings of the radioactivity in the target tissue and methods have been developed to analyze the plasma for parent compound. The combination of the two leads to the determination of rate constants. However, the physical meaning of these rate constants is confounded by the differences between FDG and glucose, which is in high concentration in the plasma. To this point, Krohn et al. state that validation of fluorinated analogs is a continuing process, less so for FDG given the years of experience, but more so for newly developed analogs (27).

Proliferation: 3′-fluorothymidine

The same authors also discuss the difference between ^{11}C thymidine and the 3′-fluoro analog, FLT, which has some of the same biochemical relationships as glucose and FDG. FLT cannot be phosphorylated at the 3′ position, which prevents incorporation into DNA unlike ^{11}C thymidine, which measures the entire metabolic pathway including DNA incorporation. The same precautions addressed for FDG are warranted here. The advantages of the longer half-life ^{18}F and metabolic trapping of the fluoro analog must be balanced by the fact that it is not thymidine. In fact, FLT may be more different than thymidine in its kinetic parameters than FDG is different from glucose (27).

The design goal has been to produce radiotracers that follow the biochemical pathway with similar kinetic parameters as thymidine. The major steps in the cellular uptake are facilitated diffusion and a carrier-mediated mechanism. Once intracellular, the nucleoside is phosphorylated primarily by thymidine kinase (TK)1. If both the 3′ and 5′ hydroxy groups are available, the radiotracer can be incorporated into DNA. FLT has a fluorine at the 3′ position and therefore 5′ phosphate is the major product in the cell. Nevertheless, a parameter related to proliferation can be measured by analyzing the pharmacokinetics of FLT. Its behavior is similar to FDG in that respect. Other ^{18}F radiolabeled nucleosides have been produced, including ^{18}F-FBAU (1-(2-deoxy-2-fluoro-1-α-D-arabinofuranosyl)-5-bromouracil), ^{18}F-FMAU (2′-fluoro-5-methyldeoxyuracil-β-D-arabinofuranosyl), and ^{18}F-FAU (2′-fluorodeoxyuracil-β-D-arabinofuranosyl), but none have progressed to the clinic as rapidly as FLT even though some follow the thymidine pathway to the point of being incorporated into DNA (28). Those compounds without an electron-withdrawing group at the 2′ or 3′ position are unstable in vivo. The metabolic decomposition of thymidine and pyrimidine 2-deoxynucleoside derivatives is initiated by thymidine phosphorylase. This cytosolic enzyme catalyzes the reversible phosphorolysis to 2-deoxy-D-ribose-1-phosphates and the pyrimidine. Therefore, the current trend is to incorporate a 2′ fluoro group as shown for FMAU and FAU and a 3′ fluoro group in FLT (Table 3). Substrates for TK1 appear to better reflect proliferation (29). But as Krohn et al. point out validation of fluorinated analogs is a continuing process (27).

FLT has been produced by several methods all of which are in low yield. Recently, a synthesis using protic solvents has been introduced for FLT. This raised the yield to more than 80%, potentially overcoming one of the impediments to large-scale synthesis (30).

Hypoxia

The National Cancer Institute (NCI) definition of hypoxia is a condition in which there is a decrease in the oxygen supply to a tissue. In cancer treatment, the level of hypoxia in a tumor may help predict the response of the tumor to the treatment. The development of radioligands to measure hypoxia by noninvasive means are based on either compounds that were developed as radiation sensitizers, or on compounds whose retention mechanism was based on a reduction of a metal core in vivo. The former is exemplified by ^{18}F]fluoromisonidazole (FMISO) and the latter by ^{64}Cu-labeled acetyl derivative of pyruvaldehyde bis[N^4-methylthiosemicarbazonato]copper(II) complex, [^{64}Cu]CuATSM. Radiation sensitizers are used to trap the free radicals produced during external beam irradiation of tumors in situations where the oxygen content is too low for it to act as a radical trap. The major use of radiolabeled agents to detect hypoxia is to identify those tumors that will not respond to radiation therapy because of low oxygen content. Alternative azomycin-based imaging agents have been developed, but FMISO remains the most studied in the clinic (31). Questions remain to be answered, on the metabolism of FMISO and the effect of metabolites on the tumor to plasma ratio. Preliminary data show that FMISO is extensively metabolized, but the effect of this on tumor uptake is not event. For example, high-performance liquid chromatography of urine demonstrated that 10% of [^{18}F]fluoroetanidazole (FETA)-derived activity was in metabolites at two hours postinjection, with 15% in metabolites by four hours; comparable values for [^{18}F]FMISO were 36% and 57%, respectively (32). FMISO has a relative low tumor to plasma ratio in hypoxic versus normoxic tumors. Using a cut-off points developed over the years, normoxic tumors have a ratio of less than 1.2 and hypoxic tumors a ratio of greater than 1.2 at 90 to 120 minutes after injection.

[^{64}Cu]CuATSM clearly is retained in hypoxic tumors and washes out of normoxic tumors at a faster rate. In

Table 3 In Vivo Behavior of a Series of Nucleosides TEXT

Nucleoside	Abbreviation	In vivo behavior
5-[^{18}F]fluoro-2′-deoxyuridine	[^{18}F]FdUrd	In vivo decomposition
5-[[124]I]iodo-2′-deoxyuridine	[[124]I]IUdR	In vivo decomposition
5-[[76]Br]bromo-2′-deoxyuridine	5-[[76]Br]BrdU	In vivo decomposition
5-[^{11}C]methyl-(2-fluoro-2-β-D-arabinofuranosyl)uracil	[^{11}C]FMAU	TK2 > TK1
5-Methyl-(2-[^{18}F]fluoro-2-β-D-arabinofuranosyl)uracil	[^{18}F]FMAU	TK2 > TK1
3′-Deoxy-3′[^{18}F]fluorothymidine	[^{18}F]FLT	TK1 > TK2
5-[[76]Br]bromo-(2-fluoro-2-β-D-arabinofuranosyl)uracil	[[76]Br]FBAU	

Abbreviation: TK, thymidine kinase.

humans, an arbitrarily selected T/M threshold of 3.5 discriminated those likely to develop recurrence; six of nine patients with normoxic tumors (T/M < 3.5) were free of disease at last follow-up (33). The major question of [^{64}Cu] CuATSM is whether the reduction process is mapping the low oxygen concentration responsible for radiation resistance. Furthermore, a fraction of [^{64}Cu]CuATSM appears to be reduced even under normoxic conditions in in vitro experiments (34). Rajendran and Krohn suggest that its retention may be related to an increased reducing agent in hypoxic tumors rather than decreased oxygen per se (31).

Apoptosis

Apoptosis is defined as programmed cell death and is an essential component of normal human growth and development, immunoregulation, and homeostasis. A failure of apoptosis and unchecked proliferation are key factors in tumor progression. Radiolabeled annexin is the compound most studied for the purpose of monitoring apoptosis. To date, annexin V has been radiolabeled with ^{99m}Tc, ^{124}I, and ^{18}F. Fluorophore and iron oxide annexin V derivatives have also been synthesized (35).

Annexin V is a 36-kDa protein that binds with high affinity to phosphatidylserine (PS), which resides on the interior surface of the cell membrane. Relatively late in the apoptosis process, the PS is redistributed to cell surface. However, other pathways, such as necrosis also expose PS to the extracellular environment (36). While apoptosis and necrosis are distinctly different modes of cell death, the use of radiolabeled annexin V detects a common molecular marker of these two processes, the exposure of anionic phospholipids (APLDs), and thereby allows their detection as a single property in dead and dying tissues.

^{18}F-labeled annexin V binds to chemically induced apoptosis with high affinity and specificity. The ^{18}F-labeled annexin V is rapidly cleared from the body via the kidneys. Apoptotic cells stain with annexin V, but do not stain with propidium iodide, since their cell membranes are still intact, whereas necrotic cells stain with both annexin V and propidium iodide. Normal cells stain with neither. The analysis of data obtained in vivo with ^{18}F-labeled annexin V is not straightforward because cell staining cannot be performed in vivo. Short of obtaining biopsy samples, annexin V will not differentiate between necrosis and apoptosis (37).

Protein Synthesis Using Amino Acids

Various amino acids have been used to monitor changes in protein synthesis. However, they do not achieve maximum sensitivity to changes in disease states because the emitted

photons are associated with various biochemical phenomena. As an example, the current amino acids labeled with positron emitting radiotracers, [^{11}C]methionine (38) and and L-2-[^{18}F]fluorotyrosine (39), are involved in several biochemical pathways. The amino acid with the highest incorporation into proteins is leucine, but its synthesis is complicated and the mathematical analysis of protein synthesis is confounded by the need to know the specific activity of the [^{11}C]leucine in the plasma and target tissue. The degradation of protein is a significant source of leucine in brain. This requires a correction for its contribution to the specific activity of the tissue precursor amino acid pool. The use of a carboxyl-labeled, aliphatic branched chain amino acid, such as L-leucine obviates the problems of extraneous biochemical reactions and the production of labeled metabolic products other than labeled protein. L-[1-^{11}C]leucine had been used as a PET tracer in monkeys, but no attempt was made to correct for recycling of amino acids (40). This PET study did not address the problem of evaluating the fraction of the precursor pool for protein synthesis derived from arterial plasma, to correct for recycling. The first PET study of protein synthesis to address the issue of recycling was published by Smith et al. (41). The goal is to understand the factors controlling the distribution so that quantitative statements can be made about protein synthesis from imaging studies.

D,L-[1-^{11}C]leucine was prepared from H^{11}CN with a modified Bucherer-Strecker reaction sequence (42). The isolation of the pure L-amino acid isomer from the enantiomeric mixture was achieved by reaction with D-amino acid oxidase/catalase enzyme complex immobilized on a Sepharose column. The L-[1-^{11}C]leucine can be obtained with a radiochemical purity of more than 99%.

An unnatural amino acid, by it nature, measures changes in transport as a function of disease. The best in terms of few radiolabeled metabolites, low background, and high tumor to background ratios is 1-amino-3-[^{18}F] fluorocyclobutane-1-carboxylic acid (FACBC) (43).

Cell Membrane Synthesis Using Radiolabeled Choline and Acetate

PET with ^{11}C-acetate shows promise for detection of recurrent prostate cancer. A review of published analyses of ^{11}C-acetate PET in prostate cancer supports the selection of this radiopharmaceutical for evaluation of its utility in radiation treatment planning for relapsed prostate cancer (44).

While the mechanism of uptake has not been fully characterized, it has been shown that tumor cells incorporate ^{14}C-acetate preferentially into lipids, and that the retention of ^{14}C in lipid-soluble fractions correlates with tumor cell growth activity. These findings support the hypothesis that acetate preferentially incorporates into the membrane lipids in tumor cells, because cell growth and proliferation require membrane constituents (45). There is a difference in the metabolism of citrate between malignant and normal prostate epithelial cells. Normal prostate epithelial cells and benign prostate hyperplastic tissue produce citrate and exhibit an extremely low capability for oxidizing citrate. Prostate cancer cells, in contrast, are citrate-oxidizing cells (46). This difference may affect lipogenesis in the prostate, but additional study is necessary. The fact remains that there are studies that suggest utility for ^{11}C-acetate PET. Moreover, there are patients who were found to have biopsy confirmed ^{11}C-acetate uptake in locally recurrent prostate cancer (47–49). This presents a need for more research in this area. The kinetics of primary prostate cancer allows for tumor response to radiation therapy, and relatively slow growth may, in fact, facilitate detectable ^{11}C-acetate uptake.

Choline radiolabeled with ^{11}C or ^{18}F has been studied as an alternate approach to measuring protein synthesis (50). ^{11}C-labeled choline (trimethyl-2 hydroxyethyl-ammonium) has shown potential in brain tumors, for which FDG has suboptimal specificity because of uptake by normal brain; prostate carcinoma, where FDG has inadequate sensitivity, and esophageal carcinoma, where background activity with FDG limits detection of neoplasms in the mediastinum (51). The short half-life of ^{11}C has led to the evaluation of a series of ^{18}F radiolabeled compounds, the first being the choline analog 2-[^{18}F]fluoroethyldimethyl-2-hydroxyethylammonium (FEC). As with FDG and FLT, the goal was to determine if the fluorinated analog resembled choline in a key biochemical step (52). FEC was found to be stable in human plasma and to be a substrate for phosphocholine. Cultured PC-3 human prostate cells accumulated fluorocholine (FCH) similar to that of CH. However, the fluoroethylated analog, FEC, showed only one-fifth of the uptake of FCH. Fluoromethylethyl choline, FMEC, showed an accumulation higher than that of FEC but lower than that of FCH. Uptake of the fluoropropyl (FPC), analog of choline, was not significantly different from that of FCH. Competitive inhibition studies documented specificity of choline transport and phosphorylation. Defluorination can be a problem with alkyl fluorides, but was not evident in this series. In the end, FCH was chosen given its biochemical properties were closest to choline.

Neuroendocrine Disease

Norepinephrine Transporter

Over the last two decades, Wieland's group at the University of Michigan has been developing radiotracers that can be used noninvasively to assess cardiac sympathetic innervation in the living human (53). Several successful sympathetic neuronal imaging agents have been produced. Each one monitors a different aspect of the norepinephrine pathway. The gamma-emitting radiotracers [^{131}I]- and [^{123}I]-*meta*-iodobenzylguanidine (MIBG), and the positron-emitting analog [^{11}C]-*meta*-hydroxyephedrine (HED) are transported efficiently by the norepinephrine transporter (NET). MIBG was taken up more efficiently by the vesicles than HED via the vesicular monoamine transporter (VMAT), but HED was released from the vesicles more efficiently. Neither were substrates for monoamine oxidase (MAO). [^{11}C]epinephrine (EPI), and [^{11}C]phenylephrine (PHEN) were weaker substrates for NET, were taken up by the vesicles, and were substrates for MAO. These studies were carried out in the heart and not in neuroendocrine tumors (54).

MIBG has been widely used in its radiolabeled forms since the early 1980s for the diagnosis and radiotherapy of various neuroendocrine tumors, such as neuroblastoma and pheochromocytoma. Clinical studies using commercially available [^{131}I]MIBG demonstrate that it undergoes little in vivo metabolism with the vast majority excreted unchanged in the urine. Up to 55% of the injected radioactivity is recovered from the urine at 24 hours and up to 90% is excreted within 4 days. At 24 hours, 60% to 96% of the [^{131}I] present in the urine is [^{131}I]MIBG with 2% to 40% [^{131}I]-*meta*-iodohippuric acid and 2% to 6% [^{131}I] iodide. Only a small portion of the injected radioactivity (1–4%) is reported to be excreted through the feces. This rapid clearance from nontarget tissues makes it an excellent agent for imaging and radiotherapy (55).

The carrier molecule MIBG is a biogenic amine, which causes hypertension as well as nausea and vomiting when administered at high mass doses. Also, the selective active uptake by the NET expressed on the cell surface is a competitive process. Thus, the presence of cold "carrier" in the injection solution can diminish the initial uptake in the target organs, cardiac tissue, or neuroendocrine tumors. Clinical studies with cardiac imaging have demonstrated twofold increases in heart to background ratios with higher specific activity (56). In addition, in vivo imaging and therapy studies in rodents confirm that target organ accumulation is at least twice as high for no-carrier added MIBG as those obtained with carrier added preparations, and tumor kill is dramatically enhanced (57).

Goldstein et al. have compared [^{123}I]MIBG with [^{18}F] fluorodopamine in pheochromocytoma. Their preliminary data suggest that [^{18}F]fluorodopamine is superior to other nuclear imaging methods, including MIBG and octreotide scintigraphy in difficult cases. Compared with MIBG scanning, the radiation risk is lower, there is no need for preoperative thyroid block, and PET scanning has high temporal and spatial resolution compared with SPECT although the differences are becoming smaller. PET scanning with 6-[^{18}F]fluorodopamine can also be carried out immediately after administration, whereas 24 to 48 hours is necessary for background radioactivity to clear after MIBG injection (58).

Somatostatin

Somatostatin binds to the five subtypes of the somatostatin receptor. This receptor is upregulated on neuroendocrine tumors and this upregulation leads to a signal to background ratio that can be detected by external imaging. It also leads to tumor selectivity in therapeutic applications. The cyclic octapeptide octreotide is the analog most frequently labeled with metal chelates, such as ^{111}In DTPA, ^{68}Ga DOTA, and various ^{99m}Tc chelates for imaging and ^{111}In DTPA and ^{90}Y DOTA for therapy, all of which were selective for the somatostatin subtype receptor 2 (SSTR2) with IC$_{50}$ values of less than 10 nM, whereas native somatostatin (SS-28) bound to all five subtypes with equally high affinity. Since these analogs have neurotransmitter properties, they are internalized which further increases the localization beneficial to imaging and therapy (59).

The design criteria of the analogs were directed toward decreasing the lipophilicity by introducing polar chelates after the first analog radiolabeled with ^{123}I-Tyr3-octreotide showed high gastrointestinal excretion. The more polar chelates did shift the biodistribution to renal excretion, but the peptides were retained in the kidney to some extent. The biodistribution was superior when 10 μg of non-radioactive material was injected, possibly because of receptors present in peritumoral vessels and in inflammatory and immune cells (e.g., activated lymphocytes), which could compete with tumor uptake.

Fani and Maecke have recently reviewed the combination of radionuclides, chelating groups attached to the amino end of the octapeptide, and variations at the 3 position of octreotide to affect the biodistribution (60). PET radionuclides used in radiolabeling somatostatin receptor positive tumors include ^{11}C, ^{18}F, ^{64}Cu, $^{68/66}$Ga, ^{94m}Tc, ^{110m}In, and ^{86}Y. The half-life of ^{11}C appears to be too short given the steady state biodistribution between 45 and 90 minutes. The radionuclides ^{66}Ga, ^{94m}Tc, ^{110m}In, and ^{86}Y all have complicated cyclotron production processes and have not been frequently employed in the clinic although ^{86}Y is the ideal imaging tracer for ^{90}Y radiotherapy. The ^{18}F analogs suffer from high lipophilicity when the 2-[^{18}F]fluoropropionylated octreotide was used and defluorination was observed in animal studies. Adding a N-(1-deoxy-D-fructose) group increased the water solubility and seems to be a competitive radioligand for the somatostatin receptor. The ^{64}Cu chelates are plagued by in vivo transchelation in the liver. The hope is that rapid labeling procedures can be produced to use the ^{64}Cu bicyclic tetraazamacrocyclic chelates, which show much

higher in vivo stability toward dissociation and binding to proteins (e.g., superoxide dismutase) (61). The bulk of the studies, both preclinical and clinical have been carried out with ^{68}Ga-labeled octreotide analogs. The one most suited for in vivo studies is TOC, the Tyr3 analog of octreotide (60). The general design criteria has been to increase the renal clearance, but minimize renal retention so that the radiolabeled probe can be used to monitor tumors anywhere in the body.

Other Peptides Targeted at Tumor Receptors

Mariani et al. have recently commented on various radiolabeled peptides that are targeted to tumors expressing upregulated receptor density. They outline the use of glucagon-like peptide-1 (GLP-1), various cholecystokinin-related peptides (CCK-A and CCK-B/gastrin, gastrin-1, gastrin-releasing peptide), vascular endothelial growth factor (VDGF, in particular VEGFR-2 and neuropilin-1), and amino acids arginine-glycine-aspartic (RGD) analogs targeted at the $\alpha_v\beta_3$ integrin receptor involved in angiogenesis. The authors outline their design parameters as predictors of successful clinical use as (a) receptor density on the target (particularly if overexpressed in a variety of cancers), (b) affinity of the ligand for receptor binding, (c) specific activity of the labeled ligand, (d) plasma half-life (short to intermediate), (e) route of metabolic degradation or excretion (renal clearance preferred), (f) ex vivo counted % ID/g tumor in adequate animal models, (g) maximum tumor-to-background ratio achievable in vivo and time at which this is achieved, and (h) time course of the tumor-to-background ratios between an early (e.g., 2 hours after injection) and a late time point (e.g., 24 hours), expressed as the ratio (62).

PET has been used frequently to radiolabel RGD analogs targeted at the $\alpha_v\beta_3$ integrin receptor (63). Angiogenesis, the growth of new blood vessels from existing vessels, plays a major role in a number of human diseases. Endothelial cells from preexisting blood vessels become activated to migrate, proliferate, and differentiate into structures with lumens, forming new blood vessels in response to hormonal cues or hypoxic or ischemic conditions (64,65). External imaging using CT, MRI, ultrasound, PET, and SPECT has been an important tool for monitoring the progress of disease and the effect of cancer treatment (66). Since external imaging can detect capillary vessel growth only in special situations because of lack of resolution, imaging has been used to determine the "leakiness" or tumor blood vessel permeability of the tumor and to monitor growth factors such as VEGF or endothelial cell markers such as the integrins and their related receptors, which are upregulated during the angiogenesis process. The α_v, β_3 integrin receptor has been a popular target for radiolabeled biochemical probes of angiogenesis (67). Antibodies against the receptor or peptides with the RGD configuration block angiogenesis in tumor models based on the high differential presence of integrin receptors on angiogenic endothelial cells and tumor cells. Early radiolabeled studies used a radioiodinated cyclic RGD peptide, but the high lipophilicity of the derivative created nonspecific uptake in the liver and intestine. Haubner et al. also radioiodinated a RGD peptide and found the lipophilicity to be too great. Adding an amino containing sugar group increased the hydrophilicity and introduced a labeling site for either ^{18}F or ^{125}I. The ^{18}F galacto-RGD showed four times the uptake in tumors containing the integrin receptor compared with the weakly expressing tumor line used as a nonspecific control. Ogawa et al. radiolabeled a cyclic peptide using electrophilic fluorination with radioactive fluorine. The lower specific activity decreased the tumor uptake (68). Chen et al. radiolabeled the D-Tyr for D-Phe analog of Haubner's cyclic peptide but conjugated fluorobenzoic acid with the epsilon amino group of lysine to produce the ^{18}F derivative rather than use a sugar derivative. Tumor to blood ratios were more than 20 at two hours after injection. The comparison with the radioiodinated compound showed faster clearance from blood, liver, kidney, and tumor. Saturable binding was demonstrated. Chen et al. had earlier compared a radiofluorinated dimer of the RGD peptide by linking a 4-[^{18}F]fluorobenzoyl moiety with the amino group of the glutamate. The dimeric RGD peptide demonstrated significantly higher tumor uptake and prolonged tumor retention in comparison with a monomeric RGD peptide analog [^{18}F]FB-c(RGDyK). The dimeric RGD peptide had predominant renal excretion, whereas the monomeric analog was excreted primarily through the biliary route. Micro-PET imaging one hour after injection of the dimeric RGD peptide-exhibited tumor to contralateral background ratio of 9.5. The synergistic effect of polyvalency and improved pharmacokinetics may be responsible for the superior imaging characteristics of [^{18}F]FB-E[c(RGDyK)]$_2$ (69).

Poethko et al. have shown that the aromatic aldehyde is also useful and is a less complicated synthesis compared with the usual procedure for introducing a ^{18}F through an active ester of 4-fluorobenzoic acid. The ^{18}F is introduced into the aromatic ring by the same method, that is, displacement of the trimethyl ammonium group. Then the aldehyde is reacted with a aminooxypeptide to form the N-(4-[^{18}F]fluorobenzylidene) oxime. This approach did require the formation of the aminooxypeptide, but this can be done in bulk before the radiosynthesis begins. This approach has been tested in vivo with a RGD analog and a somatostatin receptor binding peptide. Both showed good in vivo stability and favorable pharmacokinetics (70).

Radiolabeled Steroids

Radioligands for the estrogen, androgen, and progesterone receptor have all been radiolabeled to monitor cancers that are steroid hormone dependent (71). Although no compound is currently in clinical use, several agents have been tested for PET.

Estrogen receptor (ER) imaging, and new compounds continue to be evaluated. The analog of estradiol, 16α-[^{18}F]-fluoroestradiol-17 (FES), is the radiotracer of choice for imaging and quantifying the functional ER status of breast cancer by PET. It is prepared using the cyclic sulfate in variable yields (72,73). FES uptake in primary tumors correlates with the level of ER expression measured by in vitro radioligand binding assay. Non-invasive whole body imaging of regional estradiol binding to ER provides information not possible by biopsy and in vitro assay. FES PET can provide specific characterization of sites identified by nonspecific methods, such as CT or FDG PET (74). Another application, measuring receptor occupancy using FES before and after treatment with tamoxifen, was predictive of response (75).

Radioligands for P-Glycoprotein and The Multidrug Resistance-Associated Protein

Chemotherapeutic failure due to multidrug resistance (MDR) is a common problem in cancer treatment. In general, MDR refers to a phenotype whereby a tumor is resistant to a large number of natural chemotherapeutics of diverse structure. As a result, several inhibitors have been radiolabeled to monitor the process with the goal of preventing ineffective chemotherapy because the chemotherapeutic is pumped out of the tumor (76). ^{99m}Tc sesti-MIBI, first developed as a myocardial perfusion agent, was found to be a substrate for P-glycoprotein (P-gp) and has been used clinically to determine MDR. This represents one approach of determining the occupancy of either P-gp or multidrug resistance-associated protein (MRP) before and after chemotherapy. The second approach has been to radiolabel the chemotherapeutic, validate it as a true tracer, and then determine in vivo whether the chemotherapeutic is a substrate for P-gp or MRP. Examples of the first approach include carbon-11-labeled verapamil, examples of the second approach are ^{11}C-labeled colchicines, daunorubicin, paclitaxel, and docetaxel. Fluorine-labeled fluorouracil and fluoropaclitaxel have also been studied. In MDR1a/1b knockout mice, which have a phenotype that best simulates human MDR1 disruption, investigators have been able to quantify the effect of P-gp using biodistribution in normal and knockout mice. The increases in brain uptake are large in knockout mice. One example of the development and validation of a radiolabeled chemotherapeutic from bench to bedside was published recently by Kurdziel et al. (77).

THE IDEAL PET RADIOTRACER

Given that PET imaging does not yield an analysis of chemical structure like magnetic resonance spectroscopy does, the emitted gamma rays are an indication of the position, but not the chemical form of the tracer. The ideal then is a radiotracer that does not change chemical form extensively, yet still measures an important biochemical step. Receptor binding and enzyme inhibition have developed into two such biochemical processes that can be easily translated into biochemical terms. The best example is the development of 2-[^{18}F]FDG, which is taken up by cells via a glucose transporter and then phosphorylated, but is not metabolized further and is retained in the cell by virtue of the charged phosphate. Even though FDG follows only two of the many steps involved in glucose metabolism, its retention in the cell is related to glucose metabolism. Sokoloff and colleagues had carried out many studies validating 2-deoxy-2-[^{14}C]glucose as a measure of glucose metabolism in the brain only. In tumors, there is concern that the lumped constant, which relates the metabolic rate of FDG with that of glucose, can change as a function of the progression of the disease so that it is not a straightforward measurement of relative glucose metabolism (78).

There are several radiotracer probe design criteria that were mostly developed for PET applications in neurochemistry, but are being applied to the design of radiotracers in oncology. A simple model has been put forth by Katzenellenbogen et al. (79) and Eckelman (80) as a first approximation. At high specific activity, the maximal B/F ratio will be B_{max}/K_d. The second term in the Scatchard transformation ($B/F = B_{max}/K_d - B/K_d$) is negligible. Certainly, distribution factors, nonspecific protein binding, metabolism, and other interactions will decrease the maximal B/F ratio when the molecular probe is used in vivo. Therefore, this criterion is necessary but not sufficient. This estimation is especially important as targeting of receptor systems with low nM to pM concentration becomes more prevalent. It is incorrect to address only the issue of K_d when referring to potential targeted molecules. Only the combination of B_{max}/K_d will accurately estimate the probability of obtaining a reasonable ratio in vivo (81).

Furthermore, this B_{max}/K_d of the target protein and targeted probe cannot be considered in a vacuum. If the B_{max}/K_d for other low-density sites is comparable, there will be competition for the molecular probe. Under some conditions, even nonspecific binding can compete for the probe. Katzenellenbogen addressed this for estradiol binding nonspecifically to albumin. When the K_d is weak (5–10 μM), but the B_{max} is enormous at 400 to 650 μM, the B_{max}/K_d ratio [(400–650)/(5–10)] is competitive with so-called specific binding. As researchers tend toward more reversible ligands with slightly lower affinities, the influence of other receptors and the so-called nonspecific sites becomes more important.

Additional design criteria can be adopted from the pharmaceutical literature. Lipinski and Hopkins discussed the "rule of five" and stated that the rule applied to about 90% of the potential drug candidates (82). This rule addresses issues of oral absorption related to lipophilicity, hydrogen bond donors and acceptors, and molecular weight. There are exceptions such as the statin, atorvastatin, which has seven hydrogen bond acceptors yet is an effective drug. Nevertheless, this approach is superior to high throughput screening of a reasonable percentage of chemical space. Although the criteria for the rule of five addresses oral absorption, it is clear that these same properties affect specific and nonspecific binding, organ and lipid membrane uptake and transport, and liver metabolism, all-important to obtaining imageable target delineation and contrast in vivo. As mentioned before, none of these criteria are sufficient, but they are in most cases necessary.

REDUCTIONIST APPROACH TO IMAGING FOR SINGLE GENE DISEASES AND SINGLE CONTROL POINT

For more than 50 years, radiopharmaceutical scientists have been targeting specific proteins and therefore fall into the class of mechanistic targeting defined by Sams-Dodd (83). The first reference given for nonradioactive targeted probes is attributed to Paul Ehrlich. His concept was derived from a toxicology point of view rather than a specific target-to-nontarget advantage needed for successful external imaging of a radioligand. Ehrlich used the English expression "magic bullet" for the first time in his Harben Lectures in the early 1900s (16). This concept appeared earlier in his publications, based on his view of side chains, the precursor of our concept of receptors, and on his design criteria for drugs that attach the parasitic invader, but do not harm the normal tissue. Ehrlich's first magic bullet was Salvarsan or arsphenamine, discovered in 1909, which was the result of screening more than 600 compounds and provided the only cure for syphilis. This was not target specific as much as it was disease specific. Ehrlich also thought of attaching toxins to antibodies whereby the antibody would carry the deadly freight to the site of the invading parasite. His ideas live on in the development of immunotoxins.

Although molecular imaging with radiopharmaceuticals started somewhat later, it has a history of developing radiolabeled compounds for specific targets. Interactions at the molecular level using pregenomic techniques to identify the target include biochemical probes such as iodide (~50 years), receptor-binding radiotracers, and radiolabeled monoclonal antibodies (~25 years). The leads for this development came from autopsy samples of patient populations, genetic linkage studies, and drug efficacy, among others. The autopsy studies are often misleading, because they do not identify a control point of the disease, but rather a change in biochemistry found late in the disease. Recently, new techniques and information have been developed as a result of the progress in proteomics and genomics. Also, targeting approaches at the molecular level have more recently added postgenomic techniques such as molecular biology, nanotechnology, proteomics, genomics, antisense binding, reporter genes, and protein-protein interactions to name a few. Radiolabeled probes for genes, mRNA, antisense, and protein-protein interactions have been prepared and studied in vitro and in vivo in animals, but it is the reporter gene approach that has progressed toward clinical studies as shown by Blasberg (84) and Serganova and Blasberg (85).

Three major approaches are being pursued by those developing radiopharmaceuticals: (*i*) monitoring general disease control points such as proliferation, hypoxia, apoptosis, angiogenesis, inflammation, and metastasis; (*ii*) monitoring the targeting of radioimmunotherapeutics with the same antibody radiolabeled with an imaging radionuclide; and (*iii*) monitoring the same control point that the pharmaceutical companies are targeting using external imaging. These approaches are analogous to the pharmaceutical approach of developing a blockbuster that is therapeutically effective in a wide range of cancers as opposed to developing a targeted molecule that is effective in a small population of cancers. The latter approach is the so-called individualized or personalized medicine that is the hope of higher therapeutic efficiency.

A single disease control point must be identified as the drug target; likewise a single control point will then be available for the imaging agent. This reduces drug targeting of an organism to drug targeting a single protein expression product. This is clearly a reductionist approach to drug discovery, driven by the explosion in identification of new targets in the post-genomic era. However, since most imaging procedures are limited to a single or two scans per patient per session, it is ideal as an imaging approach and follows implicitly what radiopharmaceutical scientists have been pursuing for many years. However, following the lead of the pharmaceutical companies increases the probability that the radiotracer will have an impact on clinical studies (86). It is safe to say that earlier design criteria based on autopsy studies did not often lead to clinical use, especially in complicated neurological and psychiatric diseases.

The first approach for general disease control points is more advanced although the first generation of radiopharmaceuticals discussed above probably will undergo further validation and refinement in terms of pharmacokinetics, pharmacodynamics, and sensitivity. It is important that the research efforts demonstrate that radiotracers labeled with either a metallic radionuclide or a

radiohalogen undergo a thorough validation to demonstrate what biochemistry is accurately traced by the analog. Krohn et al. define this as an ongoing process given that using an analog as a tracer for a specific biochemical, such as glucose or thymidine is susceptible to nonparallel changes in biochemical parameters of the analog compared with the parent compound in terms of flow, permeability, metabolism, flux, receptor density and its associated binding rate constant (27). This has not been investigated uniformly for the radiotracers designed to monitor the general control point and is seldom addressed for radiometallic tracers.

The second approach is more useful if the therapeutic truly occupies a small percentage of the protein target. In that way, it can be used to judge if the biodistribution is favorable for therapeutic studies, and after treatment it can be used to monitor the effect of the radiotherapy.

The third approach to radiolabeling a key protein expression product affected by the experimental therapeutic drug requires close collaboration with either a university pharmacologist or a pharmaceutical company. Producing a radiolabeled analog of the drug with the proper validation studies will lead to an important preclinical parameter, namely, drug occupancy and the concomitant parameter of the duration of drug occupancy. However, radiolabeling an analog of the drug itself will not lead to an understanding of the effectiveness of the drug because it will be a two variable experiment that will make it difficult to interpret the changes in radioactivity at the target protein site. Unless drug washout is assured, something that is not likely to be possible during chemotherapy, changes in the radioactivity at the target could be caused by changes in the number of binding sites or changes in the drug occupancy of the target. A clearer interpretation of the imaging results is achieved if the change in the ultimate expression product is monitored by external imaging.

One example of the latter approach of targeting a single control point in a particular disease is the external imaging of HER2 expression as a function of treatment using an inhibitor of heat-shock protein 90 (HSP-90). 17-Allylaminogeldanamycin (17-AAG) is the first HSP-90 inhibitor to be tested in a clinical trial. This drug induces proteasomal degradation of HER2 by binding to HSP-90 chaperone protein. The challenge is to monitor this treatment using external imaging. The lead for targeting the HER2 protein comes from the clinical trials of an antibody to HER2. Trastuzumab is such an antibody for HER2 (also known as ErbB2 and NEU), which is a cell surface glycoprotein with tyrosine kinase activity. Based on the clinical trials, HER2 overexpression is now an entry criteria and amplification/overexpression is predictive for response in breast cancer. Larson's group at Memorial Sloan-Kettering Cancer Center has developed an antibody fragment for HER2 radiolabeled with ^{68}Ga whose physical half-life matches the biological half-life of the antibody fragment. The ^{68}Ga radiolabeled F(ab')$_2$ monitors the change in the protein expression product as a function of treatment with 17-AAG. The effectiveness of 17-AAG was demonstrated using small animal imaging in BT-474 tumor bearing mice (87). This approach does not monitor the effectiveness of 17-AAG binding to HSP-90 directly, but rather to the protein expression product and therefore does not suffer from the critique that the change in radioactivity distribution could result from either drug occupancy or reduced number of HER2 proteins per cell or a reduction in the number of cells. Only a combination of the latter two is measured with this approach.

CONCLUSION

Many probes radiolabeled with short-lived PET radionuclides are available and many more can be prepared. The key is to choose the right radiolabeled probe for the right target. This involves choosing between a single target based on either a single gene disease, or a single control point, or to choose a more general target that will be applicable to a number of treatment paradigms. But regardless of the choice, the compound must be validated as binding to the target with the appropriate pharmacokinetics and pharmacodynamics. Finally the impact on clinical care must be demonstrated. This latter aspect of probe design and development requires the utmost attention of radiopharmaceutical scientists and clinicians alike.

REFERENCES

1. Therasse P, Arbuck SG, Eisenhauer EA, et al. New guidelines to evaluate the response to treatment in solid tumors. European Organization for Research and Treatment of Cancer, National Cancer Institute of the United States, National Cancer Institute of Canada. J Natl Cancer Inst (Bethesda) 2000; 92:205–216.
2. Eckelman WC. Radiolabeling with ^{99m}Tc to study high capacity and low capacity biochemical systems. Eur J Nucl Med 1995; 22:249–263.
3. Weissleder R, Reimer P, Lee AS, et al. MR receptor imaging: ultrasmall iron oxide particles targeted to asialoglycoprotein receptors. Am J Roentgenol 1990; 155(6): 1161–1167.
4. Vera DR, Buonocore MH, Wisner ER, et al. A molecular receptor-binding contrast agent for magnetic resonance imaging of the liver. Acad Radiol 1995; 2(6):497–506.
5. Bolo NR, Brennan KM, Jones RM, et al. Fluorodeoxyglucose brain metabolism studied by NMR and PET. Ann N Y Acad Sci 1987; 508:451–459.
6. Weissleder R, Moore A, Mahmood U, et al. In vivo magnetic resonance imaging of transgene expression. Nat Med 2000; 6:351–355.
7. Carrasquillo JA. Radioimmunoscintigraphy with polyclonal or monoclonal antibodies. In: Zalutsky MR, ed. Antibodies in Radiodiagnosis and Radiotherapy. Boca Raton, Florida: CRC Press, 1989:169–198.
8. Kung HF, Kung MP, Choi SR. Radiopharmaceuticals for single-photon emission computed tomography brain imaging. Semin Nucl Med 2003; 33(1):2–13.
9. Eckelman WC, Erba PA, Schwaiger M, et al. Postmeeting summary on the round table discussion at the seventh international symposium on technetium in chemistry and nuclear medicine held in Bressanone, Italy on September 6–9, 2006. Nucl Med Biol 2007; 34(1):1–4.
10. Kung HF, Kung MP, Wey SP, et al. Clinical acceptance of a molecular imaging agent: a long march with TRODAT. Nucl Med Biol 2007; 34(7):787–789.
11. Laforest R, Rowland DJ, Welch MJ. MicroPET imaging with non-conventional isotopes. Nucl Sci Symp Conf Rec, IEEE: 2001; 3:1572–1576.
12. Hevesy G, Paneth F. A Manual of Radioactivity. 2nd ed. London: Oxford University Press, 1938.
13. Kilbourn MR. Fluorine-18 labeling of radiopharmaceuticals. Prepared for the Committee on Nuclear and Radiochemistry, National Research Council. Washington DC: National Academy Press, 1990:17–18.
14. Szajek LP, Kao CHK, Kiesewetter DO, et al. Semi-remote production of Br-76 and preparation of high specific activity radiobrominated pharmaceuticals for PET studies. Radiochim Acta 2004; 92:291–295.
15. Vuong BK, Kiesewetter DO, Lang L, et al. An automated one-step one-pot [(18)F]FCWAY synthesis: development and minimization of chemical impurities. Nucl Med Biol 2007; 34(4):433–438.
16. Ehrlich P. On immunity, with special reference to cell-life (Croonian Lecture, Royal Society of London, 1990), reprinted in Collected Papers of Ehrlich P, vol 2, Himmelweit, ed. New York: Permagon Press, 1957:178–195.
17. Fahey FH. Instrumentation in positron emission tomography. Neuroimaging Clin N Am 2003; 13(4):659–669.
18. Schmidt KC, Smith CB. Resolution, sensitivity and precision with autoradiography and small animal positron emission tomography: implications for functional brain imaging in animal research. Nucl Med Biol 2005; 32(7): 719–725.
19. Jagoda EM, Vaquero JJ, Seidel J, et al. Experiment assessment of mass effects in the rat: implications for small animal PET imaging. Nucl Med Biol 2004; 31(6): 771–779.
20. Kurdziel KA, Figg WD, Carrasquillo JA, et al. Using positron emission tomography 2-deoxy-2-[^{18}F]fluoro-D-glucose, [11]CO, and ^{15}O-water for monitoring androgen independent prostate cancer. Mol Imaging Biol 2003; 5(2): 86–93.
21. Aloj L, Jagoda E, Lang L, et al. Targeting of transferrin receptors in nude mice bearing A431 and LS 174t xenografts with [^{18}F] holo-transferrin: permeability and receptor dependence. J Nucl Med 1999; 40:1547–1555.
22. Bacharach SL, Libutti SK, Carrasquillo JA. Measuring tumor blood flow with H_2[15]O: practical considerations. Nucl Med Biol 2000; 27:671–676.

23. Miller JC, Pien HH, Sahani D, et al. Imaging angiogenesis: applications and potential for drug development. J Natl Cancer Inst 2005; 97(3):172–187.

24. Hoh CK. Clinical use of FDG PET. Nucl Med Biol 2007; 34(7):737–742.

25. Sokoloff L, Reivich M, Kennedy C, et al. The [14C] deoxyglucose method for the measurement of local cerebral glucose utilization: theory, procedure, and normal values in the conscious and anesthetized albino rat. J Neurochem 1977; 28(5):897–916.

26. Smith TA. FDG uptake, tumour characteristics and response to therapy: a review. Nucl Med Commun 1998; 19(2):97–105.

27. Krohn KA, Mankoff DA, Muzi M, et al. True tracers: comparing FDG with glucose and FLT with thymidine. Nucl Med Biol 2005; 32:663–671.

28. Couturier O, Luxen A, Chatal JF, et al. Fluorinated tracers for imaging cancer with positron emission tomography. Eur J Nucl Med Mol Imaging 2004; 31:1182–1206.

29. Toyohara J, Fujibayashi Y. Trends in nucleoside tracers for PET imaging of cell proliferation. Nucl Med Biol 2003; 30(7):681–685.

30. Kim DW, Ahn DS, Oh YH, et al. A new class of SN2 reactions catalyzed by protic solvents: facile fluorination for isotopic labeling of diagnostic molecules. J Am Chem Soc 2006; 128(50):16394–16397.

31. Rajendran JG, Krohn KA. Imaging hypoxia and angiogenesis in tumors. Radiol Clin North Am 2005; 43(1): 169–187.

32. Rasey JS, Hofstrand PD, Chin LK, et al. Characterization of [F-18] fluoroetanidazole, a new radiopharmaceutical for detecting tumor hypoxia. J Nucl Med 1999; 40(6): 1072–1079.

33. Dehdashti F, Grigsby PW, Mintun MA, et al. Assessing tumor hypoxia in cervical cancer by positron emission tomography with 60Cu-ATSM: relationship to therapeutic response—a preliminary report. Int J Radiat Oncol Biol Phys 2003; 55(5):1233–1238.

34. Lewis JS, McCarthy DW, McCarthy TJ, et al. Evaluation of Cu-64-ATSM in vitro and in vivo in a hypoxic tumor model. J Nucl Med 1999; 40(1):177–183.

35. Kelloff GJ, Krohn KA, Larson SM, et al. The progress and promise of molecular imaging probes in oncologic drug development. Clin Cancer Res 2005; 11(22):7967–7985.

36. Van Cruchen S, Van Den Broeck W. Morphological and biochemical aspects of apoptosis, oncosis, and necrosis. Anat Histol Embryol 2002; 31:214–223.

37. Yagle KJ, Eary JF, Tait JF, et al. Evaluation of 18F-annexin V as a PET imaging agent in an animal model of apoptosis. J Nucl Med 2005; 46:658–666.

38. Bustany P, Chatel M, Derlon JM, et al. Brain tumor protein synthesis and histological grade: a study by positron emission tomography (PET) with C-11-L-methionine. J Neuro-oncol 1986; 3:397–404.

39. Coenen HH, Fling P, Stocklin G. Cerebral metabolism of L-[2-18F] fluoro-tyrosine, a new PET tracer for protein synthesis. J Nucl Med 1989; 30:1367–1372.

40. Hawkins RA, Huang S-C, Barrio JR, et al. Estimation of local protein synthesis rates with L-[1-14C]leucine and

PET: methods, model, and results in animals and humans. J Cereb Blood Flow Metab 1989; 9:446–460.

41. Smith CB, Schmidt KC, Qin M, et al. Measurement of regional rates of cerebral protein synthesis with L-[1-11C] leucine and PET with correction for recycling of tissue amino acids: II. validation in rhesus monkeys. J Cereb Blood Flow Metab 2005; 25:629–640.

42. Barrio JR, Keen RE, Ropchan JR, et al. L-[1-14C]leucine: routine synthesis by enzymatic resolution. J Nucl Med 1983; 24:515–521.

43. Schuster DM, Votaw JR, Nieh PT, et al. Initial experience with the radiotracer anti-1-amino-3-18F fluorocyclobutane-1-carboxylic acid with PET/CT in prostate carcinoma. J Nucl Med 2007; 48(1):56–63.

44. Chapman JD, Bradley JD, Eary JF, et al. Molecular (functional) imaging for radiotherapy applications: an RTOG symposium. Int J Radiat Oncol Biol Phys 2003; 55(2): 294–301.

45. Yoshimoto M, Waki A, Yonekura Y, et al. Characterization of acetate metabolism in tumor cells in relation to cell proliferation: acetate metabolism in tumor cells. Nucl Med Biol 2001; 28(2):117–122.

46. Costello LC, Franklin RB. Citrate metabolism of normal and malignant prostate epithelial cells. Urology 1997; 50(1): 3–12.

47. Fricke E, Machtens S, Hofmann M, et al. Postiron emission tomography with 11C-acetate and 18F-FDG in prostate cancer patients. Eur J Nucl Med Mol Imaging 2003; 30(4): 607–611.

48. Kotzerke J, Volkmer BG, Neumaier B, et al. Carbon-11 acetate positron emission tomography can detect local recurrence of prostate cancer. Eur J Nucl Med Mol Imaging 2002; 29(10):1380–1384.

49. Oyama N, Miller TR, Dehdashti F, et al. 11C-acetate PET imaging of prostate cancer: detection of recurrent disease at PSA relapse. J Nucl Med 2003; 44(4):549–555.

50. DeGrado TR, Baldwin SW, Wang SY, et al. Synthesis and evaluation of F-18-labeled choline analogs as oncologic PET tracers. J Nucl Med 2001; 42(12):1805–1814.

51. Fowler JF, Ritter MA, Chappell RJ, et al. What hypofractionated protocols should be tested for prostate cancer? Int J Radiat Oncol Biol Phys 2003; 56(4):1093–1104.

52. DeGrado TR, Coleman RE, Wang S, et al. Synthesis and evaluation of 18F labeled choline as an oncologic tracer for positron emission tomography: initial findings in prostate cancer. Cancer Res 2001; 61:110–117.

53. Wieland DM, Wu J, Brown LE, et al. Radiolabeled adrenergic neuron-blocking agents: adrenomedullary imaging with [131I] iodobenzylguanidine. J Nucl Med 1980; 21(4):349–353.

54. Raffel DM, Wieland DM. Assessment of cardiac sympathetic nerve integrity with positron emission tomography. Nucl Med Biol 2001; 28(5):541–559.

55. Rufini V, Calcagni ML, Baum RP. Imaging of neuro-endocrine tumors. Semin Nucl Med 2006; 36:228–247.

56. Knickmeier M, Matheja P, Wichter T, et al. Clinical evaluation of no-carrier-added meta-[123I] iodobenzylguanidine for myocardial scintigraphy. Eur J Nucl Med 2000; 27:302–307.

57. Mairs RJ, Russell J, Cunningham SH, et al. Enhanced tumor uptake and in vitro radiotoxicity of no-carrier-added 131IMIBG:implications for the radiotherapy of neuroblastoma. Eur J Cancer 1995; 31:576–581.

58. Pacak K, Eisenhofer G, Carrasquillo JA, et al. Diagnostic localization of pheochromocytoma: the coming of age of positron emission tomography. Ann N Y Acad Sci 2002; 970:170–176.

59. Rufini V, Calcagni ML, Baum RP. Imaging of neuroendocrine tumors. Semin Nucl Med 2006; 36:228–247.

60. Fani M, Maecke HR. The status of diagnostic and therapeutic targeting of somatostatin receptor-positive tumours. In: Mazzi U, ed. Proceedings of the Seventh International Symposium on Technetium in Chemistry and Nuclear Medicine. Padova Italy: Servizi Grafici Editoriali snc, 2006:657–664.

61. Eiblmaier M, Andrews R, Laforest R, et al. Nuclear uptake and dosimetry of ^{64}Cu-labeled chelator somatostatin conjugates in an SSTr2-transfected human tumor cell line. J Nucl Med 2007; 48(8):1390–1396.

62. Mariani G, Erba P, Signore A. Receptor-mediated tumor targeting with radiolabeled peptides: there is more to it than somatostatin analogs. J Nucl Med 2006; 47:1904–1907.

63. Haubner R. Alphavbeta3-integrin imaging: a new approach to characterise angiogenesis? Eur J Nucl Med Mol Imaging 2006; 33(suppl 1):54–63.

64. Folkman J. Tumor angiogenesis: therapeutic implications. N Eng J Med 1971; 285:1182–1186.

65. Sanz L, Alvarez-Vallina L. The extracellular matrix: a new turn-of-the-screw for anti-angiogenic strategies. Trends Mol Med 2003; 9:256–262.

66. Schirner M, Menrad A, Stephens A, et al. Molecular Imaging of Tumor Angiogenesis. Ann N Y Acad Sci 2004; 1014:67–75.

67. Haubner R, Wester JH, Weber WA, et al. Noninvasive imaging of $\alpha_v\beta_3$ integrin expression using ^{18}F-labeled RGD-containing glycopeptide and positron emission tomography. Cancer Res 2001; 16:1781–1785.

68. Ogawa M, Hatano K, Oishi S, et al. Direct electrophilic radiofluorination of a cyclic RGD peptide for in vivo alpha(v)beta(3) integrin related tumor imaging. Nucl Med Biol 2003; 30:1–9.

69. Chen XY, Park R, Shahinian AH, et al. Pharmacokinetics and tumor retention of I-125-labeled RGD peptide are improved by PEGylation. Nucl Med Biol 2004; 31:11–19.

70. Poethko T, Schottelius M, Thumshirn G, et al. Chemoselective pre-conjugate radiohalogenation of unprotected mono- and multimeric peptides via oxime formation. Radiochim Acta 2004; 92(4–6):317–327.

71. Katzenellengoben JA. Receptor imaging of tumors (nonpepide). In: Welch MJ, Redvanly CS, eds. Handbook of Radiopharmaceuticals. London: John Wiley & Sons, Ltd., 2003:715–750.

72. Romer J, Fuchtner F, Steinbach J, et al. Automated production of 16a-[^{18}F] fluoroestradiol for breast cancer imaging. Nucl Med Biol 1999; 26:473–479.

73. Kumar P, Mercer J, Doerkson C, et al. Clinical production, stability studies and PET imaging with 16-α-[^{18}F]fluoroestradiol ([^{18}F]FES) in ER positive breast cancer patients. J Pharm Pharm Sci 2007; 10(2):256s–265s.

74. Dehdashti F, Mortimer JE, Siegel BA, et al. Positron tomographic assessment of estrogen receptors in breast cancer: comparison with FDG-PET and in vitro receptor assays. J Nucl Med 1995; 36:1766–1774.

75. Mortimer JE, Dehdashti F, Siegel BA, et al. Metabolic flare: indicator of hormone responsiveness in advanced breast cancer. J Clin Oncol 2001; 19:2797–2803.

76. Hendrikse NH. Monitoring interactions at ATP-dependent drug efflux pumps. Curr Pharm Des 2000; 6(16):1653–1668.

77. Kurdziel KA, Kalen JD, Hirsch JI, et al. Imaging multidrug resistance with 4-[^{18}F] fluoropaclitaxel. Nucl Med Biol 2007; 34(7):823–831.

78. Muzi M, Freeman SD, Burrows RC, et al. Kinetic characterization of hexokinase isoenzymes from glioma cells: implications for FDG imaging of human brain tumors. Nucl Med Biol 2001; 28(2):107–116.

79. Katzenellenbogen JA, Heiman DF, Carlson KE, et al. In vitro and in vivo steroid receptor assays in the design of estrogen radiopharmaceuticals. In: Eckelman WC, ed. Receptor Binding Radiotracers. Boca Raton, FL: CRC Press, 1982:93–126.

80. Eckelman WC. Radiolabeled adrenergic and muscarinic blockers for in vivo studies. In: Eckelman WC, ed. Receptor Binding Radiotracers. Boca Raton, FL: CRC Press, 1982: 69–92.

81. Kung MP, Choi SR, Hou C, et al. Selective binding of 2-[^{125}I] iodo-nisoxetine to norepinephrine transporters in the brain. Nucl Med Biol 2004; 31(5):533–541.

82. Lipinski C, Hopkins A. Navigating chemical space for biology and medicine. Nature 2004; 432(7019):855–861.

83. Sams-Dodd F. Drug discovery: selecting the optimal approach. Drug Discov Today 2006; 11:465–472.

84. Blasberg RG. In vivo molecular-genetic imaging: multimodality nuclear and optical combinations. Nucl Med Biol 2003; 30(8):879–888.

85. Serganova I, Blasberg R. Reporter gene imaging: potential impact on therapy. Nucl Med Biol 2005; 32:763–780.

86. Eckelman WC. Finding the right targeted probe for the right target for the right disease. In: Mazzi U, ed. Proceedings of the Seventh International Symposium on Technetium in Chemistry and Nuclear Medicine. Padova Italy: Servizi Grafici Editoriali snc, 2006:263–276.

87. Smith-Jones PM, Solit DB, Akhurst T, et al. Imaging the pharmacodynamics of HER2 degradation in response to HSP-90 inhibitors. Nat Biotechnol 2004; 22:701–706.

20

Targeted Radiolabeled Receptor-Avid Peptides

WYNN A. VOLKERT

Department of Radiology and the Radiopharmaceutical Sciences Institute, University of Missouri and H.S. Truman Memorial Veterans Administration Hospital, Columbia, Missouri, U.S.A.

INTRODUCTION

The advances in the design and development of novel molecular imaging agents continue to occur globally at an accelerating rate. Radiotracers to probe and interrogate biochemical, cellular, and genetic processes involved in a myriad of disease states are being identified and assessed in both in vitro and in vivo systems. Numerous approaches for specific in vivo targeting of cancers are being implemented to develop new radiolabeled compounds for both site-specific diagnostic and therapeutic applications. Examples of a wide variety of strategies being employed include development of radiolabeled immunologically derived targeting agents [e.g., monoclonal antibodies (MAbs)], probes for interrogating intracellular processes or markers (e.g., mRNA), and constructs that bind to specific molecular entities expressed on the surface of cells (e.g., antigens and receptors). Obviously, multiple innovative interdisciplinary paradigms must be implemented and evaluated to maximize improvement of current technologies to identify more effective tumor-specific radiotracers, if major advances in diagnostic imaging or treatment of human cancers are to be fully realized. This chapter is designed to highlight notable developments involving the design and utilization of radiolabeled peptides that bind with high affinity and specificity to cognate receptors that are uniquely expressed or overexpressed on the surface of human cancer cells and hold

potential as diagnostic and therapeutic radiopharmaceuticals. Numerous other approaches being explored to develop molecular imaging and targeted radiotherapeutic (TRT) constructs for applications in cancer are described elsewhere in this book.

DESIGN OF RADIOLABELED PEPTIDES

Over the past two decades, interest in developing radiolabeled peptides for imaging and treatment of cancers has been rapidly increasing. Technological advances in molecular biology, combinatorial chemistry, and peptide biochemistry are being used as a molecular basis to characterize receptor expression and to develop cognate receptor–avid radiolabeled peptide conjugates (1–8). To realize the potential of these advances, it is critical that the radiolabeling methodologies associated with these peptide-avid vectors be performed in a manner that minimally alters or enhances their capacity for high specificity in vivo targeting of cancer cells (9–16).

The design of effective molecular imaging and TRT agents requires optimizing the balance between specific in vivo targeting of the tumor and clearance of radioactivity from relevant nontarget tissues. Several difficulties are encountered when designing highly selective radiolabeled drug carriers and must be collectively addressed. These include problems related to the efficiency of radiotracer delivery to tumors, maximization of residence time of the radionuclide in the tumors, minimization of catabolism or metabolism of the radiotracer in the blood stream, and optimization of the relative rates of radiolabeled drug or radiolabeled metabolite clearance from nontarget organs or tissues, and maximizing the "radiotracer" specific activity, to name a few (3,10,17–25). Preparation of radiolabeled receptor-avid peptides that are or nearly approach the actual tracer levels is particularly relevant and critical when the number of cognate receptors expressed by the cancer cells is low. This is essential to minimize the potential of the "cold" unlabeled receptor-avid peptide analogue that may present in the preparation to competitively inhibit in vivo binding of the radiotracer to the targeted receptors in the tumor. Because of the multiple parameters that must be considered, developing effective cancer-specific radiolabeled peptides as in vivo radiopharmaceuticals is a complex problem, which is not accomplished by simply attaching a radionuclide to some random point on the targeting peptide-based vector (9,10,12,13). The chemistry involved in the conjugation at a specific molecular site and labeling processes, therefore, are integral and essential parts of the drug design process. For example, if a radiometal chelate is appended at a particular site on the peptide, the structure and physicochemical properties of the chelate must be compatible with and will hopefully promote high specific uptake and retention in the cancerous tumor. At the very least, the radiometal chelate should not significantly sterically interfere with binding of the peptide vector to the receptor. Thus, the selections of the appropriate radionuclide and conjugation method are critical elements in the formulation of safe and effective peptide-based radiopharmaceuticals.

Small peptides are usually rapidly excreted from the body, predominantly via renal or hepatobiliary excretion, or both, depending on their structural features. The lipophilicity/hydrophobicity contributes the pharmacokinetics and tissue distribution of peptide conjugates (3,4,13). As lipophilicity increases, a greater elimination by the hepatobiliary route is expected, while increased hydrophobicity favors preferential removal by the kidneys (10,18). It may be possible to increase tumor uptake by increasing lipophilicity causing slower blood clearance due to high plasma protein binding. However, this strategy often produces greater hepatobiliary clearance resulting in higher levels of liver and abdominal activity, which interferes with abdominal single-photon emission computed tomography (SPECT) or positron emission tomography (PET) imaging.

The utilization of receptor-avid small peptides as cancer-specific in vivo targeting vectors offers several important advantages compared to other radiolabeled constructs. However, as is the case with all drug design technologies, there are inherent limitations. Peptides consist of several covalently linked amino acids that can contain up to 50 to 100 amino acids (3,7). The majority of peptides and peptide conjugates being used as in vivo molecular imaging or TRT agents today contain less than 20 amino acids. Their relatively low molecular weight offers advantages over larger proteins (including MAbs) or other constructs (e.g., nanoparticles). For example, small peptides lack immunogenicity and can be readily and inexpensively synthesized via automated solid-state methods to produce well-defined and high-purity molecular entities, the quantitative composition can be accurately determined, exhibit relatively rapid clearance from the blood, more efficiently penetrate into most tissues (except for the normal blood-brain barrier) and tumors, and can be readily radiolabeled (3,5,6,19). There are also disadvantages associated with peptides, including the susceptibility of many naturally occurring peptides to rapid proteolysis in the blood, the potential presence of endogenous peptides that competitively inhibit receptor binding, and limitations on the magnitude of tumor uptake that is related to rapid clearance from the bloodstream (3,5,7,21).

The majority of endogenous peptides have plasma half-lives that prohibit their use in developing in vivo radiopharmaceuticals (5,7). However, syntheses of stabilized analogues can be relatively straightforward. The two most common methods to provide resistance to in vivo catabolism and metabolism are first, substitution of D-amino acids (or other pseudo-amino acids) by L-amino acids in the peptide sequence (5,6,20,26–32) and secondly, preparation of cyclized analogues to maintain the proper three-dimensional structure of the receptor-binding motif of the peptide while inhibiting proteolysis (1,11,33–36). The radiolabeled peptide conjugates described later in this chapter will provide numerous examples that demonstrate the effectiveness of these two strategies.

The receptor-avid peptide vectors used to produce cancer-specific radiotracers are generally large enough to enable conjugation of a chelate/chelator in a fashion that does not inhibit binding specificity or affinity to the receptor (3). A linker, tether, or spacer group is often required to place the radiochelate sufficiently distant from the binding sequence of the peptide so that it does not interfere with receptor binding (10,16,17). The spacer group also plays an important role in modifying the in vivo pharmacokinetics of the radio-peptide conjugate (7,10,14,16,17,37,38). Since most peptide conjugates have relatively low molecular weights, an optimum balance between the physicochemical properties reporter component (e.g., radiometal chelate), peptide targeting moiety, and the spacer group, producing a radiotracer with acceptable pharmacokinetics and tissue deposition characteristics is difficult to achieve. Considerable efforts have been and will continue to be made to develop linker

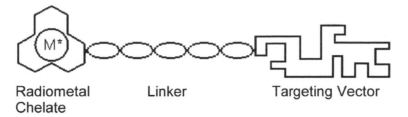

Radiometal   Linker   Targeting Vector
Chelate

Figure 1 General structure of a majority of radiometallated conjugates of receptor-avid peptides designed for in vivo targeting of their cognate receptors overexpressed on human cancer cells.

technology that has more general applicability for maximizing in vivo performance of these types of radiotracer conjugates. The general structure of many of the cancer-specific radiolabeled peptide conjugates discussed later in this chapter is shown in Figure 1. The linking group often plays a pivotal role in modifying (either positively or negatively) the binding affinity of the radiotracer to the receptor and increasing (or decreasing) trapping or residualization of the radioactive component in the tumor after it is localized on or in the cancer cells (9,10,25,39–46).

Cognate Receptor Characteristics

The majority of the radiolabeled peptide conjugates discussed in this summary are analogues of naturally occurring regulatory peptides that act on multiple cellular targets in the human body (6). These regulatory peptides control and modulate important functions of cells and organs (5,6). Their action is often mediated through specific membrane-bound receptors and most belong to the class of G protein–coupled receptors (5). Receptor subtypes exist for most regulatory peptides increasing the diversity of their mode of action and allowing for development of peptide analogue conjugates that bind preferentially to certain receptor subtypes that may be expressed by different types of cancers (3,5,6,29,47–54). The number of receptors expressed on the cancer cell surface can vary widely and range from a few thousand to over 100,000 receptors per cell (5,55). There is also considerable variation of some receptor density between cells of the same types of cancer.

An important characteristic of G protein–coupled receptors that is particularly relevant to consider during development of radiolabeled peptide receptor–avid diagnostic or TRT agents is that they are capable of efficiently transporting the radiotracer intracellularly via a receptor-mediated endocytosis mechanism (5,17,55–59). This process usually occurs following a receptor-agonist interaction on the exterior surface of the cancer cell membrane that initiates the associated signaling cascades. It must be emphasized that even though many agonists produce undesirable physiological side effects (e.g., enhancement

of tumor growth rate or toxicity) at pharmacological doses, high–specific activity radiolabeled peptide agonists are administered at "tracer" levels and produce negligible side effects. Internalization of the radiotracer provides an effective mechanism to facilitate trapping or residualization of the radioactivity following specific binding to the cancerous cells in the tumor (17,25,43,45,56,58,60). Following internalization, the receptors can be recycled back to the plasma membrane or targeted to the lysosome for degradation (55). The balance in intracellular trafficking (i.e., export, endocytosis, and degradation) dictates the level of receptor density as a function of time at the plasma membrane (55) as well as influencing the recycling rate. Similarly, internalized radiotracers may be trapped or excreted intact from the cell or degraded by intracellular processes to produce radiolabeled fragments that can also be trapped inside the cell or excreted from the cell. In most cases, the radiometal chelates have sufficient stability to "control" the radiometal, however, there may be dissociation or transchelation to intracellular proteins (e.g., as is the case with some ^{64}Cu chelates) of the radiometal. Radiolabeled peptides that bind to the receptor in an antagonistic manner are generally not transported intracellularly and are susceptible to in vivo dissociation or displacement from the cell surface receptor resulting in shorter tumor retention times. However, utility of receptor-avid radiotracers that bind to receptors in an antagonistic manner also holds important potential (61).

Targeted Radiotherapeutic Agents

A major advantage offered by radiolabeled peptides that target cell surface receptors and are used for imaging applications is that they hold important potential for development of corresponding analogues as cancer-specific targeted diagnostic and TRT pharmaceuticals (3,9,16,45,62–72). The development of radiolabeled peptide conjugates that bind to receptors that are uniquely expressed or overexpressed on the surface cancer cells provides invaluable opportunities for rapid accumulation of radioactivity with high specificity on cancer cells, and

Table 1 Receptor-Avid Peptide Analogues[a] Used as a Basis for Development of Human Cancer–Specific Radiotracers for Imaging and/or Targeted Radiotherapy

Peptide analogues	Cognate receptors[b]	Cancer cell target[c]
Octreotide	Somatostatin 1–5	Neuroendocrine tumors, SCLC, breast cancer
BB	BB 1–3	Prostate, breast, pancreatic cancers
NT	NT1,2	Prostate, breast, pancreatic cancers
α-Melanocyte stimulating hormone	MC1	Melanoma
Human ST peptide	GC-C	Colorectal cancers
VIP	VIP1/PACAP	Several cancers, including colon, GI, prostate, pancreatic, breast
CCK/gastrin	CCK2	Medullary thyroid carcinoma, SCLC, gastroenteropancreatic cancer

[a]This is a limited list of some of the more frequently used receptor-avid peptide analogues used to design promising radiotracers. Additional receptor-targeting peptides have been used as a basis to prepare potential radiolabeled imaging or targeted radiotherapeutic agents (5,171).
[b]The receptors listed may not include all of the subtypes, but represent subtypes that are frequently the most prominent that have been targeted by radiolabeled peptides.
[c]The list of human cancer cells that are listed are examples (not all inclusive) of the types of cancers that overexpress the respective "cognate receptors" and are being specifically targeted by the peptide-based radiotracers.
Abbreviations: BB, bombesin; NT, neurotensin; MC1, melanocortin-1; GC-C, guanylin/guanylate cyclase C; VIP, vasoactive intestinal peptide; PACAP, pituitary adenylate cyclase–activating polypeptide; CCK, cholecystokinin.

they behave as a therapeutic "magic bullet" (16). Peptide conjugated structures designed to selectively bind to cancer cell receptors can often be used for both molecular imaging agents and TRT pharmaceuticals, depending on the radionuclide utilized. For example, 1,4,7,10-tetraazacyclododecane-N,N′,N″,N‴-tetraacetic acid (DOTA)–peptide conjugates can be used to prepare imaging radiotracers using ^{111}In or ^{188}Ga for imaging or as TRT agents using ^{90}Y or ^{177}Lu (3,4,17,45,64,73,74). It is important to determine the degree to which the diagnostic radiolabeled analogue behaves as a "true radiotracer" for the TRT agent. Clearly, if imaging is performed with the same metal (e.g., ^{86}Y for ^{90}Y) or radiometal (e.g., using the 208-keV γ rays emitted by ^{177}Lu or the annihilation photons of ^{64}Cu) that will also be used for therapy, it will be a "true radiotracer." In contrast, if a different radiometal is used as a surrogate for the therapeutic radioisotope (e.g., ^{111}In or ^{68}Ga, in place of ^{177}Lu or ^{90}Y), the resulting radiolabeled diagnostic construct may not serve as a "true radiotracer" for the corresponding TRT agent (44). Utilization of appropriate diagnostic analogues can be and are being used not only to detect and monitor cancers but also for treatment planning dosimetry of the same peptide construct as used for TRT applications (63). In contrast, many of the molecular imaging constructs that target intracellular receptors, enzymes, mRNA, etc., without mediation of cell surface binding as an initial localizing event, will be more difficult to translate to a corresponding TRT agent. The promising future of applications of receptor-avid radiolabeled cancer-specific peptide conjugates is related predominantly to the development of their radiopharmaceuticals to treat oncological disorders in patients.

RECEPTOR-AVID PEPTIDE RADIOTRACER SYSTEMS

Numerous peptide receptors that are overexpressed in human cancer cells have been identified on a molecular basis as promising targets for sophisticated radiolabeled diagnostic imaging and TRT agents. Table 1 provides a summary of some of the most prominent receptor-avid peptide analogs that are being studied that specifically bind with their cognate receptors that are overexpressed on a wide spectrum of human cancer cell types (3,5–7). These radiotracers have been labeled with a variety of radionuclides that can be used for molecular imaging applications or for TRT applications (3,5,6,9,12,15, 16,23,29,31,45,68,73,75,76). Table 2 provides examples of radionuclides that have been used to produce peptide-based diagnostic imaging radiotracers. Table 3 summarizes examples of particle-emitting radionuclides that are used to synthesize radiolabeled peptides for TRT applications.

Somatostatin Analogues

Somatostatin receptors (SSTRs) mediate a wide spectrum of physiological functions, including endocrine and exocrine pancreatic secretion, neurotransmission, and cell proliferation (5,7,64). SSTRs are G protein–coupled receptors and expressed by a number of human cancers such as carcinoid, neuroblastoma, pheochromocytoma, gastroma, insulinoma, and medullary thyroid carcinoma (MTC) (5,6,29,40,53,56,64,70,77–79). Somatostatin (SST) inhibits release of a variety of hormones and

Table 2 Examples of Radionuclides Used to Prepare Diagnostic Receptor-avid Peptide Radiotracers

Radionuclide	Half-life	Mode of decay[a]	Photon energy (s)[b]
^{99m}Tc	6 hr	IT	140 keV (89%)
^{111}In	67.3 hr	EC	171 keV (90%)
			245 keV (94%)
^{123}I	13.2 hr	EC	159 keV (83%)
^{18}F	109 min	β^+ (97%)	511 keV
^{64}Cu	12.7 hr	β^+ (19%) EC (41%)	511 keV
^{68}Ga	1.1 hr	β^+ (90%) EC (10%)	511 keV
^{86}Y	14.7 hr	β^+ (33%) EC (66%)	511keV
^{94m}T	52 min	β^+ (62%) EC (38%)	511 keV

[a]The most prominent modes of decay including the abundance given in parenthesis. Radionuclides used for SPECT are ^{99m}Tc, ^{111}In, and ^{123}I. Radionuclides used for PET are ^{18}F, ^{64}Cu, ^{68}Ga, ^{86}Y, and ^{94m}Tc.
[b]Only the γ ray (or annihilation photon) energies used for SPECT or PET imaging, along with the abundance of each, are included in this list.
Abbreviations: SPECT, single-photon emission computed tomography; PET, positron emission tomography.

Table 3 Examples of Radionuclides Used to Prepare Therapeutic Receptor-Avid Peptide Radiotracers

Radionuclide	Half-life	Mode of decay[a]	Particle energies[b]
^{64}Cu	12.7 hr	β^+ (19%)	0.66 MeV
		β^- (40%)	0.57 MeV
^{90}Y	2.7 days	β^- (100%)	2.3 MeV
^{105}Rh	1.4 days	β^- (100%)	2.3 MeV
^{149}Pm	2.2 days	β^- (100%)	1.1 MeV
^{177}Lu	6.7 days	β^- (100%)	0.50 MeV
^{211}At	7.2 hr	α^{++}(41%)	5.9 MeV
		EC (59%)	
^{212}Bi	1 hr	α^{++} (100%)	6.1 and 8.8 MeV[c]

[a]The most prominent modes of decay via emission of a β particle (β^-), positron (β^+), or α particle (α^{++}). The abundance related to each mode is given in parenthesis.
[b]The maximum energies of the β particles and positrons emitted during the decay events are listed.
[c]^{212}Bi decays by two pathways; one is by β particle decay ($E_{max} = 2.3$ MeV) to ^{212}Po (66%) followed in 0.3 millisecond by α particle (E = 8.8 MeV) decay to ^{208}Pb; the second is by α particle decay (E = 6.1 MeV) to ^{208}Tl (34%) followed by β particle decay in 3.1 minutes ($E_{max} = 1.8$ MeV) to ^{208}Pb.

exhibits antiproliferative effects on cultured cancer cells, tumors in animal models, and neuroendocrine tumors in humans (5,6,64). Octreotide (OC) (Sando-statin®) was developed as a highly stable analogue of SST to suppress symptoms of neuroendocrine diseases (64,80). OC includes the structural motif of the four amino acids (Phe-Trp-Lys-Thr) that form the receptor-binding domain in a loop that maintains an optimal configuration for binding to SSTRs (5,6,64).

It was recognized that radiolabeled OC may selectively localize on neuroendocrine tumors and become internalized intracellularly to enable SPECT imaging (29,81). The first OC derivative studied was labeled with I-123 (Tyr^3) to produce ^{123}I-[Tyr^3]-octreotide (TOC). This radiopharmaceutical demonstrated proof of principle for imaging several different types of tumors in humans (29,81,82). However, problems associated with its high lipophilicity and dehalogenation resulted in significant accumulation of radioactivity in the liver and GI tract (7,64). Development of ^{111}In-diethylenetriamine penta acetic acid-octreotide [^{111}In-DTPA-OC], a more hydrophilic conjugate that maintained high SSTR binding affinity but cleared more rapidly and efficiently from the blood and body, subsequently occurred (83). This radiotracer (Octreoscan®) was FDA approved in 1993 and is widely used in clinical imaging of neuroendocrine as well as other tumors.

^{111}In-labeled DTPA-OC (Fig. 2A) is primarily cleared from the bloodstream via kidney with little hepatobiliary excretion, which permits visualization of abdominal tumor sites (1,6,29). ^{111}In-DTPA-OC is largely excreted intact into the urine, however, there is significant long-term retention in the kidneys, which creates a problem for tumor imaging near the kidneys and may be dose-limiting for TRT applications (6,30,63,64,84,85). The most likely mechanism for ^{111}In-DTPA-OC, like many peptides, is clearance by the glomerular filtration pathway, followed by some resorption in the proximal tubules. The resorption process involves binding of the radiolabeled peptide conjugate to a carrier on tubular cell membranes and internalization with eventual degradation in lysosomes to produce radiolabeled metabolic/catabolic products that become trapped in the proximal renal tubular cells (7,42,86,87). It is possible to partially reduce kidney uptake by pre- or coadministration of excess positively charged molecules (e.g., lysine and/or arginine) by inhibiting binding of peptides to the negatively charged sites involved in the renal uptake mechanism (42,64). While it is possible to decrease kidney uptake of radiolabeled ^{99m}Tc-DTPA-OC and other peptides using this approach, the renal retention of radioactivity remains a concern. The intracellular trapping of radiolabeled ^{111}In-DTPA-OC

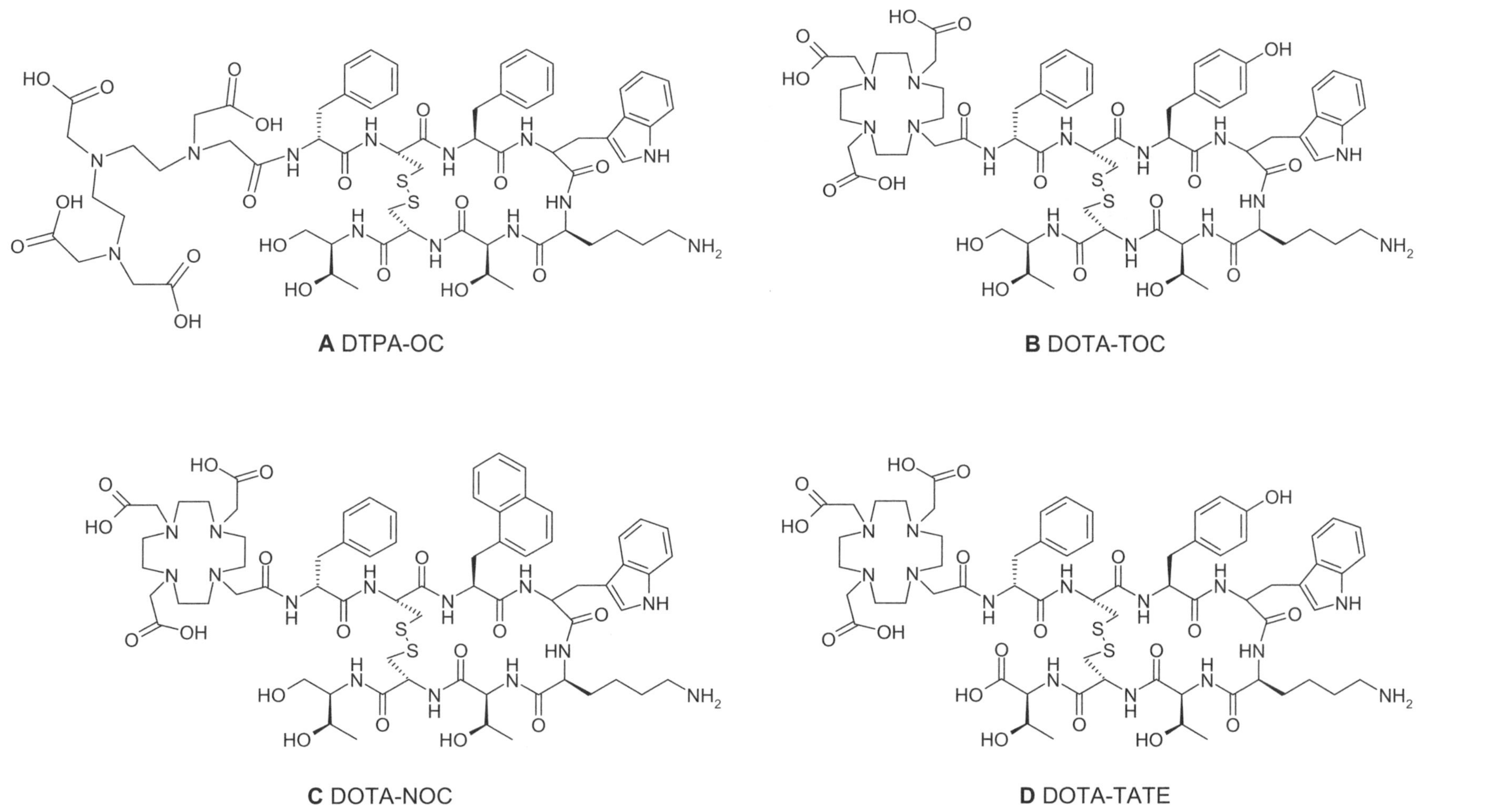

Figure 2 Examples of OC analogues conjugated with DTPA or DOTA chelating agents capable of forming stable complexes with various trivalent radiometals for in vivo targeting of somatostatin receptor-expressing cancers. (**A**) DTPA-OC, (**B**) DTPA-[Tyr³]-OC, (**C**) DOTA-[Na1³]-OC, and (**D**) DOTA-[Tyr³, Thr⁸]-OC. *Abbreviations:* OC, octreotide; DOTA, 1,4,7,10-tetraazacyclododecane-*N,N',N'',N'''*-tetraacetic acid.

metabolites in the kidney results from the lack of an efficient transport process to eliminate them from the cells (87). Development of alternative chelators and/or linking groups that facilitate efficient excretion of radiolabeled metabolites of ^{111}In-DTPA-OC and other peptide conjugates is a fruitful area of research.

Even though the development of ^{111}In-DTPA-OC for routine clinical applications was a pioneering achievement and demonstrated the immense potential of radiolabeled receptor-avid peptides for imaging cancers, ^{111}In is not the ideal radionuclide for SPECT molecular imaging. As a result, development of ^{99m}Tc-labeled SSTR targeting peptides ensued. For example, both the 6-hydrazinopyridine-3-carboxylic acid/ethylenediamine diacetic acid (HYNIC/EDDA) core (88–90) MAG$_3$ (91) and the open-chain tetraamine (1,4,8,11-tetraazaundecane) (92,93) were conjugated to OC analogues to enable production of ^{99m}Tc-labeled SSTR-specific peptides. Although these ^{99m}Tc-peptides showed promise as imaging radiotracers, they have not been developed for routine clinical use. Also, the corresponding $^{186/188}$Re analogues are not readily prepared via these chelating agents for use as potential TRT radiopharmaceuticals. ^{99m}Tc-depreotide (NeoTect®), a cyclic hexapeptide coupled to a N$_3$S chelator for ^{99m}Tc labeling, was developed for detection of malignant SSTR-expressing pulmonary nodules and is currently an FDA-approved radiopharmaceutical for routine clinical use for this application (6,38,76,94).

Since the introduction of ^{111}In-DTPA-OC, a large number of additional SSTR-targeting peptide radiotracers have been developed and studied (5,6,64). An important primary objective of the more recent basic and clinical research in this area is to identify radiolabeled OC-related constructs for TRT applications. The corresponding imaging OC analogues (e.g., labeled with ^{111}In, ^{68}Ga, ^{64}Cu, ^{86}Y, etc.) are important clinically and can be used as surrogates of therapeutic radionuclides (including ^{90}Y, ^{177}Lu, etc.) (45,64,66,68,73). Research with alternative OC analogue vectors has been conducted not only to optimize tumor uptake relative to reduced localization and retention in normal organs/tissues but also to identify structural motifs that were able to target SSTR subtypes more selectively. Five human SSTR subtypes (SSTR$_1$, SSTR$_2$, SSTR$_3$, SSTR$_4$, and SSTR$_5$) have been characterized (5,48,64,67,79,83,95,96). Some of the more extensively studied OC analogue–targeting vectors, (Fig. 2) for both diagnostic and therapeutic applications, include DOTA conjugated to TOC, [Tyr^3, Thr^8]-octreotide (TATE), [1-Nal^3]-octreotide (NOC), and lanreotide (5,6,64,67). Structures of four DTPA/DOTA conjugates based on the OC-targeting motif are shown in Figure 2. ^{111}In-DTPA-OC exhibits high affinity for SSTR$_2$ and SSTR$_5$ subtypes (64,84,95). In contrast, lanreotide binds to SSTR subtypes 3 and 4 in addition to subtypes 2 and 5 with high affinity

(6,53,83) and DOTA-NOC shows high affinity for SSTR subtypes 2, 3, and 5 (52,64). A large body of research studies with these OC analogues involves their respective conjugates with DOTA to enable labeling with trivalent radiometals (including ^{111}In, ^{68}Ga, ^{90}Y, ^{86}Y, ^{177}Lu, and other radiolanthanides) (6,64,97). Conjugates of OC, TOC, and TATE have also been synthesized where the peptide was linked to the 1,4,8,11-tetraazacyclotetradecane-N,N′, N″,N‴-tetraacetic acid (TETA) and cyclam-14-p-toluic acid (CPTA) chelation systems to produce the respective ^{64}Cu-TETA- and ^{64}Cu-CPTA-OC analogues (98–100). More recently, an ethylene cross-bridged cyclam chelator, 1,4,8,11-tetraazabicyclo[6.6.2] hexadecane-4,11-diacetic acid (CB-TE2A) was used to produce ^{64}Cu-CB-TETA-[Tyr^3] TATE, which has higher tumor uptake and lower nonspecific uptake in the liver (101,102). A wide variety of OC analogues labeled with a variety of other imaging radionuclides (including ^{18}F, ^{94m}Tc, ^{110m}In, and ^{11}C) have also been studied (64,93,103–105).

The utilization of radiolabeled DOTA-OC analogues have been tested in several clinical trials for therapeutic applications in patients with SSTR-positive tumors (mainly gastroenteropancreatic) have been performed (5,30,44,64,66,83,84,96). The radionuclides that have been predominately used in these clinical studies are ^{90}Y and ^{177}Lu. ^{90}Y is a high-energy ($E_{\beta max} = 2.27$ MeV) pure β particle emitter, and ^{177}Lu emits a moderate-energy β particle ($E_{\beta max} = 0.497$ MeV) and an imageable γ ray [E = 208 KeV (6.1%)]. The DOTA chelator conjugated to the OC analogues readily forms exceptionally stable chelates with both ^{177}Lu and ^{90}Y to minimize their in vivo dissociation or transchelation. ^{111}In-DTPA-OC, given in very high doses, to take advantage of the Auger emissions from ^{111}In, has also been used in clinical trials with limited success (64,106,107). Several studies conducted with ^{90}Y-DOTA-TOC have been conducted at multicenter sites with response rates approaching 33% (5,64,91,95). In the majority of these studies, the kidney dose was limited to 27Gy (including reduction of renal retention by infusion of basic amine acids) to minimize radiation long-term effects on the kidneys, including renal insufficiency (63,85). ^{177}Lu-DOTA-TATE has also been studied in recent years in patients producing impressive response rates (30). Results from initial studies indicate that ^{177}Lu, with its lower-energy β particle emission, has a lower potential for renal toxicity than ^{90}Y(30). These studies demonstrated that TRT agents with radiolabeled OC analogues that specifically target SSTR-expressing tumors is an effective approach for treatment of neuroendocrine tumors in human patients. A promising future goal is to develop new analogues with broader SSTR subtype profiles, coupled with strategies to reduce kidney retention and improved pharmacokinetic properties to enhance their therapeutic effectiveness.

Bombesin Analogues

The development of radiolabeled bombesin (BB) analogues for selective in vivo targeting of cancerous tumors is attractive since gastrin-releasing peptide (GRP) receptors have been shown to be overexpressed in several cancers, including prostate, breast, small-cell lung, pancreatic, and other cancers (3,17,70). In several of these human cancers (including prostate and breast cancers), GRP receptors are expressed on the surface of these cells in high density and frequency (5,50,108–112). The BB receptor family comprises four receptor subtypes,

neuromedin B (BB1), GRP (BB2), the orphan receptor subtype (BB3), and the BB receptor subtype (BB4) (49,50,54,113–115). BB is a 14–amino acid amphibian (Fig. 3A) analogue of the 27–amino acid human GRP (BB2) peptide (116). The BB2 receptor is a G protein–coupled receptor, and extensive research to characterize the receptor and subsequent cellular and physiological effects has been reported (117–119). A large number of non-radiolabeled BB2 antagonists have been synthesized and studied over the past three decades (120–124). The primary focus of this work is to use the BB antagonists to reduce or minimize the rate of tumor growth of GRP

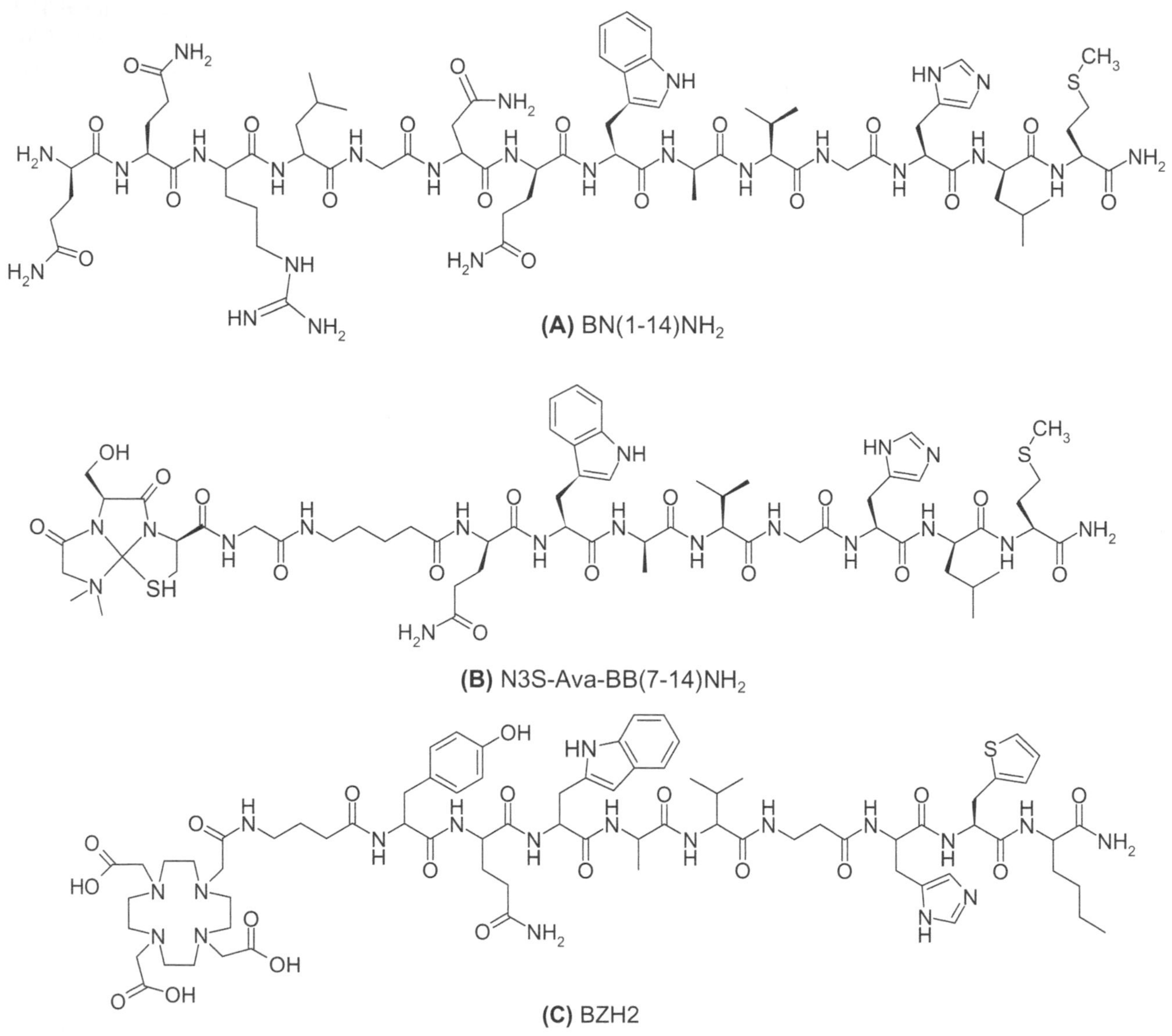

(A) BN(1-14)NH$_2$

(B) N3S-Ava-BB(7-14)NH$_2$

(C) BZH2

Figure 3 Examples of BB-based conjugates capable of chelating radiometals to produce radiotracers for in vivo targeting of human cancers. (**A**) Full-length bombesin, (**B**) N3S-Ava-BB(7–14)NH$_2$ forms stable ^{99m}Tc- and ^{188}Re-radiotracers, (**C**) BZH2, (**D**) DOTA-AOC-BB(7–14)NH$_2$, and (**E**) DOTA-AMBA. The latter three BB conjugates form stable radiotracers with ^{111}In, ^{90}Y, ^{177}Lu, ^{68}Ga, and other trivalent radiometals for targeting BB1, BB2, and/or BB3 receptor–expressing cancer cells. *Abbreviations*: BB, bombesin; Ava, aminovaleric acid; DOTA, 1,4,7,10-tetraazacyclododecane-*N,N′,N″,N‴*-tetraacetic acid; AOC, eight-amino octanoic acid.

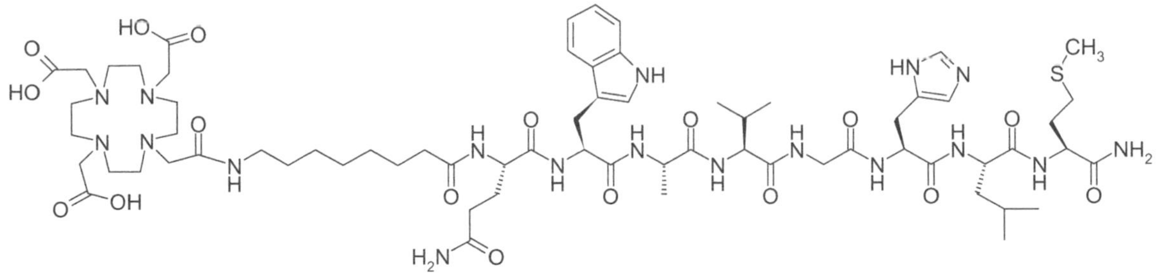

(D) DOTA-AOC-BB(7–14) NH$_2$

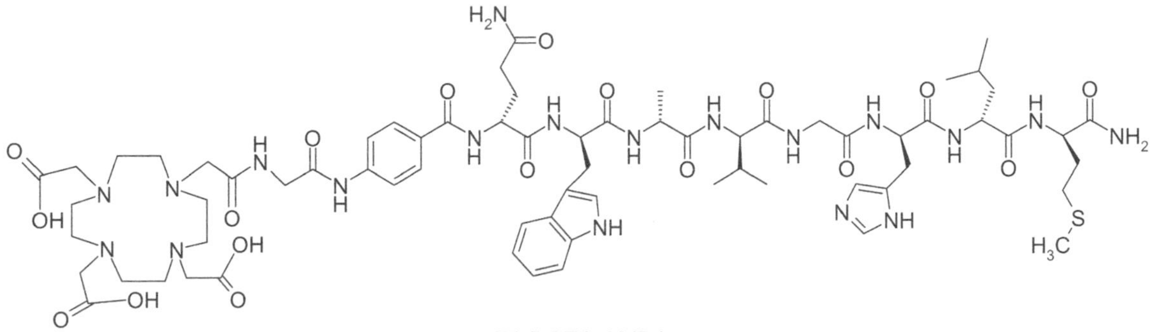

(E) DOTA-AMBA

Figure 3 (*Continued*)

receptor (BB2 receptor)–expressing cancers when administered repeatedly in large doses (120,123,124). Insights from these research efforts provided useful guidance for designing radiometallated BB derivatives that maintain high in vitro and in vivo binding affinities for BB2 receptors (17,125).

Several research groups have made important progress toward developing radiolabeled BB analogues as potential diagnostic and therapeutic radiopharmaceuticals (3,15,23,50,62,126–134). Examples of the numerous BB conjugates that were synthesized and studied have been summarized previously (3,39). While impressive success has been reported with radiolabeled derivatives of full-length BB(1–14) analogues (127,131), the majority of the research over the past decade has been directed toward development of truncated BB analogues to produce radiotracers that bind to the GRP/BB2 receptors agonistically and undergo high levels of receptor-mediated endocytosis (3,5,29,130,132). Initial studies by Hoffman and coworkers (17,135) utilized the conjugation of radiometal chelates to the N-terminal amine groups on the truncated C-terminal amidated BB(7–14)NH$_2$ sequence comprising the C-terminal binding region of native BB(1–14) via a spacer moiety.

The amino acid sequence of W-A-V-G-H-L-M (BB residues 8–14) must be maintained with the possibility of limited substitution, to confer high BB2 receptor binding affinity (17,124,129). Modification or a deletion at position 14 is important for determining properties of the peptide as an agonist or antagonist (121,124). Utilization of a spacer group or tether attached to the N-terminal end provides a mechanism to position the appended metal chelate remote from the BB2 receptor–binding sequence. The tethering group is also effective in modifying the physicochemical properties and metabolic fate of the conjugate to facilitate improvement in residualization radioactivity in the BB2-rexpressing cancer cells and clearance of the radiotracer from the blood in nontarget tissues (17,39). It was demonstrated that the BB(7–14)NH$_2$ could be readily conjugated with radiometal chelates to produce radiotracers that retain high specific BB2 receptor–binding affinities (i.e., IC$_{50}$s in the range of 1–10 nM) to human prostate, breast, and pancreatic cancer cell lines (50,88,130,133,135–138). One example of this class of BB conjugates is shown in Figure 3B. The N$_3$S-Ava-BB(7–14)NH$_2$ conjugate (Ava, aminovaleric acid), shown in Figure 3B, when labeled with ^{99m}Tc, exhibited high in vivo selectivity for BB2-expressing cancers (17,128) and was translated into clinical trials to demonstrate the potential of this and other BB-based radiotracers as effective radiopharmaceuticals for imaging BB2-expressing cancers in humans (139,140).

Over the past decade, a variety of radiolabeled conjugates using truncated BB(7–14) sequences have been synthesized to produce BB radiotracers labeled with several different radionuclides for potential use in imaging (including ^{99m}Tc, ^{111}In, ^{64}Cu, and ^{68}Ga) and TRT (including ^{188}Re, ^{177}Lu, ^{90}Y, ^{105}Rh, and ^{149}Pm) applications (23,45,54,62,71,135,141–143). Several BB(7–14) analogues conjugated with ^{99m}Tc chelators have been studied. For example, N$_4$ (136), N$_2$ (126,134), N$_3$S (128), HYNIC (88), and P$_2$S$_2$ (137) bifunctional chelating agents (BFCAs) have been appended to the N-terminal amine group to enable complexation of ^{99m}Tc(V) cores to the conjugates to form high-affinity BB receptor–targeting radiotracers. BFCAs that are able to form high–specific activity complexes with the novel M(CO)$_3^+$ [where M represents ^{99m}Tc(I) or ^{188}Re(I)] cores have also been synthesized and are capable of producing both ^{99m}Tc and ^{188}Re "matched pair" BB conjugates that exhibit exceptionally high in vitro and in vivo stability (15,138). Considerable emphasis has been placed on the synthesis of truncated BB analogue conjugates with BFCAs capable of forming high–specific activity and stable complexes with trivalent radiometals [i.e., ^{90}Y(III) and radiolanthanides] (4,9,16). The majority of these studies utilize DTPA and DOTA BFCAs for complexing these trivalent radiometals (62). For example, a series of DOTA-X-BBN(7–14)NH$_2$ (where X is the spacer group) derivatives have been used to produce the respective ^{177}Lu-, ^{149}Pm-, and ^{90}Y-labeled conjugates (141). These constructs can also be labeled with imaging radionuclides (e.g., ^{111}In, ^{86}Y, and ^{68}Ga) to produce the corresponding diagnostic BB-based radiotracers (4,5,71,74,96,130). These developments have been accompanied by efforts to develop BB sequences that target a wider spectrum of BB receptor subtypes and to improve in vivo stability. Even though the BB(7–14) NH$_2$ sequence has surprising stability in human serum and plasma (e.g., a half-life in the range of one hour), new derivatives that are less susceptible to catabolic or metabolic degradation in the blood or intracellularly may promote increased tumor uptake and/or retention. For example, Zhang et al. (45) reported the design and development of pan-BB derivatives that bind with high affinity to BB1, BB2, and BB3 receptor subtypes. The new BB conjugates are based on derivatives previously reported by Mantey, Jensen and coworkers (115) and contain the γ-aminobutyric acid, D-Tyr^6, β-Ala^{11}, Thi^{13}, Nlc^{14}-BB (6–14) sequence conjugated with either DTPA (BZH1) or DOTA (BZH2) (Fig. 3C). Both ^{111}In-BZH1 and ^{90}Y-BZH2 were found to selectively target all three BB subtypes, have improved stability toward in vivo catabolism/metabolism, and show specific in vivo targeting of AR4-2J tumors in laboratory rats (45,142). Recent studies in human patients with ^{68}Ga-BZH2 demonstrate successful imaging of prostate cancer tumors (97).

^{177}Lu-DOTA-BB analogues have demonstrated promise in preclinical rodent animal models, as effective TRT agents (45,50,144,145). Johnson et al. (146) assessed the

therapeutic effects of standard chemotherapeutic drugs, estramustine and docetaxel, in combination with ^{177}Lu-DOTA-AOC-BB(7–14)NH$_2$ (AOC, 8-amino octanoic acid), a BB2 receptor–targeting radiotracer (Fig. 3D), for treatment of antigen-independent human PC-3 tumor–bearing SCID mice. This study demonstrated that this ^{177}Lu-TRT agent provided a therapeutic response when administered alone in either single-dose or multi-dose regiments; however, an enhanced tumor control was noted when it was used in combination with the chemotherapeutic agents. Lantry et al. (50) reported that ^{177}Lu-labeled DOTA-G-(4-aminobenzoyl)-QWAVGHLM-NH$_2$ (^{177}Lu-AMBA) (Fig. 3E) binds with high affinity to both BB1 and BB2 receptors but not BB3 receptors. High specific in vivo uptake in PC-3 xenografted rodents was demonstrated, and a significant therapeutic effect on tumor control and increased survival was produced, making it a promising candidate as a TRT radiopharmaceutical for treatment of these cancers in clinical trials (45,145).

BB conjugates labeled with other radionuclides have also been studied. Several ^{64}Cu-BB analogues have been designed and assessed for potential utilization as both PET imaging and TRT radiopharmaceuticals (23,143). ^{64}Cu-DOTA-PEGylated-BB constructs have been studied by Rogers and coworkers (23) with the goal of increasing pharmacokinetics and tumor uptake. S$_4$-BB(7–14)NH$_2$ conjugates labeled with ^{105}Rh, a β particle–emitting radionuclide, have also been studied as potential candidates for TRT applications (135). Important strides have been made toward design and development of site-directed diagnostic and therapeutic BB conjugate–based radiopharmaceuticals. As a result of the promising results obtained over the past decade, efforts to develop new radiolabeled BB derivatives that are effective for treatment of human cancers are accelerating.

Neurotensin Analogues

Neutrotensin (NT) receptors are overexpressed on several human tumors, including small-cell lung, colon, exocrine pancreatic, and prostrate cancers (3,5,27,86,147). There are three NT receptor subtypes (NT1, NT2, and NT3) (5). Both the NT1 and NT2 receptors are G protein–coupled receptors (5,51,148). The expression of the NT1 receptor occurs with a high incidence rate (>75%) in exocrine pancreatic carcinoma (5,51). NT, like many small natural peptides, is metabolized rapidly in plasma by endogenous peptidases (3,5,26,149). Thus, it is critical to develop NT conjugates that have improved in vivo stability. The most prominent sites accounting for metabolism of NT(8–13), that is, Arg-Arg-Pro-Tyr-Ile-Leu, are Arg^8-Arg^9, Pro^{10}-Tyr^{11}, and Tyr^{11}-Ile^{12} (5,26,27). As a result of modification of the Arg^8-Arg^9 and Tyr^{11}-Ile^{12} sites, high plasma stability was obtained while retaining the ability of the

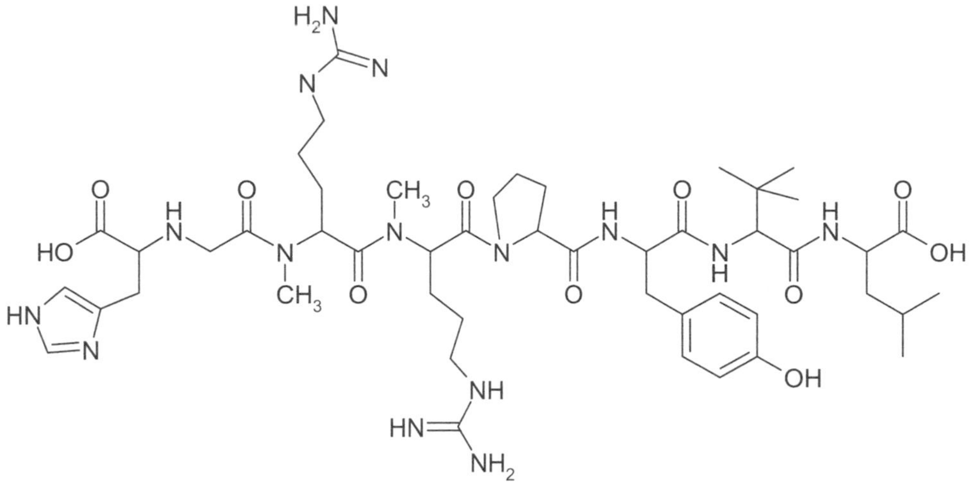

Figure 4 An example of a Nα-histinyl conjugate of a metabolically stabilized NT analog, (Nα-His)Ac-Arg-(N-CH$_3$)-Arg-Pro-Tyr-Tle-Leu. This NT conjugate, when labeled with ^{99m}Tc(CO$_3^-$), specifically binds to NT1 receptors on human cancer cells. *Abbreviation*: NT, neurotensin.

modified NT(8–13) sequence to specifically bind with high affinity to NT receptors (21,26,27,149). Several ^{99m}Tc-labeled standardized derivatives of NT have been studied (3,150). Studies with both HT-29 and PC-3 tumor xenografts in mice with one analogue, ^{99m}Tc [Nα-His]Ac-Lys-(CH$_2$NH)-Arg-Pro-Tyr-Tle-Leu, was shown to visualize a ductal pancreatic adenocarcinoma in a human patient (26). A more recent analogue labeled with ^{99m}Tc [(Nα-His)]Ac-Arg-(N-CH$_3$)-Arg-Pro-Tyr-Tle-Leu (Fig. 4) and reported by Garcia-Garayo et al. (27) showed higher specific uptake of the radiotracer (^{99m}Tc-NT-XII) in HT-29 xenografts in nude mice, along with improved pharmacokinetics and lower kidney uptake. The Nα-histinyl acetate [(Nα-His)Ac] BFCA is conjugated to the peptide to form a stable complex with the ^{99m}Tc(CO)$_3^+$ core (3,15). Impressive progress made over the past few years to develop NT1 receptor–avid radiopharmaceuticals with in vivo stability demonstrating their promise as radiolabeled peptides for imaging NT1 receptor–expressing cancers in humans.

Stabilized NT analogues were also labeled with ^{188}Re. The in vitro binding and in vivo biodistributions of the ^{99m}Tc- and ^{188}Re-NT-XII and ^{188}Re-NT-XIX matched pairs in mice with HT-29 tumor xenografts were comparable (3,151). Both of these ^{188}Re-NT peptide analogues were effective in inhibiting HT-29 tumor growth in these animal models (3,152), demonstrating the potential of these or other radiolabeled NT analogues as TRT agents.

α-MSH Analogues

Receptors for α-melanoma stimulating hormone (α-MSH) have been identified on the surface human malignant melanomas (153), making them attractive targets for

development of radiolabeled peptides that specifically target these Melanocortin (MC)1 receptor–rich tumors. The most well characterized class of anti-melanoma peptides belonging to the α-MSH family is a linear tridecapeptide (Ac-Ser-Tyr-Ser-Met-Glu-His-D-Phe-Arg-Trp-Cys-Lys-Pro-Val-NH$_2$) that binds to its cognate MC1 receptors with nanomolar affinities (32). MC1 receptors belong to the G protein–coupled receptor family, of which five (MC1 through MC5) have been isolated (154,155). Structure activity studies showed that the amino acid sequence His-Phe-Arg-Trp is sufficient for MC1 receptor recognition and replacement of Phe with D-Phe results in a 1500-fold increase in receptor binding (28,32,155). The most widely used α-MSH derivative is the linear [Nle^2-D-Phe^7] α-MSH analogue (NDP) because of its protease resistance properties (155). Several NDP analogues, labeled with diagnostic radionuclides, including ^{99m}Tc (33,36), ^{125}I (156), ^{18}F (31), and ^{111}In (157–160), have been studied, with some showing promising in vivo melanoma tumor targeting properties.

Quinn and coworkers (11,161) developed a novel class of α-MSH analogues that are cyclized via site-specific metal coordination. A rational peptide design program was employed to engineer the cyclic α-MSH analogues that coordinate ^{99m}Tc and Re into their three-dimensional structures, yielding molecules that are resistant to protolytic degradation while retaining high MC1 receptor affinities. The most promising α-MSH analogue identified was Ac-Cys^3-Cys^4-Gln^5-His^6-D-Phe^7-Arg^8-Trp^9-Cys^{10}-Lys^4-Pro^{22}-Val^{13}-NH$_2$, designated CCMSH (11). ^{99m}TcO^{+3} and ReO^{+3} were complexed into CCMSH via a glucoheptonate transchelation reaction. The structure of the DOTA conjugate of the cyclized Re-CCMSH peptide, which is capable of high-affinity binding with MC1

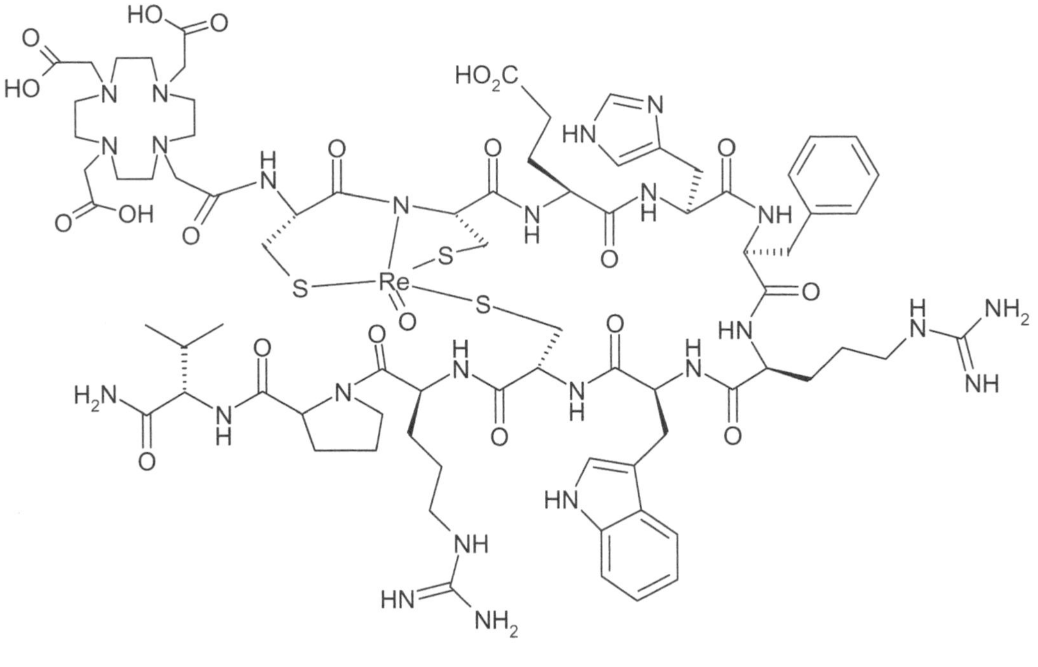

Figure 5 DOTA-Re-CCMSH, a cyclized α-melanoma stimulating hormone analogue for labeling with radiometals to produce radiotracers that bind with high specificity to MC1 receptors overexpressed on melanoma cells. *Abbreviations*: DOTA, 1,4,7,10-tetraazacyclododecane-*N,N′,N″,N‴*-tetraacetic acid; MC1, melanocortin-1.

receptors, was determined by multidimensional NMR spectroscopy, and is shown in Figure 5 (11,17). Biodistribution of ^{99m}Tc-CCMSH demonstrates surprisingly high and selective accumulation in B16-F1 melanoma–bearing CL57/Bl6 mice (11,162). Conjugation of the "cold" Re-[Cys (3,4,10), D-Phe (7)] α-MSH-[3–13] MC1 receptor–targeting vector with DOTA to the N-terminal amine allows introduction of ^{111}In (163,164) and a variety of other radiometals (including ^{64}Cu and ^{86}Y) for imaging melanoma tumors (68). This same DOTA-Re-CCMSH conjugate (Fig. 5) is also readily labeled with other β particle–emitting (e.g., ^{177}Lu) and α particle–emitting radionuclides (e.g., ^{212}Bi) and exhibit similar uptake in metastatic melanoma tissues in animal models (165). Studies with both of these compounds demonstrate their ability to provide effective therapeutic control of melanoma tumors in animal models (165).

ST$_h$ Peptide Analogues

Guanylin/guanylate cyclase C (GC-C) receptors have been shown to be expressed on virtually all of the histologically confirmed primary and metastatic colorectal cancer tumors removed from human patients (166,167). Thus, development of radiolabeled peptides that target GC-C receptors may provide new imaging radiopharmaceuticals and/or TRT agents for treatment of this disease. The GC-C receptors are single transmembrane–spanning G protein–

coupled receptors (47,168,169). The amount of work directed to development of new GC-C receptor–targeting radiopharmaceuticals has been limited. Several guanylin homologues that bind GC-C receptors have been reported (168,169), however, the heat stable (ST) bacterial peptide conjugates have been identified as a class of peptides that bind to these receptors with the highest affinity (3). The *E. coli* human ST (ST$_h$) peptide is metabolically stable and binds with nanomolar affinities in an agonist manner and undergoes receptor-mediated endocytosis (166,168). The primary structure of one of the N-terminal DOTA-conjugated *E. coli* ST$_h$ analogues reported is shown in Figure 6B. The only difference between the Phe^{19}ST$_h$(1–19)-binding moiety shown in Figure 6 and the native ST$_h$(1–19) is replacement of the Tyr^{19} residue by Phe^{19} (Fig. 6A). In the biologically active form, disulfide bridges between Cys^6 and Cys^{11}, Cys^7 and Cys^{15}, and Cys^{10} and Cys^{18} are formed (169,170). Methods to produce and purify the unique biologically active conformer have been developed (34,171,172). Several radiolabeled ST$_h$ derivatives labeled with either ^{99m}Tc or ^{111}In have been synthesized that exhibit high GC-C receptor–binding affinities and demonstrate selective in vivo targeting of human colon cancer xenografts for imaging tumors in rodent animal models (173–175). These radiolabeled ST$_h$ conjugates are cleared rapidly from the blood stream, almost exclusively via the kidney, with minimal uptake in the liver (173–175). The lack of significant liver deposition provides evidence that visualization of these

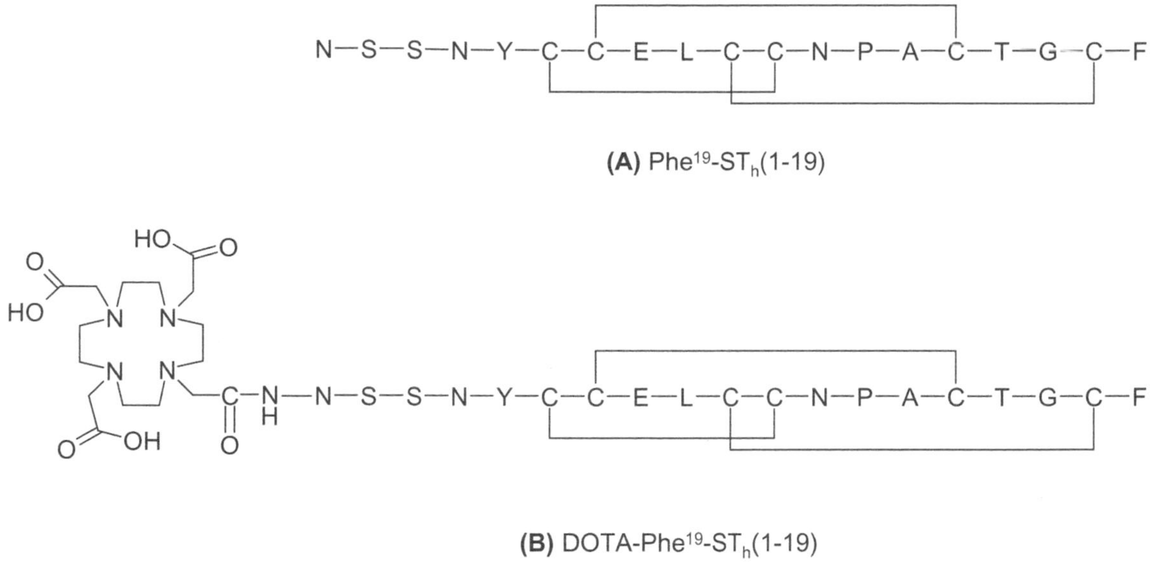

(A) Phe[19]-ST$_h$(1-19)

(B) DOTA-Phe[19]-ST$_h$(1-19)

Figure 6 (**A**) The Phe[19]-ST$_h$(1–19) peptide and (**B**) a DOTA-Phe[19]-ST$_h$(1–19) conjugate, when labeled with radiometals, specifically target guanylin/guanylate cyclase C receptors expressed on human colorectal cancer cells. *Abbreviations*: ST$_h$, human ST; DOTA, 1,4,7,10-tetraazacyclododecane-*N,N′,N″,N‴*-tetraacetic acid.

radiolabeled tracers localized on colorectal metastatic tumors in liver will be feasible.

It is important to recognize that GC-C receptors are located on the brush border domain of the enterocytes in the normal intestines but not on the basolateral domain (17,168). Mucosal cells lining the intestines are joined by tight junctions that form a barrier against exchange of molecular content in the blood (viz. radiolabeled ST$_h$ conjugates) and/or the ECF with intestinal content in the lumen of the intestines (17,169). In contrast, colorectal cancer tumors arising from colonic mucosal cells invade the surrounding tissue and establish their own blood supply, thus allowing intravenously administered radiolabeled ST$_h$ conjugates full access to the GC-C receptors expressed on invasive or metastatic colorectal cancer cells (166,167). Results with the ^{99m}Tc and ^{111}In-ST$_h$ conjugates are consistent with this hypothesis since intravenous administration of the radiotracers show impressive selective uptake in the human colon cancer xenografts in rodent

animal models but minimal deposition in the normal GI tract (172,174,175).

Giblin and coworkers (171,172,175,176) prepared a limited array of DOTA-Phe[19]-ST$_h$(1–19) conjugates, which are analogues of the structure shown in Figure 6B, to determine the effects of modifying the linking group or tether between the Phe[19]-ST$_h$(6–19) GC-C receptor–binding moiety and the ^{111}In-DOTA chelate on tumor uptake and retention and pharmacokinetics in mouse models. These studies demonstrated the utility of the N-S-S-N-Y linear sequence [i.e., ST$_h$(1–5)], as well as providing insights related to the effects of modifying the tether structure on the in vivo characteristics of the respective ^{111}In-DOTA-Phe[19]-ST$_h$(1–19) analogues (175). This group recently showed that labeling the DOTA-Phe[19]-ST$_h$(1–19) (Fig. 7) conjugate with ^{177}Lu and ^{90}Y produced a radiotracer that exhibited uptake and residualization levels in human T-84 tumor xenografts in SCID mice and pharmacokinetics, characteristics that are similar to

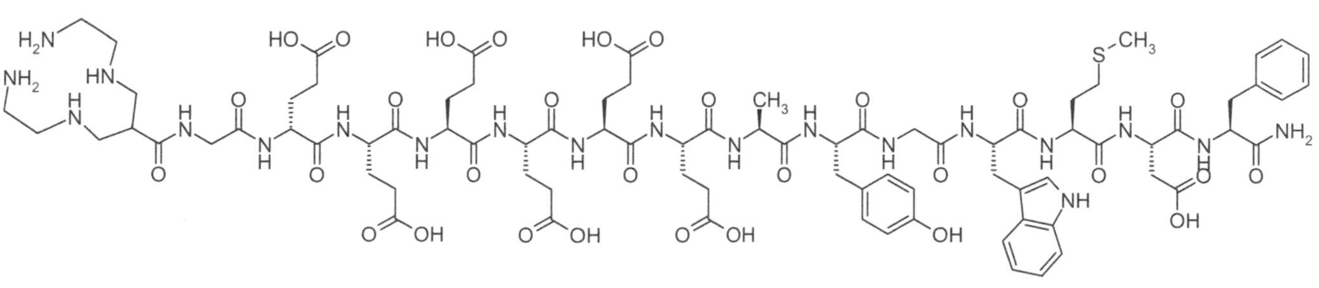

Figure 7 N$_4$-Demogastrin-2, when labeled with ^{99m}Tc(V)O$^+{}_2$, specifically targets cholecystokinin/gastrinreceptor-expressing cancers (N$_4$, 1,4,8,11-tetraazaundecane).

^{111}In-DOTA-Phe[19]-ST$_h$(1–19) (65). This indicates developing radiolabeled ST$_h$(1–19) conjugate as TRT radiopharmaceuticals for treatment of human colorectal cancers may be feasible.

In addition to utilization of radiolabeled ST$_h$(1–19) conjugates for in vivo targeting of colorectal cancers, this class of peptide radiotracers have also been shown to target an unknown cell surface moiety (not the GC-C receptor) on other human cancer cells (e.g., breast cancer) (177). Clearly, additional research is needed to identify and characterize the moiety that is expressed on these non-colorectal cancer cells and its binding properties with ST peptide–based derivatives to explore the potential utility of radiolabeled ST$_h$-based peptides for specifically targeting these additional cancers.

Vasoactive Intestinal Peptide/Pituitary Adenylate Cyclase–Activating Peptide Analogues

Vasoactive intestinal peptide (VIP) is a neuropeptide and a member of the glucagons secretion family and closely related to pituitary adenylate cyclase–activating polypeptide (PACAP) (3,5,6,178). Both are G protein–coupled receptors that can be internalized after ligand binding (179). VIP is a 28–amino acid peptide while PACAP has a similar structure with 27 or 38 amino acids (3,5,6,178). There are two VIP receptor subtypes, VIPR1 and VIPR2, both exhibiting high binding affinity for VIP and PACAP (5). VIP/PACAP receptors are found not only in brain but ubiquitously by a majority of human epithelial tissues (179,180). The VIPR1 subtype is preferentially expressed by most of these tissues, including hepatocytes, gastrointestinal mucosa, pancreatic ducts, among others (5,178–180). The presence of VIP/PACAP receptors in most normal tissue points to multiple and complex biological actions of VIP/PACAP peptides in the human body (5).

It has been shown that a large number of primary human tumors express VIP/PACAP receptors (3,6, 78,181). Most of these tumors (including lung, stomach, colon, breast, prostate, pancreatic ducts, liver, and urinary bladder) preferentially express the VIPR1 subtype (5,77). Several studies have been performed in patients with ^{123}I-VIP to determine its applicability for imaging endocrine tumors of the intestinal tract, primary adenoma, colorectal cancer, and liver (80,182,183). While these studies demonstrated that ^{123}I-VIP is able to successfully detect the tumors, residual activity in normal tissues (e.g., lung) was evident (80,183,184). Thakur et al. (91,185,186) developed two ^{99m}Tc-VIP analogues (^{99m}Tc-TP1666 and ^{99m}Tc-TP3654) to overcome difficulties in preparing ^{123}I-VIP and improve in vivo imaging capabilities. These ^{99m}Tc radiotracers were evaluated in both tumor-bearing

animal models and humans (80,183,186). These studies showed good in vivo targeting of the tumor but significant background in target tissues and organs (80,183,186). More recently, ^{64}Cu-VIP was studied in comparison with ^{99m}Tc-VIP (187). Difficulties in clearance of a radioactivity from normal tissues is likely related to the procedure of VIP receptors on numerous normal tissues and the short half-life of these radiolabeled VIP analogues that produce various radiolabeled metabolites (5,7). The identification and development of stable VIP/PACAP analogues that can be readily radiolabeled and retain high affinity for VIP/PACAP receptors is currently a challenge of potential clinical interest and a prerequisite for their successful diagnostic and radiotherapeutic applications in humans (5).

CCK2/Gastrin Receptor–Targeting Peptides

Gastrin and cholecystokinin (CCK) are gastrointestinal peptides, which exist as different peptide sequences but share the same five–amino acid sequence at the C-terminal end (3). CCK and gastrin actions are mediated by several receptor subtypes, the best characterized being CCK1 and CCK2 receptors (5,188). The CCK2/gastrin receptor has been shown to be expressed on several human tumors, including small-cell lung, stromal, ovarian, gastroenteropancreatic, neuroendocrine, and medullary thyroid cancers and astrocytomas (3,5–7). As a result, radiolabeled CCK2/gastrin peptide analogues have been prepared and studied by several research groups (8). The CCK1 receptor appears to be preferentially expressed by few human tumor types, however, those that do express CCK1 receptor also express SSTRs and can be targeted by radiolabeled OC analogues (5). The majority of radiolabeled CCK2 receptor and peptides are analogues of the C-terminus octapeptide fragment CCK8 (Gln-Ala-Tyr-Gly-Trp-Met-Asp-Phe-NH$_2$). Several CCK2[26–33] analogue conjugates labeled with ^{111}In or ^{99m}Tc have been studied and shown to target CCK2/gastrin receptor–expressing cancers in both animal models and humans. Specific uptake of ^{111}In-DTPA-[D-Asp (26), Nle (28,31)] CCK2[26–33] occurs in normal stomach (a CCK2/gastrin receptor–expressing organ), in TT cancer cell xenografted mice (30,189) and in MTC in humans (190,191). MTC is a particularly important target for these radiolabeled peptides since MTC cells have a high incidence and density of CCK2 receptor expression (5).

More recently, several ^{99m}Tc-based CCK2 receptor–avid peptides have been reported involving HYNIC/EDDA and N$_4$ chelating agents (e.g., 1,4,8,11-tetraazaundecane) conjugated to CCK2/gastrin analogues (8,31). These ^{99m}Tc radiotracers were capable of in vivo targeting of CCK2/gastrin receptor–expressing tumors. The mini-gastrin conjugates, ^{99m}Tc-N4-demogastrin-1-3, showed high CCK2/gastrin receptor affinity, high uptake in AR4-2-J tumor–bearing athymic mice. Impressive selective localization of the ^{99m}Tc labeled to the N4-demogastrin 2 conjugate shown in Figure 7 is observed in metastatic medullary thyroid cancer (MTC) tumors in a human patient, demonstrating its promise as an effective diagnostic radiopharmaceutical for imaging MTC (31). The potential for developing TRT radiopharmaceuticals based on CCK2/gastrin peptide analogues may be difficult since they show high levels of residualization of radioactivity in the kidneys (5,97).

Other Peptide Analogues

Numerous additional radiolabeled small peptides that specifically target receptors that are expressed on human cancer cells or receptor markers that are present on cells/tissues that are involved in tumor growth and/or metastasis have also been studied over the past decade (3,5–8,14). Some of these cancer cell receptor–avid peptides include radiolabeled peptide conjugates of (*i*) substance P for targeting NK1 receptors expressed on glioblastoma, astrocytomas, medullary thyroid, and breast cancers (5,7,192), (*ii*) calcitonin peptide P1410 for targeting calcitonin receptors in human breast cancer cells (193), (*iii*) neuropeptide Y for targeting NY1 receptors expressed on breast cancer (81,194), and others (3,5,7,191,195–198). A number of radiolabeled peptide analogues have also been developed that do not target the cancer cells themselves, rather target physiological processes, and tissues intimately associated with tumor growth and cancer metastases have also been reported (5). A large number of radiolabeled peptides that target markers of tumor angiogenesis have been developed and studied for imaging and TRT applications. For example, a major emphasis has been placed on targeting the V3 and V5 integrins/cell adhesion motifs, particularly the RGD (Arg-Gly-Asp)-based derivatives that bind to $\alpha_v\beta_3$ and other integrins (6,8,199–202). Utilization of other peptide vectors, for example, Annexin V for targeting phosphatidylserine (PS) featured as membrane blebs during apoptosis, to produce radiolabeled peptides for molecular imaging applications to characterize tumors has also been reported (203). Novel strategies continue to be implemented to identify peptides that hold potential as molecular vectors that can be radiolabeled for specific localization (via imaging) in cancerous tumors. For example, in vitro and in vivo phage display technologies are increasingly being utilized to produce small peptides that specifically bind to a multitude of receptors or molecular motifs overexpressed on human cancer cells and processes involved in tumor growth and metastatic processes (125,204–207).

SUMMARY

Radiolabeled receptor-avid peptide analogues are an important class of human cancer–specific targeting agents with demonstrated potential for both molecular imaging and TRT applications. The development of new radiolabeled receptor-avid peptide conjugates that selectively bind to their cognate receptors that are uniquely expressed or overexpressed on a wide spectrum of human cancers is occurring at an accelerating pace worldwide. A particularly valuable characteristic of most of these types of radiotracers is related to their ability to be transported intracellularly (via receptor-mediated endocytosis) after binding in an agonistic manner to the receptors that are expressed on the exterior surface of the cancer cell plasma membrane. Many challenges lie ahead to enable successful development of peptide-based radiopharmaceuticals as routinely available clinical diagnostic and/or TRT agents for applications in human cancer patients. Development of effective radiopharmaceuticals (particularly TRT agents) involves fundamental issues that must be recognized and optimized, including peptide receptor specificity, residualization of activity in the tumor, peptide conjugate stability in vivo, variations in radiolabeling approaches, clearance of activity of the radiotracer from nontarget tissues, among others. Tremendous progress has been made over the past decade to address these issues and design strategies implemented to produce radiolabeled peptide conjugates that hold important promise for the near future. With priority investments being made at the corporate, federal, and academic levels and the increased rate of translation of receptor-avid peptide radiotracers into the clinical settings, a tremendous growth in the number of new radiotracers introduced and in their applicability for imaging and targeted therapy of human cancer patients is expected over the next decade.

REFERENCES

1. Boerman OC, Oyen WJ, Corstens FHM. Radiolabeled receptor-binding peptides: a new class of radiopharmaceuticals. Semin Nucl Med 2000; 30:195–208.
2. Buchsbaum DJ, Chandhuri TR, Yamamoto M, et al. Gene expression imaging with radiolabeled peptides. Ann Nucl Med 2004; 18:275–283.
3. Garcia-Garayo E, Schubiger PA. Peptide-based radiopharmaceuticals radiolabelled with Tc-99m and Re-188 as potential diagnostic and therapeutic agents. In: Mazzi U, ed. Technetium, Rhenium and Other Metals in Chemistry and Nuclear Medicine. 7th ed. Padova, Italy: S.G. Editoriali, 2006:247–262.
4. Ginj M, Maecke HR. Radiometallo-labeled peptides in tumor diagnosis and therapy. Met Ions Biol Syst 2004; 42:109–142.

5. Reubi JC. Peptide Receptors in molecular targets for cancer diagnosis and therapy. Endocr Rev 2003; 24: 389–427.

6. Weiner RE, Thakur ML. Radiolabeled peptides: role in diagnosis and treatment. BioDrugs 2005; 19:145–163.

7. Knight LC. Radiolabeled peptides for tumor imaging. In: Welch MJ, Redvanly CS, eds. Handbook of Radiopharmaceuticals. West Sussex, England: John Wiley & Sons, Ltd., 2003:643–684.

8. Mariani G, Erba PA, Signore A. Receptor-mediated tumor targeting with radiolabeled peptides: there is more to it than somatostatin analogs. J Nucl Med 2006; 47: 1904–1907.

9. Anderson CJ, Welch MJ. Radiometal-labeled agents (Non-Technetium) for diagnostic imaging. Chem Rev 1999; 99:2235–2268.

10. Beneditt E, Morelli E, Accardo G, et al. Criteria for the design and biological characterization of radiolabeled peptide-based pharmaceuticals. BioDrugs 2004; 18: 279–295.

11. Giblin MF, Wang N, Hoffman TJ, et al. Design and characterization of alpha-melanotropin peptide analogs cyclized through rehenium and technetium metal coordination. Proc Natl Acad Sci U S A 1998; 95:12814–12818.

12. Jurisson SS, Lydon JD. Potential technetium small molecule radiopharmaceuticals. Chem Rev 1999; 99: 2005–2018.

13. Liu S. The role of coordination chemistry in development of target-specific radiopharmaceuticals. Chem Soc Rev 2004; 33:1–18.

14. Okarvi SM. Peptide-based radiopharmaceuticals: future tasks as diagnostic imaging of cancer and other diseases. Med Res Rev 2004; 24:357–397.

15. Schibli R. Organometallic precursors of technetium and rhenium: unique opportunities for radiotracer development due to chemical diversity. In: Mazzi U, ed. Technetium, Rhenium and Other Metals in Chemistry and Nuclear Medicine. 7th ed. Padova, Italy: S.G. Editoriali, 2006:25–34.

16. Volkert WA, Hoffman TJ. Therapeutic radiopharmaceuticals. Chem Rev 1999; 99:2269–2292.

17. Hoffman TJ, Quinn TP, Volkert WA. Radiometallated receptor-avid peptide conjugates for specific *in vivo* targeting of cancer cells. Nucl Med Biol 2001; 28: 527–539.

18. Akazawa H, Arano Y, Mifune M, et al. Effect of molecular charges on renal uptake of ^{111}In-DTPA conjugated peptides. Nucl Med Biol 2001; 28:761–768.

19. Eberle AN, Mild G, Froidevaux S. Receptor-mediated tumor targeting with radiopeptides. Part 1: general concepts and methods: applications to somatostatin receptor-expressing tumors. J Recept Signal Transduct Res 2004; 24:319–455.

20. Fujimori K, Covell DG, Fletcher JE, et al. A modeling analysis of monoclonal antibody percolation through tumors: a binding-site barrier. J Nucl Med 1990; 31: 1191–1198.

21. Garcia-Garayoa E, Blaeuenstein P, Bruehlmeier M, et al. Preclinical evaluation of a new, stabilized neurotensin

22. Jain RK. Physiological barriers to delivery of monoclonal antibodies and other macromolecules in tumors. Cancer Res 1990; 50S:814s–819s.

23. Rogers BE, Manna DD, Safavy S. *In vitro* and *in vivo* evaluation of a ^{64}Cu-labeled polyethylene glycol-bombesin conjugate. Cancer Biother Radiopharm 2004; 19:25–34.

24. Wester HJ, Kessler H. Molecular targeting with peptides or peptide-polymer conjugates: just a question of size? J Nucl Med 2005; 46:1940–1945.

25. Whetstone PA, Akazawa H, Meares CF. Evaluation of clearable (TYR3) octreotate derivatives for longer intracellular probe residence. Bioconjug Chem 2004; 15:647–657.

26. Buchegger F, Bonvin B, Kosinski M, et al. Stabilization of neurotensin analogues: effect on peptide catabolism, biodistribution and tumor binding. J Nucl Med 2003; 44:1649–1654.

27. Garcia-Garayo E, Maes V, Blauenstein P, et al. Double-stabilized neurotensin analogues as potential radiopharmaceuticals for NTR-positive tumors. Nucl Med Biol 2006; 33:495–503.

28. Hruby VJ, Sharma SD, Toth K, et al. Design, synthesis, and conformation of superpotent and prolonged acting melanotropins. Ann N Y Acad Sci 1993; 680:51–63.

29. Krenning EP, Kwekkeboom DJ, Bakker WH, et al. Somatostatin receptor scintigraphy with [^{111}In-DTPA-D-Phe[1]]- and [^{123}I-Tyr[3]]-octreotide: the Rotterdam experience with more than 1000 patients. Eur J Nucl Med 1993; 20: 716–731.

30. Kwekkeboom DJ, Teunissen JJ, Bakker WH, et al. Radiolabeled somatostatin analog [^{177}Lu-DOTAO,Tyr[3]]octreotate in patients with endocrine gastroenteropancreatic tumors. J Clin Oncol 2005; 23:2754–2762.

31. Nock B, Maina T, Behe M, et al. CCK-2/gastrin receptor-targeted tumor imaging with ^{99m}Tc-labeled minigastrin analogs. J Nucl Med 2005; 46:1727–1736.

32. Sawyer TK, Sanfilippo PJ, Hruby VJ. A [Nle[4]-D-Phe[7]]α-melanocyte stimulating hormone: a highly potent α-melanotropin with ultralong biological activity. Proc Natl Acad Sci U S A 1980; 77:5788.

33. Chen J, Giblin MF, Wang N, et al. *In vivo* evaluation of Tc-99m/Re-188-labeled linear alpha-melanocyte stimulating hormone analogs for specific melanoma targeting. Nucl Med Biol 1999; 26:687–693.

34. Gali H, Hoffman TJ, Sieckman GL, et al. Chemical synthesis of *escherichia coli* ST$_h$ analogs by regioselective disulfide bond formation: biological evaluation of an ^{111}In-DOTA-Phe[19]-ST$_h$ analog for specific targeting of human colon cancers. Bioconjug Chem 2002; 13: 224–231.

35. Giblin MF, Veerendra B, Smith CJ. Radiometallation of receptor specific peptides for diagnosis and treatment of human cancer. In Vivo 2005; 19:9–29.

36. Miao Y, Gallazzi F, Figueroa SD, et al. A novel ^{111}In labeled DOTA conjugated amino acid bridge cyclized alpha-MSH peptide for melanoma imaging. In: Mazzi U, ed. Technetium, Rhenium and Other Metals in Chemistry

and Nuclear Medicine. 7th ed. Padova, Italy: S.G. Editoriali, 2006:491–494.

37. Fritzberg AR, Gustavson LM, Hylarides MD, et al. In: Weiner DB, Williams MV, eds. Chemical and Structural Approaches to Rational Drug Design. Boca Raton, FL: CRC Press, 1994:125.

38. Lister-James J, Moyer BR, Dean RT. Pharmacokinetic considerations in the development of peptide-based imaging agents. Q J Nucl Med 1997; 41:111–118.

39. Smith CJ, Volkert WA, Hoffman TJ. Gastrin releasing peptide (GRP) receptor targeted radiopharmaceuticals: a concise update. Nucl Med Biol 2003; 30:861–868.

40. Cescato R, Schulz S, Waser B, et al. Internalization of sst$_2$, sst$_3$ and sst$_5$, receptors: effects of somatostatin agonists and antagonists. J Nucl Med 2006; 47:511.

41. Meares CF, McCall MJ, Deshpande SV, et al. Chelate radiochemistry: cleavable linkers lead to altered levels of radioactivity in the liver. Int J Cancer 1988; 2:99–102.

42. deJong M, Barone R, Krenning E, et al. Megalin is essential for renal proximal tubule resorption of ^{111}In-DTPA-octreotide. J Nucl Med 2005; 46:1696–1700.

43. Ginj M, Hinni K, Tshumi S, et al. Trifunctional somatostatin-based derivatives designed for targeted radiotherapy using auger emitters. J Nucl Med 2005; 46:2097–2103.

44. Heppeler A, Froidevaux S, Maacke HR, et al. Radiometal-labelled macrocyclic chelator-derivatised somatostatin analogue with superb tumour-targeting properties and potential for receptor-mediated internal radiotherapy. Chem A Eur J 1999; 5:1016–1023.

45. Zhang H, Chen J, Waldherr C, et al. Syntheses and evaluation of bombesin derivatives on the basis of pan-bombesin peptides labeled with indium-111, lutetium-177, and yttrium-90 for targeting bombesin receptor expressing tumors. Cancer Res 2004; 64:6707–6715.

46. Tian XB, Arnva MR, Qin WY, et al. External imaging of CCNDI cancer gene activity in experimental human breast cancer xenografts with ^{99m}Tc-peptide-peptide-nucleic acid-peptide chimeras. J Nucl Med 2004; 45:2070–2082.

47. Drewett JG, Garbers DL. The family of guanylyl cyclase receptors and their ligands. Endocr Rev 1994; 15:135–162.

48. Reubi JC, Schaer JC, Laissue JA, et al. Somatostatin receptors and their subtypes in human tumors and peritumoral vessels. Metabolism 1996; 45:39–41.

49. Sun B, Halmos G, Schally AV, et al. Presence of receptors for bombesin/gastrin-releasing peptide and MRNA for three receptor subtypes in human prostate cancers. Prostate 2000; 42:295–303.

50. Lantry LE, Cappelletti E, Maddalena ME, et al. Synthesis and characterization of a selective ^{177}Lu-labeled GRP-R agonist for systemic radiotherapy of prostate cancer. J Nucl Med 2006; 47:1144–1152.

51. Vincent JP, Mzella P, Kitabgi P. Neurotensin and neurotensin receptors. Trends Pharmacol Sci 1999; 20:302–309.

52. Wild D, Schmitt JS, Ginj M, et al. DOTA-NOC, a high affinity ligand of somatostatin receptor subtypes 2, 3 and 5 for labelling with various radiometals. Eur J Nucl Med Mol Imaging 2003; 30:1338–1347.

53. Virgolini I, Traub T, Leimer M, et al. New radiopharmaceuticals for receptor scintigraphy and radionuclide therapy. Q J Nucl Med 2000; 44:50–58.

54. Smith CJ, Volkert WA, Hoffman TJ. Radiolabeled peptide conjugates for targeting of the bombesin receptor superfamily subtypes. Nucl Med Biol 2005; 32:733–740.

55. Duvernay MT, Filipeanu CM, Wu GY. The regulatory mechanisms of export trafficking of G-protein-coupled receptors. Cell Signal 2005; 17:1457–1465.

56. deJong M, Bernard BF, DeBruin E, et al. Internalization of radiolabeled [DTPA] octreotide and [DOTA$_8$Tyr$_3$] octreotide: peptides for somatostatin receptor-targeted scintigraphy and radionuclide therapy. Nucl Med Commun 1998; 19:283–288.

57. Fraser CM. Structure and functional analysis of G-protein-coupled receptors and potential diagnostic ligands. J Nucl Med 1995; 36S:17S–21S.

58. Bijsterbosch MK. Selective drug delivery by means of receptor-mediated endocytosis. Q J Nucl Med 1995; 39: 4–19.

59. Harden TK, Boyer JL, Dougherty RW. Drug analysis based on signaling response to G-protein-coupled receptors. In: Leff P, ed. Receptor-Based Drug Design. New York, NY: Marcel Dekker, 1998:79–105.

60. Chen P, Wang J, Hope K, et al. Nuclear localizing sequences promote nuclear translocation and enhance radiotoxicity of the anti-CD33 monoclonal antibody HuM195 labeled with ^{111}In in human myeloid leukemia cells. J Nucl Med 2006; 47:827–836.

61. Ginj M, Zhang H, Waser B, et al. Radiolabeled somatostatin receptor antagonists are preferable to agonist for *in vivo* peptide receptor targeting of tumors. Proc Natl Acad Sci U S A 2006; 103:16436–16441.

62. Breeman WAP, Hofland LJ, deJong M, et al. Evaluation of radiolabelled bombesin analogues for receptor-targeted scintigraphy and radiotherapy. Int J Cancer 1999; 81:658–665.

63. Cremonesi M, Ferrari M, Bodei L, et al. Dosimetry in peptide radionuclide receptor therapy: a review. J Nucl Med 2006; 47:1467–1525.

64. Fani M, Maecke HR. The status of diagnostic and therapeutic targeting of somatostatin receptor-positive tumors. In: Mazzi U, ed. Technetium, Rhenium and Other Metals in Chemistry and Nuclear Medicine. 7th ed. Padova, Italy: S.G. Editoriali, 2006:263–276.

65. Giblin MF, Sieckman GL, Shelton TD, et al. *In vitro* and *in vivo* evaluation of Lu-177 and Y-90-labeled *E. coli* heat-stable enterotoxin for specific targeting of uroguanylin receptors on human colon cancers. Nucl Med Biol 2006; 33:481–488.

66. Krenning EP, Kwekkeboom DJ, Volkema R, et al. Peptide receptor radionuclide therapy. Ann N Y Acad Sci 2004; 1014:234–245.

67. Kwekkeboom DJ, Mueller-Brand J, Paganelli G, et al. Overview of results of peptide receptor radionuclide therapy with three radiolabeled somatostatin analogs. J Nucl Med 2005; 46S:62S–66S.

68. McQuade P, Miao Y, Yoo J, et al. Imaging of Melanoma Using [64]Cu- and [86]Y-DOTA-ReCCMSH(Arg[11]), a

cyclized peptide analogue of α-MSH. J Med Chem 2005; 48:2985–2992.

69. Paganelli G, Zoboli S, Cremonesi M, et al. Receptor-mediated radiotherapy with ^{90}Y-DOTA-D-Phe^1-Tyr^3-octreotide. Digestion 1996; 27(suppl 1):57–61.

70. Reubi JC, Maecke HR, Krenning EP. Candidates for peptide receptor radiotherapy today and in the future. J Nucl Med 2005; 46S:67S–75S.

71. Smith CJ, Gali H, Sieckman GL, et al. Radiochemical investigations of ^{177}Lu-DOTA-8-AOC-BBN(7-14)NH$_2$: an in vitro/in vivo assessment of the targeting ability of this new radiopharmaceutical for PC-3 human prostate cancer cells. Nucl Med Biol 2003; 30:101–109.

72. Wang X, Ginj M, Zhang H, et al. NLS-modified somatostatin-based radiopeptides with enhanced potential for imaging and targeted therapy of tumors. In: Mazzi U, ed. Technetium, Rhenium and Other Metals in Chemistry and Nuclear Medicine. 7th ed. Padova, Italy: S.G. Editoriali, 2006:531–534.

73. Breeman WAP, deJong M, deBlois E, et al. Radiolabeling DOTA-peptides with ^{68}Ga. Eur J Nucl Med 2005; 32:478–485.

74. Rossin R, Azhdarinia A, Mendez R, et al. Evaluation of commercially available ^{68}Ge/^{68}Ga-generators for the synthesis of high specific activity ^{68}Ga-radiotracers. In: Mazzi U, ed. Technetium, Rhenium and Other Metals in Chemistry and Nuclear Medicine. Padova, Italy: S.G. Editoriali, 2006:239–240.

75. Erba PA, Signore A, Mariani G. Prospective molecular targets for the development of ^{99m}Tc-labeled agents with potential clinical use. In: Mazzi U, ed. Technetium, Rhenium and Other Metals in Chemistry and Nuclear Medicine. 7th ed. Padova, Italy: S.G. Editoriali, 2006:665–682.

76. Blum J, Handmaker H, Lister-James J, et al. A multicenter trial with a somatostatin analog ^{99m}Tc-depreotide in the evaluation of solitary pulmonary nodules. Chest 2000; 117:1232–1238.

77. Oberg K, Erickson B. Nuclear medicine in detection, staging and treatment of gastrointestinal carcinoid tumors. Best Pract Res Clin Endocrinol Metab 2005; 19:265–276.

78. Reubi JC. Neuropeptide receptors in health and disease: the molecular basis for in vivo imaging. J Nucl Med 1995; 36:1825–1835.

79. Teunissen JJ, Kwekkeboom DJ, Krenning EP. Staging and treatment of differentiated thyroid carcinoma with radiolabeled somatostatin analogs. Trends Endocrinol Metab 2006; 17:19–25.

80. Virgolini I, Kurtaran A, Raderer M, et al. Vasoactive intestinal peptide receptor. J Nucl Med 1995; 36:1732–1739.

81. Krenning EP, Bakker WH, Breeman WAP, et al. Localization of endocrine-related tumours with radioiodinated analogue of somatostatin. Lancet 1989; 1:242–244.

82. Krenning EP, Kwekkeboom DJ, Pauwels S, et al. Somatostatin receptor scintigraphy. In: Freeman LM, ed. Nuclear Medicine Annual. New York: Raven Press, 1995:1–50.

83. Virgolini I, Traub T, Novotry C, et al. Experience with indium-111 and yttrium-90-labeled somatostatin analogs. Curr Pharm Des 2002; 8:1781–1787.

84. Krenning EP, Teunissen JJ, Valkema R, et al. Molecular radiotherapy with somatostatin analogs for neuroendocrine tumors. J Endocrinol Invest 2005; 28:146–150.

85. Lambert B, Cybulla M, Weiner SM, et al. Renal toxicity after radionuclide therapy. Radiat Res 2004; 1611:607–611.

86. deJong M, Rolleman EJ, Bernard BF, et al. Inhibition of renal uptake of Indium-111-DTPA-octreotide in vivo. J Nucl Med 1996; 37:1388–1392.

87. Duncan JR, Stephenson MT, Wu HP, et al. Indium-111-dithylenetriaminepentaacetic acid-octreotide is delivered in vivo to pancreatic, tumor cell, renal, and hepatocyte lysosomes. Cancer Res 1997; 57:659–671.

88. Faintuch BL, Santos RLSR, Souza ALFM, et al. ^{99m}Tc-HYNIC-Bombesin(7-14)NH$_2$: radiochemical evaluation with co-ligands EDDA (EDDA = ethyledediamine-N, N'diacetic acid), tricine, and nicolinic acid. Synth React Inorg Met-Org Nano-Met Chem 2005; 35:43–51.

89. Liu S, Edwards DS. ^{99m}Tc-labeled small peptides as diagnostic radiopharmaceuticals. Chem Rev 1999; 99:2235–2268.

90. Plachenska A, Mikolajczah R, Maecke HR, et al. Efficacy of ^{99m}Tc-EDDA.HYNIC-TOC scintigraphy in differential diagnosis of solitary pulmonary nodules. Cancer Biother Radiopharm 2004; 19:613–620.

91. Thakur ML, Kolan H, Li R, et al. ^{99m}Tc-labeled vasoactive intestinal peptide: analog for rapid localization of tumors in humans. J Nucl Med 2001; 41:107–110.

92. Maina T, Nock B, Nikolopoulou A, et al. [99mTc]Demotate, a new ^{99m}Tc-based [Tyr^3]octreotate analogue for the detection of somatostatin receptor-positive tumours: synthesis and preclinical results. Eur J Nucl Med Mol Imaging 2002; 29:742–753.

93. Decristoforo C, Maina T, Nock B, et al. ^{99m}Tc-Demotate 1: first data in tumour patients-results of a pilot/phase I study. Eur J Nucl Med Mol Imaging 2003; 30:1211–1219.

94. Blum J, Handmaker H, Rinne NA. The utility of a somatostatin-type receptor binding peptide radiopharmaceutical (P829) in the evolution of solitary pulmonary nodules. Chest 1999; 115:224–232.

95. van der Hoek J, Hofland LJ, Lamberts S. Novel subtype specific and universal somatostatin analogues: clinical potential and pitfalls. Curr Pharm Des 2005; 11:1573–1592.

96. Wild D, Maecke HR, Waser B, et al. ^{68}Ga-DOTANOC: a first compound for PET imaging with high affinity somatostatin receptor subtypes 2 and 5. Eur J Nucl Med Mol Imaging 2005; 32:724.

97. Maecke HR, Hofman M, Haberkorn U. Ga-68-labeled peptides in tumor imaging. J Nucl Med 2005; 46S:172S–178S.

98. Anderson CJ, Pajeau TS, Edwards W, et al. In vitro and in vivo evaluation of copper-64-octreotide conjugates. J Nucl Med 1995; 36:2315–2325.

99. Lewis JS, Laforest R, Lewis MR, et al. Comparative dosimetry of copper-64 and yttrium-90 labeled somatostatin analogs in a tumor-bearing rat model. Cancer Biother Radiopharm 1995; 15:593–604.

100. Li WP, Lewis JS, Kim J, et al. DOTA-D-Tyr(1)-octreotate: a somatostatin analogue for labeling with

metal and halogen radionuclides for cancer imaging and therapy. Bioconjug Chem 2002; 13:721–728.

101. Boswell CA, Sun X, Nin W, et al. Comparative *in vivo* stability of copper-64-labeled cross-bridged and conventional tetraazamacrocyclic complexes. J Med Chem 2004; 47:1465–1474.

102. Anderson CJ, Wadas TJ, Wong EH, et al. Development of chelators for copper-64 radiopharmaceuticals: optimizing for *in vivo* stability. In: Mazzi U, ed. Technetium, Rhenium and Other Metals in Chemistry and Nuclear Medicine. 7th ed. Padova, Italy: S.G. Editorali, 2006: 215–218.

103. Wester HJ, Schottelius KS, Scheidhauer K, et al. PET imaging of somatostatin receptors: design, synthesis and preclinical evaluation of a novel ^{18}F-labelled, carbohydrated analogue of octreotide. Eur J Nucl Med Mol Imaging 2003; 30:117–122.

104. Henriksen G, Schottelius M, Poethko T, et al. Proof of principle for the use of ^{11}C-labelled peptides in tumour diagnosis with PET. Eur J Nucl Med Mol Imaging 2004; 31:1653–1657.

105. Lubbrink M, Tolmachev V, Widstrom C, et al. ^{110m}In-DTPA-D-Phe^{1}-octreotide for imaging of neuroendocrine tumors with PET. J Nucl Med 2002; 43:1391–1397.

106. Valkema R, deJong M, Bakker WH, et al. Phase I study of peptide receptor radionuclide therapy with [In-DTPA]octreotide: the Rotterdam experience. Semin Nucl Med 2002; 32:110–122.

107. Anthony L, Woltering E, Espeuan G, et al. Indiana-III-pentetreotide prolongs survival in gastroenteropancreatic malignancies. Semin Nucl Med 2002; 32:123–132.

108. Fleischmann A, Laderach U, Friess H, et al. Bombesin receptors in distinct tissue compartments of human pancreatic diseases. Lab Invest 2000; 80:1807–1817.

109. Giacchetti S, Gauville C, de Cremoux P, et al. Characterization, in some human breast cancer cell lines, of gastrin-releasing peptide-like receptors which are absent in normal breast epithelial cells. Int J Cancer 1990; 46: 293–298.

110. Gugger M, Reubi JC. GRP receptors in non-neoplastic and neoplastic human breast. Am J Pathol 1999; 155:2067–2076.

111. Halmos G, Wittliff JL, Schally AV. Characterization of bombesin/gastrin-releasing peptide receptors in human breast cancer and their relationship to steroid receptor expression. Cancer Res 1995; 55:280–287.

112. Markwalder R, Reubi JC. Gastrin-releasing peptide receptors in the human pancreatic cancers. Ann Surg 2000; 231:838–848.

113. Fathi Z, Grjar MH, Shapira H, et al. BRS-3 novel bombesin receptor subtype selectively expressed in testes and lung carcinoma cells. J Biol Chem 1993; 268:5974–5984.

114. Maina T, Nock B, Zhang H, et al. Species differences of bombesin analog interactions with GRP-R define the choice of animal models in the development of GRP-R-targeting drugs. J Nucl Med 2005; 46:823–830.

115. Mantey SA, Weber HC, Sainz E, et al. Discovery of a high affinity radioligand for the human orphan receptor, bombesin receptor subtype 3, which demonstrates that it has a

116. Anastosi A, Espamer V, Nucci M. Isolation and aminoacid sequence of alytesin and bombesin, two analogous active tetradecapeptides from the skin of European discoglossid frogs. Arch Biochem Biophys 1972; 148:443–446.

117. Battey JF, Way JM, Corjay MH, et al. Molecular cloning of the bombesin/gastrin-releasing peptide receptor from Swiss 3T3 cells. Proc Natl Acad Sci U S A 1991; 88:395–399.

118. McDonald TJ, Jorvall H, Nilsson G, et al. Characterization of a gastrin releasing peptide from porcine non-antral gastric tissue. Biochem Biophys Res Commun 1979; 90:227–233.

119. Spindel ER, Giladi E, Brehm P, et al. Cloning and functional characterization of a complementary DNA encoding the murine fibroblast bombesin/gastrin-releasing peptide receptor. Mol Endocrinol 1990; 4:1956–1963.

120. Cutitta F, Carney DN, Mulshine J, et al. Bombesin-like peptides can function as autocrine growth factors in human small-cell lung cancer. Nature 1985; 316:823–826.

121. Moody TW, Bertness V, Carney DN. Bombesin-like peptides and receptors in human tumor cell lines. Peptides 1983; 4:483–486.

122. Yano T, Pinski J, Groot K, et al. Stimulation by bombesin and inhibition by bombesin/gastrin-releasing peptide antagonist RC-3095 of growth of human breast cancer cell lines. Cancer Res 1992; 52:4545–4547.

123. Yano T, Pinski J, Szepeshazi K, et al. Inhibitory effect of bombesin/gastrin-releasing peptide antagonist RC-3095 and luteinizing hormone-releasing hormone antagonist SB-75 on the growth of MCF-7 MIII human breast cancer xenografts in athymic nude mice. Cancer 1994; 73:1229–1238.

124. Coy DH, Jensen RT, Jiang NY. Systematic development of bombesin/gastrin-releasing peptide antagonists. NCI Monogr 1992; 133–139.

125. Landon LA, Zou J, Deutscher SL. An effective combinatorial strategy to increase affinity of carbohydrate binding by peptides. Mol Divers 2004; 1:113–132.

126. Alves S, Paulo A, Correia JDG, et al. Pyrazolyl derivatives as bifunctional chelators for labeling tumor-seeking peptides with the *fac*[M(CO)3]+ moiety (M=Tc-99m, Re): synthesis, characterization and biological behaviour. Bioconjug Chem 2005; 16:438–449.

127. Baido KE, Lin KS, Zhan Y, et al. Design, synthesis, and initial evaluation of high-affinity technetium bombesin analogues. Bioconjug Chem 1998; 9:218–225.

128. Smith CJ, Gali H, Sieckman GL, et al. Radiochemical investigations of ^{99m}Tc-N$_3$S-X-BBN(7-14)NH$_2$: an *in vitro*/*in vivo* structure-activity relationship study where X = 0, 3, 5, 8, and 11-carbon tethering moieties. Bioconjug Chem 2003; 14:93–102.

129. Chen X, Park R, Hou Y, et al. MicroPET and autoradiographic imaging of GRP receptor expression with ^{64}Cu-DOTA-[Lys^3]bombesin in human prostate adenocarcinoma xenografts. J Nucl Med 2004; 45:1397.

130. Hoffman TJ, Gali H, Smith CJ, et al. Novel series of indium-111 labeled bombesin analogs as potential

radiopharmaceuticals for specific targeting of gastrin releasing peptide (GRP) receptors expressed on human prostate cancer cells. J Nucl Med 2003; 44:823–831.

131. Lin KS, Liu A, Baido KE, et al. A new high affinity technetium-99m-bombesin analogue with low abdominal accumulation. Bioconjug Chem 2005; 16:43–50.

132. Nock B, Nikolopoulou A, Galanis A, et al. Potent bombesin-like peptides for GRP-receptor targeting of tumors with ^{99m}Tc: a preclinical study. J Med Chem 2005; 48:100–110.

133. Rogers BE, Rosenfeld ME, Khazaeli MB, et al. Localization of Iodine-125-mIP-Des-Met14-bombesin(7-13)NH$_2$ in ovarian carcinoma induced to express the gastrin releasing peptide receptor by adenoviral vector-mediated gene transfer. J Nucl Med 1997; 38:1221–1229.

134. Smith CJ, Sieckman GL, Owen NK, et al. Radiochemical investigations of GRP receptor-specific [^{99m}Tc(X)(CO)$_3$-Dpr-Ser-Ser-Ser-Gln-Trp-Ala-Val-Gly-His-Leu-Met-(NH$_2$)]: in PC$_3$, tumor-bearing, rodent models: syntheses, radiolabeling, and *in vitro/in vivo* studies where Dpr=2,3-diamino-propionic acid and X=H2$_O$ or P(CH$_2$OH)$_3$. Cancer Res 2003; 63:4082–4088.

135. Hoffman TJ, Li N, Volkert WA, et al. Synthesis and characterization of Rh-105 labeled bombesin analogues: enhancement of GRP receptor binding affinity utilizing aliphatic carbon chain linkers. J Labelled Comp Radiopharm 1997; 40(S):490–493.

136. Nock B, Nikolopoulou A, Chiotellis E, et al. [^{99m}Tc] Demobesin 1, a novel potent bombesin analogue for GRP receptor-targeted tumour imaging. Eur J Nucl Med 2003; 30:247–258.

137. Karra SR, Schibli R, Gali H, et al. ^{99m}Tc-labeling and *in vivo* studies of a bombesin analogue with a novel water-soluble dithia-diphosphine based bifunctional chelating agents. Bioconjug Chem 1999; 10:254–260.

138. Smith CJ, Sieckman GL, Owen NK, et al. Radiochemical investigations of ^{188}Re(H$_2$O)(CO)$_3$-diaminopropionic acid-sss-bombesin (7-14)NH$_2$; synthesis, radiolabeling and *in vitro/in vivo* GRP receptor targeting studies. Anticancer Res 2003; 23:63–70.

139. Van de Wiele C, Dumont F, Broecke RV, et al. Technetium-99m RP527, a GRP analogue for visualization of GRP receptor-expressing malignancies: a feasible study. Eur J Nucl Med 2000; 27:1694–1699.

140. Van de Wiele C, Phillippe P, Pauwels P, et al. Gastrin-releasing peptide receptor imaging in human breast carcinoma versus immunohistochemistry. J Nucl Med 2008; 49:260–264.

141. Hu F, Cutler C, Hoffman TJ, et al. Pm-149-DOTA bombesin analogs for potential radiotherapy, *in vivo* comparison with Sm-153 and Lu-177 labeled DO3A-amide-βAla-BBN(7-14)NH$_2$ Nucl Med Biol 2002; 29:423–430.

142. Schumacker J, Zhang H, Doll J, et al. GRP receptor-targeted PET of a rat pancreas carcinoma xenograft in nude mice with a ^{68}Ga-labeled bombesin (6-14) analog. J Nucl Med 2005; 46:691–699.

143. Rogers BE, Bigott HM, McCarthy DW, et al. Micro-PET imaging of gastrin-releasing peptide receptor positive tumor in a mouse model of human prostate cancer using a ^{64}Cu-labeled bombesin analogue. Bioconjug Chem 2003; 14:756–763.

144. Johnson CV, Shelton TD, Smith CJ, et al. Evaluation of combined ^{177}Lu-DOTA-8-AOC-BBN(7-14)NH$_2$ GRP receptor-targeted radiotherapy and chemotherapy in PC-3 human prostate tumor cell xenografted SCID mice. Cancer Bioether Radiopharm 2006; 21:155–166.

145. Pangione S, Nunn AD. Luteium-177-labeled gastrin releasing peptide receptor binding analogs: a novel approach to radionuclide therapy. Q J Nucl Med Mol Imaging 2006; 50:310–321.

146. Johnson CV, Shelton TD, Smith CJ, et al. Evaluation o combined ^{177}Lu-DOTA-8-AOC-BBN(7-14)NH$_2$ GRP receptor-targeted radiotherapy and chemotherapy in PC-3 human prostate tumor cell xenografted SCID mice. Cancer Bioether Radiopharm 2006; 21:155–166.

147. Reubi JC, Waser B, Friess H, et al. Neurotensin receptors: a new marker for human ductal pancreatic adenocarcinoma. Gut 1998; 42:546–550.

148. Mule F, Serio R, Postorino A, et al. Antagonism by SR-48692 of mechanical responses to neurotensin in rat intestine. Br J Pharmacol 1996; 117:488–492.

149. Garcia-Garayoa E, Allemann-Tannahill L, Blauenstein P, et al. *In vitro* and *in vivo* evaluation of new radiolabeled neurotensin(8-13) analogues with high affinity for NT1 receptors. Nucl Med Biol 2001; 28:75–84.

150. Zhang K, An R, Gao Z, et al. Radionuclide imaging of small-cell lung cancer (SCLC) using ^{99m}Tc-labeled neurotensin peptide 8-13. Nucl Med Biol 2006; 33:505–512.

151. Blauenstein P, Garcia-Garayo E, Rueegg D, et al. Improving tumor uptake of Tc-99m-labeled neuropeptides using stabilized peptide analogs. Cancer Biother Radiopharm 2004; 19:181–188.

152. Garcia-Garayoa E, Blauestein P, Blanc A, et al. Preclinicale evaluation of a new, stabilized neurotensin (8–13) pseudopeptide labeled with Tc-99m. J Nucl Med 2002; 43:374–383.

153. Siegrist W, Solca F, Stutz S, et al. Characterization of receptors for alpha-melanocyte-stimulating hormone on human melanoma cells. Cancer Res 1989; 49: 6352–6358.

154. Cone RD, Lu D, Koppula S, et al. The melanocortin receptors: agonists, antagonists, and the hormonal control of pigmentation. Recent Prog Horm Res 1996; 51:287–317.

155. Mountjoy KG, Robins LS, Mortrud MT, et al. The cloning of a family of genes that encode the melanocortin receptors. Science 1992; 257:1248–1251.

156. Garg PK, Alston KL, Welsh PC, et al. Enhanced binding and inertness to dehalogenation of α-melanotropic peptides labeled using N-succinimidyl 3-iodobenzoate. Bioconjug Chem 1996; 7:233–239.

157. Bagutti C, Stolz B, Albert R, et al. ^{111}In-DTPA-labeled analogs for alpha-melanocyte-stimulating hormone for melanoma targeting: receptor binding *in vitro* and *in vivo*. Int J Cancer 1994; 58:749–755.

158. Bard DR, Knight CG, Page-Thomas DP. A chelating derivative of α-melanocyte stimulating hormone as a potential imaging agent for malignant melanoma. Br J Cancer 1990; 62:919–922.

159. Wraight EP, Bard DR, Maughan TS, et al. The use of a chelating derivative of alpha melanocyte stimulating hormone for the clinical imaging of malignant melanoma. Br J Radiol 1992; 6:112–118.

160. Froidevaux S, Calame-Christe M, Schuhmacher J, et al. A gallium-labeled DOTA-α-melanocyte-stimulating hormone analog for imaging of melanoma metastases. J Nucl Med 2004; 45:116–123.

161. Giblin MF, Jurisson SS, Quinn TP. Synthesis and characterization of rhenium-complexed α-melanotropin analogs. Bioconjug Chem 1997; 8:347–353.

162. Chen J, Cheng Z, Hoffman TJ, et al. Melanoma-targeting properties of ^{99m}Technetium-labeled cyclic α-melanocyte-stimulating hormone peptide analogues. Cancer Res 2000; 60:5658.

163. Chen J, Cheng Z, Owen NK, et al. Evaluation of an ^{111}In-DOTA-rhenium cyclized alpha-MSH analog: a novel cyclic peptide analog with improved tumor targeting properties. J Nucl Med 2001; 42:1847–1855.

164. Miao Y, Whitener D, Feng W, et al. Evaluation of the human melanoma targeting properties of radiolabeled alpha-melanocyte stimulating hormone peptide analogues. Bioconjug Chem 2003; 14:1177–1184.

165. Miao Y, Hylarides M, Fisher DR, et al. Melanoma therapy via peptide-targeted alpha-radiation. Clin Cancer Res 2005; 11:5616–5626.

166. Carrithers SL, Parkinson SJ, Goldstein S, et al. *Escherichia coli* heat-stable toxin receptors in human colonic tumors. Gastroenterology 1994; 107:1653–1661.

167. Carrithers SL, Barber MT, Biswas S, et al. Guanylyl cyclase C is a selective marker for metastatic colorectal tumors in human extraintestinal tissues. Proc Natl Acad Sci U S A 1996; 93:14827–14832.

168. Forte LR, London RM, Freeman RH, et al. Guanylin peptides: renal actions mediated by cyclic GMP. Am J Physiol Renal Physiol 2000; 278:F180–F191.

169. Forte LR. Uroguanylin and guanylin peptides: pharmacology and experimental therapeutics. Pharmacol Ther 2004; 104:137–162.

170. Ozaki H, Sato T, Kubota H, et al. Molecular structure of the toxic domain of heat-stable enterotoxin produced by a pathogenic strain of *Escherichia coli*. J Biol Chem 1991; 266:5934–5941.

171. Giblin MF, Sieckman GL, Gali H, et al. Selective *in vitro* and *in vivo* targeting of human *E. coli* ST peptide analogs to human pancreatic cancer cells. J Labelled Comp Radiopharm 2003; 46:S101.

172. Giblin MF, Gali H, Sieckman GL, et al. *In vitro* and *in vivo* evaluation of In-111-labeled human *E. coli* heat-stable enterotoxin analogs for specific targeting of human breast cancers. Bioconjug Chem 2004; 15:872–880.

173. Gali H, Sieckman GL, Hoffman TJ, et al. Synthesis and *in vitro* evaluation of ^{111}In-labeled heat-stable enterotoxin (ST) analogue for specific targeting of guanylin receptors on human colonic cancers. Anticancer Res 2006; 21:2785–2792.

174. Wolfe HR, Mendizabal M, Lleong E, et al. *In vivo* imaging of human colon cancer xenografts in immunodeficient mice using a guanylyl cyclase C-specific ligand. J Nucl Med 2002; 43:392–399.

175. Giblin MF, Sieckman GL, Watkinson LD, et al. Selective targeting of E. coli heat-stable enterotoxin analogs to human colon cancer cells. Anticancer Res 2006; 26:3243–3252.

176. Giblin MF, Sieckman GL, Owen NK, et al. Radiolabeled *Escherichia coli* heat-stable enterotoxin analogs for *in vivo* imaging of colorectal cancer. Nucl Instrum Methods Phys Res B 2005; 241:689–692.

177. Giblin MF, Gali H, Sieckman GL, et al. *In vitro* and *in vivo* evaluation of In-111-labeled E. coli heat-stable enterotoxin analogs for specific targeting of human breast cancers. Breast Cancer Res Treat 2006; 98:7–15.

178. Magistretti PJ, Journot L, Bockaert J. Brain PACAP/VIP receptors: regional distribution functional properties and physiological relevance. In: Quirion R, Bjorklund A, Holefelt T, eds. Handbook of Chemical Neuroanatomy. Amsterdam: Elsevier Science, 2000:45–77.

179. Reubi JC. *In vitro* evaluation of VIP/PACAP receptors in healthy and diseased human tissues: clinical implications. Ann N Y Acad Sci 2000; 921:1–25.

180. Basto R, Prieto JC, Bodega G, et al. Immunohistochemical localization and distribution of VIP/PACAP receptors in human lung. Peptides 2000; 21:265–269.

181. Reubi JC. *In vitro* identification of vasoactive intestinal peptide receptors in human tumors: implications for tumor imaging. J Nucl Med 1995; 36:1846–1853.

182. Wu Y, Zhang XZ, Xiong ZM, et al. MicroPET imaging of glioma alphaV-integrin expression using ^{64}Cu-labeled tetrameric RGD peptide. J Nucl Med 2005; 46:1707–1718.

183. Roderer M, Kurtaran A, Yang Q, et al. Iodine-123-vasoactive intestinal peptide receptor scanning in patients with pancreatic cancer. J Nucl Med 1998; 39:1570–1575.

184. Weiner RE, Thakur ML. Radiolabeled peptides in the diagnosis and therapy of oncological diseases. Appl Radiat Isot 2002; 57:749–763.

185. Thakur ML. Imaging tumors in humans with Tc-99m-VIP. Ann N Y Acad Sci 2000; 921:37–44.

186. Thakur ML, Marcus CS, Saeed S, et al. ^{99m}Tc-labeled vasoactive intestinal peptide receptor analog for rapid localization of tumors in humans. J Nucl Med 2000; 41:107–110.

187. Thakur ML, Arnva MR, Gariepy J, et al. PET imaging of oncogene overexpression using ^{64}Cu-vasoactive intestinal peptide (VIP) analog: comparison with ^{99m}Tc-VIP analog. J Nucl Med 2004; 45:1318–1319.

188. Noble F, Wank SA, Crawley JN, et al. Structure, distribution, and functions of cholecystokinin receptors. Pharmacol Rev 51; 1999:745–781.

189. Reubi JC, Waser B, Schaer JC, et al. Unsulfated DTPA- and DOTA-CCK analogs as specific high affinity ligands for CCK-B receptor-expressing human and rat tissues *in vitro* and *in vivo*. Eur J Nucl Med 1998; 25:481–490.

190. Kwekkeboom DJ, Bakker WH, Kooij PP. Cholecystokinin receptor imaging using an octapeptide DTPA-CCK analogue in patients with medullary thyroid carcinoma. Eur J Nucl Med 2000; 27:1312–1317.

191. Wild D, Behe M, Wicki A, et al. [Lys^{40}(Ahx-DTPA^{111}-In) NH$_2$] Exendin-4, a very promising ligand for glucagon-like

peptide-1 (GLP-1) receptor targeting. J Nucl Med 2006; 47:2025–2033.

192. Ozku KS, Krasnow AZ, Hellman RS. Tc-99m-labelled substance P(SP) analogues for SP receptor imaging. J Nucl Med 2000; 41:246P.

193. Nelson CA, Moyer BR, Pearson DA, et al. Radiolabeled P1470, a calcitonin analog, targets human breast cancer xenografts in nude mice. Nucl Med Commun 2000; 21:575–577.

194. Langer M, LaBella R, Garcia-Garayoa E, et al. Tc-99m-labelled neuropeptide Y with a preference for the Y1 receptor. Eur J Biochem 2001; 268:2828–2837.

195. Reilly RM, Kiarash R, Cameron RG, et al. ^{111}In-labeled EGF is selectively radiotoxic to human breast cancer cells overexpressing EGER. J Nucl Med 2000; 41:429–438.

196. Rusckowski M, Qu T, Chang F, et al. Technetium-99m-labeled epidermal growth factor-tumor imaging in mice. J Pept Res 1997; 50:393–401.

197. Blower PJ, Puncher MR, Kettle AG, et al. Iodine-123 salmon calcitonin, an imaging agent for calcitonin receptors: synthesis, biodistribution, metabolism and dosimetry in humans. Eur J Nucl Med 1998; 25:101–108.

198. Alekic S, Szabo Z, Scheffel U, et al. *In vivo* labeling of endothelin receptors with ^{11}C-L-753,037: studies in mice and a dog. J Nucl Med 2001; 42:1274–1280.

199. Chen X, Hou Y, Tohme M, et al. Pegylated Arg-Gly-Asp peptide: [64]Cu labeling and PET imaging of brain tumor alpha v beta3-integrin expression. J Nucl Med 2004; 45:1776–1783.

200. Beer AJ, Haubner R, Goebel M, et al. Biodistribution and pharmacokinetics of the alpha(v)beta(3)-selective tracer F-18-galacto-RGD in cancer patients. J Nucl Med 2005; 46:1333–1341.

201. Wester HJ. Present status and future trends of tracers for clinical use: oncology. Eur J Nucl Med 2004; 31:S241–S141.

202. Haubner R, Wester HJ, Weber WA, et al. Radiotracer-based strategies to image angiogenesis. Q J Nucl Med 2003; 47:189–199.

203. Cardio-Vila M, Arap W, Pasqualini R. Alpha v beta5 integrin-dependent programmed cell death triggered by a peptide mimic of annexin V. Mol Cell 2003; 11:1151–1162.

204. Pasqualini R. Vascular targeting with phage peptide libraries. Q J Nucl Med 1999; 43:159–162.

205. Peletskaya EN, Glinsky GV, Deutscher SL, et al. Identification of peptide sequences that bind the Thomsen–Friedenreich cancer-associated glycoantigen from bacteriophage peptide display libraries. Mol Divers 1996; 2:13–18.

206. Landon LA, Zou J, Deutscher SL. Is Phage display technology on target for developing peptide-based drugs? Curr Drug Discov Technol 2004; 1:113–132.

207. Zurith AJ, Arap W, Pasqualini R. Mapping of tumor vascular diversity by screening phage display libraries. J Control Release 2003; 91:183–186.

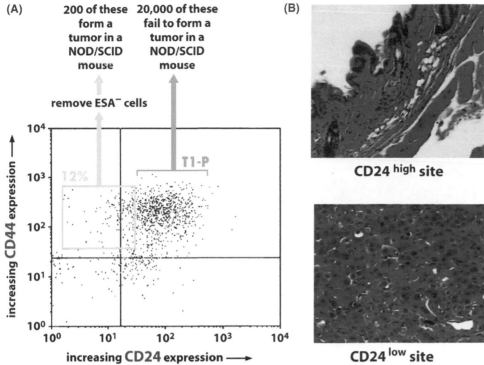

(A)

200 of these form a tumor in a NOD/SCID mouse

20,000 of these fail to form a tumor in a NOD/SCID mouse

remove ESA⁻ cells

12%

T1-P

increasing CD44 expression ⟶

increasing CD24 expression ⟶

(B)

CD24 ^high^ site

CD24 ^low^ site

Figure 1.10 (*see page 18*).

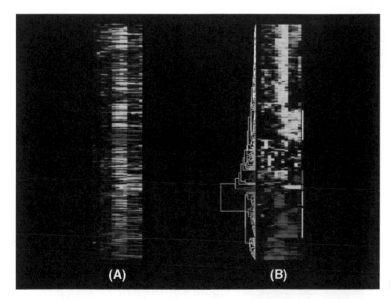

(A) **(B)**

Figure 4.3 (*see page 57*).

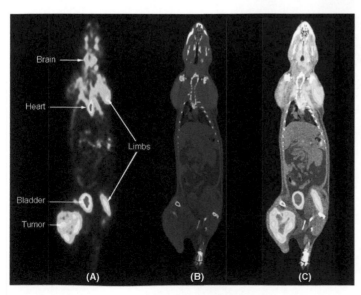

Brain

Heart

Limbs

Bladder

Tumor

(A) **(B)** **(C)**

Figure 5.13 (*see page 83*).

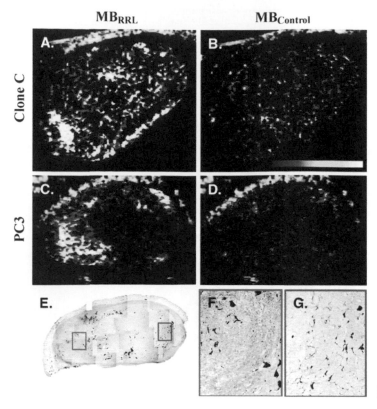

Figure 7.5 *(see page 116).*

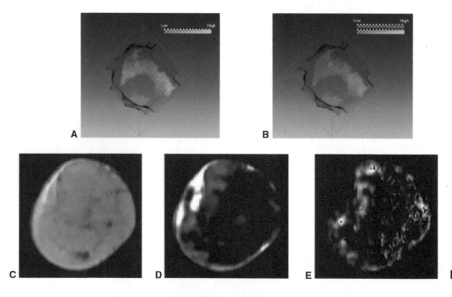

Figure 8.5 *(see page 127).*

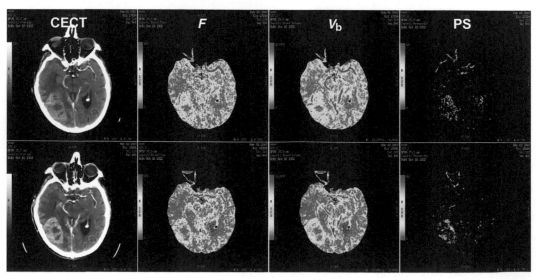

Figure 9.8 *(see page 149).*

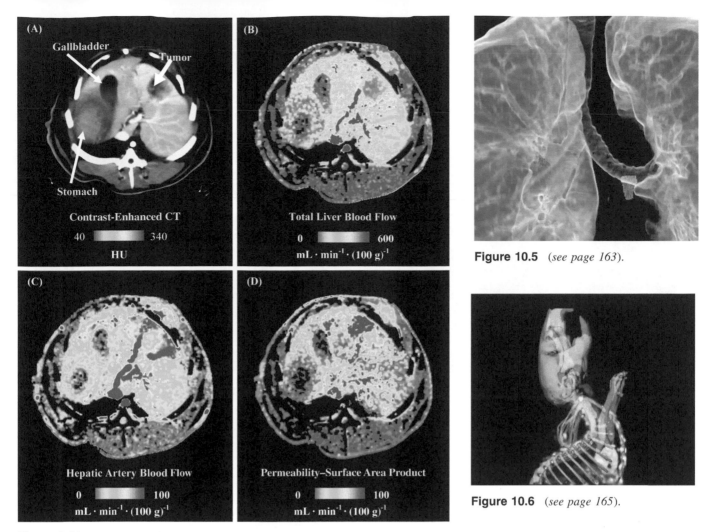

Figure 9.11 (*see page 151*).

Figure 10.5 (*see page 163*).

Figure 10.6 (*see page 165*).

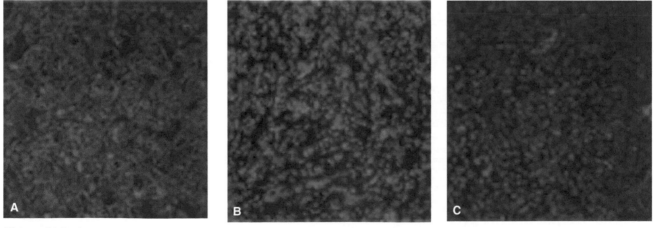

Figure 11.2 (*see page 173*).

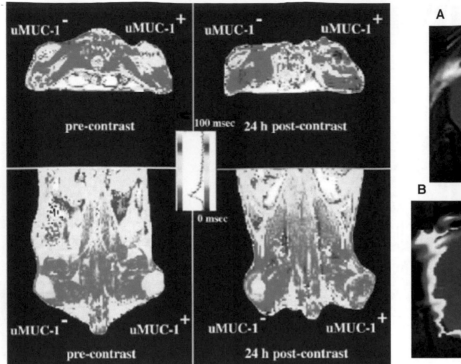

Figure 11.3 *(see page 174)*.

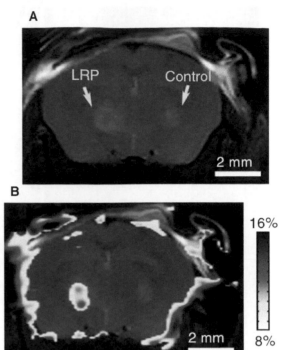

Figure 15.5 *(see page 238)*.

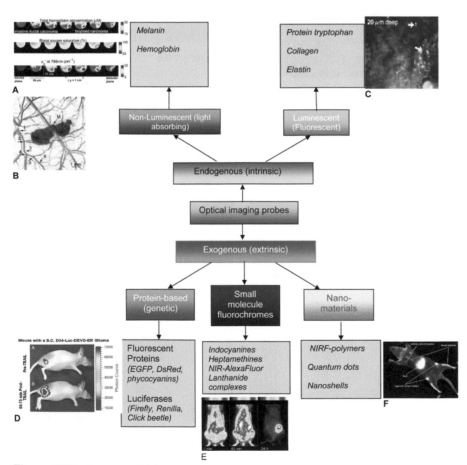

Figure 16.1 *(see page 247)*.

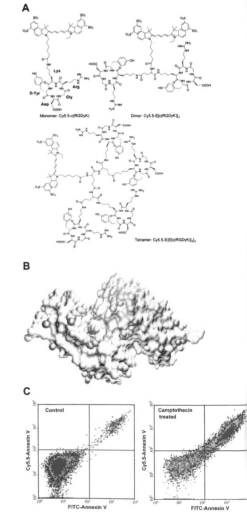

Figure 16.3 *(see page 253)*.

Quantum Dots

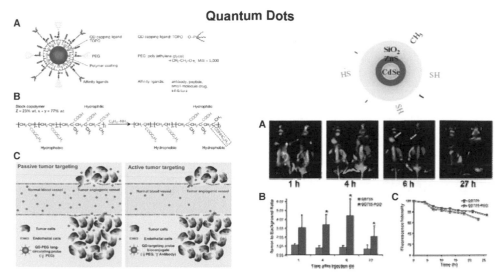

Figure 17.3 (*see page 266*).

Single-walled Carbon Nanotubes

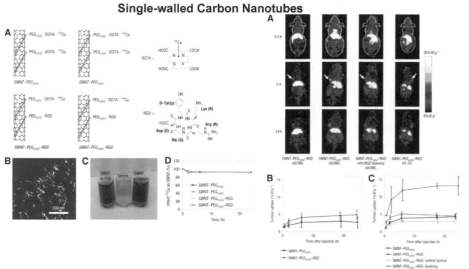

Figure 17.4 (*see page 269*).

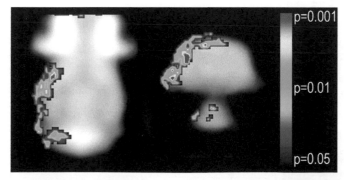

Figure 22.2 (*see page 349*).

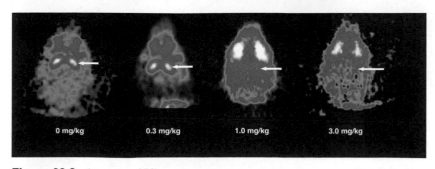

Figure 22.3 (*see page 350*).

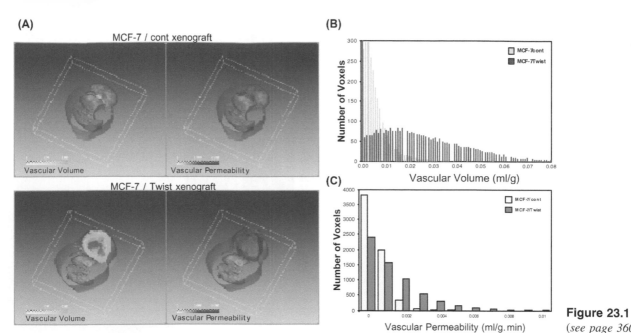

(A)

MCF-7 / cont xenograft

Vascular Volume — Vascular Permeability

MCF-7 / Twist xenograft

Vascular Volume — Vascular Permeability

(B)

(C)

Figure 23.1 (*see page 360*).

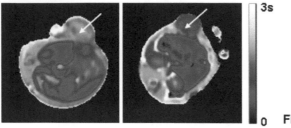

Figure 23.2 (*see page 361*).

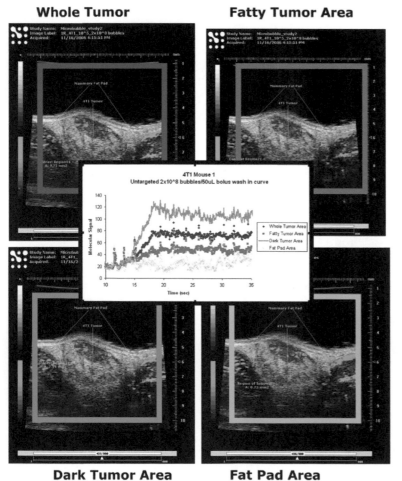

Whole Tumor   **Fatty Tumor Area**

4T1 Mouse 1
Untargeted 2x10^8 bubbles/50uL bolus wash in curve

Dark Tumor Area   **Fat Pad Area**

Figure 23.3 (*see page 363*).

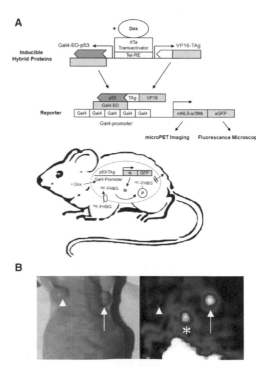

Figure 25.1 (*see page 393*).

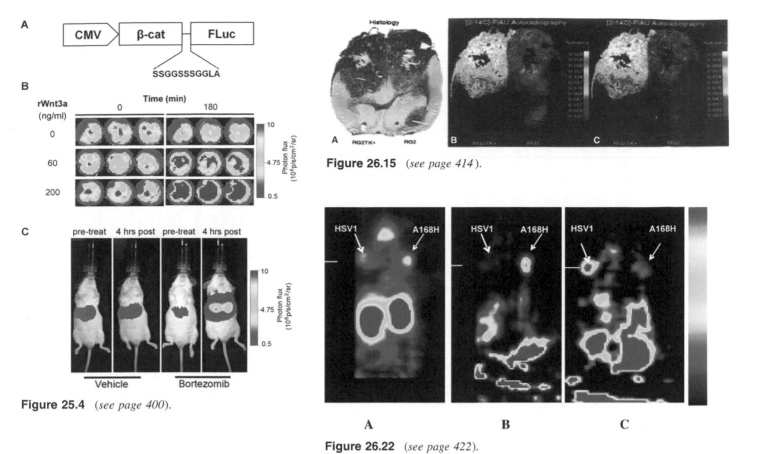

Figure 25.4 (*see page 400*).

Figure 26.15 (*see page 414*).

Figure 26.22 (*see page 422*).

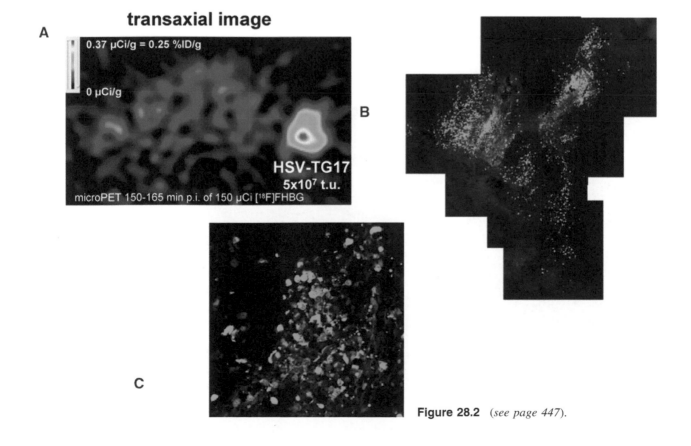

Figure 28.2 (*see page 447*).

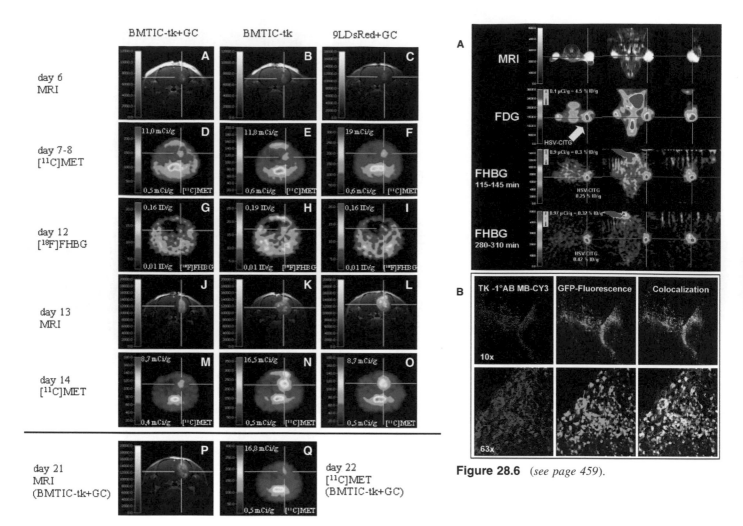

Figure 28.5 (see page 458).

Figure 28.6 (see page 459).

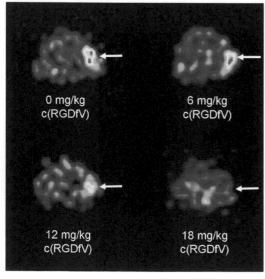

Figure 29.6 (see page 482).

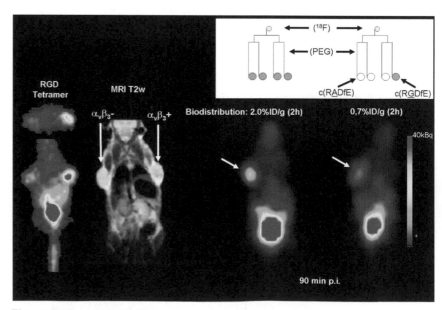

Figure 29.7 (see page 483).

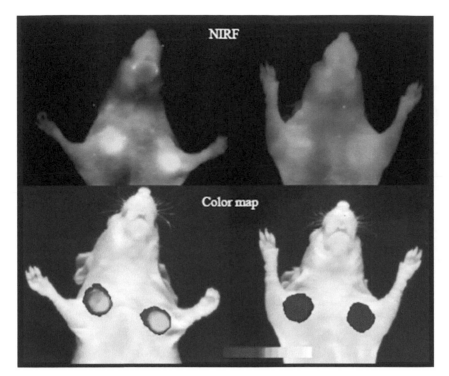

Figure 29.10 *(see page 486).*

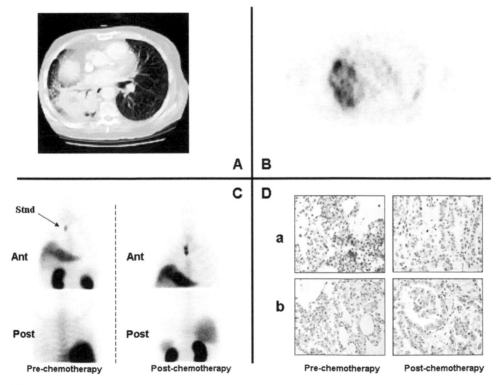

Figure 30.5 *(see page 498).*

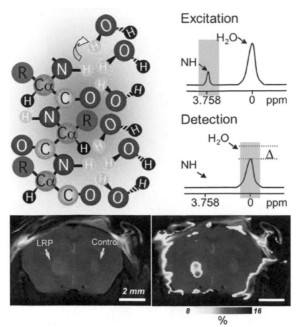

Excitation

Detection

Figure 31.3 (*see page 506*).

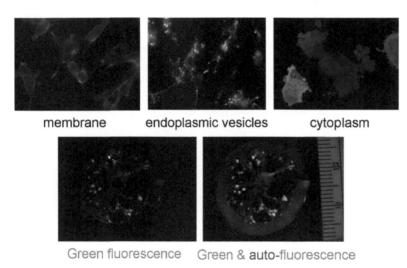

membrane   endoplasmic vesicles   cytoplasm

Green fluorescence   Green & auto-fluorescence

Figure 32.8 (*see page 518*).

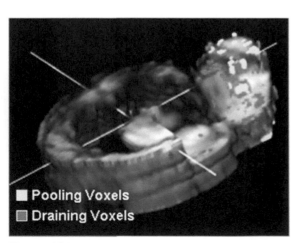

■ Pooling Voxels
■ Draining Voxels

Figure 33.2 (*see page 526*).

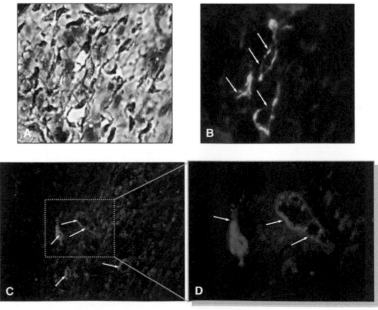

Figure 33.3 (*see page 526*).

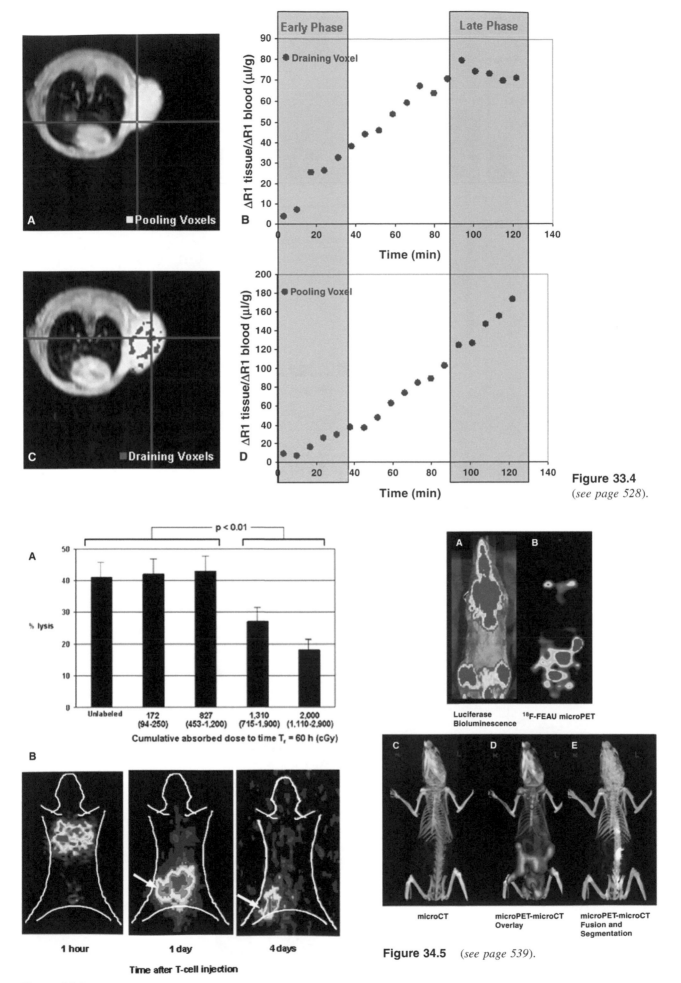

Figure 33.4 (*see page 528*).

Figure 34.2 (*see page 534*).

Figure 34.5 (*see page 539*).

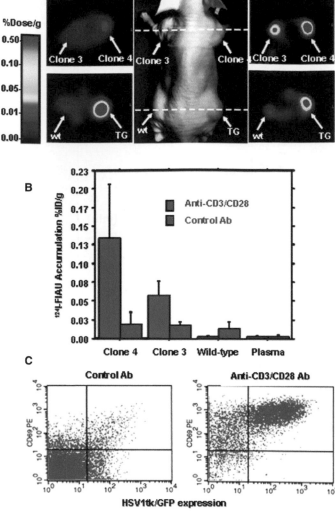

Figure 34.6 (*see page 540*).

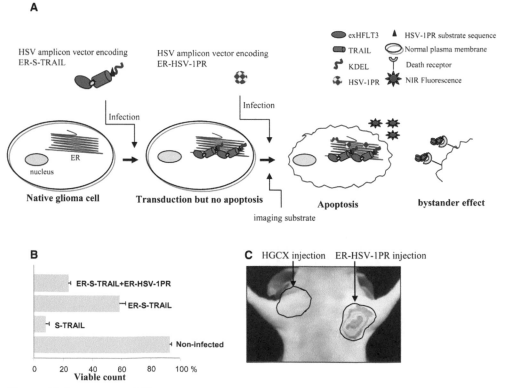

Figure 35.3 (*see page 548*).

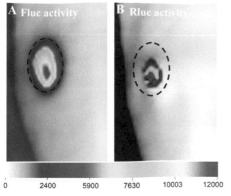

Figure 35.4 *(see page 550)*.

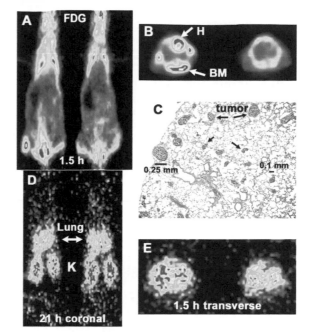

Figure 37.4 *(see page 579)*.

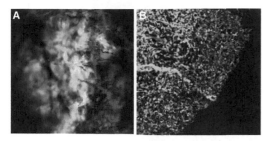

Figure 35.7 *(see page 554)*.

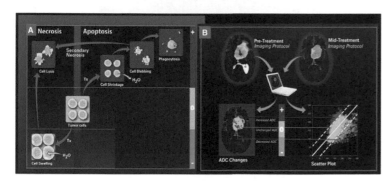

Figure 38.4 *(see page 588)*.

Week 2   Week 8

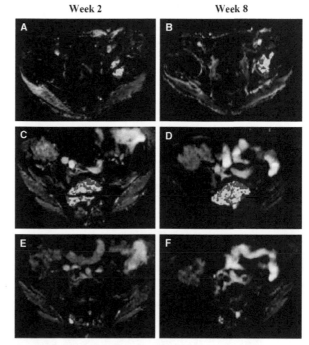

Figure 38.6 *(see page 590)*

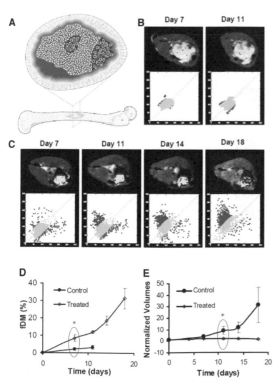

Figure 38.5 *(see page 589)*

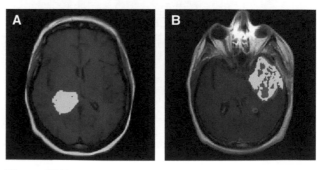

Figure 38.7 *(see page 591)*

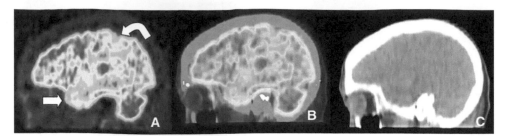

Figure 40.1 (*see page 607*).

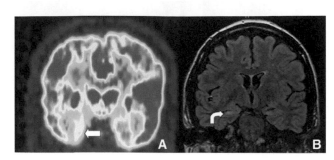

Figure 40.2 (*see page 607*).

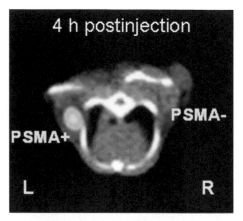

Figure 41.9 (*see page 637*).

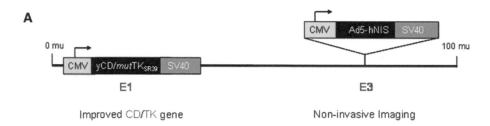

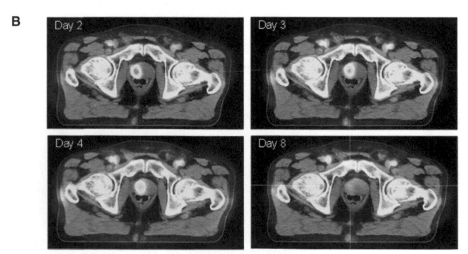

Figure 41.10 (*see page 638*).

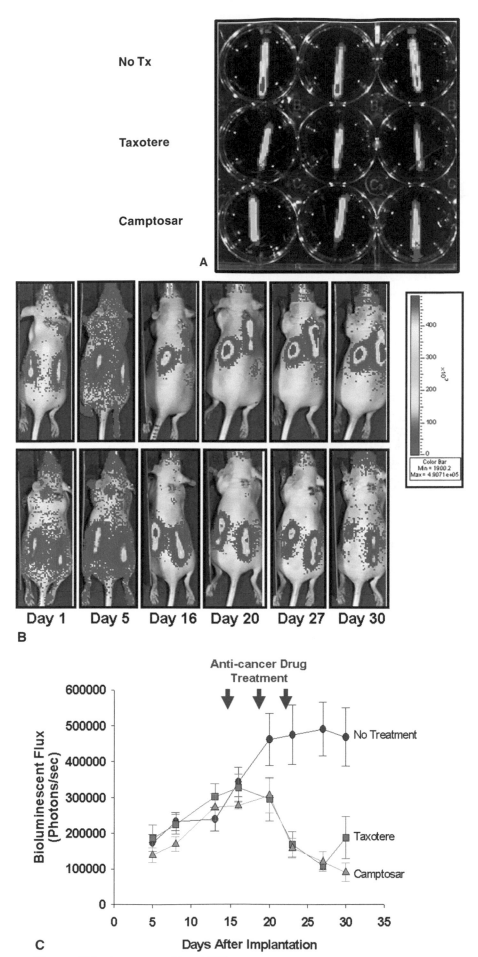

No Tx

Taxotere

Camptosar

A

Day 1   Day 5   Day 16   Day 20   Day 27   Day 30

B

Anti-cancer Drug Treatment

No Treatment

Taxotere

Camptosar

Bioluminescent Flux (Photons/sec)

Days After Implantation

C

Figure 42.1 *(see pages 647 and 648).*

PDGFR inhibition

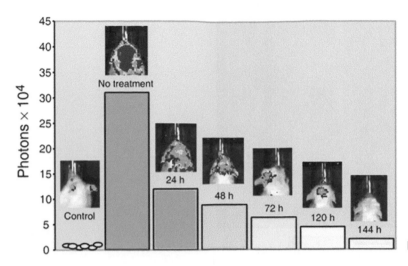

Figure 42.7 (*see page 656*).

FLT images of Mel-28 SQ tumor-bearing mice untreated/treated with PD901

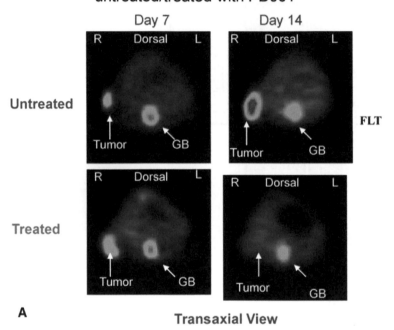

A   **Transaxial View**

Mel-28 xenografts treated/untreated with PD901

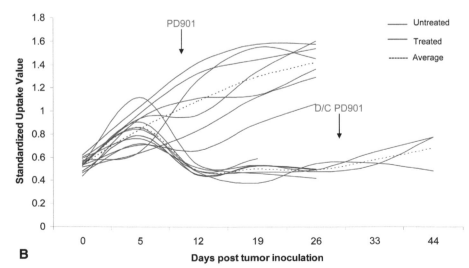

B

Figure 47.5 (*see page 701*).

21

Targeted Ultrasound Contrast Agents

MARK A. BORDEN

Department of Chemical Engineering, Columbia University, New York, New York, U.S.A.

PAUL A. DAYTON

Joint Department of Biomedical Engineering, University of North Carolina at Chapel Hill and North Carolina State University, Raleigh, North Carolina, U.S.A.

INTRODUCTION

Contrast agents are an essential part of ultrasound molecular imaging. The contrast agent serves to recognize the molecule of interest through ligand-receptor binding and then acts as an echo responder for detection with the ultrasound scanner. Without the targeted contrast agent, ultrasound molecular imaging would not be possible. Below, a brief discussion is given to illustrate important concepts regarding the targeted contrast agent and its use for ultrasound molecular imaging. Our goal is to inform the molecular imaging team of the important insights into the rational engineering design of the contrast agent. More detailed information can be found in the cited references.

TYPES OF ULTRASOUND CONTRAST AGENTS

Unlike other imaging modalities, which primarily use electromagnetic waves to see inside the body, ultrasound uses only acoustic waves. High-frequency sound waves are generated by the ultrasound transducer, and the image is reconstructed based on the received acoustic echoes. The backscattered energy in this case is better described by classical continuum mechanics rather than quantum mechanics. Because a scattering surface is necessary, colloidal constructs are preferred over single molecules for use as ultrasound contrast agents. Colloids formed by biocompatible materials (biocolloids) are used.

Ultrasound contrast agents were first proposed almost four decades ago. Gramiak and Shah are credited with having first discovered ultrasound contrast through a serendipitous injection of indocyanine green (1). Since that groundbreaking work, research efforts have focused on formulating ultrasound contrast agents that are both stable and multifunctional. Several types of biocolloids have been used, and these can be classified into two general classes: nanoparticles and microbubbles. A brief description of various nanoparticle formulations is given below, followed by a more detailed discussion of the most commonly employed biocolloid—the microbubble. Emphasis is given to rational design of the physicochemical properties of microbubbles to control their echogenic properties and targeting behavior in vivo.

Nanoparticles

Nanoparticles are defined here as liquid or solid colloids in the 10- to 1000-nm diameter size range. In general, nanoparticles are difficult to detect by ultrasound without high accumulation at a target surface, necessitating copious and densely confined receptors. This is largely due to their relatively incompressible core and small size, which results in nanoparticles acting as simple Rayleigh scatterers without the resonance behavior of microbubbles. High-speed videomicroscopy has been used to visualize the differences in oscillation between gas- and liquid-filled biocolloids (Fig. 1). What nanoparticles lose in their ability to oscillate and generate loud echoes, they gain in their reach. Their small size provides long circulation times and the ability to enter cells and extravascular space. These properties make nanoparticle ultrasound contrast agents interesting for targeting tumors, owing to the enhanced permeability and retention (EPR) effect (2).

Liquid Fluorocarbon Nanoparticles

Liquid-liquid nanoparticle emulsions have been used as ultrasound contrast agents (3–5). Often, the dispersed phase is a fluorocarbon liquid encapsulated by a monomolecular surfactant adlayer that stabilizes the tiny droplet from coarsening effects. The surfactant layer also serves to passivate the surface from immunogenic and thrombogenic effects, and it provides a platform on which to attach targeting ligands. Molecular contrast agents from other imaging modalities, such as MRI or optical tomography, can be incorporated into the shell. The dispersed phase can be engineered to vaporize through the energy transfer induced by heating or insonation (6,7). This combines the high stability of liquid droplets with the exceptional echogenicity of gas bubbles (3).

Liposomes

A liposome is a vesicle formed by a lipid bilayer membrane, which separates the interior aqueous phase from the exterior aqueous environment. The lipids self-assemble into the bilayer membrane, so that their hydrophilic headgroups face the aqueous interior and exterior, while the hydrocarbon tails form the hydrophobic core. Liposomes can be unilamellar or multilamellar, and their size can range from ~20-nm to >10-μm diameter. Studies have shown moderate echogenicity for certain liposome formulations (8,9). The mechanism of echo contrast appears to be the backscatter from entrapped pockets of air within the liposomes that form during rehydration of the liposomes (10).

Solid Nanoparticles

Solid nanoparticles with moderate echogenicity have been described. Bubblicles, for example, are amorphous solid particles that contain gas pockets in their pores and fissures (11). Such particles can be submicrometer in size and the gas pockets can be highly stable due to pinning of the interfacial contact lines within the solid crevices. Silica nanoparticles have also been tested as ultrasound contrast agents (12). In general, solid and liquid nanoparticles offer little contrast as individual ultrasound scatterers.

Microbubbles

Microbubbles are the most commonly used ultrasound contrast agents for both blood pool imaging and molecular imaging. The gas core has low density and high compressibility, allowing it to shrink and expand with the passage of an acoustic wave. This is shown with high-speed videomicroscopy in Figure 1. Fortuitously, the resonance frequency of a microbubble lies within the acoustic bandwidth of typical clinical diagnostic scanners (1–10 MHz). This yields exceptional contrast backscatter, not only at the fundamental frequency but also at harmonics and in nonlinear imaging modes. The extraordinary sensitivity of ultrasound to microbubbles is demonstrated by the ability to detect individual microbubbles (~0.004-pL gas volume) with an ultrasound scanner (13). The remainder of the discussion will focus on these highly echogenic biocolloids.

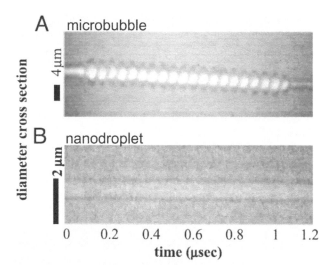

Figure 1 (**A**) Radius–time oscillation of a 2-μm-radius microbubble in response to a 180-kPa acoustic pulse at 2.25 MHz. Displacement by ultrasound radiation force is also observed. (**B**) Radius–time oscillation of a 450-nm-radius liquid nanoparticle in response to a 3-MPa acoustic pulse at 10 MHz. *Source*: Adapted from Ref. 5.

Microbubbles are gas spheres between 0.1 and 10 μm in diameter and are much smaller than the wavelength of diagnostic ultrasound, which is typically ∼100 μm. Because of their size, they are restricted to the intravascular space and in most circumstances do not reach the extravascular space. Current ultrasound molecular imaging technology for oncology is therefore restricted to receptors expressed in the vessel lumen, such as integrins associated with angiogenesis.

The physicochemical aspects of the microbubble can be quite complex. This complexity, however, lends itself to greater functionality. Through elucidation of the thermodynamics and kinetics controlling assembly and subsequent dynamics, microbubble formulations can be engineered to be more useful and reliable. Next generation microbubble constructs will be valuable tools for improving our understanding of molecular events in cancer research. In this light, some important physicochemical aspects of the microbubble are introduced below.

Microbubble Stability

The microbubble formulation is a gas-in-liquid emulsion. As such, it is thermodynamically unstable and will coarsen over time to form bulk liquid and gas phases. It is therefore important to kinetically trap the emulsion long enough to prevent coarsening over the time frame needed for fabrication, storage, and use. The microbubble shell offers a means of obtaining sufficient metastability.

Dissolution

The most obvious mechanism of microbubble instability is surface-tension-induced dissolution. A microbubble with surface tension (σ) is inherently unstable owing to the high pressure inside, which is a manifestation of the highly curved surface. The overpressure inside the microbubble (ΔP) was given by Young and Laplace [14]:

$$\Delta P = P_b - P_a = \frac{2\sigma}{r}, \qquad (1)$$

where P_b is the total pressure inside the bubble, P_a is the ambient pressure, and r is the bubble radius. For a microbubble, the overpressure is on the order of an atmosphere. According to Henry's Law, the overpressure increases the local solubility of the gas at the microbubble surface, thus creating a chemical potential gradient (i.e., a concentration gradient) over which gas diffuses into the surroundings.

An ordinary differential equation has been derived to describe the transport of gaseous species into and out of the shell [15,16]. The model is formulated by taking a mass balance over the microbubble and coupling it to the

diffusion equation to arrive at the following expression for the microbubble radius as a function of time (t).

$$-\frac{dr}{dt} = \frac{L}{r/D_w + R_{shell}} \left(\frac{1 + (2\sigma_{shell}/P_a r) - f}{1 + 3\sigma_{shell}/4P_a r} \right), \qquad (2)$$

where L is volume of dissolved gas per volume of water at equilibrium, D_w is the gas diffusivity in water, R_{shell} is the resistance of the shell to gas permeation, σ_{shell} is the surface tension of the shell, and f is the ratio of the gas concentration in the bulk medium versus that at saturation. Gas permeation through the shell and diffusion into the surrounding medium are modeled here as resistances in series, analogous to electrical circuits. The shell resistance is a function of both the permeating gas species and the shell composition. R_{shell} becomes the dominant resistance term for high molecular weight gases and in convective flow, where the diffusive boundary layer becomes thin [17].

Table 1 shows the parameters for various filling gases. The modified Epstein-Plesset equation predicts that a "clean" air microbubble will completely dissolve within a second, even in fully saturated water. One approach to increase stability has been to use hydrophobic gases, such as perfluorocarbons, which have water permeation resistances ($L^{-1}D_w^{-1}$) that are several orders of magnitude higher than air [18,19]. The water permeation resistance of C_4F_{10}, for example, is about 100 times greater than that of air. Although this may increase the microbubble lifetime by an order of magnitude or more, the surface tension effect drives complete microbubble dissolution to within a minute, which is far too short for a molecular imaging study.

Encapsulation of the gas core by a shell is required to stabilize the microbubble. Ideally, the microbubble shell should eliminate surface tension and impart a significant permeation resistance. Thus, the shell must have solid-like character. Interestingly, this can be achieved with surfactants, such as lipids below their main phase transition temperature, due to jamming of the interface [20]. Removing the overpressure term eliminates the driving force for dissolution in saturated media. This allows long-term storage of microbubbles, which are stable for months in a sealed vial [21].

Table 1 Physical Parameters for Various Filling Gases Used to Make Ultrasound Contrast Agents

Gas	M (g/mol)	$L \times 10^3$ (cm^3/cm^3)	$D_w \times 10^6$ (cm^2/sec)
Air (N$_2$)	(28)	15	20
n-C$_3$F$_8$	188	4.5	7.7
n-C$_4$F$_{10}$	238	0.51	6.9

Abbreviations: M, molecular weight; L, Ostwald's coefficient; D_w, gas diffusivity in water.

Coalescence and popping

Coalescence can lead to large changes in microbubble size distribution during fabrication and storage and can also lead to embolism in vivo. Microbubble fusion can be inhibited by the presence of the shell, which requires fracture to allow the gas surfaces to come into contact. Addition of a hydrophilic polymer brush layer, such as that formed by grafted polyethylene glycol (PEG), can provide repulsive steric and osmotic forces that prevent microbubble shells from contact during a collision.

As microbubbles rise, they accumulate into a foam at the suspension surface that separates the bulk gas and liquid phases. In this state, microbubble "popping" can be a significant problem, because one event can induce others in a chain reaction. When a microbubble approaches the suspension surface, a thin liquid layer is present between the two gas phases. Film drainage and rupture can be hindered by solid-like character in the microbubble shell and the presence of a grafted PEG layer, as a corollary to reducing coalescence.

In vivo stability

Another important factor for a microbubble placed into a new environment (i.e., blood) is gas exchange, which involves the influx of ambient gas species into the microbubble and the accompanying outflux of the original encapsulated gas. Gas exchange is driven by the difference in partial pressures for each gas species between the inside and the outside of the microbubble. A microbubble containing only fluorocarbon gas, for example, will experience a net influx of nitrogen and metabolic gases when injected into the blood stream, which will cause it to grow. At the same time, the fluorocarbon gas experiences a concentration gradient in the opposite direction. Eventually, the microbubble will completely dissolve regardless of these factors, but gas exchange can significantly alter the dissolution kinetics and protective ability of the shell.

Finally, microbubbles are highly susceptible to instability through hydrostatic pressure fluctuations. Microbubbles experience high pressures as they are pushed through the syringe needle. On entering the blood stream, microbubbles experience blood pressures as high as a few hundred mmHg. These pressures can cause the microbubble to dissolve. The shell can stabilize the gas core by inhibiting lateral compression and gas escape.

Microbubble Composition and Fabrication

The discussion above points to the need for a solid-like shell coating the microbubble for the purposes of stability. The shell also provides functionality through the attachment of targeting ligands, imaging molecules for other modalities, and therapeutic agents. The shell also passivates the surface against thrombogenic and immunogenic effects. Various biocompatible shell materials have been tested, including sugars, surfactants, lipids, proteins, biopolymers, and their combinations. Of the shell materials tested thus far, lipids provide the most convenience and versatility, as well as compliance and stability during insonification.

Sugar matrices

Galactose-based agents were among the first ultrasound contrast agents (22). In these systems, echogenic gas pockets are entrapped in the matrix of galactose microparticulate granules. The gas microbubbles are released as the sugar matrix dissolves in blood, allowing for a brief ultrasound contrast effect. Later galactose-based agents included palmitic acid (0.1%) for greater stability. Similar sugar matrices can provide an excellent stabilizing matrix for the long-term storage of microbubble contrast agents in the dried state.

Surfactant shells

Surfactants, such as the polysorbates Span and Tween, have been used to stabilize microbubble contrast agents (23). Interestingly, certain surfactant ratios and processing conditions were found to provide optimal stability, lending support to stabilization through surfactant complexation and kinetic entrapment (23,24). More recently, Span and Tween were used to create submicron bubbles (25) and as a substrate for polyelectrolyte multilayer formation (26).

Protein shells

Early ultrasound contrast agents were coated with an adsorbed layer of albumin protein (27). The albumin-coated microbubbles Albunex® and Optison™ (GE Healthcare, Princeton, New Jersey, U.S.) were the first commercially available, Food and Drug Administration (FDA)-approved contrast agents. More recently, protein-shelled microbubbles have been functionalized to carry targeting ligands (28). Albumin shells tend to be rigid and less stable to ultrasound (29), however, and introduce the typical immunogenicity issues associated with animal-derived materials. Albumin shells are also known to bind complement proteins (30).

Polymer shells

Several methods have been described to encapsulate gas in a polymer shell. Ionic gelation was used to create alignate-shelled microbubbles (31). Double emulsion methods have been used to create a variety of hollow polymer capsules (32–34). Polymerization of microbubbles at the gas-liquid interface during high sheer agitation has also been described (35). Each of these methods has produced microbubbles with enhanced stability. One drawback of polymer shells is their rigidity and, thus,

insensitivity to ultrasound. Chain entanglement and covalent bonds inherent in the polymer shells severely dampen
oscillation of the gas core (36,37), thus reducing echogenicity. The impact of the polymer shell on oscillation can
be easily shown during microbubble destruction, as in
Figure 2. Whereas a lipid-shelled microbubble fragments
symmetrically at lower acoustic pressures, the gas core of
the polymer-shelled agent is expelled through a single
fracture only at high acoustic pressures. The resulting
clean microbubble can be highly echogenic.

Lipid shells

Phospholipids are the most commonly used microbubble
shell materials for ultrasound molecular imaging. Several
phospholipid-based ultrasound contrast agents are commercially available worldwide for contrast echocardiography (38). Lipid-stabilized microbubbles are easy to
manufacture, biocompatible, and echogenic. The lipid
shell is a self-assembled structure that is oriented similarly
to the outer leaflet of a liposome membrane. The microbubble has a gas core and a monolayer membrane,
whereas the liposome has an aqueous core and a bilayer
membrane. The lipid shell is essentially a spherical
Langmuir monolayer held in a state of high compression.
As such, the mechanisms of microbubble shell formation
and dissolution are governed by the physics of lipid
adsorption and self-organization, as well as those of
monolayer collapse. A broad library of different lipids is
available to provide stability and functionality. Most
formulations for targeted microbubbles consist of three
components: a matrix lipid, an emulsifying lipid (or
surfactant), and a targeted lipid. The matrix lipid stabilizes
the shell by providing cohesion and is often chosen to be
below the main phase transition temperature (39). The
emulsifying lipid usually contains a polymeric group, such
as PEG, that aids in lipid adsorption and assembly (40).
The brush also inhibits coalescence and passivates the
surface. On the targeting lipid, a polymer spacer is used to
extend the ligand past the brush (41).

Lipid composition can have a dramatic effect on
microbubble properties. Longer chains provide more
cohesion through enhanced van der Waals and hydrophobic interactions, which increases the shear viscosity
(42) and decreases the gas permeability (43). Longer
chains also change the mechanism and kinetics of lipid
collapse and shedding from vesiculation to fracture and
folding (44). This is evident as morphological changes in
the microbubble during dissolution (15). Shell composition also affects the kinetics of microbubble destruction
during high-power insonification (45).

Microbubble fabrication

The most common method of microbubble fabrication has
been simple emulsification through high shear. This

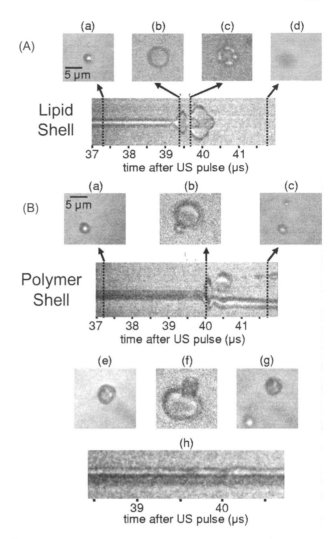

Figure 2 High-speed observations of polymer versus lipid-
shelled microbubble oscillation and destruction during insonification. Panel (**A**) shows the lipid-shelled agent BR14 (Bracco
Research SA, Geneva, Switzerland) being fragmented symmetrically. Still images depict the agent before, during, and after
exposure to a two-cycle, 2.25-MHz, 920-kPa ultrasound pulse.
Streak image shows one line of sight through the agent versus
time, with the acquisition times of the still images indicated by
dotted lines. The agent is observed to expand and collapse in
response to the ultrasound pulse. During the second cycle,
fragments of the agent expand again around the position of the
original agent. Panel (**B**) shows the polymer-shelled agent
BG1135 (Bracco Research SA) being fragmented asymmetrically. Image depicts the agent before, during, and after exposure
to a two-cycle, 2.25-MHz, 1.4-MPa ultrasound pulse. The agent
did not exhibit significant oscillation at lower acoustic pressures.
The microbubble is observed to acquire a shell defect and
subsequently to eject a gas bubble some distance from the
original shell. *Source*: Adapted from Ref. 37.

method involves the entrainment of a gaseous hood into
the aqueous phase by mechanical agitation of the gas-
liquid interface. Methods of diminution include shaking

(amalgamation) and sonication, both of which occur at 10 to 100 kHz frequencies. These techniques rely on stochastic events that produce a polydispersed size distribution, generally ranging between submicrometers to tens of micrometers in diameter. Size fractionation techniques can be employed to isolate sizes based on buoyancy (46). Emulsification techniques provide rapid and cost-effective microbubble generation that can be done at the bedside.

Microfluidic techniques are currently being explored for controlled production of contrast agents. Methods such as flow focusing can result in a contrast agent population with a precise size distribution (Fig. 3A). Flow focusing utilizes micron-sized channels to precisely mix the gas and lipid solution through a micron-sized orifice in a manner which results in nearly identical encapsulated microbubbles. In this way, a population of contrast agents can be tailored to match the desired imaging frequency (47,48). T-junctions (49), jetting (50), and electrohydrodynamic atomization (51) have also been used. Microfluidic technologies will need to show similar robustness and ease of preparation in generating a sufficient microbubble dose. However, the potential gains in control over the size and microbubble surface chemistry could significantly enhance quantification in molecular imaging studies.

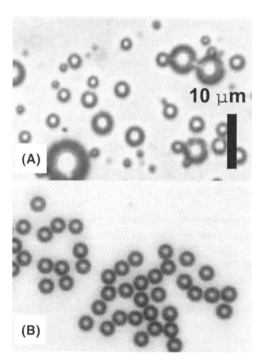

Figure 3 Control of microbubble size distribution. (**A**) Current diminution techniques result in a polydispersed size distribution. (**B**) Monodisperse microbubbles can be created by microfluidic methods, such as flow focusing. *Source*: Adapted from Ref. 105.

DESIGN OF TARGETED CONTRAST AGENTS

General design criteria can be outlined for targeted biocolloids used as ultrasound contrast agents. First, the biocolloid must be capable of backscattering a detectable acoustic signal. Second, the biocolloid should be biologically inert. It must be safe to administer to the patient with no undesirable or toxic side effects. It should not be immunogenic or thrombogenic; the biocolloid should not interfere with the physiological process under study. Third, the biocolloid must be capable of reaching and adhering to its target. It should remain stably adhered and echogenic for the duration of the imaging exam. Finally, it should be economical, robust, and easy to handle and administer to the patient (52).

Microbubbles are inherently more complex than molecules. The criteria for designing a targeted microbubble formulation include not only consideration of ligand-receptor interactions but also other factors such as stability, echogenicity, and immunogenicity. Perhaps the most facile means of engineering the microbubble shell is simply changing the shell constituents. Various formulations have been optimized in this vein. However, it is becoming increasingly clear that microbubbles should be designed with a physicochemical outlook, i.e., with an understanding of the underlying thermodynamics and kinetics of surface-related phenomena.

Selection of Ligand Chemistry

The ability to detect molecular events from ultrasonic echoes is possible through the adhesion of microbubbles to a receptor-bearing surface. Although individual microbubbles can be imaged, a robust ultrasound signal requires the adhesion of several microbubbles to the target. Microbubbles (or other biocolloids) can adhere to endothelial targets through either nonspecific or specific interactions. Studies of the former have shown accumulation to sites of ischemia/reperfusion (53) and atherosclerosis (30). These interactions can be mediated through charge or complement protein attachment. However, to achieve high selectivity of the contrast agent for the target, specific ligand-receptor interactions are desired.

Firm biocolloid adhesion is mediated by many ligand-receptor interactions and depends on the kinetics and thermodynamics of bond formation and rupture in a multivalent system. Knowing the equilibrium binding constant (affinity) of the ligand-receptor pair is not enough. Bond formation depends on the collision time, the loading force, and the intermolecular interactions (54). Bond rupture depends on the pulling force (55). These factors can be lumped into a kinetic rate constant for bond formation (k_{on}) and rupture (k_{off}), the ratio of which gives the bond dissociation constant (K_D). In situations with high flow, such as in larger vessels, a very high k_{on} is desired (56). In addition, firm adhesion requires that the paired bonds have sufficient strength to overcome the dislodging force. The magnitude of this force depends on the fluid shear stress and microbubble size (57,58). Multiple ligand-receptor pairs can act in concert to enhance bond stability (59), leading to firm adhesion. The use of ligand combinations, which combine a high k_{on} with a large adhesion strength, can be used for high shear flow (60). Shells with excess area that maximize ligand-receptor contact have also been described (61).

Ligand Conjugation

Depending on the needs of the specific targeting application, ligands can be incorporated into the shell during microbubble formation, or they can be attached to the previously formed shell. For the former, the targeting ligand is conjugated to a lipopolymer and then added into the lipid mixture before producing the microbubbles. This can be done before or after lipid hydration. The hydrophobic anchor of the lipid moiety will ensure that the targeting molecule self-inserts into micelles and vesicles that are present in the premicrobubble lipid mixture. This process is facilitated by heating above the main phase transition temperature of the matrix lipid species (62). With the targeting molecule now interdispersed within the lipid mixture, it will become incorporated into the shell of a freshly formed microbubble. This allows rapid production of targeted microbubbles without the need for subsequent chemical modifications. The microbubble suspension should be washed, however, to avoid competitive binding effects from the free lipid.

Free lipid can constitute more than 90% of the total lipid following microbubble production. Microbubble washing is done simply through centrifugation-flotation. Lipid-coated microbubbles can survive centrifugation up to several hundred equivalent gravity (63). The microbubbles rise to form a thick cake on the top of the centrifuge vessel. The infranatant is removed and replenished with fresh medium, and the microbubbles are redispersed by gentle agitation.

Fragile ligands, such as antibodies, can be easily denatured by the high shear stresses and temperatures involved with microbubble production. Furthermore, in cases where the ligand is precious, it may be necessary to conserve and prevent waste during postmicrobubble washing. Therefore, it is often desired to conjugate the ligand onto the shells of preformed microbubbles. The most common method to achieve this has been biotin-avidin cross-linking (64,65). This simple method involves a stepwise labeling process. First, biotin is added to the premicrobubble lipid mixture by conjugating it to the distal end of a lipopolymer. Second, avidin (or one of its analogs) is added to coat the biotinylated microbubbles. It is very important to add avidin in excess to prevent microbubble aggregation. Finally, the biotinylated ligand is added, which becomes immobilized onto the microbubble through binding to free pockets on the avidin. Washing is performed between each step to maximize efficiency. One drawback of biotin-avidin linkage is the immunogenicity of the resulting surface (66).

Postproduction conjugation of ligands to microbubbles can also be achieved through covalent binding (64). Amine groups on the ligand can be attached to carboxylic acid groups exposed on the microbubble shell, or vice versa. These reactions often produce unwanted side products that can limit the conjugation efficiency. The maleimide-thiol approach offers an attractive alternative. In this approach, a thiol-containing targeting ligand binds to a maleimide group that is exposed on the microbubble shell (64,65). This reaction is more stable in aqueous buffer and exhibits fewer side reactions, thus improving overall efficiency. Employment of "click chemistry" (67) approaches may provide other valuable means of attaching ligands to microbubbles and other ultrasound contrast agents.

Engineering the Microbubble Shell

Microstructure

Microstructure refers to the size and shape of domains (or grains) that form within the shell by self-aggregation phenomena (Fig. 3B). Lipid-coated microbubbles have been shown to exhibit elegant microstructures (42,68). Microscopy and spectroscopy evidence indicates that the lipid monolayer shell consists of two or more distinct phases (20,68). Dark domains of matrix lipid are seen dispersed in a bright interdomain region. The interdomain region is enriched in lipopolymer and bulky molecules that are excluded from the crystalline domains.

Microstructure is governed by the underlying thermodynamic phase behavior as well as kinetic processes. Thus, microstructure of the microbubble shell can be controlled through composition and processing (20,42,68). Thermal effects can change the morphology of the ordered and disordered phases (Fig. 3C). The ordered phase can be melted by heating above the main phase transition temperature of the matrix lipid. Cooling through the transition at different rates leads to differences in domain density, shape, and size. For example, slow annealing can yield very large domains on the shell. These domains can provide compartments on which to load targeting ligands or other molecules (Fig. 4). The domains are not rigid plates, they can bend to accommodate the spherical surface (20).

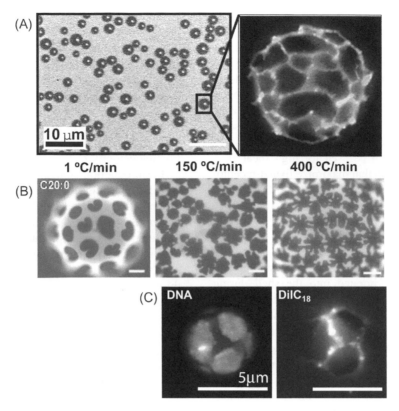

Figure 4 Microstructure of lipid-shelled microbubbles. (**A**) Microbubbles appear as simple gas spheres under bright field microscopy (*left*), but the complexity of the microbubble shell structure is revealed by fluorescence microscopy (*right*). (**B**) Microstructure can be controlled by means of thermal treatment. Shown here are microbubbles after shell melting and then cooling at different rates through the main phase transition temperature of the matrix lipid. (**C**) Phase separation phenomena and thermal control of microstructure can be used to create compartmentalized microbubbles. Shown here are domains of DNA (*left*) and the membrane probe DiIC$_{18}$ (*right*) on the same microbubble. *Source*: Adapted from Refs. 20, 68, and 75.

Microstructure affects several physicochemical properties. For example, increasing the defect density, through smaller and more ramified domains, leads to an increase in microbubble shell gas permeability (43,69) and a decrease in the surface shear viscosity (42). Therefore, shell microstructure affects many performance characteristics of the microbubble, including stability, ligand presentation, and immunogenicity.

Architecture

In addition to binding kinetics and bond strength, ligand presentation is an important property to consider for targeting applications. Clearly, ligand presentation will depend on microstructure, since the lateral spatial distribution of the ligand is fixed by the underlying phase partitioning behavior. In addition, the presentation of the ligand depends on the surface architecture, or the vertical arrangement of molecules on the surface.

For microbubbles and other biocolloids, the PEG brush layer provides the basis for understanding the ligand architecture (Fig. 5A). Microbubble stability is enhanced by the incorporation of a PEG brush layer. Ligands are typically conjugated to the distal ends of the polymer chains. Architecture thus refers to the internal structure of the brush layer on the microbubble shell, which depends on the lateral chain-chain interactions, the grafting density, and the chain lengths of the constituent polymers.

Macromolecular ligands, such as monoclonal antibodies (~ 100 kDa), have a much greater mass than the PEG chains (2–5 kDa). Therefore, these larger molecules are somewhat restricted on the surface. Immobilization of the ligand is further enhanced by avidin-biotin cross-linking, owing to the large size (~ 60 kDa) and multiple binding pockets on the avidin molecule (70). In contrast, small molecule ligands (~ 100 Da) that are conjugated to the distal end of the PEG chains will exhibit dynamics primarily determined by the thermal motion of the polymer spacer (71). In the latter case, polymer stretching and tiered-layer architectures can have a profound effect on microbubble adhesion.

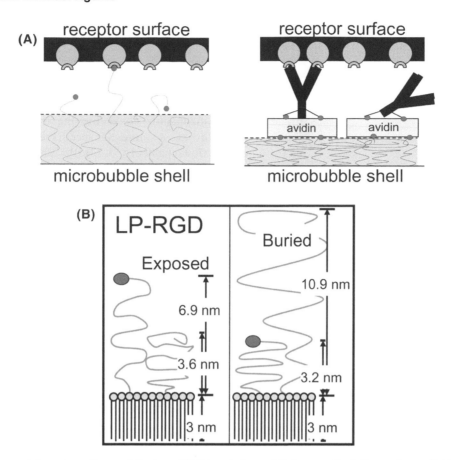

Figure 5 Ligand presentation via surface architecture. (**A**) Ligand size and linkage method dictate the availability of the ligand for binding. Small molecule ligands can be attached to the polymer tether and move according to the polymer dynamics (*left*). Large ligands (e.g., antibodies) attached through biotin-avidin linkage are less mobile (*right*). (**B**) The ligand tether can be longer than the surrounding brush (*left*) or shorter than the surrounding brush (*right*). The relative equilibrium brush heights are calculated from self-consistent field theory. Thermal motion allows for transient stretching of the polymer chains well beyond these equilibrium values. *Source*: (**A**) Adapted from Ref. 17 and (**B**) adapted from Ref. 73.

Bimodal brushes (i.e., two different chain lengths) can be used. The ligand can be tethered to the shell by a spacer arm that is longer than surrounding chains in order to increase the ligand availability and adhesion strength (41). Alternatively, the ligand can be conjugated to a shorter spacer arm in order to decrease immunogenicity (72,73). The buried-ligand architecture is shown in Figure 5B. Importantly, the buried ligand can be revealed by ultrasound oscillation and radiation force (Fig. 6).

Construction

Construction entails the addition of shell components after formation and stabilization of the initial microbubble. It therefore adds another layer of architectural complexity. Avidin-biotin cross-linking was introduced above as a simple method of postproduction construction. Other

materials have been constructed onto microbubbles. Polymers with clustered ligands, for example, were used to enhance adhesion in high-shear flow (74).

A popular means of construction for biocolloids involves the sequential addition of oppositely charged polyelectrolytes, as in layer-by-layer (LbL) assembly. LbL assembly is possible through ionic cross-linking and charge overcompensation, which allows several paired layers to be added in a stepwise fashion (Fig. 7). This technique has been applied to microbubbles. Multilayer shells were shown to enhance the stability of the gas core against dissolution (26). Further, multilayer shells were shown to increase DNA-loading capacity (75). Multilayers can slightly dampen the microbubble oscillation over the first few cycles (75), and they may provide a means of improving the overall stability and adhesion efficiency of targeted microbubbles.

Targeting of a Stealth Agent by Ultrasound

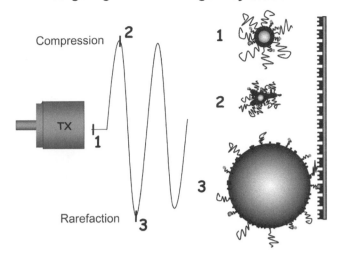

Figure 6 Targeted adhesion of a stealth microbubble by ultrasound radiation force. The microbubble oscillates and translates during insonification to reveal the ligand. The ligand architecture is designed to allow firm adhesion after the ultrasound pulse. *Source*: Adapted from Ref. 72.

TESTING CONTRAST AGENT ADHESION

Standard methods have been developed for testing the adhesion efficiency of targeted ultrasound contrast agents to model receptor surfaces. Adhesion testing is generally done in vitro. Perhaps the most simple method is the parallel-plate static chamber (76,77). In this method, targeted contrast agents are allowed to contact a receptor-coated surface without the presence of flow, either by buoyancy or ultrasound radiation force. The surface is then gently washed to remove free contrast agent, and the amount of adherent contrast agent is quantified by optical microscopy or acoustic backscatter. This method provides information on specificity (with appropriate controls), but it does not account for the fluid mechanics governing the dynamics of the adhesion event. A more advanced method is the parallel-plate flow chamber (63,72). By tuning the flow rate, the wall shear stress can be controlled to look for the effects of inertial forces on capture probability and adhesion strength. Finally, it is often useful to consider an acoustically transparent chamber with cylindrical coordinates to assess targeted contrast agent adhesion kinetics and the interplay with ultrasound. Hollow fibers make excellent environments for testing targeted adhesion in a high-throughput format (78,79). The wall shear stress can be controlled, and the effects of ultrasound radiation forces on adhesion efficiency can be examined. Acoustic methods can be used to quantify adhesion efficiency (80).

CONSIDERATIONS FOR IN VIVO MOLECULAR IMAGING

The methods for detecting targeted contrast agents in ultrasound molecular imaging have been treated in a previous chapter. Here, we consider the fate of the contrast agent once injected. Because of the infancy of the field, much of the discussion centers on studies of blood pool contrast agents. We treat targeted microbubbles where data is available.

Layer-by-Layer Assembly Scheme

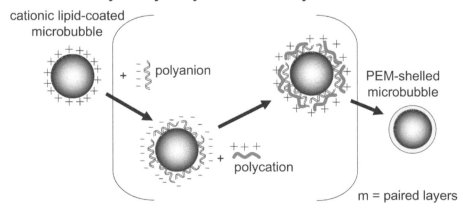

Figure 7 Surface construction through layer-by-layer assembly. The charged microbubble (cationic shown here) can be loaded with an oppositely charged polyelectrolyte. Ionic complexation leads to irreversible adsorption and charge overcompensation, which allows subsequent deposition of an oppositely charged polyelectrolyte. Multilayers can be built up with intermediate washing steps. *Source*: Adapted from Ref. 75.

Biodistribution

Little is currently known about the pharmacology of targeted microbubbles for use in molecular imaging. Guidelines can be sought from contrast agents used in echocardiography, with the caveat that changing the surface chemistry through the addition of targeting ligands will likely change the pharmacokinetics and biodistribution. For blood pool microbubble agents, the typical circulation half-life is on the order of minutes (72). Once injected, the gas core of the microbubble dissolves due to concentration gradients, pressurization, shear forces, and convective transport. Experiments have shown that the gas is eliminated through the lungs within minutes (81–84). The lipid, protein, or biopolymer shell is handled through normal metabolic routes (85).

Microbubbles have a similar size and deformability as erythrocytes and therefore exhibit similar rheological properties in the blood. Such particles tend to migrate to the center in parabolic, steady flow (86). Intravital microscopy studies have shown that microbubbles have similar velocities to red blood cells in arterioles, venules, and capillaries (87–89). In the microcirculation, they can become lodged and then dislodged without significant vascular effects, as is observed for normal leukocyte plugging (89,90).

Microbubbles tend to be opsonized and eliminated from circulation via the reticuloendothelial system (RES). Early studies with protein-coated microbubbles showed clearance by macrophages (91,92). As with liposomes, the mechanism of clearance for lipid-coated microbubbles depends on the surface chemistry. For example, anionic microbubbles exhibit different pharmacology than cationic microbubbles (53,93). Phagocytosis by Kupffer cells is different for SonoVue® (Bracco Diagnostics, Inc., Princeton, New Jersey, U.S.) (94) than for Sonazoid™ (GE Healthcare, Oslo, Norway) (95); both are lipid-coated microbubble agents.

Immunogenicity

An important concern for contrast agents, in general, and targeted microbubbles, in particular, is the response of the immune system. Complement activation may stimulate inflammation and hypersensitivity and is thus a major concern. For successful molecular imaging, it is paramount to have a minimal affect on the underlying physiology. Likewise, rapid clearance from the circulation can preclude microbubble adherence to the target site.

The innate immune system is highly adept at detecting and removing foreign pathogens and particles from the bloodstream. The complement proteins play a crucial role. The immunity pathways converge on the complement protein C3, which is converted to the fragments C3b and C3a by C3 convertase (96). The C3b fragment contains an unstable thioester bond that may bind to nucleophilic groups on the particle surface (97). The complement system is activated through a positive feedback loop when C3b is attached to the particle's surface. Immobilized C3b can be recognized by phagocytic cells, and it can interact with the other complement proteins to stimulate humoral immunity and form the membrane attack complex (MAC).

Increased complement attachment has been observed for lipid-shelled microbubbles with a net negative charge (93). Likewise, increased C3b binding, C3a production, and neutrophil attachment has been observed in vitro and in vivo for microbubbles exposing biotin or peptide ligands (72,73). Complement C3 has also been shown to bind to albumin-encapsulated microbubbles, mediating adherence of the microbubble to the vascular endothelium (30). Surface passivation with methyl-terminated poly(ethylene glycol) (mPEG) chains has been a major advance in biomaterials science. On liposomes, for example, the mPEG brush has been shown to significantly increase particle circulation half-life (98). On microbubbles, the PEG brush plays a similar role in reducing immunogenicity.

Ligand groups present on the microbubble surface can lead to opsonization and complement activation (73). Ideally, the targeting ligand would be hidden from the milieu until the contrast agent reaches the target site, where it is exposed for binding and results in adhesion (72). The unique properties of microbubbles (expansion and contraction in response to an ultrasound field) have been shown to facilitate a stealth ligand (72,73). With the use of ultrasound radiation force, adhesion efficiency for a buried ligand has been shown to be equivalent to that of an exposed ligand (Fig. 5B). This opens up the possibility of triggering the adhesion event through the use of a focused ultrasound transducer.

Safety

In humans, adverse reactions to ultrasound contrast agents have been rare, and these have typically been transient and mild. According to a recent study by the Contrast Media Safety Committee (CMSC) of the European Society of Urogenital Radiology (ESUR) (99), ultrasound contrast agents are generally safe. Ultrasound contrast agents approved for clinical use are well tolerated, and serious adverse reactions are rarely observed. Adverse events are usually minor (e.g., headache, nausea, altered taste, sensation of heat) and self-resolving. Generalized allergy-like reactions occur rarely. The rate of adverse reactions has been comparable to, or lower than, those reported for contrast agents associated with other imaging modalities, such as CT or MRI (100,101). A few serious reactions have been reported, which include severe hypotension, bradicardia, anaphylactic shock, and fatal outcome in patients undergoing contrast echocardiography (102,103). Recently, steps have been taken by the U.S. FDA and the European Agency for the Evaluation of Medicinal Products (EMEA) to limit the use of microbubbles in patients with acute coronary syndrome and other conditions (100,102). For imaging, ultrasound power output should be minimized to reduce cavitation-related bioeffects (104), although these may be useful for applications requiring localized enhancement of vascular permeability.

CHALLENGES AND LIMITATIONS

While targeted ultrasound contrast agents have come a long way in the past decade, there remains much room for improvement. Below are listed some of the current challenges and limitations:

Immune stealthiness: Reducing the immunogenicity of contrast agents by further optimizing the PEG brush layer or utilizing other biocompatible materials will improve safety and reduce loss to degradation of the agents by phagocytic cells.

Instability and short circulation persistence: Increasing the half-life by an order of magnitude, to tens of minutes, will significantly improve the ability to quantify receptor density based on echo intensity.

Limited receptor reach: Decreasing microbubble size or promoting active transport, while maintaining high echogenicity, will be a significant challenge for ultrasound molecular imaging.

Multimodal imaging: Biocolloids can be multifunctional and engineered to provide contrast in not only ultrasound but also MRI, CT, PET, OT, and other imaging modalities. Additionally, microbubble-induced cavitation may allow localized penetration of other molecular imaging agents into the extravascular space.

Poor adhesion efficiency: Design of better ligands and microbubble shell properties will improve adhesion efficiency. The use of radiation force and other ultrasound effects to improve microbubble-endothelium contact will also improve adhesion efficiency and drastically reduce the accumulation period.

Size polydispersity: The ability to generate dose quantities of monodisperse targeted contrast agents quickly and economically, possibly by microfluidic methods, will substantially improve the conspicuity and quantification of ultrasound molecular imaging.

REFERENCES

1. Gramiak R, Shah PM. Echocardiagraphy of the aortic root. Invest Radiol 1968; 3(5):356–366.
2. Maeda H. SMANCS and polymer-conjugated macromolecular drugs—advantages in cancer-chemotherapy. Adv Drug Deliv Rev 1991; 6(2):181–202.
3. Mattrey RF. The potential role of perfluorochemicals (Pfcs) in diagnostic-imaging. Artif Cells Blood Substit Immobil Biotechnol 1994; 22(2):295–313.
4. Morawski AM, Lanza GA, Wickline SA. Targeted contrast agents for magnetic resonance imaging and ultrasound. Curr Opin Biotechnol 2005; 16(1):89–92.
5. Dayton PA, Zhao SK, Bloch SH, et al. Application of ultrasound to selectively localize nanodroplets for targeted imaging and therapy. Mol Imaging 2006; 5(3):160–174.
6. Correas JM, Quay SD. EchoGen(TM) emulsion: a new ultrasound contrast agent based on phase shift colloids. Clin Radiol 1996; 51:11–14.
7. Kripfgans OD, Fowlkes JB, Miller DL, et al. Acoustic droplet vaporization for therapeutic and diagnostic applications. Ultrasound Med Biol 2000; 26(7):1177–1189.
8. AlkanOnyuksel H, Demos SM, Lanza GM, et al. Development of inherently echogenic liposomes as an ultrasonic contrast agent. J Pharm Sci 1996; 85(5):486–490.
9. Huang SL, Hamilton AJ, Nagaraj A, et al. Improving ultrasound reflectivity and stability of echogenic liposomal dispersions for use as targeted ultrasound contrast agents. J Pharm Sci 2001; 90(12):1917–1926.
10. Huang SL, Hamilton AJ, Pozharski E, et al. Physical correlates of the ultrasonic reflectivity of lipid dispersions suitable as diagnostic contrast agents. Ultrasound Med Biol 2002; 28(3):339–348.
11. Parker KJ, Tuthill TA, Lerner RM, et al. A particulate contrast agent with potential for ultrasound imaging of liver. Ultrasound Med Biol 1987; 13(9):555–566.
12. Liu J, Levine AL, Mattoon JS, et al. Nanoparticles as image enhancing agents for ultrasonography. Phys Med Biol 2006; 51(9):2179–2189.
13. Klibanov AL, Rasche PT, Hughes MS, et al. Detection of individual microbubbles of ultrasound contrast agents—imaging of free-floating and targeted bubbles. Invest Radiol 2004; 39(3):187–195.
14. Hunter RJ. Foundations of colloid science. Oxford: Oxford University Press, 1986.
15. Borden MA, Longo ML. Dissolution behavior of lipid monolayer-coated, air-filled microbubbles: effect of lipid hydrophobic chain length. Langmuir 2002; 18(24): 9225–9233.
16. Epstein PS, Plesset MS. On the stability of gas bubbles in liquid-gas solutions. J Chem Phys 1950; 18(11): 1505–1509.
17. Ferrara KW, Pollard RE, Borden MA. Ultrasound microbubble contrast agents: fundamentals and application to drug and gene delivery. Annu Rev Biomed Eng 2007; 9:415–447.
18. Kabalnov A, Klein D, Pelura T, et al. Dissolution of multicomponent microbubbles in the bloodstream: 1. Theory. Ultrasound Med Biol 1998; 24(5):739–749.
19. Kabalnov A, Bradley J, Flaim S, et al. Dissolution of multicomponent microbubbles in the bloodstream: 2. Experiment. Ultrasound Med Biol 1998; 24(5):751–760.
20. Borden MA, Martinez GV, Ricker J, et al. Lateral phase separation in lipid-coated microbubbles. Langmuir 2006; 22(9):4291–4297.

21. Klibanov AL. Ultrasound contrast agents: development of the field and current status. In: Krause W, ed. Contrast Agents II. New York: Springer-Verlag, 2002:73.

22. Schlief R. Galactose-based echo-enhancing agents. In: Goldberg BB, ed. Ultrasound Contrast Agents. St. Louis, MO: Mosby, 1997.

23. Singhal S, Moser CC, Wheatley MA. Surfactant-stabilized microbubbles as ultrasound contrast agents—stability study of Span-60 and Tween-80 mixtures using a Langmuir trough. Langmuir 1993; 9(9):2426–2429.

24. Wang WH, Moser CC, Wheatley MA. Langmuir trough study of surfactant mixtures used in the production of a new ultrasound contrast agent consisting of stabilized microbubbles. J Phys Chem 1996; 100(32):13815–13821.

25. Oeffinger BE, Wheatley MA. Development and characterization of a nano-scale contrast agent. Ultrasonics 2004; 42(1–9):343–347.

26. Shchukin DG, Kohler K, Mohwald H, et al. Gas-filled polyelectrolyte capsules. Angew Chem Int Ed Engl 2005; 44:3310–3314.

27. Feinstein SB, Cheirif J, Tencate FJ, et al. Safety and efficacy of a new transpulmonary ultrasound contrast agent—initial multicenter clinical-results. J Am Coll Cardiol 1990; 16(2):316–324.

28. Korpanty G, Grayburn PA, Shohet RV, et al. Targeting vascular endothelium with avidin microbubbles. Ultrasound Med Biol 2005; 31(9):1279–1283.

29. Dayton PA, Morgan KE, Klibanov AL, et al. Optical and acoustical observations of the effects of ultrasound on contrast agents. IEEE Trans Ultrason Ferroelectr Freq Control 1999; 46(1):220–232.

30. Anderson DR, Tsutsui JM, Xie F, et al. The role of complement in the adherence of microbubbles to dysfunctional arterial endothelium and atherosclerotic plaque. Cardiovasc Res 2007; 73(3):597–606.

31. Wheatley MA, Schrope B, Shen P. Contrast agents for diagnostic ultrasound - development and evaluation of polymer-coated microbubbles. Biomaterials 1990; 11(9): 713–717.

32. Schneider M, Arditi M, Barrau MB, et al. Br1—a new ultrasonographic contrast agent based on sulfur hexafluoride-filled microbubbles. Invest Radiol 1995; 30(8):451–457.

33. Bjerknes K, Braenden JU, Braenden JE, et al. Air-filled polymeric microcapsules from emulsions containing different organic phases. J Microencapsul 2001; 18(2):159–171.

34. Narayan P, Wheatley MA. Preparation and characterization of hollow microcapsules for use as ultrasound contrast agents. Polymer Eng Sci 1999; 39(11):2242–2255.

35. Cavalieri F, El Hamassi A, Chiessi E, et al. Stable polymeric microballoons as multifunctional device for biomedical uses: synthesis and characterization. Langmuir 2005; 21(19):8758–8764.

36. Leong-Poi H, Song J, Rim SJ, et al. Influence of microbubble shell properties on ultrasound signal: implications for low-power perfusion imaging. J Am Soc Echocardiogr 2002; 15(10):1269–1276.

37. Bloch SH, Wan M, Dayton PA, et al. Optical observation of lipid- and polymer-shelled ultrasound microbubble contrast agents. Appl Phys Lett 2004; 84(4):631–633.

38. Kaufmann BA, Lankford M, Behm CZ, et al. High-resolution myocardial perfusion imaging in mice with high-frequency echocardiographic detection of a depot contrast agent. J Am Soc Echocardiogr 2007; 20(2):136–143.

39. Klibanov AL. Targeted delivery of gas-filled microspheres, contrast agents for ultrasound imaging. Adv Drug Deliv Rev 1999; 37(1–3):139–157.

40. Klibanov AL. Ultrasound contrast agents: development of the field and current status. In: Contrast Agents II. Berlin, Heidelberg: Springer, 2002:73–106.

41. Kim DH, Klibanov AL, Needham D. The influence of tiered layers of surface-grafted poly(ethylene glycol) on receptor-ligand-mediated adhesion between phospholipid monolayer-stabilized microbubbles and coated class beads. Langmuir 2000; 16(6):2808–2817.

42. Kim DH, Costello MJ, Duncan PB, et al. Mechanical properties and microstructure of polycrystalline phospholipid monolayer shells: novel solid microparticles. Langmuir 2003; 19(20):8455–8466.

43. Borden MA, Longo ML. Oxygen permeability of fully condensed lipid monolayers. J Phys Chem B 2004; 108(19):6009–6016.

44. Pu G, Borden MA, Longo ML. Collapse and shedding transitions in binary lipid monolayers coating microbubbles. Langmuir 2006; 22(7):2993–2999.

45. Borden MA, Kruse D, Caskey C, et al. Influence of lipid shell physicochemical properties on ultrasound-induced microbubble destruction. IEEE Trans Ultrason Ferroelectr Freq Control 2005; 52(11):1992–2002.

46. Kvale S, Jakobsen HA, Asbjornsen OA, et al. Size fractionation of gas-filled microspheres by flotation. Separations Technol 1996; 6(4):219–226.

47. Ganan-Calvo AM, Gordillo JM. Perfectly monodisperse microbubbling by capillary flow focusing. Phys Rev Lett 2001; 87(27 pt 1):274501.

48. Talu E, Lozano MM, Powell RL, et al. Long-term stability by lipid coating monodisperse microbubbles formed by a flow-focusing device. Langmuir 2006; 22(23):9487–9490.

49. Xu JH, Li SW, Wang YJ, et al. Controllable gas-liquid phase flow patterns and monodisperse microbubbles in a microfluidic T-junction device. Appl Phys Lett 2006; 88(13):A133506.

50. Bohmer MR, Schroeders R, Steenbakkers JAM, et al. Preparation of monodisperse polymer particles and capsules by ink-jet printing. Colloids Surf A 2006; 289 (1–3):96–104.

51. Farook U, Stride E, Edirisinghe MJ, et al. Microbubbling by co-axial electrohydrodynamic atomization. Med Biol Eng Comput 2007; 45(8):781–789.

52. Klibanov AL. Ultrasound molecular imaging with targeted microbubble contrast agents. J Nucl Cardiol 2007; 14, 876–884.

53. Lindner JR, Coggins MP, Kaul S, et al. Microbubble persistence in the microcirculation during ischemia/reperfusion and inflammation is caused by integrin- and complement-mediated adherence to activated leukocytes. Circulation 2000; 101(6):668–675.

54. Zhu C. Kinetics and mechanics of cell adhesion. J Biomech 2000; 33(1):23–33.

55. Leckband D, Israelachvili J. Intermolecular forces in biology. Q Rev Biophys 2001; 34(2):105–267.

56. Dayton PA, Rychak JJ. Molecular ultrasound imaging using microbubble contrast agents. Front Biosci 2007; 12, 5124–5142.

57. Alon R, Hammer DA, Springer TA. Lifetime of the P-selectin-carbohydrate bond and its response to tensile force in hydrodynamic flow. Nature 1995; 374(6522): 539–542.

58. Patil VRS, Campbell CJ, Yun YH, et al. Particle diameter influences adhesion under flow. Biophys J 2001; 80(4): 1733–1743.

59. Sulchek TA, Friddle RW, Langry K, et al. Dynamic force spectroscopy of parallel individual Mucin1-antibody bonds. Proc Nat Acad Sci U S A 2005; 102(46):16638–16643.

60. Rychak JJ, Klibanov AL, Leppanen A, et al. Enhanced binding of ultrasound contrast microbubbles targeted to P-selectin using a physiological capture ligand. FASEB J 2004; 18(4):A446.

61. Rychak JJ, Lindner JR, Ley K, et al. Deformable gas-filled microbubbles targeted to P-selectin. J Control Release 2006; 114(3):288–299.

62. Uster PS, Allen TM, Daniel BE, et al. Insertion of poly (ethylene glycol) derivatized phospholipid into pre-formed liposomes results in prolonged in vivo circulation time. FEBS Lett 1996; 386(2–3):243–246.

63. Takalkar AM, Klibanov AL, Rychak JJ, et al. Binding and detachment dynamics of microbubbles targeted to P-selectin under controlled shear flow. J Control Release 2004; 96(3):473–482.

64. Klibanov AL. Ligand-carrying gas-filled microbubbles: ultrasound contrast agents for targeted molecular imaging. Bioconjug Chem 2005; 16(1):9–17.

65. Lanza GM, Wickline SA. Targeted ultrasonic contrast agents for molecular imaging and therapy. Prog Cardio-vasc Dis 2001; 44(1):13–31.

66. Phillips NC, Emili A. Immunogenicity of immunolipo-somes. Immunol Lett 1991; 30(3):291–296.

67. Kolb HC, Finn MG, Sharpless KB. Click chemistry: diverse chemical function from a few good reactions. Angew Chem Int Ed 2001; 40(11):2004–2021.

68. Borden MA, Pu G, Runner GJ, et al. Surface phase behavior and microstructure of lipid/PEG-emulsifier monolayer-coated microbubbles. Colloids Surf B 2004; 35(3–4):209–223.

69. Pu G, Longo ML, Borden MA. Effect of microstructure on molecular oxygen permeability through condensed phospholipid monolayers. J Am Chem Soc 2005; 127:6524–6525.

70. Lin JJ, Silas JA, Bermudez H, et al. The effect of polymer chain length and surface density on the adhesiveness of functionalized polymersomes. Langmuir 2004; 20(13): 5493–5500.

71. Jeppesen C, Wong JY, Kuhl TL, et al. Impact of polymer tether length on multiple ligand-receptor bond formation. Science 2001; 293(5529):465–468.

72. Borden MA, Sarantos MR, Stieger SM, et al. Ultrasound radiation force modulates ligand availability on targeted contrast agents. Mol Imaging 2006; 5(3):139–147.

73. Borden MA, Zhang H, Gillies RJ, et al. A stimulus-responsive contrast agent for ultrasound molecular imaging. Biomaterials 2008;29:597–606.

74. Klibanov AL, Rychak JJ, Yang WC, et al. Targeted ultrasound contrast agent for molecular imaging of inflammation in high-shear flow. Contrast Media Mol Imaging 2006; 1(6):259–266.

75. Borden MA, Caskey CF, Little E, et al. DNA and poly-lysine adsorption and multilayer construction onto cationic lipid-coated microbubbles. Langmuir 2007; 23(18): 9401–9408.

76. Klibanov AL, Hughes MS, Marsh JN, et al. Targeting of ultrasound contrast material. An in vitro feasibility study. Acta Radiol Suppl 1997; 412:113–120.

77. Shortencarier MJ, Dayton PA, Bloch SH, et al. A method for radiation-force localized drug delivery using gas-filled liposphere. IEEE Trans Ultrason Ferroelectr Freq Control 2004; 51(7):822–831.

78. Dayton PA, Morgan KE, Klibanov ALS, et al. A preliminary evaluation of the effects of primary and secondary radiation forces on acoustic contrast agents. IEEE Trans Ultrason Ferroelectr Freq Control 1997; 44(6):1264–1277.

79. Zhao S, Borden MA, Bloch S, et al. Radiation-force assisted targeting facilitates ultrasonic molecular imaging. Mol Imaging 2004; 3(3):135–148.

80. Zhao S, Kruse DE, Ferrara KW, et al. Selective imaging of adherent targeted ultrasound contrast agents. Phys Med Biol 2007; 52(8):2055–2072.

81. Hutter JC, Luu HMD, Mehlhaff PM, et al. Physiologically based pharmacokinetic model for fluorocarbon elimination after the administration of an octafluoropropane-albumin microsphere sonographic contrast agent. J Ultrasound Med 1999; 18(1):1–11.

82. Schneider M. Characteristics of SonoVuetrade mark. Echocardiography 1999; 16(7, pt 2):743–746.

83. Straub JA, Chickering DE, Hartman TG, et al. AI-700 pharmacokinetics, tissue distribution and exhaled elimination kinetics in rats. Int J Pharm 2007; 328(1):35–41.

84. Toft KG, Hustvedt SO, Hals PA, et al. Disposition of perfluorobutane in rats after intravenous injection of Sonazoid (TM). Ultrasound Med Biol 2006; 32(1):107–114.

85. Walday P, Tolleshaug H, Gjoen T, et al. Biodistributions of air-filled albumin microspheres in rats and pigs. Biochem J 1994; 299(pt 2):437–443.

86. Goldsmith H, Mason SG. Axial migration of particles in Poiseuille flow. Nature 1961; 190(478):1095–1096.

87. Feinstein SB, Shah PM, Bing RJ, et al. Microbubble dynamics visualized in the intact capillary circulation. J Am Coll Cardiol 1984; 4(3):595–600.

88. Keller MW, Segal SS, Kaul S, et al. The behavior of sonicated albumin microbubbles within the microcirculation—a basis for their use during myocardial contrast echocardiography. Circ Res 1989; 65(2):458–467.

89. Lindner JR, Song J, Jayaweera AR, et al. Microvascular rheology of definity microbubbles after intra-arterial and intravenous administration. J Am Soc Echocardiogr 2002; 15(5):396–403.

90. Braide M, Rasmussen H, Albrektsson A, et al. Micro-vascular behavior and effects of Sonazoid microbubbles in

the cremaster muscle of rats after local administration. J Ultrasound Med 2006; 25(7):883–890.

91. Killam AL, Mehlhaff PM, Zavorskas PA, et al. Tissue distribution of I-125-labeled albumin in rats, and whole blood and exhaled elimination kinetics of octafluoropropane in anesthetized canines, following intravenous administration of OPTISON (R) (FS069). Int J Toxicol 1999; 18(1):49–63.

92. Walday P, Tolleshaug H, Gjoen T, et al. Biodistributions of air-filled albumin microspheres in rats and pigs. Biochem J 1994; 299:437–443.

93. Fisher NG, Christiansen JP, Klibanov A, et al. Influence of microbubble surface charge on capillary transit and myocardial contrast enhancement. J Am Coll Cardiol 2002; 40(4):811–819.

94. Yanagisawa K, Moriyasu F, Miyahara T, et al. Phagocytosis of ultrasound contrast agent microbubbles by Kupffer cells. Ultrasound Med Biol 2007; 33(2):318–325.

95. Kindberg GM, Tolleshaug H, Roos N, et al. Hepatic clearance of Sonazoid perfluorobutane microbubbles by Kupffer cells does not reduce the ability of liver to phagocytose or degrade albumin microspheres. Cell Tissue Res 2003; 312(1):49–54.

96. Sahu A, Lambris JD. Structure and biology of complement protein C3, a connecting link between innate and acquired immunity. Immunol Rev 2001; 180:35–48.

97. Janssen BJC, Huizinga EG, Raaijmakers HCA, et al. Structures of complement component C3 provide insights into the function and evolution of immunity. Nature 2005; 437(7058):505–511.

98. Klibanov AL, Maruyama K, Torchilin VP, et al. Amphipathic polyethyleneglycols effectively prolong the circulation time of liposomes. FEBS Lett 1990; 268(1): 235–237.

99. Jakobsen JA, Oyen R, Thomsen HS, et al. Safety of ultrasound contrast agents. Eur Radiol 2005; 15(5):941–945.

100. Torzilli G. Adverse effects associated with SonoVue use. Expert Opin Drug Saf 2005; 4(3):399–401.

101. Wink MH, Wijkstra H, De la Rosette J, et al. Ultrasound imaging and contrast agents: a safe alternative to MRI? Minim Invasive Ther Allied Technol 2006; 15(2): 93–100.

102. Correas JM, Bridal L, Lesavre A, et al. Ultrasound contrast agents: properties, principles of action, tolerance, and artifacts. Eur Radiol 2001; 11(8):1316–1328.

103. Blomley M, Claudon M, Cosgrove D. WFUMB safety symposium on ultrasound contrast agents: clinical applications and safety concerns. Ultrasound Med Biol 2007; 33(2):180–186.

104. Dalecki D. WFUMB safety symposium on echo-contrast agents: bioeffects of ultrasound contrast agents in vivo. Ultrasound Med Biol 2007; 33(2):205–213.

105. Dayton PA, Rychak JJ. Molecular ultrasound imaging using microbubble contrast agents. Front Biosci 2007; 12(51):124–142.

22

Quantification in Small-Animal PET and SPECT Imaging

PAUL D. ACTON

Johnson & Johnson Pharmaceutical R&D, Spring House, Philadelphia, Pennsylvania, U.S.A.

INTRODUCTION

While the technological developments in positron emission tomography (PET) (1–4) and single-photon emission computerized tomography (SPECT) (5–11) scanners for small-animal imaging have been impressive, methods for extracting quantitative information from these systems have lagged behind. The majority of imaging studies simply present images or organ uptake of radioactive tracers as arbitrary counts or as a fraction of the injected dose. This is subject to considerable fluctuations and is dependent on many factors, such as blood flow, metabolism, and enzyme activity, which may be unrelated to the physiological parameter of interest. The field of small-animal imaging has now matured sufficiently where simple measures of uptake, such as percentage of the injected dose per gram of tissue (%ID/g), are inadequate and may give misleading or inaccurate results. Indeed, recent applications of small-animal imaging are demanding the use of more quantitative methods for determining organ or tissue function, particularly where longitudinal studies are required to monitor changes in function over time resulting from disease progression or therapy. It is the role of quantitative imaging studies to provide the link between simple measures of radioactivity in an organ or tissue and meaningful parameters that represent the underlying physiology.

Accurate quantification is vital in a multitude of applications, from the correct dosing of an experimental therapeutic to the monitoring of disease progression in an animal model. The true power of molecular imaging is the ability to perform longitudinal studies on individual animals, allowing the acquisition of multiple time points, and where each animal can act as its own control. Using quantitative imaging studies, investigators can track changes in organ or tissue function in response to treatment and be confident that the alterations observed truly represent a measure of the underlying physiology.

TRACER KINETIC MODELING

Tracer kinetic modeling provides the mathematical description that converts activity levels measured in the functional scan into quantitative physiological parameters associated with the particular organ or function being studied. These models generally describe the behavior of a tracer in terms of a number of compartments, each of which represent distinct anatomical, physiological, or biochemical stages in the behavior of the tracer (12).

The pioneering work on tracer kinetic modeling (13–18) was developed to describe the uptake mechanisms of the glucose analogues [^{11}C]deoxyglucose and [^{18}F]-2-fluoro-2-deoxyglucose (FDG). In the case of FDG, the tracer is transported from the blood pool across the cell membrane, where it is phosphorylated by the enzyme hexokinase, and trapped in tissue. Unlike glucose, FDG-6-phosphate does not undergo further glycolytic pathways, so cellular FDG uptake reflects the overall rate of transmembranous exchange of glucose and the availability of the enzyme hexokinase. Dephosphorylation of FDG-6-phosphate is slow and is generally ignored.

Changes in %ID/g with FDG could be misinterpreted as variations in delivery of the tracer in the vasculature, active transport of the probe across the cell membrane, or hexokinase enzyme activity, or combinations of all three. This has been illustrated in a study of the effects of different anesthetics on FDG uptake (19,20). The effects of anesthesia on blood glucose or FDG levels include a complex interaction of multiple mechanisms, such as insulin levels, hepatic and renal metabolism, and uptake by peripheral tissues, all of which can have effects on simple measures such as %ID/g, and none of which represent a change in tumor metabolism.

For this reason, quantitative studies require tracer kinetic compartmental models to determine FDG metabolism. In this example, the compartments describe both physical processes, in the active transport across the cell membrane, and biochemical pathways in the phosporylation and subsequent trapping of FDG. Dynamic measurement of the uptake, retention, and washout of the tracer in tissue, using PET, can be used to provide quantification of glucose metabolism with a compartmental model, leading to absolute measures such as the rate of glucose metabolism (MRGlc in units of μmol/min/g). Potentially this technique allows the separate quantification of glucose transporter activity and hexokinase enzyme levels, with no dependency on peripheral plasma clearance or scanning time (21).

Much of the pioneering research in the development of tracer kinetic models was performed in studies of the brain. FDG uptake in the brain follows the same compartmental kinetic model described previously, with the exception that the simple cell membrane is replaced by the blood-brain barrier (BBB). Kinetic modeling of the uptake of FDG in the brain yields the absolute rate of cerebral glucose metabolism in different brain regions, which can be a powerful probe of brain activity and function.

More recently, radiolabeled ligands have been developed to study specific cell types or neurotransmitters in the brain. The compartmental model for these ligands is similar to FDG, with the tracers crossing the intact BBB into a brain tissue compartment. From this pool of available tracer, it can specifically bind to the receptor site under study, which describes another distinct compartment in the model. In this case, the different compartments are both physical and biochemical, representing the diffusion from the vasculature into the brain, followed by chemical binding to the receptor.

QUANTIFICATION IN SMALL-ANIMAL IMAGING

Quantitative imaging generally requires rapid arterial blood sampling to measure the input function to the tracer kinetic model. Blood samples are withdrawn, spun down to separate plasma, and tested for radioactive metabolites. The metabolite-corrected plasma curve is used to drive the kinetic model, and rate constants are calculated from fitting to the imaging data.

For a single bolus injection of tracer, the most critical time for blood collection is immediately after injection, when the concentration of radioactivity in blood is changing the fastest. Generally, for the first one to two minutes samples must be drawn every few seconds to capture fully the peak of the arterial curve. Manual extraction of such rapid samples can be extremely difficult, and automated techniques, such as fraction collectors or microvolumetric samplers (22), are preferable. Thereafter, blood collection can be slowed, with later samples drawn many minutes apart. Care must be taken with dead space in arterial lines, as blood samples can become contaminated by residual activity remaining in the line from the previous sample.

In humans and larger animals, the use of arterial lines is invasive, but relatively straightforward. However, in smaller animals, particularly mice, the routine use of arterial lines is extremely difficult. The total blood volume in a mouse is approximately 2 mL, and in order not to alter the hemodynamic either after an injection of tracer or during blood withdrawal, sample volumes are limited. The amount of blood permitted to be withdrawn from a mouse is generally <10% of the total blood volume, and the repeated puncture of arteries in longitudinal studies of the same animal results in considerable tissue and vessel damage. Implanted arterial catheters provide a useful means of access, but it is difficult to keep the lines patent over extended periods of time. Some success with absolute quantification has been achieved using arterial lines in mice (23,24) and rats (25–28), but it remains a complex and invasive procedure. Direct puncture of the left ventricle or exposing a femoral artery through skin incision is possible in small animals (29), but both remain terminal experiments best suited to validating other less-invasive techniques.

Consequently, the development of noninvasive methods for obtaining the arterial input function is vital. Image-derived methods for obtaining the input function from the imaging data alone are highly desirable. Some groups have used the blood pool activity in the left ventricle or other organs measured on the PET scanner (24,29–33), although this is limited by partial volume effects resulting from the relatively poor spatial resolution of the animal scanner. Further, this provides a measurement of whole-blood activity, with no information on plasma or metabolites. Additional blood samples may be required for certain tracers to determine plasma-to-whole-blood ratio at different time points and for correction of radiolabeled metabolites. Also, it is difficult to get both the heart and the brain in the field of view simultaneously, unless the animal scanner has a long axial bore (33). In addition, this requires very rapid time frames on the PET scans to capture fully the shape of the input function—in general, these images have very low counting statistics and give poor quality fits. Performing this type of study with small-animal pinhole SPECT would be even more difficult, with lower sensitivity, fewer counts, and a small field of view. However, a more recent small-animal SPECT system, based on slit apertures rather than pinholes, may provide an opportunity for larger field-of-view imaging in this application (34).

Different approaches for obtaining the arterial input function include inserting a β microprobe into the femoral artery of rats (35) or to run an arteriovenous shunt through an external counter (36). Although these techniques provide excellent temporal resolution, their applicability is limited by their complexity and invasiveness. Also, like measuring ventricular activity in the scanner, these methods are limited in that they acquire whole blood, not plasma, activity. Various methods for extracting arterial time–activity curves in small animals have been compared recently (37), with factor analysis of the ventricular images leading to the most accurate input function.

SIMPLIFIED METHODS OF QUANTIFICATION

The most difficult aspect of performing fully quantitative imaging studies is the difficulty in obtaining rapid arterial blood samples from small animals. Consequently, simplified imaging and analysis protocols have been developed, in the hope that accurate and quantitative results can be obtained without the need for arterial blood sampling.

One accepted method for simplifying the acquisition protocol is to use a population-based input function, in which the arterial input function for individual subjects is replaced by a general curve based on the average of a large sample of measurements (38–42). This removes the need for rapid arterial blood sampling, which simplifies the technique and reduces the invasiveness of the procedure. Generally, a single late blood sample (possibly venous) is taken to normalize the population curve to the individual. However, it is important to validate that a population curve is a suitable replacement for individual measurements. This technique has been validated recently for FDG in rats, where a scaled population-based input function was found to replicate each individual arterial blood curve to an accuracy of about 1.3% (Fig. 1) (28). While this is an important first step in simplifying quantitative small-animal imaging, it should be stressed that these results may vary depending on the species, strain, disease model, treatment group, tracer used, and anesthetic.

Many of the techniques for simplifying the acquisition and analysis protocols were pioneered in the field of neuroimaging, and specifically for the study of neurotransmitters. One of the most successful techniques uses a reference tissue approach, which removes the need for any blood sampling by identifying a reference region in the imaging data, which can provide the necessary input function to the kinetic model (43). The reference tissue

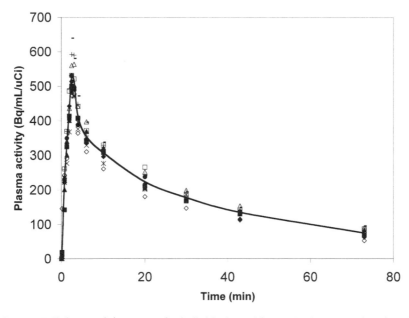

Figure 1 Normalized plasma FDG time–activity curves for individual rats (*data points*) compared against the population mean (*line*) (28). *Abbreviation*: FDG, [¹⁸F]-2-fluoro-2-deoxyglucose. *Source*: Data courtesy of Dr. Philipp Meyer, University Hospital Aachen.

model is based on the same description of the dynamics of radiotracer as the full three-compartment model, but the key is the identification of a valid background region that is devoid of the target sites. Many tracers have been validated using a reference tissue model in the brain (44–52). This model is now routinely applied in small-animal PET and SPECT imaging studies of neurotransmitter-binding sites, such as the dopamine transporter (DAT) (53,54) and postsynaptic dopamine receptors (54–60).

This model can be simplified still further if the tracer attains an equilibrium state between the background and specifically bound compartments (61). The main difficulty with this simplified protocol is the identification of a stable equilibrium level, however short-lived, which is consistent across subjects and across diseases. Infusion of the tracer over an extended period of time, or a combined bolus-plus-slow-infusion protocol, can be used to obtain a true equilibrium state (62–65), although the rate of infusion may not be optimal for all subjects and the bolus-to-infusion ratio requires optimization (66,67).

In many cases, normalization can be made relative to the total uptake of tracer. This is analogous to measuring standardized uptake values (SUVs) in clinical FDG PET, where the tissue or tumor activity is quantified in terms of the injected dose and a factor such as body weight (68), surface area (69), or lean body mass (70). SUV analysis is attractive as it requires only a single static scan and no blood sampling. However, SUVs are only semiquantitative at best, and do not account for the injected dose which is lost during the injection, or changes in plasma clearance resulting from disease, treatment, or animal handling. In addition, the various methods for normalization have not been tested or validated in small animals.

An even simpler model uses the uptake in a background organ or region, such as the contralateral muscle tissue, to normalize tumor uptake. While this removes the complications arising from activity remaining in the interstitial space at the injection site, it introduces further potential confounds such as variable background tissue uptake. This background normalization, which is analogous to the equilibrium model in brain imaging, is the most widely used method for quantifying FDG in mouse tumor models, mainly due to its simplicity.

Simplified models of tracer behavior generally represent a compromise between model accuracy and parameter identification. Simplified models tend to reduce the total number of parameters, resulting in smaller variance and covariance in the derived values, but may introduce bias with an oversimplified model (71). It is always vital that the simplification process is validated against the full model to determine if bias has been introduced into the system. Because of their reduced statistical noise, the simplified methods of analysis are often utilized in voxel-based techniques.

VOXEL-BASED ANALYSIS

Conventional analysis methods use manually drawn regions of interest (ROIs) to extract counts. This is particularly difficult in small-animal images, where it is often impossible to identify specific organs or subregions of the brain. Hence, drawing ROIs on small-animal PET or SPECT images can be highly subjective, time consuming, and inaccurate. Automated methods of drawing ROIs on PET or coregistered PET-CT images of mice have been developed using a digital mouse atlas (72,73), which is useful for quantifying tracer uptake in multiple organs throughout the body or in different brain regions. However, reducing regions to single voxels may be the most accurate and objective method of analysis. Instead of drawing regions and using those counts as inputs to a mathematical model of tracer behavior, it is possible to apply the kinetic modeling equations at every voxel independently, thereby generating a parametric image of quantitative parameters (74–76).

The real power of imaging is the ability to follow individual animals over extended periods, looking for changes as a result of disease progression or treatment. Having obtained quantitative imaging data, the next step is to analyze those data and detect the subtle alterations in signal resulting from these processes. This illustrates a further disadvantage of ROI analysis methods. Small ROIs are capable of resolving localized focal changes between images, although they are subject to a loss of specificity due to the problems associated with multiple comparisons. Alternatively, large ROIs encompassing an entire brain structure may dilute small activation foci, with a subsequent loss of sensitivity. Unless a study is very strongly hypothesis driven and comparisons between images are only being made in highly specific regions, ROI analysis lacks the power to accurately distinguish regional variations between a set of images (77).

The solution to this problem in human imaging, particularly in the brain, has been the development of pixel-based statistical analyses, where the regions are effectively reduced to single pixels, such as statistical parametric mapping (SPM) (77,78). Applying SPM to the parametric images of quantitative binding parameters would allow highly accurate, unbiased, automated analysis in longitudinal animal studies.

An example of this technique is shown in Figure 2, where voxel-based statistical analysis has been performed on quantitative FDG images in the rat brain. In this study, vibrissae stimulation was initiated during FDG uptake and changes in cerebral glucose metabolism compared against control studies of the same animals without the stimulus. These results indicated unilateral increases in glucose metabolism in response to the stimulus, on the side contralateral to the whiskers that were manipulated.

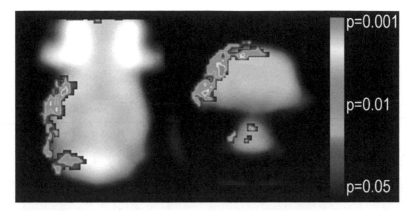

Figure 2 Voxel-based statistical parametric mapping showing cerebral hypermetabolism resulting from vibrissae stimulation in rats. Transverse and coronal slices through the mean template image (*gray scale*) show statistically significant regions of hypermetabolism (*color*). The two hot regions on the left image correspond to uptake in the Harderian glands (*See Color Insert*).

Voxel-based techniques, such as SPM, are becoming utilized only recently in the field of small-animal imaging, but it is clear they are going to be the way forward for objective analysis of imaging data, particularly in multiple studies of the same animals.

APPLICATIONS OF QUANTITATIVE SMALL-ANIMAL IMAGING

Drug Occupancy

Small animal molecular imaging has been proposed as an important tool in the development of novel therapeutics, potentially reducing both the time and the cost of bringing new drugs to the marketplace (79–81). Quantitative imaging is vital in this endeavor, enabling the effects of a new drug to be assessed using meaningful physiological parameters. In fact, quantification of the imaging data has been recognized as one of the main prerequisites for applying imaging in drug discovery (82). It is likely that imaging of biomarkers, such as the drug target, and surrogate endpoints, such as glucose metabolism in a tumor, may become more widespread and accepted during the development phase of a new drug. Furthermore, the development of new radiotracers and quantitative methods of analysis will go hand-in-hand with the new drugs they are designed to test, and track the drugs throughout their development cycle, including preclinical studies and clinical trials.

The most significant potential barrier to this role is the development and validation of imaging biomarkers, and their application as surrogate endpoints (81). However, the rewards are profound, particularly as PET and SPECT studies in small animals are readily translatable to the clinic, with little or no modification to the imaging procedure. In fact, the translation of imaging biomarkers to humans is one of the main aims in personalized medicine, leading to better patient selection for specific treatments and earlier prediction of response.

So far, the primary role of imaging in preclinical drug development has been to determine the relationship between the drug dose and occupancy of the target binding site, particularly in the brain. Small-animal imaging is a powerful tool to assist in the understanding of the interaction of drugs at cerebral binding sites in vivo. Although this type of study is possible using other methods, such as quantitative autoradiography, imaging does not necessitate the sacrifice of multiple animals at each dose point. In addition, the dynamic data provided by PET and SPECT imaging give unique information on the target sites and their interaction with competing ligands.

Quantitative [^{123}I]IBF SPECT studies of the occupancy of competing antagonists at the dopamine D2 receptor have been performed in mice to demonstrate the ability of small-animal imaging to generate dose-occupancy data using a bolus-infusion paradigm (Fig. 3) (83). A saturation curve was used for a single receptor site model, and gave an excellent fit, with an ED_{50} (the dose of competing antagonist required to reduce the tracer binding by 50%) of 0.26 mg/kg. This information could be used to optimize the drug dose of a novel medication for maximum efficacy. Using imaging techniques, one can obtain dose-occupancy curves with many fewer animals and provide increased statistical power since each animal can receive multiple doses and act as its own control. Similarly, occupancy of DAT in rats by methylphenidate has been demonstrated using SPECT (84). In the brain, SPECT offers certain advantages over PET, including higher spatial resolution and tracers with higher specific activities (85). For some PET tracers, particularly those labeled with ^{11}C, low specific activity can lead to high occupancy of the binding site by the ligand itself, causing

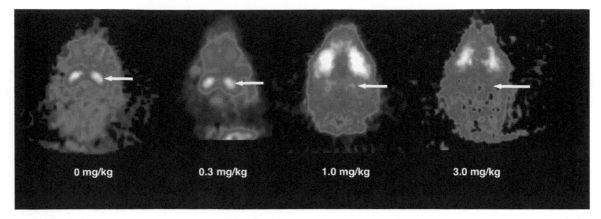

Figure 3 Changes in dopaminergic binding for [^{123}I]IBF resulting from competition with an antagonist at the D2 receptor. Shown are progressively larger doses of the competing antagonist, from 0 up to 3 mg/kg, with a concomitant decrease in tracer binding in the striatum (*arrowed*) (*See Color Insert*).

pharmacological reactions in the animals being studied, and violates assumptions underlying tracer kinetic modeling (59,86,87).

Photodynamic Therapy Response

The response of an organ or tissue to some kind of therapeutic intervention is an important application of imaging biomarkers and surrogate endpoints. Imaging plays an important role in measuring response and efficacy of a treatment and in assessing safety, where it can ensure that the therapy is hitting the correct target, and provide information on dosing. Longitudinal imaging studies are able to provide three of the most important pieces of information on the effects of treatment on a tumor; regression of the tumor, recurrence after the cessation of treatment, and the development of resistance to the therapy.

Photodynamic therapy (PDT) is a promising treatment for tumors located on or near the surface, using photosensitive drugs to activate cell death only in those regions that receive light irradiation (88–90). Imaging tumors in mice using FDG and PET could provide important information on the mechanisms of action of PDT and allow rapid evaluation of novel photosensitizers (22,91). However, simple semiquantitative SUV analysis would mask much of the available information, particularly involving the time course of the effects of the treatment. This has led some investigators to study a slow infusion of FDG into the animals, allowing transient changes in glucose metabolism to be measured almost in real time (92). During the infusion, changes in FDG uptake by the tumor cells were interpreted as the metabolic response to treatment. Any changes in tracer uptake over time are a complex interaction of variations in tumor metabolism and the kinetics of FDG. This is further complicated by the time-varying

nature of the photosensitizer drugs, which evolve continuously throughout the experiment (Fig. 4).

Despite the complexity of the data, semiquantitative analysis of the infusion images reveals the modes of action of the different classes of PDT drugs. Drugs that induce direct cell death, such as the more hydrophobic or amphiphilic photosensitizers, resulted in rapid reduction in FDG uptake by the tumor, which recovered relatively quickly, suggesting reversible damage. Conversely, drugs that act on the tumor vasculature caused a delayed reduction in FDG, which appeared to be irreversible. Dynamic imaging with a continuous infusion of tracer has provided vital information on changes in transient metabolic processes inside tumors and even revealed an unexpected systemic response in control tumors, which were not exposed to light. While these data are not fully quantitative and would have benefited from full kinetic modeling, they could provide vital information on optimization of treatment regimen and for the screening of new drugs (93).

Gene Expression

Imaging reporter gene expression has become one of the fastest growing fields in small-animal radionuclide imaging. A variety of reporter genes have been developed, including herpes simplex virus type 1 thymidine kinase (HSV1-tk) (24,94–103), dopamine D2 receptor (104,105), DAT (106), somatostatin receptor (107), and the sodium-iodide symporter (108–111), which are imaged with the appropriate PET or SPECT reporter probe. However, a common theme with all these studies is the lack of quantification of the reporter probe uptake beyond simple measures of %ID/g. Consequently, monitoring changes in expression of the gene are impossible, since variations in %ID/g can be a result of multiple factors, such as blood flow,

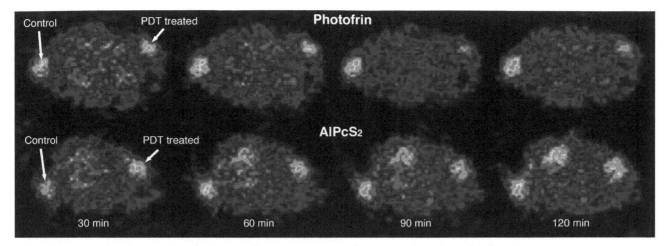

Figure 4 Tumor glucose metabolism measured by FDG and PET in a rat study of the effects of two different PDT drugs. The times indicate the period between the start of FDG infusion and the beginning of the PET scan. PDT illumination occurred immediately prior to the scan at 30 minutes and ended at 60 minutes. The top row shows the effects of photofrin, which is known to be deposited in the vascular stroma of the tumor, acting indirectly on the tumor by inducing vascular stasis shortly after treatment. In the bottom row, the amphophilic photosensitizer AlPcS$_2$ is taken up by the tumor, inducing direct cell death, which comes into effect later in the imaging sequence. Quantitative analysis of these images shows the varying modes of action of the two different classes of drugs (92). *Abbreviations*: FDG, [^{18}F]-2-fluoro-2-deoxyglucose; PET, positron emission tomography; PDT, photodynamic therapy. *Source*: Image courtesy of Dr. Roger Lecomte, University of Sherbrooke.

transport mechanisms, and peripheral clearance, none of which give any indication of how the gene is being expressed.

Recently, however, studies have been performed to develop and validate a compartmental model of tracer uptake, using the PET reporter probe 9-(4-^{18}F-fluoro-3-[hydroxymethyl]butyl)guanine (FHBG) for the mutant HSV1-tk gene, HSV1-sr39tk (24). The gene, driven by a constitutive promoter, was delivered by adenoviral vector to mouse liver. On the basis of the known biochemistry of the phosphorylation of FHBG by the enzyme HSV1-sr39TK, a three-compartment model was used to fit the dynamic PET imaging data. Quantitative PET results were compared against independent measures of reporter gene activity, such as mRNA assay and enzyme activity. While the kinetic rate parameters derived from the compartmental analysis compared favorably with enzyme activity, the conventional value %ID/g did not. This suggests that measuring the full arterial input function normalizes for differences between experiments and animals, while using injected dose normalization alone leads to errors. Since it was shown that FHBG rapidly equilibrates between whole blood and plasma, the blood pool measured by PET in the left ventricle may be adequate to describe the kinetics of the input function, without the need for arterial blood sampling.

CONCLUSION

The importance of quantification of small-animal PET and SPECT imaging data is being recognized, particularly in longitudinal experiments where multiple scans of the same animal are performed to monitor changes in disease progression or response to therapy. As was the case in human imaging, studies of the brain in rats and mice are leading the way in the development of fully quantitative methods of analysis. However, techniques are being developed for quantification in other applications, particularly tumor imaging, and the field of drug discovery and development will likely be taking a leading role. Effort is still required in the simplification of protocols, but at least now the developments in quantitative analysis will parallel the impressive strides taken in small-animal imaging instrumentation.

ACKNOWLEDGMENTS

The author is indebted to Dr. Philipp Meyer, University Hospital Aachen, and Dr. Roger Lecomte, University of Sherbrooke, for kindly providing some of the figures. This work was supported in part by grants from the National Institutes of Health (R01-EB001809 and R01-NS048315).

REFERENCES

1. Cherry SR, Shao Y, Silverman RW, et al. MicroPET: a high resolution PET scanner for imaging small animals. IEEE Trans Nucl Sci 1997; 44:1161–1166.
2. Chatziioannou AF, Cherry SR, Shao Y, et al. Performance evaluation of microPET: a high resolution lutetium oxyorthosilicate PET scanner for animal imaging. J Nucl Med 1999; 40:1164–1175.

3. Surti S, Karp JS, Freifelder R, et al. Design evaluation of A-PET: a high sensitivity animal PET camera. IEEE Trans Nucl Sci 2003; 50:1357–1364.

4. Yang Y, Tai YC, Siegel S, et al. Optimization and performance evaluation of the microPET II scanner for in vivo small animal imaging. Phys Med Biol 2004; 49: 2527–2545.

5. MacDonald LR, Patt BE, Iwanczyk JS, et al. Pinhole SPECT of mice using the LumaGEM gamma camera. IEEE Trans Nucl Sci 2001; 48:830–836.

6. Weber DA, Ivanovich M. Pinhole SPECT: ultra-high resolution imaging for small animal studies. J Nucl Med 1995; 36:2287–2289.

7. Ishizu K, Mukai T, Yonekura Y, et al. Ultra-high resolution SPECT system using four pinhole collimators for small animal studies. J Nucl Med 1995; 36:2282–2287.

8. Wirrwar A, Schramm NU, Vosberg H, et al. High resolution SPECT in small animal research. Rev Neurosci 2001; 12:187–193.

9. Yokoi T, Kishi H. Development of a high resolution pinhole SPECT system using dual-head gamma camera for small animal studies. Jpn J Nucl Med 1998; 35:901–907.

10. McElroy DP, MacDonald LR, Beekman FJ, et al. Performance evaluation of A-SPECT: a high resolution desktop pinhole SPECT system for imaging small animals. IEEE Trans Nucl Sci 2002; 49:2139–2147.

11. Cao Z, Bal G, Accorsi R, et al. Optimal number of pinholes in multi-pinhole SPECT for mouse brain imaging—a simulation study. Phys Med Biol 2005; 50:4609–4624.

12. Gunn RN, Gunn SR, Cunningham VJ. Positron emission tomography compartmental models. J Cereb Blood Flow Metab 2001; 21:635–652.

13. Sokoloff L, Reivich M, Kennedy C. The [^{14}C]deoxyglucose method for the measurement of local cerebral glucose utilisation: theory, procedure, and normal values in the conscious and anesthetised albino rat. J Neurochem 1977; 28:897–916.

14. Reivich M, Alavi A, Greenberg J. Mapping of functional cerebral activity in man using the ^{18}F-2-Fluoro-2-deoxyglucose technique. J Comput Assist Tomogr 1978; 2:656–660.

15. Reivich M, Kuhl DE, Wolf AP. The [^{18}F]fluorodeoxyglucose method for the measurement of local cerebral glucose utilisation in man. Circ Res 1979; 44:127–137.

16. Reivich M, Alavi A, Greenberg J. Use of 2-deoxy-D-[1-11C]glucose for the determination of local cerebral glucose metabolism in humans: variation within and between subjects. J Cereb Blood Flow Metab 1979; 6:371–388.

17. Phelps M, Huang S-C, Hoffman E, et al. Tomographic measurement of cerebral glucose metabolic rate in humans with [$^{F-18}$]2-fluoro-2-deoxy-D-glucose: validation of method. Ann Neurol 1979; 6:371–388.

18. Huang S-C, Phelps M, Hoffman E, et al. Noninvasive determination of local cerebral metabolic rate of glucose in man. Am J Physiol 1980; 238:B69–B82.

19. Lee KH, Ko BH, Paik JY, et al. Effects of anesthetic agents and fasting duration on 18F-FDG biodistribution and insulin levels in tumor-bearing mice. J Nucl Med 2005; 46:1531–1536.

20. Fueger BJ, Czernin J, Hildebrandt I, et al. Impact of animal handling on the results of 18F-FDG PET studies in mice. J Nucl Med 2006; 47:999–1006.

21. Lammertsma AA, Hoekstra CJ, Giaccone G, et al. How should we analyse FDG PET studies for monitoring tumour response? Eur J Nucl Med 2006; 33:S16–S21.

22. Lapointe D, Brasseur N, Cadorette J, et al. High resolution PET imaging for in vivo monitoring of tumor response after photodynamic therapy in mice. J Nucl Med 1999; 40: 876–882.

23. Toyama H, Ichise M, Liow JS, et al. Absolute quantification of regional cerebral glucose utilization in mice by 18F-FDG small animal PET scanning and 2-14C-DG autoradiography. J Nucl Med 2004; 45:1398–1405.

24. Green LA, Nguyen K, Berenji B, et al. A tracer kinetic model for 18F-FHBG for quantitating herpes simplex virus type 1 thymidine kinase reporter gene expression in living animals using PET. J Nucl Med 2004; 45:1560–1570.

25. Nakao Y, Itoh Y, Kuang TY, et al. Effects of anesthesia on functional activation of cerebral blood flow and metabolism. Proc Natl Acad Sci U S A 2001; 98:7593–7598.

26. Shimoji K, Ravasi L, Schmidt K, et al. Measurement of cerebral glucose metabolic rates in the anesthetized rat by dynamic scanning with 18F-FDG, the ATLAS small animal PET scanner, and arterial blood sampling. J Nucl Med 2004; 45:665–672.

27. Fujita M, Zoghbi SS, Crescenzo MS, et al. Quantification of brain phosphodiesterase 4 in rat with (R)-[11C]rolipram-PET. Neuroimage 2005; 26:1201–1210.

28. Meyer PT, Circiumaru V, Cardi C, et al. Simplified quantification of small animal 18FDG PET studies using a standard arterial input function. Eur J Nucl Med 2006; 33:948–954.

29. Green LA, Gambhir SS, Srinivasan A, et al. Noninvasive methods for quantitating blood time-activity curves from mouse PET images obtained with fluorine-18-fluorodeoxyglucose. J Nucl Med 1998; 39:729–734.

30. Huang S-C, Wu HM, Shoghi-Jadid K, et al. Investigation of a new input function validation approach for dynamic mouse microPET studies. Mol Imag Biol 2004; 6:34–46.

31. Yee SH, Jerabek PA, Fox PT. Non-invasive quantification of cerebral blood flow for rats by microPET imaging of 15O labeled water: the application of a cardiac time-activity curve for the tracer arterial input function. Nucl Med Commun 2005; 26:903–911.

32. Kim J, Herrero P, Sharp T, et al. Minimally invasive method of determining blood input function from PET images in rodents. J Nucl Med 2006; 47:330–336.

33. Yee SH, Lee K, Jerabek PA, et al. Quantitative measurement of oxygen metabolic rate in the rat brain using microPET imaging of briefly inhaled 15O-labeled oxygen gas. Nucl Med Commun 2006; 27:573–581.

34. Walrand S, Jamar F, de Jong M, et al. Evaluation of novel whole-body high-resolution rodent SPECT (Linoview) based on direct acquisition of linogram projections. J Nucl Med 2005; 46:1872–1880.

35. Pain F, Laniece P, Mastrippolito R, et al. Arterial input function measurement without blood sampling using a beta-microprobe in rats. J Nucl Med 2004; 45:1577–1582.

36. Weber B, Burger C, Biro P, et al. A femoral arteriovenous shunt facilitates arterial whole blood sampling in animals. Eur J Nucl Med 2002; 29:319–323.

37. Laforest R, Sharp TL, Engelbach JA, et al. Measurement of input functions in rodents: challenges and solutions. Nucl Med Biol 2005; 32:679–685.

38. Takikawa S, Dhawan V, Spetsieris PG, et al. Noninvasive quantitative fluorodeoxyglucose PET studies with an estimated input function derived from a population-based arterial blood curve. Radiology 1993; 188:131–136.

39. Eberl S, Anayat AR, Fulton RR, et al. Evaluation of two population-based input functions for quantitative neurological FDG PET studies. Eur J Nucl Med 1997; 24:299–304.

40. Shiozaki T, Sadato N, Senda M, et al. Noninvasive estimation of FDG input function for quantification of cerebral metabolic rate of glucose: optimzation and multicenter evaluation. J Nucl Med 2000; 41:1612–1618.

41. Takagi S, Takahashi W, Shinohara Y, et al. Quantitative PET cerebral glucose metabolism estimates using a single non-arterialized venous blood sample. Ann Nucl Med 2004; 18:297–302.

42. Brock CS, Young H, Osman S, et al. Glucose metabolism in brain tumors can be estimated using [18F]2-fluorodeoxyglucose positron emission tomography and a population-derived input function scaled using a single arterialized venous blood sample. Int J Onc 2005; 26:1377–1383.

43. Lammertsma AA, Hume SP. Simplified reference tissue model for PET receptor studies. Neuroimage 1996; 4:153–158.

44. Acton PD, Kushner SA, Kung MP, et al. Simplified reference region model for the kinetic analysis of [99mTc]TRODAT-1 binding to dopamine transporters in non-human primates using SPET. Eur J Nucl Med 1999; 26:518–526.

45. Acton PD, Meyer PT, Mozley PD, et al. Simplified quantification of dopamine transporters in humans using [99mTc]TRODAT-1 and single photon emission tomography. Eur J Nucl Med 2000; 27:1714–1718.

46. Acton PD, Choi SR, Hou C, et al. Quantification of serotonin transporters in nonhuman primates using [123I]ADAM and single photon emission tomography. J Nucl Med 2001; 42:1556–1562.

47. Parsey RV, Slifstein M, Hwang DR, et al. Validation and reproducibility of measurement of 5-HT1A receptor parameters with [carbonyl-11C]WAY-100635 in humans: comparison of arterial and reference tissue input functions. J Cereb Blood Flow Metab 2000; 20:1111–1133.

48. Lammertsma AA, Bench CJ, Hume SP, et al. Comparison of methods for analysis of clinical [11C]raclopride studies. J Cereb Blood Flow Metab 1996; 16:42–52.

49. Ichise M, Fujita M, Seibyl JP, et al. Graphical analysis and simplified quantification of striatal and extrastriatal dopamine D2 receptor binding with [123I]epidepride SPECT. J Nucl Med 1999; 40:1902–1912.

50. Gunn RN, Sargent PA, Bench CJ, et al. Tracer kinetic modeling of the 5-HT1A receptor ligand [carbonyl-11C]WAY-100635 for PET. Neuroimage 1998; 8:426–440.

51. Ichise M, Ballinger JR, Vines D, et al. Simplified quantification and reproducibility studies of dopamine D2-receptor binding with iodine-123-IBF SPECT in healthy subjects. J Nucl Med 1997; 38:31–37.

52. Farde L, Ito H, Swahn CG, et al. Quantitative analyses of carbonyl-carbon-11-WAY-100635 binding to central 5-hydroxytryptamine-1A receptors in man. J Nucl Med 1998; 39:1965–1971.

53. Acton PD, Choi SR, Plössl K, et al. Quantification of dopamine transporter in mouse brain using ultra-high resolution single photon emission tomography. Eur J Nucl Med 2002; 29:691–698.

54. Inaji M, Okauchi T, Ando K, et al. Correlation between quantitative imaging and behavior in unilaterally 6-OHDA-lesioned rats. Brain Res 2005; 1064:136–145.

55. Morris ED, Yoder KK, Wang C, et al. ntPET: a new application of PET imaging for characterizing the kinetics of endogenous neurotransmitter release. Mol Imag 2005; 4:473–489.

56. Honer M, Bruhlmeier M, Missimer JH, et al. Dynamic imaging of striatal D2 receptors in mice using quad-HIDAC PET. J Nucl Med 2004; 45:464–470.

57. Thanos PK, Taintor NB, Alexoff D, et al. In vivo comparative imaging of dopamine D2 knockout and wild-type mice with 11C-raclopride and microPET. J Nucl Med 2002; 43:1570–1577.

58. Ishiwata K, Ogi N, Hayakawa N, et al. Positron emission tomography and ex vivo and in vitro autoradiography studies on dopamine D2-like receptor degeneration in the quinolinic acid-lesioned rat striatum: comparison of [11C]raclopride, [11C]nemonapride and [11C]N-methylspiperone. Nucl Med Biol 2002; 29:307–316.

59. Alexoff DL, Vaska P, Marsteller D, et al. Reproducibility of 11C-raclopride binding in the rat brain measured with the microPET R4: effects of scatter correction and tracer specific activity. J Nucl Med 2003; 44:815–822.

60. Nikolaus S, Larisch R, Beu M, et al. Bilateral increase in striatal dopamine D2 receptor density in the 6-hydroxy-dopamine-lesioned rat: a serial in vivo investigation with small animal PET. Eur J Nucl Med 2003; 30:390–395.

61. Farde L, Eriksson L, Blomqvist G, et al. Kinetic analysis of central [^{11}C]raclopride binding to D$_2$-dopamine receptors studied by PET: a comparison to the equilibrium analysis. J Cereb Blood Flow Metab 1989; 9:696–708.

62. Laruelle M, Abi-Dargham A, Rattner Z, et al. Single photon emission tomography measurement of benzodiazepine receptor number and affinity in primate brain: a constant infusion paradigm with [123I]iomazenil. Eur J Pharmacol 1993; 230:119–123.

63. Ito H, Hietala J, Blomqvist G, et al. Comparison of the transient equilibrium and continuous infusion method for quantitative PET analysis of [11C]raclopride binding. J Cereb Blood Flow Metab 1998; 18:941–950.

64. Laruelle M, Abi-Dargham A, Al-Tikriti MS, et al. SPECT quantification of [I-123] iomazenil binding to benzodiazepine receptors in nonhuman primates. 2. Equilibrium analysis of constant infusion experiments and correlation with in vitro parameters. J Cereb Blood Flow Metab 1994; 14:453–465.

65. Seibyl JP, Zea-Ponce Y, Brenner L, et al. Continuous intravenous infusion of iodine-123-IBZM for SPECT

determination of human brain dopamine receptor occupancy by antipsychotic agent RWJ-37796. J Nucl Med 1996; 37:11–15.

66. Carson RE, Channing MA, Blasberg RG, et al. Comparison of bolus and infusion methods for receptor quantitation: application to [18F]cyclofoxy and positron emission tomography. J Cereb Blood Flow Metab 1993; 13:24–42.

67. Carson RE. PET physiological measurements using constant infusion. Nucl Med Biol 2000; 27:657–660.

68. Wahl RL, Cody RL, Hutchins GM, et al. Primary and metastatic breast carcinoma: initial clinical evaluation with PET with the radiolabeled glucose analogue 2-[F-18]-fluoro-2-deoxy-D-glucose. Radiology 1991; 179: 765–770.

69. Kim CK, Gupta NC, Chandramouli B, et al. Standardized uptake values of FDG: body surface area correction is preferable to body weight correction. J Nucl Med 1994; 34:164–167.

70. Zasadny KR, Wahl RL. Standardized uptake values of normal tissues at PET with 2-[fluorine-18]-fluoro-2-deoxy-D-glucose: variations with body weight and a method for correction. Radiology 1993; 189:847–850.

71. Slifstein M, Parsey RV, Laruelle M. Derivation of [11C] WAY-100635 binding parameters with reference tissue models: effect of violations of model assumptions. Nucl Med Biol 2000; 27:487–492.

72. Rubins DJ, Melega WP, Lacan G, et al. Development and evaluation of an automated atlas-based image analysis method for microPET studies of the rat brain. Neuroimage 2003; 20:2100–2118.

73. Kesner AL, Dahlbom M, Huang SC, et al. Semiautomated analysis of small animal PET data. J Nucl Med 2006; 47:1181–1186.

74. Gunn RN, Lammertsma AA, Hume SP, et al. Parametric imaging of ligand-receptor binding in PET using a simplified reference region model. Neuroimage 1997; 6:279–287.

75. Ma Y, Dhawan V, Mentis M, et al. Parametric mapping of [18F]FPCIT binding in early stage Parkinson's disease: a PET study. Synapse 2002; 45:125–133.

76. Rakshi JS, Bailey DL, Ito K, et al. Methodology for statistical parametric mapping of [18F]fluorodopa uptake rate using three-dimensional PET. In: Carson RE, Daube-Witherspoon ME, Herscovitch P, ed. Quantitative Functional Brain Imaging with Positron Emission Tomography. San Diego: Academic Press, 1998:117–123.

77. Acton PD, Friston KJ. Statistical parametric mapping in functional neuroimaging: beyond PET and fMRI activation studies. Eur J Nucl Med 1998; 25:663–667.

78. Friston KJ, Holmes AP, Worsley KJ, et al. Statistical parametric maps in functional imaging: a general linear approach. Hum Brain Map 1995; 2:189–210.

79. Burns HD, Hamill TG, Eng W, et al. Positron emission tomography neuroreceptor imaging as a tool in drug discovery, research and development. Curr Opin Chem Biol 1999; 3:388–394.

80. Roselt P, Meikle SR, Kassiou M. The role of positron emission tomography in the discovery and development of new drugs; as studied in laboratory animals. Eur J Drug Metab Pharmacokinet 2004; 29:1–6.

81. Richter WS. Imaging biomarkers as surrogate endpoints for drug development. Eur J Nucl Med 2006; 33:S6–S10.

82. Rudin M, Weissleder R. Molecular imaging in drug discovery and development. Nat Rev Drug Discov 2003; 2:123–131.

83. Acton PD, Hou C, Kung MP, et al. Occupancy of dopamine D2 receptors in the mouse brain measured using ultra-high resolution single photon emission tomography and [123I]IBF. Eur J Nucl Med 2002; 29:1507–1515.

84. Nikolaus S, Wirrwar A, Antke C, et al. Quantitation of dopamine transporter blockade by methylphenidate: first in vivo investigation using [123I]FP-CIT and a dedicated small animal SPECT. Eur J Nucl Med 2004; 32:308–313.

85. Acton PD, Kung HF. Small animal imaging with high resolution single photon emission tomography. Nucl Med Biol 2003; 30:889–895.

86. Hume SP, Brown DJ, Ashworth S, et al. In vivo saturation kinetics of two dopamine transporter probes measured using a small animal positron emission tomography scanner. J Neurosci Methods 1997; 76:45–51.

87. Hume SP, Gunn RN, Jones T. Pharmacological constraints associated with positron emission tomography scanning of small laboratory animals. Eur J Nucl Med 1998; 25:173–176.

88. Dougherty TJ. Photosensitizers: therapy and detection of malignant tumors. Photochem Photobiol 1987; 45:879–889.

89. Henderson BW, Dougherty TJ. How does photodynamic therapy work? Photochem Photobiol 1992; 55:145–157.

90. Dougherty TJ, Marcus SL. Photodynamic therapy. Eur J Cancer 1992; 28A:1734–1742.

91. Moore JV, Waller ML, Zhao S, et al. Feasibility of imaging photodynamic injury by high resolution positron emission tomography. Eur J Nucl Med 1998; 25:1248–1254.

92. Berard V, Rousseau JA, Cadorette J, et al. Dynamic imaging of transient metabolic processes by small animal positron emission tomography for the evaluation of photosensitizers in photodynamic therapy of cancer. J Nucl Med 2006; 47:1119–1126.

93. Acton PD. Dynamic imaging of transient metabolic processes: PDT is just the beginning. J Nucl Med 2006; 47:1067–1069.

94. Gambhir SS, Barrio JR, Phelps ME, et al. Imaging adenoviral-directed reporter gene expression in living animals with positron emission tomography. Proc Natl Acad Sci U S A 1999; 96:2333–2338.

95. Gambhir SS, Barrio JR, Wu L, et al. Imaging of adenoviral-directed herpes simplex virus type 1 thymidine kinase reporter gene expression in mice with radiolabeled ganciclovir. J Nucl Med 1998; 39:2003–2011.

96. Haubner R, Avril N, Hantzopoulos PA, et al. In vivo imaging of herpes simplex virus type 1 thymidine kinase gene expression: early kinetics of radiolabelled FIAU. Eur J Nucl Med 2000; 27:283–291.

97. Herschman HR, MacLaren DC, Iyer M, et al. Seeing is believing: non-invasive, quantitative and repetitive imaging of reporter gene expression in living animals, using positron emission tomography. J Neurosci Res 2000; 59:699–705.

98. Gambhir SS, Barrio JR, Herschman HR, et al. Assays for noninvasive imaging of reporter gene expression. Nucl Med Biol 1999; 26:481–490.

99. Iyer M, Barrio JR, Namavari M, et al. 8-[18F]fluoropenciclovir: an improved reporter probe for imaging HSV1-tk reporter gene expression in vivo using PET. J Nucl Med 2001; 42:96–105.

100. MacLaren DC, Toyokuni T, Cherry SR, et al. PET imaging of transgene expression. Biol Psychiatry 2000; 48: 337–348.

101. Gambhir SS, Herschman HR, Cherry SR, et al. Imaging transgene expression with radionuclide imaging technologies. Neoplasia 2000; 2:118–138.

102. Gambhir SS, Bauer E, Black ME, et al. A mutant herpes simplex virus type 1 thymidine kinase reporter gene shows improved sensitivity for imaging reporter gene expression with positron emission tomography. Proc Natl Acad Sci U S A 2000; 97:2785–2790.

103. Tjuvajev JG, Doubrovin M, Akhurst T, et al. Comparison of radiolabeled nucleoside probes (FIAU, FHBG, and FHPG) for PET imaging of HSV1-tk gene expression. J Nucl Med 2002; 43:1072–1083.

104. MacLaren DC, Gambhir SS, Satyamurthy N, et al. Repetitive, non-invasive imaging of the dopamine D2 receptor as a reporter gene in living animals. Gene Ther 1999; 6: 785–791.

105. Liang Q, Satyamurthy N, Barrio JR, et al. Noninvasive, quantitative imaging in living animals of a mutant dopamine D2 receptor reporter gene in which ligand binding is uncoupled from signal transduction. Gene Ther 2001; 8:1490–1498.

106. Auricchio A, Acton PD, Hildinger M, et al. In vivo quantitative non-invasive imaging of gene transfer with single-photon emission computerized tomography. Hum Gene Ther 2003; 14:255–261.

107. Zinn KR, Buchsbaum DJ, Chaudhuri TR, et al. Noninvasive monitoring of gene transfer using a reporter receptor imaged with a high-affinity peptide radiolabeled with 99mTc or 188Re. J Nucl Med 2000; 41:887–895.

108. Chung JK. Sodium iodide symporter: its role in nuclear medicine. J Nucl Med 2002; 43:1188–1200.

109. Shin JH, Chung JK, Kang JH, et al. Feasibility of sodium/iodide symporter gene as a new imaging reporter gene: comparison with HSV1-tk. Eur J Nucl Med 2004; 31:425–432.

110. Cho JY, Shen DH, Yang W, et al. In vivo imaging and radioiodine therapy following sodium iodide symporter gene transfer in animal model of intracerebral gliomas. Gene Ther 2002; 9:1139–1145.

111. Niu G, Gaut AW, Ponto LL, et al. Multimodality noninvasive imaging of gene transfer using the human sodium iodide symporter. J Nucl Med 2004; 45:445–449.

23

In Vivo Imaging Mouse Models of Breast Cancer

KATHLEEN GABRIELSON, TERESA SOUTHARD, and YI XU

*Department of Molecular and Comparative Pathobiology, Johns Hopkins University
School of Medicine, Baltimore, Maryland, U.S.A.*

FRANK C. MARINI

M.D. Anderson Cancer Center, University of Texas, Houston, Texas, U.S.A.

BRETT M. HALL

*Department of Pediatrics, Columbus Children's Research Institute, The Ohio State University School of Medicine,
Columbus, Ohio, U.S.A.*

ROBERT D. CARDIFF

Department of Pathology, School of Medicine, University of California, Davis, California, U.S.A.

VENU RAMAN

Department of Radiology, Johns Hopkins University School of Medicine, Baltimore, Maryland, U.S.A.

INTRODUCTION

Mouse models of breast cancer have been used as models of human breast cancer since the 1890s (1). The landmark description of the histopathology of "spontaneous" mouse mammary cancer was written in 1906 (2) and reviewed in the English literature in 1911 (3). Coupled with Jensen's transplantable mammary cancer line, these papers were the foundations of experimental cancer research (4). The experimental era leading up to modern times used the mouse to establish the role of hormones, transplantation biology, and neoplastic progression (1). However, "spontaneous" mammary cancer in mice proved to be virus

induced and initiated by insertion activation of developmental genes not directly related to human breast cancer, and the tumors were not morphologically similar to human.

INTRODUCTION TO GENETICALLY ENGINEERED MICE MODELS OF BREAST CANCER

A new era was introduced by genetic engineering that has modeled human breast cancer in well over 200 types of genetically engineered mice (GEM). The advent of genetic engineering has created GEM with unique biological and morphological characteristics that have never been found in the virus-induced mice (1). Thus, the mouse became the mammalian model to test the oncogenicity of genes associated with human breast cancer.

The models were formally reviewed at a 1999 NIH-sponsored meeting in Annapolis, Maryland, where a panel of pathologists reviewed about 80% of the then existing models (5). The panel developed standard protocols and recommended a hierarchical diagnostic terminology. Although a large number of new models of human breast cancer have been added to the list, the basic principles outlined by the Annapolis Pathology Panel still apply.

The histopathology of GEM models of breast cancer proved to be unique (6). Most GEM tumors do not resemble the spontaneous tumors induced by the mouse mammary tumor virus (MMTV) or by carcinogenic agents. The GEM tumors closely resemble that seen in human breast cancers. The most thoroughly studied GEM group belongs to the ErbB2 (HER2) signal transduction pathway. GEM bearing erbB2, various forms of mutated erbB2 and erbB2-related genes produce tumors via similar molecular mechanisms, and also have a remarkable morphological resemblance to some forms of human breast cancer, particularly lobular and some forms of ductal carcinoma in situ (DCIS) (6). Tumors that are associated with tumor suppressor genes, such as BrCa1 and SV40-tag (that suppresses expression of Rb and p53) tend to resemble poorly differentiated tumors and, in some cases, medullary carcinoma of the human breast (6). The combined knockout of e-cadherin and p53 leads to the classic single file infiltrates of human lobular carcinoma (7).

Most GEM develop mammary tumors with characteristic or unique gene-specific "signature" microscopic phenotypes. Mammary tumors induced in myc, erbB2, and wnt1 transgenics can be easily distinguished by their growth patterns and cytological detail (8). The principle that genotype predicts phenotype has been applied to other GEM and extended to include entire molecular pathways, referred to as "Pathway Pathology" (8). The Wnt and the ErbB signal transduction pathways have been the most thoroughly dissected using a variety of targeted transgenics. The tumors arising in the same pathway share identifiable morphological characteristics and differ from those induced in another pathway. The erbB2/ras pathway can be readily separated from the wnt pathway on the basis of microscopic anatomy. Further, molecular analysis has shown that the expression profiles of erbB tumors can be separated from those of SV40-tag and myc (9).

MMTV infection activates the notch, wnt, and fibroblast growth factor (FGF) family of genes. These tumors have been traditionally classified as "spontaneous". When FGF family members are used in GEM, wnt1, wnt 10b, and FGF all induce the classical type A, B, or P tumors that were described in MMTV-induced tumors by Dunn (10). Further, the two MMTV-activated genes, wnt and FGF are complementary (11,12). That is, when mice

transgenic for wnt are infected with MMTV, the virus activates FGF (12). When a mouse transgenic for FGF is MMTV infected, the virus activates a wnt family member (11). In all cases, the phenotype is consistent with the classical "spontaneous" tumors of MMTV infection.

The majority of murine breast cancer models have been induced using the MMTV-LTR as a promoter, however, C3 (1), WAP, and BLG promoters frequently have been used. These promoters introduce a slightly different biology to the system. However, the tumors retain the phenotype characteristic of the oncogene, suggesting that the oncogene controls the phenotype. Insertion of the transgene behind the native promoter or "knocking-in" an oncogenic variant at the normal gene locus has resulted in identical tumors (13). This suggests that the tumor phenotype is not regulated by the promoter (6).

The knockout mice provided the opportunity to study the phenotype associated with tumor suppressor genes. GEM with inactivation of tumor suppressor genes follow a different set of rules. Mice with generalized "knocked-out" tumor suppressor genes generally die with tumors other than mammary tumors. The mammary tumors developed using conditional or mammary-targeted knockouts tend to be more poorly differentiated, aneuploid tumors with a wider range of phenotypes. However, when crossed with GEM bearing activated transgenes, the tumors resemble the phenotype of the transgene. The tumors in bigenic mice do, however, exhibit more pleomorphism and aneuploidy (6).

Conditional activation with either doxycycline or tamoxifen has introduced the concept of "oncogene addiction" (14). Under these conditions, the induction of the oncogene leads to dramatic and rapid tumor development (15–17). Deinduction (that is turning off the oncogene) leads to the equally dramatic reversion of the tumors to morphologically normal mammary glands. These tumors are addicted to the expression of a single oncogene. However, some tumors persist or recur (15–17). Several mechanisms for oncogene evasion have been identified. The most intriguing evasive tumor is the epithelial-mesenchymal transition (EMT) tumor that involves the activation of the Snail transcription gene (18). While not readily appreciated in human breast cancer, EMT has long been known in the mouse. Both, the Jensen and the Ehrlich sarcoma lines originated in the early 1900s as mammary tumor transplants that underwent EMT. Sarcomatous transformation has long been considered an artifact of mammary tumor transplantation (10).

Premalignancy, carcinoma in situ, has received considerable attention in mouse and human breast disease (19). The Annapolis pathologists chose to regard the focal dysplastic lesions of the GEM mammary gland as mammary intraepithelial neoplasms (MIN) (5). When the topic was reviewed in 2005, another panel recommended that the traditional test-by-transplantation be used (19). By definition, a premalignant lesion is a focal atypia associated with increased risk of malignancy (5,19,20). The operational definition is that MIN will grow as a transplant in the gland-cleared mammary fat pad (orthotopic) but not as a subcutaneous (ectopic) transplant (19). Several recent studies have now verified that the focal dysplastic lesions found in some GEMs are premalignant MIN (21). These models are of interest because the premalignant stage can be imaged using microPET (22,23).

Since the field is concerned with the use of GEMs as models of human breast cancer, considerable attention has been focused on the similarities between the mammary cancers of the two species. It is true that genes that cause cancer of the human mammary epithelium cause cancer of the mouse mammary epithelium. In some cases, there is a remarkable morphological similarity of the cancers from the two species. However, the mouse and human are different species with different biological systems. It is, therefore, not surprising that the biology of their tumors is different (24). One of the chief differences is that most mouse mammary tumors, in contrast to 50% of human breast cancers, are hormone independent. Therefore, the mouse is primarily a model for estrogen receptor negative, hormone-independent breast cancer. However, new GEM models are apparently overcoming this objection (25). The biology of metastasis is also quite different with the mouse displaying a hematogenous spread almost exclusively to the lung, and with the human displaying regional lymph node involvement with preferential spread to bone, brain and liver. The use of in vivo imaging has not been applied to the study metastasis in breast cancer in GEM. In fact, GEM models have not been used extensively in imaging studies, in contrast to xenograft models of breast cancer.

MICE XENOGRAFT MODELS OF BREAST CANCER

The xenograft models of human breast cancers have been used primarily in molecular imaging studies especially for preclinical drug trials. Direct transplantation of primary human breast cancers into mice is accompanied by rare successful takes, less than 10% in most hands. The transplants of standard cell lines into immunologically impaired mice results in a mass that can be easily observed and easily imaged. However, the cell lines have spent many years in culture and do no remotely resemble the original tumors. These xenografts, although useful, are generally not considered as "predictive" models for drug trials. One the other hand, proof of principal experiments with GEM have begun to suggest that they can be used as models of molecularly defined human disease (26,27).

Because of the shortcoming of the traditional xenograft models, investigators have been developing other models. Repasky, for example, has shown a high rate of primary tumor graft takes using the periovarian gonadal fat pad (28). The biology of the transplant appears to correspond to the clinical biology. The recombination of human cancer–associated fibroblasts and malignant epithelium also results in a human-like tumorous growth (29). As these and other techniques are developed and exploited, the xenograft models will return to their previous prominence.

Besides the obvious benefits of generating transgenic mice, one would have to consider the cost factor and the probability of the lack of a functional phenotype. An alternative approach to test the functionality of the gene of interest would be to use a xenograft model (30,31). The use of a xenograft model does have several advantages. First, the generation of the xenograft is relatively easy and inexpensive. This feature of the xenograft model would permit the testing of multiple gene functions, or the effects of carcinogens, or the beta testing of new chemotherapeutic drugs (32). Second, the incubation time to generate solid tumors is relatively short. Subcutaneous or orthotopic injection of breast cancer cell lines, such as MDA-MB-231 or Hs578t will result in solid tumors with a short latency period (33). Third, these xenograft models are reproducible making it a useful tool for longitudinal studies (34). Besides the advantages of using xenograft models, there are limitations such as it cannot mimic the ontogeny of breast tumor formation in patients (35). The human mammary neoplasia is characterized by multiple alterations both biochemically and genetically either through mutations or by dysregulation of genes or in combination (36–39). Furthermore, the development of breast cancer is rather a slow process, which indicates that the majority of aberrant cellular pathways resulting from deletions or mutations (as well as other factors) do not initiate tumor biogenesis. As xenografts are formed by cancer cell lines, attributing the observed phenotype to the introduced or silenced gene could be an oversimplification of the functional roles of these genes. In addition, the lack of stromal interactions in tumor formation is definitely minimized. As in human breast cancer patients, the long latency period could be influenced by the stromal fraction preventing neoplastic growth and proliferation (40,41). This is very difficult to recapitulate in a xenograft model. Furthermore, the involvement of any stromal cells will be that of murine origin resulting in a chimeric tumor.

Most xenograft models of breast cancer are initiated from well-established breast cancer cell lines grown on plastic over a long period of time (33). As such only a small percentage of breast cancer cells can establish in tissue culture, which underscores the need for appropriate genetic alteration that needs to take place within cancer cells for it to establish and grow on plastic. In addition, genetic drifts are common in these cell lines when grown on plastic for extended periods of time (42). Besides altered growth properties of these cells, the environment is vastly different from that of the in situ tumor. Also, the use of immunodeficient (SCID/Nude) mice to generate xenografts disregards the role of the immune system to curtail tumor growth and proliferation (43,44). An alternative to using cell lines is direct implantation of the primary breast tumor within the mammary fat pad of SCID/Nude mice (31). This definitely is a better model at the onset, but the success rate for serial implantations has been very poor. Subsequent growth of the cancer cells from the mammary fat pad onto tissue culture dish brings into question the above- mentioned concerns of tissue culture cells. Still given the caveats of xenograft breast cancer models, it is robust enough to address the effects of various biochemical and physiological factors on tumor growth and progression.

MAGNETIC RESONANCE IMAGING IN BREAST CANCER MODELS

Breast cancer xenograft models have been used extensively to study the effects of gene functions as well as to understand the tumor microenvironment. Most of the initial xenograft models generated where to analyze the functional role of genes either in promoting tumor growth or suppressing it (45–47). With the advent of molecular imaging techniques, these same models could now be used to study and characterize physiological parameters such as gradients of pH, oxygen, lactate etc., within the tumor microenvironment (48–52). In addition, the use sophisticated techniques like magnetic resonance imaging (MRI) could provide vital information with respect to the blood flow volume or vascular permeability surface area product within the tumor (48,53–55). As shown in Figure 1, xenografts generated from a breast cancer cell line overexpressing Twist exhibits elevated vascular flow volume and vascular permeability when compared with the parental cells (47). This in combination with multiple parametric imaging modalities has enabled us to better understand the dynamic tumor microenvironment.

The use of MRI to validate functional endpoints in transgenic mouse model of cancers has gained a lot of prominence. For example, sequential volumetric MRI scans were acquired to follow prostate cancer growth in an autochthonous transgenic mouse model (56). Similarly, MRI was used to detect gliomas in a RasB8 glioma-prone mice and submillimeter size primary lung tumors in a

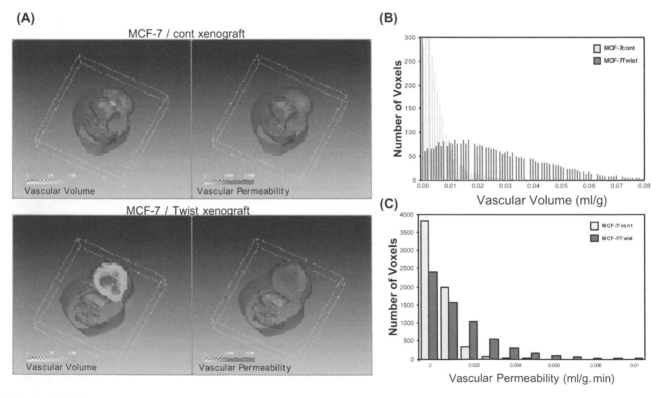

Figure 1 Determination of vascular volume and vascular permeability surface area product by magnetic resonance images of MCF-7/cont and MCF-7/Twist xenografts in SCID mice. (**A**) Representation of three-dimensional volume rendering of vascular volume (red) and vascular permeability surface area product (green) of the tumors obtained with in vivo dynamic MRI. (**B**) Histogram of the vascular volume in MCF-7/cont and MCF-7/Twist xenografted tumors (pooled data for 5 animals in each group). (**C**) Histogram of the vascular permeability in MCF-7/cont and MCF-7/Twist xenografted tumors (pooled data for 5 animals in each group) (*See Color Insert*).

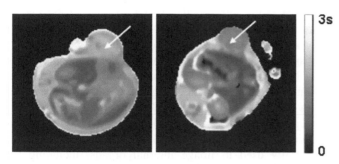

Figure 2 Quantitative T_1 maps reconstructed from MR images of female SCID mice. Axial T_1 maps of mice bearing orthotopic Her-2/neu positive BT-474 human breast cancer xenograft. Images were acquired 24 hours following injection of avidin-(DTPA-Gd) (500 mg/kg). The contrast agent was administered 48 hours following injection of Herceptin (left, tumor $T_1 = 1.9 \pm 0.1$ second) and biotinylated Herceptin (right, tumor $T_1 = 1.6 \pm 0.1$ second). Strong positive contrast enhancement (shorter T_1) is detected in the tumor prelabeled with biotinylated primary mAbs that are recognized by the contrast agent. Tumor locations are marked by arrows (*See Color Insert*).

transgenic mice (57). As depicted in Figure 2, mice bearing orthotopic HER-2/neu positive BT-474 human breast cancer xenograft could be detected by MRI via a cascade signal amplification mechanism (Dmitri Artemov, personal communication). Increased sensitivity of detection was obtained by the binding of the contrast agent to the biotinylated primary antibody bound to the receptor. Such phenotypic information obtained by MRI using mouse models of cancer will help in the critical development and preclinical testing of therapeutic drugs. Besides identifying gross morphological changes of the tumor, techniques such as magnetic resonance angiography (MRA) and micro-magnetic resonance lymphangiography are used to detect changes in the vasculature and the lymphoid system respectively in mouse models (58).

In recent times, the imaging technology has enabled us to track the migration of cancer cells using a variety of techniques. For example, fluorescent-labeled cancer cells can be tracked following injection into an orthotopic site (59). This is accomplished by establishing a transgenic cell line expressing a given fluorescent protein. Based on the excitation and emission wavelength and on the animal model used, one can noninvasively track these engineered cells by optical imaging. However, no anatomical information can be obtained by optical imaging. An alternative is to use MRI to circumvent some of the caveats of optical imaging. In addition, the recent advances in the field of MRI have enhanced the three-dimensional image acquisitions and reconstruction of tumor phenotype in a noninvasive manner (60,61). Also, the generation of new contrast agents is beginning to address the low signal–

sensitivity issue, which is a major limitation of MRI. Earlier work to track migration, angiogenesis, apoptosis, and gene expression was facilitated by the use of iron oxide nanoparticles (62–66). Albeit very useful and informative, the use of iron oxide nanoparticles did not provide the increased sensitivity of detection compared with fluorescence and positron emission tomography (PET). Continuing research on the development of contrast agents have led to the generation of new molecules such as submicron particles of iron oxide (MPIOs) that project as negative contrast and could be useful to image tumor xenografts from engineered cell lines loaded with MPIOs (67,68).

The need to increase the detection limits and sensitivity by MRI of contrast agents has led to the generation of imaging agent such as magnetism-engineered iron oxide (MEIO) nanoparticles (69). The unique combinatorial chemistry used enhanced the magnetic characteristics and the tunability of these nanoparticles, thus greatly increasing the sensitivity of detection. The feasibility of detection using MEIO particles was recently demonstrated by the detection of biomolecules present within cancer cell. Herceptin, an antibody against HER2/neu marker, was conjugated to nanoparticles and used to detect the expression of HER2/neu cell surface marker both in vitro and in vivo.

The ability to conjugate biomolecules as well as other fluorescent tags to these contrast agents truly provides multimodalilty imaging to study biological processes. In addition, the attachment of a therapeutic arm to these contrast agents provides unique opportunities to validate the efficacy of these drugs in a longitudinal study. A recently published paper took advantage of the ability to link small interfering RNA (siRNA) molecules to these contrast agents to determine both the delivery rate and the functional effect of siRNA. The dextran-coated superparamagnetic nanoparticles where linked with Cy5.5 optical dye, membrane translocation peptides (MPAP) and siRNA molecules targeting green fluorescence protein (GFP). Following generation of tumor xenografts with GFP-expressing gliosarcoma cell (9L), the animals were injected with the above contrast agent and imaged using both MRI and optical methods (70). The observation of the delivery of the contrast agent to the tumor site and the decreased GFP expression in these xenografts clearly points to the feasibility of using such contrast agents in patients to monitor the efficacy of chemotherapeutic drugs. An extension of this study demonstrated the knockdown of a functional gene such as Survivin (antiapoptotic gene), in a xenograft model, which exhibited increase apoptosis and could be imaged using both optical and MR imaging (70). Such advances in the area of tracking delivery as well as characterizing functional utility of molecules, noninvasively, by different imaging techniques will provide a pivotal platform to test and design regimens for drugs for cancer treatment.

The use of exogenous contrast agents has tremendous advantages with respect to studying tumor biogenesis and to determine treatment efficacy. However, it does have its limitations as well. The major concern is the delivery of the contrast agent to the tumor site. Insufficient amount of the contrast agents within the tumor environment can make data interpretation difficult. An alternative is to use engineered cell lines that express resonance reporter gene that utilizes water relaxation to achieve contrast. For example, xenografts using transgenic 9L glioma cell lines expressing a non-metallic biodegradable lysine-rich protein (LRP) was imaged by MRI (71). The use of frequency-specific reporter genes such as LRP can be modified to produce multiple labeling signals to study different parameters simultaneously in a given experimental setting.

ULTRASOUND IMAGING RODENT MODELS OF BREAST CANCER

Small-animal ultrasonography is rapidly becoming a cornerstone in biomedical investigation in cancer biology, serving as an important inexpensive translation tool between cancer model research and clinical application. In vivo imaging with ultrasound has been improved recently due to high-frequency capabilities (40 MHz) allowing resolution of structures up to 30 microns. This resolution is now in the realm of MRI resolution, yet ultrasonography takes seconds to acquire an image with a fraction of the cost of MRI. This allows for the ability to probe complex tumor host interactions dynamically, and to study disease and treatment responses over time noninvasively in the same animal, thus offering the potential to accelerate basic research and drug discovery using fewer animals. Ultrasound directed to the heart, called echocardiography, has been an important tool to help identify the harmful effects of cancer therapy on the heart (72).

Ultrasound imaging is the most frequently used clinical imaging modality in humans, accounting for almost 25% of all imaging procedures (73). In cancer research, ultrasound imaging is used to image primary tumors, tumor metastases, blood vessels, blood flow, and molecular targets of endothelial cells lining tumor vessels. Ultrasound imaging has been applied in the fields of developmental and tumor biology (74), monitoring anticancer treatment effects (75), and tumor cell death characterization (76). Ultrasound techniques are capable of distinguishing tumor morphology, for example, benign fibroadenomas versus mammary carcinomas in rodent models of breast cancer (76), or carcinomas versus sarcomas in mouse models of mammary cancer (77).

The term "ultrasound" applies to all acoustic energy with a frequency above human hearing (20,000 Hz or 20 kHz). Typical diagnostic sonography scanners used in hospitals on patients operate in the frequency range of 2 to 15 MHz. The choice of frequency is a trade-off between spatial resolution of the image and imaging depth. The lower frequencies produce less resolution but image deeper into the body thus applicable to humans. In smaller patients, like mice and rats, 15 to 40 MHz transducers are typically used to image internal organs, including the heart (echocardiography), lymph nodes, or breast tissue. Ultrasound imaging can be used to image the thorax, abdomen or subcutaneous tissues. In contrast, ultrasound will not penetrate bone and performs very poorly when there is a gas between the transducer and the organ of interest, due to the extreme differences in acoustical impedance.

Ultrasound machines are portable, built on wheels and can be moved easily within the animal facility, and decontaminated (from infectious agents) with MB-10 or hydrogen peroxide vapor. Transducers can be extended into a biosafety hood allowing animals to be imaged without breaking the biosafety barrier. The time required to acquire an image is also relatively short (minutes) compared with magnetic resonance (MR) or nuclear imaging (30–60 minutes). Images are viewed in real time, saved, and stored in multiple-frame files that can be analyzed at a later date. Ultrasound is less forgiving to motion artifacts. Since motion of the animal during MR or nuclear imaging adversely affects image quality, anesthesia is always necessary. Ultrasound imaging without anesthesia eliminates the effects of anesthesia on heart function and tumor blood flow and reduces the total time needed to cycle through each animal to acquire images. To reduce the stress of handling, when not using anesthesia, animals are habituated to ultrasound before the study.

Ultrasound is used to track location of metastases and measure tumor burden in mice. Preclinical mouse models have been imaged by three-dimensional high-frequency ultrasound to noninvasively track the longitiudinal growth of breast cancer liver metastases and evaluate potential chemotherapeutics in experimental liver metastasis models (78,79). Tumor volumes are calculated from the three-dimensional volumetric data. Tumor volume measurement during treatment additionally allows for the establishment of humane endpoints for euthanasia.

Doppler sonography employs the Doppler effect to assess whether blood in blood vessels is moving toward or away from the probe, and its relative velocity (80). By calculating the frequency shift of a particular sample volume, like a jet of blood flow over a heart valve, its speed and direction can be determined and visualized. This is particularly useful in cardiovascular studies or in tumor

blood-flow studies. Doppler sonography depicting the morphology of the vessels at the periphery of tumors or within tumors, has been recently recognized for its accuracy in providing data on blood-flow velocity from microvessels (54). The recent development of high-frequency probes makes power Doppler sonography suitable for its use in small animals or in small tumors (74). Microbubbles are used as contrast media in medical and in research sonog-

raphy to improve ultrasound signal backscatter, known as contrast-enhanced ultrasound. Figures 3 and 4 demonstrate various capabilities of ultrasonography in mouse breast cancer studies, including tumor volume assessment, morphology of tumors, and blood vessels.

Targeted contrast-enhanced high-frequency ultrasonography has been successfully used to image vascular endothelial growth factor receptor 2 (VEGFR2) expression on

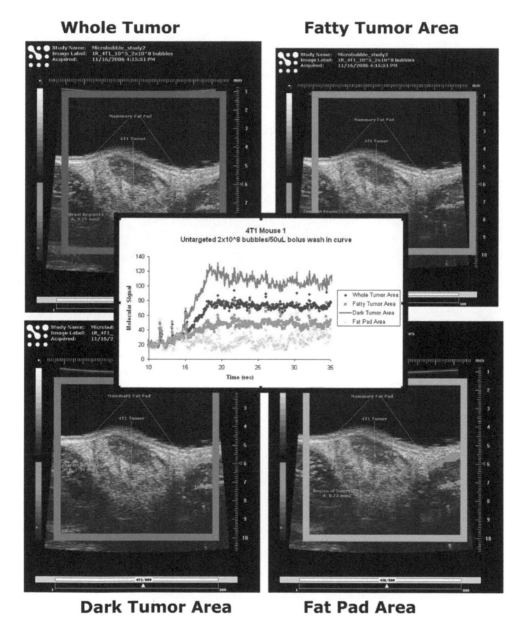

Figure 3 Regions of interest within a mammary tumor to quantify vascular patterning. The vascular patterns for four regions of interest were compared: the whole tumor, fatty tumor area, dark tumor area, and the fat pad area. The untargeted contrast agent was injected through the tail vein of the mouse and the cine loop was acquired when the contrast agent entered the tumor vasculature. Postprocessing was performed to generate the green contrast overlay after reference subtraction was done. Regions of interest were drawn over the tumor. The tumor itself is heterogenous with a dark tumor core and an echogenic fatty area composed of both tumor and fat cells. The graph in the center shows the wash-in curves for the various regions of interest (contrast intensity versus time). The plateau of each graph indicates blood volume. *Source*: Courtesy of Fenster A et al., Robarts Research, London, Ontario (*See Color Insert*).

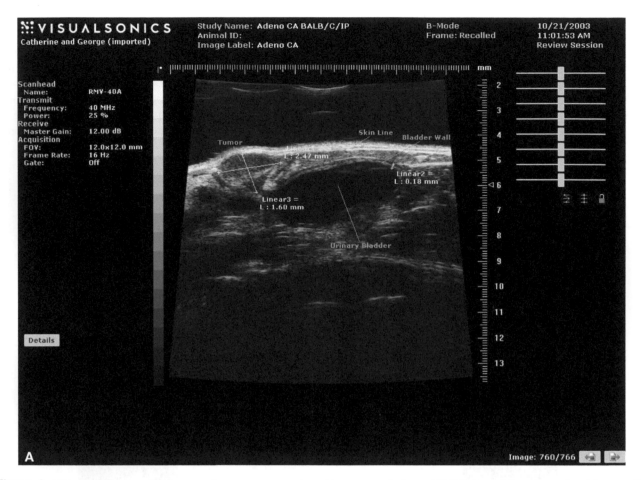

Figure 4 Ultrasound images for tumor volume measurement and tumor morphology. (**A**) Ultrasound two-dimensional image of a mouse lower abdomen demonstrating an inguinal subcutaneous xenograft implant. Images are used to measure tumor dimensions and calculate tumor volumes. Urinary bladder is in the field of view for comparison. (**B**) Mammary tumors have heterogenous signals that represent live tumor and necrotic tumor tissue.

tumor vascular endothelium in murine models of breast cancer. A 50 to 100 µL bolus of ultrasound contrast agent conjugated with an anti-VEGFR2 monoclonal antibody is injected through a tail vein catheter and tumors are quickly imaged to provide useful noninvasive longitudinal evaluations of tumor angiogenesis in preclinical studies (81). A second approach to imaging the vasculature of tumors is directed to altered expression of molecular markers on tumor endothelium. Numerous peptides have been identified that specifically bind tumor angiogenic endothelium, including the tripeptide arginine-arginine-leucine (RRL). Ultrasound imaging of tumor angiogenesis using contrast microbubbles targeted via the tumor-binding peptide arginine-arginine-leucine also has shown much promise (82).

The imaging ability of dynamic microbubble contrast-enhanced sonography, dynamic contrast-enhanced MRI, and fluorodeoxyglucose positron emission tomography (FDG-PET) has been compared to quantitate tumor perfusion in implanted murine tumors before and after treatment with a variety of regimens (83). Microbubble contrast-enhanced sonography showed that intratumoral perfusion, blood volume, and blood velocity were highest in the untreated control group and successively lower in each of the treatment groups: radiation therapy alone resulted in a two-thirds reduction of perfusion; antiangiogenic chemotherapy resulted in a relatively larger reduction, and combined chemoradiotherapy resulted in the largest reduction. Microbubble contrast-enhanced sonography revealed longitudinal decreases in tumor perfusion, blood volume, and microvascular velocity over the five-day course of chemoradiotherapy. Dynamic contrast-enhanced MRI showed a smaller and statistically insignificant average decrease in relative tumor perfusion for treated tumors. Dynamic PET revealed delayed uptake of FDG in the tumors that underwent chemoradiotherapy. In comparison to MRI and PET, microbubble contrast-enhanced sonography has considerable potential in the clinical assessment of tumor vascularization and in the assessment of the response to treatment. In a second study, tumor perfusion from

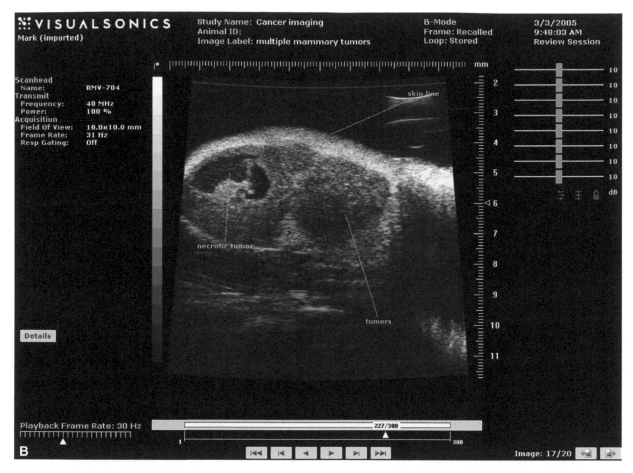

Figure 4 (*Continued*)

microbubble contrast-enhanced sonography and dynamic contrast-enhanced MRI revealed a correlation ($r^2 = 0.57$) with a statistical significant relationship ($P < 002$) between the estimates of perfusion obtained by the two modalities (84). Tumor vascularization has also been compared between ultrasound and micro-computed tomography (micro-CT) modalities. In a third study, a comparison of ultrasound and contrast enhanced micro-CT analysis revealed that both methods demonstrate the anti-angiogenesis effects of DC101, a highly specific VEGFR2-targeting antibody, in inducing growth inhibition and functional vascular changes in established melanoma (MeWo) xenografts in mice (85).

Ultrasound has been used to investigate dynamically whether changes in tumor vasculature implicate tumor tissue degeneration during antiangiogenic therapies (86). This study identified essential parameters needed to quantify specifically and sensitively the number of microvessels, and the extent of necrosis in xenografted human carcinomas during natural tumor evolution, using contrast-enhanced high-frequency ultrasonography with or without color Doppler. Unlike X-ray, there is no ionizing radiation exposure with the ultrasound approach; yet,

prolonged ultrasound (1 MHz for 3 minutes) to a tissue does induce hyperthermia, vascular and tumor injury inducing cell death demonstrating a therapeutic application of ultrasound (87,88).

Multifunctional nanoparticles that are tumor-targeted drug carriers, long-lasting ultrasound contrast agents, and enhancers of ultrasound-mediated drug delivery have been developed (89). Drug delivery of doxorubicin in polymeric micelles and perfluoropentane (PFP) nano/microbubbles has been combined with tumor irradiation by ultrasound resulting in effective drug targeting to tumors. The effect of the nano/microbubbles on the ultrasound-mediated cellular uptake of doxorubicin in MDA-MB-231 breast tumors xenograft was determined. Upon intravenous injection into mice, doxorubicin-loaded micelles and nanobubbles extravasated selectively into the tumor interstitium, where the nanobubbles coalesced to produce microbubbles with a strong, durable ultrasound contrast. Doxorubicin was strongly retained in the microbubbles but released in response to therapeutic ultrasound microbubble rupture.

Ultrasound has been used to guide site-specific gene delivery system using adenoviral vectors and commercial ultrasound contrast agents (90). The contrast agents were tested for their ability to enclose and to protect an adenoviral vector carrying the GFP marker gene (Ad-GFP) into the microbubbles. Systemic delivery through the mouse tail vein of Ad-GFP enclosed into microbubbles resulted in specific targeting of the GFP transgene. Target specificity of microbubbles and their contents is induced by ultrasound pulses directed at the desired target, which cause bubble destruction and delivery of the viral-mediated gene transfer.

Ultrasound can be applied during cancer drug therapy to induce additional cell death of tumors. Therapeutic ultrasound enhances the cell death effects of doxorubicin (91) or docetaxel (92) against murine tumors. Ultrasound has also been used to guide cryoablation of a tumor, or to guide the deposition of microencapsulated 5-fluorouracil in prostate tumors in mouse models (93).

In summary, ultrasound is useful in both cancer diagnostics and cancer therapeutics. Ultrasound has been successfully used in mouse breast cancer models to assess the location and volume of primary tumors or metastases, assess tumor blood flow, induce tumor cell death, and guide the deposition of cancer drugs to tumor sites.

NUCLEAR IMAGING MOUSE MODELS OF BREAST CANCER

Nuclear imaging is a powerful and versatile tool in detecting tumors and monitoring progression and response to therapy. The basic premise of nuclear imaging is that the subject is injected with a radionuclide-labeled compound, which preferentially distributes to tissues of interest. The radionuclide emits gamma rays, which readily penetrate tissue and can be detected by external imaging systems. Single-photon emission computed tomography (SPECT) and PET are two forms of nuclear imaging used in vivo.

With SPECT, the radionuclide emits single gamma rays that are detected by gamma cameras. A lead collimator filters out any gamma rays not arriving perpendicular to the camera face. These gamma rays create a two-dimensional image, but if the camera is rotated around the subject, or the subject is rotated in front of the camera, a three-dimensional image can be constructed. Radionuclides used for SPECT include ^{99m}Tc, ^{123}I, ^{201}Tl, and ^{111}In.

For breast cancer imaging, radionuclides have been linked to a variety of compounds that accumulate in tumors, including sestamibi, tetrofosmin, glucarate, methylene diphosphonate, octreotide, and monoclonal antibodies. The most widely used radionuclide in breast cancer is ^{99m}Tc-sestamibi (94). Sestamibi is a lipophilic cation that reversibly accumulates in mitochondria. Uptake in breast cancer has been correlated to inflammation, vascularity, cellular density, and tumor size (95). Sestamibi and tetrafosmine are

substrates of the multidrug resistance P-glycoprotein and are expelled from drug-resistant tumors. This washout effect can be used to identify tumors that may be resistant to chemotherapy (96). Other tracers that are not expelled from drug-resistant tumors, such as glucarate, have also been identified. In mice with xenografted BT20 tumors, ^{99m}Tc-labeled glucarate has a higher uptake than ^{99m}Tc-sestamibi and in mice with MCF-7 tumor xenografts, ^{99m}Tc-glucarate was shown to be retained in tumors from which sestamibi was rapidly expelled (97).

For more specific labeling of proteins produced by breast cancer cells, radionuclides can be linked to antibodies or to synthetic antibodies called Affibodies. The HER2 receptor, which has low or undetectable expression in normal tissue, is overexpressed in some human breast cancers with implications for treatment and prognosis. Orlova et al. (98) used affibodies for the HER2 receptor labeled with ^{99m}Tc or ^{125}I and found that both provided clear imaging of breast tumor xenographs in nude mice, although the iodinated conjugate had a higher tumor to liver ratio.

PET differs from SPECT in both type of radionuclide and detection system used. The radionuclides used in PET emit positrons, which travel a short distance and undergo an annihilation reaction. The annihilation reaction produces two gamma rays that travel at the same speed in opposite directions. A scintillator (either a series of crystals or a continuous sheet) converts the gamma rays to photons, which are then converted to electrons by a photomultiplier tube. The resulting current pulses are used to determine the location of the annihilation reaction and a cross sectional image is created by the same method used in computed tomography. Positron-emitting radionuclides include ^{11}C, ^{13}N, ^{15}O, ^{18}F, ^{76}Br, and ^{124}I. These radionuclides can be incorporated into almost any biologically relevant compound, including monoclonal antibodies, receptor ligands, and oligonucleotides.

The resolution of PET scanners allows detection of tumors before they can be seen or palpated. Abbey et al. (23) used ^{18}F-fluorodeoxyglucose to detect and quantify premalignant mammary neoplasia in mice, and to document the transformation into invasive malignancy. This methodology is an alternative to the standard histological methods, which require sequential sacrifice of animals with the advantage of using fewer animals and comparing tumor progression within single animals rather than between groups of animals.

PET scans can provide functional, as well as anatomic information. For example, ^{15}O can be used to measure blood flow in tumors and ^{18}F-fluorodeoxyglucose can evaluate tumor metabolic rate (94). Labeled ligands for sigma receptors, which are overexpressed up to 10-fold in proliferating mouse adenocarcinoma cells, provide both anatomic and proliferative information in nude mice with tumor xenografts (99). 16α-^{18}F-fluoroestradiol has been used to monitor estrogen positive tumors in human and murine tumor cells transplanted into nude mice (100). Sun et al. (101) used PET to image unr mRNA in MCF-7 tumors in mice. Since naturally occurring oligonucleotides are rapidly degraded, they used peptide nucleic acids (sugar-phosphate backbone replaced by peptide bonds) labeled with ^{64}Cu.

Both SPECT and PET have advantages and disadvantages in small-animal imaging. The major limitation of SPECT is the sensitivity of the gamma camera. New camera technology, including a cadmium-zinc-telluride semiconductor detector and better collimators, have evolved to improve the sensitivity for detecting small lesions using SPECT, but the sensitivity of PET imaging is still better. The evolution of small-animal PET scanners has led to improvements in sensitivity and reductions in size. A system developed at Sherbrooke University uses solid state photon detectors instead of the larger photomultiplier tubes. A system developed at University of California, Los Angeles (UCLA) uses a new scintillator material, optical fibers, and multichannel photomultiplier tubes to improve resolution. Limitations to the ultimate resolution of PET scanners include the distance the positron travels before the annihilation reaction, and minor alterations in the paths of the gamma rays (102).

Another advantage of PET imaging is that the agents generally have better tumor specificity than SPECT agents. In mice implanted with human breast cancer cells, L-^{18}F-α-methyltyrosine and ^{11}C-methionine had higher tumor-to-muscle ratios than ^{18}F-fluorodeoxyglucose, and all three had a more specific tumor distribution than the SPECT radiopharmaceuticals, ^{99m}Tc-sestamibi, ^{201}Tl-chloride, and ^{99m}Tc-tetrofosmin, (103). In 31 HH-16 mammary tumors implanted into immunocompromised rats, ^{18}F-fluorodeoxyglucose had higher tumor uptake than ^{99m}Tc-sestamibi or ^{99m}Tc (V)DMSA (104).

The major disadvantage of PET imaging is the cost of the equipment and the short half-life of many of the radionuclides. Once synthesized, the radiolabeled molecules should be used within two half-lives. ^{15}O has a half-life of 122 seconds and is therefore only available to facilities with an on-site cyclotron. A few radionuclides used in PET are commercially available. ^{18}F has a half-life of 110 minutes, and can be shipped from regional distribution centers. ^{64}Cu and ^{124}I have half-lives of 13 hours and 4 days, and can therefore be shipped to more distant locations (102).

OPTICAL IMAGING FOR BREAST CANCER MOUSE MODELS

Fluorescence and bioluminescence imaging (BLI) are the two approaches used to track and identify cells in small-animal optical imaging studies. Each approach relies on detecting electromagnetic emissions within a defined spectrum of visible light. Fluorescence imaging modalities require an external light source to excite a given fluorophor, which emits light at a longer wavelength (i.e., lower energy). On the other hand, BLI utilizes an enzymatic oxidation reaction that results in emission of visible light, and bioluminescence does not need external light stimulus. Herein, we describe some basic concepts and current applications of fluorescence and bioluminescence for small-animal imaging. In addition, we will outline some of the inherent strengths and weaknesses of each optical imaging modality.

Multiple fluorophors are commercially available for use in fluorescence imaging studies. Fluorescent proteins (e.g., EGFP, EYFP, and dsRed), fluorescent membrane dyes (PKH-26, DiI, and CFSE), vital fluorescent dyes (e.g., Calcein-AM and PI), fluorophors conjugated to antibodies or other protein carriers (e.g., Alexa 488, FITC, PE, Cy3, or Annexin-V), and quantum dots (Q-dots) are a few examples of commonly used fluorescent materials (105–109). The breadth of fluorescence imaging is far greater than BLI with respect to the number of fluorophor options available. In fluorescence imaging, it is essential to fully understand the fluorophor excitation and emission spectra as well as inherent biological properties of each fluorophor prior to initiating in vitro, in vivo, or ex vivo imaging studies. The major caveat, for fluorescence whole body imaging, is that one must consider the ability to detect fluorescent output through tissue, as tissue depth and concentration of the fluorophor will impact fluorescence images and determine whether the fluorescence target can be adequately resolved. Given that fluorescence emission relies on excitation from an external light source, tissue attenuation of the excitatory signal and emitted light, particularly at wavelengths in the near ultraviolet (NUV) to green light spectrum, can drastically impact sensitivity and overall image quality. Autofluorescence in the green light spectra, which is due primarily to collagen, elastin, NADH, and FMN (110) can also contribute to high backgrounds, especially in the blue to green light wavelengths. Fluorescence substances in the red to near infrared spectrum (i.e., 570–800 nm) tend to outperform shorter wavelengths in the NUV to green spectrum (i.e., 350–570 nm) in vivo, whereas in vitro, the entire spectrum of visible light can be readily utilized. Another important consideration when choosing a fluorophor in fluorescence imaging is whether the target of interest (e.g., tumor cell or immune cell) will need to be visualized for a short period of time (e.g., hours to days), or for longer periods of time (e.g., a few weeks to months). If rapid cell growth is expected, stable cell lines that produce a given fluorescent protein may be a better option when compared with fluorescence membrane dyes or quantum dots, where cell division decreases fluorescence intensity by twofold with every cell division.

How to Detect Fluorescence

In general terms, fluorescently labeled cells will be most visible when placed subcutaneously under the skin of a nude mouse or rat. Deeper tissues within the peritoneal cavity will be considerably less visible, and in a hair-covered animals, the fluorescence signal can be even more difficult to detect. Interestingly, white hair absorbs less energy than black hair, and yet it is frequently suggested that one shaves the regions of interest on animals with dark fur to improve detection. Best results for fluorescence imaging are obtained with nude mice on iso-Blox™ (Harlan Teklad; www.harlan.com) or similar bedding. Fluorescence imaging of mice from cages with corncob or similar bedding will display a significant amount of punctuate skin autofluorescence due to the dust and particulate matter of this bedding. Finally, if ex vivo fluorescence imaging of tumor sections is desired, perfusion fixation with ice-cold 4% paraformaldehyde (PFA) is recommended prior to tissue resection in order to preserve optimal cellular compartmentalization of fluorescence proteins. Following resection, fix small sections of each tissue in 4% PFA then cryopreserve in Tissue-Tek® O.C.T. Compound (ProSciTech, Australia).

Pros/Cons of Fluorescence

Pros

1. Easy to establish and use
2. Sequential noninvasive longitudinal imaging
3. Ability to detect in vivo gene expression
   (i) Superficial tissue imaging tends to outperform deep tissue imaging
4. Ability to detect multiple cell populations emitting unique light wavelengths
5. High structural resolution in vitro and ex vivo of whole organs down to individual cells
6. Reduced attenuation of fluorophors with emission spectra in the red to near infrared range
7. Low cost of excitation substrate (i.e., cost of electricity to power excitation lamp/laser)
8. Chemical or nonprotein fluorophors are not a subject to transcriptional regulation
   (i) Diminished fluorescence intensities can be directly equated to cell proliferation
9. Fluorescence microscopy and sterile flow cytometric cell sorting

Cons

1. Higher background noise in vivo (compared with bioluminescence)
   (i) Primarily due to tissue autofluorescence following excitation at 488 nm

(ii) Less pronounced when using excitation light at wavelengths more than 510 nm or fluorophors with red to near infrared spectral emissions
2. Attenuation of light emission in tissue (both excitory and emission light is attenuated)
   (i) More pronounced in fluorophors with blue to green light emissions
3. Alterations in gene expression impact detection (i.e., only for fluorescent proteins)
   (ii) Does not apply to fluorescent dyes, quantum dots, and chemical-based fluorophors
4. Although less than bioluminescence, fluorescence imaging equipment can be expensive

Bioluminescence Imaging

Bioluminescence is a process in which living organisms convert chemical energy into light. In most bioluminescence systems, light arises from the oxidation of an organic substrate, such as luciferin, which is catalyzed by an enzyme called luciferase. In nature, there is an assortment of organisms that emit light, including bacteria, fungi, crustaceans, mollusks, fishes, and insects. While the specific biochemistries of bioluminescence are diverse, all include an enzyme-mediated reaction between molecular oxygen and an organic substrate. Bioluminescence (in vivo) must be distinguished from chemiluminescence (the emission of light from a chemical reaction in vitro), and fluorescence (the emission of light as a result of light excitation). In 1985, the first ATP-dependent firefly luciferase was cloned (111), and subsequently many other luciferases have been identified, including the sea pansy *Renilla reniformis* luciferase (112) and the South American click beetle luciferase (113).

During the bioluminescence chemical reaction, light is emitted as the result of generating an electronically excited state. Electrons in higher energy orbitals decay to the ground state and emit a photon of light. The emission of light resulting from the electronic transition is the same process as fluorescent or phosphorescent light emission in vitro. That is, once the excited state is created, it undergoes a transition similar to that created by light absorption in fluorescence. The end product of a bioluminescent reaction is visible light. The emitted light has very precise characteristics in terms of color, intensity, polarization, and timing.

The visible area of the spectrum is 400 to 700 nm and the emission maxima of most marine species falls within the range of 450 to 490 nm. Species found in the pelagic environment (i.e., mid-ocean) are mostly blue-emitting, whereas terrestrial organisms are predominantly yellow-green emitting. Firefly bioluminescence is a multistep process that is outlined in (Fig. 5). Luc represents firefly

A

$$Luc + LH_2 + ATP \xrightarrow{Mg^{2+}} Luc \cdot LH_2 \text{-} AMP + PP_i \quad (\textbf{Eq. 1})$$

$$Luc \cdot LH_2 \text{-} AMP + O_2 \rightarrow Luc \cdot Oxyluciferin^* + AMP + CO_2 \quad (\textbf{Eq. 2})$$

$$Luc \cdot Oxyluciferin^* \rightarrow Luc \cdot Oxyluciferin + light \quad (\textbf{Eq. 3})$$

$$Luc + L + ATP \xrightarrow{Mg^{2+}} Luc \cdot L \text{-} AMP + PP_i \quad (\textbf{Eq. 4})$$

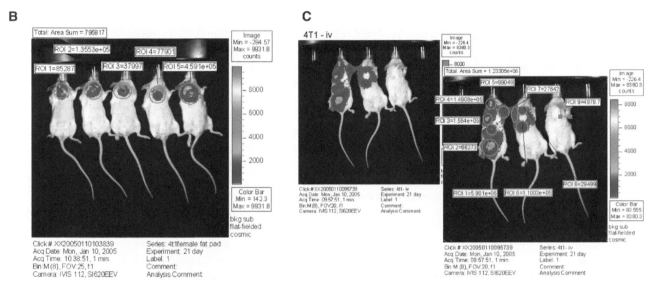

Figure 5 In vivo analysis of Luciferase-labeled 4T1 mouse mammary carcinoma cells. (**A**) Firefly luciferase bioluminescence chemical reactions generate light (note: light emissions are generated in Eq. 3). (**B**) Orthotopic 4T1 xenografts were well established in female immunocompetent Balb/c mice three weeks after 4T1^{luc} challenge. Bioluminescence photon quantitation using the Xenogen IVIS 200 Imaging System (Caliper LifeSciences, Cranbury, New Jersey) is illustrated. (**C**) Decreasing numbers of 4T1^{luc} were injected into the lateral tail vein of female immunocompetent Balb/c mice. Three weeks later, mice receiving the highest number of injected 4T1^{luc} cells had extensive metastasis, including lesions in the lung, brain, liver, and ovaries. Mice receiving the middle and lowest number of injected 4T1^{luc} cells had less extensive metastasis. However, all regions of interest (ROI) generated quantifiable photon emissions.

luciferase, ATP is adenosine triphosphate, PP$_i$ is inorganic pyrophosphate, and the structures that correspond to the other abbreviations are shown below. In the first step (Eq. 1), luciferase converts firefly D-luciferin into the corresponding enzyme-bound luciferyl adenylate. Firefly luciferase has extraordinary specificity for this nucleotide triphosphate. The adenylate is the true substrate of the subsequent oxidative chemistry. In fact, D-LH$_2$-AMP produced synthetically reacts with oxygen in the presence of luciferase to produce light emission identical to that obtained with the natural substrates D-luciferin and Mg-ATP.

How to Detect Bioluminescence

The detection of Luc signal in vivo is straightforward and user friendly, early work used little more than a dark sealed box (to omit light), and a very sensitive camera system. After injection of substrate into an animal bearing Luc positive cells, light emitted from the anesthetized animal was collected over one to five minutes and the psuedocolored image was overlayed over a black and white photographic image. Data was collected as photons per second. The newer devices that detect BLI have incorporated the older concept with some improved technology. The camera systems are now charged couple cooled camera (CCD) with a 3 to 4 log dynamic range. These cameras can detect a few photons of light deep with most mouse and rat tissues (Fig. 5B, C). Additionally, spectral filter sets are now incorporated to improve emission detection and prevent overlap of neighboring light sources. Similar to fluorescent imaging, the limitation of this technique is the ability of the bioluminescent light to penetrate tissue and is the main factor that limits the sensitivity of BLI. Currently, Luc positive cells can be detected anywhere in mice and rats, and for subcutaneous applications, Luc positive cells can be detected in rabbits, and chinchillas, and cats.

Pros/Cons of Bioluminescence

Pros

1. Easy to establish and use
2. Low background noise in vivo
3. Sequential longitudinal imaging
4. Ability to detect in vivo gene expression
   (*i*) Deep tissue imaging outperforms fluorescence imaging
5. Ability to detect low numbers of photons (i.e., low numbers of transduced cells)
6. Ability to detect multiple cell populations emitting unique bioluminescent wavelengths

Cons

1. Attenuation of light emission through tissues
2. Alterations to gene expression decrease detection
3. High cost of substrate (e.g., luciferin)
4. Substrate half-life limits imaging window time
5. Substrate must be intravenously injected prior to imaging
6. Poor structural imaging capabilities at the cellular level
7. High cost of imaging and detection equipment
8. Limited number of enzyme-substrate options
   (*i*) Fluorescence excitation and emission spectra limited to blue-green spectral range
9. Stable expression of enzyme required
10. Limited potential for direct clinical application in humans

BIOLUMINESCENCE AND FLUORESCENCE IMAGING APPLICATIONS IN BREAST CANCER MODELS

Whole body optical imaging is a sensitive tool for molecular imaging in rodents. Disadvantages of optical imaging include limited spatial resolution and depth sensitivity, thus limiting this method to rodents or smaller models (114). Bioluminescence and fluorescence optical imaging have been applied to breast cancer biology within the same animal (115). SKBr3-luc xenografts, tumor cells with a high overexpression of erbB2, were implanted and detected by BLI. A dual-labeled (anti-erbB2) trastuzumab-based imaging agent was then injected into mice to

detect erbB2 overexpressing cells. This imaging agent was labeled with a near-infrared (NIR) fluorescent dye (IRDye 800CW) and (^{111}In-DTPA) and was able to specifically label cells overexpressing erbB2 in vivo by both SPECT and optical imaging methods.

Dual probes have also been developed for MR and optical imaging (116). One example is a dual probe with fluorescent and magnetic reporter groups constructed by linkage of the NIR fluorescent transferrin conjugate on the surface of contrast agent-encapsulated cationic liposome. This probe was successfully used for MRI and optical imaging of MDA-MB-231-luc breast cancer xenografts in nude mice.

Optical imaging has been used to track tumor metastases in mice. Methods to image lymph nodes are now being developed and compared. A dendrimer-based nano-sized contrast agent dual labeled for MR and optical fluorescence imaging was used to localize the sentinel lymph node (SLN) in mice (117). A macromolecular MR/ NIR optical contrast agent was synthesized based on an approximately ^{191}gadolinium-labeled contrast agent using generation-6 polyamidoamine dendrimer (G6), which is also labeled with 2 Cy5.5, a NIR fluorophore. After establishing the optimal dose, the agent was injected into mammary glands of 10 normal mice to examine the lymphatic drainage from the breast using a 3 T clinical scanner. Immediately after the MRI scan, NIR optical imaging and image-guided surgery were performed to compare the two imaging modalities. All SLNs could be easily identified and resected under NIR optical imaging-guided surgery. Although external NIR optical imaging failed to identify SLNs close to the injection site, MR lymphography consistently identified all SLNs regardless of their location.

The Xenogen IVIS 200 imaging system for real-time fluorescence protein-based optical imaging has been applied to metastatic progression in live animals (59). Green fluorescent protein–expressing cells (100×10^6) were not detectable in a mouse cadaver phantom experiment. However, a 10-fold lower number of tdTomato-expressing cells were easily detected. Mammary fat pad xenografts of stable MDA-MB-231-tdTomato cells were generated for the imaging of metastatic progression. At two weeks postinjection, barely palpable tumor burdens were easily detected at the sites of injection. At 8 weeks, a small contralateral mammary fat pad metastasis was imaged, and by 13 weeks, metastases to lymph nodes were detectable. Metastases with nodular composition were detectable within the rib cage region at 15 weeks. Three-dimensional image reconstructions indicated that the detection of fluorescence extended to approximately 1 cm below the surface. A combination of intense tdTomato fluorescence, imaging at $\geq$ 620 nm (where autofluorescence is minimized), and the sensitivity of the

Xenogen imager allowed tumor metastatic progression in live animals to be evaluated.

With a growing appreciation that the tumor microenvironment is a critical and often dominant factor in breast cancer tumorigenesis and metastasis (118), development of more complex in vitro systems (e.g., 3D, coculture, etc.) that better mimic more complex in vivo tumor microenvironments are essential. Fluorescence and bioluminescence reporters represent a viable solution to cell tracking in complex multicell systems in vitro and in vivo. For example, xenograft model systems can be developed to utilize fluorescent or bioluminescent breast cancer cells (Figs. 5 and 6). Subsequently, coinjection of tumor microenvironment cells (i.e., stromal cells) labeled

with a second yet distinct optical reporter [e.g., enhanced green fluorescence protein (EGFP) in opposition to dsRed] allows for simultaneous investigation of at least two independent cell populations within a given experiment (119,120). Alternatively, cellular homing and engraftment within established tumors can be accomplished using multioptical reporter systems (121). These approaches are amendable to various systems and allow for noninvasive observation as well as easy manipulation of multiple cell types within complex biological systems, both in vitro and in vivo.

In summary, mouse models of human cancer continue to become more sophisticated and more refined to better model human disease. The uncertainty of cancer progression

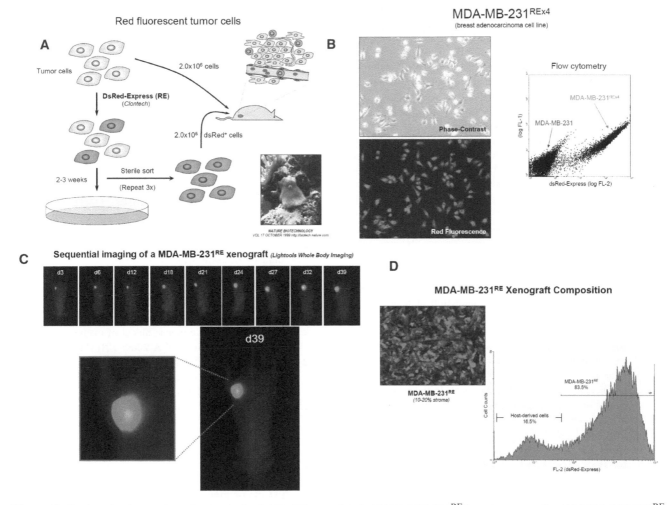

Figure 6 In vitro, in vivo, and ex vivo analysis of dsRed-Express-labeled MDA-MB-231RE breast cancer cells. (**A**) MDA-MB-231RE cells were generated by lipid-based transfections followed by two- to three-week selection in the presence of G418. (**B**) MDA-MB-231RE cells then underwent multiple rounds of flow-based sterile cell selection to obtain a pure population of stable, bright dsRed-Express (RE) positive MDA-MB-231RE cells. (**C**) MDA-MB-231RE xenografts growth rates were compared with parental (nonfluorescent) cells, and identical growth rates were observed. In addition, MDA-MB-231RE cells were imaged using a Lightools Macro-Imaging System (Encinitas, CA) (every 3–6 days to monitor tumor growth. (**D**) Tumors were resected and then bisected. Half of the tumor was fixed in 4% paraformaldehyde, and embedded in O.C.T. embedding compound prior to sectioning, and the other half was digested in collagenase prior to performing flow cytometry. On an average, 80% to 90% of all MDA-MB-231RE tumor xenografts were composed of tumor cells and only 10% to 20% of tumor stroma.

and cancer location in these models has necessitated the development of small-animal imaging modalities. Fortunately, the rapid advancement of in vivo imaging technologies in the last decade has revealed important cellular and molecular features of cancer biology, leading to better cancer therapy with improved patient outcomes.

REFERENCES

1. Cardiff RD, Kenney N. Mouse mammary tumor biology: a short history. Adv Cancer Res 2007; 89:53–116.
2. Apolant H. Die epithelialen Geschwülste der Maus. Arbeiten a.d. Koniglchn Inst. F.Expt.Ther. zu Frankfurt a.M., 1906; 1:7–68.
3. Haaland M. Spontaneous tumours in mice. In: Bashford EF, ed. Fourth Scientific Report on the Investigations of the Imperial Cancer Research Fund. London: Imperial Cancer Research Fund, 1911:1–113.
4. Dunn TB. Morphology and histogenesis of mammary tumors. In: Moulton FR, ed. Symposium on Mammary Tumors in Mice. Washington, D.C.: Am. Assoc. Adv. Sci, 1945:13–38.
5. Cardiff RD, Anver MR, Gusterson BA, et al. The mammary pathology of genetically engineered mice: the consensus report and recommendations from the Annapolis meeting. Oncogene 2000; 19(8):968–988.
6. Cardiff RD, Munn RJ, Galvez JJ. The tumor pathology of genetically engineered mice: a new approach to molecular pathology. In: Fox JG, Davisson MT, Quimby FW, et al., eds. The Mouse in Biomedical Research: Experimental Biology and Oncology. New York: Elsevier, Inc., 2006:581–622.
7. Derksen PW, Liu X, Saridin F, et al. Somatic inactivation of E-cadherin and p53 in mice leads to metastatic lobular mammary carcinoma through induction of anoikis resistance and angiogenesis. Cancer Cell 2006; 10(5):437–449.
8. Rosner A, Miyoshi K, Landesman-Bollag E, et al. Pathway pathology: histological differences between ErbB/Ras and Wnt pathway transgenic mammary tumors. Am J Pathol 2002; 161(3):1087–1097.
9. Desai KV, Xiao, N, Wang, W, et al. Initiating oncogenic event determines gene-expression patterns of human breast cancer models. Proc Natl Acad Sci U S A 2002; 99(10):6967–6972.
10. Dunn TB. Morphology of mammary tumors in mice. In: Homburger F, ed. The Physiopathology of Cancer. New York: Paul B. Hoeber, Inc., 1958:38–84.
11. Lee FS, Lane TF, Kuo A, et al. Insertional mutagenesis identifies a member of the Wnt gene family as a candidate oncogene in the mammary epithelium of int-2/Fgf-3 transgenic mice. Proc Natl Acad Sci U S A 1995; 92(6):2268–2272.
12. Shackleford GM, MacArthur CA, Kwan HC, et al. Mouse mammary tumor virus infection accelerates mammary carcinogenesis in Wnt-1 transgenic mice by insertional activation of int-2/Fgf-3 and hst/Fgf-4. Proc Natl Acad Sci U S A 1993; 90(2):740–744.
13. Andrechek ER, Hardy WR, Siegel PM, et al. Amplification of the neu/erbB-2 oncogene in a mouse model of mammary tumorigenesis. Proc Natl Acad Sci U S A 2000; 97(7):3444–3449.
14. Giuriato S, Ryeom S, Fan AC, et al. Sustained regression of tumors upon MYC inactivation requires p53 or thrombospondin-1 to reverse the angiogenic switch. Proc Natl Acad Sci U S A 2006; 103(44):16266–16271.
15. Gunther EJ, Moody SE, Belka GK, et al. Impact of p53 loss on reversal and recurrence of conditional Wnt-induced tumorigenesis. Genes Dev 2003; 17(4):488–501.
16. Moody SE, Sarkisian CJ, Hahn KT, et al. Conditional activation of Neu in the mammary epithelium of transgenic mice results in reversible pulmonary metastasis. Cancer Cell 2002; 2(6):451–461.
17. D'Cruz CM, Gunther EJ, Boxer RB, et al. c-MYC induces mammary tumorigenesis by means of a preferred pathway involving spontaneous Kras2 mutations. Nat Med 2001; 7(2):235–239.
18. Moody SE, Perez D, Pan TC, et al. The transcriptional repressor Snail promotes mammary tumor recurrence. Cancer Cell 2005; 8(3):197–209.
19. Cardiff RD, Anver MR, Boivin GP, et al. Precancer in mice: animal models used to understand, prevent, and treat human precancers. Toxicol Pathol 2006; 34(6):699–707.
20. Cardiff RD, Moghanaki D, Jensen RA. Genetically engineered mouse models of mammary intraepithelial neoplasia. J Mammary Gland Biol Neoplasia 2000; 5(4):421–437.
21. Maglione JE, McGoldrick ET, Young LJ, et al. Polyomavirus middle T-induced mammary intraepithelial neoplasia outgrowths: single origin, divergent evolution, and multiple outcomes. Mol Cancer Ther 2004; 3(8):941–953.
22. Abbey CK, Borowsky AD, Gregg JP, et al. Preclinical imaging of mammary intraepithelial neoplasia with positron emission tomography. J Mammary Gland Biol Neoplasia 2006; 11(2):137–149.
23. Abbey CK, Borowsky AD, McGoldrick ET, et al. In vivo positron-emission tomography imaging of progression and transformation in a mouse model of mammary neoplasia. Proc Natl Acad Sci U S A 2004; 101(31):11438–11443.
24. Cardiff RD. Validity of mouse mammary tumour models for human breast cancer: comparative pathology. Microsc Res Tech 2001; 52(2):224–230.
25. Lin SC, Lee KF, Nikitin AY, et al. Somatic mutation of p53 leads to estrogen receptor alpha-positive and -negative mouse mammary tumors with high frequency of metastasis. Cancer Res 2004; 64(10):3525–3532.
26. Namba R, Young LJ, Abbey CK, et al. Rapamycin inhibits growth of premalignant and malignant mammary lesions in a mouse model of ductal carcinoma in situ. Clin Cancer Res 2006; 12(8):2613–2621.
27. Namba R, Young LJ, Maglione JE, et al. Selective estrogen receptor modulators inhibit growth and progression of premalignant lesions in a mouse model of ductal carcinoma in situ. Breast Cancer Res 2005; 7(6):R881–R889.
28. Sakakibara T, Xu Y, Bumpers HL, et al. Growth and metastasis of surgical specimens of human breast carcinomas in SCID mice. Cancer J Sci Am 1996; 2(5):291–300.

29. Kuperwasser C, Chavarria T, Wu M, et al. Reconstruction of functionally normal and malignant human breast tissues in mice. Proc Natl Acad Sci U S A 2004; 101(14): 4966–4971.

30. Wagner KU. Models of breast cancer: quo vadis, animal modeling? Breast Cancer Res 2004; 6(1):31–38.

31. Kim JB, O'Hare MJ, Stein R. Models of breast cancer: is merging human and animal models the future? Breast Cancer Res 2004; 6(1):22–30.

32. Vanderhyden BC, Shaw TJ, Ethier JF. Animal models of ovarian cancer. Reprod Biol Endocrinol 2003; 1:67.

33. Lacroix M, Leclercq G. Relevance of breast cancer cell lines as models for breast tumours: an update. Breast Cancer Res Treat 2004; 83(3):249–289.

34. Smith LP, Thomas GR. Animal models for the study of squamous cell carcinoma of the upper aerodigestive tract: a historical perspective with review of their utility and limitations. Part A. Chemically-induced de novo cancer, syngeneic animal models of HNSCC, animal models of transplanted xenogeneic human tumors. Int J Cancer 2006; 118(9):2111–2122.

35. Brunner N, Osborne CK, Spang-Thomsen M. Endocrine therapy of human breast cancer grown in nude mice. Breast Cancer Res Treat 1987; 10(3):229–242.

36. Visvader JE, Lindeman GJ. Transcriptional regulators in mammary gland development and cancer. Int J Biochem Cell Biol 2003; 35(7):1034–1051.

37. Fendrick JL, Raafat AM, Haslam SZ. Mammary gland growth and development from the postnatal period to postmenopause: ovarian steroid receptor ontogeny and regulation in the mouse. J Mammary Gland Biol Neoplasia 1998; 3(1):7–22.

38. Lochter A, Bissell MJ. Involvement of extracellular matrix constituents in breast cancer. Semin Cancer Biol 1995; 6(3):165–173.

39. O'Connell P, Pekkel V, Fuqua S, et al. Molecular genetic studies of early breast cancer evolution. Breast Cancer Res Treat 1994; 32(1):5–12.

40. Hunter K. Host genetics influence tumour metastasis. Nat Rev Cancer 2006; 6(2):141–146.

41. Mueller MM, Fusenig NE. Tumor-stroma interactions directing phenotype and progression of epithelial skin tumor cells. Differentiation 2002; 70(9–10):486–497.

42. Masramon L, Vendrell E, Tarafa G, et al. Genetic instability and divergence of clonal populations in colon cancer cells in vitro. J Cell Sci 2006; 119(pt 8):1477–1482.

43. Cespedes MV, Casanova I, Parreno M, et al. Mouse models in oncogenesis and cancer therapy. Clin Transpl Oncol 2006; 8(5):318–329.

44. Dewan MZ, Terunuma H, Ahmed S, et al. Natural killer cells in breast cancer cell growth and metastasis in SCID mice. Biomed Pharmacother 2005; 59(suppl 2): S375–S379.

45. Wallden B, Emond M, Swift ME, et al. Antimetastatic gene expression profiles mediated by retinoic acid receptor beta 2 in MDA-MB-435 breast cancer cells. BMC Cancer 2005; 5:140.

46. Monsky WL, Mouta Carreira C, Tsuzuki Y, et al. Role of host microenvironment in angiogenesis and microvascular functions in human breast cancer xenografts: mammary fat pad versus cranial tumors. Clin Cancer Res 2002; 8(4):1008–1013.

47. Mironchik Y, Winnard PT Jr, Vesuna F, et al. Twist overexpression induces in vivo angiogenesis and correlates with chromosomal instability in breast cancer. Cancer Res 2005; 65(23):10801–10809.

48. Raman V, Artemov D, Pathak AP, et al. Characterizing vascular parameters in hypoxic regions: a combined magnetic resonance and optical imaging study of a human prostate cancer model. Cancer Res 2006; 66(20): 9929–9936.

49. Fischer DR, Reichenbach JR, Rauscher A, et al. Application of an exogenous hyperoxic contrast agent in MR mammography: initial results. Eur Radiol 2005; 15(4): 829–832.

50. Ntziachristos V, Yodh AG, Schnall MD, et al. MRI-guided diffuse optical spectroscopy of malignant and benign breast lesions. Neoplasia 2002; 4(4):347–354.

51. Bhujwalla ZM, Artemov D, Ballesteros P, et al. Combined vascular and extracellular pH imaging of solid tumors. NMR Biomed 2002; 15(2):114–119.

52. Sijens PE, van Dijk P, Oudkerk M. Correlation between choline level and Gd-DTPA enhancement in patients with brain metastases of mammary carcinoma. Magn Reson Med 1994; 32(5):549–555.

53. Hayes C, Padhani AR, Leach MO. Assessing changes in tumour vascular function using dynamic contrast-enhanced magnetic resonance imaging. NMR Biomed 2002; 15(2):154–163.

54. Brix G, Kiessling F, Lucht R, et al. Microcirculation and microvasculature in breast tumors: pharmacokinetic analysis of dynamic MR image series. Magn Reson Med 2004; 52(2):420–429.

55. Turetschek K, Preda A, Novikov V, et al. Tumor microvascular changes in antiangiogenic treatment: assessment by magnetic resonance contrast media of different molecular weights. J Magn Reson Imaging 2004; 20(1):138–144.

56. Shukla S, Maclennan GT, Marengo SR, et al. Constitutive activation of P I3 K-Akt and NF-kappaB during prostate cancer progression in autochthonous transgenic mouse model. Prostate 2005; 64(3):224–239.

57. Wei Q, Clarke L, Scheidenhelm DK, et al. High-grade glioma formation results from postnatal pten loss or mutant epidermal growth factor receptor expression in a transgenic mouse glioma model. Cancer Res 2006; 66(15): 7429–7437.

58. Brubaker LM, Bullitt E, Yin C, et al. Magnetic resonance angiography visualization of abnormal tumor vasculature in genetically engineered mice. Cancer Res 2005; 65(18): 8218–8223.

59. Winnard PT Jr., Kluth JB, Raman V. Noninvasive optical tracking of red fluorescent protein-expressing cancer cells in a model of metastatic breast cancer. Neoplasia 2006; 8(10):796–806.

60. Klifa CS, Shimakawa A, Siraj Z, et al. Characterization of breast lesions using the 3D FIESTA sequence and contrast-enhanced magnetic resonance imaging. J Magn Reson Imaging 2007; 25(1):82–88.

61. Dougherty L, Isaac G, Rosen MA, et al. High frame-rate simultaneous bilateral breast DCE-MRI. Magn Reson Med 2007; 57(1):220–225.

62. Artemov D, Mori N, Okollie B, et al. MR molecular imaging of the Her-2/neu receptor in breast cancer cells using targeted iron oxide nanoparticles. Magn Reson Med 2003; 9(3):403–408.

63. Artemov D, Mori N, Ravi R, et al. Magnetic resonance molecular imaging of the HER-2/neu receptor. Cancer Res 2003; 63(11):2723–2727.

64. Blankenberg F, Mari C, Strauss HW. Imaging cell death in vivo. Q J Nucl Med 2003; 47(4):337–348.

65. Partlow KC, Chen J, Brant JA, et al. 19F magnetic resonance imaging for stem/progenitor cell tracking with multiple unique perfluorocarbon nanobeacons. FASEB J 2007; 21(8):1647–1654.

66. Verdijk P, Scheenen TW, Lesterhuis WJ, et al. Sensitivity of magnetic resonance imaging of dendritic cells for in vivo tracking of cellular cancer vaccines. Int J Cancer 2007; 120(5):978–984.

67. Rodriguez O, Fricke S, Chien C, et al. Contrast-enhanced in vivo imaging of breast and prostate cancer cells by MRI. Cell Cycle 2006; 5(1):113–119.

68. Shapiro EM, Skrtic S, Koretsky AP. Sizing it up: cellular MRI using micron-sized iron oxide particles. Magn Reson Med 2005; 53(2):329–338.

69. Lee JH, Huh YM, Jun YW, et al. Artificially engineered magnetic nanoparticles for ultra-sensitive molecular imaging. Nat Med 2007; 13(1):95–99.

70. Medarova Z, Pham W, Farrar C, et al. In vivo imaging of siRNA delivery and silencing in tumors. Nat Med 2007; 13(3):372–377.

71. Gilad AA, McMahon MT, Walczak P, et al. Artificial reporter gene providing MRI contrast based on proton exchange. Nat Biotechnol 2007; 25(2):217–219.

72. Gabrielson K, Bedja D, Pin S, et al. Heat shock protein 90 and ErbB2 in the cardiac response to doxorubicin injury. Cancer Res 2007; 67(4):1436–1441.

73. Forsberg F. Ultrasonic biomedical technology; marketing versus clinical reality. Ultrasonics 2004; 42(1–9):17–27.

74. Foster FS, Pavlin CJ, Harasiewicz KA, et al. Advances in ultrasound biomicroscopy. Ultrasound Med Biol 2000; 26(1):1–27.

75. Czarnota GJ, Kolios MC, Abraham J, et al. Ultrasound imaging of apoptosis: high-resolution non-invasive monitoring of programmed cell death in vitro, in situ and in vivo. Br J Cancer 1999; 81(3):520–527.

76. Oelze ML, O'Brien WD Jr, Blue JP, et al. Differentiation and characterization of rat mammary fibroadenomas and 4T1 mouse carcinomas using quantitative ultrasound imaging. IEEE Trans Med Imaging 2004; 23(6):764–771.

77. Oelze ML, Zachary JF. Examination of cancer in mouse models using high-frequency quantitative ultrasound. Ultrasound Med Biol 2006; 32(11):1639–1648.

78. Graham KC, Wirtzfeld LA, MacKenzie LT, et al. Three-dimensional high-frequency ultrasound imaging for longitudinal evaluation of liver metastases in preclinical models. Cancer Res 2005; 65(12):5231–5237.

79. Wirtzfeld LA, Graham KC, Groom AC, et al. Volume measurement variability in three-dimensional high-frequency ultrasound images of murine liver metastases. Phys Med Biol 2006; 51(10):2367–2381.

80. Coatney RW. Ultrasound imaging: principles and applications in rodent research. ILAR J 2001; 42(3):233–247.

81. Lyshchik A, Fleischer AC, Huamani J, et al. Molecular imaging of vascular endothelial growth factor receptor 2 expression using targeted contrast-enhanced high-frequency ultrasonography. J Ultrasound Med 2007; 26(11):1575–1586.

82. Weller GE, Wong MK, Modzelewski RA, et al. Ultrasonic imaging of tumor angiogenesis using contrast microbubbles targeted via the tumor-binding peptide arginine-arginine-leucine. Cancer Res 2005; 65(2):533–539.

83. Niermann KJ, Fleischer AC, Huamani J, et al. Measuring tumor perfusion in control and treated murine tumors: correlation of microbubble contrast-enhanced sonography to dynamic contrast-enhanced magnetic resonance imaging and fluorodeoxyglucose positron emission tomography. J Ultrasound Med 2007; 26(6):749–756.

84. Yankeelov TE, Niermann KJ, Huamani J, et al. Correlation between estimates of tumor perfusion from microbubble contrast-enhanced sonography and dynamic contrast-enhanced magnetic resonance imaging. J Ultrasound Med 2006; 25(4):487–497.

85. Cheung AM, Brown AS, Cucevic V, et al. Detecting vascular changes in tumour xenografts using micro-ultrasound and micro-ct following treatment with VEGFR-2 blocking antibodies. Ultrasound Med Biol 2007; 33(8):1259–1268.

86. Magnon C, Galaup A, Rouffiac V, et al. Dynamic assessment of antiangiogenic therapy by monitoring both tumoral vascularization and tissue degeneration. Gene Ther 2007; 14(2):108–117.

87. Bunte RM, Ansaloni S, Sehgal CM, et al. Histopathological observations of the antivascular effects of physiotherapy ultrasound on a murine neoplasm. Ultrasound Med Biol 2006; 32(3):453–461.

88. Wood AK, Bunte RM, Cohen JD, et al. The antivascular action of physiotherapy ultrasound on a murine tumor: role of a microbubble contrast agent. Ultrasound Med Biol 2007; 33(12):1901–1910 [Epub 2007 Aug 27].

89. Rapoport N, Gao Z, Kennedy A. Multifunctional nanoparticles for combining ultrasonic tumor imaging and targeted chemotherapy. J Natl Cancer Inst 2007; 99(14): 1095–1106.

90. Howard CM, Forsberg F, Minimo C, et al. Ultrasound guided site specific gene delivery system using adenoviral vectors and commercial ultrasound contrast agents. J Cell Physiol 2006; 209(2):413–421.

91. Saad AH, Hahn GM. Ultrasound-enhanced effects of adriamycin against murine tumors. Ultrasound Med Biol 1992; 18(8):715–723.

92. Mohamed F, Stuart OA, Glehen O, et al. Docetaxel and hyperthermia: factors that modify thermal enhancement. J Surg Oncol 2004; 88(1):14–20.

93. Le Pivert P, Haddad RS, Aller A, et al. Ultrasound guided combined cryoablation and microencapsulated

5-fluorouracil inhibits growth of human prostate tumors in xenogenic mouse model assessed by luminescence imaging. Technol Cancer Res Treat 2004; 3(2):135–142.

94. Cho RC, Khalkhali I, Gregory ME, et al. A vision for nuclear imaging in breast cancer care. Med Solut 2005:1–18.

95. Tiling R, Stephan K, Sommer H, et al. Tissue-specific effects on uptake of 99mTc-sestamibi by breast lesions: a targeted analysis of false scintigraphic diagnoses. J Nucl Med 2004; 45(11):1822–1828.

96. Liu Z, Stevenson GD, Barrett HH, et al. Imaging recognition of inhibition of multidrug resistance in human breast cancer xenografts using 99mTc-labeled sestamibi and tetrofosmin. Nucl Med Biol 2005; 32(6):573–583.

97. Liu Z, Stevenson GD, Barrett HH, et al. Imaging recognition of multidrug resistance in human breast tumors using 99mTc-labeled monocationic agents and a high-resolution stationary SPECT system. Nucl Med Biol 2004; 31(1):53–65.

98. Orlova A, Magnusson M, Eriksson TL, et al. Tumor imaging using a picomolar affinity HER2 binding affibody molecule. Cancer Res 2006; 66(8):4339–4348.

99. Mach RH, Huang Y, Buchheimer N, et al. [(18)F]N-(4'-fluorobenzyl)-4-(3-bromophenyl) acetamide for imaging the sigma receptor status of tumors: comparison with [(18)F]FDG, and [(125)I]IUDR. Nucl Med Biol 2001; 28(4):451–458.

100. Aliaga A, Rousseau JA, Ouellette R, et al. Breast cancer models to study the expression of estrogen receptors with small animal PET imaging. Nucl Med Biol 2004; 31(6):761–770.

101. Sun X, Fang H, Li X, Rossin R, et al. MicroPET imaging of MCF-7 tumors in mice via unr mRNA-targeted peptide nucleic acids. Bioconjug Chem 2005; 16(2):294–305.

102. Cherry SR, Gambhir SS. Use of positron emission tomography in animal research. ILAR J 2001; 42(3):219–232.

103. Amano S, Inoue T, Tomiyoshi K, et al. In vivo comparison of PET and SPECT radiopharmaceuticals in detecting breast cancer. J Nucl Med 1998; 39(8):1424–1427.

104. Palmedo H, Hensel J, Reinhardt M, et al. Breast cancer imaging with PET and SPECT agents: an in vivo comparison. Nucl Med Biol 2002; 29(8):809–815.

105. Ballou B, Fisher GW, Hakala TR, et al. Tumor detection and visualization using cyanine fluorochrome-labeled antibodies. Biotechnol Prog 1997; 13(5):649–658.

106. Jaiswal JK, Simon SM. Potentials and pitfalls of fluorescent quantum dots for biological imaging. Trends Cell Biol 2004; 14(9):497–504.

107. Oksvold MP, Skarpen E, Widerberg J, et al. Fluorescent histochemical techniques for analysis of intracellular signaling. J Histochem Cytochem 2002; 50(3):289–303.

108. Studeny M, Marini FC, Champlin RE, et al. Bone marrow-derived mesenchymal stem cells as vehicles for interferon-beta delivery into tumors. Cancer Res 2002; 62(13):3603–3608.

109. Tsien RY. Building and breeding molecules to spy on cells and tumors. FEBS Lett 2005; 579(4):927–932.

110. Andersson-Engels S, Klinteberg C, Svanberg K, et al. In vivo fluorescence imaging for tissue diagnostics. Phys Med Biol 1997; 42(5):815–824.

111. de Wet JR, Wood KV, Helinski DR, et al. Cloning of firefly luciferase cDNA and the expression of active luciferase in Escherichia coli. Proc Natl Acad Sci U S A 1985; 82(23):7870–7873.

112. Lorenz WW, McCann RO, Longiaru M, et al. Isolation and expression of a cDNA encoding Renilla reniformis luciferase. Proc Natl Acad Sci U S A 1991; 88(10):4438–4442.

113. Viviani VR, Silva AC, Perez GL, et al. Cloning and molecular characterization of the cDNA for the Brazilian larval click-beetle Pyrearinus termitilluminans luciferase. Photochem Photobiol 1999; 70(2):254–260.

114. Henriquez NV, van Overveld PG, Que I, et al. Advances in optical imaging and novel model systems for cancer metastasis research. Clin Exp Metastasis 2007; 24(8):699–705.

115. Sampath L, Kwon S, Ke S, et al. Dual-labeled trastuzumab-based imaging agent for the detection of human epidermal growth factor receptor 2 overexpression in breast cancer. J Nucl Med 2007; 48(9):1501–1510.

116. Shan L, Wang S, Sridhar R, et al. Dual probe with fluorescent and magnetic properties for imaging solid tumor xenografts. Mol Imaging 2007; 6(2):85–95.

117. Koyama Y, Talanov VS, Bernardo M, et al. A dendrimer-based nanosized contrast agent dual-labeled for magnetic resonance and optical fluorescence imaging to localize the sentinel lymph node in mice. J Magn Reson Imaging 2007; 25(4):866–871.

118. Roskelley CD, Bissell MJ. The dominance of the microenvironment in breast and ovarian cancer. Semin Cancer Biol 2002; 12(2):97–104.

119. Sasser AK, Mundy BL, Smith KM, et al. Human bone marrow stromal cells enhance breast cancer cell growth rates in a cell line-dependent manner when evaluated in 3D tumor environments. Cancer Lett 2007; 254(2):255–264.

120. Sasser AK, Sullivan NJ, Studebaker AW, et al. Interleukin-6 is a potent growth factor for ER-alpha-positive human breast cancer. FASEB J 2007; 21(13):3763–3770.

121. Hall B, Andreeff M, Marini F. The participation of mesenchymal stem cells in tumor stroma formation and their application as targeted-gene delivery vehicles. Handb Exp Pharmacol 2007;(180):263–283.

24

Basics of Small Animal Handling for In Vivo Imaging

LAURENCE W. HEDLUND

Center for In Vivo Microscopy, Department of Radiology, Duke University Medical Center, Durham, North Carolina, U.S.A.

TRACY L. GLUCKMAN

Department of Molecular and Comparative Pathobiology, Johns Hopkins University, Baltimore, Maryland, U.S.A.

INTRODUCTION

For successful imaging of live, small animals, several basic issues must be addressed, regardless of the specific experimental goals. To begin with, the animal must be restrained from making gross body movements that would degrade image quality; this is usually accomplished by using drugs such as anesthetics and sedatives. The use of these drugs, particularly anesthetics, raises the next major issue for small-animal imaging, which is, the effects these drugs have on temperature control and cardiopulmonary function. Anesthetics used for restraint result in loss of temperature control. Because of the small size of rats and mice, loss of body heat can occur quickly, requiring artificial support of body temperature. Artificial support requires knowledge of the exact status of the animal during imaging, which is accomplished by physiologic monitoring (e.g., body temperature, breathing, and cardiac activity). Finally, for survival studies, proper post-procedure care is essential. The goal of this support and monitoring is to maintain a near-normal physiologic status of the animal during the imaging session, which helps ensure survival. Achieving these goals is no small task, but is absolutely necessary for quality science and repeatability of results from animal to animal.

In this chapter, we consider the possible solutions to these problems of handling small animals for in vivo imaging. Since this area of small-animal imaging research is dynamic and rapidly developing, our methods to overcome the problems can help meet the immediate needs of researchers and can also serve as starting points to develop even better methods. This area is very much the merger of biology and technology, with its progress and perfection being highly dependent on development of "new technology." Because specific solutions to the basic physiologic problems such as temperature support may vary for different imaging modalities, here we only provide some insight into the nature of the problems and offer specific solutions for some modalities. An encouraging recent development is that some imaging vendors deliver their systems with instrumentation for small-animal support and monitoring.

OVERVIEW

First, we will consider the issue of selecting drugs for restraint of animals during imaging; this is perhaps one of the most significant issues faced by the investigator. The choices made have consequences on temperature control, respiration, cardiac performance, and ultimate survival of the animal from the imaging experience. Next, we consider the issues of physiologic support and monitoring in relation to the particular constraints imposed by various imaging modalities. Finally, we turn to the issues of post-imaging care and recovery of the animal.

CHEMICAL RESTRAINT

Anesthesias

Relatively few drugs are commonly used for chemical restraint of rodents during survival imaging studies. The selection of agents we discuss is based partly on availability, ease of use, chemical stability, lack of carcinogenicity, relative safety, and cost. For these reasons, some agents will not be considered here, for example, halothane (hepatotoxic) (1), sevoflurane (costly), nitrous oxide (minimal anesthetic effect, no second gas effect in rodents) (2), ether (hazardous) (2), tribromoethanol, chloral hydrate, and chloralose (adverse postanesthetic effects such as peritonitis) (3), and urethane (hazardous, carcinogenic, and mutagenic) (1). Superior alternatives to all these agents are available; some of these will be discussed later in the chapter.

Selection of a particular anesthetic agent or combination depends on several criteria determined by the investigator—specific physiologic parameter(s) being measured, duration of imaging, need for rapid recovery such as for longitudinal studies, and need for high throughput. The focus of the following discussion is limited strictly to maintaining chemical restraint for survival imaging, a most challenging goal. If imaging is immediately preceded by surgery or potentially painful manipulations, additional pre- and post-imaging analgesics must also be considered.

Inhalational anesthesias, because of their relative safety and ease of delivery, are a popular choice for chemical restraint. As a result of rapid uptake, systemic distribution, and subsequent rapid elimination by the lungs, predictable adjustments to the anesthetic state can be made quickly, including rapid recovery once delivery is stopped (2). With continuous pulmonary uptake, inhaled anesthesias are rapidly distributed to the central nervous system resulting in brain concentration closely approximating the inhaled concentration (2). However, the actual effect of inhaled agent is influenced by the rate of breathing, pulmonary function, and vascular perfusion. In contrast, responses to most injectable agents are slower because they first distribute in nonneural tissue, and are eliminated more slowly by the liver and/or kidneys (1), making recovery slower. However, both types of anesthesia have their advantages and disadvantages in the context of specific imaging needs.

Assessing Level of Anesthesia

Assessing the level of anesthesia is a difficult and critical issue (4). Ideally, depth of anesthesia for restraint during imaging should be just sufficient to keep the animal nonreactive to the environment. The difficulty is in judging the level of anesthesia to achieve this nonreactive state and not unsafely exceeding it. The absence of response to noxious stimulus, such as a toe and/or skin pinch, is the initial method for assessing anesthetic depth. Critical for this assessment is careful and continuous observation of physiologic signs such as respiratory quality and rate, cardiac activity, and body temperature (4). Under conditions of constant, normal body temperature, changes in heart and breathing rates can be indices of altered anesthetic depth. For example, increasing rates may suggest a diminishing anesthesia depth. Ideally, these physiologic measurements should be performed noninvasively, such as using ECG electrodes taped to the paws for heart rate, a rectal thermistor for temperature, and a pneumatic pillow for breathing. Finally, it is critical that the person in charge of animal care identifies the relationships between variation of the physiologic parameters and the appropriate anesthetic levels.

The most challenging imaging situation is when direct contact with the animal is not possible and remote monitoring must be used to assess the state of the animal, such as with magnetic resonance (MR) imaging. Also, direct testing of reflexes may be undesirable because of the possibility of producing image-degrading motion. In these situations, a reasonable practice is to establish level of anesthesia on the bench top by using reflex tests (toe pinch) and then noting breathing and heart rates. These observations must be made after normal body temperature has been established and is constant. Then, changes in heart and breathing rates from the baseline rates can be used to adjust anesthetic level. Elevation of heart and breathing rates can indicate reduced anesthetic depth, but such elevations could also be related to other causes, for example, stress or discomfort. To detect such physiologic changes, monitoring equipment should continuously plot data so that trends of temperature, breathing, and heart rates can be easily observed. With careful observation, experience can be gained to make anesthesia management a predictable and routine process.

Inhalational Anesthesia

Isoflurane

A commonly used inhalational anesthetic in research is isoflurane (Halocarbon Products Corporation, River Edge, New Jersey, U.S.) typically administered with oxygen as the carrier gas. Isoflurane can be delivered to the animal using a calibrated, commercial vaporizer in three ways—to a chamber containing the animal (used for anesthetic induction), by a nose cone, or by an endotracheal tube with or without mechanical ventilation. During imaging, anesthetic depth can be quickly altered by changing the percentage of vaporization based on changes in physiologic parameters, as previously described. Ideally, anesthesia should be maintained at the lowest level necessary to ensure nonreactivity of the animal. Using isoflurane also requires a scavenging system for waste gas removal to protect laboratory staff from exposure.

Using a closed chamber containing a known percentage of isoflurane is useful for very short procedures requiring anesthesia and for anesthetic induction. Based on the vaporizer setting, the operator can be confident of the concentration of anesthesia and thus avoid overdose. This type of gas-flow anesthesia system can then be easily adapted for use with nose cone or for delivery by mechanical ventilation using an endotracheal tube. Most commercially available small-animal ventilators have provisions for using inhalational gases such as isoflurane.

Isoflurane produces dose-dependent depression of the central nervous system in rats and mice, but it also produces depression of the respiratory system (5). Mechanical ventilation, with an endotracheal tube, is an option to preemptively address the consequences of respiratory depression. With isoflurane, cardiovascular depression also occurs in a dose-dependent manner. Although a range of mechanisms are in play, direct myocardial depression predominates (5). But certainly, one of the great advantages of isoflurane anesthesia is rapid recovery once delivery is stopped.

Injectable Anesthesia

Very few injectable agents, when used alone, produce all of the components of general anesthesia, such as central nervous system depression and muscle relaxation. Most agents induce either a state of sedation or hypnosis in a dose-dependent manner, and thus, a combination of drugs is usually required for complete anesthesia (1). Unlike inhalational anesthesia, injectable anesthesias can be delivered by a number of routes. Perhaps the most common route is by intraperitoneal (IP) injection. However, the IP route can be associated with prolonged induction and delay of time of peak effect, because drug absorption is less predictable and occurs across the serosal surfaces of the abdominal organs and is subject to early metabolism (6,7). An indwelling IP catheter is a convenient way to deliver maintenance doses of anesthesia during longer imaging studies, rather than repeated IP injections.

The intravenous route is more effective for systemic delivery of both anesthetics and contrast agents (used in MR, X-ray) or radiolabeled compounds [used for positron emission tomography (PET), single-photon emission computed tomography (SPECT)]. The lateral tail veins are readily accessible for either direct injection or percutaneous catheterization in both rats and mice, although mice less than 20 g can be very challenging. In difficult cases, tail vein cutdown may be required for catheterization. The key to success with tail vein injection or catheterization is main-

taining good peripheral circulation by keeping the animal body and tail warm. For longitudinal studies, especially in rats, tail veins in the same animal can be repeatedly catheterized over periods of weeks without adverse effect.

Common Injectable Drugs

The following is a general summary of some of the more common injectable anesthetic agents for immobilizing rodents during imaging. For information concerning specific dose, route, and mechanism of action, see Refs. 1 and 7–12.

Pentobarbital sodium (Nembutal, Abbott Labs, North Chicago, Illinois, U.S.) is a frequently used barbiturate, which has rapid anesthetic onset with short duration, although it is a relatively poor analgesic. IP injections are well tolerated. Cardiac and respiratory depression occurs in a dose-dependent manner.

Methohexital sodium (Brevital, King Pharmaceuticals, Inc., Bristol, Tennessee, U.S.) is a very short-acting barbiturate providing 5 to 10 minutes of anesthesia followed by rapid recovery. This drug is useful for short, noninvasive procedures, such as endotracheal intubation, in preparation for mechanical ventilation and for being subsequently established on another anesthetic, such as isoflurane.

Ketamine HCl (Ketaset, Fort Dodge Animal Health, Fort Dodge, Iowa, U.S.), a dissociative anesthetic, is widely used in rodents combined with other agents to produce a range from sedation to general anesthesia. When used alone, muscle tone is present or increased. Ketamine also produces mild visceral analgesia. Respiration is transiently depressed with ketamine, while heart rate, myocardial contractility, and blood pressure typically increase. Also associated with ketamine is a significant rise in cerebral blood flow and intracranial pressure, and cerebrospinal fluid pressure. This property can make ketamine less desirable in brain kinetic studies.

Ketamine (Ketaset, Fort Dodge Animal Health, Fort Dodge, Iowa, U.S.) *and xylazine* (AnaSed®, Lloyd Laboratories, Shenandoah, Iowa, U.S.) combination is commonly used for short-term, general anesthesia (25–40 minutes). Xylazine has muscle relaxation and analgesic properties. It also initially increases systemic blood pressure associated with peripheral vasoconstriction followed by a longer period of lower pressure, and reduced heart rate and cardiac output. With this drug combination, the effect of ketamine diminishes more rapidly than xylazine, thus when re-dosing, ketamine alone should be given to avoid the possibility of severe bradycardia associated with additional doses of xylazine. Respiratory effects are not clinically significant.

Ketamine and diazepam (Hospira, Inc., Lake Forest, Illinois, U.S.) is another popular drug combination for general anesthesia. Diazepam is an anxiolytic muscle relaxant and hypnotic, but has fair-to-poor analgesic properties, and thus, this drug is not recommended for painful procedures. This combination also produces minor respiratory and cardiovascular depression in rodents.

Other dissociative anesthetics are used in rodents, such as ketamine in combination with acetylpromazine, medetomidine, and tiletamine plus zolazepam.

ANIMAL SUPPORT

Body Temperature

Once the decision has been made about which chemical-restraint drugs to use, the next major issue is how to maintain body temperature of these small animals. The combination of the depressive effects of anesthetics and the large ratio of body surface area to body mass promotes rapid loss of body heat (9,10), thus requiring an artificial heat source during animal setup, imaging, and recovery. We cannot overstress the importance of maintaining proper body temperature of the small animals at all times; maintaining stable, normal body temperature is fundamental for success for many reasons.

Excessive heat loss not only alters cardiovascular function, it can also lead to prolonged recovery and, in extreme cases, death. Body temperature should be monitored continuously with rectal, esophageal, or skin surface sensors to provide feedback for maintenance of normal body temperature. The exact placement of temperature sensors depends on potential to cause artifacts; this varies with the specific modality and region of the body being imaged. For example, if imaging involves flank tumors, rectal probes may cause artifacts in MR and X-ray computed tomography (CT); esophageal placement may be more appropriate. However, nonmetallic or fiber-optic-based thermometers may be needed when exact temperature is required from the region being imaged.

In practice, maintaining normal body temperature of small animals after anesthesia is a most challenging task, especially when there is a rush to image. Particularly with the anesthetized mouse, body heat can be lost quickly on the preparation table and temperatures can drop within minutes to unacceptable levels. This temperature drop can result in delays of start of imaging to allow for return of stable, normal temperature. A major consequence of low body temperature is abnormally low heart rates, along with reduced cardiac performance and peripheral blood flow. Therefore, abnormally low body temperatures can significantly affect imaging studies, for example, vascular flow in peripheral tumors and MR diffusion imaging.

In the animal preparation area, heat lamps can help maintain body temperature during setup. While using benchtop heat lamps, feedback controllers (Digi-Sense, Cole-Parmer Instrument Company, Vernon Hills, Illinois, U.S.) using rectal thermistors can help avoid overheating the animal. However, working under hot lamps can be

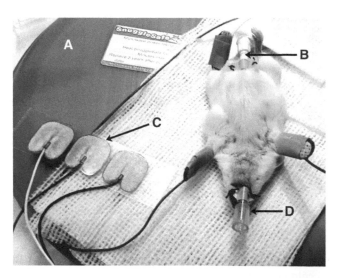

Figure 1 An anesthetized mouse is placed on a microwavable heating disk (**A**) (SnuggleSafe, Littlehampton, West Sussex, U.K.) to keep warm during setup for imaging. The mouse was intubated with an endotracheal tube (**D**), and an intraperitoneal catheter (**B**) was inserted for anesthesia maintenance. ECG electrodes were taped to the paws. (**C**) The type of electrodes used (Blue Sensor Electrodes, Ambu, Glen Burnie, Maryland, U.S.).

uncomfortable. An alternative heat source is to use microwavable heat disks (Fig. 1) (SnuggleSafe, Littlehampton, West Sussex, U.K.). When the animal is properly shielded from direct contact with the warmed surfaces, these disks can be a great advantage when used in conjunction with body temperature monitoring. Electrically silent microwavable heating pads have a significant advantage over electric (AC) heating pads, which interfere with cardiac monitoring using ECG.

Several vendors are also addressing animal temperature–support issues by including anesthesia and temperature-support instrumentation in their products. As an example, an ultrasound imaging system (VisualSonics, Toronto, Ontario, Canada) includes an animal platform with DC-heating elements to keep the animal warm by feedback control using rectal temperature (Fig. 2). However, some imaging modalities may require custom solutions for control of animal temperature, for example, for X-ray CT and digital subtraction angiography (DSA), heat lamps controlled by the Digi-Sense system previously described (13,14). However, to keep animals warm during PET imaging, heat lamps may not be desirable because they may nonuniformly heat the sensitive radiation detectors. One solution to avoid considerable heating effects is to use two water-heating pads (20 × 23 cm, Duo-Therm Pads, Allegiance Healthcare Corporation, McGraw Park, Illinois, U.S.) wrapped around a plastic cylinder with water circulated from temperature-controlled baths (Fig. 3) (T/Pump, Gaymar Industries, Inc., Orchard Park,

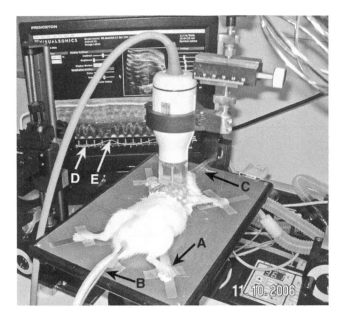

Figure 2 Example of an ultrasound imaging system that includes animal support and monitoring (VisualSonics, Toronto, Ontario, Canada). The paws of the supine rat are taped to ECG electrodes embedded in the platform (**A**), which also provide heat by feedback control from the rectal thermistor (**B**). The rat was anesthetized with isoflurane delivered by nose cone (**C**). Both cardiac (**D**) and breathing rates (**E**) are recorded from this platform and displayed on a monitor.

New York, U.S.). When the room temperature is stable, the circulated warm water keeps animals at a stable normal body temperature. The water pads of this type do not attenuate radiation of isotopes commonly used for PET imaging.

For MR imaging systems, temperature-controlled warm air circulating through the bore is an effective method for controlling body temperature. Air temperature can be controlled by feedback from rectal, esophageal, or surface probes (15) (SA Instruments, Inc., Stony Brook, New York, U.S.).

Respiration

To address the respiratory-depressive effects of anesthesias (1,2), mechanical ventilation may be needed. The use of mechanical ventilation requires endotracheal intubation, which can be performed either perorally or by tracheostomy. For survival studies, intubation should be done perorally. Peroral intubation is relatively easy to do in rats (16,17). The anesthetized rat is placed supine on a 45° slant board, held by the upper incisor; a laryngoscope blade is used to hold open the mouth, and a fiber-optic pipe at the tip illuminates the oropharynx (Fig. 4a). The endotracheal tube is then inserted between the vocal cords

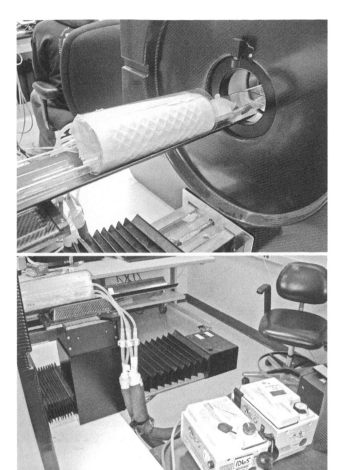

Figure 3 An example of temperature control for a microPET system (Concorde Microsystems Rodent 4, Knoxville, Tennessee, U.S.). An anesthetized rat in a hemispherical cradle is surrounded by two water-heating pads that are wrapped around a plastic cylinder (*top*). Pads are fed by two temperature-controlled water baths (*bottom*). *Abbreviation*: PET, positron emission tomography.

when they separate during inspiration. The small mouth of the mouse makes insertion of a laryngoscope blade extremely difficult and, in fact, unnecessary. Instead, a strong fiber-optic light can be directed on to the ventral surface of the neck while the mouse is lying supine on the slant board, and this illuminates the back of the mouth, even through pigmented skin. As the mouth is held open with forceps, the endotracheal tube is inserted between the vocal cords. Visualization of the oropharynx can be aided significantly using magnifying loupes. Especially for the novice, it is critical to determine if the endotracheal tube is in the trachea and not in the esophagus. To confirm correct placement in the trachea, use a cotton swab with some fibers teased free at the tip, then hold the tip close to the endotracheal tube opening and observe movement of the fibers as the animal breathes (Fig. 4b). Do not inject air into the endotracheal tube to confirm placement,

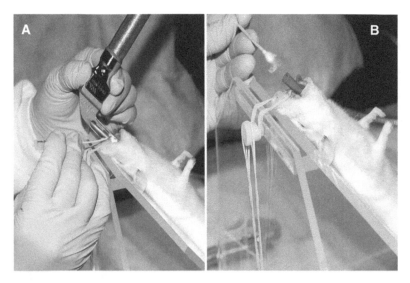

Figure 4 (**A**) Rat (200 g) anesthetized with methohexital (45 mg/kg, intraperitoneal) on a 45° slant board held by upper incisor. The rat is being perorally intubated with shortened 18-gauge intracath using a laryngoscope (Welch Allyn Medical Products, Skaneateles Falls, New York, U.S.) with a Miller 0 blade that has been cut to fit into the rat's mouth. The light from the bulb in the handle is projected to the mouth with a fiber-optic pipe. (**B**) Endotracheal intubation is confirmed by observing the teased fibers of a cotton swab blown back on exhalation.

because this risks inflating the stomach, and excess air in the stomach can interfere with breathing. Vascular intra-catheters (BD intracatheters), cut to the proper length, can be used as endotracheal tubes. However, for MR imaging of the head, catheters without metal inserts should be used (Sherwood Medical, Tullamore, Ireland). For rats, 14- to 18-gauge catheters (Quick-Cath, Baxter Healthcare Corporation, Deerfield, Illinois, U.S.) provide good fit, and for mice, 20- to 24-gauge catheters can be used. The endotracheal tube is secured by suturing it to the muzzle on either side of the Luer connector.

In addition to supporting gas exchange, mechanical ventilation can also be used to deliver inhalational anesthesia, alter inspired oxygen concentration (FiO_2), and control lung volume for pulmonary/thoracic imaging (18–21). Some ventilators can produce a triggering signal to initiate imaging at specific phases of the breathing cycle and thus eliminate the degrading effects of breathing motion on the image (18). Exact control of breathing is particularly important for cardiopulmonary imaging using MR (18), CT (22), and DSA (13).

There are numerous vendors of small-animal ventilators; however, in specific imaging environments, a specialized ventilator may be required. For example, in MRI, a conventional ventilator would require many meters of hose between the animal, and the ventilator controller and pump. This amount of hose results in unacceptably large ventilator dead space and compliance, which can result in poor anesthetic delivery and rebreathing of waste gases. A specially designed ventilator is required for MRI (23). An MR-compatible ventilator (Fig. 5) (MRI-1, CWE, Inc.,

Ardmore, Pennsylvania, U.S.) consists of two major components: (*i*) a controller (not MR-compatible), which is a stand-alone solid-state device or a computer positioned a safe distance from the magnet, beyond the 10-gauss line, and (*ii*) a breathing valve (MR-compatible) for pneumatically controlling inspiration and expiration that is attached either directly to the endotracheal tube or is very close to the animal inside the magnet. The controller is connected to the breathing valve by several meters of hose, which supply breathing gas and anesthesia to the animal, and pneumatic power to control the valve. This type of ventilator addresses all the major problems of mechanically ventilating small animals for MR imaging, and may be useful for other imaging modalities where physical configuration prevents placement of a controller close to the animal.

Hydration

In addition to heat loss during anesthesia, dehydration may also occur, especially during prolonged studies. Dehydration can affect all body systems secondary to hypovolemia, including reduction in cardiac performance and extended recovery time (7). To compensate for dehydration, pre-warmed (37°C), sterile, 0.9% (NaCl) saline or lactated ringers can be given subcutaneously (SC) or intraperitoneally. These fluids can be injected either at the beginning or at the end of the study. If dehydration is a concern, it can be estimated by checking for weight loss after the study. Possible losses can be estimated based on

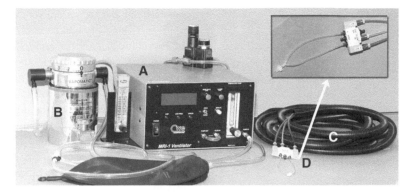

Figure 5 MR-compatible ventilator for small animals showing the important components (CWE, Inc., Ardmore, Pennsylvania, U.S.). A controller with inspiratory pump (**A**), which can be positioned safely beyond the magnetic field; isoflurane vaporizer for anesthesia delivery (**B**); 5 m of hose (**C**) connecting the controller to the breathing valve (**D**); and a short 6-cm pair of hoses connecting the breathing valve to the animal's endotracheal tube. Inset shows the MR-compatible breathing valve (1 × 2 × 5.5 cm) with the three hoses—outer hoses provide power to control inspiration/expiration position of the valve, and the middle hose supplies breathing gas/isoflurane. The two hoses (*left*) coming from the valve attach to the endotracheal tube for inspiration and exhalation. *Abbreviation*: MR, magnetic resonance.

daily fluid requirements (9), which, on average, in a four-hour period are expected to be equal to about 2.5 ml for a 250-g rat or about 15% of its blood volume. Similarly for a 25-g mouse, fluid requirement is about 0.25 ml over four hours, or, again, about 15% of its blood volume. Dehydration during the postanesthetic period should be considered because most animals may not drink water for several hours. Those animals with concurrent cardiovascular disease (e.g., valvular dysfunction or reduced ejection fractions) or with ongoing hypoproteinemia (e.g., hepatic, renal, or gastrointestinal losses) should be administered one-quarter to one-third of the recommended daily maintenance volume (50–100 ml/kg of body weight) (9,24,25). These values provide a guide for potential dehydration in small animals during extended studies.

However, losses could be much greater with mechanical ventilation with dry air or may be less in animals receiving drug injections in a saline/aqueous vehicle.

Physical Support

For many imaging systems, the animal needs to be physically supported to maintain the body in a stable and repeatable position using a bed or platform. The configuration of such a support device is highly dependent on the architecture of the imaging system. For instance, tubular cradles work well with systems that have circular bores, such as PET, MR (Figs. 3 and 6), and CT. Such cradles can be constructed to be compatible with all these modalities to

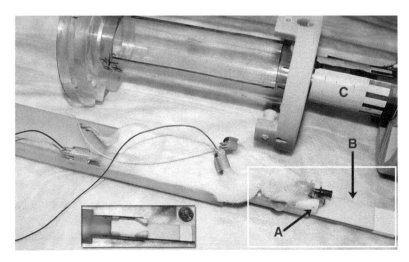

Figure 6 An example of a custom-made cradle and head holder (Quickparts, Atlanta, Georgia, U.S.) for head MR imaging. The intubated rat is placed supine on the cradle with the head in the head holder (*inset*) and stabilized by a Q-tip stick (**A**) against the upper incisor. ECG electrodes are taped to the paws. The extension of the cradle (**B**) is for positioning a ventilator valve (Fig. 7, *inset*) for MR imaging. The animal is placed in the cylinder, and then the head is moved into the imaging coil (**C**). *Abbreviation*: MR, magnetic resonance.

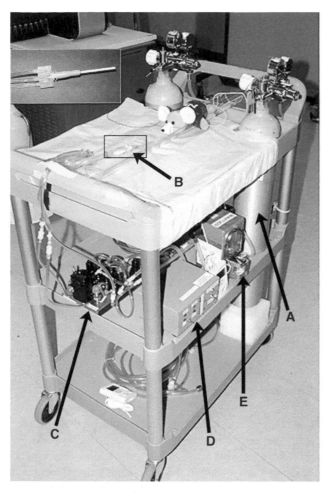

Figure 7 A custom-made, MR-compatible cart supporting multimodality imaging for transporting small animals between MR, positron emission tomography, digital subtraction angiography, and ultrasound imaging systems. This includes a battery-powered microcomputer controller (**D**) programmed to ventilate rats (60 breaths/min) and mice (90 breaths/min), and provide anesthesia by an isoflurane vaporizer (**E**). The breathing valve (**B**, *inset*) (0.5 × 1 × 1.5 cm) attaches directly to the endotracheal tube. Inset shows the breathing valve with an endotracheal tube attached. Electropneumatic circuitry (**C**) interfaces the controller with the breathing valve. Compressed air for breathing and power are supplied by aluminum e-tanks (**A**). *Abbreviation*: MR, magnetic resonance.

allow multimodality imaging. Thus, once the animal is stabilized in the cradle, it can be moved from one system to another without alteration of the animal's position with respect to the cradle. Moving the anesthetized animal between systems can be done safely, for example, by using an animal transport cart equipped with a battery-operated ventilator and anesthesia system (Fig. 7) (26). Cradles can also incorporate devices for physiologic monitoring such as ECG electrodes, temperature probes, and pneumatic pillows for breathing, and nose cones for inhalational anesthesia delivery (Figs. 8 and 9). In addition to physical stability and capabilities for monitoring/support, such cradles can significantly shorten setup time, improve consistency of positioning, and reduce animal handling. When multiple animal platforms are available, additional animals can be set up, while others are being imaged, significantly increasing imaging throughput. Or as in the special case of a multiple-mouse MR coil, several animals are set up for simultaneous imaging (27). These same principles of animal platform design incorporating monitoring and anesthesia capabilities could also be applied to imaging systems having a flat bed configuration, such as ultrasound and bioluminescence imaging. An additional use of custom-designed small animal cradles is in facilitating handling of immunocompromised rodents for imaging studies outside the barrier housing facilities. This can be accomplished safely by placing the animal in an isolation chamber, equipped with a nose cone for isoflurane delivery, transferring animals using sterile technique inside a biosafety cabinet (28). The chambers can be sized to fit into PET, CT, or MR systems for multimodality imaging. This type of isolation chamber could also be fitted with monitoring devices as described above.

PHYSIOLOGIC MONITORING

During imaging, monitoring is critical to maintain physiologic stability for animal health, survival, and data reproducibility, and this requires checking vital signs and depth of anesthesia. How this is accomplished depends on the nature of the study such as the time required, general health status of the animal, and modality being used. For example, short, inhalational anesthetic events in young healthy animals may require minimal monitoring, while animals with poor health status or preexisting disease undergoing prolonged anesthesia will require extensive support and assessment.

In recent years, imaging has been made easier by vendors that offer the basic instrumentation needed for monitoring and support of small animals that is compatible with a variety of modalities. This instrumentation typically includes monitoring of cardiac activity, breathing, and body temperature and support needed to maintain body temperature. The ideal monitoring should use noninvasive probes/detectors—ECG pads (cardiac), rectal or oral thermistors (temperature), pneumatic pillows or exhaled CO_2 (breathing), or peripheral oximetry (pulse pressure). The ideal monitoring display should show waveforms, digital values, and cumulative plots to show trends, and record and display other parameters, such as those related to the imaging process (Fig. 10).

Optical pulse oximetry has had the potential for being a valuable, noninvasive method for detecting peripheral

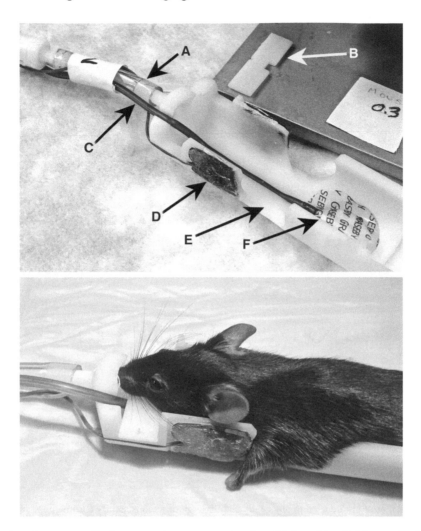

Figure 8 A custom-designed mouse cradle for magnetic resonance imaging, fabricated by Quickparts (Atlanta, Georgia, U.S.), for nose cone delivery of isoflurane, along with ECG and breathing monitoring (*top*). Hose for air/isoflurane delivery (**A**); tooth bar, upper and lower incisor notches (**B**); tube for pneumatic breathing pillow (**C**); ECG electrodes (**D**) for left and right paws, cemented to the sides of the cradle; cutout for upper limbs (**E**); pneumatic pillow (**F**). Mouse with tooth bar in place holding the head centered to the nose cone, lying on the breathing pillow, and paws on the sides ready to be taped to the electrodes using a small amount of conductive electrode jelly (*bottom*). Physiologic monitoring uses instruments from SA Instruments, Inc. (Stony Brook, New York, U.S.A.).

arterial pulse and oxygenation. However, this potential has historically not been met for small animals because of small sampling area, physical instability of the probes, inconsistency of attachment, and pigmentation problems with hair and skin. Systems are now available that provide cardiac pulse, breathing rate, and oxygen saturation from a single sensor applied to the thigh or tail of a mouse or rat (Starr Life Sciences Corporation, Oakmont, Pennsylvania; SA Instruments, Inc., Stony Brook, New York, U.S.). But, because the probe attachment depends on slight pressure, the probes may interfere with blood flow distal to the sensor. Also, any process that interferes with peripheral blood flow may preclude the use of peripheral pulse

oximetry. Devices of this type provide a convenient and valuable addition to noninvasive monitoring of the small animals.

Cardiac Monitoring

Cardiac monitoring, using ECG electrodes taped to the paws of the animal (Figs. 1c and 8) (Blue Sensor Electrodes, Ambu, Glen Burnie, Maryland, U.S.), has been simplified by using either two electrodes (one forepaw and one hindpaw or two forepaws) or three electrodes (two forepaws and one hindpaw), which are sufficient for QRS detection for heart rate and irregularities of the RR

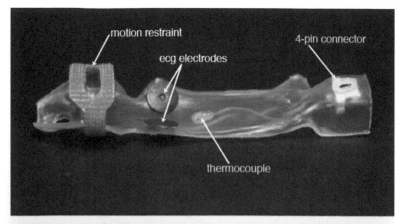

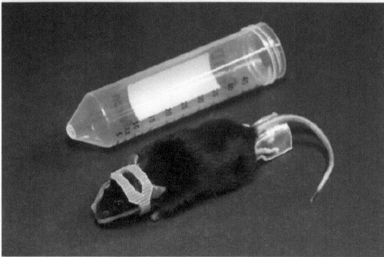

Figure 9 An example of a mouse cradle used to physically stabilize a mouse consistently for imaging, administer inhalant anesthesia, and monitor ECG and body temperature. Top panel shows a molded cradle with head restraint and ECG electrodes and thermocouple embedded in the base, along with a connector for ECG and temperature leads. Bottom panel show the mouse positioned on the cradle and ready to be inserted into a 50 ml centrifuge tube. A hole in the conical end of the tube serves as a nose cone for inhalant anesthesia delivery. This type of cradle improves efficiency of animal setup for high throughput imaging. *Source*: From Ref. 30.

interval. Diagnostic-quality ECG is not needed for cardiac monitoring, but ECG recording from the small animal does require electronic amplification and processing capable of detecting sub-millivolt signals and processing heart rates up to 600 and 700 beats/minute. These requirements are met by a number of vendors (such as SA Instruments, Inc., Stony Brook, New York, U.S.).

Body Temperature

Rectal or esophageal temperature probes (thermistor or thermocouple) are suitable for monitoring body temperature. Temperature can also be measured from the surface by positioning the animal on the probe (Fig. 9) and then correcting this measurement based on the core body temperature. As previously mentioned, there are several types of heat sources and methods for feedback control of body temperature.

Respiration

Respiration can be monitored by recording breathing movement based on the pressure changes from a pneumatic pillow placed under the animal (Fig. 8) or from a pneumatic belt around the thorax. These devices indicate mechanical performance of breathing, both frequency and magnitude of inspiration. Respiration can also be monitored by measuring exhaled carbon dioxide using a capnometer, which also provides breathing frequency, and can indicate the adequacy of breathing or ventilation, based on measurement of end-tidal CO_2. Normal end-tidal CO_2 ranges from 35 to 45 mmHg; below 20 mmHg indicates hyperventilation associated with a respiratory alkalosis, while values above 60 mmHg indicate hypoventilation, respiratory acidosis, and hypoxemia. Blood gas analysis of arterial samples can also be used to assess effectiveness of gas exchange as it yields information on

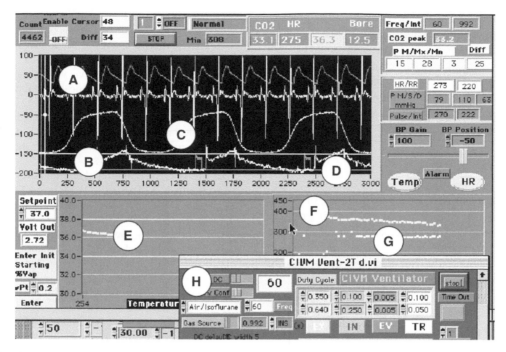

Figure 10 The video monitor display of custom-built physiologic monitoring system, which shows a variety of important parameters as waveforms, digital values, and cumulative records. ECG from foot-pad electrodes, arterial pressure from the carotid artery (**A**); airway pressure (**B**); exhaled CO_2 (**C**) showing end-tidal CO_2 values in a digital display (*top right*); a square wave pulse representing a scan trigger pulse synchronous with the ventilation cycle (**D**); and cumulative records of body temperature (**E**), exhaled CO_2 (**F**), and heart rate (**G**). Inset shows the ventilator control panel (**H**). *Source*: From Ref. 18.

circulating PaO_2, $PaCO_2$, and acid/base status (29). Since this method is invasive, it is not appropriate for routine monitoring.

MR imaging poses unique challenges for physiologic monitoring. The use of strong magnetic and radiofrequency (RF) fields makes most conventional physiologic monitoring equipment basically incompatible, with some exceptions—those devices that use pneumatics, such as breathing pillows (Fig. 8) and capnography. However, for capnography, the length of tubing needed to sample exhaled CO_2 from an animal in an imaging magnet may dampen the waveform sufficiently to prevent accurately estimating end-tidal CO_2, but capnography can still be used for monitoring breathing frequency. In addition to the fundamental magnetic/RF incompatibilities, the animal is no longer directly visually and physically accessible because it is within the bore of the magnet. Thus, the animal must be completely instrumented for physiologic recording before being put in the magnet. The animal is then connected to signal-processing and display instrumentation located a safe distance from the magnet. Care must be taken to ensure that wires and other metallic components are out of the imaging field to avoid image artifacts. Any wires coming from the animal in the bore of the magnet must be shielded and signals filtered to avoid introducing noise into the image and minimize noise

in the recording. An alternative to metallic wires is to use fiber-optic cables for ECG and body temperature (SA Instruments, Inc., Stony Brook, New York, U.S.).

POST-IMAGING CARE

For post-imaging recovery, several issues must be considered. With an animal anesthetized by nose cone delivery of inhaled anesthetics, recovery should occur very quickly when delivery is stopped. However, for animals on mechanical ventilation that are anesthetized with inhalants or injectables, the major issue is when to extubate. If extubation occurs before deep spontaneous breathing has been established, the animal may stop breathing when the endotracheal tube is removed, requiring reintubation. If extubation is delayed, there is a risk of tracheal damage if the animal struggles.

Extubation should be safe when a swallow reflex is present following mild stimulation of the tongue or mouth, which indicates pharyngeal tone has returned. For added assurance of an unobstructed airway and subsequent survival, any accumulated fluid should be aspirated from the back of the animal's mouth. Dehydration may be an issue depending on the duration of the study, and fluid therapy may be needed during recovery (see the section on hydration).

Essential to recovery is maintenance of body temperature. Low body temperature will certainly prolong recovery. To provide temperature support, a heat lamp could be used over the cage or the cage could be placed on a histology slide warmer. To avoid overheating, the temperature of the animal should continue to be monitored. Exogenous heat support should be maintained until the animal is ambulatory and able to generate endogenous heat.

CONCLUSION

This textbook is testimony to the importance of small-animal imaging in cancer research. The impressive physics and engineering advancements that enabled the realization of these marvelous advanced imaging machines have traditionally overshadowed importance of the animal side of this biomedical evolution, that is, the technology and methodology that enable the imaging of live, very small animals, in these complex machines. In this chapter, we have emphasized the importance of attending to the small-animal issues involved with in vivo imaging. Similar to any patient being imaged in a radiology department, small animals must be "still," must be kept physiologically stable during imaging, and must survive the experience. The most expensive and sophisticated imaging system is worthless for this type of small-animal research if the investigator cannot ensure that the animal survives. We hope this chapter highlights the importance of attending to the significant needs of these small animals during imaging and provides some guidance for success in this effort.

ACKNOWLEDGMENTS

The authors thank the many investigators who have challenged us to develop solutions to the many difficult problems of handling small animals in an imaging environment. Thanks to T. Wheeler BS, B. Fubara BS, and Y. Qi MD for their expertise in small-animal handling; J. Nouls MS, G. Cofer MS, and J. Pollaro MS for technical contributions; and F. J. Sun DVM, DACLAM for helpful veterinary discussions. And special thanks to S. Zimney MEd for final editing and production of this manuscript. Support was provided by NIH/NCRR (P41 RR005959) and NCI/SAIRP (U24 CA092656) for development of technology, methods, and the applications described.

REFERENCES

1. Wixson SK, Smiler KL. Chapter 9: anesthesia and analgesia in rodents. In: Kohn DF, Wixson SK, White WJ, et al. eds. Anesthesia and Analgesia in Laboratory Animals. San Diego: Academic Press, 1997:165–203.
2. Brunson DR. Chapter 2: pharmacology of inhalational anesthetics. In: Kohn DF, Wixson SK, White WJ, et al. eds. Anesthesia and Analgesia in Laboratory Animals. San Diego: Academic Press, 1997:29–41.
3. Meyer RE, Fish RE. A review of tribromoethanol anesthesia for production of genetically engineered mice and rats. Lab Animal (NY) 2005; 34(10):47–52.
4. Mason DE, Brown MJ. Chapter 5: monitoring of anesthesia In: Kohn DF, Wixson SK, White WJ, et al. eds. Anesthesia and Analgesia in Laboratory Animals. San Diego: Academic Press, 1997:73–82.
5. Steffey EP. Chapter 11: inhalation anesthetics. In: Thurmon J, Tranquilli W, Benson GJ, eds. Lumb and Jones' Veterinary Anesthesia. 3rd ed. Baltimore: Williams & Wilkins, 1996:297–329.
6. Corcoran AC, Page IH. Effects of anesthetic dosage of pentobarbital sodium on renal function and blood pressure in dogs. Am J Physiol 1943; 140:234.
7. Thurmon J, Tranquilli W, Benson GJ, eds. Lumb and Jones' Veterinary Anesthesia. 3rd ed. Baltimore: Williams & Wilkins, 1996:928.
8. Plumb DC. Plumb's Veterinary Drug Handbook. 5th ed. Ames: Blackwell Publishing, 2005:929.
9. Flecknell PA. Laboratory Animal Anesthesia: An Introduction for Research Workers and Technicians. 1st ed. San Diego: Academic Press, Ltd., 1987:156.
10. Meyer RE, Braun RD, Dewhirst MW. Anesthetic considerations for the study of murine tumors. In: Teicher BA, ed. Tumor Models in Cancer Research. Totowa: Humana Press Inc., 2002:407–431.
11. Harkness JE, Wagner JE. The Biology and Medicine of Rabbits and Rodents. 4th ed. Baltimore: Williams and Wilkins, 1995:392.
12. Hawk CT, Leary SL, Morris T. Formulary for Laboratory Animals. Ames: Blackwell Publishing, 2005:216.
13. Lin MD, Samei E, Badea CT, et al. Optimized radiographic spectra for small animal digital subtraction angiography. Med Phys 2006; 33(11):4249–4257.
14. Badea CT, Hedlund LW, Lin MD, et al. Tumor imaging in small animals with a combined micro-CT/micro-DSA system using iodinated conventional and blood pool contrast agents. Contrast Media Mol Imaging 2006; 1(4):153–164.
15. Qiu H, Cofer GP, Hedlund LW, et al. Automated feedback control of body temperature for small animal studies with MR microscopy. IEEE Trans Biomed Eng 1997; 44(11):1107–1113.
16. Thet LA. A simple method of intubating rats under direct vision. Lab Anim Sci 1983; 33(4):368–369.
17. Costa DL, Lehmann JR, Harold WM, et al. Transoral tracheal intubation of rodents using a fiberoptic laryngoscope. Lab Anim Sci 1986; 36(3):256–261.
18. Hedlund LW, Johnson GA. Mechanical ventilation for imaging the small animal lung. ILAR J 2002; 43(3):159–174.
19. Driehuys B, Cofer GP, Pollaro J, et al. Imaging alveolar-capillary gas transfer using hyperpolarized 129Xe MRI. Proc Natl Acad Sci U S A 2006; 103(48):18278–18283.
20. Driehuys B, Hedlund LW. Imaging techniques for small animal models of pulmonary disease: MR microscopy. Toxicol Pathol 2007; 35(1):49–58.

21. Chen BT, Yordanov AT, Johnson GA. Ventilation-synchronous MR microscopy of pulmonary structure and ventilation in mice. Magn Reson Med 2005; 53(1):69–75.

22. Badea CT, Hedlund LW, Johnson GA. Micro-CT with respiratory and cardiac gating. Med Phys 2004; 31(12): 3324–3329.

23. Hedlund LW, Cofer GP, Owen SJ, et al. MR-compatible ventilator for small animals: computer-controlled ventilation for proton and noble gas imaging. Magn Reson Imaging 2000; 18(6):753–759.

24. Oglesbee B. Emergency medicine of pocket pets. In: Bonagura JD, ed. Current Veterinary Therapy XII: Small Animal Practice. Philadelphia: W.B. Saunders, 1995: 1328–1331.

25. DiBartola SP. Fluid Therapy in Small Animal Practice. Philadelphia: W.B. Saunders, 2000:611.

26. Bowsher J, Yuan H, Hedlund L, et al. Using a priori MRI information to estimate F18-FDG distributions in rat flank tumors. IEEE Nuclear Science Symposium and Medical Imaging Conference. Rome, Italy: October 16-22, 2004.

27. Bock NA, Nieman BJ, Bishop JB, et al. In vivo multiple-mouse MRI at 7 Tesla. Magn Reson Med 2005; 54(5): 1311–1316.

28. Stout DB, Chatziioannou AF, Lawson TP, et al. Small animal imaging center design: the facility at the UCLA crump institute for molecular imaging. Mol Imaging Biol 2005; 7(6):393–402.

29. McDonell W. Chapter 6: respiratory system. In: Thurmon J, Tranquilli W, Benson GJ, eds. Lumb and Jones' Veterinary Anesthesia. 3rd Ed. Baltimore: Williams & Wilkins, 1996:115–147.

30. Dazai J, Bock NA, Nieman BJ, et al. Multiple mouse biological loading and monitoring system for MRI. Magn Reson Med 2004; 52(4):709–715.

25

Imaging Cellular Networks and Protein-Protein Interactions In Vivo

SNEHAL NAIK, BRITNEY L. MOSS, and DAVID PIWNICA-WORMS

Molecular Imaging Center, Mallinckrodt Institute of Radiology and Department of Molecular Biology and Pharmacology, Washington University School of Medicine, St. Louis, Missouri, U.S.A.

ANDREA PICHLER-WALLACE

Molecular Imaging Center, Mallinckrodt Institute of Radiology, Washington University School of Medicine, St. Louis, Missouri, U.S.A.

INTRODUCTION

One goal of molecular imaging is to advance the understanding of biology and medicine through noninvasive in vivo investigation of the cellular and molecular events mediating normal physiology and pathological processes (1). While some aspects of molecular imaging relate to clinical applications, a great deal of basic research is performed with cellular and animal models of disease. In practice, molecular imaging can complement, and in some cases, replace conventional laboratory techniques. Routinely used methodologies in the laboratory and in vitro settings are based on destructive sampling of cells or tissue samples, which yield only a static snapshot at a given experimental endpoint. New molecular imaging technologies now allow for noninvasive, repetitive in vivo imaging of dynamic biological processes.

In this regard, one fundamental area of active molecular imaging research that was not thought possible a few years ago, focuses on interrogation of signal transduction pathways and protein-protein interactions in live cells and animals.

Regulation of gene expression and protein function in normal physiology is complex and occurs at multiple stages. Messenger RNA (mRNA) levels are controlled both at the transcriptional (gene expression) and posttranscriptional (mRNA processing) phases. In addition, translating mRNA into the protein of interest contains several potential levels of regulation. Once translated, protein and enzyme activities and subcellular localization are controlled by processes known collectively as posttranslational modifications, which result in phosphorylation, nitrosylation, ubiquitination, and acylation of the protein of interest. The protein, both in its native state or modified, can reversibly associate with a diverse family of protein partners that regulate the subcellular localization, catalytic function, and biological activity of the protein of interest. Multiple extracellular stimuli often impact gene expression and protein function through these coordinated modifications to dynamically control protein levels and bioactivity within the cell, constituting a diverse array of communication and regulatory networks within the cell termed signal transduction pathways. Evidence is accumulating that pathways of protein interactions in specific tissues produce regional effects that cannot be investigated fully with in vitro systems and thus, there is considerable interest in evaluating protein interactions in living animals in vivo and in real time using molecular imaging strategies.

Overall, imaging reagents can comprise injectable radiopharmaceuticals and contrast agents, with or without activation strategies, or genetically encoded reporters. Both types of reagents are useful in biological studies, but injectable agents have the potential to directly translate to the clinic. Except in the context of gene therapy, genetically encoded reporters are less likely to be used in humans, but possess a fundamental advantage in basic research in that once validated, a genetically encoded reporter can theoretically be cloned into a variety of vectors and a broad array of regulatory pathways can be interrogated with the same validated reporter. For radiopharmaceuticals, this eliminates constraints inherent to traditional routes of synthesizing, labeling and validating a new and different radioligand for every new receptor or protein of interest. Genetically encoded imaging reporters also provide the potential for a stable source of signal, enabling longitudinal studies in living organisms with high temporal resolution and, in some cases, high spatial resolution.

These reporters can be easily introduced into cells and transgenic animals to enable noninvasive, long-term studies of dynamic biological processes in intact cells and living animals (1). These reporters can produce signal intrinsically (e.g., fluorescent proteins), through enzymatic activation of an inactive substrate (luciferases), by enzymatic modification of an active (e.g., radiolabeled) substrate with selective retention in reporter cells, or by direct binding or import of an active (e.g., radiolabeled) reporter substrate or probe. The most common reporters include firefly luciferase (FLuc) (bioluminescence imaging), green fluorescent protein (GFP) (fluorescence imaging), transferrin receptor (magnetic resonance imaging), Herpes Simplex Virus-1 thymidine kinase (HSV-1-TK) (positron emission tomography, PET) and variants with enhanced spectral and kinetic properties optimized for use in vivo. When cloned into promoter/enhancer sequences or engineered into fusion proteins, imaging reporters enable fundamental processes, such as transcriptional regulation, signal transduction cascades, protein-protein interactions, protein degradation, oncogenic transformation, cell trafficking, and targeted drug action to be temporally and spatially registered in vivo. Ideally, the magnitude and time course of reporter gene activity should parallel the strength and duration of expression of the endogenous target gene. This chapter focuses on the use of luciferase-based reporter systems in the context of transcriptional or posttranscriptional events to monitor protein-protein interactions and dynamic signaling in complex cellular networks.

IMAGING TRANSCRIPTIONAL EVENTS

Genetically encoded molecular imaging reporters offer the ability to indirectly monitor protein-protein interactions, or to directly monitor the transcriptional responses occurring downstream of signal transduction cascades. Furthermore, these techniques can be used to dynamically monitor signaling events within live cells and/or live animals noninvasively (1–3).

Compared with studies of protein interactions in cultured cells, strategies to interrogate protein-protein interactions in living organisms impose even further constraints on reporter systems and mechanisms of detection. Most strategies for detecting protein-protein interactions in intact cells are based on fusion of the pair of interacting molecules to defined protein elements to reconstitute a biological or biochemical function. Examples of reconstituted activities include activation of transcription, repression of transcription, activation of signal transduction pathways, or reconstitution of a disrupted enzymatic activity (4). A variety of these techniques have been developed to investigate protein-protein interactions in cultured cells. The two-hybrid system is the most widely applied method to identify and characterize protein interactions.

Two-hybrid systems exploit the modular nature of transcription factors, many of which can be separated into discrete DNA-binding and activation domains (5). Proteins of interest are expressed as fusions with either a DNA-binding domain (BD) or an activation domain (AD), creating hybrid proteins. As a result of an interaction between the proteins of interest, the separate BD and AD of the transcription factor are brought together within the cell nucleus to drive expression of a reporter gene. In the absence of specific interaction between the hybrid proteins, the reporter gene is not expressed because the BD and AD do not associate independently. Two-hybrid assays can detect transient and/or unstable interactions between proteins, and the technique is reported to be independent of expression of endogenous proteins (6). Although the two-hybrid assay originally was developed in yeast, commercial systems (BD Biosciences, Clontech) are now available for studies in bacteria and mammalian cells. Two-hybrid systems can successfully be used to image protein interactions in living mice with PET (7,8) or bioluminescence imaging (9).

For example, p53 and large T antigen (TAg) were fused to the Gal4 DNA-BD from *Saccharomyces cerevisiae* (Gal4-BD-p53) and the VP16 AD from HSV-1 (VP16-TAg), respectively (8). The specific binding of p53 to SV40 TAg leads to reconstitution of the Gal4/VP16 activator that can then induce expression of a reporter gene composed of a novel mutant HSV-1-TK/GFP fusion reporter driven by a promoter composed of five copies of Gal4 DNA-binding sequences and a minimal TATA box promoter (Gal4 → mNLS-sr39TK-EGFP). In the absence of interacting proteins, or in the presence of proteins that did not bind, only basal reporter activity was detected in cultured cells and in tumors in vivo. By using micro-PET imaging with 9-(4-[^{18}F]fluoro-3-hydroxymethylbutyl)guanine (^{18}F-FHBG), which TK can phosphorylate, thus trapping the radioactive product within cells, we detected binding of p53 and TAg in living mice and quantified an approximately sixfold enhancement of mNLS-sr39TK activity in response to interactions of these two proteins in vivo. Furthermore, the GFP component of the fusion reporter gene could also be imaged upon binding of p53 and SV40 TAg in vitro and in vivo (Fig. 1). Further work demonstrated that this imaging-based two-hybrid system responds in a proportional fashion to increasing amounts of interacting proteins in vivo (7). Thus, use of this technique allows protein complexes to be studied in the context of the regulatory pathways that modulate protein interactions in living animals and can potentially facilitate studies of pharmacokinetics, pharmacodynamics, and overall efficacy of drugs targeted to specific protein-protein interactions.

However, the two-hybrid method has some limitations. Some types of proteins do not lend themselves to study by the two-hybrid method. For example, because production of signal in the two-hybrid method requires nuclear localization of the hybrid proteins, membrane proteins cannot be studied in their intact state (though other techniques exist that may be more suitable for these types of proteins, see below). Also, the time delay associated with both transcriptional activation of the reporter gene and degradation of the reporter protein and mRNA limits kinetic analysis of protein interactions (10).

Other transcriptional read-out strategies exist that offer variations on the system described above that may be better suited to the properties of the proteins of interest. The split-ubiquitin system enables signal amplification from a transcription factor-mediated reporter readout (11,12). In one application, the interaction of two membrane proteins forces reconstitution of two halves of ubiquitin, leading to a cleavage event mediated by ubiquitin-specific proteases that release an artificial transcription factor to activate an imageable reporter gene. In the cytokine-receptor-based interaction trap method, a signaling-deficient receptor provides a scaffold for recruitment of interacting fusion proteins that phosphorylate endogenous signal transducers and activators of transcription-3 (STAT3). Activated STAT complexes then drive a nuclear reporter (13). This system permits detection of both modification-independent and phosphorylation-dependent interactions in intact mammalian cells, but the transcriptional readout again limits kinetic analysis.

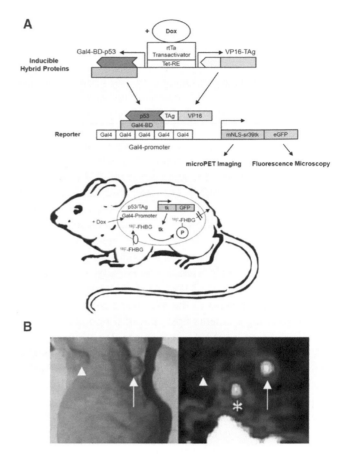

Figure 1 Imaging protein-protein interactions in vivo. (**A**) Treatment with doxycycline activates a constitutively expressed reverse tetracycline-responsive transactivator to induce bidirectional transcription of Gal4-BD-p53 and VP16-TAg, hybrid proteins containing the target proteins p53 and TAg fused to the yeast Gal4 DNA-BD and the HSV-1 VP16 AD, respectively. Interaction of p53 and TAg assembles the hybrid transcriptional activator on the Gal4 promoter, inducing transcription of the mNLS-sr39TK-EGFP fusion reporter. The fusion reporter protein can be detected by micro-PET imaging of living mice by using TK-mediated phosphorylation (P) and intracellular trapping of the positron-emitting radiopharmaceutical ^{18}F-FHBG or by fluorescence imaging of GFP. (**B**) Photograph (*left*) of the anterior thorax of a *nu/nu* mouse with axillary xenograft tumors of control negative, noninteracting coat protein cells (*arrowhead*) and positive-interacting TAg cells (*arrow*). Coronal micro-PET image (*right*) of the same mouse 48 hours after starting treatment with i.p. injections of doxycycline (dox; 60 μg/g body weight × six doses) showing accumulation of ^{18}F-FHBG only in the TAg tumor (*arrow*) expressing the interacting proteins Gal4-BD-p53 and VP16-TAg. Asterisk denotes radiotracer in the gallbladder. Intestinal activity from normal hepatobiliary clearance of the radiotracer is observed in the lower portion of the image. *Abbreviations*: BD, binding domain; AD, activation domain; GFP, green fluorescence protein. *Source*: From Ref. 8 (*See Color Insert*).

As mentioned above for conventional two-hybrid systems, the indirect readout of the reporter limits kinetic analysis, and the released transcription factor must translocate to the nucleus.

Genetically encoded imaging reporters can also be used to directly measure the downstream effects of signal transduction cascades. This is typically done by placing the reporter under the control of a promoter containing response elements specific to the signaling pathway of interest. This technique is compatible with many different genetically encoded imaging reporters (fluorescent proteins, luciferases, HSV1-TK, etc.) and can be used to noninvasively, nondestructively study signaling networks in cellulo or in vivo. Reporter vectors and stable cell lines have been developed for numerous signaling pathways and are commercially available from many vendors. An example of a widely used, commercially available transcriptional reporter is TOPFLASH (Upstate), which contains multiple repeats of the Wnt responsive T-cell factor (TCF)-binding elements upstream of a minimal promoter driving FLuc (14). As a control for this reporter, FOPFLASH was generated containing mutated TCF-binding motifs rendering it unresponsive to Wnt signaling. Furthermore, a stable cell line expressing a Super-TOPFLASH reporter (STF293 cells) exhibits over 1000-fold induction over basal luciferase signal upon Wnt stimulation (15).

Other pathways can be interrogated using genetically encoded reporters engineered to express multiple imaging agents under the control of specific promoters. For example, a retroviral vector containing the dual reporter gene HSV1-TK-GFP regulated by an upstream p53 response element (p53 → TK-GFP) was used to transduce U87 glioma (p53+/+) and SaOS osteosarcoma (p53−/−) cells that were implanted into rats to establish tumor xenografts (16). Whole body PET imaging and fluorescence microscopy demonstrated DNA damage–induced upregulation of TK-GFP in a p53-dependent manner and this increase in activity correlated with upregulation of downstream p53-regulated genes as measured by independent assays.

To analyze the dynamics of estrogen receptor (ER) transcriptional activity in vivo, a transgenic mouse model was generated (17) wherein FLuc is expressed under transcriptional control of the ER (ERE → FLuc). As expected, in reproductive organs and in the liver, luciferase activity paralleled circulating estrogen levels, peaking at proestrus. However, in nonreproductive organs, such as bone and brain, peak transcriptional activity of ERs was observed in diestrus. It was further demonstrated that these tissue-specific responses are masked when mice undergo conventional hormone treatment, and that ERs are transcriptionally active even in immature mice (before gonadal production of sex hormones) and in ovariectomized mice. Overall, this study emphasizes the importance of estrogen-independent activation of ER, especially in nonreproductive organs, and provides far-reaching implications for hormone replacement therapy and cancer risk.

Tissue-specific and temporal changes in transcriptional regulation also have been shown to be resolved by reporter gene imaging in transgenic mouse models. For instance, a transgenic mouse has been generated wherein FLuc is expressed under the regulation of an NF-κB response element and used to study time and organ-dependent changes in bioluminescence after administration of classical stressors, such as tumor necrosis factor-α (TNF-α), interleukin-1α (IL-1α), lipopolysaccharide (LPS), or after inducing genotoxic stress by UV irradiation (18). It was demonstrated in this study that in the absence of extrinsic stimuli, strong NF-κB activity was evident in cervical lymph nodes, thymus and Peyer's patches. However, treatment with TNF-α, IL-1α, or LPS increased the NF-κB-dependent bioluminescent signal in an organ-specific manner with the strongest activity observed in skin, lungs, spleen, Peyer's patches, and the wall of the small intestines. It was further shown that induction of chronic inflammation resembling rheumathoid arthritis produced a strong signal in affected joints.

IMAGING POSTTRANSCRIPTIONAL MOLECULAR EVENTS

Imaging posttranscriptional events such as translational regulation, protein-protein interactions, protein processing or protein degradation is primarily obtained by fusing the reporter gene, a partial reporter fragment or an upstream transactivator to the protein of interest, thereby generating a molecular sensor that activates (or deactivates) the reporter in response to a given protein interaction or modification.

Split-Luciferase Strategies

A split reporter protein approach using either complementation or reconstitution strategies can circumvent limitations of conventional transactivation strategies for studying protein-protein interactions. These include the requirement for protein translocation and stable protein interactions in the nucleus as well as temporal delays inherent to transcriptional readouts. Complementation strategies do not require the formation of an intact protein from split fragments as opposed to reconstitution strategies that attempt to reconstitute the mature reporter protein. Reporter complementation is based on the principle that reporter activity (e.g., enzymatic activity) is regained when its split fragments are brought in close proximity due to a specific protein-protein interaction. Fundamentally, the detection of physical interaction among two or more proteins can be assisted if association between the interactive partners leads to the production of a readily observed biological or physical readout.

Most reporter complementation strategies used in optical imaging are based on either *Renilla* luciferase (coelenterazine substrate), or firefly and click beetle luciferases (D-luciferin substrate) (19–21). *Renilla* luciferases generally emit in the blue range ($\lambda_{max} = 475$ nm) of the visible spectrum, a property less favorable for in vivo imaging, while FLucs generally emit yellow to red ($\lambda_{max} = 575$–600 nm), enhancing their utility in vivo. Both types of luciferases have been utilized in intein-mediated protein complementation assays for detection of protein-protein interactions, developed to overcome limitations inherent to two-hybrid and fluorescence resonance energy transfer systems, such as the need for partners to be in exacting close proximity to each other or detecting interaction occurring only in the nucleus. This technique relies on posttranslational protein splicing reactions that facilitate precise excision of an intein (internal protein segment) followed by ligation of flanking exteins (external proteins) (22). The intein peptide itself is split into N- and C-terminal halves and fused in frame to each half of a reporter gene that are in turn fused in frame to protein partners of interest (23). When the two interacting proteins come together, the intein is reconstituted and spliced out, leading to reconstruction of an intact luciferase reporter gene.

One intein-mediated split-FLuc reporter system is based on DnaE, a naturally split intein derived from a strain of *Cyanobacterium synechocystis* that can be reconstituted in *trans* to ligate N and C terminals of exteins (23–25). Two interacting proteins were fused, one to a fusion protein consisting of the N-terminal of DnaE and an N-terminal fragment of firefly luciferase (N-FLuc) and the other to a fusion protein consisting of the C-terminal of DnaE and a C-terminal fragment of firefly luciferase (C-FLuc). An interaction between the two proteins of interest allows for formation of an intact DnaE, leading to protein splicing and formation of a mature FLuc. This technique was used to study insulin-stimulated phosphorylation of insulin receptor substrate 1 (IRS-1) and its target, PI3-kinase-derived SH2N (p85 subunit of phosphatidylinositol 3-kinase) domain, in living cells (23). The next generation of split-intein-mediated luciferases used split *Renilla* luciferase (RLuc), instead of FLuc (25), to study ligand-induced protein trafficking into the nucleus both via cell-based in vitro assays and in vivo imaging of mice. Specifically, translocation of the androgen receptor (AR) from the cytosol to the nucleus was monitored upon stimulation with 5α-dihydrotestosterone (DHT) by fusing the N-terminus of RLuc to the N-terminus of DnaE and a nuclear localization sequence (NLS). The AR was fused to the C-terminus of RLuc, which in turn was fused in frame to the C-terminus of DnaE. Upon DHT stimulation, AR would translocate to the nucleus, allowing the split inteins to associate, and resulting in formation of an active RLuc protein. Addition of DHT showed two- to eightfold induction in signal in a concentration-dependent manner, which could be inhibited using antagonists. The potential utility of this bioluminescence-based technique for high-throughput screening of chemicals was simulated using 13 different chemicals and its in vivo application was demonstrated using either subcutaneous (s.c.) or intracranial (i.c.) implantation of cells cotransfected with each split fusion protein. Using this technique in combination with animals that are genetically engineered to express split fragments in specific tissues, it may be possible to monitor translocations of proteins of interest in target tissues as well as monitor activity of agonist and antagonist drugs mediating those translocations specifically in various organs.

The salient limitations of the split-intein-based luciferase complementation systems arise from the self-catalytic nature of the DnaE gene, which, while forming the basis of the trans splicing, also results in very high-background luminescence, purportedly due to the splicing event occurring even when there is partial association of the DnaE fragments (23). In addition, reconstitution of spliced luciferase is permanent, providing only an "on" signal. Even a fleeting interaction of the proteins of interest will result in luminescence signal and furthermore, disassociation of the protein complexes of interest occurring subsequent to their association cannot be monitored. Thus, while certain initial rates of kinetic reactions could be estimated, quantitative titration curves of protein- and drug-mediated equilibrium reactions cannot be accurately measured. Finally, the truly important aspects of studying protein-protein interactions in living cells or animals lie in the ability to do so in real time. The inevitable delay in the ability to detect an interaction using this strategy can be attributed to the time required for the splicing reaction. While this may not be a factor for slow reactions occurring over long time frames, numerous drugs, chemicals and natural ligands exert their effects in seconds to minutes, and the split-intein strategy precludes the study of these important protein-protein interactions in cells and live animals.

Studies using split *Renilla* luciferase have been successfully used to capture signal transduction events occurring over shorter time courses, such as a phosphorylation-dependent interaction between SH2N domain, and a peptide derived from IRS-1 (26). Peak protein interaction, as captured by bioluminescence imaging, was seen at five minutes post-induction with slow degradation of signal, even with very low levels of insulin (10 pM–100 nM). In addition, sites of interactions within cells were mapped as occurring primarily on the plasma membrane using a supercooled CCD camera and Zeiss microscopic optics. This split *Renilla* luciferase shows significant promise for use in in cellulo assays as a measure of protein interactions.

However, several coelenterazines have been found to be substrates for the efflux transporter MDR1 P-glycoprotein, including native coelenterazine and synthetic coelenterazine analogs f, h, and hcp (27). This raises general concern for the indiscriminate use of coelenterazine and *Renilla* luciferase reporters in live-cell assays and noninvasive whole animal imaging. The photon output of the reporter can be impacted by changes in P-glycoprotein transport activity that alter substrate availability within the cells, thereby introducing signal artifacts not related to the biological process under investigation. Furthermore, coelenterazine cannot be used in experimentation involving transport across the blood brain barrier, since brain capillaries are rich in outwardly directed P-glycoprotein, effectively excluding coelenterazine from the central nervous system.

These limitations can be overcome using split-luciferase complementation systems based on firefly and click beetle red (CBR) and click-beetle green (CBG) luciferases. This group of enzymes generates light by oxidizing the substrate, luciferin, in the presences of Mg, ATP, and O_2 (20,21). According to crystal structure data (28), FLuc is composed of two distinct domains, a large N-terminal and small C-terminal domain. These domains encompass a large cleft within the active site and are hypothesized to work as a clamshell mechanism, opposing each other to exclude water upon the binding of the substrate D-luciferin and cofactors, thereby enabling the bioluminescent reaction. Various sites for creating two individually inactive, but reconstitutable halves of the FLuc enzyme have been tested, including the tether region between the two domains of intact luciferase (23) to study interaction between myoD and Id, members of the helix-loop-helix family of nuclear proteins (29), and a series of overlapping sequences that were able to self-associate to produce highlight output (30). The self-associating split-luciferase could potentially be used to elucidate macromolecular delivery vehicles, measure bilayer transport of tagged proteins, and explore protein compartmentalization. These self-associating constructs, however, are not intended for and have limited utility in the measurement of regulated or titratable protein-protein interactions.

To identify an enhanced pair of FLuc fragments that reconstituted an active (bioluminescent) heterodimer only upon association, a well-characterized protein interaction system, rapamycin-mediated association of the FKBP-rapamycin-binding (FRB) domain of human mTOR (residues 2024–2113) with FKBP-12 (FK506 binding protein), was employed in a genetic screen of incrementally truncated luciferase fragments (31,32). Optimal bioluminescence was seen with the FRB-N-FLuc (2–416) and C-FLuc (398–550)-FKBP pair, netting greater than 1200-fold signal over background, while the individual fragments exhibited undetectable signal compared with background. The rapamycin-inducible FRB-FKBP interaction was titrated as a function of rapamycin concentration yielding values for apparent K_d of rapamycin binding (1.5 nM $\pm$ 0.3 nM) comparable with literature values for the isolated protein in vitro. Furthermore, inhibition of rapamycin-induced interactions with FK506, a potent inhibitor of rapamycin binding to FKBP, yielded an apparent K_i value (4.2 nM) that was also comparable with literature values, demonstrating that this reporter equilibrium interaction is reversible and quantitative (31). Drug-induced protein interactions were readily visualized in mice in vivo by generating intraperitoneal pseudotumors of cells transiently transfected with the fusion constructs and treating the mice systemically with rapamycin. Real-time measurement of rapamycin-induced FRB/FKBP association over time provided a noninvasive readout of target-specific rapamycin pharmacodynamics with 23-fold signal amplification upon treatment in vivo (Fig. 2).

The versatility and strength of this split-FLuc system as a tool to visualize inducible protein-protein interaction was demonstrated via the detection of a phosphorylation-dependent interaction of Cdc25C and 14-3-3ε, members of the DNA replication and damage checkpoint pathways. Up to 50% inhibition of this interaction could be measured using a staurosporine analogue, UCN-01 (33), and the signal was totally abrogated by a S216A mutation in Cdc25C, a substitution known to block 14-3-3ε binding to Cdc25C. This reporter now allows for real-time assessment of cellular protein-protein interactions in their normal environment, regardless of subcellular localization of the binding partners, and can also be performed in living animals. The fold-induction of this enhanced split-luciferase system is exceptional, while the background activity of the individual fragments is indistinguishable from untransfected background when used properly at low to modest (i.e., physiological) expression levels, thereby providing a powerful tool for elucidating protein function and kinetics in living systems.

Reporter Fusion Strategies

An intricate interplay of signal relay mechanisms controls normal physiological processes at both the cellular and organismal levels. Yet, disrupting the function of a single key protein can often be the precipitating event leading to complex diseases, such as cancer. The ability to monitor such events in real time, and in relevant physiological contexts, is tremendously important to gain an in-depth understanding of disease-related signaling networks and target them with effective therapeutics.

Imaging Caspase-3 Activation

The cysteine protease caspase-3 is an effector caspase activated during apoptotic cell death by upstream initiator caspases (i.e., caspases 8, 9, 10, and 12). Once activated,

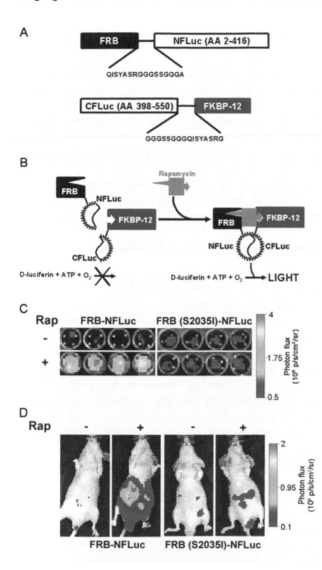

Figure 2 Firefly luciferase protein-fragment complementation imaging. (**A**) Schematic representation of the optimized N- and C-terminal fragments of luciferase (as revealed by screening of incremental truncation libraries), fused to FRB and FKBP-12, respectively. (**B**) Luciferase protein-fragment complementation imaging is rapamycin (rap)-dependent. Rapamycin induces the association of proteins FRB and FKBP-12 bringing the inactive fragments of luciferase into close proximity, thereby producing bioluminescence activity. (**C**) Monitoring rapamycin-induced FRB/FKBP12 association in live cells. HEK-293 cells transfected with FRB-NFLuc + C-FLuc-FKBP-12 (*left*) or S2035I FRB-N-FLuc + C-FLuc-FKBP-12 (*right*) were treated for six hours with 50 nM rapamycin. Note that the S2035I mutation of mTOR/FRB is known to abrogate the rapamycin-induced association of FRB and FKBP-12. (**D**) Luciferase complementation imaging of two representative *nu/nu* mice, one implanted with HEK-293 cells expressing FRB-N-FLuc + CFLuc-FKBP-12 (*left pair*) and the other with cells expressing mutant S2035I FRB-N-FLuc + C-FLuc-FKBP-12 (*right pair*). Images were taken 18 hours before treatment with rapamycin (*left panel*) and 2.5 hours after receiving a single dose of rapamycin (4.5 mg/kg, i.p., *right panel*). *Abbreviation*: HEK-293, Human embryonic kidney -293. *Source*: From Refs. 1, 31.

caspase-3 executes apoptosis by cleaving cellular proteins at a specific DEVD consensus motif. To enable non-invasive and repetitive imaging of apoptosis in living animals, a reporter was engineered (34) for bioluminescence imaging wherein the estrogen receptor regulatory domain was fused to FLuc, thereby sterically silencing FLuc catalytic activity. Inclusion of a DEVD sequence between these two moieties allowed for caspase-3-mediated restoration of luciferase activity, enabling real-time monitoring of apoptotic activation. Using this reporter, the investigators demonstrated activation of caspase-3 in intact cells and living animals in response to treatment with TNF-α-related apoptosis-inducing ligand (TRAIL). Furthermore, ZVAD-fmk, a general caspase inhibitor, was shown to abrogate TRAIL-induced reporter activation, thus confirming the role of caspases for regulating activity of this reporter.

Imaging Total Proteasome Inhibition

The ubiquitin-proteasome pathway is the central mediator of regulated proteolysis, an instrumental switch for a variety of signaling cascades. Several important proteins that are regulated by the proteasome include inhibitor of nuclear factor κB (IκB) (35), β-catenin (36), tumor suppressor p53 (37), cyclin-dependent kinase inhibitors p21 (38) and p27 (39), hypoxia-inducible transcription factor HIF-1α (40), pro-apoptotic protein Bax (41), and to some extent epidermal growth factor receptor ErbB1 (42). Deregulation of proteasomal activity or improper substrate recognition and processing by the ubiquitin-proteasome machinery may lead to cancer, stroke, chronic inflammation, and neurodegenerative diseases (43). Of note, the proteasome inhibitor bortezomib (Velcade®) was recently approved by the FDA for treatment of multiple myeloma (44).

To monitor total proteasomal activity, an ubiquitin-luciferase bioluminescence imaging reporter was developed by fusing the N-terminus of FLuc to four copies of a mutant ubiquitin (Ub^{G76V}) (45). The tetraubiquitin fusion degradation motif has been shown to significantly destabilize heterologous proteins in cultured cells, while the glycine to valine substitution at the C-terminus of ubiquitin limits cleavage by ubiquitin hydrolases (46,47). Both in cultured cells and in tumor xenografts, the 4xUb-FLuc reporter was degraded rapidly under steady-state conditions and stabilized in a concentration- and time-dependent manner in response to various proteasome inhibitors. Bioluminescence imaging revealed that proteasome function in tumor xenografts was blocked as soon as 30 minutes after administration of a single dose of the chemotherapeutic proteasome inhibitor bortezomib and returned to nearly baseline by 46 hours. However, after a two-week regimen of bortezomib, imaging of target tumors showed significantly enhanced proteasome inhibition that no longer returned to baseline (45). These types of data may be critical in designing clinical dosing regimens of a variety of drugs.

This Ub-FL reporter enables repetitive tissue-specific analysis of 26S proteasome activity in vivo and should facilitate development and validation of proteasome inhibitors in mouse models as well as investigations of the ubiquitin-proteasome pathway in disease pathogenesis. However, when imaging drug-induced stabilization and accumulation of Ub-FL, functional readout is coupled to transcription and translation of the reporter. Consequently, the temporal changes in bioluminescence do not necessarily accurately reflect relevant kinetic aspects of drug pharmacodynamics. Therefore, Ub-FL is appropriate for assaying proteasomal degradation and for comparing the potency of different proteasome inhibitors in vitro and in vivo, but extracting meaningful rate constants for drug action or upstream regulators in vitro or temporally resolving rapid pharmacodynamic data in vivo from such data sets are impractical. Hence, the next section is focused on strategies to overcome this problem by introducing methods for uncoupling the bioluminescence readout from reporter transcription/translation, thereby enabling real-time imaging of proteasomal substrates.

Imaging IKK-Regulated Degradation of IκBα

The transcription factor NF-κB is a key regulator of cellular activation, proliferation, and apoptosis. Defects in the NF-κB pathway contribute to cancer, neurodegenerative diseases, rheumatoid arthritis, asthma, inflammatory bowel disease, and atherogenesis, thus representing important targets for drug development. In resting cells, inactive NF-κB dimers reside in the cytoplasm, bound to members of the IκB family, thereby masking NF-κB nuclear localization signals and preventing nuclear uptake and DNA binding of NF-κB (48–50). Activation of NF-κB depends on induced degradation of IκBs in a phosphoserine-dependent manner (35). This stimulus-induced phosphorylation is executed by an upstream trimeric kinase complex (IKK). Phosphorylation of IκBα by IKK renders IκBα a substrate for rapid polyubiquitination by β-TrCP, a specific E3-ligase, and targeted degradation by the 26S proteasome (35).

Using an IκBα-FLuc fusion reporter, IKK activity and pharmacological modulation can be monitored in real time (51). Reporter degradation was recorded in cultured cells after treatment with TNF-α, reaching a minimum value of ~30% of initial, 20 minutes after addition of TNF-α. A slow signal rebound, up to 60% of initial at 120 minutes after addition of TNF-α was observed, which can be attributed to resynthesis of IκBα-FLuc and is in a good agreement with the previously reported ligand-induced stabilization of newly-synthesized endogenous IκBα (52). In addition, the effect of IKK or proteasome inhibitors

could be tested and were shown to inhibit the TNF-α-induced degradation of IκBα-FLuc in a time- and concentration-responsive manner.

IκBα-FLuc can generate functional readouts reflecting native IκBα status noninvasively in living animals. IκBα stabilization and accumulation in a tumor model can be imaged using tumor xenografts after administration of a single dose of the proteasome inhibitor bortezomib. One can also use the reporter to study acute liver inflammation rapidly induced (within minutes) by a single systemic administration of LPS (53), wherein the IκBα-FLuc reporter was delivered to liver hepatocytes by hydrodynamic somatic gene transfer (Fig. 3).

Imaging Stabilization of β-Catenin

The highly conserved Wnt/β-cat signal transduction pathway has been studied extensively for its key role in metazoan development (54), and aberrant expression of its various vital components in colorectal tumors (14,55), gastric cancer, and other carcinomas (56). The key signaling molecule in the pathway, β-cat, can be found mainly at the plasma membrane in the absence of Wnt, whereas Wnt signaling results in its cytoplasmic and nuclear accumulation (56). Nuclear β-cat forms a complex with TCF or lymphoid enhancer-binding factor (LEF) (57) to activate transcription of more than 50 genes, including c-MYC, cyclin D1, gastrin, and matrilysin (58).

The use of bioluminescence-based β-cat reporters (β-cat-FLuc and β-cat-CBG) facilitated in cellulo and in vivo analysis of signal transduction via regulation of post-transcriptional stabilization of β-cat (59). Quantification of signal from β-cat-FLuc in response to various known modulators of Wnt signaling, including activating Wnt ligand, proteasome inhibition, and inhibition of an upstream kinase, glycogen synthase kinase 3β, not only matched the overall predicted outcome, that is, stabilization or destabilization, but also provided detailed temporal information about the effect of each compound. To date, the Wnt pathway could only be interrogated singularly, either at the level of β-cat stabilization or transcription of target genes of the TCF-β-cat complex. The development of a new technique, spectral unmixing of multicolored luciferases (60), allowed simultaneous monitoring of both β-cat accumulation (β-cat-CBG) and TCF transactivation (using TOP-FLASH-FLuc) in the same cells in real time (59). This technique allows for signal capture from multiple luciferases of different color, followed by deconvolution of the total light to determine the individual contribution of each distinct luciferase. In additional to providing a means of simultaneously capturing both an upstream and a downstream event in the same signaling cascade, this approach was used to determine the mechanism of inhibition of Wnt signaling by epigallocatechin gallate (61), a natural

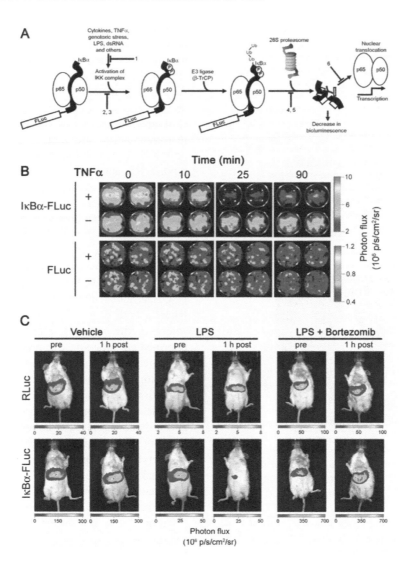

Figure 3 Stimulus-induced degradation of IκBα-FLuc. (**A**) In resting cells, IκBα-FLuc binds NF-κB (p50:p65 dimer). Upon stimulation (e.g., TNF-α, LPS, etc.), the IκB kinase complex (IKK) is activated and in turn phosphorylates IκBα-FLuc. This double phosphorylation renders IκBα-FLuc a substrate for the specific E3-ligase (β-TrCP) that polyubiquitinates IκBα-FLuc. Polyubiquitinated IκBα-FLuc is then selectively degraded by the 26S proteasome, producing a decrease in bioluminescence. NF-κB then freely translocates to the nucleus to promote κB-dependent gene transcription. (1–6) Molecular targets of various NF-κB pathway modulators: 1, IKK-NBD peptide; 2, Bay 11-7085; 3, PS-1145; 4, MG-132; 5, bortezomib; 6, SN-50 peptide. (**B**) Bioluminescence imaging of HeLa^IκBα-FLuc (*upper panel*) and control HeLa^FLuc (*lower panel*) cells before and at the indicated time points after addition of TNF-α (10 ng/mL) or vehicle (phosphate buffered saline). Images show color-coded maps of photon flux superimposed on black and white photographs of the 24-well assay plates. (**C**) Representative bioluminescence images of RLuc (*upper panels*) and IκBα-FLuc (*lower panels*) taken before (*left panels*) or one hour after treatment (*right panels*). Images are ordered in four-panel sets each corresponding to one mouse. Treatments are listed on top of each set (vehicle; 4 μg/g LPS; 1 μg/g bortezomib). *Source*: From Ref. 51.

antioxidant that is under investigation as a chemopreventive agent in a variety of cancers (62).

In vivo pharmacological characterization of drugs targeting β-cat, such as the proteasome inhibitor bortezomib, has also been demonstrated using the β-cat-FLuc reporter (44). Noninvasive imaging of intact mice whose hepatocytes were transfected with the reporter was used for single time point pharmacodynamic analysis as well as

for temporal profiling of targeted drug action (Fig. 4). Thus, luciferase fusion strategies offer several advantages, including the ability to monitor events in real-time instead of a delayed response of transcriptionally-dependent reporters, conducting live-cell assays instead of analysis of lysates or fixed cells, and independence from use of additional reagents that require extensive optimization, such as antibodies.

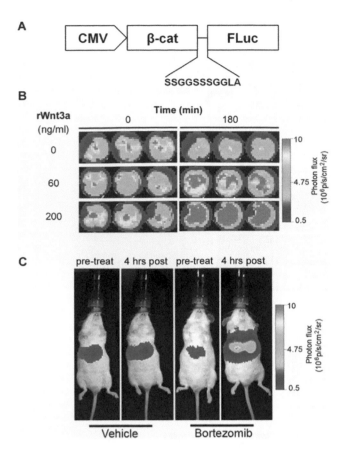

Figure 4 Validation of β-cat-FLuc as a reporter for posttranslation stabilization of total β-cat protein levels in cellulo. (**A**) Schematic representation of the reporter construct with the cytomegalovirus promoter driving β-cat fused to FLuc via a short linker. (**B**) Triplicate bioluminescent images of β-cat-FLuc response to vehicle or representative concentrations (60 or 200 ng/mL) of rWnt3a at representative time points (0 and 180 minutes after treatment). (**C**) Imaging pharmacological modulation of β-cat in living mice. Following somatic gene transfer of β-cat-FLuc into mouse livers, bioluminescent images of vehicle- (saline) or bortezomib-treated (1 μg/g) mice were taken before (*first and third panels*) or four hours after treatment (*second and fourth panels*). *Source*: From Ref. 59 (*See Color Insert*).

IMAGING ONCOGENIC TRANSFORMATION NETWORKS AND SPONTANEOUS TUMORIGENESIS

The use of transgenic animal models of human diseases promises to extend our understanding of the mechanisms of pathogenesis by placing target genes and processes in the appropriate physiological milieu. However, until recently, analysis of these animal models was limited by the ability to monitor only obvious phenotypic changes or perform destructive analyses at defined time points. In cancer research, this pitfall becomes a major drawback because almost all aspects of tumorigenesis, tumor growth, invasion, metastatic potential and response to therapy are dynamic in time and space. Moreover, while it is clear that the closest approximation of human cancers are attained by spontaneous transformation models, the stochastic nature of spontaneous tumors complicates and thereby severely limits the application of these models. Consequently, recent advances in small animal imaging instrumentation, molecular genetics and reporter gene design have yielded the ability to integrate an "imageable" reporter capacity into transgenic models of human diseases. Such aptitude not only refines the data by allowing each animal to serve as its own control, but also permits in vivo high-throughput analyses of drugs for preclinical trials. Consecutive analysis of the same animal means that fewer animals are needed for each study and experimental uncertainties arising from inter-animal variations are greatly reduced (63).

Of particular interest is a transgenic mouse model (64) wherein both FLuc and Cre recombinase were expressed solely in the pituitary gland under the control of the intermediate lobe-specific pro-opiomelanocortin (POMC) promoter. These mice were crossed with mice carrying conditional lox-Rb-lox alleles, thereby coupling luciferase activation to deletion of Rb and development of pituitary-specific melanotrophic tumors. This sophisticated model allowed the researchers to monitor, by bioluminescence imaging, tumor onset, progression and response to antineoplastic therapy, thereby generating temporally resolved, statistically significant data from a relatively small cohort of animals.

There is no doubt that conditional activation or deletion of an oncogene or a tumor suppressor gene, coupled with reporter gene expression (e.g., by using Cre/loxP conditional recombination technology) is indispensable for longitudinal studies of the role of a specific transformation event for tumorigenesis. However, to limit the need to generate, optimize and validate novel independent transgenic luciferase mouse strains for each conditional transformation model, a ubiquitously expressing conditional luciferase reporter mouse was developed that can be used to render a wide range of Cre/loxP mouse tumor models for bioluminescence imaging (65). Herein, a β-actin promoter drives FLuc in a Cre-dependent manner. To illustrate the usefulness of this model, the investigators coupled luciferase activation with lung tumorigenesis, induced by $Kras2^{v12}$ (a constitutively active ras mutant) in a preexisting mouse model of non–small cell lung cancer and followed onset and progression of the spontaneously generated lung tumors. An improved version of a conditional loxP-luciferase mouse was recently described (66) where a true knock-in was generated by introducing a lox-stop-lox cassette upstream to FLuc cDNA under the control of the ubiquitous ROSA26 promoter. Another advantage of this model over previous attempts (65) is the use of codon-optimized FLuc, thereby increasing its activity by two orders of magnitude.

In the studies mentioned above, luciferase activation was regionally coupled to Cre-mediated Rb knockout (64) or Cre-mediated Kras2^{v12} expression (65), but not biochemically dependent on the molecular transformation event, that is, luciferase did not serve as a downstream target reporter of Rb or Kras function. In contrast, a recent transgenic mouse model to study gliomagenesis by bioluminescence imaging was reported (67), wherein luciferase activation is not only coupled, but dependent upon platelet-derived growth factor (PDGF)-induced loss of Rb. This mouse (Ef-FLuc) expresses luciferase under the control of the E2F1 promoter, which is negatively regulated by Rb under normal conditions, and thus luciferase activity increases upon loss of Rb in tumors, regardless of mitotic status. These mice were crossed with N-tv-a mice that express the viral receptor tv-a from the nestin promoter, thereby restricting retroviral transactivation of E2F1 → FLuc to glial progenitor cells using viral PDGF-RCAS vectors (68). This strategy enables spontaneous gliomagenesis and tumor progression to be followed noninvasively and repetitively over time. Furthermore, the bioluminescent signal correlates in this model to both tumor cell number and loss of Rb control, thereby enabling analyses of the potency and pharmacodynamics of drugs that interfere with tumor maintenance and proliferation (i.e., PDGFR and mTOR inhibitors) as well as cytotoxic drugs.

CONCLUSION

Integration of genetically encoded imaging reporters into intact cells and small animal models of cancer has provided powerful tools to monitor cellular networks and protein-protein interactions in vivo. These molecular imaging strategies are gaining widespread acceptance within the scientific community and therefore could be considered, in some cases, as the method of choice for deciphering complex biological responses in a living animal.

ACKNOWLEDGMENTS

We thank colleagues of the Molecular Imaging Center, past and present, for their outstanding contributions and spirited discussions. This educational project was funded by National Institutes of Health grant P50 CA94056.

REFERENCES

1. Gross S, Piwnica-Worms D. Spying on cancer: molecular imaging in vivo with genetically encoded reporters. Cancer Cell 2005; 7(1):5–15.

2. Tsien RY. Imagining imaging's future. Nat Rev Mol Cell Biol 2003; (suppl):SS16–SS21.

3. Contag CH, Bachmann MH. Advances in vivo bioluminescence imaging of gene expression. Annu Rev Biomed Eng 2002; 4:235–260.

4. Toby G, Golemis E. Using the yeast interaction trap and other two-hybrid-based approaches to study protein-protein interactions. Methods 2001; 24:201–217.

5. Fields S, Song O. A novel genetic system to detect protein-protein interaction. Nature 1989; 340:245–246.

6. von Mering C, Krause R, Snel B, et al. Comparative assessment of large-scale sets of protein-protein interactions. Nature 2002; 471:399–403.

7. Luker G, Sharma V, Pica C, et al. Molecular imaging of protein-protein interactions: controlled expression of p53 and large T antigen fusion proteins in vivo. Cancer Res 2003; 63:1780–1788.

8. Luker G, Sharma V, Pica C, et al. Noninvasive imaging of protein-protein interactions in living animals. Proc Natl Acad Sci U S A 2002; 99:6961–6966.

9. Ray P, Pimenta H, Paulmurugan R, et al. Noninvasive quantitative imaging of protein-protein interactions in living subjects. Proc Natl Acad Sci U S A 2002; 99: 2105–3110.

10. Rossi F, Blakely B, Blau H. Interaction blues: protein interactions monitored in live mammalian cells by beta-galactosidase complementation. Trends Cell Biol 2000; 10(3):119–122.

11. Johnsson N, Varshavsky A. Split ubiquitin as a sensor of protein interactions in vivo. Proc Natl Acad Sci U S A 1994; 91:10340–10344.

12. Stagljar I, Korostensky C, Johnsson N, et al. A genetic system based on split-ubiquitin for the analysis of interactions between membrane proteins in vivo. Proc Natl Acad Sci U S A 1998; 95:5187–5192.

13. Eyckerman S, Verhee A, Van der Heyden J, et al. Design and application of a cytokine-receptor-based interaction trap. Nat Cell Biol 2001; 3:1114–1119.

14. Korinek V, Barker N, Morin PJ, et al. Constitutive transcriptional activation by a beta-catenin-Tcf complex in APC-/- colon carcinoma. Science 1997; 275(5307):1784–1787.

15. Xu Q, Wang Y, Dabdoub A, et al. Vascular development in the retina and inner ear: control by Norrin and Frizzled-4, a high-affinity ligand-receptor pair. Cell 2004; 116(6): 883–895.

16. Doubrovin M, Ponomarev V, Beresten T, et al. Imaging transcriptional regulation of p53-dependent genes with positron emission tomography in vivo. Proc Natl Acad Sci U S A 2001; 98:9300–9305.

17. Ciana P, Raviscioni M, Mussi P, et al. In vivo imaging of transcriptionally active estrogen receptors. Nat Med 2003; 9:82–86.

18. Carlsen H, Moskaug JO, Fromm SH, et al. In vivo imaging of NF-kappa B activity. J Immunol 2002; 168(3):1441–1446.

19. Wilson T, Hastings JW. Bioluminescence. Annu Rev Cell Dev Biol 1998; 14:197–230.

20. Wood KV, Lam YA, McElroy WD. Introduction to beetle luciferases and their applications. J Biolumin Chemilumin 1989; 4(1):289–301.

21. Wood K. The chemical mechanism and evolutionary development of beetle bioluminescence. Photochem Photobiol 1995; 62:662–673.

22. Chen L, Pradhan S, Evans TC Jr. Herbicide resistance from a divided EPSPS protein: the split Synechocystis DnaE intein as an in vivo affinity domain. Gene 2001; 263(1–2): 39–48.

23. Ozawa T, Kaihara A, Sato M, et al. Split luciferase as an optical probe for detecting protein-protein interactions in mammalian cells based on protein splicing. Anal Chem 2001; 73:2516–2521.

24. Ozawa T, Umezawa Y. Detection of protein-protein interactions in vivo based on protein splicing. Curr Opin Chem Biol 2001; 5(5):578–583.

25. Kim SB, Ozawa T, Watanabe S, et al. High-throughput sensing and noninvasive imaging of protein nuclear transport by using reconstitution of split Renilla luciferase. Proc Natl Acad Sci U S A 2004; 101(32):11542–11547.

26. Kaihara A, Kawai Y, Sato M, et al. Locating a protein-protein interaction in living cells via split Renilla luciferase complementation. Anal Chem 2003; 75(16):4176–4181.

27. Pichler A, Prior J, Piwnica-Worms D. Imaging reversal of multidrug resistance in living mice with bioluminescence: *MDR1* P-glycoprotein transports coelenterazine. Proc Natl Acad Sci U S A 2004; 101:1702–1707.

28. Nakatsu T, Ichiyama S, Hiratake J, et al. Structural basis for the spectral difference in luciferase bioluminescence. Nature 2006; 440(7082):372–376.

29. Paulmurugan R, Umezawa Y, Gambhir SS. Noninvasive imaging of protein-protein interactions in living subjects by using reporter protein complementation and reconstitution strategies. Proc Natl Acad Sci U S A 2002; 99(24): 15608–15613.

30. Paulmurugan R, Gambhir SS. Firefly luciferase enzyme fragment complementation for imaging in cells and living animals. Anal Chem 2005; 77(5):1295–1302.

31. Luker KE, Smith MC, Luker GD, et al. Kinetics of regulated protein-protein interactions revealed with firefly luciferase complementation imaging in cells and living animals. Proc Natl Acad Sci U S A 2004; 101(33): 12288–12293.

32. Luker K, Piwnica-Worms D. Optimizing luciferase protein fragment complementation for bioluminescent imaging of protein-protein interactions in live cells and animals. Methods Enzymol 2004; 385:349–360.

33. Fuse E, Kuwabara T, Sparreboom A, et al. Review of UCN-01 development: a lesson in the importance of clinical pharmacology. J Clin Pharmacol 2005; 45(4):394–403.

34. Laxman B, Hall D, Bhojani M, et al. Noninvasive real-time imaging of apoptosis. Proc Natl Acad Sci U S A 2002; 99:16551–16555.

35. Karin M, Ben-Neriah Y. Phosphorylation meets ubiquitination: the control of NF-[kappa]B activity. Annu Rev Immunol 2000; 18:621–663.

36. Aberle H, Bauer A, Stappert J, et al. Beta-catenin is a target for the ubiquitin-proteasome pathway. EMBO J 1997; 16(13): 3797–3804.

37. Moll UM, Petrenko O. The MDM2-p53 interaction. Mol Cancer Res 2003; 1(14):1001–1008.

38. Blagosklonny MV, Wu GS, Omura S, et al. Proteasome-dependent regulation of p21WAF1/CIP1 expression. Biochem Biophys Res Commun 1996; 227(2):564–569.

39. Pagano M, Tam SW, Theodoras AM, et al. Role of the ubiquitin-proteasome pathway in regulating abundance of the cyclin-dependent kinase inhibitor p27. Science 1995; 269(5224):682–685.

40. Maxwell PH, Wiesener MS, Chang GW, et al. The tumour suppressor protein VHL targets hypoxia-inducible factors for oxygen-dependent proteolysis. Nature 1999; 399 (6733):271–275.

41. Li B, Dou QP. Bax degradation by the ubiquitin/proteasome-dependent pathway: involvement in tumor survival and progression. Proc Natl Acad Sci U S A 2000; 97(8): 3850–3855.

42. Levkowitz G, Waterman H, Zamir E, et al. c-Cbl/Sli-1 regulates endocytic sorting and ubiquitination of the epidermal growth factor receptor. Genes Dev 1998; 12(23): 3663–3674.

43. Voorhees PM, Dees EC, O'Neil B, et al. The proteasome as a target for cancer therapy. Clin Cancer Res 2003; 9(17): 6316–6325.

44. Bross PF, Kane R, Farrell AT, et al. Approval summary for bortezomib for injection in the treatment of multiple myeloma. Clin Cancer Res 2004; 10(12 pt 1):3954–3964.

45. Luker G, Pica C, Song J, et al. Imaging 26S proteasome activity and inhibition in living mice. Nat Med 2003; 9:969–973.

46. Stack J, Whitney M, Rodems S, et al. A ubiquitin-based tagging system for controlled modulation of protein stability. Nat Biotechnol 2000; 18(12):1298–1302.

47. Johnson E, Bartel B, Seufert W, et al. Ubiquitin as a degradation signal. EMBO J 1992; 11:497–505.

48. Ghosh S, Karin M. Missing pieces in the NF-kappaB puzzle. Cell 2002; 109(suppl):S81–S96.

49. Karin M, Cao Y, Greten FR, et al. NF-kappaB in cancer: from innocent bystander to major culprit. Nat Rev Cancer 2002; 2:301–310.

50. Li Q, Verma IM. NF-kappaB regulation in the immune system. Nat Rev Immunol 2002; 2(10):725–734.

51. Gross S, Piwnica-Worms D. Real-time imaging of ligand-induced IKK activation in intact cells and in living mice. Nat Methods 2005; 2:607–614.

52. Place RF, Haspeslagh D, Hubbard AK, et al. Cytokine-induced stabilization of newly synthesized I(kappa)B-alpha. Biochem Biophys Res Commun 2001; 283(4):813–820.

53. Streetz KL, Wustefeld T, Klein C, et al. Lack of gp130 expression in hepatocytes promotes liver injury. Gastroenterology 2003; 125(2):532–543.

54. McCrea PD, Turck CW, Gumbiner B. A homolog of the armadillo protein in Drosophila (plakoglobin) associated with E-cadherin. Science 1991; 254(5036):1359–1361.

55. Nishisho I, Nakamura Y, Miyoshi Y, et al. Mutations of chromosome 5q21 genes in FAP and colorectal cancer patients. Science 1991; 253(5020):665–669.

56. Clevers H. Wnt/beta-catenin signaling in development and disease. Cell 2006; 127(3):469–480.

57. Korinek V, Barker N, Willert K, et al. Two members of the Tcf family implicated in Wnt/beta-catenin signaling during

embryogenesis in the mouse. Mol Cell Biol 1998; 18(3): 1248–1256.

58. Willert J, Epping M, Pollack JR, et al. A transcriptional response to Wnt protein in human embryonic carcinoma cells. BMC Dev Biol 2002; 2:8.

59. Naik S, Piwnica-Worms D. Real-time imaging of beta-catenin dynamics in cells and living mice. Proc Natl Acad Sci U S A 2007; 104(44):17465–17470.

60. Gammon ST, Leevy WM, Gross S, et al. Spectral unmixing of multicolored bioluminescence emitted from heterogeneous biological sources. Anal Chem 2006; 78:1520–1527.

61. Kim J, Zhang X, Rieger-Christ KM, et al. Suppression of Wnt signaling by the green tea compound (-)-epigallocatechin 3-gallate (EGCG) in invasive breast cancer cells. Requirement of the transcriptional repressor HBP1. J Biol Chem 2006; 281(16):10865–10875.

62. Khan N, Afaq F, Saleem M, et al. Targeting multiple signaling pathways by green tea polyphenol (-)-epigallocatechin-3-gallate. Cancer Res 2006; 66(5):2500–2505.

63. Herschman HR. Molecular imaging: looking at problems, seeing solutions. Science 2003; 302(5645):605–608.

64. Vooijs M, Jonkers J, Lyons S, et al. Noninvasive imaging of spontaneous retinoblastoma pathway dependent tumors in mice. Cancer Res 2002; 62:1862–1867.

65. Lyons SK, Meuwissen R, Krimpenfort P, et al. The generation of a conditional reporter that enables bioluminescence imaging of Cre/loxP-dependent tumorigenesis in mice. Cancer Res 2003; 63(21):7042–7046.

66. Safran M, Kim WY, Kung AL, et al. Mouse reporter strain for noninvasive bioluminescent imaging of cells that have undergone Cre-mediated recombination. Mol Imaging 2003; 2(4):297–302.

67. Uhrbom L, Nerio E, Holland EC. Dissecting tumor maintenance requirements using bioluminescence imaging of cell proliferation in a mouse glioma model. Nat Med 2004; 10(11):1257–1260.

68. Holland EC. Gliomagenesis: genetic alterations and mouse models. Nat Rev Genet 2001; 2(2):120–129.

26

Novel Reporter Probes for *HSV1-tk* Gene Expression

MIAN M. ALAUDDIN and JURI G. GELOVANI

Department of Experimental Diagnostic Imaging, Center for Advanced Biomedical Imaging Research, The University of Texas M.D. Anderson Cancer Center, Houston, Texas, U.S.A.

INTRODUCTION

Herpes simplex virus type 1 thymidine kinase (*HSV1-tk*) gene is being used as a suicide gene for gene therapy of cancer (1–4). Cancer cells are transduced with a retroviral vector carrying *HSV1-tk* gene. The gene expressed in the transduced cells produces the HSV1-TK enzyme that selectively phosphorylates a guanosine derivative, ganciclovir, to its monophosphate. The ganciclovir monophosphate is then converted to its diphosphate by the cellular kinases and/or HSV1-TK, and finally to the triphosphate form by the cellular kinases. The ganciclovir triphosphate becomes a prodrug and inhibits DNA polymerase, and thus kills the tumor cells. Malignant tumors have been successfully treated in animal models with suicide gene therapy using *HSV1-tk* gene and ganciclovir (1,2). However, clinical results with this method showed that gene delivery to the tumor cell in human was not sufficient (3,4). Therefore, an in vivo method to assess the HSV1-TK enzyme activity after gene transfer is required for the optimization of gene delivery and establishment of treatment efficacy. Positron emission tomography (PET) is a noninvasive modality for in vivo imaging of *HSV1-tk* gene expression using reporter gene and reporter probe, and can provide repeated and quantitative assessment of the expression of genes in tissues and organs (5,6).

Noninvasive imaging of transgene expression involves the appropriate combination of a reporter gene and a reporter probe (5–10). The application of reporter gene and reporter probe with PET in noninvasive imaging of gene expression is now well documented by various groups (11–17). Model systems have been established and validated by *HSV1-tk* gene as a reporter gene, and radiolabeled pyrimidine nucleoside and acycloguanosine analogues as reporter probes (6–17). Reporter genes can be used (*i*) to image vector targeting and level of suicide gene (*HSV1-tk*) expression (10), (*ii*) to image the regulation of endogenous genes and signal-transduction pathways (6,10,14,18,19), and (*iii*) to monitor and quantitatively assess the expression of a second transgene that is cis-linked to the reporter gene by an internal ribosome entry site sequence (14,19). Figure 1 represents the paradigm of molecular PET imaging of *HSV1-tk* gene expression.

Imaging of *HSV1-tk* gene expression was first reported by Tjuvajev J (aka Gelovani J) et al. in 1995 using radiolabeled pyrimidine nucleoside analogue, 2′-deoxy-2′-fluoro-5-iodo-1-β-D-arabinofuranosyluracil (^{14}C-FIAU) and quantitative autoradiography (8). The *HSV1-tk* gene was selected as an example of a marker gene and radiolabeled compounds, such as ^{14}C-FIAU, ^{3}H-5-iodo-2′-deoxyuridine and ^{3}H-ganciclovir used as marker substrates.

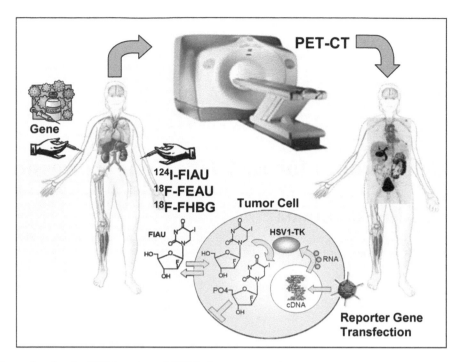

Figure 1 A paradigm of molecular PET imaging of *HSV1-tk* gene expression.

The recombinant STK retrovirus containing *HSV1-tk* was used to transduce RG2 glioma cells. RG2TK⁺ cell lines expressing the *HSV1-tk* gene and these three potential marker substrates for HSV1-TK enzyme were evaluated in vitro and in vivo. Incorporation of these radiotracers into the transduced cells was normalized to thymidine uptake into the cells. It was demonstrated that FIAU is a substantially better marker substrate for HSV1-TK enzyme than 5-iodo-2′-deoxyuridine and ganciclovir. The magnitude of FIAU accumulation in different RG2TK+ clones corresponded to their sensitivity to ganciclovir and to the level of HSV1-TK mRNA expression. 2-^{14}C-FIAU accumulation was shown to be high in RG2TK⁺ brain tumors compared to the control non-transduced tumors. This report opened a new avenue for noninvasive imaging of *HSV1-tk* gene expression in gene therapy of cancer.

While imaging of *HSV1-tk* was demonstrated by quantitative autoradiography (8), a radiofluorinated analogue of ganciclovir, 9-{[3-(^{18}F)-fluoro-1-hydroxy-2-propoxy] methyl}guanine (^{18}F-FHPG) was synthesized and reported by Alauddin et al. in 1996 (20). Subsequently the same compound (^{18}F-FHPG) was also synthesized and reported by others (21,22). The biological results of ^{18}F-FHPG as a marker for noninvasive PET imaging of *HSV1-tk* gene expression in animal models encouraged to expand the field of molecular imaging of *HSV1-tk*. As a continuing effort for development of imaging agents for *HSV1-tk* gene expression, the penciclovir analogue, 9-{[4-(^{18}F)-fluoro-3-hydroxymethyl-butyl]guanine}

([^{18}F]-FHBG) was also reported for the first time by Alauddin et al. in 1998 (12). During this time period several other acycloguanosine derivatives radiolabeled with ^{18}F in the C$_8$-position, such as 8-[^{18}F]-fluoroacyclovir (^{18}F-FACV), 8-[^{18}F]-fluoroganciclovir (^{18}F-FGCV), and 8-[^{18}F]-fluoropenciclovir (^{18}F-FPCV) were developed by others (23). While ^{18}F-labeled acycloguanosine derivatives were under investigation, radio-iodinated FIAU was available for noninvasive imaging of *HSV1-tk* gene expression using gamma camera (19) and PET (5,24). However, radioiodinated FIAU always has been suffering from in vivo de-iodination, therefore, there was a great desire for FIAU radiolabeled with ^{18}F as well as other fluorinated thymidine analogues, radiolabeled with ^{18}F. 2′-Deoxy-2′-fluoro-5-methyl-1-β-D-arabinofuranosyluracil (FMAU), another fluorinated analogue of thymidine is not only a substrate for HSV1-TK but also a substrate for cellular thymidine kinase, TK1 (25–28), as a result there was a great demand for FMAU radiolabeled with PET isotope. FMAU was first radiolabeled with ^{11}C for imaging tumor proliferation (29). Subsequently, FMAU and some other analogues, such as 2′-deoxy-2′-fluoro-5-substituted-1-β-D-arabinofuranosyluracil were labeled with ^{18}F (30,31). During the past decade many radiotracers have been developed and tested for noninvasive imaging of *HSV1-tk*. This chapter will describe the novel reporter probes radiolabeled with various radioisotopes that are recently developed and currently used in the laboratory research and preclinical and clinical trials for imaging *HSV1-tk*.

REPORTER PROBES FOR IMAGING *HSV1-tk* GENE EXPRESSION

Figure 2 represents a list (with chemical structure) of ^{18}F-labeled probes that have been developed for imaging *HSV1-tk* gene expression with PET. These imaging agents have been developed during the last 15 years, some of them are in the preclinical investigations, and some of them have not yet been evaluated for their biological properties. Many of these agents (radiotracers) have been developed based on their antiviral properties against

herpes simplex virus reported in mid 1980s for treatment of herpes simplex virus encephalitis. Basically there are two classes of probes for imaging *HSV1-tk* gene expression; these are primarily nucleoside analogues: (*i*) pyrimidine nucleoside analogues and (*ii*) acycloguanosine analogues, both are radiolabeled with different radioisotopes. The pyrimidine nucleoside analogues are fluorinated derivatives of thymidine and deoxy uridine, and most of them are 2′-fluoro-arabinofuranisyl-uarcil derivatives, which have been radiolabeled with ^{18}F for PET or other isotopes for other modalities. Beside these,

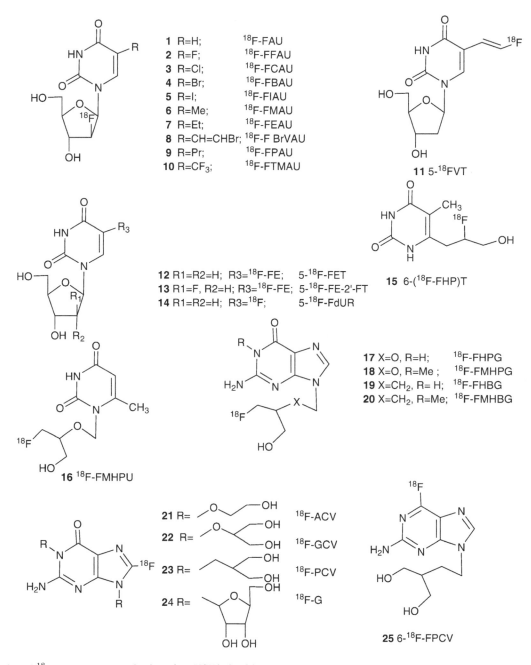

Figure 2 List of ^{18}F-labeled probes for imaging *HSV1-tk* with PET.

a few other 5-substituted pyrimidine analogues and 6-substituted uracil derivative have been developed. The acycloguanosine analogues are also fluorinated derivatives of guanosine with an open chain substituted for the sugar moiety, which have been radiolabeled with ^{18}F for PET or other isotopes for other modalities. Similar to the acycloguanososine analogues, at least one pyrimidine analogue 17 with an acyclic group has been developed. A brief description of methods on chemical and radiochemical syntheses of these compounds and their detailed biological properties will be discussed in this chapter.

PYRIMIDINE-BASED PROBES FOR IMAGING *HSV1-tk* BY PET: SYNTHESIS AND RADIOSYNTHESIS

A series of ^{18}F-labeled pyrimidine nucleoside analogues were developed by Alauddin et al. including 2'-deoxy-2'-[^{18}F]fluoro-1-β-D-arabinofuranosyluracil (^{18}F-FAU) 1, 2'-deoxy-2'-[^{18}F]fluoro-5-fluoro-1-β-D-arabinofuranosyluracil (^{18}F-FFAU) 2, 2'-deoxy-2'-[^{18}F]fluoro-5-chloro-1-β-D-arabinofuranosyluracil (^{18}F-FCAU) 3, 2'-deoxy-2'-[^{18}F]fluoro-5-bromo-1-β-D-arabinofuranosyluracil (^{18}F-FBAU) 4, 2'-deoxy-2'^{18}F]fluoro-5-iodo-1-β-D-arabino-furanosyluracil (^{18}F-FIAU) 5, 2'-deoxy-2'-[^{18}F]fluoro-5-methyl-1-β-D-arabinofuranosyluracil (^{18}F-FMAU) 6, and 2'-deoxy-2'-[^{18}F]fluoro-5-ethyl-1-β-D-arabinofuranosyluracil (^{18}F-FEAU) 7 (Fig. 1) (30,31). Some of these compounds were also synthesized and reported later by others (32,33). Similarly, 2'-deoxy-2'-[^{18}F]fluoro-5-bromovinyl-1-β-D-

arabinofuranosyluracil (^{18}FBrVAU) 8, 2'-deoxy-2'-[^{18}F]fluoro-5-propyl-1-β-D-arabinofuranosyluracil (^{18}FPAU) 9, and 2'-deoxy-2'-[^{18}F]fluoro-5-trifluoromethy-1-β-D-arabinofuranosyluracil (^{18}FTMAU) 10 were synthesized by others following the same methodology (31). The synthetic method for these fluorinated compounds was similar as those reported earlier (25–28), however, radiosynthetic method has been developed with major modifications of the old method (25–28). Figure 3 represents the radiosyntheses of compounds 1 to 10.

The commercially available sugar derivative, 1,3,5-tri-O-benzoyl-2-hydroxy-ribose was converted to the 2-trifluoromethasulfonyl-1,3,5-tri-O-benzoyl-ribose in high yields, which was then radiolabeled with ^{18}F-fluoride using either Bu$_4$N^{18}F or K^{18}F/kryptofix to the corresponding 2-^{18}F-fluoro-arabinose (30,31). The 2-^{18}F-labeled sugar is the key intermediate for radiosyntheses of all these pyrimidine nucleoside analogues. The protected ^{18}F-fluoro-sugar was then converted to its 1-bromo-derivative, which was subsequently condensed with the respective protected pyrimidine base in order to get the desired protected nucleoside. Finally, hydrolysis of the protecting groups in the sugar moiety with a strong base produced the desired radiolabeled nucleoside, which was purified by high performance liquid chromatography (HPLC). The decay corrected (d. c.) radiochemical yields of these compounds were 20% to 30% from the end of bombardment (EOB). The purified products were generally evaporated to dryness and then re-constituted in saline and filtered through a 0.22 micron Millipore filter for in vitro cell uptake studies or in vivo animal studies. This synthetic

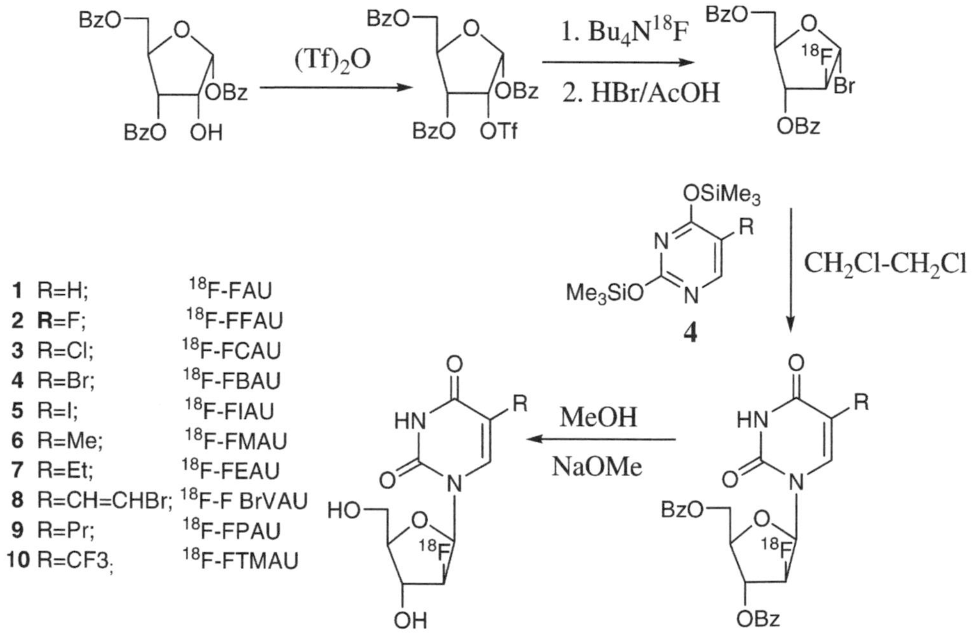

1 R=H; ^{18}F-FAU
2 R=F; ^{18}F-FFAU
3 R=Cl; ^{18}F-FCAU
4 R=Br; ^{18}F-FBAU
5 R=I; ^{18}F-FIAU
6 R=Me; ^{18}F-FMAU
7 R=Et; ^{18}F-FEAU
8 R=CH=CHBr; ^{18}F-F BrVAU
9 R=Pr; ^{18}F-FPAU
10 R=CF3; ^{18}F-FTMAU

Figure 3 Radiosynthesis of ^{18}F-labeled pyrimidine nucleoside analogues.

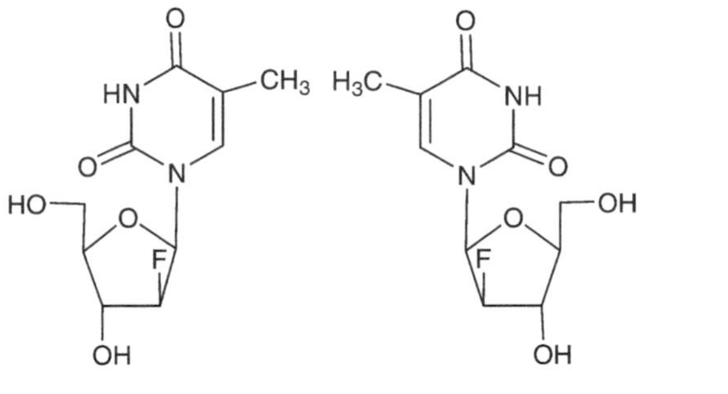

Figure 4 The chemical structures of L-FMAU and D-FMAU.

method is a multi-step synthesis after radiolabeling of the sugar, and the method is not convenient, especially for radiosynthesis, because of short half-life of ^{18}F ($t_{1/2}$ = 110 minutes) and manipulation of the process in different steps after radiolabeling. However, this is the only method to synthesize these compounds, since a direct fluorination on a nucleoside to its 2′-fluoro-arabino nucleoside has not been successful yet (34,35). Because of the multiple steps in production of these compounds, no automated commercial box for routine production of these compounds has been developed yet.

An unnatural analogue of FMAU, called L-FMAU has been radiolabeled with ^{18}F following the same method as the natural isomer D-FMAU, **6** (36) and tested for imaging *HSV1-tk* gene expression (37). Figure 4 represents the structural difference between L-FMAU and D-FMAU. The radiochemical yields, purity and specific activity of ^{18}F-L-FMAU were similar to those of ^{18}F-D-FMAU.

5-^{18}F-Fluorovinyl-2′-deoxyuridine (5-^{18}FVDU) **11** and 5-^{18}F-fluoroethyl-2′-deoxyuridine (5-5-^{18}FEDU) **12** have been synthesized recently by a one-step fluorination reaction on the intact nucleoside precursors (38). Figure 5 represents the synthesis of the compounds **11** and **12**.

Compound **11** was synthesized by using a stanylated precursor and ^{18}F-F$_2$ as a fluorinating agent following an electrophilic substitution, and the product was obtained as a mixture of two isomers (cis and trans). The protecting groups (acetate) were not removed in these compounds, and the final product was isolated as protected compound. The radiochemical yield for **11** was 7.5%, and the product was a mixture in the ratio of 3:1 (E:Z), and synthesis time was seven minutes from the EOB. Since this method produces a mixture of two isomeric compounds, which is difficult to separate, this method may not be ideal. Furthermore, this is a carrier-added synthesis, therefore, specific activity of the product is low.

Compound **12** was prepared by nucleophilic substitution of a tosyl group with ^{18}F-fluoride, and the product was purified by HPLC with an isolated radiochemical yield of 9.5% in two hours from the EOB. The radiochemical yields for both compounds **11** and **12** were low, however, the product should be enough for biological studies in vitro and in vivo in animal models.

Figure 6 represents the synthesis of 2′-fluoro-2′-deoxy-1-β-D-arabinofuranosyl-5-(2-[^{18}F]fluoroethyl)-uracil (F^{18}FEAU), compound **13** (39). The precursor compounds with two different leaving groups, mesylate and tosylate, were synthesized in multiple steps.

2′-Fluoro-2′-deoxy-1-β-D-arabinofuranosyl-5-(2-^{18}F-fluoroethyl)-uracil (F^{18}FEAU) **13** was prepared by

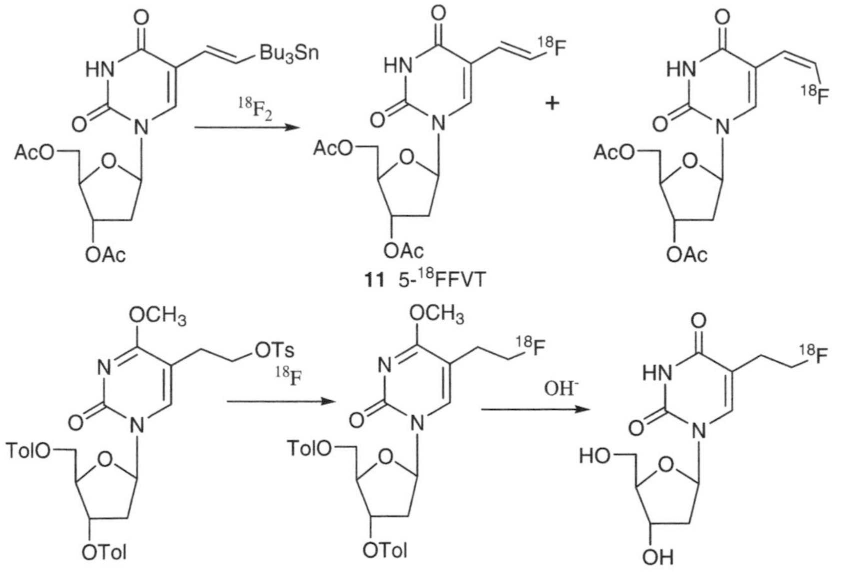

Figure 5 Radiosynthesis of 5-^{18}F-fluorovinyl-2′deoxyuridine and 5-^{18}F-fluoroethyl-2′-deoxyuridine.

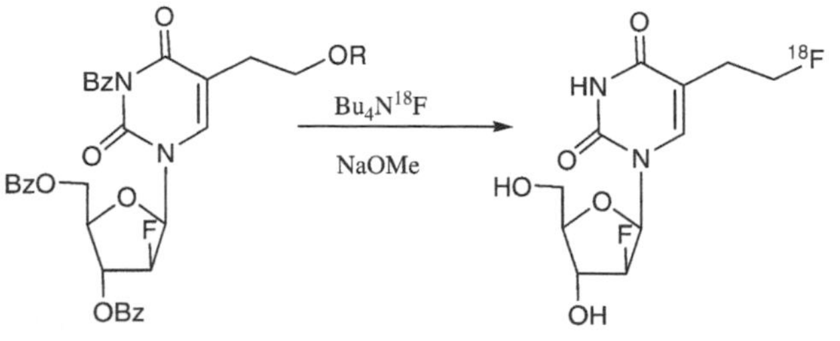

Figure 6 Radiosynthesis of 2′-fluoro-1-β-D-arabinofuranosyl-5-(2-[^{18}F]fluoroethyl)-uracil.

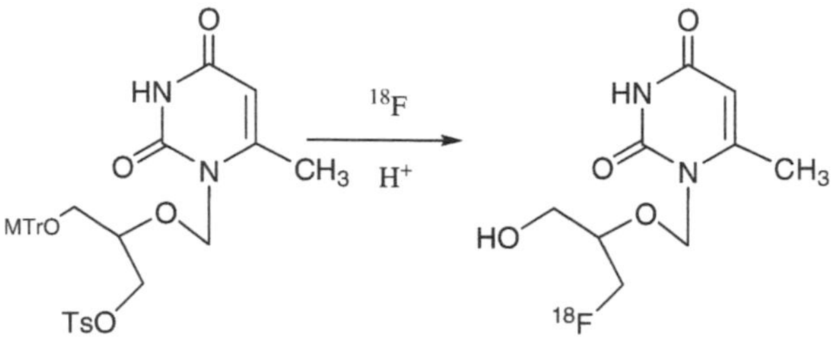

Figure 8 Radiosynthesis of 1-{[3-(^{18}F)fluoro-1-hydroxy-2-propoxy]methyl}-6-methyluracil.

nucleophilic substitution of the corresponding tosyl or trifluoroethanesulfonyl derivative with *n*-Bu$_4$N^{18}F. Base hydrolysis was used to remove the benzoyl protecting groups, then the product was purified by HPLC to afford **13**. The trifluoroethanesulfonyl substrate appeared to be the better labeling precursor. The average radiochemical yield was 0.5% in six runs. With the tosylate precursor the yield was <0.1% in a single run. Carrier *n*-Bu$_4$NF was added to the labeling reaction, which resulted in specific activities of 40 to 70 Ci/mmol (estimated). Radiochemical purity was averaged to 94 ± 4%. Although F^{18}FEAU was obtained in low radiochemical yield, sufficient product was available for a series of in vitro and in vivo studies.

Compound **14** was synthesized from a stannylated precursor, such as 3′,5′-O-diacetyl-5-tributylstannyl-2′-deoxyuridine by fluorination with ^{18}F-F$_2$ (40). Synthesis of this compound is identical to that of compound **11**. Since this is a carrier-added synthesis, the specific activity of this product was low.

Figure 7 represents the synthesis of the 6-substituted thymine, 6-(3-hydroxy-2-[^{18}F]fluoropropyl)thymine (H^{18}FPT), compound **15** (41). A precursor compound with mesylate as the leaving group was synthesized from thymine in a multi-step process. Fluorination and radiofluorination were performed on the precursor compound using K^{18}F/kryptofix or Bu$_4$N^{18}F, following which hydrolysis was performed using acid to remove the protecting groups. The product was purified by HPLC. The radiochemical yield of this compound was 1% from the EOB.

Figure 8 represents the synthesis of the 6-substituted acyclouracil derivative, 1-{[3-(^{18}F)fluoro-1-hydroxy-2-propoxy]methyl}-6-methyluracil (^{18}F-FHPMU) **16** (42,43). The precursor compound with a tosylate group was synthesized in multiple steps starting from 6-methyl uracil, then fluorination and radiofluorination were performed on the precursor compound using K^{18}F/kryptofix as fluorinating agent.

After radiofluorination the intermediate compound (protected fluoro-compound) was hydrolyzed by acid then the product was purified by HPLC. The radiochemical yield was 10%, synthesis time was 90 to 110 minutes from the EOB. Radiochemical purity was >98% and specific activity was 19 GBq/μmol.

PURINE-BASED PROBES FOR IMAGING *HSV1-tk* BY PET: SYNTHESIS AND RADIOSYNTHESIS

The purine nucleoside analogues radiolabeled for imaging *HSV1-tk* gene expression includes primarily acycloguanosine analogues, and only one compound with the cyclic sugar (23). Among these analogues, acyclovir, ganciclovir, and penciclovir were previously developed as antiviral agents for herpes simplex virus (44–46). Based on the antiviral property of these compounds, the fluorinated analogues as well as their radiolabeled versions were developed for PET imaging of *HSV1-tk* gene expression (12,20,23,47). The first compound synthesized in this series is an analogue of ganciclovir, FHPG (47), and its radiolabeled analogue, ^{18}F-FHPG was reported by

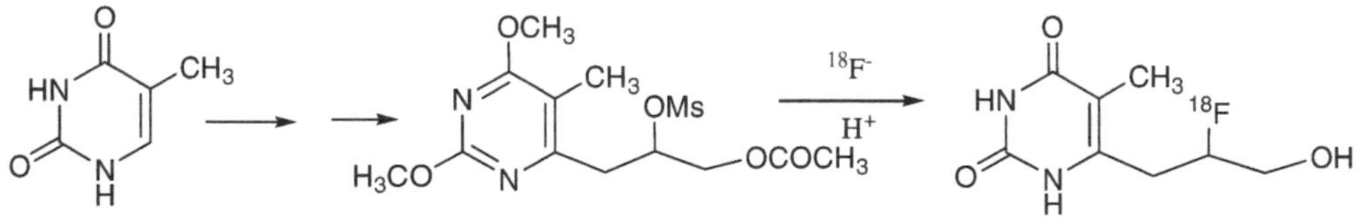

Figure 7 Radiosynthesis of 6-(3-hydroxy-2-[^{18}F]fluoropropyl)thymine.

Alauddin et al. (20). The radiosynthetic method for
^{18}F-FHPG is different than the original nonradioactive
FHPG synthesis. A precursor compound carrying a tosylate group was synthesized from ganciclovir in multiple
steps. The tosylate was replaced by ^{18}F-fluoride using a
nucleophilic substitution reaction. Following the synthesis
of ^{18}F-FHPG, the penciclovir analogue, 9-[4-^{18}F-fluoro-
3-hydroxymethyl-butyl)guanine] (^{18}F-FHBG) was also
reported for the first time by Alauddin et al. (12). Figure 9
represents a synthetic scheme for preparation and production of ^{18}F-FHPG and ^{18}F-FHBG.

The precursor compounds (tosylates) were prepared
from the respective nucleoside analogues, ganciclovir
and penciclovir, respectively, which were shelve compounds. Radiofluorination reactions were performed using
K[18]F/kryptofix in dry MeCN. The radiolabeled intermediate compounds were then hydrolyzed with acid (HCl in
MeOH) to produce the desired compounds, **17** and **19,** and
the products were purified by HPLC. The radiochemical
yields for these compounds, ^{18}F-FHPG and ^{18}F-FHBG
were 10% to 15% from the EOB. The specific activity for
these compounds was estimated to be >2 Ci/μmol at the
end of synthesis. Preliminary work demonstrated that the
fluoro-analogue of penciclovir, FHBG, gets selectively
phosphorylated by HSV1-TK, and with a higher accumulation in transduced cells compared to the fluoro-analogue

of ganciclovir (12,13). Because of the better efficacy of
^{18}F-FHBG, attention was drawn towards this compound,
and radiosynthesis of ^{18}F-FHBG has been repeated by
many other groups with minor modifications, including
one pot–simplified method (48), employment of dual sep-
pack techniques instead of HPLC purification (49), a fully
automated one pot synthesis (50), rapid reproducible
method (51) and a robotic synthesis (52). All these
methods involve technical modifications in one way or
other; however, none of these methods demonstrated
any significant improvement in radiochemical yields or
any better quality. Beside the method reported by
Alauddin et al., ^{18}F-FHPG was also synthesized by others
using a ditosylate derivative of ganciclovir (21,22). The
disadvantage of using a ditosylate is that, a difluorinated
compound can also be produced, and thus reduced radiochemical yields of the product (2%) as opposed to 10% to
15% from the monotosylate (20).

The *N*-methyl derivatives of FHPG, 9-{[(3-(^{18}F)fluoro-
1-hydroxy-2-propoxy]methyl}-N[3]-methyl-guanine
(^{18}F-FHPMG) **18**, and that of FHBG, 9-[4-([^{18}F]-fluoro-3-
hydroxymethyl-butyl)-N[3]-methyl]guanine (^{18}F-FHBMG)
20 were synthesized following the method similar as
those for ^{18}F-FHPG and ^{18}F-FHBG. The syntheses of
these compounds as reported by the authors are represented in Figure 10 (42,43).

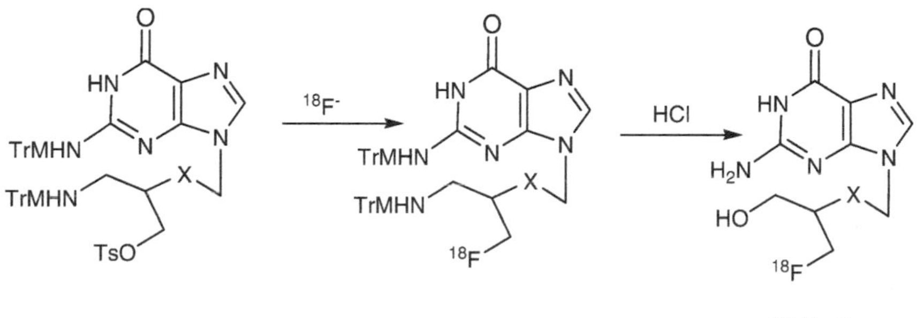

Figure 9 Radiosynthesis of ^{18}F-FHPG and ^{18}F-FHBG.

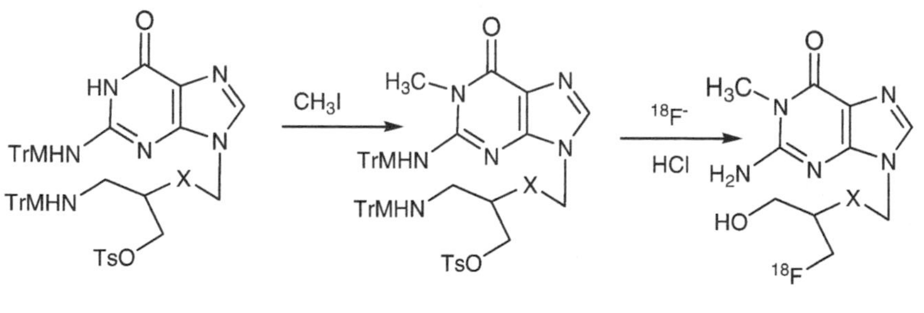

Figure 10 Radiosynthesis of ^{18}F-FMHPG and ^{18}F-FMHBG.

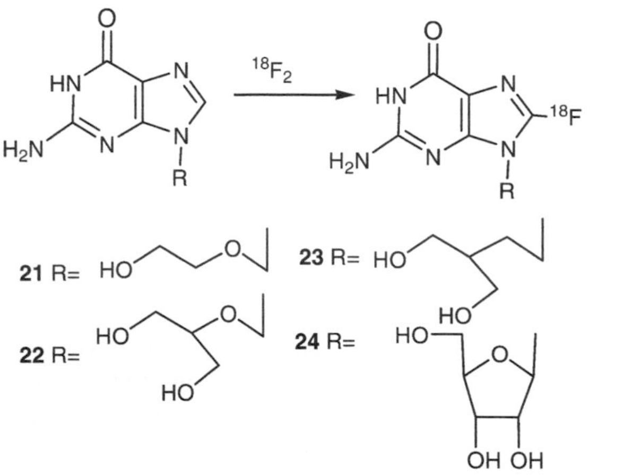

Figure 11 Radiosynthesis of C_8-fluoro-acyclovir, ganciclovir, penciclovir and guanosine.

Precursor compounds were synthesized from the tosylate derivatives of FHPG and FHBG by *N*-methylation with methyl iodide. The radiofluorination reactions, hydrolysis and purification methods were identical to those used for radiosyntheses of ^{18}F-FHPG and ^{18}F-FHBG. The radiochemical yields and purity of the products were comparable with those of ^{18}F-FHPG and ^{18}F-FHBG (12,20).

While the ^{18}F-labeled analogues of ganciclovir and penciclovir have been developed by Alauddin et al., the parent compounds, such as acyclovir, ganciclovir, penciclovir as well as guanosine were also radiolabeled with ^{18}F in the C_8-position using ^{18}F$_2$ as fluorinating agent (23). Figure 11 represents the radiochemical syntheses of the C_8-fluorinated analogues of acyclovir (^{18}F-ACV) **21**, ganciclovir (^{18}F-GCV) **22**, penciclovir (^{18}F-PCV) **23**, and guanosine (^{18}F-G) **24**. The parent compounds can be labeled without any manipulation, such as protection of the functional groups and their de-protection after radiolabeling are not necessary. However, their radiochemical yields are very low in the range of 0.9% to 1.2% from the EOB. The other disadvantage in this synthesis is carrier-added synthesis, and therefore, these products had low specific activity. Although radiochemical yields in these products were quite low, sufficient amount of the radiotracer was produced for cell uptake studies as well as small-animal imaging studies.

Another analogue of acycloguanosine, C_6-fluoropenciclovir **25**, radiolabeled in the C_6-position, has been reported recently (53). The synthesis of this compound is represented in Figure 12. The precursor compound was synthesized from a 6-chloro-derivative of penciclovir to a 6-trimethyl-ammonium salt in multiple steps. Radiofluorination was performed using K^{18}F/kryptofix in N, N-dimethylformamide (DMF) at a relatively low temperature (60°C). The radiochemical yields were 45% to 55%, much higher compared to those for the other radiotracers. The synthesis time was also shorter, 35 to 42 minutes, since there were no other steps involved, such as de-protection etc. The product was purified by solid-phase extraction using a Sep-pack cartridge, and the isolated product was analyzed by HPLC on an analytical column using 90% MeCN/water solvent system.

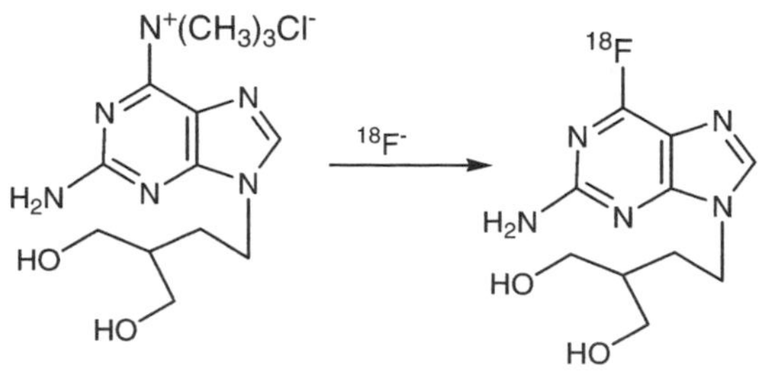

The product was co-injected with cold standard compound, which eluted with the radioactive product in less than four minutes. The chromatograms (UV and radioactivity) are presented side by side, and the exact retention times are not shown, therefore, it is difficult to judge whether two peaks have exactly same retention time. From the data on ^{18}F-FHPG and ^{18}F-FHBG the HPLC solvent used for analysis of these compounds appears to have a very high concentration of MeCN (90% vs. 10% for FHPG), therefore, resolution of peaks is poor, and multiple peaks can be eluted together without any resolution. It would be worth to analyze the sample using 10% to 12% MeCN/water to confirm the presence or absence of any unknown impurity. This method is a one-step synthesis, quite convenient to perform in any commercial automated production box.

Compared to the syntheses of the pyrimidine nucleoside analogues, syntheses of the purine nucleoside analogues are much simpler, such as one-step fluorination followed by hydrolysis of the protecting groups. Therefore, synthesis of the acycloguanosine analogues, such as ^{18}F-FHPG, ^{18}F-FHBG, and C_6-fluoro-penciclovir **25** can be easily adapted for routine production in a commercial radiosynthesis box, such as ^{18}F-FDG box. On the other hand, use of such a box for routine production of the pyrimidine nucleoside analogues such as ^{18}F-FEAU or ^{18}F-FMAU requires further developments.

PROBES RADIOLABELED WITH ISOTOPES OTHER THAN ^{18}F

Besides the ^{18}F-labeled pyrimidine and purine nucleoside analogues described above, a very limited number of probes radiolabeled with other isotopes have been reported. Among these, the most popular one is the

Figure 12 Radiosynthesis of C_6-fluoro-penciclovir.

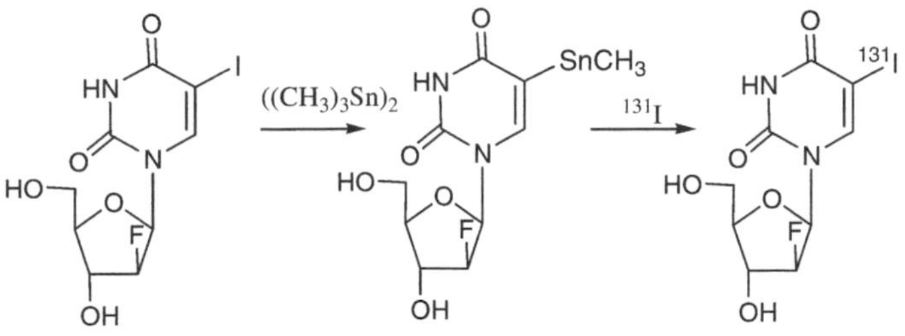

Figure 13 Radiosynthesis of ^{131}I-FIAU.

FIAU labeled with various isotopes of iodine, such as ^{123}I, ^{124}I, ^{125}I, and ^{131}I (5,24,40,54–56). Radioiodinated FIRU has also been known as a probe for imaging *HSV1-tk* (57). Various isotopes of iodine offer a variety of imaging modality, such as planner gamma camera, single photon emission tomography (SPECT), and PET. The radiolabeling procedure for all isotopes of iodine is similar, either exchange of cold iodine with radioiodine or using a precursor such as stanylated derivative for displacement with radioiodine. Figure 13 shows an example of radio-iodination of FIAU.

For the synthesis of ^{125}I-FIRU, the same methodology was used, i.e., a precursor 2′-deoxy-2′-fluoro-5-tributyl-stannyluracil was radiolabeled with ^{125}I-iodide (57). The only difference between FIAU and FIRU is the fluorine in the down position in FIRU.

Compounds, such as (E)-5-(2-iodovinyl)-2′-deoxyuridine (IVDU) and (E)-5-iodovinyl)-2′-fluoro-2-deoxyuridine have been radiolabeled with ^{125}I and ^{131}I by iodination of a 5-(2-trimethylsilyl derivative (58). Na^{125}I or Na^{131}I, were placed in a reaction vial, and ICl (in 20% acetic acid) in acetonitrile were added to the above as carrier. Carrier-free radioiodinated IVDU and IVFRU were prepared by iodo-destannylation using Na^{125}I and H_2O_2 oxidizing agent. Subsequently, 5-(2-trimethylsilylvinyl)-2′-deoxyuridine

(SiMe3-VDU) or 5-(2-trimethylsilylvinyl)-2′-fluorodeoxy-yuridine (SiMe3-VFRU) was added. The reaction was allowed to proceed for 15 minutes at 25°C. The radio-labeling efficiencies of the carrier-added compounds were over 98% and no carrier–added compounds, approximately 70%. The labeled compounds were separated, collected, and analyzed by using reverse phase HPLC with UV detector and radioactivity detector.

Bromine-76-labeled FBAU is also known for PET imaging of *HSV1-tk* gene expression (59). The synthesis of this compound is similar as iodination of FIAU in fifth position (Fig. 13). Thus, 1-(2-fluoro-2-deoxy-β-D-araba-nofuranosyl)-5-trimethyl-stannyluracil (100 µg), water (30 µL), and peracetic acid (30 µL, 0.3% v/v in acetic acid) were added to dry ^{76}Br-NH$_4$Br. The solution was vortexed and allowed to stand at room temperature for 20 minutes. Then 0.1 mol/L NaH$_2$PO$_4$ (40 µL) was added to the reaction mixture and the entire solution was purified on a analytic HPLC column eluting with phosphate buffer (pH 5, 0.05 mol/L) and 9% ethanol at 1 mL/min. The product eluting at nine minutes was collected and passed through a 0.2-µm sterile filter (59).

In one exploration of the Tc-99m-labeled HSV1-TK substrates for nuclear gene imaging of *HSV1-tk* is tricyclic ganciclovir (TGCV) (60). Precursor compound was synthesized in multi-step process, then labeled with Tc99m. Radiometal labeling was accomplished through a neutral bisaminoethanethiol (N$_2$S$_2$)-based chelating moiety attached in the precursor. The synthesis of this compound is shown in Figure 14.

The precursor compound with an N$_2$S$_2$ functional group was taken in aqueous methanol in the presence of Sn-glucoheptonate, and then 2.1 mCi of ^{99m}Tc pertechne-tate in PBS buffer was added. The mixture was purified by HPLC on a C$_{18}$ reversed-phase Econosphere column to obtain 1.5 mCi of the target radiochemical **26**.

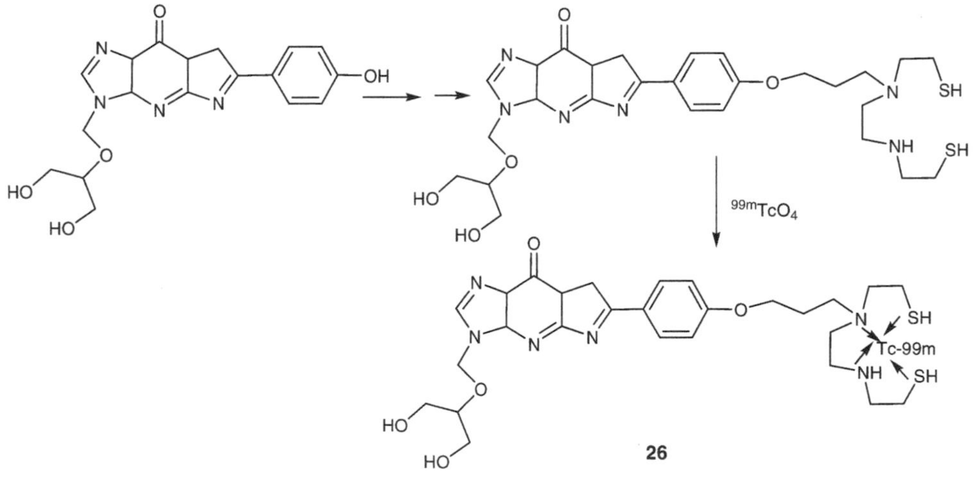

Figure 14 Synthesis of Tc-99m-labeled probe for *HSV1-tk* gene expression.

The radiotracer was collected with retention time at 10.38 minutes with radiochemical yield of 73%. To characterize the chemical structure of the radiochemical **26**, a rhenium conjugated analog of **26** was synthesized by adding tetrabutylammonium tetrachlorooxorhenate (V) into precursor compound in methanol and stirring for 12 hours. The rhenium conjugated **26** was purified by flash chromatography and characterized with ^{1}H NMR and mass spectrum. Finally the characterization of Tc-99m tracer **26** was carried out by co-injection with rhenium analog of **26** using reverse phase HPLC (60).

Another Tc-99m-labeled probe, ^{99m}Tc-Demotate 2, was reported (61) and prepared as follows: 20 μg Demotate 2 (10^{-3} mol/L), in 50 μL 0.5 mol/L phosphate buffer (pH 10.5), and 5 μL (0.1 mol/L) Na$_3$-citrate and 410 μL ^{99m}TcO$_4$ were mixed, and the reaction was started by the addition of 20 μg SnCl$_2$ (2 mg SnCl$_2$ per mL ethanol, freshly made) at room temperature. After 15 minutes, another 20 μg SnCl$_2$ in ethanol was added and mixed. After 30 minutes, 8 μL of 1M HCl and 50 μL of ethanol were added and the solution was sterilized by filtration through a Millex 0.22-μm GV filter (Millipore). The radiochemical purity was tested by high-performance liquid chromatography and found to be >90%. The mean specific activity of ^{99m}Tc-Demotate 2 was 40 to 200 MBq/μg (61).

PYRIMIDINE-BASED PROBES FOR IMAGING *HSV1-tk* BY PET: BIOLOGICAL STUDIES

In the 1980s many pyrimidine nucleoside analogues were developed as antiviral drugs against herpes simplex virus. Most of these compounds are fluorinated analogues of thymidine with fluorine in the 2′-position with an arabino (up) configuration in the sugar moiety, and with various elements and alkyl groups substituted at the 5-position of the pyrimidine ring (25–28). Thymidine is the natural nucleo-side that is an integral part of DNA of the cells, incorporated through mono-phosphorylation by cellular thymidine kinases, TK1 and TK2. These enzymes have preferential ability to phosphorylate thymidine into its monophosphate form. In contrast to the mammalian kinase, which phosphorylates thymidine preferentially, HSV1-TK is less discriminative and phosphorylates a wide range of nucleoside analogues such as acycloguanosines and 2′-fluoro-2′-deoxyuridine derivatives that are not phosphorylated efficiently by the native enzyme (7,8,11,13,15,16). More specifically, 5-substituted 2′-fluoro-2′-deoxy-arabinofuranosyluracil nucleosides are efficiently phosphorylated by HSV1-TK. This property together with the presence of fluorine in the 2′-arabino-position endows the 2′-fluoro-2′-deoxyuridines with antiviral activity against HSV type 1 and type 2 (25,28). Among the pyrimidine nucleoside analogues ^{14}C-FMAU was first used for imaging HSV encephalitis in rat brain by quantitative autoradiography (62). Later on, the expression of *HSV1-tk* was imaged in transducer RG2 glioma cells using radiolabeled FIAU (^{14}C-FIAU) as marker probe and *HSV1-tk* as marker gene in rat brain (8). Figure 15 shows images produced by autoradiography using ^{14}C-FIAU.

FMAU, another analogue of thymidine, is phosphorylated by cellular thymidine kinase, TK1 as well as HSV1-TK. ^{11}C-FMAU was first developed for PET imaging of tumor proliferation (29). Since FMAU is also phosphorylated by the HSV1-TK, ^{11}C-FMAU was also used for imaging *HSV1-tk* gene expression (63). With the development of the ^{18}F-labeled FMAU **6** and the other analogues **1** to **10**, interests were increased for imaging *HSV1-tk* gene expression using these ^{18}F-labeled radiotracers. Although the primary focus on development of ^{18}F-FMAU was to use it as a cell proliferation marker; it has been used for PET imaging of *HSV1-tk* gene expression, and shown to be a good PET imaging agent for *HSV1-tk* in transduced human colon cancer model (64,65).

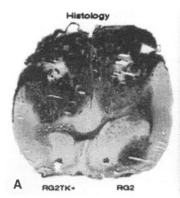
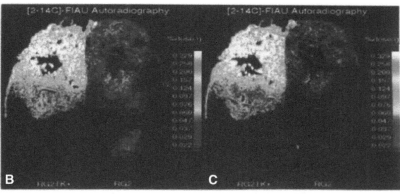

Figure 15 Imaging *HSV1-tk* gene expression using ^{14}C-FIAU and quantitative autoradiography. (**A**) Toluidine blue-stained histological section. (**B**) Color-coded quantitative autoradiographic image of 2-^{14}C-FIAU accumulation 24 hour after administration, expressed as % ID/g tissue. (**C**) Color-coded image of an adjacent section to that shown in (**B**) that was rinsed in 10% TCA for 4 h prior to autoradiographic exposure. *Source*: From Ref. 8 (*See Color Insert*).

Table 1 Comparative Biodistribution Results Between ^{18}F-FBAU, ^{18}F-FCAU, and ^{14}C-FMAU in Tumor Xenografts Implanted with HT-29 Cells (Wild-Type) and HT-29 Cells (Transduced) in Mice

Organs	^{18}F-FBAU		^{18}F-FCAU		^{14}C-FMAU	
	%ID/g[a]	Tum (tk+)/org	%ID/g[a]	Tum (tk+)/org	%ID/g[a]	Tum (tk+)/org
Blood	1.41 ± 0.56	9.6	1.92 ± 0.95	7.2	1.97 ± 0.35	6.7
Skin	1.37 ± 0.77	9.9	1.59 ± 0.76	8.7	2.04 ± 0.52	6.5
Muscle	0.85 ± 0.33	15.9	1.47 ± 0.49	9.4	2.18 ± 0.44	6.1
Bone	0.90 ± 0.41	15.1	1.44 ± 0.49	9.6	2.20 ± 0.76	6.1
Heart	1.34 ± 0.58	10.2	1.95 ± 0.93	7.1	2.17 ± 0.76	6.1
Lung	1.12 ± 0.43	12.2	1.80 ± 0.93	7.6	2.26 ± 0.45	5.9
Liver	1.83 ± 0.53	7.5	2.27 ± 1.51	6.1	2.93 ± 0.54	4.5
Spleen	3.23 ± 1.39	4.5	2.42 ± 0.86	5.7	2.92 ± 0.45	4.6
Pancreas	0.94 ± 0.35	14.5	1.61 ± 1.02	8.6	2.21 ± 0.26	6.0
Stomach	0.84 ± 0.29	16.3	1.26 ± 0.72	10.9	2.95 ± 0.25	7.2
Intestine	3.25 ± 1.41	4.2	3.37 ± 1.07	4.1	3.17 ± 0.76	4.2
Kidney	6.24 ± 1.74	2.2	6.92 ± 2.08	2.0	2.82 ± 0.23	4.7
Tumor (wild)	1.74 ± 0.51	7.8	2.43 ± 0.84	5.7	3.52 ± 0.96	5.2
Tumor (tk+)	13.63 ± 3.88		13.84 ± 2.61		13.34 ± 2.54	

[a]Average of five animals ± SD.

The other compounds, **2** to **7** had also been investigated in human colon cancer cell line, HT-29, and in vivo in nude mice bearing xenografts with transduced and non-transduced HT-29 cells (66–68). Compound **2** (^{18}F-FFAU) has been demonstrated as an excellent PET imaging agent in vitro and in vivo for *HSV1-tk* gene expression (67). Uptake (%ID/g, percentage injected dose per gram) of ^{18}F-FFAU in transduced and wild-type tumors were 30.75 ± 7.43 and 3.87 ± 1.80, respectively. Uptake in other organs including blood was quite low except kidney, which was slightly higher with renal clearance being the primary route of radiotracer excretion. Uptake ratio between transduced and wild-type tumor was 7.9, while the transduced tumor/blood was 10.4. In vivo data was consistent with cell uptake studies. As opposed to ^{18}F-FMAU (65) no significant uptake of ^{18}F-FFAU in wild-type tumor was observed suggesting that ^{18}F-FFAU undergoes only minimal phosphorylation by the host kinase over the two-hour period studied (67). Similarly, ^{18}F-FCAU **3** and ^{18}F-FBAU **4** were also shown to be very good PET imaging agents in cell culture and animal imaging (66). By quantitative measurement (%ID/g) both ^{18}F-FCAU and ^{18}F-FBAU hade exactly similar incorporation in transduced tumors, however, the uptake ratio between the transduced and non-transduced tumors were higher in ^{18}F-FBAU than ^{18}F-FCAU, which was higher than FMAU (66). Table 1 represents the comparative results between ^{18}F-FBAU, ^{18}F-FCAU and ^{14}C-FMAU, and these results suggest that ^{18}F-FBAU and ^{18}F-FCAU have better selectivity and specificity than ^{14}C-FMAU toward HSV1-TK enzyme. Compounds **5** (^{18}F-FIAU) and **7** (^{18}F-FEAU) were also investigated in the same cell line HT-29 in vitro and in vivo in animals

bearing xenografts with transduced and non-transduced cell (68). Biodistribution studies were performed using ^{14}C-FIAU and ^{3}H-FEAU, and micro-PET imaging studies were performed by using ^{18}F-FIAU and ^{18}F-FEAU (68). The %ID/g of FIAU was higher than FEAU, and the ratio of tumor uptake between the transduced and wild-type cells for FIAU was also slightly higher than that of FEAU. Table 2 represents biodistribution of FEAU and FIAU in tumor-bearing animals.

Table 2 Comparative Biodistribution Results Between ^{14}C-FIAU and ^{3}H-FEAU in Tumor Xenografts Implanted with HT-29 Wild-Type Cells and HT-29 Transduced Cells in Mice

Organs	^{14}C-FIAU		^{3}H-FEAU	
	%ID/g[a]	tum (tk+)/org	%ID/g[a]	tum (tk+)/org
Blood	2.09 ± 0.70	7.4	1.89 ± 0.35	5.2
Skin	1.84 ± 0.32	8.4	1.79 ± 0.18	5.6
Muscle	2.18 ± 0.57	7.1	1.98 ± 0.28	5.0
Bone	1.59 ± 0.27	9.7	1.71 ± 0.29	5.9
Heart	2.39 ± 0.42	6.5	1.94 ± 0.28	5.1
Lung	2.36 ± 0.39	6.6	2.48 ± 0.23	4.0
Liver	3.18 ± 0.68	4.9	3.16 ± 0.37	3.2
Spleen	3.19 ± 0.33	4.8	2.02 ± 0.35	4.9
Pancreas	2.14 ± 0.29	7.2	3.13 ± 0.42	3.2
Stomach	1.61 ± 0.08	9.6	2.11 ± 0.49	4.7
Intestine	2.89 ± 0.72	5.4	2.48 ± 0.52	4.0
Kidney	5.69 ± 1.13	2.7	3.48 ± 0.69	2.9
Tumor (wild)	2.32 ± 0.26	6.7	1.97 ± 0.33	5.0
Tumor (tk+)	15.48 ± 3.94		9.98 ± 1.99	

[a]Average of six animals ± SD.

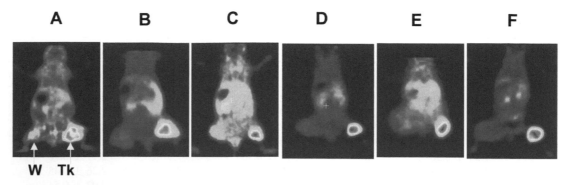

Figure 16 PET images of nude mice bearing xenografts produced with HT-29 cells and transduced with *HSV1-tk* (*right flank*) and wild-type cells (*left flank*), using ^{18}F-labeled radiotracers: (**A**) ^{18}F-FFAU, (**B**) ^{18}F-FCAU, (**C**) ^{18}F-FBAU, (**D**) ^{18}F-FIAU, (**E**) ^{18}F-FMAU, and (**F**) ^{18}F-FEAU.

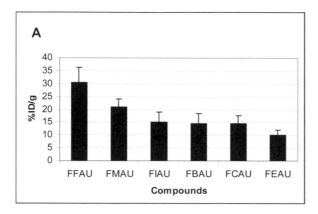

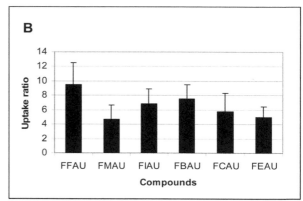

Figure 17 Comparative uptake results of ^{18}F-labeled pyrimidine nucleoside analogues in *HSV1-tk*-expressing tumors. (**A**) Quantitative uptake (%ID/g), (**B**) ratio of uptake between transduced tumor and wild-type tumor.

Since two different isotopes were used in two different groups of animals, a direct comparison between FIAU and FEAU may not be quite reasonable. However, as the PET images show both tracers have minimal background radioactivity uptake.

Figure 16 represents PET images of nude mice bearing xenografts produced with HT-29 cells transduced with *HSV1-tk* (right flank) and wild-type cells (left flank) using ^{18}F-FFAU (**A**), ^{18}F-FCAU (**B**), ^{18}F-FBAU (**C**), ^{18}F-FIAU (**D**) and ^{18}F-FMAU (**E**) and ^{18}F-FEAU (**F**).

Based on the PET images, all compounds **2** to **7** seem to be good PET imaging agents (Fig. 16) although there is some nonspecific tumor uptake for ^{18}F-FMAU and ^{18}F-FIAU. The quantitative measurement (%ID/g) provides better comparison, which shows nonspecific uptake of the tracer. Since these images do not have normalized background, it is difficult to judge the efficacy and specificity of these compounds toward *HSV1-tk* just by comparing the PET images.

A comparison between compounds **2** to **7** was reported earlier in HT-29 cells as presented here in Figure 17.

Figure 17**A** represents the quantitative uptake (%ID/g), i.e., sensitivity in transduced tumors across the compounds, and **B** represents the ratio of uptake between transduced tumor and wild-type tumor, i.e., specificity, of the compounds (68). In HT-29 cells, FFAU has been shown to be the most potential compound for PET imaging of *HSV1-tk* gene expression (68).

In this series of compounds, **2** to **7**, the rate of phosphorylation of ^{18}F-FMAU by TK1 is quite low compared to that by HSV1-TK; therefore, this compound could be used for PET imaging of *HSV1-tk* gene expression by neglecting the uptake because of mono-phosphorylation by TK1. The only drawback is its lower specificity compared to the other similar analogues, such as compounds **2**, **3**, **4**, and **7**. ^{18}F-FIAU has also some specificity problem like ^{18}F-FMAU, i.e., it is also phosphorylated by cellular kinase TK1, however, much lower than ^{18}F-FMAU. The biological evaluation of all these pyrimidine nucleosides labeled with ^{18}F suggest that all these compounds can be used as marker for *HSV1-tk* gene expression (65–68), however, ^{18}F-FMAU and ^{18}F-FIAU have low levels of incorporation because of cellular proliferation. All other compounds have been shown to be specific for *HSV1-tk*. In one cancer cell line, HT-29, ^{18}F-FFAU has been shown to be the best radiotracer for *HSV1-tk* (68), however, in another cell line, MDA-MB-468, uptake of this compound was quite low, which may be because of some other factors involved (69). Since the method of production of all these compounds is same, one can chose a probe suitable for imaging *HSV1-tk* gene expression from this series, however, it will be advisable to use ^{18}F-FEAU, since much work has been done on this compound for imaging *HSV1-tk* gene expression as described below.

Recently ^{18}F-FEAU has been extensively investigated and shown to have highest uptake ratio between tk-positive transduced cells and wild-type cells compared to FHBG, FIAU, FMAU, FHPG, and ^{18}F-FLT (70). In cellular accumulation experiments, the potential of ^{18}F-FEAU as a PET tracer for *HSV1-tk* was compared to the known acyclic guanosine derivatives ^{18}F-FHPG and ^{18}F-FHBG, and the thymidine derivatives ^{18}F-FLT, ^{18}F-FMAU, and ^{18}F-FIAU. For this purpose, C6 control cells and *HSV1-tk*-expressing C6tk cells were incubated with the different tracers for various periods of time and cellular uptake and initial uptake rates were analyzed. The initial rate of tracer uptake was determined from the slope of the plot of tracer uptake versus incubation time. After two hours of tracer incubation, the C6tk/C6 accumulation ratio was 1.6 for ^{18}F-FLT, 2.4 for ^{18}F-FMAU, 5.5 for ^{18}F-FHPG, 10.3 for ^{18}F-FIAU, 40.8 for ^{18}F-FHBG and 84.5 for ^{18}F-FEAU. This study indicates that the high uptake rate of ^{18}F-FEAU together with its high selectivity make this tracer an excellent candidate as a PET tracer for *HSV1-tk* gene expression.

To assess the optimal reporter probe/reporter gene combination for monitoring *HSV1-tk* gene expression, the cellular uptake of FMAU, FEAU, FIAU, and PCV were studied in both *HSV1-tk* and *HSV1-sr39tk*-expressing cells (71). For stably transfected cell studies, C6 rat glioma cells, C6 *HSV1-tk* transfectant, C6 mutant *HSV1-sr39tk* transfectant, rat Morris hepatoma cells (MH3924A), and MH3924A *HSV1-tk* transfectant cells were used. For adenoviral infection studies, C6 rat glioma cells were exposed to serial titers of AdCMV-*HSV1-tk*, AdCMV-*HSV1-sr39tk*, or AdCMV-fluc for 24 hours. FEAU exhibited the highest or second highest accumulation and the most selectivity regardless of the mode of gene transfer for both *HSV1-tk* and mutant *HSV1-sr39tk* reporter genes. It has been reported that combination of high accumulation and high selectivity for both *HSV1-tk* and *HSV1-sr39tk* makes ^{18}F-FEAU a promising candidate for PET imaging of *HSV1-tk* gene expression (71).

^{18}F-FEAU has also been used for monitoring treatment response of tumor using PET after systemic Sindbis/tk (vector) treatment as a basis for determining the levels of tissue distribution of vectors in living animals (72).

Sindbis/tk vectors were harvested from the supernatant of in vitro cultures of a packaging cell produced by electroporation of both replicon RNA (SinRep5/tk) and helper RNA (DH-BB) into baby hamster kidney (BHK) cells. The therapeutic effect of GCV was determined by incubation of transfected tumor cells with increasing concentrations of GCV. BHK tumors growing as xenografts in severe combined immunodeficiency disease (SCID) mice were transfected by parenteral administration of the vector. Imaging was performed using small-animal PET at 2 hour after injection of ^{18}F-FEAU and 24 hour after the final parenteral injection of Sindbis/tk viral vector. The vector efficiently expresses the *HSV1-tk* enzyme in infected tumor cells, both in vitro and in vivo. High levels of *HSV1-tk* expression ensure sufficient prodrug GCV conversion and activation for bystander effects that kill the surrounding untransduced tumor cells. Tumor localization of intravenously administered ^{18}F-FEAU after two and three parenteral vector treatments of Sindbis/tk demonstrated uptake of 1.7 and 3.1 %ID/g, respectively. The *HSV1-tk* activities in tumors could be noninvasively monitored using PET after systemic Sindbis/tk treatments as a basis for determining the levels and tissue distribution of vector, noninvasively in living animals, and for optimizing in vivo transfection rates of tumor.

Most recently a novel phage-based targeted vector, a genetic chimera of filamentous phage and recombinant adenoassociated virus (AAV), termed as adenoassociated virus phase (AAVP), has been developed, and it has been demonstrated that it is possible to assess noninvasively targeted AAVP vectors in experimental tumors using ^{18}F-FEAU and PET in preclinical tumor models (73,74). The tracer ^{18}F-FEAU could be used for imaging the *HSV1-tk* gene delivered through the targeted vector into tumor xenogafts in mice. Following the gene expression, the animals were treated with ganciclovir for three days, and ganciclovir treated animals were imaged again with PET using ^{18}F-FEAU, and found that cells expressing the *HSV1-tk* were killed, and no ^{18}F-FEAU uptake was observed. Imaging the same animals on the following day with ^{18}F-FDG showed some viable cells that are not transfected with the vector suggesting that ^{18}F-FEAU can be used for monitoring gene therapy with ganciclovir and AAVP vector. Figure 18 represents micro-PET images of tumor xenografts on nude mice targeted with AAVP and imaged with ^{18}F-FDG and ^{18}F-FEAU prior and post treatment with ganciclovir. As the images show, untargeted tumor (upper panel) can be visualized with ^{18}F-FDG before and after ganciclovir treatment, without any tumor uptake of ^{18}F-FEAU. The targeted tumors (lower panel) can be visualized with both ^{18}F-FDG and ^{18}F-FEAU before treatment, however, could not be visualized well with ^{18}F-FEAU after treatment, which suggests that the cancer cells targeted with the AAVP were killed by

FDG/PET   FEAU/PET   FEAU/PET   FDG/PET

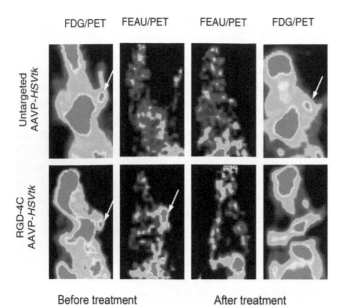

Before treatment   After treatment

Figure 18 Micro-PET images of tumor-bearing nude mice targeted with AAVP using ^{18}F-FEAU prior and posttreatment with ganciclovir.

ganciclovir treatment. This result demonstrates that ^{18}F-FEAU is a good probe for *HSV1-tk* and can be used for assessment of treatment response with targeted AAVP and ganciclovir.

^{18}F-L-FMAU, an unnatural nucleoside analogue has been tested for PET imaging of *HSV1-tk* gene expression, and reported to be a good PET imaging agent for *HSV1-tk* (37). The selectivity of L-FMAU for *HSV1-tk* was shown to be higher than the D-FMAU, and thus claimed to be a better PET imaging agent for *HSV1-tks* gene expression compared to the D-FMAU. L-FMAU is known to be a substrate for cellular kinase TK1 and deoxycytidine kinase dCK (72), therefore its selectivity for *HSV1-tk* is expected to be lower compared to the other existing tracers such as ^{18}F-FEAU. Further studies are necessary to identify ^{18}F-L-FMAU to be PET imaging agent for *HSV1-tk* gene expression, however, it may not be a good agent because of its lower selectivity.

5-Bromovinyl-2'-^{18}F-fluoro-deoxy-arabinofuranosyl-uracil (^{18}F-FBrVAU) **8**, 5-propyl-2'-[^{18}F]fluoro-deoxy-arabino-furanosyuracil (^{18}F-FPAU) **9** and 5-trifluoro-methyl-2'-[^{18}F]fluoro-deoxy-arabinofuranosyluracil (^{18}F-FTMAU) **10** have recently been developed for imaging *HSV1-tk* gene expression (33). In vitro uptake studies of [^{18}F]FBrVAU **8**, ^{18}F-FPAU **9**, and [^{18}F]FTMAU **10** were performed concurrently in *HSV1-tk*-expressing RG2TK+ cells and in wild-type RG2 cells (negative control). Two reference tracers, ^{3}H-TdR (for cell viability) and ^{14}C-FIAU (for *HSV1-tk* expression), were also included in the incubation medium for paired comparisons. The results of these uptake studies suggest that **8**, **9**, and **10**

are accumulated only in RG2TK+ cells and not in RG2 cells. The uptake rates for, **8**, **9**, and **10** in RG2TK+ and RG2 cells were calculated from the slopes of the plots and normalized to that of TdR. The rate of uptake follows the order **10** > **8** > **9**. These in vitro uptake results suggest that ^{18}F-FBrVAU **8** and ^{18}F-FTMAU **10** have better uptake profiles in comparison to ^{18}F-FPAU **9**, therefore, have efficacy as PET probes for imaging *HSV1-tk* gene expression. Further in vivo studies are required to compare these new radiotracers with the in vitro data and for comparison with other existing radiotracers, such as ^{18}F-FEAU or ^{18}F-FFAU.

Compounds **11** and **12** have been synthesized and reported just recently as new radiotracers for PET imaging of *HSV1-tk* gene expression (38), and no biological studies have been performed yet, therefore, it is premature to consider whether these compounds will be useful as imaging agents. Compound **13**, ^{18}F-FE-2'-FAU, was directly compared with ^{3}H-TdR in a series of in vitro accumulation studies involving a *HSV1-tk* stably trans-duced cell line, RG2TK+ and a nontransduced, wild-type RG2 cells (39). The initial in vitro and in vivo imaging studies are promising; ^{18}F-FE-2'-FAU has in vitro accu-mulation and sensitivity characteristics similar to that previously reported for FIAU, and greater selectivity than FIAU because of lower uptake and retention in nontrans-duced cells and tissues. The animal imaging experiment showed low levels of radioactivity in the lungs, with little or no radioactivity seen in the heart, liver, spleen, and intestines, therefore, this agent has greater potential in PET imaging of *HSV1-tk* gene expression, however, additional detailed studies are necessary to establish this probe.

Compound **14**, ^{18}F-FUdR, was used for imaging *HSV1-tk* gene expression (40), accumulation in all *HSV1-tk*-expressing tumors was very similar before GCV therapy, decreased significantly at day 4 of GCV therapy ($P < 0.005$), and had a tendency to decrease slightly further at day 7 of GCV therapy ($P < 0.005$) compared with pretreatment levels. The overall magnitude of decrease in ^{18}F-FUdR accumulation was independent of the per-centage of *HSV1-tk*-expressing cells, at least down to 25% of *HSV1-tk*-expressing cells in tumors. Analysis of the tumor-to-blood ratios demonstrated a more significant decrease in ^{18}F-FUdR accumulation in tumors with a higher percentage of *HSV1-tk*-expressing cells. It was concluded that repetitive PET of nucleoside utilization and tumor proliferative activity with ^{18}F-FUdR or other suitable radiotracers can provide additional information about the localization of tumor responses to GCV therapy. ^{18}F-FUdR is more sensitive than some other radiotracers such as ^{18}F-FDG for monitoring tumor responses to prodrug activation gene therapy of sarcomas with *HSV1-tk* and GCV (40), however, in NG4TL4 tumors, no statis-tically significant differences in ^{18}F-FUdR accumulation were observed between GCV-treated and non-treated groups. PET with ^{18}F-FUdR reliably visualizes proliferating tumor tissue and is most suitable for the assessment of responses in tumors undergoing *HSV1-tk* plus GCV prodrug activation gene therapy.

Compound **15** was synthesized and radiolabeled with ^{18}F recently (41), and only the nonradioactive compound was tested in vitro. The compound (40 μM) showed better binding affinity for HSV1-TK than acyclovir [ACV (acyclovir; (9-(2-hydroxyethoxymethyl)guanine)), 170 mM] and ganciclovir (GCV, 48 μM). Catalytic turnover constant (Kcat) of **15** (0.08/sec) was close to the Kcat values of ACV (0.10/Sec) and GCV (0.10/sec). This compound did not show any antiviral activity against HSV1 and HSV2. Further animal biodistrbution and imaging studies are necessary to assess the efficacy of this compound. Compound **16** also has not been tested for biological evaluations (42,43).

Radioiodinated (^{125}I and ^{131}I) IVDU and IVFRU were shown to monitor enzyme activity of *HSV1-tk* in gene expressing cells in vitro and in vivo. Although IVDU could not efficiently evaluate *HSV1-tk*-expressing tumor in vivo, IVFRU exhibited stable in vivo characteristics with less deiodination and could discriminate *HSV1-tk*-expressing tumor from non-expressing cells (58).

PURINE-BASED PROBES FOR IMAGING *HSV1-tk* BY PET: BIOLOGICAL STUDIES

Among the purine nucleoside analogues, the acycloguanosine derivative ^{18}F-FHPG **18** was developed first and a significant number of studies were performed both in vitro and in vivo including PET imaging (13,22,24,63,76). In vitro studies in human colon cancer cells, HT-29, transduced with the retroviral vector G1Tk1SvNa and nontransduced (wild-type) showed 4, 8, 12, and 15 times higher uptake of the probe in one, three, five, and seven hours, respectively in transduced cells compared to the controls. In vivo studies in tumor-bearing nude mice with HT-29 cells demonstrated that the tumor uptake of the radiotracer in transduced cells was three- and sixfold higher in two and five hours, respectively compared to the control cells (13). In vivo studies including PET were performed in rats bearing xenografts produced by using rat glioma C6 cells transduced with *HSV1-tk* and wild-type cells (76). The dynamic PET images with ^{18}F-FHPG showed that the majority of ^{18}F-FHPG was incorporated into the tranduced cells without any significant uptake in the controlled cells. The results of both static ROI analysis of tracer uptake at two hours postinjection and dynamic Patlak analysis closely correlated with the percentage of *HSV1-tk* expressing cells implanted, but not with the amount of HSV-tk protein in the tumor. HSV1-TK enzyme activity was underestimated, possibly because of the rate limiting transport of the radiotracer across the cell membrane (76). Figure 19 represents the PET image of rat bearing four different tumors with various amounts of *HSV1-tk*-expressing C6tk cells.

Because of the presence of a chiral center in the molecule (FHPG) it forms two different enantiomers (R and S), and these enatiomers of ^{18}F-FHPG were separated and isolated. These isomers were tested in vitro, and no difference of incorporation of these isomers into transduced

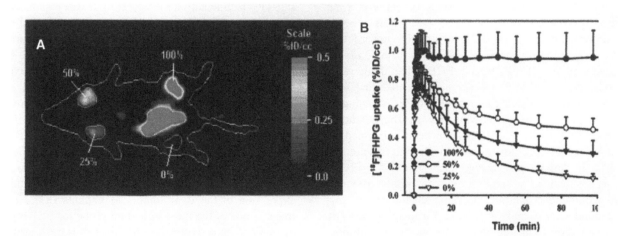

Figure 19 PET image of rat bearing four different tumors with various amounts *HSV1-tk*-expressing C6tk cells. (**A**) Coronal cross-section of a nude rat bearing four tumors containing various amounts of *HSV1-tk*-expressing C6 cells. ROIs defining the four tumors are shown with labels that indicate the percentage of C6tk cells injected at the tumor site. The image is color coded and scaled to level of accumulated activity as %ID/cc. (**B**) The mean time-activity curves (*n* = 3) for tumor growth from various portions of *HSV1-tk*-expressing C6tk cells.

cells was observed. This suggests that the HSV1-TK cannot differentiate these isomers, therefore, phosphorylates them in the same rate (22).

Compared to ^{18}F-FHPG much attention has been given to the penciclovir analogue ^{18}F-FHBG **20** (Fig. 1) in terms of its synthesis as well as biological studies both in vitro and in vivo (6,11,14,15,24,49–52,73,74,77,79–83) because of the fact that the efficacy of penciclovir as an antiviral drug is higher than that of ganciclovir (46). Beside labeling on the side chain, the parent compounds, ganciclovir and penciclovir were labeled with ^{18}F by replacing the C_8-hydrogen with ^{18}F; and a comparative study between ^{18}F-fluoropenciclovir (^{18}F-FPCV) and ^{18}F-fluoroganciclovir (^{18}F-FGCV) were performed for monitoring the expression of *HSV1-tk* reporter gene in cell culture and in vivo. C6 Rat glioma cells stably transfected with *HSV1-tk* (C6-stb-tk+) and control C6 cells were evaluated for their ability to accumulate ^{18}F-FGCV versus ^{18}F-FPCV. For in vivo studies, 15 mice were injected by tail vein with increasing levels of an adenoviral vector carrying *HSV1-tk*. Forty-eight hours later the mice were injected with ^{18}F-FPCV and killed three hours later. The %ID/g liver was then determined. Two additional mice were studied by micro-PET and autoradiography using ^{18}F-FPCV to image adenoviral-mediated hepatic *HSV1-tk* reporter gene expression. A tumor-bearing mouse (C6 control and C6-stb-tk+) was imaged with ^{18}F-FDG, ^{18}F-FGCV, and ^{18}F-FPCV. It was demonstrated that ^{18}F-FPCV had a significantly greater accumulation in C6-stb-tk+ cells than does FGCV ($P < 0.05$). Over identical ranges of adenoviral administration, mouse liver shows a higher %ID/g liver for FPCV (0–9%) compared with results with FGCV (0–3%). In C6 control and C6-stb-tk+ tumor-bearing mice, ^{18}F-FPCV has a greater accumulation than does ^{18}F-FGCV for equal levels of *HSV1-tk* gene expression. It was concluded that ^{18}F-FPCV is a better reporter probe than is ^{18}F-FGCV for imaging lower levels of *HSV1-tk* gene expression in vivo.

Compared to ^{18}F-FPCV, ^{18}F-FHBG had high radio chemical yields and high specific activity, therefore, it is a more useful and better radiotracer for PET imaging of *HSV1-tk* gene expression. Majority of these studies including PET with ^{18}F-FHBG have been performed by Gambhir et al. including human dosimetry studies (77–83). In human pharmacokinetic studies ^{18}F-FHBG has been shown as a safe tracer with highly desirable pharmacokinetic properties. Its rapid clearance and low background activity make it suitable for imaging *HSV1-tk* gene expression in all regions except the brain and, possibly, the lower abdomen. ^{18}F-FHBG has been shown to have high affinity for HSV1-TK in cell culture and animal studies and is now ready for testing on patients who express *HSV1-tk* (77).

A tracer kinetic model for ^{18}F-FHBG for quantitating *HSV1-tk* reporter gene expression in living animals using PET has been reported by Green et al. (82). ^{18}F-FHBG ($\sim$7.4 MBq) was injected into four mice; ^{18}F-FHBG concentrations in plasma and whole blood were measured from mouse heart left ventricle (LV) direct sampling. Replication-incompetent adenovirus (0–2 × 10^9 plaque-forming units) with the E1 region deleted or replaced by *HSV1-sr39tk* was tail vein injected into mice. Mice were dynamically scanned using micro-PET over one hour. Serial whole blood ^{18}F-FHBG concentrations were measured in six of the mice by LV sampling, and one least-squares ratio of the heart image to the LV time–activity curve was calculated for all six mice. For two control mice and nine mice expressing *HSV1-sr39tk*, heart image (input function) and liver image time–activity curves (tissue curves) were fit to 2- and 3-compartment models using Levenberg–Marquardt nonlinear regression. The models were compared using an F statistics. HSV1-sr39TK enzyme activity was determined from liver samples and compared with model parameter estimates. For another three control mice and six *HSV1-sr39tk*-positive mice, the model-predicted relative percentage of metabolites was compared with HPLC analysis. The ratio of ^{18}F-FHBG in plasma to whole blood was 0.84 ± 0.05 by 30 seconds after injection. The least-squares ratio of the heart image time–activity curve to the LV time–activity curve was 0.83 ± 0.02, consistent with the recovery coefficient for the partial-volume effect (0.81) based on independent measures of heart geometry. A three-compartment model best described ^{18}F-FHBG kinetics in mice expressing *HSV1-sr39tk* in the liver; a two-compartment model best described the kinetics in control mice. The three-compartment model parameter, k_3, correlated well with the HSV1-sr39TK enzyme activity ($r^2 = 0.88$). It was concluded that ^{18}F-FHBG equilibrates rapidly between plasma and whole blood in mice. Heart image time–activity curves corrected for partial-volume effects well approximate LV time–activity curves and can be used as input functions for two- and three-compartment models. The model parameter k_3 from the three-compartment model can be used as a noninvasive estimate for HSV1-sr39TK reporter protein activity and can predict the relative percentage of metabolites.

^{18}F-FHBG has also been approved by the U.S. food and drug administration as an investigational new imaging agent and has been shown to detect *HSV1-tk* transgene expression in the liver tumors of patients (83). So, this tracer is one of the most important probe for PET imaging of *HSV1-tk* gene expression, however, it is most useful for mutated *HSV1-tk* gene as opposed to the native *HSV1-tk* gene, and detailed comparison of this difference between ^{18}F-FHBG vs. ^{18}F-FEAU is discussed in the following section.

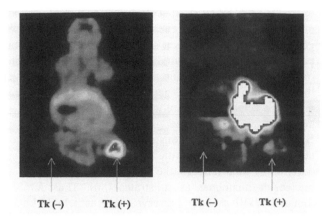

Figure 20 PET images of tumor xenografts with ^{18}F-FMAU and ^{18}F-FHBG.

COMPARISON BETWEEN PYRIMIDINE-BASED PROBES AND GUANOSINE-BASED PROBES

A comparative study on ^{18}F-FMAU with ^{18}F-FHPG and ^{18}F-FHBG suggested that uptake (%ID/g) of ^{18}F-FMAU was 16-fold higher than that of ^{18}F-FHBG in one hour. However, tumor-blood ratio for ^{18}F-FMAU was 4.27, much less than that for ^{18}F-FHBG (9.21) (65). Figure 20 represents PET images of tumor xenografts produced in nude mice using transduced and wild-type HT-29 cells and imaged with ^{18}F-FMAU and ^{18}F-FHBG on the same animal at two hours postinjection.

Tumor xenograft grown with transduced cells on the right flank has a very high accumulation of ^{18}F-FMAU compared to the tumor with non-transduced cells on the left flank. The image with ^{18}F-FHBG shows uptake in the tumor with transduced cells on the right flank, however, the intensity of activity accumulation is quite low compared that of ^{18}F-FMAU. Although PET images show excellent image for ^{18}F-FMAU and the quantitative uptake (%ID/g) is also very high, the ratio of uptake between the transduced tumor and non-transduced tumor was lower for ^{18}F-FMAU (4.27) than that of ^{18}F-FHBG (9.21). These results are in agreement that ^{18}F-FMAU is not only phosphorylated by HSV1-TK but also phosphorylated by mammalian thymidine kinase TK1, as a result total incorporation for ^{18}F-FMAU is very high, but the ratio between TK+ and wild-type tumor is lower than that of ^{18}F-FHBG.

In another study [124]I-FIAU was compared with ^{18}F-FHPG and ^{18}F-FHBG in rats bearing tumors using transduced RG2 cells and wild-type cells on the same animal (24), and [124]I-FIAU has been shown to be 12- to 14-fold more sensitive than ^{18}F-FHPG or ^{18}F-FHBG. Figure 21 shows comparative images in rats bearing transduced RG2 cells using [124]I-FIAU and ^{18}F-FHBG. In general the pyrimidine nucleoside analogues have very high phosphorylation rates by the native HSV1-TK enzyme compared to the acycloguanosine analogues (24,62–65). On the other hand, ^{18}F-FHBG has been shown to be more sensitive, and gets phosphorylated in higher rates by the mutated HSV1-TK, HSV1-sr39TK (77–83). All these radiotracers, pyrimidine derivatives, and acycloguanosine derivatives were investigated in human colon cancer cells, HT-29 to compare their efficacies in vitro and in vivo (65–68). Results from in vitro and in vivo studies suggested that the pyrimidine derivatives have two advantages over the acycloguanosine derivatives: (*i*) Pyrimidine nucleosides are much more sensitive (in the order of magnitude) than ^{18}F-FHPG and ^{18}F-FHBG. (*ii*) Pyrimidine derivatives follow renal clearance as a

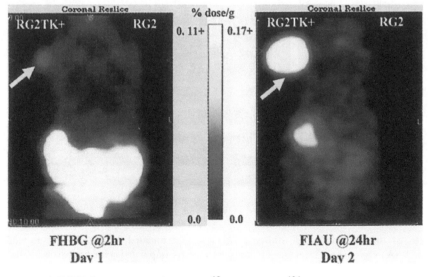

Figure 21 PET images with of *HSV1-tk* gene expression in rat ^{18}F-FHBG and [124]I-FIAU.

result the background activity is negligible, while ^{18}F-FHBG is cleared through a hepatobiliary pathway, resulting in retention of radioactivity in the intestine and other organs (6,77). Among the pyrimidine nucleosides, ^{18}F-FFAU has the highest sensitivity and specificity for HSV1-TK in HT-29 cells, however, uptake of ^{18}F-FFAU in *HSV1-tk*-expressing human breast cancer MDA-MB-468 cells was 150-fold less than ^{18}F-FEAU (67). From these studies it appears that ^{18}F-FEAU had very high selectivity for *HSV1-tk*, and high sensitivity. ^{18}F-FEAU has also been shown to have highest uptake ratio between *HSV1-tk*-expressing cells and wild-type cells compared to ^{18}F-FHBG, ^{18}F-FIAU, ^{18}F-FMAU, ^{18}F-FHPG, and ^{18}F-FLT (70). Recent studies suggest that combination of high accumulation and high selectivity for both *HSV1-tk* and *HSV1-sr39tk* makes ^{18}F-FEAU a promising candidate for PET imaging of *HSV1-tk* gene expression (71).

The mutated *HSV1-tk* gene was developed to enhance suicide gene therapy of cancer, and the sensitivity of ^{18}F-FHBG for PET imaging of *HSV1-tk* was improved by using the mutant *HSV1-tk* gene, *HSV1-sr39tk* (6,83). The mutant *HSV1-sr39tk* gene was generated by semi-random mutagenesis of the *HSV1-tk* gene, changing five codons that resulted in increased GCV sensitivity of C6 glioma cells and tumor xenografts expressing it (84). In addition, *HSV1-sr39tk* was selected from a library of mutants that were less efficient than *HSV1-tk* in phosphorylation of thymidine (85). It was demonstrated that C6 cells expressing *HSV1-sr39tk* accumulated approximately twice as much ^{18}F-FHBG as *HSV1-tk*-

expressing C6 cells (6). Success of gene therapy depends on the level of *HSV1-tk* gene expression; and the mutated gene *HSV1-sr39tk* has been shown to have higher incorporation of FHBG compared to the native *HSV1-tk* gene (6), suggesting that the mutated gene has higher potential than the native gene in gene therapy of cancer. This prompted scientists to explore mutations of the *HSV1-tk* gene that would enhance ganciclovir phosphorylation. Balzarini et al. have demonstrated that *HSV1-tk* mutation at A168H makes the enzyme more specific for the purine derivatives and reduces the specificity for pyrimidine nucleoside analogues as substrates (86). Thus A168H-mutated *HSV1-tk* fully preserves its ganciclovir kinase activity (fourfold higher than wild-type *HSV1-tk*) while showing a diminished thymidine kinase (TK1) activity (3–4 orders of magnitude lower than wild-type *HSV1-tk*) (86). Most recently, it has been demonstrated that HSV1-A168HTK selectively phosphorylates the purine derivative ^{18}F-FHBG without any phosphorylation of the pyrimidine nucleoside ^{18}F-FEAU (87).

Figure 22 represents PET images of tumors expressing wild-type *HSV1-tk* and mutated *HSV1-A168Htk* in nude mice using ^{18}F-FDG (A), ^{18}F-FHBG (B) and ^{18}F-FEAU (C).

Figure 22A is the image taken with ^{18}F-FDG, which shows the presence of viable cells in the tumors generated from cells transduced with wild-type *HSV1-tk* (left shoulder) and mutated *HSV1-tk*, *HSV1-A168Htk* (right shoulder). Figure 22B shows image with ^{8}F-FHBG, which only shows the tumor with *HSV1-A168Htk*, and does not show the other tumor expressing the wild-type *HSV1-tk*.

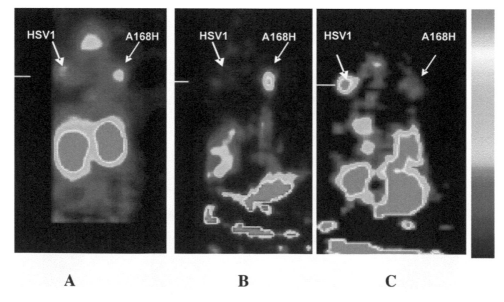

Figure 22 PET images of tumors expressing wild-type *HSV1-tk* and mutated *HSV1-A168Htk* in nude mice using ^{18}F-FDG, ^{18}F-FHBG, and ^{18}F-FEAU. (**A**) Coronal PET images of tumor xenografts implanted with transduced cells using wild-type *HSV1-tk* gene (*left shoulder*) and mutated *HSV1-tk* gene, *HSV1-A168Htk*, (*right shoulder*) in nude mice using ^{18}F-FDG, (**B**) coronal PET images of the same tumor-bearing mice using ^{18}F-FHBG, (**C**) coronal PET images of the same tumor-bearing mice using ^{18}F-FEAU (*See Color Insert*).

Figure 22C is the PET image with ^{8}F-FEAU, which shows only the wild-type *HSV1-tk*-expressing tumor. These results suggest that ^{18}F-FHBG is very useful for PET imaging of mutated *HSV1-tk* gene expression in cancer gene therapy. Furthermore, ^{18}F-FHBG has been approved as an investigational new drug (IND) by the U.S. food and drug administration (83).

PROBES RADIOLABELED WITH ISOTOPES OTHER THAN ^{18}F

The most common and popular probe radiolabeled with isotope other than ^{18}F for imaging *HSV1-tk* gene expression is radioiodinated FIAU (5,10,19,24,54–56). This compound has been extensively used by labeling with ^{131}I for imaging on a gamma camera (19,54), ^{124}I for PET (10,24) and ^{123}I for SPECT (40,55). Highly specific images were obtained noninvasively using radioiodinated ^{131}I-FIAU and a clinical gamma camera (19,54) or ^{124}I-FIAU and PET (5,24). ^{123}I-FIAU brain SPECT imaging was performed in eight patients receiving intra-temporal injection of HSV1716, before and after administration of the virus. Baseline images were acquired three days prior to virus administration and between one and five days following virus administration. Increased ^{123}I-FIAU accumulation because of *HSV1-tk* expression was not detected in this study (55).

The efficacy of SPECT with ^{123}I-FIAU and PET with 5-^{18}F-fluoro-2′-deoxyuridine (^{18}F-FUdR), 2-^{18}F-fluoroethyl-L-tyrosine (^{18}F-FET), and ^{18}F-FDG were tested for monitoring tumor responses during prodrug activation gene therapy with *HSV1-tk* and ganciclovir (GCV) (40,55). In the flanks of FVB/N female mice, four tumors per animal were established by subcutaneous injection of 1×10^5 cells of NG4TL4 sarcoma cells, *HSV1-tk*-transduced NG4TL4-STK cells, or a mixture of these cells in different proportions to model different efficacies of transfection and *HSV1-tk* gene expression levels in tumors. Ten days later, the animals were treated with GCV (10 mg/kg/d intraperitoneally) for seven days. γ-Imaging with ^{123}I-FIAU and PET with ^{18}F-FUdR, ^{18}F-FET, and ^{18}F-FDG were performed before and after initiation of therapy with GCV in the same animal. Before GCV treatment, no significant difference in weight and size was found in tumors that expressed different *HSV1-tk* levels, suggesting similar in vivo proliferation rates for NG4TL4 and NG4TL4-STK sarcomas. The accumulation of ^{123}I-FIAU at 24 hours after injection was directly proportional to the percentage of NG4TL4-STK cells in the tumors. The ^{123}I-FIAU accumulation at fourth and seventh day of GCV therapy decreased significantly compared with pretreatment levels and was proportional to the percentage of *HSV1-tk*–positive tumor cells. It was

shown that γ-camera imaging with ^{123}I-FIAU was the most reliable method for prediction of tumor response to GCV therapy, which was proportional to the magnitude of *HSV1-tk* expression in tumor tissue. ^{123}I-FIAU imaging can be used to verify the efficacy of elimination of *HSV1-tk*-expressing cells by therapy with GCV (40).

Recently 1-(2′-fluoro-2′-deoxy-β-D-ribofuranosyl)-5-*I-iodouracil (FIRU) labeled with ^{125}I was used to compare uptake of the tk-substrate and the somatostatin analog ^{111}In-DOTA-Tyr3-octreotate in several glioma cell lines after infection with Ad5.tk.sstr. Uptake of ^{125}I-FIRU was measured in rat 9L-tk glioma cells without infection with Ad5.tk.sstr. Results showed that the uptake of ^{125}I-FIRU was concentration and time dependent. In all cell lines, the uptake of ^{125}I-FIRU increased with increasing multiplicity of infection of virus (57).

(E)-5-(2-Iodovinyl)-2′-deoxyuridine (IVDU) and (E)-5-(2-iodovinyl)-2′-fluoro-2′-deoxyuridine (IVFRU) have been used as substrates of HSV1-TK (58). Cellular uptake of radioiodinated substrates was found to be low in wild-type MCA cells, but high in *HSV1-tk* gene expressing cells. Biodistribution showed that the %ID/g of the MCA-TK/MCA tumor ratio of IVDU injected at 1, 4, and 24 hours were 1.1, 0.9, and 1.3, and those of IVFRU were 1.7, 1.7, and 1.8, respectively. Therefore, both IVDU and IVFRU could possibly be used as radiopharmaceuticals to evaluate reporter gene expression. However, IVFRU was more specific and stable than IVDU for selective noninvasive imaging of *HSV1-tk* expression (58).

The utility of 5-^{76}Br-bromo-2′-fluoro-2′-deoxyuridine (^{76}Br-FBAU) **4**, a uracil analog, as a PET reporter probe for use with the *HSV1-tk* reporter gene system for gene expression imaging was evaluated in vivo and in vitro using human and rat glioma cells (59). Human glioma cell lines U87 and U251 were transduced with replication-defective adenovirus constitutively expressing *HSV1-tk* or a control expressing green fluorescent protein. In vitro uptake of equimolar concentrations (1.8×10^{-8} mol/L) of ^{76}Br-FBAU and 2′-fluoro-2′-deoxy-5-iodouracil-β-D-arabinofuranoside (^{14}C-FIAU) was also determined in RG2-TK rat glioma cells stably expressing *HSV1-tk* and in control RG2 cells at 30 to 120 minutes. In vivo uptake of ^{76}Br-FBAU was determined in subcutaneous U87 tumor intratumorally transduced with *HSV1-tk* by ex vivo biodistribution. Uptake in intracranial U87 tumors expressing *HSV1-tk* was measured by brain autoradiography. In vivo PET was performed on subcutaneous and intracranial U87 tumors transduced with *HSV1-tk* and on subcutaneous and intracranial stably expressing RG2-TK tumors. U87 and U251 cells transduced with *HSV1-tk* had significantly increased uptake of ^{76}Br-FBAU compared with cells transduced with green fluorescent protein (GFP) over 20 to 120 minutes. In stably expressing cells at 120 minutes, ^{14}C-FIAU uptake in RG2-TK tumor cells was 11.3%ID/g and in

RG2 control cells was 1.7 %ID, and [76]Br-FBAU uptake in RG2-TK tumor cells was 14.2 %ID and in RG2 control cells was 1.5 %ID. Biodistribution of subcutaneous U87 tumors transduced with *HSV1-tk* accumulated [76]Br-FBAU significantly more than in the control GFP transduced tumor and normal tissue, with the lowest uptake in brain. Autoradiography showed localized uptake in intracranial U87 and U251 cells transduced with *HSV1-tk*. PET image analyses of mice with RG2-TK tumors resulted in an increased tumor-to-background ratio of 13 and 26 from two to six hours after injection, respectively, in intracranial tumors. [76]Br-FBAU accumulates in glioma cells constitutively expressing *HSV1-tk* by either adenoviral transduction or in stably expressing cell lines both in vitro and in vivo. It was concluded that [76]Br-FBAU is a promising agent for PET imaging of *HSV1-tk* in vivo gene expression, which is consistent with the ^{18}F-FBAU.

In one exploration of the Tc-99m-labeled HSV1-TK substrate for nuclear gene imaging (60), tricyclic ganciclovir (TGCV) was selected for imaging of *HSV1-tk* gene expression. However, no biological data is available; therefore, it is difficult to comment whether this tracer will be useful at all. Another study was performed with [^{99m}Tc-N(4)(0-1),Asp(0),Tyr(3)]octreotate (^{99m}Tc-Demotate 2) to evaluate intratumoral delivery of adenoviral vectors and compare it with single injection (SI) and multiple injection (4x, MI) (61). A replication-deficient adenoviral vector encoding the *HSV1-tk* and the human somatostatin receptor subtype 2 [sst(2)] was administered into nude mice bearing subcutaneous U87 xenografts. Tumors were injected with $1.5 \times 10(9)$ plaque-forming units of Ad5.tk.sstr by CED, SI, or MI. Three days later, ^{99m}Tc-Demotate 2 was injected intravenously to monitor the virus-induced sst(2) expression. Gamma-camera imaging was performed for in vivo imaging, and the tumor uptake of ^{99m}Tc-Demotate 2 was determined by gamma-counter. Transfected xenograft tissues showed high sst(2) expression and were clearly visualized with a gamma-camera. Accumulation of radioactivity was twofold higher in the tumors that were injected with MI compared with CED and SI ($P = 0.01$). CED and SI resulted in equal uptake of radioactivity in the tumors. The measured areas of transduction in ex vivo and in vitro autoradiographs showed a high concordance [$r(2) = 0.89, P < 0.0001$]. The maximum area of transfection was significantly larger after MI than after CED ($P < 0.05$) or SI ($P = 0.05$). Also, the measured volume of distribution was twice as high after administration of Ad5.tk.sstr by MI [56.6 mm(3)] compared with SI [25.3 mm(3)] or CED [26.4 mm(3)]. CED does not increase adenoviral vector distribution in a glioma xenograft model compared with SI. Therefore, in the clinic MI is probably the most effective delivery method for the large adenoviral particle (70 nm) in malignant glioma (61).

SUMMARY AND CONCLUSION

Two classes of compounds have been radiolabeled for imaging *HSV1-tk* gene expression, and most of them are labeled with [18]F. These are pyrimidine nucleoside analogues, primarily thymidine analogues; and guanosine analogues, especially acycloguanosine derivatives. Among the pyrimidine nucleoside analogues, most compounds are 2′-deoxy-2′-fluoro-arabinofuranosyluracil derivatives with a variety of substitution in the 5-position. These analogues are excellent substrates for HSV1-TK, however, some of them such as FMAU and FIAU are also substrates for cellular thymidine kinase TK1, therefore, their selectivity toward the *HSV1-tk* is lower than the other analogues. Based on the available data, ^{18}F-FEAU has been acknowledged to be the best radiotracer for imaging the native *HSV1-tk* gene expression. Among the guanosine analogues ^{18}F-FHBG has been acknowledged as the best imaging agent for *HSV1-tk*, although its sensitivity toward the native *HSV1-tk* is much less than that of the pyrimidine nucleoside analogues. Since mutation of the *HSV1-tk* has been achieved by changing the amino acid sequence on different location of the enzyme, the sensitivity of ^{18}F-FHBG has been improved significantly in imaging the mutated *HSV1-tk* gene, and in one case ^{18}F-FHBG has been shown to be the only substrate for that mutated *HSV1-tk* (*HSV1-A168Htk*) without any incorporation of the pyridine nucleoside analogue, such as ^{18}F-FEAU. Therefore, the choice of the probes for imaging the mutated *HSV1-tk* is ^{18}F-FHBG; and that for the native *HSV1-tk* is ^{18}F-FEAU. Although other imaging agents are available, such as radioiodinated agents and Tc-99m-labeled agents, the application of those agents will be quite limited. For example, iodinated compounds have the major drawback of in vivo deiodination; and also their long half-life may restrict in clinical applications of these products. Bromine-76-labeled FBAU may suffer because of the longer half-life of the isotope. The Tc-99m-labeled agent has very limited study done, and more studies are required to show more biological data before approval for clinical application. The most advantage with ^{18}F-FHBG is its approval by the FDA for its clinical applications; and ^{18}F-FEAU is under the process of submission for an IND. Therefore, ^{18}F-FHBG and ^{18}F-FEAU are the choices of radiotracers for imaging *HSV1-tk* gene expression, and the selection of the radiotracer will depend on the type of *HSV1-tk*, such ^{18}F-FHBG is used for mutated gene; and ^{18}F-FEAU is used for native gene. It can be summarized that the pyrimidine nucleoside analogues, such as ^{18}F-FEAU is the choice of radiotracer for imaging the expression of the native *HSV1-tk* gene. On the other hand, ^{18}F-FHBG is the choice of the radiotracer for imaging the expression of the mutated *HSV1-tk* gene such as *HSV1-sr39tk* and *HSV1-A168Htk*.

REFERENCES

1. Moolten FL, Wells JM, Heyman RA, et al. Lymphoma regression induced by ganciclovir in mice bearing a herpes thymidine kinase transgene. Hum Gene Therapy 1990; 1:125–134.

2. Culver KW, Ram Zvi, Wallbridge S, et al. In vivo gene transfer with retroviral vector-producer cells for treatment of experimental brain tumors. Science 1992; 256:1550–1552.

3. Oldfield EH, Ram Zvi, Culver K, et al. Clinical protocols: gene therapy for the treatment of brain tumors using intra-tumoral transduction with the thymidine kinase gene and intravenous ganciclovir. Human Gene Therapy 1993; 4:39–69.

4. Ram Zvi, Culver KW, Oshiro EM, et al. Therapy of malignant brain tumors by intratumoral implantation of retroviral vector producing cells. Nat Med 1997; 3:1354–1361.

5. Tjuvajev JG, Avril N, Oku T, et al. Imaging herpes virus thymidine kinase gene transfer and expression by positron emission tomography. Cancer Res 1998; 58:4333–4341.

6. Gambhir SS, Barrio JR, Phelps ME, et al. Imaging adenoviral-directed reporter gene expression in living animals with positron emission tomography. Proc Natl Acad Sci, U S A 1999; 2333–2338.

7. Urbain JC. Reporter genes and imagene. J Nucl Med 2001; 42:106–109.

8. Tjuvajev JG, Stockhammer G, Desai R, et al. Imaging the expression of transfected genes in vivo. Cancer Res 1995; 55:6126–6132.

9. Gambhir SS, Barrio JR, Herschman HR, et al. Assays for non-invasive imaging of reporter gene expression. Nucl Med Biol 1999; 26:481–490.

10. Tjuvajev JG, Chen SH, Joshi A, et al. Imaging adenoviral-mediated herpes virus thymidine kinase gene transfer and expression in vivo. Cancer Res 1999; 59:5186–5193.

11. Alauddin MM, Shahinian A, Gordon EM, et al. Evaluation of 9-(4-[^{18}F]-fluoro-3-hydroxymethyl-butyl)guanine ([^{18}F]-FHBG) as a probe for PET imaging of gene expression in tumor-bearing nude mice. Anticancer Res 1998; 18:4992–4993.

12. Alauddin MM, Conti PS. Synthesis and preliminary evaluation of 9-(4-[^{18}F]-fluoro-3-hydroxymethyl-butyl)guanine ([^{18}F]-FHBG): a new potential imaging agent for viral infection and gene therapy using PET. Nucl Med Biol 1998; 25:175–180.

13. Alauddin MM, Kundu R, Gordon EM, et al. Evaluation of 9-(3-[^{18}F]-fluoro-1-hydroxy-2-propoxymethyl)guanine ([^{18}F]-FHPG) in vitro and in vivo as a probe for PET imaging of gene incorporation and expression in tumors. Nucl Med Biol 1999; 26:371–376.

14. Yu Y, Annala AJ, Barrio JR, et al. Quantification of gene expression by imaging reporter gene expression in living animals. Nat Med 2000; 6:933–937.

15. Alauddin MM, Shahinian A, Gordon EM, et al. Preclinical evaluation of the penciclovir analog 9-(4-[^{18}F]-fluoro-3-hydroxymethyl-butyl)guanine ([^{18}F]-FHBG for in vivo measurement of suicide gene expression with PET. J Nucl Med 2001; 42:1682–1690.

16. Iyer M, Barrio JR, Namavari M, et al. 8-[^{18}F]-fluoropenciclovir: an improved reporter probe for imaging HSV1-tk reporter gene expression in vivo using PET. J Nucl Med 2001; 42:96–105.

17. Jacobs A, Tjuvajev JG, Dubrovin M, et al. Positron emission tomography-based imaging of transgene expression mediated by replication conditional, oncolytic herpes simplex virus type-1 mutant vectors of cancer. Cancer Res 2001; 61:2983–2995.

18. Haberkorn U, Khazaie K, Morr I, et al. Ganciclovir uptake in human mammary carcinoma cells expressing herpes simplex virus thymidine kinase. Nucl Med Biol 1998; 25:367–373.

19. Tjuvajev JG, Joshi A, Callegari J, et al. A general approach to the non-invasive imaging of transgene using cis-linked herpes virus thymidine kinase. Neoplasia 1999; 1:315–320.

20. Alauddin MM, Conti PS, Mazza SM, et al. Synthesis of 9-[(3-[^{18}F]fluoro-1-hydroxy-2-propoxy)methyl]guanine ([^{18}F]FHPG): a potential imaging agent of viral infection and gene therapy using PET. Nucl Med Biol 1996; 23:787–792.

21. Monclus M, Lauxen A, Van Noemen J, et al. Development of PET radiopharmaceuticals for gene therapy: synthesis of 9-[(3-[^{18}F]fluoro-1-hydroxy-2-propoxy)methyl]guanine. J Labelled Compd Radiopharm 1995; 37:193–195.

22. Monclus M, Damhaut P. Lauxen A, et al. In vitro validation of (R)- and (S)- 9-[(3-[^{18}F]fluoro-1-hydroxy-2-propoxy) methyl]guanine as radiopharmaceuticals for gene therapy. J Labelled Compd Radiopharm 1999; 42:S627–S629.

23. Namavari M, Barrio JR, Toyokuni T, et al. Synthesis of 8-[^{18}F]-fluoroguanine derivatives: in vivo probes for imaging gene expression with PET. Nucl Med Biol 2000; 27:157–162.

24. Tjuvajev JG, Doubrovin M, Akhurst T, et al. Comparison of radiolabeled nucleoside probes (FIAU, FHBG, and FHPG) for PET imaging of HSV1-tk gene expression. J Nucl Med 2002; 43:1072–1083.

25. Watanabe KA, Reichman W, Hirota K, et al. Nucleosides 110. Synthesis and herpes virus activity of some 2′-fluoro-2′-deoxyarabinofuranosyl pyrimidine nucleosides. J Med Chem 1979; 22:21–24.

26. Perlman ME, Watanabe KA, Schinazi RF, et al. Nucleoside 133. Synthesis of 5-alkenyl-1-(2-deoxy-2-fluoro-β-D-arabinofuranosyl)cytocines and related pyrimidine nucleosides as potential antiviral agents. J Med Chem 1985; 28:741–748.

27. Tann CH, Brodfuehrer PR, Brundidge SP, et al. Fluorocarbohydrates in synthesis. An efficient synthesis of 1-(2-deoxy-2-fluoro-β-D-arabinofuranosyl)-5-iodouracil (β-FIAU) and 1-(2-deoxy-2-fluoro-β-D-arabinofuranosyl) 5-methyluracil (β-FIAU). J Org Chem 1985; 50: 3644–3647.

28. Watanabe KA, Su T-L, Reichman U, et al. Nucleosides. 129. Synthesis of antiviral nucleosides: 5-alkenyl-1-(2-deoxy-2-fluoro-β-D-arabinofuranosy)uracis. J Med Chem 1984; 27:91–94.

29. Conti PS, Alauddin MM, Fissekis JD, et al. Synthesis of 2′-fluoro-5-[^{11}C] methyl-1-β-D-arabinofuranosyluracil ([^{11}C]-FMAU): a potential nucleoside analogue for in vivo study of cellular proliferation with PET. Nucl Med Biol 1995; 22:783–789.

30. Alauddin MM, Fissekis JD, Conti PS. Synthesis of [^{18}F]-labeled 2'-deoxy-2'-fluoro-5-methyl-1-β-D-arabinofuranosyluracil ([^{18}F]-FMAU). J Labelled Compd Radiopharm 2002; 45:583–590.

31. Alauddin MM, Fissekis JD, Conti PS. A general synthesis of 2'-deoxy-2'-[^{18}F]fluoro-5-methyl-1-β-d-arabinofuranosyluracil and its 5-substituted nucleosides). J Labelled Compd Radiopharm 2003; 46:285–289.

32. Mangner TJ, Klecker RW, Anderson L, et al. Synthesis of 2'-deoxy-2'-[^{18}F]fluoro-1-β-D-arabinofuranosyl nucleosides, [^{18}F]FAU, [^{18}F]FMAU, [^{18}F]FBAU and [^{18}F]FIAU, as potential PET agents for imaging cellular proliferation. Nucl Med Biol 2003; 30:215–224.

33. Pillarsetty N, Cai S, Ageyeva L, et al. Synthesis and evaluation of [^{18}F] labeled pyrimidine nucleosides for positron emission tomography imaging of herpes simplex virus 1 thymidine kinase gene expression. J Med Chem 2006; 49(17):5377–5381.

34. Reichman U, Watanabe KA, Fox JJ. A practical synthesis of 2-deoxy-fluoro-D-arabinofuranose derivatives. Carbohydrate Res 1975; 42:233–240.

35. Pankiewicz KW, Nawrot B, Gadler H, et al. Nucleosides 146. 1-Methyl-5-(2-deoxy-2-fluoro-arabinofuranosyl)uracil, the C-nucleoside isoster of the potent antiviral agent 1-(2-deoxy-2-fluoro-β-D-arabinofuranosyluracil)thymine (FMAU). Studies towards the synthesis of 2'-deoxy-2' substituted arabino nucleosides. J Med Chem 1987; 30:2314–2316.

36. Mukhopadhyay U, Pal A, Gelovani JG, et al. Radiosynthesis of 2'-deoxy-2'-[^{18}F]-fluoro-5-methyl-1-β-L-arabinofuranosyluracil ([^{18}F]-L-FMAU) for PET. Appl Radiat Isot 2007; 65(8):941–946.

37. Hong SH, Choi TH, Kim EJ. Biological evaluation of D- and L-form 5-methyl-2'-deoxy-2'-[^{18}F]fluoroarabinofuranosyluracil (D-FMAU and L-FMAU) in HSV1-tk gene expression cell line bearing mice. Joint Molecular Imaging Conference, Providence, Rhode Island, Sept 8–11, 2007.

38. Yu C-H, Eisenbarth J, Runz A, et al. Synthesis of 5-(2-radiohaloethyl)- and 5-(2-radiohalovinyl)-2'-deoxyuridines. Novel types of radiotracer for monitoring cancer gene therapy with PET. J Labelled Compd Radiopharm 2003; 46:421–439.

39. Balatoni JA, Doubrovin M, Ageyeva L, et al. Imaging herpes viral thymidine kinase-1 reporter gene expression with a new ^{18}F-labeled probe: 2'-fluoro-2'-deoxy-5-[^{18}F]fluoroethyl-1-β-D-arabinofuranosyluracil. Nucl Med Biol 2005; 32(8):811–819.

40. Wang HE, Yu HM, Liu RS, et al. Molecular imaging with ^{123}I-FIAU, ^{18}F-FUdR, ^{18}F-FET, and ^{18}F-FDG for monitoring herpes simplex virus type 1 thymidine kinase and ganciclovir prodrug activation gene therapy of cancer. J Nucl Med 2006; 47:1161–1171.

41. Raic-Malic S, Johayem A, Ametamey SM, et al. Synthesis, ^{18}F-radiolabeling and biological evaluation of C-6 alkylated pyrimidine nucleoside analogues. Nucleosides Nucleotides Nucleic acids 2004; 23:1707–1721.

42. Grote M, Noll S, Noll B. Synthesis of ^{18}F-labeled acyclic purine and pyrimidine nucleosides intended for monitoring gene expression. Radiochimica Acta 2005; 93 (9–10):585–588.

43. Grote M, Noll B, Noll S. Syntheses of novel modified acyclic purine and pyrimidine nucleosides as potential substrates of herpes simplex virus type-1 thymidine kinase for monitoring gene expression. Can J Chem 2004; 82 (4):513–523.

44. Elion GB, Furman PA, Fyfe JA, et al. Selectivity of action of an antiherpetic agent, 9-(2-hydroxy-ethoxymathyl)guanine. Proc Natl Acad Sci U S A 1977; 74:5716–5720.

45. Cheng Y-C, Grill SP, Dutschman GE, et al. Metabolism of 9-(1, 3-dihydroxy-2-propoxymethyl)guanine, a new antiherpes virus compound in herpes simplex virus-infected cells. J Biol Chem 1983; 258:12460–12464.

46. Boyd MR, Bacon TH, Sutton D, et al. Antiherpes virus activity of 9-(4-hydroxy-3-hydroxymethylbut-1-yl)guanine (BRL 39123) in cell culture. Antimicrob Agents Chemother 1987; 31:1238–1242.

47. Martin JC, McGee D, Jeffrey G, et al. Synthesis and anti-herpes-virus activity of acyclic 2'-deoxyguanosine analogues related to 9-[(1, 3-dihydroxy-2-propoxy)methyl]guanine. J Med Chem 1986; 29:1384–1389.

48. Shiue GG, Shiue CY, Lee RL, et al. A simplified one-pot synthesis of 9-[(3-[^{18}F]fluoro-1-hydroxy-2-propoxy) methyl]guanine ([^{18}F]FHPG) and 9-(4-[^{18}F]fluoro-3-hydroxymethylbutyl)-guanine ([^{18}F]FHBG) for gene therapy. Nucl Med Biol 2001; 28(7):875–883.

49. Wang JQ, Zheng QH, Fei X, et al. Novel radiosynthesis of PET HSV1-tk gene reporter probes [^{18}F]FHPG and [^{18}F]FHBG employing dual Sep-Pak SPE techniques. Bioorg Med Chem Lett 2003; 13:3933–3938.

50. Penuelas I, Boán JF, Marti-Climent JM, et al. A fully automated one pot synthesis of 9-(4-[^{18}F]fluoro-3-hydroxymethylbutyl) guanine for gene therapy studies. Mol Imaging Biol 2002; 4:415–424.

51. Ponde DE, Dence CS, Schuster DP, et al. Rapid and reproducible radiosynthesis of [^{18}F] FHBG. Nucl Med Biol 2004; 31:133–138.

52. Chang CW, Lin M, Wu SY, et al. A high yield robotic synthesis of 9-(4-[18F]-fluoro-3-hydroxymethylbutyl)guanine ([^{18}F]FHBG) and 9-[3-[^{18}F]fluoro-1-hydroxy-2-propoxy)methyl]guanine([^{18}F]-FHPG) for gene expression imaging. Appl Radiat Isot 2007; 65:57–63.

53. Cai H, Yin D, Zhang L, et al. Preparation and biological evaluation of 2-amino-6-[^{18}F]fluoro-9-(4-hydroxy-3-hydroxy-methylbutyl) purine (6[^{18}FFPCV] as a novel PET probe for imaging HSV1-tk reporter gene expression. Nucl Med Biol 2007; 34:717–725.

54. Schipper ML, Goris ML, Gambhir SS. Evaluation of herpes simplex virus 1 thymidine kinase-mediated trapping of (131)I FIAU and prodrug activation of ganciclovir as a synergistic cancer radio/chemotherapy. Mol Imaging Biol 2007; 9(3):110–116.

55. Dempsey MF, Wyper D, Owens J, et al. Assessment of 123I-FIAU imaging of herpes simplex viral gene expression in the treatment of glioma. Nucl Med Commun 2006; 27(8):611–617.

56. Hsieh CH, Liu RS, Wang HE, et al. In vitro evaluation of herpes simplex virus type 1 thymidine kinase reporter system in dynamic studies of transcriptional gene regulation. Nucl Med Biol 2006; 33(5):653–660.

57. Verwijnen SM, Sillevis Smith PA, Hoeben RC, et al. Molecular imaging and treatment of malignant gliomas following adenoviral transfer of the herpes simplex virus-thymidine kinase gene and the somatostatin receptor subtype 2 gene. Cancer Biother Radiopharm 2004; 19(1): 111–120.

58. Choi TH, Ahn SH, Kwon HC, et al. In vivo comparison of IVDU and IVFRU in HSV1-TK gene expressing tumor bearing rats. Appl Radiat Isot 2004; 60(1):15–21.

59. Cho SY, Ravasi L, Szajek LP, et al. Evaluation of ^{76}Br-FBAU as a PET reporter probe for HSV1-tk gene expression imaging using mouse models of human glioma. J Nucl Med 2005; 46:1923–1930.

60. Zhang Y, Lin J, Pan D. Synthesis of a technetium-99m labeled tricyclic ganciclovir analog for non-invasive reporter gene expression imaging. Bioorg Med Chem Lett 2007; 17:741–744.

61. ter Horst M, Verwijnen SM, Brouwer E, et al. Locoregional delivery of adenoviral vectors. J Nucl Med 2006; 47 (9):1483–1489.

62. Satio Y, Price RW, Rottenberg DA. Quantitative autoradiographic maping of herpes simplex virus encephalitis with radiolabeled antiviral drug. Science 1982; 217:1151–1153.

63. deVries EFJ, Waarde A, Harmsen MC, et al. [^{11}C]FMAU and [^{18}F]FHPG as PET tracers for herpes simplex virus thymidine kinase enzyme activity and human cytomegalovirus infections. Nucl Med Biol 2000; 27:113–119.

64. Alauddin MM, Shahinaian A, Gordon EM, et al. Evaluation of 2'-deoxy-2'-fluoro-5-methyl-1-β-D-arabinofuranosyluracil as a potential gene imaging agents for HSV1-tk expression in vivo. Mol Imaging 2002; 1:74–81.

65. Alauddin MM, Shahinaian A, Gordon EM, et al. Direct comparison of radiolabeled probes FMAU, FHBG and FHPG as PET imaging agents for HSV1-tk gene expression in human breast cancer model. Mol Imaging 2004; 3: 76–84.

66. Alauddin MM, Shahinian A, Park R, et al. Synthesis of 2'-deoxy-2'-[^{18}F]fluoro-5-bromo-1-β-D-arabinofuranosyluracil ([^{18}F]FBAU) and 2'-deoxy-2'-[^{18}F]fluoro-5-chloro-1-β-D-arabinofuranosyluracil ([^{18}F]FCAU), and their biological evaluation as markers for gene expression. Nucl Med Biol 2004; 31:399–405.

67. Alauddin MM, Shahinian A, Park R, et al. Synthesis and evaluation of 2'-deoxy-2'-[^{18}F]fluoro-5-fluoro-1-β-D-arabinofuranosyluracil as a potential PET imaging agent for gene expression. J Nucl Med 2004; 45:2063–2069.

68. Alauddin MM, Shahinian A, Park R, et al. In vivo evaluation of 2'-deoxy-2'-[^{18}F]fluoro-5-iodo-1-β-d-arabinofuranosyluracil ([^{18}F]-FIAU) and 2'-deoxy-2'-[^{18}F]fluoro-5-ethyl-1-β-d-arabinofuranosyluracil ([^{18}F]-FEAU) as markers for suicide gene expression. Eur J Nucl Med Mol Imaging 2007; 34:822–829.

69. Alauddin MM, Shahinian A, Conti PS. Evaluation of 2'-deoxy-2'-fluoro-5-substituted-1-β-D-arabinofuranosyluracils as markers for suicide gene expression in breast cancer cells. J Nucl Med 2005; 46:35.

70. Buurnsma AR, Rutgers V, Hospers GAP, et al. ^{18}F-FEAU as a radiotracer for Herpes simplex virus thymidine kinase gene expression: in-vitro comparison with other PET tracers. Nucl Med Commun 2006; 27:25–30.

71. Kang KW, Min JJ, Chen X, et al. Comparison of [^{14}C]FMAU, [^{3}H]FEAU, [^{14}C]FIAU and [^{3}H]PCV for monitoring reporter gene expression with wild type and mutated herpes simplex virus type 1 thymidine kinase in cell culture. Mol Imaging Biol 2005; 7:296–303.

72. Tseng JC, Zanzonico PB, Levin B, et al. Tumor specific in vivo transfection with HSV-1 thymidine kinase gene using a Sindbis viral vector as a basis for prodrug ganciclovir activation and PET. J Nucl Med 2006; 47:1136–1143.

73. Hajitou A, Trepel M, Lilley CE, et al. A hybrid vector for ligand-directed tumor targeting and molecular imaging. Cell 2006; 125:385–398.

74. Soghomonyan S, Hajitou AE, Rangel R, et al. Molecular PET Imaging of HSV1-tk Reporter Gene Expression using [^{18}F]-FEAU. Nat Protoc 2007; 2:416–423.

75. Nishii R, Volgin AY, Mawlawi O, et al. Evaluation of 2'-deoxy-2'[^{18}F]fluoro-5-methyl-1-β-L-arabinofuranosyluracil ([^{18}F]-L-FMAU) as a PET imaging agent for cellular proliferation: comparison with [^{18}F]-D-FMAU and [^{18}F]FLT. Eur J Nucl Med Mol Imaging 2008; 35:990–998.

76. deVries EFJ, van Dillen IJ, Waarde A, et al. Evaluation of [^{18}F]FHPG as PET tracer for HSV1-tk gene expression. Nucl Med Biol 2003; 30:651–660.

77. Yaghoubi S, Barrio JR, Dahlbom M, et al. Human pharmacokinetic and dosimetry studies of [^{18}F]FHBG: a reporter probe for imaging herpes simplex virus Type-1 thymidine kinase reporter gene expression. J Nucl Med 2001; 42:1225–1234.

78. Herschman HR, MacLaren DC, Iyer M, et al. Seeing is believing: non-invasive, quantitative and repetitive imaging of reporter gene expression in living animals, using positron emission tomography. J Neurosci Res 2000; 59:699–705.

79. Gambhir SS, Barrio JR, Herschman HR, et al. Assays for noninvasive imaging of reporter gene expression. Nucl Med Biol 1999; 26:481–490.

80. Yu Y, Annala AJ, Barrio JR, et al. Quantification of target gene expression by imaging reporter gene expression in living animals. Nat Med 2000; 6:933–937.

81. Yaghoubi SS, Wu L, Liang Q, et al. Direct correlation between positron emission tomographic images of two reporter genes delivered by two distinct adenoviral vectors. Gene Ther 2001; 8:1072–1080.

82. Green LA, Nguyen K, Berenji B, et al. A tracer kinetic model for ^{18}F-FHBG for quantitating herpes simplex virus type 1 thymidine kinase reporter gene expression in living animals using PET. J Nucl Med 2004; 45: 1560–1570.

83. Yaghoubi SS, Gambhir SS. PET imaging of herpes simplex virus type 1 thymidine kinase (HSV1-tk) or mutated HSV1-sr39tk reporter gene expression in mice using [^{18}F]FHBG. Nat Protocols 2006; 1:3069–3075.

84. Black ME, Newcomb TG, Wilson HM, et al. Creation of drug-specific herpes simplex virus type 1 thymidine kinase mutants for gene therapy. Proc Natl Acad Sci U S A 1996; 93:3525–3529.

85. Black ME, Kokoris MS, Sabo P. Herpes simplex virus-1 thymidine kinase mutants created by semi-random sequence mutagenesis improve prodrug-mediated tumor cell killing. Cancer Res 2001; 61:3022–3026.

86. Bazarini J, Liekens S, Solaroli N, et al. Engineering of a single conserved amino acid residue of herpes simplex virus type 1 thymidine kinase allows a predominant shift from pyrimidine to purine nucleoside phosphorylation. J Biol Chem 2006; 281:19273–19279.

87. Najjar A, Nishii R, Maxwell D, et al. PET imaging with a novel mutant HSV1-tk reporter gene with enhanced specificity to acycloguanosine nucleoside analogs. J Nucl Med 2007, (submitted).

27

Clinical Potential of Gene Expression Imaging

VIKAS KUNDRA

Departments of Diagnostic Radiology and Experimental Diagnostic Imaging, University of Texas M.D. Anderson Cancer Center, Houston, Texas, U.S.A.

INTRODUCTION

Methods for monitoring and specifically imaging expressed genes are poised to benefit gene therapy. There is great promise for gene and cellular therapies to treat a variety of diseases such as cardiovascular diseases, genetic diseases, diabetes, neurodegenerative diseases, and cancer. Among the over 1300 gene therapy clinical trials already completed or ongoing worldwide (1), most focus on cancer (66%) and cardiovascular diseases (9%), whereas others focus on monogenic diseases, infectious diseases, gene marking, neurologic diseases, ocular diseases, other diseases, or healthy volunteers (2). Because of the broad scope of the technology, a variety of genes have been transferred, including those for antigens (20%), cytokines (19%), tumor suppressors, growth factors, suicide, receptors, and markers, among others. A great majority of such trials have been/are performed in the United States (66%) or Europe (27%), and almost all have been either phase I or II studies (96%). There was great excitement during the origins of this relatively young field. The number of gene therapy clinical trials steadily increased from 1989 to 1999 and then plateaued at approximately 95/yr. Reasons for drop-off in expansion in the number of new trials included concern for safety and questions regarding expression. Newer technologies addressing the former have reignited interest, whereas noninvasive metrics for the latter are beginning to be addressed by molecular imaging.

Gene therapy may consist of delivering a gene to a specific tissue by direct injection into the tissue or via systemic delivery. Many different vectors may be applied. Clinically, for delivery, the most common vectors are adenovirus (25%), retroviruses (23%), naked/plasmid DNA (18%), lipofection, vaccinia virus, pox virus, adeno-associated virus (AAV), herpes simplex virus, among others (1). The choice of vector can influence the location of delivery. For example, naked/plasmid DNA tends to express better upon injection into muscle. The location of delivery may also be driven by the biologic process. For example, for treating Parkinson's disease, the substantia nigra is a target, and in cancer, the tumor is a target. Thus, most gene therapies target specific tissues. However, it remains difficult to locate gene expression in the body without performing a biopsy.

Although target presence may be evaluated by biopsy, there is a low rate of complications, and some structures such as the brain are more difficult to access. To follow expression serially, multiple biopsies would be needed over time. This can lower patient compliance. In many instances, biopsy may not be the ideal test. For example, in larger tumors, sampling error can limit evaluation of the heterogeneity of expression within the mass. Delivery to multiple sites is difficult to assess by biopsy because of practical issues of the number of sites that can be sampled and because of patient compliance. For example, in patients with metastases, heterogeneity of expression in the different metastases is difficult to assess by biopsy and there may be greater expression in some metastases, but not others. Further, this limits evaluation of biodistribution because one cannot sample all organs of interest. In some situations, the biopsy itself can alter underlying tissue, limiting secondary evaluation, such as ^{18}F fluorodeoxyglucose (^{18}F-FDG) uptake, and limiting evaluation of clinical therapeutic effect since lesions created by biopsy may be of clinical significance, such as in the brain.

Although studying delivery is important, to evaluate success of the entire process, evaluation of the protein product is desirable. One may attempt to image the product directly or make imaging agents that bind, and thus allow visualization of the imaging product. As can be seen above, a large number of genes have therapeutic potential. Attempting to make imaging systems for each would be a daunting task. This is exemplified by the limited number of imaging agents that have been approved for clinical use.

Alternatively, a reporter may be used. In this case, a reporter gene may be developed whose product binds an imaging agent. This reporter gene may then be used to follow expression via a delivery vehicle, or its expression may be linked to that of a therapeutic gene; and, in the latter case, imaging of the reporter gene can be used to gauge expression of the linked therapeutic gene. Because the reporter gene may be considered a movable cassette, it may be placed in a variety of delivery vectors or linked to a variety of therapeutic genes; thus, one reporter gene system can be applied to numerous gene therapies, providing versatility.

Clearly, tagging a gene with a reporter that can be noninvasively imaged will benefit monitoring efficacy and toxicity. One would then be able to determine whether expression is achieved in the target tissue and, with the appropriate reporter, determine whether the necessary level of expression is achieved for therapeutic effect. Additionally, if the reporter could be repeatedly visualized (3), the duration and level of expression in a particular location could be repeatedly monitored, aiding dosing regimens. Maintaining long-term expression is presently a challenge for the field of gene therapy. In addition, following expression in nontarget tissues should also prove fruitful because of its potential to impact toxicity.

Thus, imaging methods designed to detect gene expression in vivo will be needed, both for further development of gene delivery systems and for monitoring clinical efficacy and toxicity. Further, a number of imaging systems will be needed for monitoring either single gene therapy or multiple gene therapies in a patient. For example, a patient with diabetes and cancer may benefit from two different gene therapy interventions that can be monitored independently by two separate reporters. If an inducible promoter is used, it may be advantageous to also transfer a constitutively active promoter inducing a different reporter to gauge whether gene transfer occurred in case induction fails.

Although a few gene expression imaging systems have been designed, many do not sufficiently penetrate human tissues [those based on light such as green fluorescent protein (GFP) or luciferase]. Light-based systems are useful in small animals and may prove useful clinically for evaluating expression in or near external epithelial structures, such as the skin, or in or near internal epithelium interrogated by endoscopy. For percutaneous imaging, currently, radiopharmaceutical-based techniques are the nearest to clinical use owing to the sensitivity of nuclear medicine cameras. There have also been positive developments for MR-based imaging of gene expression, although sensitivity of MR for imaging agents is comparatively less.

UNMET NEEDS FOR GENE THERAPY—CHARACTERIZING EXPRESSION: LOCATION, QUANTIFICATION, AND DURATION

Gene therapy has enjoyed limited success. Most of the clinical trials to date have primarily assessed safety in phase I or II studies. A major limitation has been characterizing expression. Expression of an introduced gene tends to increase, plateau, and then commonly wane. The relative duration of each of these cycles varies depending on the delivery vehicle, delivered gene, and the patient. For efficacy, one needs to express the gene in the appropriate amount, in the appropriate location, and for an appropriate duration of time. Thus, gene therapy like drug therapy requires development of dosing schedules. Clinical trials incorporating multiple doses of gene therapy have been performed (4). To understand toxicity, one also needs to assess expression in nontarget tissues.

When deciding on a gene therapy trial, one has to select not only the appropriate gene for therapy but also the appropriate vector. Briefly, viral vectors tend to provide greater expression, but tend to have greater immunogenicity and may have greater cell type restriction. Immune responses tend to be greater toward the commonly utilized adenovirus. This virus tends to be episomal and results in the greatest amount of expression among delivery vehicles, but the expression is transient, usually lasting a few days to weeks because integration into the genome is uncommon. In comparison, other viral vectors such as retroviruses, AAVs, or lentivirus-based vectors tend to be relatively less immunogenic; tend to have less expression, but due to integration, expression is commonly of long duration; and may be cell type restricted, but usually less than adenovirus. Liposomal delivery tends to result in low levels of expression, less immunogenicity, and may be cell type restricted. Naked DNA tends to result in good expression in muscle, but not in tumors.

Many of the new gene therapies will target particular locations. Strategies for targeted expression include altering the binding domains of the delivery vehicle or using tissue-specific promoters. Clinical trials have already attempted to exploit such targeting strategies; for example, "pathotropic" systems based on von Willebrand's clotting factor were used to target exposed collagen in tumors (5), and the osteocalcin promoter was used to attempt to drive expression in prostate cancer cells and adjacent stroma (6). As such targeted systems are developed, confirmation of expression in target and nontarget tissues will be needed.

In the case of systemic therapy, such as production of insulin, each cell in a particular location need not express. Assessing overall expression levels is adequate. In other instances, heterogeneity of expression at a local site may be problematic, for example, in the case of cancer. Although target presence may be evaluated by biopsy, the distribution of expression is not evaluated. Sampling error may give a false idea of expression since only sites of greatest or least expression may be sampled. Without bystander effect, areas of tumor without expression may not respond to the targeted therapy. In patients with metastases, heterogeneity of expression in different metastases may be limiting. If expression is present in some metastases, but not others, there may be a mixed response to the therapy, suggesting that improved delivery, adding a chemotherapeutic, or adding local therapy such as radiation, may be useful to enhance efficacy. Thus, evaluation within and among tumors is needed.

Another issue limiting gene therapy may be lack of a receptor for internalization of the delivery vehicle into the target cell. This is exemplified by adenovirus, which prefers infecting cells expressing coxsackie-adenovirus receptor (CAR domain) and integrins such as $\alpha_v\beta_3$ and $\alpha_v\beta_5$. Expression of the CAR domain is variable and some cells lack its expression, furthermore, heterogeneity of its expression as well as that of integrins can be variable within the same tumor (7). Additionally, systemic adenovirus delivery results in a large amount of infection of the liver, resulting in less availability for other target sites. To redirect "tropism" of the virus, it has been decorated, for example, with peptides, antibodies, or growth factors. With such vector manipulations, the question remains, did the manipulation improve targeted expression and decrease the "natural tropism" to nonspecific tissues such as the liver?

When performing therapy, it is common to ask what is the best route of administration: systemic, such as intra-

arterial, intravenous, intraperitoneal; or local, which may be the aforementioned routes, but may also include intratumoral, subcutaneous, intramuscular, or inhalational? There is overlap since local delivery of a gene can result in a product secreted into the blood stream that can have systemic effects. The route of delivery can be dictated by the vector. For example, naked/plasmid DNA express more in muscle, systemic delivery of adenovirus tends to result in expression in the liver, and lipid-based formulations tend to result in expression in the lungs.

In many instances, the disease will dictate a preferred route of delivery. For example, cystic fibrosis is an autosomal recessive disease caused by mutations of the cystic fibrosis transmembrane regulator (CFTR) gene. It provides instructions for making a channel that transports negatively charged chloride ions into and out of cells, which in turn helps control the movement of water, thus affecting the consistency of mucus. Mutations in the CFTR gene result in thick, sticky mucus that first clogs the respiratory tract and later digestive organs, particularly the pancreas. Signs and symptoms of cystic fibrosis presenting in childhood tend to be related to respiratory infections secondary to mucus obstructing the airways. Later in life, both exocrine and endocrine pancreatic functions may fail. Because the first organ to be affected by potentially life-threatening infections is the lungs, gene therapy to provide the wild-type CFTR gene has been attempted using adenovirus delivered by inhalation (8). With new conventional therapies, patients with cystic fibrosis are now often living longer and may experience pancreatic failure. Thus, selective intra-arterial routes via the celiac axis for selective delivery to the pancreas or systemic delivery such as intravenously for delivery to the lungs and pancreas may be evaluated in the future. Expression after delivery by these routes needs to be tested.

Ovarian cancer arises within the abdomen and, except for late-stage disease, metastases tend to occur within the abdomen, most commonly within the peritoneum and less commonly within retroperitoneal lymph nodes. Because of the biology of this disease, an intraperitoneal route of therapy administration has been attempted (9). Theoretically, intraperitoneal delivery should result in homogeneous distribution of the vector throughout the abdomen, but entry into the abdomen can result in adhesions, particularly with long-term catheter placement, which can result in sequestering of virus in pockets created by the adhesions. Further, infection may occur not only of targeted ovarian cells but also of normal cells such as mesothelial cells. Adenovirus may potentially become systemic since the peritoneal cavity can serve as a route for vascular delivery. Another issue is depth of penetration of the virus into the target organ/tumor with such a surface delivery approach. Studies with conventional cytotoxic agents have suggested that the effectiveness of intraperitoneal treatment is highly dependent on the diameter of the residual tumor nodules and that the best responses are noted in tumors less than 0.5 cm in diameter (10,11). This may be addressed by appropriate dosing, continuous infusion, or supplementation with systemic delivery for delivering virus to the tumor via the vasculature. In this case, assessments of distribution of expression within the abdomen, between normal abdominal structures and the tumor, between the peritoneum and retroperitoneum, among sites outside the abdomen, and three-dimensionally within the target are needed.

Even with localized delivery, host factors may limit expression. Immune and decoy mechanisms may restrict delivery. For example, virus-neutralizing antibodies may be present, and these have been noted in ovarian cancer-related ascites. Matrix proteins that bind integrins, such as fibronectin and fibrinogen, may compete with or obstruct vector binding and internalization; and potentially secreted CAR domains may compete with and thus block adenovirus binding (9).

Expression in clinical trials has been determined primarily by biopsy. There are a variety of difficulties with biopsy as mentioned above, including access to certain sites, potential alteration of the underlying tissue, heterogeneity among sites delivered such as within a tumor and among metastases, need for longitudinal evaluation to assess expression over time, practical limitations in the number of organs that can be sampled, patient compliance, and uncommonly complications such as hemorrhage or infection that may be more devastating in particular locations such as the brain.

Noninvasive methods for imaging gene expression are needed. The approach of making an imaging agent for each delivery vehicle or gene of interest is not practical because it would be time consuming, expensive, and in some cases, technically exceptionally difficult. An alternative approach is to use a reporter gene that can be inserted into delivery vehicles and/or linked to a gene of interest, and whose product can be visualized and quantified directly or indirectly. This provides versatility. One reporter may be used for a variety of applications.

Because patients often suffer from more than one disease, multiple reporters will be needed to visualize and quantify the different gene therapies that a patient may receive. In some situations, a single gene target may not be effective by itself, therefore multiple genes may be delivered. In this case, multiple different reporters would be needed, each linked to a different therapeutic gene, to assess relative expression because the ratio of expression may dictate efficacy. More than one reporter may also be needed within a single delivery vehicle when analyzing two separate promoters or genes of interest, such as inducible promoter activity and constitutive reporter activity.

For most reporter technologies, the reporter gene encodes a protein product that binds a systemically introduced imaging agent. The most commonly introduced imaging agents are radiopharmaceuticals owing to the exquisite sensitivity of nuclear medicine imaging cameras. In one example of a reporter imaging experiment, the subject has the reporter gene introduced into the body and after a certain time period to allow for transcription and translation, a radiopharmaceutical is introduced systemically intravenously. After another defined period of time (minutes to days), the subject is placed in front of or within a planar/single-photon emission computed tomography (SPECT) camera or a positron emission tomography (PET) camera. Radioactive decay is then counted and spatially encoded for image reconstruction. The image can be used to localize the activity. Nuclear medicine is a functional technique. Combining nuclear medicine data with anatomic data, such as by magnetic resonance or CT, can aid both signal localization and quantification. Alternative technologies such as MR may also be used for reporter imaging; however, using conventional proton MR, the relative concentration of imaging agent needs to be higher (usually mM instead of nM) and there may be a longer delay in the time between introduction of the imaging agent and imaging. Other imaging modalities, such as CT and ultrasound, require even higher concentrations of imaging agent.

PHYSICS

Radionuclides are unstable atoms. Nucleons in their ground state are stable, but if the ratio of neutrons to protons is not optimal or the nucleons are not in their ground state, they may release energy/particles, including gamma rays with characteristic energy. The de-excitation may occur immediately or be delayed. If the latter, the nucleus is said to be in a metastable state. The decay of ^{99m}Tc (m for metastable) is commonly imaged in nuclear medicine. Gamma rays usually arise from nucleon energy changes; in nuclear medicine imaging, they usually arise from radiopharmaceuticals delivered into the body. The characteristic energy signature is used to distinguish radioactive decay arising directly from the radionuclide from background/scatter reactions that result in different energies from the source of interest. Gamma cameras are used in nuclear medicine to image gamma rays from radiopharmaceuticals administered to patients. Spectral analysis can be used to distinguish the characteristic energies of different radionuclides. This permits distinction of radiopharmaceuticals labeled with different radionuclides, theoretically permitting distinction of different reporter gene products simultaneously. A gamma camera may form a two-dimensional or planar image, or the camera may rotate around, more commonly than encircle, the patient to obtain multiple planar images in different projections that can be processed into 3D images as in SPECT.

A particular type of nucleon decay is positron emission, which reduces the number of protons in the nucleus by transforming a proton to a neutron and ejecting both a positron and a neutrino from the nucleus. A positron has the same mass as an electron, but opposite charge. After traveling a short distance (usually millimeters), it loses kinetic energy and collides with an electron in an annihilation reaction that transforms their combined mass into energy, releasing two gamma-ray photons (each of 511 keV) traveling in opposite trajectories. This allows coincidence detection, for localizing an annihilation event along a line called the line of response (LOR) that connects the two detectors. In PET imaging, a ring of radiation detectors encircles the patient and detect the gamma rays on opposite sides within a specified period of time. Positron decay results in photons with a characteristic energy of 511 keV, therefore different PET radiopharmaceuticals cannot be distinguished by spectral gating. If more than one radiopharmaceutical is to be imaged, they must be distinguished over time. This is aided by the fact that most clinically useful radionuclides that decay by positron emission have short half-lives in the order of minutes. Because positrons travel a short distance before decay, resolution and magnification is theoretically limited. In comparison, gamma cameras attempt to image single gamma rays from the atom itself and can theoretically be used for infinite magnification. Gamma cameras distinguish gamma rays from scatter by characteristic energy windows and collimators designed to filter scatter. Unlike SPECT, PET imaging does not require a collimator to help identify the source of activity and clinically, currently, has higher sensitivity. Both SPECT and PET cameras have large linear ranges for quantifying the amount of radioactive decay.

MR is both a functional and high-resolution anatomic technique. Because of its natural abundance, nonzero nuclear spin (odd number of protons, neutrons, or both), and available imaging coils, hydrogen is most commonly imaged. In a strong static magnetic field, a very small net excess of protons preferentially align with the magnetic field. Additional time-varying magnetic fields are applied to encode spatial information, and the signals created are reconstructed into the MR image. Most commonly, clinical MR images are either T_1-weighted or T_2-weighted. In the case of the T_1-weighted images, the image contrast depends primarily on the T_1 (spin-lattice) relaxation times, with substances having short T_1 relaxation times, such as fat, appearing hyperintense (brighter). Most MR contrast agents are based on the gadolinium atom (seven unpaired electrons), which causes shortening of T_1 relaxation times of water protons in its local vicinity, resulting in hyperintense areas on T_1-weighted images. T_2-weighted

image contrast depends primarily on the T_2 (spin-spin) relaxation times, and substances with long T_2 relaxation times, such as more hydrated material, appear hyperintense. Ferromagnetic substances, such as iron-based contrast agents, decrease T_2 relaxation times of adjacent water molecules, causing hypointense (dark) signal on T_2-weighted images. Note that traditional MR contrast agents affect signal by altering adjacent water molecules. Thus, the local environment can influence the amount and appearance of MR signal, which limits signal quantification.

REPORTER GENES

Reporter genes include those encoding for receptors, such as somatostatin receptor type 2 (SSTR2)-based (12,13) or dopamine receptor type 2 (D2R)-based (3); enzymes, such as herpes simplex virus type 1 thymidine kinase (HSV1-TK)-based (14,15); and transporters, such as sodium-iodide symporter (NIS)-based (16). Other reporter systems have also been suggested.

An ideal reporter should be amenable to imaging in vivo, small, amenable to imaging by a variety of methods, amenable to repetitive imaging in an appropriate timescale, nonimmunogenic, should not perturb the cellular milieu, should not interfere with endogenous cellular signaling or function, should not interfere with the products of introduced (therapeutic) genes, and should be quantifiable in vitro, in vivo, and ex vivo. Ideally, the reporter probe should accumulate proportional to the magnitude of the reporter gene product, be nontoxic, have access to the organ of interest, have low background (particularly in the organ of interest), and be FDA approved for use in humans. Quantification of reporter expression in the patient should be possible using noninvasive imaging.

The reporter needs to fit into a vector using as little of the limited insert space available as possible. This is more important for certain vectors such as AAV, which commonly support inserts of only approximately 3 kb (17). This leaves little room for insertion of both a therapeutic gene and a reporter gene, and since the phenotypic benefit will come from the therapeutic gene, the reporter gene needs to be of minimal size. The size of more extensively studied reporter genes are approximately 1100 kb for human SSTR2 (18) and HSV1-TK (19), 1250 kb for the rat D2R (20), and 2000 kb for the human NIS (21).

Most reporter gene systems are currently unimodal and primarily nuclear medicine-based. MR-based reporter gene imaging has been performed, for example, using the transferin receptor with iron-based MR contrast agents (22), and a β-galactosidase-based system with a gadolinium-based imaging agent in animals (23). With appropriate imaging agents, multimodal imaging of a given reporter should be possible.

Immunogenicity of the reporter is not desirable in most circumstances since it may result in an immune response and potentially kill transduced cells, prevent repeated administration of the therapy, and worse, possibly cause an anaphylactic reaction. Nonimmunogenic reporters are desirable for many applications, but may not be needed if a goal of the gene therapy is to induce an immune response, as may be the case for some cancer therapies. It has been noted that donor lymphocytes transduced to express HSV-TK elicit a strong immune response to this transgene and the response increases with repeated exposure (24). Berger et al. (25) also found that the T-cell response to HSV-TK recognized multiple epitopes, suggesting modifications of immunogenic sequences in the transgene are unlikely to be effective in humans, where the diversity of human leukocyte antigen (HLA) alleles will allow the recognition of multiple immunogenic epitopes and intimates that introduction of HSV-TK may be used to boost immunity to transduced cells or contemporaneously introduced therapeutic genes. Predictably, Traversari et al. suggest that the immune response is dependent on the degree of immunocompetence, with greater response occuring with greater immunocompetence, and that immunogenic reporter genes may be useful in appropriately immunocompromised patients (26). Such findings suggest that using immunogenic reporters will limit not only cell-trafficking studies, particularly of autologous stem cells for tissue repair and regeneration, but may also lead to the death of transduced cells when such a reporter is used with another gene. This is a problem for nonlethal gene therapies such as for diabetes or X-linked severe combined immunodeficiency, where the goal is to maintain expression of the gene of interest. It may also be a problem for interpretation of lethal gene therapies, because one has to separate the effect of the reporter from that of the therapeutic gene. Inflammation can also interfere with assessment of other modalities for analyzing efficacy, including CT, MR, and more so ^{18}F-FDG PET. In addition, immunogenicity may limit repetitive dosing, which will be desirable in many gene therapy situations since gene expression very commonly wanes with time, particularly with popular vectors such as adenovirus or lipid-based formulations. Use of human genes as reporters is desirable. Traversari et al. found that cells expressing foreign genes are targets of an immune response, whereas endogenous proteins commonly are not, even if ectopically expressed in a context otherwise extremely immunogenic (26). The D2R reporter system described is based on the rat sequence, thus, has potential for immunogenicity. A new system based on human mitochondrial TK expression in the cytosol has been recently described. A truncated form of the TK functioned as a superior reporter compared with the nontruncated form (27), but the truncated form phosphorylated the substrate FIAU approximately five times less than did HSV1-TK; yet, it could be imaged in vivo (28). Since it is a human protein, it may be less immunogenic; however, this needs further study since inappropriate subcellular localization of proteins can lead to immunogenicity. Fortunately, both the SSTR2 and the NIS are human proteins.

The goal of reporter imaging is not phenotypic change. Most reporter systems are biologically active molecules such as receptors, enzymes, and transporters. All three categories may affect intracellular signaling. Expression of biologically active molecules such as enzymes or transporters can affect the cellular milieu. Toxic or unwanted side effects in transduced cells may be seen; and, alterations in the expression of various cellular regulatory proteins, including oncogenes, have been noted after exogenous NIS expression (29). Biologic activity needs also to be considered not only for endogenous cell function, but also among exogenously introduced genes. For example, two expressed genes may compete with each other. When expressing both hNIS and rat D2R mutant R80A, the reporting capability of each competed with each other (30). On ligand stimulation, cell membrane receptors induce multiple signaling pathways. Signaling-deficient receptors are preferable as reporters of gene expression. A mutated rat dopamine receptor, D2R-R80A, has been shown to be deficient in regulating cAMP (31). It has recently been shown that signaling can be uncoupled from imaging of SSTR2. Using a truncated SSTR2, it was demonstrated at the biochemical level that both cAMP and cGMP levels were not altered on ligand stimulation, and at the cellular level that ligand stimulation did not induce growth inhibition. In comparison, wild-type SSTR2 modulated cAMP and cGMP and inhibited growth. Significantly, the mutant receptor could be imaged in vivo (32). This truncated human receptor is promising as a signaling-deficient reporter of gene expression.

Subcellular localization can be important when considering a reporter. For example, transmembrane localization, such as that of receptors and transporters, allows live cell sorting (fluorescence-activated cell sorting, FACS) of expressing cells, for example, when using the reporter for cell-trafficking studies. Light-emitting proteins such as GFP may be used for FACS. Intracellularly located HSV-TK-GFP or HSV-TK-GFP-luciferase fusion proteins have been produced. Such nuclear with optical reporter fusion proteins are useful preclinically since the sensitivity of luciferase imaging is often significantly greater and luciferase imaging is less expensive in animal models. Clinically, GFP and or luciferase may result in an immune response, and neither GFP nor luciferase is expected to be valuable for percutaneous imaging of patients due to poor tissue penetration. The potential lack of useful function in

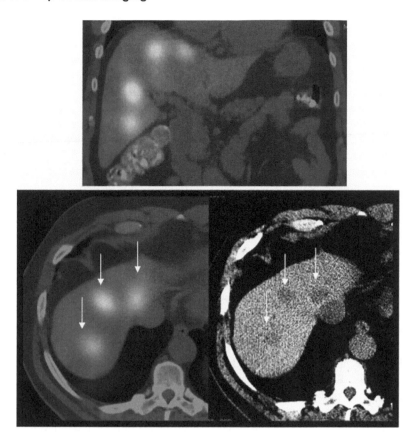

Figure 1 SPECT-CT of somatostatin receptor expression. A patient with carcinoid tumor, which endogenously express SSTR2, was injected systemically with ^{111}In-octreotide. Note that the apparent sizes of the lesions (*arrow*) on the functional nuclear medicine portion of the fused image appear larger than on the anatomic CT image. Coronal SPECT-CT, top; axial SPECT-CT, bottom left; axial noncontrast CT, bottom right. *Abbreviations*: SPECT-CT, single-photon emission computed tomography–computed tomography; SSTR2, somatostatin receptor type-2.

many situations, potential immunogenicity, and increase in insert size may limit clinical utility of nuclear with optical reporter fusion proteins. Moreover, cell sorting is now commonly done using magnetic beads, which requires cell surface expression and is not amenable to intracellular proteins.

For rapid translation to the clinic, a reporter such as human SSTR2 or NIS that can be imaged using FDA-approved agents is advantageous (Fig. 1). Such ligands are not currently available for the TK-based reporters or the D2R. The fact that there are several FDA-approved imaging agents for SSTR2, such as ^{111}In and ^{99m}Tc somatostatin analogues, and NIS, such as iodine isotopes and ^{99m}Tc-pertechnetate, has great value because it shortens the time for translation to the clinic given that most imaging agents and drugs; do not pass clinical trials due to toxicity; are not deemed financially worthy of the millions of dollars required for further development; for clinical radiopharmaceuticals in particular and especially for PET agents, require development of infrastructure, including an economical production and distribution system, or

require each facility to acquire a generator or cyclotron and develop synthesis expertise; and if approved, new agents are often significantly more expensive than established agents.

Imaging agents for both SSTR2 and NIS are safe at tracer doses used for imaging. For example, at the tracer doses used for imaging, no side effects greater than placebo are found with ^{111}In-labeled octreotide (33–36), and patients are routinely imaged serially. Clinically, increased SSTR2 expression renders even small tumors detectable. Other somatostatin-based radiopharmaceuticals have been described (37,38) and PET-based agents are being developed (39–44), but the new agents are not currently clinically available, thus their use will delay translation.

However, new imaging agents are worth pursuing since they may provide greater sensitivity and specificity. Recently, Hoffman et al. described that PET imaging in patients using ^{68}Ga-DOTATOC[^{68}Ga-DOTA-d-Phe(1)-Tyr(3)-octreotide] identified 100% of carcinoid tumors (endogenously express SSTR2) compared with 85% by ^{111}In-octreotide planar and SPECT imaging and noted higher tumor to nontumor contrast as well as lower kidney accumulation by the new imaging agent (45). Others have also noted increased sensitivity (46,47). Imaging agents for HSV1-TK have undergone toxicity studies in man, including the ^{18}F-labeled penciclovir derivative 9-(4-[18F] fluoro-3-hydroxymethylbutyl)-guanine (^{18}F-FHBG) and the 124I-labeled uracil derivative 5-[124I]iodo-2′-fluoro-2′-deoxy-1-β-D-arabinofuranosyl-5-iodouracil (^{124}I-FIAU). The HSV1-TK mutant, HSV1-sr39tk, has higher affinity for ^{18}F-FHBG. The restricted availability and longer four day half-life of ^{124}I-FIAU may impede serial imaging and increase radiation exposure (48–51), but the longer half-life may turn out to be useful since substrate phosphorylation by TK, thus accumulation, can increase over days (52). In a study with a small number of patients, improved signal-to-noise ratio was noted 6.5 hours versus 1.5 hours after ^{18}F-FHBG injection (50,51).

Increased signal-to-noise ratio is important. The process of converting a gene to a protein provides an amplification scheme. Two copies of DNA produce tens to hundreds of copies of mRNA, which in turn produces thousands of copies of protein. The latter are targeted by the imaging agent in most reporter systems. Receptors can amplify signal by sequestering imaging by pinocytosis or endocytosis. Transporters can also sequester imaging agent, but commonly when the gradient decreases, the agent leaves the cell. Enzymes alter their substrate one after another and if appropriately designed, the product of the enzymatic reaction will become entrapped. For example, HSV1-TK entraps various radiolabeled substrates by phosphorylation, thereby adding a charge that prevents escape from the cell. Yet, Sun et al. suggested that %ID/g (percentage of the injected dose per gram of tissue) of D$_2$R with ^{18}F 3-N-(2-fluoroethyl) spiperone (^{18}F-FESP) was greater than HSV-TK with ^{18}F-FHBG (53). However, given potential variables, such as tumor type and various potential substrates, the comparative sensitivity of various reporter systems is as yet unclear.

In terms of quantification, that of NIS expression may be limited because the degree of NIS expression is not the sole reason dictating the degree of radioiodide uptake, the degree of sodium iodide uptake is saturable and therefore not linear beyond a certain degree of expression, and further, the maximal radioiodide uptake induced by NIS gene transfer differs among different cells (54). Although HSV-TK activity appears to be quantifiable in vivo, it has been suggested that HSV-TK does not show good correlation between the number of gene copies and signal when compared with SSTR2 (55).

QUANTIFYING GENE EXPRESSION

To optimally utilize reporter technology for gene therapy, methods for noninvasively quantifying expression are

needed. After gene transfer, the degree of expression changes as a function of time. On transduction, there is a lag period. Expression then increases and may plateau before it wanes. Tracking such changes will prove fruitful because similar to drug therapy, a certain amount of the gene product will be needed to obtain a therapeutic effect. Reporter systems closest to the clinic are primarily nuclear medicine-based, which although powerful, lack true anatomic detail (Fig. 1). These functional methods rely on detecting a radiopharmaceutical for localizing the reporter, not on the underlying anatomy. On such functional images, the size of the object may vary by the amount of radiopharmaceutical present. In addition, machines may be used near the limit of their anatomic resolution either due to the size of the underlying object or due to morphology where only a thin portion of the object of interest is in the field of view. Thus, the machines are prone to volume averaging artifacts that occur when the object of interest is less than 2.7 times the resolution of the imaging system (56). Currently, PET and gamma cameras have resolutions in the order of 0.5 to 1 cm. In comparison, anatomic imaging can now be routinely performed at submillimeter resolution.

Using functional imaging alone is not sufficient for imaging gene transfer in many instances, for example, in growing children and in the setting of many illnesses, such as infection, where organ size or morphology may change. This is particularly true in the setting of cancer because unlike organs in adults, tumors grow, and if therapy is successful, they regress, sometimes rather quickly. This change in size poses a problem for quantifying gene expression because the signal change may be due to the number of cells present instead of the efficiency of induction. For example, over time, apparently decreased uptake at a subsequent time point may be due to a smaller tumor, less expression, or both.

Combining functional and anatomic imaging affords the ability to distinguish these possibilities by normalizing uptake to tumor size (57). This will benefit using reporters for assessing the efficacy of dosing regimens of conventional therapy or of gene therapy. Common in vivo gene delivery vectors result in relatively inhomogeneous and temporally variable expression. For example, using an AAV for delivery, onset of expression may require two to six weeks (58,59). In comparison, using adenovirus for delivery, expression occurs in days, but then often decreases after approximately two to three weeks (60); however, multiple temporally separated injections can improve therapeutic effectiveness (61). During this time and upon subsequent examinations, the mass may grow or regress. In the setting of multiple targets within a patient, normalization is also needed. For example, at any one point in time, metastases are almost always of varying sizes and for evaluating clinical efficacy, each may need to be assessed. Similarly, when comparing among individuals, variability in the size of organs will also require normalization.

This concept is also important for in vivo assessment of promoter activity. Preclinically, HSV-TK reporter expression has been used to image induction of a tetracycline responsive promoter (53) and to demonstrate tumor-specific targeting by the carcinoembryonic antigen (CEA) promoter (62), implying that in vivo assessment of transcriptional regulation is possible. To assess changes in expression over time in order to compare among promoters, functional assays need to be normalized to cell number or target size.

Unlike many other diseases, the ultimate aim of oncology is to kill the cancer. Tomographic techniques allow interrogation of the inside of a structure and can demonstrate heterogeneity. In large tumors that outgrow their blood supply, or as therapy is effective, tumor necrosis occurs. After gene therapy, the portion of the tumor undergoing necrosis will not be expressing the reporter, thus, should be excluded in the assessment of expression. Using anatomic techniques, such as MR, these areas can be excluded when assessing size or weight. Thus, those areas not contributing to the functional signal may be excluded. Using a combination of noninvasive gamma camera and MR imaging, quantification of exogenous somatostatin receptor-based reporter expression correlated with that of excised tumors in a preclinical model (57). Previously, quantification of this reporter in vitro was shown to correlate with expression in animal models (13). For confirming imaging findings of reporter expression, a reporter that is distinguishable ex vivo, such as at the time of biopsy, is desirable. In the case of human proteins, it can be of value to include an epitope tag (13,32,57) to distinguish the exogenous gene product from the endogenous gene product.

An interesting new reporter is a metalloprotein from the ferritin family, which accumulates endogenous iron in the cell for MR imaging (63). Addition of an imaging agent is not needed. This may be useful for following cell trafficking after iron is accumulated in vitro. Since the gene is continuously expressed in live cells, theoretically, trafficking may be followed long term. Because it takes about five days to accumulate iron in vivo, it may not be useful in short-term imaging studies evaluating change in expression over days. The rate of washout may be slow and this may limit evaluation of whether expression is waning, and in live versus dead cells depending on the speed of removal of accumulated iron. Another issue to address is the effect of accumulation of large amounts of iron in different cell types since hemochromatosis type I and II (primary or secondary iron overload) are known diseases. Even given these potential limitations, this is an interesting new reporter and paradigm.

POTENTIAL USES OF REPORTER GENE IMAGING

Reporter gene imaging can be used to test an end goal of gene therapy, expression of the gene of interest in order to cure a disease. Preclinically, evaluation of vector targeting has been performed, such as demonstrating enhanced infectivity of ovarian cells using an adenovirus containing an alteration of the H1 loop compared with wild-type virus (64). Tumor-specific targeting has also been visualized using the CEA promoter and HSV-TK as the reporter (62). Linking two separate genes and evaluation of promoter activity have also been performed, such as for in vivo visualization of the induction of two separate genes using a tetracycline-promoter system (53), suggesting that in vivo monitoring of gene transfer can be approached using reporter genes either alone or in conjunction with a gene of interest. In expressing two different genes, the therapeutic gene may be fused to the reporter or be produced as a separate protein. For example, the gene of interest and reporter may be induced by separate promoters in separate delivery vehicles by cotransfection (coinfection) (65) or by separate promoters in the same delivery vehicle (55). In addition, the two genes may be linked to the same promoter by, for example, an internal ribosome entry site (66,67) or a bidirectional promoter (53). Using such techniques, expression of the gene of interest and reporter correlate (53,55,65–67). Thus, one may gauge the location, amount, and duration of expression of the gene of interest using the reporter.

Because cells can be transfected with reporter genes, the reporter may be used to follow cell trafficking. For example, in vitro, specific cells may be transfected/infected with a reporter and then returned to an animal to assess homing. Using PET, Koehne et al. demonstrated in vivo that Epstein-Barr virus (EBV)-specific T cells expressing HSV-TK selectively traffic to EBV$^+$ tumors. Furthermore, these T cells retain their capacity to eliminate targeted tumors (68). HSV-TK has also been used to image stem cells in vivo (69,70). As mentioned above, HSV-TK may not be ideal for cellular trafficking studies in immunocompetent patients due to a potential immune response and alteration in cell function. Nonimmunogenic and signaling/functionally deficient reporters are preferable.

Both gene and cellular therapies may be given by direct injection, such as for Parkinson's disease, intraprostatic prostate cancer, or claudication; or systemically given with or without targeting for localization. The pharmacokinetics of expression may then be evaluated, for example, to locate the site of target and nontarget expression and to determine dosing, such as how much to give and how often to give it. Such analysis will require correlation of reporter imaging studies with clinical outcome. Appropriate localization and amount of expression may serve as an early predictor of response in the appropriate clinical context. It may also serve to determine when to give a prodrug in the case of suicide gene therapy in order to avoid toxicity by giving a prodrug in the setting of no or low expression of the suicide gene. If therapy is effective, no target may remain. Serial monitoring may also be used to determine when and if to re-dose with the prodrug versus re-dose with gene therapy before again instilling prodrug is appropriate. Reevaluation after the second or subsequent doses of gene therapy may also be helpful because many events may interfere with expression of the second dose, such as an immune response to the vector or inserted genes, selection of cells less permissive to infection, and remaining lesions consisting of nonviable cells or cells in the process of dying.

Evaluating expression in nontarget locations can be beneficial for assessing toxicity. A clinical example of this is a patient who died from multiorgan failure within four days of gene therapy in 1999 (71). Although this may have been an unusual reaction, it highlights issues of safety. The patient received 3.8×10^{12} adenovirus particles with an ornithine-transcarbamylase gene insert to treat his ornithine-transcarbamylase deficiency. Viral particles were identified not only in the liver, the target organ, but also in multiple nontarget organs, and the patient had "a systemic inflammatory response" followed by multiorgan failure. In this particular study, minimal gene expression was noted and only 1% of the transferred genes reached target cells, highlighting the problem of achieving high levels of expression in the target and not in nontarget organs. It also highlights the potentially fatal outcomes of an immune response and suggests that using nonimmunogenic material, including vectors, products of genes of interest, and reporter gene products, is desirable in many circumstances.

Some considerations in choosing a reporter for a particular clinical context are described above. Other relevant factors may include: how long after gene delivery should the tracer be injected, how long after tracer delivery should imaging be performed, and how often should imaging be performed. In addition, there may be a low level of expression that cannot be detected. This may or may not be relevant depending on whether such low level of expression is thought to be sufficient for clinical benefit. Multiple reporter systems are needed because, in addition to the considerations above such as evaluation of constitutive and inducible promoters and patients needing treatment for more than one disease, having a choice of reporter systems will allow selection tailored to the clinical question/situation including the cellular context, imaging agent access to the site of interest (may be limited in the brain due to the blood-brain barrier), and the background signal produced by the imaging agent. For example, an imaging agent eliminated by renal excretion

may not be ideal for monitoring gene therapy to the kidney. Gene expression imaging does not directly evaluate vector distribution, but rather the end outcome of expression. Many of the delivered vectors may not express, so for assessing vector distribution, it may be more appropriate to label the vector directly as has been done for herpes simplex virus (72) and adenovirus (73,74). Variability in expression may not only be due to the vector but also due to host factors, for example, gene silencing, differential perfusion, health of the underlying cells in a tumor, effect of other therapies including local therapies such as radiation; these may alter morphology and function. In a clinical study utilizing intramuscular delivery of AAV, expression of the factor IX gene was noted on muscle biopsy (75). In one patient who received the lowest dose of AAV, factor IX levels were highest, and this was at least in part attributed to the patient also taking zidovudine, which can increase transgene expression in vitro. The findings point out interpatient variability and the influence of other compounds, known or unknown, which a patient may be taking, on gene expression. It also highlights the need for "personalized medicine" to dose patients individually and not just as a population. This may be afforded by noninvasive reporter imaging.

Reporter gene imaging has been tested in clinical trials. For example, HSV-TK expression was noted by increased ^{124}I-FIAU uptake in one out of five patients with glioblastoma (Fig. 2). In this study, a lipid formulation including a plasmid containing a HSV-tk insert was infused into the tumor. In this patient, treatment response after gancyclovir treatment was noted at the site of ^{124}I-FIAU uptake (50,51). Although one cannot draw conclusions from a single patient, the finding suggests that noninvasive imaging has the potential to select patients for prodrug treatment and to predict treatment response. No expression was noted in another study using HSV-tk and ^{123}I-FIAU to noninvasively monitor a selectively replication competent mutant of HSV1, HSV1716, administered intratumorally to patients with high-grade glioma (76). In a phase I study of seven patients with hepatocellular carcinoma (Fig. 3), escalating doses of adenovirus with an HSV-tk insert were delivered into the tumor. Two days after vector delivery, transgene expression could be imaged in all patients who received 10^{12} viral particles (4 of 7 patients), using ^{18}F-FHBG as a probe. Treatment with valganciclovir was begun immediately after imaging. At day 30, no tumor progression was seen in patients receiving 10^{12} viral particles and tumor necrosis was seen in 2 of 4 of these patients (50,51). Because of the small numbers of patients, definite conclusions cannot be made, but this study also suggests that noninvasive imaging has the potential to select patients for prodrug treatment and to predict treatment response. One patient who had demonstrated uptake was reinjected with

Pre-gene delivery Post-gene delivery

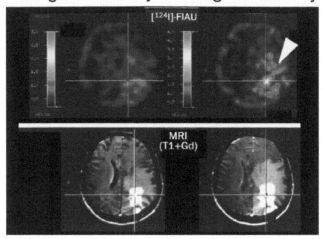

Figure 2 PET imaging of HSV-TK expression in a patient with gliobastoma. A lipid formulation including a plasmid with an HSV-tk insert was delivered into the tumor. Three days later, PET imaging was performed after systemic delivery of the substrate [124]I-FIAU. Axial images, [124]I-FIAU-PET top, intravenous contrast-enhanced MR, bottom. Arrowhead points to the tumor and crossbars indicate site of gene expression noted on the posttherapy [124]I-FIAU-PET. *Abbreviations*: PET, positron emission tomography; HSV-TK, herpes simplex virus thymidine kinase; [124]I-FIAU, 5-[124I]iodo-2'-fluoro-2'-deoxy-1-β-D-arabinofuranosyl-5-iodouracil. *Source*: Modified from Ref. 51.

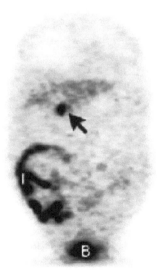

Figure 3 PET imaging of HSV-TK expression in a patient with hepatocellular carcinoma; 10^{12} viral particles of adenovirus containing an HSV-tk insert were injected into the tumor. Two days later, PET imaging was performed after systemic delivery of the substrate ^{18}F-FHBG. Coronal image at the level of the tumor (*arrow*) in the liver. *Abbreviations*: I, intestines; B, bladder; PET, positron emission tomography; HSV-TK, herpes simplex virus thymidine kinase; ^{18}F-FHBG, 9-(4-[18F]fluoro-3-hydroxymethylbutyl)-guanine. *Source*: Modified from Ref. 50.

adenovirus one month later, but repeat imaging did not show increased uptake (50, 51). Although this may be due to various reasons in this patient (see above), it intimates the value of repeat imaging after an additional dose of gene therapy to verify expression. The serial imaging data and variability in ^{18}F-FHBG uptake in the four patients who initially received 10^{12} viral particles imply that following gene expression in each patient "personally" will be of value.

CONCLUSION

Imaging of reporter gene expression has a very promising future for clinical applications. Multiple reporter systems are now available for selection of either single or multiple gene therapies based on clinical need. Often, a nonimmunogenic reporter that does not perturb the intracellular milieu, for example, is signaling deficient, will be preferred. The technology enables evaluation of expression not only in the target for efficacy, but also in non-target tissues, which may be involved in toxicity. Monitoring gene expression will compliment clinical evaluations of therapeutic response and has the potential to predict response. Waning clinical response to initially successful gene therapy may be due to loss of expression, and this too may be assessed by reporter systems. Noninvasive, image-based quantification of expression can be performed by incorporating both functional and anatomic data. Clinically, variability in expression among patients is expected. By performing quantification in individual patients, reporter systems will enable "personalizing" gene therapy for each patient.

REFERENCES

1. Edelstein ML, Abedi MR, Wixon J. Gene therapy clinical trials worldwide to 2007—an update. J Gene Med 2007; 9:833–842.
2. Journal of Gene Medicine. Gene Therapy Clinical Trials Worldwide. John Wiley and Sons Ltd. Available at: http://www.wiley.co.uk/genmed/clinical/. Cited December 4, 2007.
3. MacLaren DC, Gambhir SS, Satyamurthy N, et al. Repetitive, non-invasive imaging of the dopamine D2 receptor as a reporter gene in living animals. Gene Ther 1999; 6: 785–791.
4. Fujiwara T, Tanaka N, Kanazawa S, et al. Multicenter phase I study of repeated intratumoral delivery of adenoviral p53 in patients with advanced non-small-cell lung cancer. J Clin Oncol 2006; 24:1689–1699.
5. Gordon EM, Lopez FF, Cornelio GH, et al. Pathotropic nanoparticles for cancer gene therapy Rexin-G IV: three-year clinical experience. Int J Oncol 2006; 29:1053–1064.

6. Kubo H, Gardner TA, Wada Y, et al. Phase I dose escalation clinical trial of adenovirus vector carrying osteocalcin promoter-driven herpes simplex virus thymidine kinase in localized and metastatic hormone-refractory prostate cancer. Hum Gene Ther 2003; 14:227–241.

7. Zeimet AG, Muller-Holzner E, Schuler A, et al. Determination of molecules regulating gene delivery using adenoviral vectors in ovarian carcinomas. Gene Ther 2002; 9:1093–1100.

8. Perricone MA, Morris JE, Pavelka K, et al. Aerosol and lobar administration of a recombinant adenovirus to individuals with cystic fibrosis. II. Transfection efficiency in airway epithelium. Hum Gene Ther 2001; 12:1383–1394.

9. Zeimet AG, Marth C. Why did p53 gene therapy fail in ovarian cancer? Lancet Oncol 2003; 4:415–422.

10. Pujade-Lauraine E, Guastalla JP, Colombo N, et al. Intraperitoneal recombinant interferon gamma in ovarian cancer patients with residual disease at second-look laparotomy. J Clin Oncol 1996; 14:343–350.

11. Alberts DS, Liu PY, Hannigan EV, et al. Intraperitoneal cisplatin plus intravenous cyclophosphamide versus intravenous cisplatin plus intravenous cyclophosphamide for stage III ovarian cancer. N Eng J Med 1996; 335:1950–1955.

12. Zinn KR, Buchsbaum DJ, Chaudhuri TR, et al. Noninvasive monitoring of gene transfer using a reporter receptor imaged with a high-affinity peptide radiolabeled with 99mTc or 188Re. J Nucl Med 2000; 41:887–895.

13. Kundra V, Mannting F, Jones AG, et al. Noninvasive monitoring of somatostatin receptor type 2 chimeric gene transfer. J Nucl Med 2002; 43:406–412.

14. Tjuvajev JG, Stockhammer G, Desai R, et al. Imaging the expression of transfected genes in vivo. Cancer Res 1995; 55:6126–6132.

15. Gambhir SS, Barrio JR, Wu L, et al. Imaging of adenoviral-directed herpes simplex virus type 1 thymidine kinase reporter gene expression in mice with radiolabeled ganciclovir. J Nucl Med 1998; 39:2003–2011.

16. Mandell RB, Mandell LZ, Link CJ Jr. Radioisotope concentrator gene therapy using the sodium/iodide symporter gene. Cancer Res 1999; 59:661–668.

17. Matsushita T, Elliger S, Elliger C, et al. Adeno-associated virus vectors can be efficiently produced without helper virus. Gene Ther 1998; 5:938–945.

18. Yamada Y, Post SR, Wang K, et al. Cloning and functional characterization of a family of human and mouse somatostatin receptors expressed in brain, gastrointestinal tract, and kidney. Proc Natl Acad Sci U S A 1992; 89:251–255.

19. Gompels U, Minson A. The properties and sequence of glycoprotein H of herpes simplex virus type 1. Virology 1986; 153:230–247.

20. Bunzow JR, Van Tol HH, Grandy DK, et al. Cloning and expression of a rat D2 dopamine receptor cDNA. Nature 1988; 336:783–787.

21. Smanik PA, Liu Q, Furminger TL, et al. Cloning of the human sodium iodide symporter. Biochem Biophys Res Comm 1996; 226:339–345.

22. Weissleder R, Moore A, Mahmood U, et al. In vivo magnetic resonance imaging of transgene expression. Nat Med 2000; 6:351–355.

23. Louie AY, Huber MM, Ahrens ET, et al. In vivo visualization of gene expression using magnetic resonance imaging. Nat Biotechnol 2000; 18:321–325.

24. Burt RK, Drobyski WR, Seregina T, et al. Herpes simplex thymidine kinase gene-transduced donor lymphocyte infusions. Exp Hematol 2003; 31:903–910.

25. Berger C, Flowers ME, Warren EH, et al. Analysis of transgene-specific immune responses that limit the in vivo persistence of adoptively transferred HSV-TK-modified donor T cells after allogeneic hematopoietic cell transplantation. Blood 2006; 107:2294–2302.

26. Traversari C, Marktel S, Magnani Z, et al. The potential immunogenicity of the TK suicide gene does not prevent full clinical benefit associated with the use of TK-transduced donor lymphocytes in HSCT for hematologic malignancies. Blood 2007; 109:4708–4715.

27. Ponomarev V, Doubrovin M, Shavrin A, et al. A human-derived reporter gene for noninvasive imaging in humans: mitochondrial thymidine kinase type 2. J Nucl Med 2007; 48:819–826.

28. Ponomarev V, Doubrovin M, Serganova I, et al. Cytoplasmically retargeted HSV1-tk/GFP reporter gene mutants for optimization of noninvasive molecular-genetic imaging. Neoplasia 2003; 5:245–254.

29. Gol Choe J, Kim YR, Kim KN, et al. Altered gene expression profiles by sodium/iodide symporter gene transfection in a human anaplastic thyroid carcinoma cell line using a radioactive complementary DNA microarray. Nucl Med Commun 2005; 26:1155–1162.

30. Hwang do W, Kang JH, Chang YS, et al. Development of a dual membrane protein reporter system using sodium iodide symporter and mutant dopamine D2 receptor transgenes. J Nucl Med 2007; 48:588–595.

31. Liang Q, Satyamurthy N, Barrio JR, et al. Noninvasive, quantitative imaging in living animals of a mutant dopamine D2 receptor reporter gene in which ligand binding is uncoupled from signal transduction. Gene Ther 2001; 8:1490–1498.

32. Han L, Yang D, Kundra V. Signaling can be uncoupled from imaging of the somatostatin receptor type-2. Mol Imaging 2007; 6:427–437.

33. Krenning EP, Bakker WH, Kooij PP, et al. Somatostatin receptor scintigraphy with indium-111-DTPA-D-Phe-1-octreotide in man: metabolism, dosimetry and comparison with iodine-123-Tyr-3-octreotide. J Nucl Med 1992; 33:652–658.

34. Bajc M, Palmer J, Ohlsson T, et al. Distribution and dosimetry of 111In DTPA-D-Phe-octreotide in man assessed by whole body scintigraphy. Acta Radiol 1994; 35:53–57.

35. Stabin MG, Kooij PP, Bakker WH, et al. Radiation dosimetry for indium-111-pentetreotide. J Nucl Med 1997; 38:1919–1922.

36. Inoue T, Ootake H, Hirano T, et al. [Clinical evaluation of safety, pharmacokinetics and dosimetry of the somatostatin analog 111In-DTPA-D-Phe-octreotide–report of the phase 1 study]. Kaku Igaku 1995; 32:511–521.

37. Gabriel M, Decristoforo C, Donnemiller E, et al. An intrapatient comparison of 99mTc-EDDA/HYNIC-TOC

with 111In-DTPA-octreotide for diagnosis of somatostatin receptor-expressing tumors. J Nucl Med 2003; 44:708–716.

38. Reubi JC, Schar JC, Waser B, et al. Affinity profiles for human somatostatin receptor subtypes SST1-SST5 of somatostatin radiotracers selected for scintigraphic and radiotherapeutic use. Eur J Nucl Med 2000; 27:273–282.

39. Anderson CJ, Dehdashti F, Cutler PD, et al. 64Cu-TETA-octreotide as a PET imaging agent for patients with neuroendocrine tumors. J Nucl Med 2001; 42:213–221.

40. Eisenwiener KP, Prata MIM, Buschmann I, et al. NODA-GATOC, a new chelator-coupled somatostatin analogue labeled with [$^{67/68}$Ga] and [^{111}In] for SPECT, PET, and targeted therapeutic applications of somatostatin receptor (hsst2) expressing tumors. Bioconjug Chem 2002; 13: 530–541.

41. Wester HJ, Schottelius M, Scheidhauer K, et al. PET imaging of somatostatin receptors: design, synthesis and preclinical evaluation of a novel 18F-labelled, carbohydrated analogue of octreotide. Eur J Nucl Med Mol Imaging 2003; 30:117–122.

42. Kowalski J, Henze M, Schuhmacher J, et al. Evaluation of positron emission tomography imaging using [68Ga]-DOTA-D Phe(1)-Tyr(3)-Octreotide in comparison to [111In]-DTPAOC SPECT. First results in patients with neuroendocrine tumors. Mol Imaging Biol 2003; 5:42–48.

43. Schottelius M, Poethko T, Herz M, et al. First (18)F-labeled tracer suitable for routine clinical imaging of sst receptor-expressing tumors using positron emission tomography. Clin Cancer Res 2004; 10:3593–3606.

44. Wild D, Mäcke HR, Waser B, et al. 68Ga-DOTANOC: a first compound for PET imaging with high affinity for somatostatin receptor subtypes 2 and 5. Eur J Nucl Med Mol Imaging 2005; 32:724–724.

45. Hofmann M, Maecke H, Borner R, et al. Biokinetics and imaging with the somatostatin receptor PET radioligand (68)Ga-DOTATOC: preliminary data. Eur J Nucl Med 2001; 28:1751–1757.

46. Buchmann I, Henze M, Engelbrecht S, et al. Comparison of 68Ga-DOTATOC PET and 111In-DTPAOC (Octreoscan) SPECT in patients with neuroendocrine tumours. Eur J Nucl Med Mol Imaging 2007; 34:1617–1626.

47. Gabriel M, Decristoforo C, Kendler D, et al. 68Ga-DOTA-Tyr3-octreotide PET in neuroendocrine tumors: comparison with somatostatin receptor scintigraphy and CT. J Nucl Med 2007; 48:508–518.

48. Yaghoubi S, Barrio JR, Dahlbom M, et al. Human pharmacokinetic and dosimetry studies of [(18)F]FHBG: a reporter probe for imaging herpes simplex virus type-1 thymidine kinase reporter gene expression. J Nucl Med 2001; 42:1225–1234.

49. Jacobs A, Braunlich I, Graf R, et al. Quantitative kinetics of [124I]FIAU in cat and man. J Nucl Med 2001; 42:467–475.

50. Penuelas I, Mazzolini G, Boan JF, et al. Positron emission tomography imaging of adenoviral-mediated transgene expression in liver cancer patients. Gastroenterology 2005; 128:1787–1795.

51. Jacobs A, Voges J, Reszka R, et al. Positron-emission tomography of vector-mediated gene expression in gene therapy for gliomas. Lancet 2001; 358:727–729.

52. Tjuvajev JG, Avril N, Oku T, et al. Imaging herpes virus thymidine kinase gene transfer and expression by positron emission tomography. Cancer Res 1998; 58:4333–4341.

53. Sun X, Annala AJ, Yaghoubi SS, et al. Quantitative imaging of gene induction in living animals. Gene Ther 2001; 8:1572–1579.

54. Vadysirisack DD, Shen DH, Jhiang SM. Correlation of Na+/I- symporter expression and activity: implications of Na+/I- symporter as an imaging reporter gene. J Nucl Med 2006; 47:182–190.

55. Zinn KR, Chaudhuri TR, Krasnykh VN, et al. Gamma camera dual imaging with a somatostatin receptor and thymidine kinase after gene transfer with a bicistronic adenovirus in mice. Radiology 2002; 223:417–425.

56. Kessler RM, Ellis JR Jr., Eden M. Analysis of emission tomographic scan data: limitations imposed by resolution and background. J Comput Assist Tomogr 1984; 8:514–522.

57. Yang D, Han L, Kundra V. Exogenous gene expression in tumors: noninvasive quantification with functional and anatomic imaging in a mouse model. Radiology 2005; 235:950–958.

58. Herzog RW, Hagstrom JN, Kung SH, et al. Stable gene transfer and expression of human blood coagulation factor IX after intramuscular injection of recombinant adeno-associated virus. Proc Natl Acad Sci U S A 1997; 94:5804–5809.

59. Flotte TR, Beck SE, Chesnut K, et al. A fluorescence video-endoscopy technique for detection of gene transfer and expression. Gene Ther 1998; 5:166–173.

60. Zsengeller ZK, Wert SE, Hull WM, et al. Persistence of replication-deficient adenovirus-mediated gene transfer in lungs of immune-deficient (nu/nu) mice. Hum Gene Ther 1995; 6:457–467.

61. Lin SH, Pu YS, Luo W, et al. Schedule-dependence of C-CAM1 adenovirus gene therapy in a prostate cancer model. Anticancer Res 1999; 19:337–340.

62. Qiao J, Doubrovin M, Sauter BV, et al. Tumor-specific transcriptional targeting of suicide gene therapy. Gene Ther 2002; 9:168–175.

63. Genove G, DeMarco U, Xu H, et al. A new transgene reporter for in vivo magnetic resonance imaging. Nat Med 2005; 11:450–454.

64. Hemminki A, Belousova N, Zinn KR, et al. An adenovirus with enhanced infectivity mediates molecular chemotherapy of ovarian cancer cells and allows imaging of gene expression. Mol Ther 2001; 4:223–231.

65. Yaghoubi SS, Wu L, Liang Q, et al. Direct correlation between positron emission tomographic images of two reporter genes delivered by two distinct adenoviral vectors. Gene Ther 2001; 8:1072–1080.

66. Tjuvajev JG, Joshi A, Callegari J, et al. A general approach to the non-invasive imaging of transgenes using cis-linked herpes simplex virus thymidine kinase. Neoplasia 1999; 1:315–320.

67. Liang Q, Gotts J, Satyamurthy N, et al. Noninvasive, repetitive, quantitative measurement of gene expression from a bicistronic message by positron emission tomography, following gene transfer with adenovirus. Mol Ther 2002; 6:73–82.

68. Koehne G, Doubrovin M, Doubrovina E, et al. Serial in vivo imaging of the targeted migration of human HSV-TK-transduced antigen-specific lymphocytes. Nat Biotechnol 2003; 21:405–413.

69. Hung SC, Deng WP, Yang WK, et al. Mesenchymal stem cell targeting of microscopic tumors and tumor stroma development monitored by noninvasive in vivo positron emission tomography imaging. Clin Cancer Res 2005; 11:7749–7756.

70. Cao F, Lin S, Xie X, et al. In vivo visualization of embryonic stem cell survival, proliferation, and migration after cardiac delivery. Circulation 2006; 113:1005–1014.

71. Marshall E. Gene therapy death prompts review of adenovirus vector. Science 1999; 286:2244–2245.

72. Schellingerhout D, Bogdanov A Jr., Marecos E, et al. Mapping the in vivo distribution of herpes simplex virions. Hum Gene Ther 1998; 9:1543–1549.

73. Zinn KR, Douglas JT, Smyth CA, et al. Imaging and tissue biodistribution of 99mTc-labeled adenovirus knob (serotype 5). Gene Ther 1998; 5:798–808.

74. Lerondel S, Le Pape A, Sene C, et al. Radioisotopic imaging allows optimization of adenovirus lung deposition for cystic fibrosis gene therapy. Hum Gene Ther 2001; 12:1–11.

75. Manno CS, Chew AJ, Hutchison S, et al. AAV-mediated factor IX gene transfer to skeletal muscle in patients with severe hemophilia B. Blood 2003; 101:2963–2972.

76. Dempsey MF, Wyper D, Owens J, et al. Assessment of 123I-FIAU imaging of herpes simplex viral gene expression in the treatment of glioma. Nucl Med Commun 2006; 27:611–617.

28

Molecular-Genetic Imaging

YANNIC WAERZEGGERS, ALEXANDRA WINKELER, and ANDREAS H. JACOBS
Laboratory for Gene Therapy and Molecular Imaging at the Max Planck Institute for Neurological Research with Klaus-Joachim-Zülch-Laboratories of the Max Planck Society and the Faculty of Medicine of the University of Cologne, Cologne, Germany

INTRODUCTION

Molecular-genetic imaging is a fascinating novel technology that aims at unraveling and visualizing detailed information on cellular and molecular mechanisms in vivo in real time. It permits close monitoring of complex biological pathways involved in normal development and disease progression. The ability to address basic scientific questions e.g., transcriptional regulation, signal transduction, or protein/protein interaction, makes molecular imaging an important tool for the development and validation of molecular-targeted and disease-tailored treatment strategies. This chapter introduces the basic principles of molecular-genetic imaging and summarizes some recent applications in preclinical research.

In vivo molecular-genetic imaging is a rapidly evolving field based on concerted research and technical developments spanning multiple disciplines such as molecular biology, cell biology, chemistry, and imaging technology. The ultimate goal of molecular-genetic imaging is to provide noninvasive visualization in space and time of normal as well as abnormal cellular processes at the molecular or genetic level (1). This is in contrast to traditional imaging methodologies that rather provide visualization at the anatomical level.

There exist certain prerequisites for visualizing specific molecules or molecular mechanisms in vivo, which can be summarized as follows: (*i*) the availability of stable, nontoxic, and high-affinity probes; (*ii*) the ability of these probes to overcome biological delivery barriers such as the blood-brain barrier; (*iii*) the use of amplification strategies to increase the signal-to-background ratio; and (*iv*) the availability of fast and high-resolution imaging techniques (2).

Different approaches and technologies for noninvasive high-resolution imaging of mammalian gene expression have been developed more or less in parallel during the last decades using either radionuclide, magnetic resonance or optical imaging techniques. Novel imaging paradigms are being developed to monitor molecular-genetic and cellular processes in vivo over time with the potential of a detailed kinetic analysis. These noninvasive and versatile paradigms will complement and eventually abolish the need of established in vitro and in situ molecular assays requiring invasive sampling procedures to provide spatial as well as temporal information on various molecular-genetic and cellular processes in animal models of human disease as well as in human subjects. Moreover, the ability to longitudinally image the same subject over time abolishes the need for time course studies requiring large numbers of animals that are sacrificed at specific time points in order to achieve a statistically significant temporal profile.

Molecular imaging will substantially speed up development and validation of new drugs and treatment protocols. Molecular events that can be noninvasively localized and quantified in vivo include endogenous or exogenous gene expression (including oncogenic transformation, cell trafficking, and targeted drug action), signal transduction, protein-protein interaction, transcriptional, and posttranscriptional regulation. As such, in vivo molecular-genetic imaging will have great implications for the identification of potential molecular therapeutic targets, in the development of new treatment strategies and in their successful translation into clinical application. In the clinical setting, molecular imaging can significantly aid in early lesion detection, patient stratification, and treatment monitoring, which can allow for much earlier diagnosis, earlier treatment, better prognosis, and individualized patient and disease management.

MOLECULAR IMAGING TECHNOLOGIES

Various imaging technologies for noninvasive in vivo molecular imaging have been developed (3). These technologies differ in a number of aspects like spatial (microns to centimeters) and temporal (milliseconds to hours) resolution, tomographic potential, depth penetration, energy needed for image generation, availability of imaging probes and detection threshold (sensitivity), throughput, cost, ease of operation, and clinical translatability. Therefore, the use of a specific imaging modality will depend on the molecular event in question. As no single modality addresses all aspects of molecular imaging, there is increasing interest in multimodality imaging, either on a hardware (PET/CT, PET/MR) (4–7) or on a software basis (image coregistration, multimodality gene reporter constructs) (8,9).

Radionuclide imaging [positron emission tomography (PET) and single photon emission tomography (SPECT)] (10,11) enables the assessment and quantification of the intensity and regional/spatial distribution of gene expression in vivo. Nuclear imaging is highly sensitive (detecting fmole levels of probe), quantitative, and inherently tomographic. However, nuclear imaging has only moderate spatial resolution when compared with MR imaging (in the range of 1–2 mm), demands sophisticated instrumentation, committed personnel, readily available in-house production of radiopharmaceuticals, and stringent dependency on tracer pharmacokinetics. PET uses decaying nuclides such as ^{11}C, ^{13}N, ^{18}F, ^{15}O, ^{64}Cu, ^{124}I and images the distribution of trace quantities of positron-emitting molecular probe administered. Molecular probes labeled with positron-emitting isotopes are used to detect biologically active molecules, as a result of the target-dependent sequestration of the systemically administered positron-emitting probes. Positrons emitted from the probe travel a few millimeters in tissue before being annihilated by collision with an electron, resulting in a pair of high-energy (511 keV) photons or gamma rays. The two gamma rays are emitted at nearly 180° from one another and are detected by the scintillation crystals of the PET detector by producing light flashes that are converted to electronic signal by the photomultiplier tubes surrounding the scintillation crystals. These data are corrected for signal attenuation due to absorption by tissue and then used to reconstruct volumetric images of the positron-emitting probe. Positron-emitting radionuclides are primarily used to tag small molecules that are recognized by enzymes or bind to receptors or membrane transporters. SPECT acquires information on the concentration of gamma-emitting radionuclides, such as ^{111}In, ^{123}I, ^{201}Tl, or ^{99}mTc introduced into an organism. These radionuclides emit a single photon. In SPECT imaging, the rotation of a photon detector array around the body of the subject tracks the position and concentration of radionuclide distribution from multiple angles. Some advantages of SPECT over PET are its ability to measure relatively slow kinetic processes because of the long half-life of the commonly used isotopes (hours to days, compared with minutes to hours in PET), and its ability to probe two or more molecular pathways simultaneously by detecting isotopes with different emission energies.

MRI's fundamental principle is the alignment of unpaired nuclear spins (such as hydrogen atoms in water and organic compounds) when placed into a magnetic field, forming a net effect called net magnetization. A temporary radiofrequency pulse is then given to disturb this equilibrium state by changing the alignment of the spins. The relaxation back to the equilibrium state is recorded as a change in electromagnetic flux, and the relaxation time depends on the physicochemical environment. Atoms in different physicochemical environment will have different relaxation times, and thus generate different MR signals and image contrast (12).

MRI has a number of important advantages over other noninvasive imaging modalities: it has relatively high three-dimensional spatial resolution when compared with PET and SPECT; it has very good sample penetration with complete body coverage (when compared with optical imaging methods); and it has the ability to measure more than one physiological parameter using different radiofrequency pulse sequences, no radioactivity is involved and it is already widely used in the clinic. The drawback is its low sensitivity compared with the aforementioned methods (approximately micromolar concentrations of an imaging probe within a given voxel, which is three to six orders of magnitude lower than the sensitivity of optical imaging for detection of fluorochromes in vivo), and this requires the development of powerful signal amplification strategies for instance by using smart contrast agents (2).

Optical imaging modalities (13) are based on very sensitive devices capable of detecting and quantifying bioluminescent or fluorescent light that is transmitted through tissues from internal sources. This imaging of very weak visible light is rendered possible by the use of charged coupled device (CCD) cameras that include microchannel plate intensifiers and liquid nitrogen–cooled detectors and aim at enhancing the signal-to-noise ratio by decreasing the background (cooling) or amplifying the signal (intensifiers). Optical imaging can be divided in fluorescence and bioluminescence imaging (BLI). In fluorescence imaging, an external light source excites a fluorochrome and the transferred energy is emitted at a different wavelength when the fluorochrome returns to its ground state. In BLI, the energy is obtained from a chemical reaction and light is released enzymatically at a specific wavelength. No external light source is necessary. The major drawbacks of optical imaging are limited light transmission through tissue and light scatter and absorption limiting depth of imaging and signal quantification.

It should be pointed out that with these advantages and disadvantages, the various imaging modalities should be used in concerted action to serve complementary information on a specific molecular process of interest to get the best possible answer to a certain scientific question.

MOLECULAR IMAGING STRATEGIES

Three different molecular imaging strategies have been identified: direct, indirect, and surrogate (1,14).

Direct molecular imaging generally involves direct probe-target interaction. Image probe localization and accumulation is directly related to the interaction of the image probe with its target epitope, transporter, or enzyme. This strategy can be used by all three imaging technologies: nuclear, MR, and optical by the use of paramagnetic, fluorescent, or radionuclide-labeled probes. The target-specific probe can be a monoclonal antibody or a genetically engineered antibody fragment (e.g., minibody) directed against a cell surface–specific antigen or epitope. Imaging cell surface–specific antigens or epitopes with radionuclide-labeled antibodies was the first strategy to be used for direct molecular imaging application in clinical nuclear medicine research. Other examples of direct imaging paradigms include PET imaging of receptor density or occupancy using small radionuclide–labeled molecular probes, PET imaging of glucose utilization using the radiolabeled analogue of naturally occurring fluorodeoxyglucose (FDG), or PET imaging of a particular transporter (e.g., hNIS or human sodium iodide symporter) with a transport-specific probe. More recent research focused on the development of small radiolabeled or fluorescent probes and paramagnetic nanoparticles that

target specific receptors (e.g., estrogen or androgen receptors), that are activated by specific endogenous proteases (smart contrast agents), or that target mRNA or proteins [antisense or aptamer oligonucleotide probes (15) or magnetic nanosensors (16–18)]. Direct imaging strategies are constrained by the necessity to develop a specific probe for each molecular target and then to validate both sensitivity and specificity in the application of each newly developed probe-target imaging paradigm. This can be very time consuming and costly. However, direct imaging remains widely used as the traditional approach, and to develop new probes for imaging specific molecular-genetic targets using radionuclide-labeled, paramagnetic, or fluorescent small molecular probes.

Indirect imaging strategies are more complex as they involve pretargeting components that function as molecular-genetic sensors. This strategy is mostly used for radionuclide-based and optical molecular imaging and to a lesser extent for MRI. Most indirect molecular-imaging paradigms involve the coupling of a reporter gene with a complementary reporter probe (reporter gene imaging). The reporter gene must be delivered (pretargeted) to the target tissue by the use of transfection or transduction. Imaging the level of reporter gene product activity— through the level of reporter probe accumulation or the level of emitted light—provides indirect information that reflects the level of reporter gene expression as well as the levels of endogenous signaling and transcription factors that drive reporter gene expression. Reporter transgenes can encode for an enzyme [e.g., herpes simplex virus type 1 thymidine kinase (HSV-1-TK), luciferase], a receptor [e.g., human dopamine type 2 receptor (hD2R), human somatostatin receptor subtype-2 (hSSTR2)], a transporter (e.g., hNIS), an antigen or a fluorescent protein [e.g., enhanced fluorescencent green protein (eGFP)] (see more in detail below) (Figs. 1 and 2). An advantage of reporter gene imaging is the ability to develop and validate indirect imaging strategies more rapidly and at considerably lower costs than direct imaging strategies as only a small number of well-characterized and validated reporter gene-reporter probe pairs need to be established that can be used in many different reporter constructs to image many different biological and molecular-genetic processes.

The third imaging strategy, surrogate marker imaging, reflects the down-stream effects of one or more endogenous molecular-genetic processes. This approach is particularly attractive for potential clinical translation as radiopharmaceuticals and imaging paradigms that are already established in the clinic can be used in surrogate imaging. However, surrogate imaging is less specific and more limited with respect to the number of molecular-genetic processes that can be studied. Surrogate imaging may be useful for monitoring down-stream effects of specific molecular-genetic pathways that are

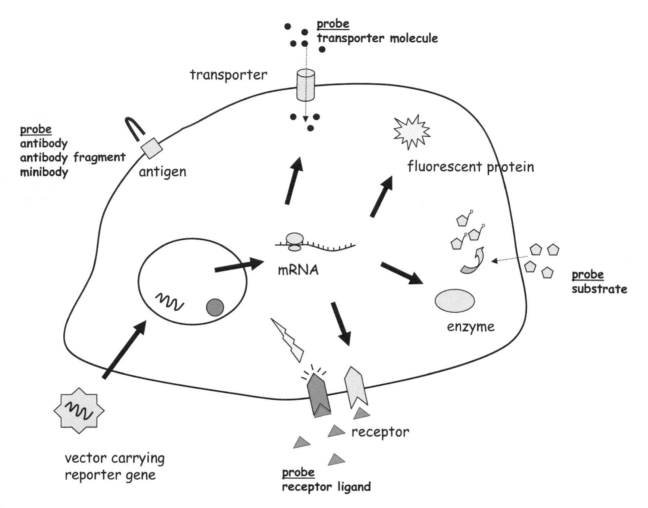

Figure 1 General paradigms for reporter gene imaging. First, the reporter gene complex is transduced into target cells by a vector (viral or nonviral). Inside the transduced cell, the reporter gene may integrate into the host genome or remain episomal. After initiation of reporter gene transcription, the reporter gene product is expressed. The reporter gene product can be an enzyme, a membrane transporter, a membrane receptor, an artificial cell surface antigen, or a fluorescent protein. A complementary reporter probe (a radiolabeled, paramagnetic or bioluminescent molecule) has to be administered and concentrates or emits light at the site of reporter gene expression. The level of reporter probe concentration or the intensity of emitted light is usually proportional to the level of reporter gene expression.

altered in diseases such as cancer or that are targeted by novel pathway-specific drugs. Assessment of the therapy response of noncytotoxic, cytostatic drugs, such as antiangiogenic drugs can be problematic when only based on tumor volume assessment. Surrogate imaging markers of tumor vascularity can be used for assessing anti-angiogenesis treatment response prior to tumor volume changes (19–21). Other examples of clinically useful surrogate markers are FDG and FLT (3-deoxy-3-fluorothymidine) for imaging glucose metabolism and DNA synthesis in the assessment of early treatment response. This has been shown impressively in gastrointestinal stromal tumors (GIST) where responders to imatinib/Gleevec treatment can be distinguished from non-responders within six days by a conventional FDG PET measurement, in contrast to CT imaging that requires over

four months to distinguish imatinib responders from non-responders (22,23) and in breast cancer where FLT imaging can predict longer term clinical outcome after the first course of chemotherapy (24).

REPORTER GENES

There has been a "high speed" development in the field of gene expression imaging with the availability of a variety of cloning vectors and animal models, the ease of recombinant DNA technology, and the importance for preclinical evaluation and clinical application. Different classes of marker genes encoding proteins, enzymes, transporters or cell-surface receptors have been developed and characterized (25).

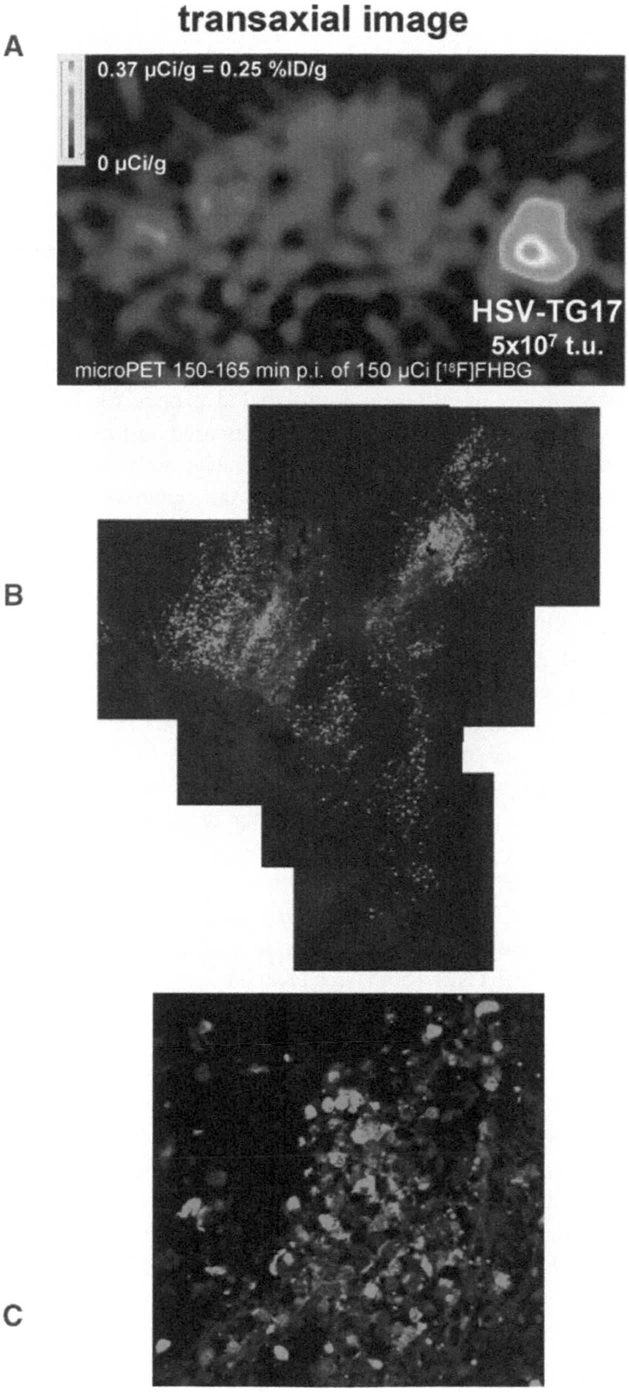

transaxial image

Figure 2 Indirect imaging of any proportionally coexpressed gene of interest. Coregistration between HSV-TG17–mediated *tg17*-gene expression in vivo as assessed by [^{18}F]FHBG-PET (**A**) and histology/fluorescence microscopy (**B** and **C**). After PET imaging, the animal was killed and the HSV-TG17-transduced tumor processed for fluorescence microscopy. In **B**) a set of representative pictures (10×) acquired at the laser scanning microscope (LSM) in the same transaxial plane was put together; (**C**) demonstrates a part at higher magnification (63×). Both PET and fluorescence microscopy demonstrate efficient *tg17*-gene transduction within the tumor. *Source*: From Ref. 34 (*See Color Insert*).

The paradigm for quantitative imaging of transgene expression involves several key steps, including the transfer of the reporter construct into target tissue or cells, the initiation of transcription (that can be controlled by specific promoter/enhancer elements), the process of DNA transcription, and the subsequent translation of mRNA into gene product (26). All of these key events can be specifically visualized in vivo by utilizing reporter gene imaging.

A common feature of all reporter constructs is the cDNA expression cassette containing the reporter gene of interest. The versatility of reporter gene imaging results in part from the flexibility to tailor the expression cassette to an individual need. The reporter genes can be placed under the control of specific promoter-enhancer elements. By the use of constitutive promoters [such as cytomegalovirus (CMV), long terminal repeat (LTR), Rous sarcoma virus (RSV), phosphoglycerate kinase (PGK), elongation factor (EF1), etc.] the reporter genes are always active. This approach is mainly used in gene therapy paradigms where the constitutively driven reporters are used to identify the site, extent and duration of vector delivery, and monitor the efficiency of tissue and cell transduction as well as for cell trafficking experiments to label the cells for long-term monitoring. Alternatively, the promoter-enhancer elements can be constructed to be inducible and sensitive to activation and regulation by specific endogenous pathways, or exogenous drugs, or to be tissue specific and activated by transcription factors that are overexpressed in specific tissues [e.g., the prostate-specific membrane antigen (PSMA) promoter in prostate cancer cells, the albumin promoter in liver cells, and the carcinoembryonic antigen (CEA) promoter in colorectal cancer cells]. Furthermore, multimodality reporter constructs can be created containing two or more different (reporter) genes with a proportional and constant relationship in their coexpression over a wide range of expression levels, underlining the versatility of reporter gene imaging. Many reports on the construction and validation of several multimodality bifusion and triple fusion reporter genes in living animals exist (9,27–32). Such double or triple reporter gene constructs can be particularly useful in gene therapy protocols by linking a therapeutic gene to a reporter gene. In principle, direct measure of the expression and activity of the reporter gene gives indirect evaluation of the expression and activity of the therapeutic gene of interest. In principle, proportional coexpression of two genes can be achieved by two coordinately acting promoters, by gene fusion or by certain translational linkers, such as the internal ribosomal entry site sequence (IRES) (33,34). The versatility of promoter and transgene variations introduced in reporter vectors reflects the investigator's imaging goals or the combination of imaging and therapeutic goals. Ideal vectors for targeting reporter constructs to specific organs or tissue in patients do not exist at this time and are an active area of human gene therapy research. An ideal transduction vector will contain at least two different reporter constructs (Fig. 2). One will be a constitutive reporter that will be used to identify the site, extent and duration of vector delivery, and monitor the efficiency of tissue transduction (the normalizing term) for subsequent image and data analysis. A second reporter will be inducible and sensitive to endogenous transcription factors as well as posttranscriptional processing, and will be used to monitor functional status and characteristics of the transduced target cells (35,36).

One major disadvantage of reporter gene imaging is the need to transduce or transfect the target tissue, which hampers its widespread clinical use. The cDNA containing vector can be used directly to transfect the cells, mostly facilitated by cationic lipid-based transfection agents or electroporation; or the vectors can be wrapped into a recombinant viral vector, which is then used to transduce the cells. Several currently available vector types can be used (e.g., retrovirus, adenovirus, adeno-associated virus, lentivirus, Herpes simplex virus). In general, viral vectors result in higher transfection efficiency as nonviral system but are limited in their use due to immunogenicity, manufacturing difficulties and size limitations of the DNA insert, in contrast to nonviral systems that are less immunogenic, easier to manufacture and do not have size limitations for DNA inserts (2,34).

For years, in vitro and ex vivo assays have used the reporter gene technology to image the production of a protein (e.g., eGFP, β-galactosidase, choline-phenylacetyltransferase, or luciferase) stoichiometrically linked to a gene of interest (37). In recent years, many reporter gene-reporter probe systems for noninvasive molecular-genetic imaging have been developed and validated.

An ideal reporter gene is not (or only limited) endogenously expressed in the host tissue and codes for a receptor, a transporter, an enzyme, an antigen, or a protein. Expression of the reporter in the transduced cells must be nontoxic to the host cells, not perturb normal cell function, and lead to accumulation of reporter substrate or reporter probe by (*i*) binding to the receptor or antigen, (*ii*) transport of the compound into the cell, or (*iii*) metabolizing and trapping of the probe by the reporter enzyme (38). The use of extracellular receptors or cell membrane transporters as reporter genes eliminates the need of the reporter probes to cross the cell membrane.

Essential for reporter gene imaging is the fact that reporter probe accumulation or light emission should directly reflect the activity of the reporter and thereby expression of the reporter gene.

Several genes have been proposed as potential genes for radiotracer-based molecular imaging (35,39,40). The most commonly used reporter genes for molecular imaging studies using radiolabeled probes and PET imaging

are wild-type HSV-1-*tk* (41–43) and mutant HSV-1-*sr39tk* (44). HSV-1-TK can, like mammalian thymidine kinase 1 (TK1), convert thymidine to its phosphorylated form. However, HSV-1-TK has less substrate specificity than mammalian TK1 and can moreover convert acycloguanosines [like ganciclovir, acyclovir, penciclovir, and FHBG (9-[4-fluoro-3-(hydoxy-methyl)butyl]guanine)] as well as 2′-fluoronucleoside analogues of thymidine such as FIAU (5-iodo-2′-fluoro-2′deoxy-1-β-D-arabino-furanosyl-uracil). The second-generation HSV-1-*sr39tk* are better able to utilize positron-emitting acycloguanosine substrates, most commonly FHBG. The advantages and disadvantages of different radiolabeled probes for imaging viral TK expression have been compared and extensively discussed in the literature (45,46). The advantage of the use of HSV-1-*tk* is the fact that this gene cannot only be used as an imaging gene but also as a therapeutic gene. The phosphorylated acycloguanosines, following conversion to their di- and tri-phosphate forms by HSV-1-TK, can kill cells either by blocking DNA synthesis or by causing chain termination. Most commonly ganciclovir is used as prodrug in this suicide gene therapy paradigm. However, at the trace levels utilized for PET reporter gene imaging, no physiological consequences of radiolabeled acycloguanosine administration are observable.

Other molecular-genetic nuclear reporter systems that utilize enzymatic signal amplification and trapping mechanisms include *Escherichia coli* and yeast cytosine deaminases (yCD) (47,48), *E. coli* xanthine phosphoribosyl transferase (49), and human mitochondrial thymidine kinase 2 (hTK2) (50,51). hTK2 has several biochemical features that make it an attractive PET reporter gene. The hTK2 enzyme has a spectrum of substrate specificity similar to that of viral thymidine kinase. A truncated version of hTK2 (ΔhTK2), which lacks the 18 N-terminal amino acids that are responsible for the mitochondrial localization of this protein, has been recently shown to function as an improved reporter gene than native hTK2 (52).

Other PET reporter gene-reporter probe systems that have been implemented to image and quantify exogenous gene delivery utilize genes encoding a receptor and a positron-emitting PET reporter ligand. The dopamine D2 receptor (D2R), primarily expressed in the striatum, has been one of the most well-studied receptors in nuclear neurosciences research. A number of positron-emitting probes have been developed to noninvasively image the endogenous striatal D2R and can also be used to non-invasively image ectopic expression of D2R as a PET reporter gene. A second-generation D2R reporter gene, D2R80A, has been generated to prevent ligand-induced activation of a G-protein-coupled response resulting in decreased intracellular cAMP levels (53,54). The level of adenovirus vector-mediated expression of a wild type (55–57) or mutated (54) D2R by using the specific D2R binding compounds [^{11}C]raclopride (56,57) and 3-(2'-[^{18}F]fluoroethyl)-spiperone (54,55) have been quantified with PET. After injection into the rat striatum, a kinetic analysis revealed the maximum level of D2R expression two to three days after vector application with a decline to basal levels at day 16 (56,57), indicating that various levels of D2R expression can be differentiated by PET. By placing the D2R gene and a mutated HSV-1-*tk* gene under transcriptional control of a bidirectional, tetracycline-responsive element, Sun et al. (58) could demonstrate that various levels of PET marker gene expression can be differentiated by PET in cell lines stably expressing these constructs, depending on the state of induction (58). These data indicate that PET can monitor time-dependent variations of gene expression mediated by inducible promoters.

Another example of a receptor as a reporter gene for radionuclide-based imaging is the somatostatin receptor. Radionuclide-labeled derivatives of somatostatin receptor agonists and antagonists have been developed that permit the noninvasive imaging of ectopically expressed somatostatin receptors (59–61).

A third possibility for nuclear marker gene/marker substrate combinations employs reporter genes encoding a transporter. The human thyroid sodium/iodide symporter (hNIS) gene encoding an endogenous membrane glycoprotein uses the transmembrane sodium gradient maintained by the sodium/potassium ATPase to cotransport iodine and sodium across the thyroid cell membrane. Expression of this symporter in extrathyroidal tumor tissue has been employed to facilitate radioiodine therapy (62–64), to image gene transfer, (65) and to image the transcriptional activity of human telomerase promoter fragments in tumor cells (59). Some of the drawbacks of this system are that (radiolabeled) the iodide is not metabolically trapped within transduced tissues resulting in the lack of retention of radioactivity in nonthyroid tissues. Therefore, quantification of gene expression is not possible and the use of NIS as a suicide protein is limited. However, the lack or retention of radioactivity in nonthyroid tissues can be overcome by coexpression of both NIS and thyroperoxidase (TPO), which catalyzes iodination of proteins and subsequent iodide retention within thyroid cells, thus resulting in enhanced tumor cell apoptosis consequent to increased radioiodide uptake and retention (66). Another human gene encoding for a transporter that can be used for reporter gene imaging is the human norepinephrine transporter (hNET) gene, a transmembrane protein that mediates the transport of norepinephrine, dopamine, and epinephrine across the cell membrane and that is exclusively located in the central and peripheral sympathetic nervous system (67,68).

Human-derived imaging genes have the advantage over nonhuman genes to reduce the risk of generating a potential immune response. However, HSV-1-*tk* has been used as a therapeutic gene and reporter gene in the clinical setting. It has been shown to be essentially nontoxic in humans and has been used in clinical gene therapy protocols as a prodrug-activating gene for treating cancer in combination with ganciclovir (69,70) and for imaging the location of transduced tumor cells with FIAU or FHBG (71,72). One important advantage of HSV-1-*tk* or HSV-1-*sr39tk* is this ability to function as suicide genes as well as reporter genes. Vector-safety and vector-monitoring are the important features of this dual reporter-suicide.

Optical-based reporter gene systems are receiving increasing attention because of their operational ease, cost benefit, and high-throughput potential. Most commonly used bioluminescence reporter gene systems utilize *Firefly luciferase* (*Fluc*) from the North American firefly *Photinus Pyralis* or *Renilla luciferase* (*Rluc*) from the seapansy *Renilla Reniformis*. Fluorescent protein-based reporter systems mostly use different spectral shifted variants of *Aequorea victoria* green fluorescent protein (GFP) (including an enhanced eGFP) or a number of red fluorescent proteins (RFPS), including *Discosoma* species (dsRed 1 and 2) and *Heteractis crispa* (HcRed) (26). BLI depends on the delivery of a specific substrate to the reporter gene product in transduced cells (as with nuclear and magnetic resonance reporter systems) and further requires the presence of oxygen, and in the case of firefly luciferase additionally ATP. This is in contrast to fluorescence reporter gene imaging where light emission is only dependent on illumination by an external source of light. Autobioluminescence in most cases is essentially nonexistent and results in very low background light emission, contributing to the very high sensitivity and specificity of this optical imaging technique. Under the conditions that the level of substrate, oxygen and ATP are not rate limiting but rather in excess, photon emission is directly related to reporter gene expression and the level of the reporter gene product. Fluorescent protein-based reporter systems are frequently limited by endogenous tissue autofluorescence resulting in substantial background emission, limiting the sensitivity, and specificity of these reporter systems.

Because of better spectral properties of near-infrared light leading to increased tissue penetration and reduced autofluorescence, near-infrared fluorescence (NIRF) is gaining increased attention. Whereas visible light penetration in tissues is only 1 to 2 mm, near-infrared light with wavelengths of 700 to 1.2 nm enables better penetration into tissues (73). The recent advances in NIRF imaging have been accelerated by the development of NIR fluorochromes coupled to quenching peptides that are activated by specific proteases at the target site (26). Such proteases can also be used as reporter genes as was demonstrated by Shah et al. (74) for the viral HIV-1 protease (HIV-1 PR). The authors showed specific fluorescence activation of a HIV-1 PR specific NIRF probe in human Gli36 gliomas after injection with an HSV-1 amplicon vector expressing HIV-1 PR. Essential for the development of reporter protease/substrate systems is the fact that the protease is not ubiquitously expressed in mammalian tissue as is the case by the use of viral proteases.

The sensitivity of different luciferase systems has been compared (75) and dual BLI has been performed enabling the monitoring of two different biological processes in a single animal over time (76,77). Dual luciferase imaging takes advantage of the substrate specificity of *Firefly* and *Renilla* luciferase, luciferin and coelenterazine, respectively. Luciferase may be well suited to monitor transcription due to its relatively fast induction (78) and to the considerable short biological half-life of luciferin and luciferase (79). This is an advantage compared with the longer-lived eGFP. However, short-lived variants of eGFP have been developed, and eGFP can be used for higher-resolution imaging in cells in vitro. Combining these reporter genes into a single gene provides additional tools for the analysis of cells in vivo and ex vivo (80). A detailed review on in vivo BLI of gene expression has been published by Contag and Bachmann (13). BLI has been used mainly to monitor tumor cell growth (exogenously induced or after spontaneous oncogenic transformation in transgenic animal models) (81,82) and the kinetics of tumor regression in response to therapy (83,84). Constitutive expression of luciferase has rendered many different xenograft tumor cell lines stably luminescent, and tight correlations have been demonstrated between photon emission and tumor burden (85) making BLI particularly useful to quantify the growth of primary tumor and spontaneous metastasis and to evaluate the efficacy of cancer therapeutics, especially in the case of firefly luciferase that can only detect viable cells, as for light emission ATP and oxygen are required in addition to the substrate luciferin. Other commonly used applications of BLI are cell trafficking [immune cells or stem/progenitor cells (86)] and tracking of gene expression (12).

A novel technology, quantum dot imaging, comprises a near-infrared imaging platform with great potential for noninvasive in vivo imaging. Quantum dots (QDs) are nanosized particles that fluoresce brightly when excited, and possess tight, highly specific emission wavelength properties (ranging from visible to near-infrared portions of the spectrum) that are directly proportional to the size of their photoexcitable core (87). QDs have been targeted to tumor-specific targets such as human epidermal growth factor receptor 2 (HER2) or prostate-specific membrane antigen (PSMA) using antibody conjugates (88,89) and to specific organs, such as the lungs, tumor-associated vasculature, and lymph in living mice using short peptide conjugates (90). A recent review addresses the application of QDs for molecular and cellular imaging (91).

Efforts toward the development of MR reporter genes have been made for at least a decade (92). MR reporter genes have the potential to monitor transgene expression noninvasively in real time at high resolution.

Imaging of gene expression using MRI may be achieved by two approaches: (*i*) imaging of the translated protein introduced by the reporter gene, which can be a membrane-bound receptor binding a targeted contrast agent, an enzyme converting a substrate or a metalloprotein, or (*ii*) imaging of a unique spectroscopic signature by means of MR spectroscopy (MRS) (12). MRS shares the same principle as MRI; in MRS, the signal obtained from a single element is further separated into its different chemical forms. With MRS, a spectrum of nuclear magnetic resonance signals is defined in which the several chemical forms of an element peak in specific positions and thus offer the potential to measure gene expression. MRS has been used for quantitative noninvasive imaging of tumors expressing cytosine deaminase (*cd*) as a combined reporter and therapeutic gene (48). Animals bearing tumors expressing the cDNA encoding for yCD were treated with nontoxic 5-fluorocytosine (5-FC) prodrug. The yCD-catalyzed conversion of 5-FC to the chemotherapeutic agent 5-fluorouracil (5-FU) was quantified in vivo using ^{19}F MRS. Another study using MRS to quantify deoxycytidine kinase (cDK) transgene expression confirmed the use of MRS as a noninvasive tool to determine efficacy of prodrug conversion (93). In this study, human colon carcinoma xenografts in mice were infected with a retroviral vector containing the cDK gene. cDK catalyzes the phosphorylation of gemcitabine (dFdCyd) to the triphosphate derivative dFdCTP, which is cytotoxic and incorporates into DNA. 19F MRS could detect the increased incorporation of dFdCTP in these cells. Other examples of detection of genetically encoded reporter genes using MRS are based on the expression of enzymes that catalyze the conversion of ATP into ADP, and therefore, are detectable with 31P MRS, such as creatine kinase (94,95) or arginine kinase (96).

MR reporter genes encode for receptors, enzymes or metalloproteins. An example of a cell surface imaging receptor is the transferrin receptor (TfR). It has been shown that receptor expression and regulation can be visualized with MRI when an engineered TfR is probed with a superparamagnetic transferrin probe (97,98). In this system, an engineered human transferrin receptor (ETR) that lacks feedback downregulation of receptor expression in response to iron uptake due to the absence of the iron-regulatory region and mRNA destabilization motifs in the 3′ untranslated region, and therefore, constitutively overexpressing high levels of receptor protein is used as MR reporter gene and probed with a human holo-transferrin covalently conjugated with monocrystalline iron oxide nanoparticles (MION), sterically protected by a layer of low-molecular-weight dextran (Tf-MION). It could be shown that in rat 9L gliosarcoma cells stably expressing the ETR, the MR signal intensity was related to cellular Tf-MION concentrations and correlated with ETR expression. As more and more cell-surface proteins are shown to be upregulated in different human diseases (e.g., cancer), it is conceivable that specific superparamagnetic markers for each cell-surface protein might be used to enhance tumor detection and imaging. Other examples of cell-surface proteins that can be targeted with MR contrast probes are Her2/NeuR (99), endothelial vascular cell adhesion molecule-1 (VCAM-1) (100) and inflammatory adhesion molecule ICAM-1 (101), among many others.

A frequently used marker enzyme in molecular biology, β-galactosidase, has been explored as MR imaging reporter. In this system, β-galactosidase is used to enzymatically cleave an inactive contrast agent (a paramagnetic chelate) resulting in activation of the contrast agent, which in turn decreases $T1$ relaxation and thus increases signal in $T1$-weighted images. The feasibility of detecting β-galactosidase activity noninvasively in vivo could be demonstrated using this approach (102). In this study, the contrast agent (1-(2-(β-galactopyranosyloxy)propyl)-4,7,10-tris(carboxymethyl)-1,4,7,10-tetraazacyclododecane)gadolinium (III) (EgadMe) consists of (*i*) a chelator with high-affinity binding to gadolinium that occupies eight of the nine coordination sites on gadolinium and (*ii*) a galactopyranose residue positioned to block the remaining coordination site on the gadolinium ion from water. In this water-inaccessible conformation, the contrast agent is "inactive" and does not strongly modulate $T1$. β-Galactosidase enzymatically cleaves the galactopyranose from the chelate, freeing a coordination site and causing the irreversible transition of the contrast agent to an "active" state. ^{19}F MRS has also been used to probe the enzyme activity of β-galactosidase. This enzyme has been shown to liberate aglycone from the substrate 4-fluoro-2-nitrophenyl-β-D-galactopyranoside, leading to a ^{19}F NMR chemical shift of 5 to 10 ppm, depending on the pH value (103). Other substrates for β-galactosidase-based ^{19}F chemical shift imaging are 2-fluoro-4-nitrophenol-β-D-galactopyranoside (104) or the iron-based commercial substrate S-gal (3,4-cyclohexenoesculetin-β-D-galactopyranoside), which demonstrated T2* shortening in cultured cells and in tumors (105). Examples of MRI reporter genes based on engineered iron-binding metalloproteins (and which are independent of the delivery of exogenously injected contrast agents) are overexpression of the TfR leading to increased iron accumulation, the tyrosinase enzyme, and the ferritin protein. Iron enters cells through the TfR that binds the transferrin (Tf) protein containing two iron atoms. Upon binding of two iron-loaded Tf

molecules (but not apotransferrin, which does not contain iron), the receptor internalizes rapidly, after which the TfR-Tf complex dissociates in endosomes and the iron is released. As ferric iron is paramagnetic, overexpression of the TfR and increased iron accumulation generates MR contrast (106). However, the very high levels of TfR expression that are required and the relatively small relaxation time changes have limited the application of this approach to measure gene expression but inspired the use of the tyrosinase enzyme and the ferritin protein. Tyrosinase is a part of the melanin synthesis pathway. Specifically, it catalyzes the hydroxylation of tyrosine-yielding dioxyphenlyalanine (dopa) and its subsequent oxidation to dopaquinone. DOPAquinone is then converted into melanin, which has a high affinity for iron and counts for the iron-induced $T1$ hyperintensities of melanin. MR imaging of tyrosinase expression has been demonstrated in transfected mouse fibroblast, human embryonal kidney cells, and in an inducible way in breast cancer cells (107,108). However, melanin and melanin precursors catalyzing and binding iron produce highly reactive oxygen species, and thus exhibit significant toxic effects, which could limit their clinical application.

Ferritin is another metalloprotein that can contain up to 4000 Fe atoms in the form of an iron oxyhydroxide core and servers as the body's iron depot. The feasibility of using ferritin as a MRI reporter gene has been demonstrated in a C6 rat glioma cell line overexpressing the heavy chain of murine ferritin under a conditional tetracycline promoter (109) as well as by injecting an adenoviral vector encoding ferritin into the mouse brain (110). Furthermore, Deans et al. (111) used the human TfR and a human ferritin H-subunit combined in one coexpression vector to image a mouse neural stem cell line. One possible drawback for the use of the ferritin reporter may be the fact that, unlike other reporter genes, the ferritin reporter may not be able to differentiate between live or death cells. When cells die, the ferritin-based iron particles will remain for some time and provide MR contrast until they are degraded in lysosomes or further metabolised.

IMAGING OF EXOGENOUS GENE EXPRESSION

Numerous examples of noninvasive imaging of exogenously introduced marker gene expression have already been addressed above. Many of these examples are based on constitutive or tissue-specific gene expression. However, constitutive expression of proteins, which may be toxic or have a negative effect on cell growth, may not always be desirable. For instance, in gene therapy protocols, constitutive expression of therapeutic genes at all stages of therapeutic application may not be desirable, or in transgenic

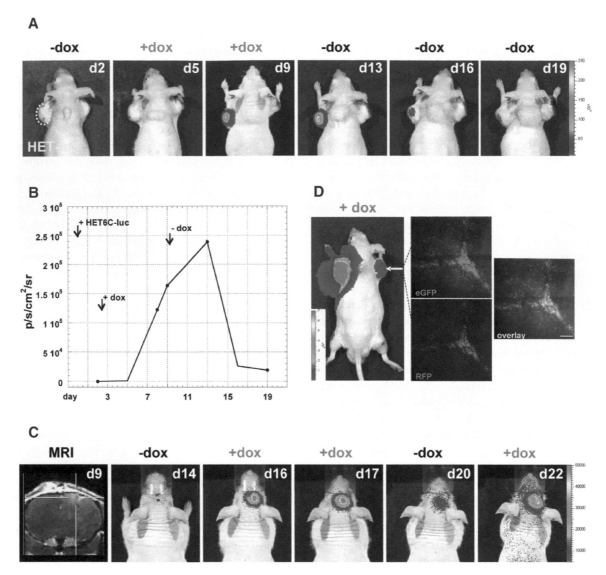

Figure 3 Imaging exogenous gene regulation. In vivo BLI of induced LUC expression and image validation by histology. Unit for all color scales as well as the histogram on temporal analysis was defined as photons per second per cm^2 pre steradian (p/sec/cm^2/sr). (**A**) Temporal analysis of up- and downregulation of LUC expression. HET-6C injection was performed intratumorally at day 0. Days where bioluminescent images were obtained are indicated at the upper right corner, days of doxycycline treatment at the top. (**B**) Quantitative analysis of luciferase signal (OFF-ON-OFF) in response to doxycycline. (**C**) Temporal analysis of up- and downregulation of LUC expression in the intracranial glioma model (OFF-ON-OFF-ON). Indicated are the days of tumor growth. (**D**) Image validation by histology. BLI of a mouse bearing a subcutaneous glioma stably expressing LUC on its left shoulder after in vivo transduction with HET6C-luc in the tumor on the right shoulder. Representative histological sections taken from the in vivo transduced tumor showing colocalization of eGFP, expressed constitutively from the herpes viral immediate early 4/5 promoter, and *rfp*, expressed from the bidirectional regulated promoter (scale bar overlay: 150 mm, exposure time: 0.5 seconds). *Abbreviations*: BLI, bioluminescence imaging; LUC, luciferase; rfp, red fluorescence protein. *Source*: From Ref. 121.

animals gene expression may only be desirable after the embryos or fetuses have reached a certain developmental stage. In such cases, inducible gene expression systems could be of great value. Several laboratories have reported the design of inducible eukaryotic gene expression systems regulated by, for example, antibiotics, hormones, heat shock, or heavy metal ions (112–119) and these systems have been

used to serve induced expression of imagable reporter genes. Yu et al. (120) used the mifepristone-regulated two-plasmid-based GeneSwitch promoter activation system to noninvasively study the induction and expression of a *Renilla* luciferase-*gfp* fusion gene construct. Using this activation system, the authors observed a 10- to 25-fold activation, depending on the mifepristone dose, of both luciferase and

GFP expression in transiently transfected cells in comparison with cells that were not exposed to the inducer. Furthermore, they could show activation of gene expression in live animals. Cohen et al. (109) demonstrated the dynamic detection of tetracycline-regulated ferritin gene expression with MRI. Our group also could demonstrate the feasibility of noninvasive imaging of regulated gene expression after in vivo transduction (121). For this purpose, we generated regulatable Herpes simplex virus type 1 (HSV-1) amplicon vectors carrying hormone (mifepristone) or antibiotic (tetracycline)-regulated promoters driving the proportional coexpression of a PET (HSV-1-*tk* or HSV-1-*tkgpf*), fluorescent (*rfp*), or bioluminescent (*FLuc*) marker gene (Fig. 3). Regulated gene expression was monitored by fluorescence microscopy in culture and by PET or BLI in vivo. The induction levels evaluated in glioma models varied depending on the dose of inductor up to 200-fold. With fluorescence microscopy and BLI being the tools for assessing gene expression in culture and animal models, and with PET being the technology for possible application in humans, the generated vectors may serve to noninvasively monitor the dynamics of any gene of interest, which is proportionally coexpressed with the respective imaging marker gene in research applications aiming toward translation into clinical application.

In gene therapy protocols, besides controlling the expression of the therapeutic genes such inducible systems also have the possibility to regulate the expression of suicide genes as "artificial death switches": when the gene therapy is satisfactory or its continuation is undesirable for the host, the treatment can be terminated by activating the expression of the suicide proteins and initiate cell death.

IMAGING OF ENDOGENOUS GENE EXPRESSION

Imaging the transcriptional regulation of endogenous genes or the activity of specific signaling pathways in living subjects using noninvasive imaging techniques can provide better understanding of normal and disease-related biological processes. However, imaging endogenous gene expression may be limited when weak promoters in their usual *cis*-configuration are activated and used to induce reporter gene expression resulting in low transcriptional activity of the reporter gene and a low or nondetectable level of probe accumulation. Several approaches have been used to enhance the transcriptional activity of weak promoters, either by the use of a two-step transcriptional amplification (TSTA) system (122) or by the use of a *trans* system (123). To amplify the transcriptional activity of the tissue-specific androgen-responsive prostate-specific antigen promoter (PSA) and hence, amplify the expression of the reporter genes *FLuc* and HSV-1-*sr39tk*, in the TSTA system, the first step involves tissue-specific expression of the GAL4-

VP16 fusion protein and the second step involves GAL4-VP16 induction of target gene expression under the control of GAL4 response elements in a minimal promoter. Transcription of the reporter gene, either *FLuc* or HSV-1-*sr39tk*, then leads to a detectable signal in the presence of the appropriate probe with a 12- (HSV-1-*sr39tk*) to 50-fold (*FLuc*) enhancement of reporter activity using this two-step approach. Furthermore, it could be shown that the TSTA system was androgen concentration sensitive, suggesting a continuous rather than a binary reporter response (122).

To increase the transcriptional activity of the CEA while maintaining tissue specificity, in the *trans* system a recombinant adenovirus was constructed that contained a TSTA system with a tumor-specific CEA promoter driving a transcription transactivator, which then activates a minimal promoter to drive the expression of the HSV-1-*tk* suicide/reporter gene. This adenovirus/CE-binary-tk system resulted in equal or greater killing of transduced cells by ganciclovir in a CEA-specific manner, compared with killing by ganciclovir of cells transduced with a CEA-independent vector containing a constitutive viral promoter driving HSV-1-*tk* expression (adenovirus/RSV-*tk*). The use of this recombinant adenovirus led to a tumor-specific transcriptional targeting of the applied suicide gene therapy protocol and to reduced side effects. After intratumoral injection of adenovirus/CE-binary-tk, there was significantly less spread to adjacent normal liver tissue and reduced liver toxicity than after administration of the universally expressed adenovirus/RSV-*tk* (123).

IMAGING OF SIGNAL TRANSDUCTION PATHWAYS/BIOLOGICAL PROCESSES

To examine a specific molecular target or pathway with a reporter probe, at least two strategies can be used: (*i*) one would be to place the reporter under the control of a transcriptional promoter that is responsive to the molecule or pathway of interest and (*ii*) the other would be to discover or reengineer reporter probes such that their activity is quantitatively or qualitatively altered by the molecule or pathway under study.

The status of p53, for example, can be monitored by placing luciferase (124) or TKeGFP under the control of a p53-responsive promoter (125). Using a retroviral vector containing a *cis*-p53/TKeGFP dual-reporter gene under control of a p53-specific response element, PET imaging was sufficiently sensitive to detect upregulation of genes in the p53 signal transduction pathway in response to DNA damage induced by BCNU chemotherapy. In a similar approach, the transcriptional regulation of nuclear factor of activated T cells (NFAT) could be noninvasively imaged (126). In this study, activation of Jurkat T-cells stably expressing an HSV-1-TK/GFP fusion protein under control of the T-cell-specific

NFAT promoter after systemic administration of anti-CD3 and anti-CD28 antibodies could be visualized with [^{124}I]FIAU PET. In another study by Serganova (36), the dynamics and spatial heterogeneity of hypoxia-inducible factor-1 (HIF-1)-specific transcriptional activity in tumors was measured repetitively and noninvasively with PET and [^{18}F]2′fluoro-2′deoxy-1β-D-arabinofuranosyl-5-ethyl-uracil (FEAU). In this study, a retroviral vector bearing a dual reporter gene cassette (the Red2XPRT beacon gene under control of the constitutive CMV promoter, and the HIF-inducible TKGFP sensor gene) was developed for imaging of transduced cell localization and HIF-1 transcriptional activity, respectively, in chemical as well as low atmospheric oxygen-induced hypoxia. Noninvasive imaging of ligand-induced or drug-mediated modulation of the NF-κB pathway has been achieved by the development of an IκBα-*Firefly* luciferase fusion reporter (127). The transcription factor NF-κB is a key regulator of cellular activation, proliferation, apoptosis, and IKK-dependent IκBα degradation is a critical upstream NF-κB regulatory control point, which is emerging as an important target for drug development.

Over the past decade, a number of genetically engineered reporters have been made that respond to phosphorylation by particular kinases or cleavage by specific proteases to noninvasively image a specific endogenous molecular target or pathway. Some examples of such targets are protein tyrosine kinase (128), protein kinase A (129), cyclin-dependent kinase2 (130), and Akt kinase (131).

In recent years also, an increasing number of transgenic mouse models that express luciferase reporter genes under control of various promoters and transcription factor binding sites have been developed. Such mouse models can serve to monitor gene expression in vivo and to screen exogenous factors, such as nutrients, pharmaceuticals, pollutants, etc. for modulation of gene expression. Carlsen et al. (132) have developed transgenic mice that express luciferase under the control of NF-κB, enabling real-time in vivo imaging of NF-κB activity in intact animals as a function of cytokines (TNF-α, IL-1α), endotoxin (LPS), physical agent (UVB treatment), and state of disease (chronic rheumatoid arthritis model). A similar transgenic mouse model expresses eGFP under control of NF-κB (133). Cytochrome P450 enzymes are a superfamily of heme-containing proteins involved in the metabolism of a variety of structurally diverse substances, including endogenous chemicals and xenobiotics such as drugs, carcinogens, and environmental pollutants. The cytochrome P450 3A4 (CYP3A4) is responsible for oxidation of 50% to 60% of clinical drugs. To efficiently study CYP3A4 regulation in vivo, a transgenic mouse model was developed consisting of the human CYP3A4 promoter controlling expression of the firefly luciferase gene. Regulation of the reporter gene in whole animals in response to CYP3A4 inducers could rapidly be assessed allowing the noninvasive study of the time course of drug response (134). Other transgenic mouse models expressing a regulated imagable reporter are sensitive to Smad2- and Smad3-dependent signaling (135), serum amyloid A (136), p21 signaling (137), E2F1 signaling (138), serum albumin (139), lactase (140), bone morphogenic protein (BMP4) (141) or metalloporphyrins (142).

Various signaling cascades depend on the HER-kinase axis. The HER family of receptor tyrosine kinases controls critical pathways involved in epithelial cell differentiation, growth, division, and motility. The HER family consists of four closely related members, namely, EGFR (HER1 or ErbB1), HER2 (ErbB2), HER3 (ErbB3), and HER4 (ErbB4), and controls a complex network of ligand-receptor interactions and cellular responses known as the HER-kinase axis. This axis is now a validated target for the treatment of cancer patients (143). Multimodality noninvasive imaging of the HER-kinase axis in cancer has been reported using various targeting ligands (small molecules, peptides, proteins, antibodies, and antibody fragments) and a variety of labels (radionuclides, fluorescent dyes and a number of magnetic nanoparticles). In-depth reviews covering the complete axis (144) as well as specific parts (145) have been published. Many of the targeting ligands used for HER-kinase axis imaging are analogues of a drug or the drugs themselves with a radiolabel. The first quantitative PET imaging of EGFR expression was reported in xenograft-bearing mice using ^{64}Cu-labeled cetuximab (146). Using seven xenograft tumor models, the tumor uptake of [^{64}Cu]DOTA-cetuximab measured by PET was correlated with the EGFR expression level quantified by Western blotting, and [^{64}Cu]DOTA-cetuximab had increasing tumor activity accumulation over time in EGFR-positive tumors but relatively low uptake in EGFR-negative tumors. Sampath et al. (147) developed a dual-labeled antibody based imaging agent ([^{111}In]DTPA)n-trastuzumab-(IRDye800)m) for targeting HER2 in cell lines as well as in a standard subcutaneous animal model of human breast cancer and demonstrated a statistical correlation between nuclear and optical imaging results.

IMAGING PROTEIN-PROTEIN INTERACTION

The interaction of specific cellular proteins forms the basis of many biological processes, including transcription, translation, and various signal transduction and hormone activation pathways involved in cell proliferation, cell differentiation, regulation of cell death, inflammation, tumorigenesis, and metastasis. Several approaches have been developed for studying protein-protein interactions in cells based on transcriptional (two-hybrid system and split ubiquitin system) or posttranslational strategies

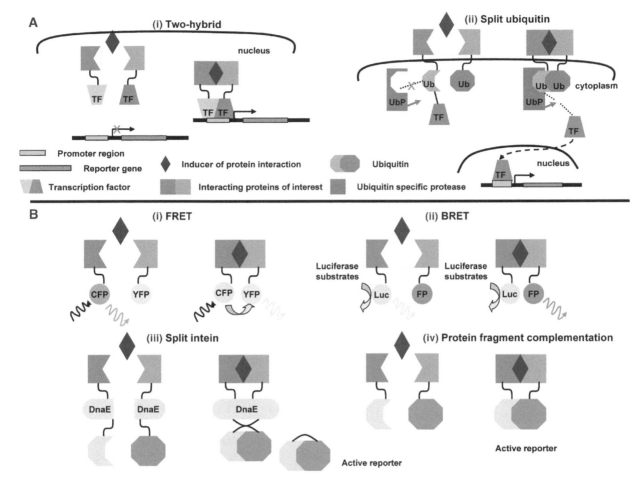

Figure 4 Strategies for imaging protein-protein interaction. (**A**) Transcriptional strategies. (*i*) Two-hybrid systems are applicable to protein interactions that can translocate to the nucleus. When a protein interaction is induced, the fusion proteins bring together transactivator and DNA binding domains of a TF, which can then induce reporter transcription. (*ii*) The split Ub system bypasses the nuclear translocation requirement by taking advantage of UBP that recognize only intact Ub. One fragment of the split Ub is fused to a TF that under basal conditions remains tethered outside the nucleus. Upon protein interaction and cleavage by UBP, the TF localizes to the nucleus and induces reporter gene transcription. (**B**) Posttranslational strategies. (*i*) FRET monitors the degree of protein interaction as a change in color caused by nonradiative light transfer from the donor fluorophore (CFP) to the acceptore fluorophore (YFP) when the proteins are within proximity to each other. (*ii*) BRET displays the same characteristics as FRET except the donor is a bioluminescence protein (LUC), which only requires a substrate and no excitation light. (*iii*) Self-splicing split inteins (DnaE) will splice the reporter protein together when brought within close proximity of each other. The splicing reaction is covalent and produces an intact, active reporter protein. (*iv*) Protein fragment complementation monitors protein interactions as an increase in reporter activity caused by reversible approximation of two fragments, which when separate are inactive, yet brought together reconstitute activity. *Abbreviations*: TF, transcription factor; Ub, ubiquitin; UBP, ubiquitin-specific proteases; FRET, fluorescence resonance energy transfer; BRET, bioluminescence resonance energy transfer. *Source*: From Ref. 148.

[fluorescence resonance energy transfer (FRET), bioluminescence resonance energy transfer (BRET), self-splicing split inteins, protein fragment complementation] (Fig. 4). A comprehensive review on the current state of imaging protein-protein interactions in vivo has been recently published (148). The major disadvantage of transcriptional strategies is the fact that they do not allow for real-time measurements of protein interactions as their readout is based on transcriptional activity, and therefore, the measurement of these assays is delayed by several hours, depending on the reporter being used. Furthermore, in the two-hybrid strategy, membrane proteins cannot be studied in their intact state as this system requires target protein interactions that are localized within the nucleus or that are at least compatible with nuclear translocation of the complexes because proximity to DNA and the transcriptional machinery is needed for reporter expression. Posttranslational strategies do not have these limitations and have increasingly gained attention. Resonance energy transfer monitors the degree of protein interaction as a change in color caused by nonradiative light transfer form a donor fluorophore (FRET) or bioluminescence protein (BRET) to an acceptor fluorophore when the proteins are within proximity to each other. These strategies have been mainly used for live-cell imaging but have many disadvantages for use in vivo. Protein fragment complementation assays, sometimes called split reporter strategies, depend on division of a monomeric reporter protein into two separate inactive components that can reconstitute function upon association. When these reporter fragments are fused to interacting proteins, the reporter is reactivated upon association of the interacting proteins. For in vivo imaging, mainly the split luciferase strategy is used, most commonly with the reporters *Renilla* or *Firefly* luciferase (149,150). Other proteins and enzymes that can be used for the split reporter strategy are dihydrofolate reductase, β-galactosidase, β-lactamase, and GFP. The use of most of the developed strategies to study protein interactions has been limited to assays in vitro and in cultured cells. However, these strategies can also be used for in vivo detection of protein-protein interaction by the use of reporters suitable for imaging.

Several studies have shown that it is possible to image protein-protein interactions in vivo using PET (151) and optical techniques (152,153), as well as MRI (17). Ray et al. have used the two-hybrid system and modified it to be inducible. They used the NF-κB promoter to drive expression of two fusion proteins (VP16-MyoD and GAL4-Id), and modulated the NF-κB promoter through TNF-α. *FLuc* reporter gene expression was driven by the interaction of MyoD and Id through a transcriptional activation strategy. A similar strategy by Luker et al. involved interactions between the p53 tumor suppressor and the large T antigen of simian virus 40 (SV40). Specific binding of p53 to SV40 TAg induced expression of a reporter gene composed of a mutant HSV-1-*tk* fused to *gfp*. By using microPET imaging with [^{18}F]FHBG the authors could detect binding of p53 and TAg in living mice and quantified a sixfold enhancement of tk activity in response to interaction of these two proteins in vivo in tumor xenografts of HeLa cells stably transfected with the imaging construct. In a proof-of-principle study De et al. demonstrated that BRET can be used for interrogating and observing protein-protein interactions directly at limited depths in living mice (153). They used the BRET^2 system, which utilizes *hRenilla* luciferase protein and its protein DeepBlueC as an energy donor and a mutant GFP^2 as the acceptor. These donor and acceptor proteins were fused to FKBP12 [the 12 kDa FK506 (=Tacrolimus) binding protein] and FRB [the rapamycin binding domain of FRAP (FKBP rapamycin-associated protein)], respectively, which are known to interact only in the presence of the small molecule mediator rapamycin. BRET^2-specific GFP^2 signal could only be detected in the presence of rapamycin, validating the use of BRET^2 to noninvasively detect protein-protein interaction.

IMAGING APOPTOSIS

Apoptosis is a physiological form of programmed cell death and is critical for organ development, tissue homeostasis, and removal of defective cells in vivo without inducing a concomitant inflammatory response. A deficiency or excess in apoptosis is an integral component of autoimmune disorders, transplant rejection, neurodegenerative disorders, and cancer. Apoptosis depends on the recognition of multiple extracellular and intracellular signals, integration and amplification of signals, and sequential activation of initiator (e.g., caspase-1) and effector caspases (e.g., caspase-3) (154,155). Once the apoptotic pathway is activated, caspase-mediated proteolysis is irreversible and ultimately leads to the typical cellular changes, such as cell shrinkage, plasma membrane blebbing, nuclear chromatin condensation and aggregation, and nuclear fragmentation. One of the earliest indications of apoptosis is the translocation of the membrane phospholipid phosphatidylserine (PS) from the inner to the outer plasma membrane. Once exposed to the extracellular environment, binding sites on PS become available for Annexin V, a Ca^{2+}-dependent phospholipid binding protein with high affinity for PS. Modulating the apoptotic pathway by caspase inhibitors or activators represents special opportunities for therapeutic intervention and underline the need for noninvasive monitoring of early drug response at the molecular level. This can be achieved by direct imaging of caspase activity [e.g., caspase peptide substrates containing either a nuclear or a bioluminescence label (156) or a near-infrared optical fluorochrome (157)] or by imaging the downstream effects on surface PS expression [e.g., radionuclide (158,159), paramagnetic (160), or fluorochrome labeled Annexin V (161)]. By means of these imaging paradigms, the effect of apoptotic pathway regulating drugs can been identified (162). This is particularly important as there is already an evidence, both from the laboratory and the clinic, that an early apoptotic response to therapy is a good prognostic indicator for treatment outcome (163).

Several imaging paradigms have been developed to noninvasively measure the activity of numerous other proteases (as a proof of principle or in response to therapy), such as cathepsins (cathepsin-B, -H, -D) (164–167), metalloproteinases (168), lipases (169), urokinases (170), the ubiquitin-proteasome pathway (171,172), and many others.

IMAGING ANGIOGENESIS

Angiogenesis, defined as the growth and remodeling of a primitive vascular network into a complex one, occurs physiologically during embryonic development, the female reproductive cycle, wound healing, and hair growth. In adults, except during the menstrual cycle, the vascular network is quiescent and tightly regulated by angiogenic inducers and inhibitors. Under certain pathological conditions (like cancer, cardiovascular disease, immunological disease, and diabetes), this tight control of the vascular network becomes deregulated. Key endogenous angiogenesis agonists include vascular endothelial growth factor (VEGF), basic fibroblast growth factor (bFGF), angiopoietins, matrix metalloproteases (MMP), integrins, and catherins, among others. Key endogenous angiogenesis inhibitors are thrombospondins, endostatins, angiostatins, troponins, metallospondins, interleukins and tissue inhibitors of matrix metalloproteinases, among others (2). Currently, some biological or small synthetic angiogenesis inhibitors are in clinical trials. Noninvasive monitoring of drug effect plays an important role in assessing response to therapy. Conventional imaging techniques like MRI and PET focus on the measurement of physiological parameters, such as blood flow, blood volume, vascular perfusion, permeability, and/or structure. However, a more specific approach to image antiangiogenesis is to target with an imaging probe the same molecular events that are targeted with the therapeutic drug, enabling early assessment of response to therapy, before physiological changes become apparent. Specific examples include targeting of endothelial integrin $\alpha(v)\beta 3$ by using targeted paramagnetic nanoparticles for MR imaging (173–175) or radiolabeled glycosylated RGD-containing peptides for PET imaging (176,177), targeting of E-selectin by attaching a cross-linked iron oxide or a NIRF probe to a high-affinity antibody (178,179), respectively, targeting of the angiogenesis-associated fibronectin isoform by using optical probes (180), radiolabeled peptidomimetics of a urokinase plasminogen activator receptor antagonist (181), peptides adhering to the glycoprotein IIb/IIIa receptor on the surface of activated platelets (182), and antibodies against the tumor growth factor β receptor (183). Ongoing tumor angiogenesis and neovascularization can also be noninvasively imaged by magnetically labeled endothelial precursor cells (184), which are known to home to site of angiogenesis and are being investigated as angiogenesis-selective gene-targeting vectors (185).

The VEGF/VEGFR signaling pathway plays a pivotal role in regulating angiogenesis and many therapeutic agents targeting VEGF and VEGFR are currently in preclinical and clinical development. The ability to quantitatively image VEGF/VEGFR expression in a noninvasive and multimodal manner has been recently reviewed (186).

IMAGING CELL-BASED THERAPY

Cell-based therapies (187) have received great attention as novel therapeutics for the treatment of cancer, autoimmune,

cardiovascular, inflammatory, and degenerative diseases. A number of native cells, antigen-specific T-lymphocytes, or, more recently, stem and progenitor cells have been used for these approaches. Noninvasive and repetitive imaging of adoptively administered cells provides the opportunity to study trafficking, homing, tumor targeting, activation, proliferation, and persistence of adoptively transferred cells.

T cells are an important component of the immune response and noninvasive imaging of this complex and highly dynamic immune response can provide accurate and detailed information on the regulatory dynamics of the immune system in real time (188). Imaging the trafficking of T lymphocytes has been performed using nuclear (189,190), optical- (191) and MR-based (192) techniques. The first experiments for noninvasive imaging of lymphocyte trafficking date back to the early 1970 and used ex vivo cell labeling (193,194). However, ex vivo labeling of cells with MR contrast agents or radiotracers does not provide an opportunity to monitor their functional status, such as activation upon antigen recognition or cell proliferation at specific target sites, and has limited temporal resolution due to radiotracer decay or label washout. Therefore, stable genetic labeling of cells to be administered for adoptive therapy with reporter genes has gained increasing attention and confirm the targeted migration of these cells (195–197). T-cell activation is an essential component of the immune response in many normal and disease states and noninvasive monitoring of T-cell receptor-dependent activation in vivo using PET has been performed (126).

Numerous studies have demonstrated the potential use of stem cells for the repair and regeneration of injured (198,199) or degenerated (200–202) tissue or as tumor targeting vehicles (203,204). Many reports on noninvasive imaging of the migratory capacity of stem cells toward ischemic lesions (205–208) and experimental tumors (86,184,209,210) in real time exist. Stem cells have been used as gene delivery vectors and response to therapy has been monitored noninvasively. Miletic et al. (211) together with our group used a multimodal imaging protocol to demonstrate that a subpopulation of bone marrow–derived mesenchymal stem cells can be used as tumor-infiltrating therapeutic cells against malignant glioma. The stem cells genetically engineered to express HSV-1-*tk* were injected into rat intracranial 9L gliomas. After transplantation, stem cell localization and distribution could be monitored noninvasively by means of [^{18}F] FHBG-PET. In addition, the therapeutic effect of ganciclovir treatment could be monitored sequentially by MRI and [^{11}C]methionine-PET and strongly correlated with histological analysis (Fig. 5).

Simultaneous tracking transplanted stem cell fate and function in vivo noninvasively has gained increased attention as it can address many safety aspects of the use of these cells as targeting vehicles for gene therapy (stem cell

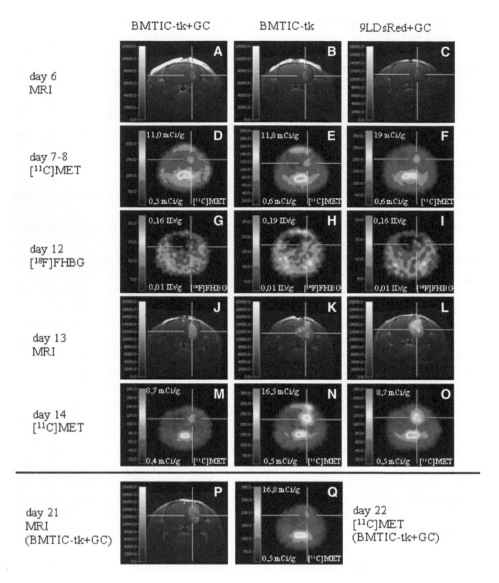

Figure 5 Multimodal imaging of cell-based therapy. Representative three-dimensional MRI [*T*1-weighted FLASH, echo time = 5 milliseconds, repetition time = 70 milliseconds, 60° pulse, resolution 121 × 121 × 242 μm, post-administration of gadopentetic acid (Gd-DTPA)], [11C]MET-PET and [18F]FHBG-PET scans. Time points after tumor implantation: (**A–C**) 6 days, MRI before ganciclovir (GC) treatment; (**D–F**) seven to eight days, [11C]MET-PET before GC treatment; (**G–I**) 12 days, [18F]FHBG-PET during GC treatment; (**J–L**) 13 days, MRI during GC treatment; (**M–O**) 14 days, [11C]MET PET during GC treatment; (P) 21 days, MRI after GC were treated as described for the survival study: (**A, D, G, J, M, P, Q**) bone-marrow derived tumor- infiltrating cells expressing thymidine kinase and green fluorescent protein (BM-TIC-tk-GFP) injection with GC treatment; (**B, E, H, K, N**) BM-TIC-tk-GFP injection without GC treatment; (**C, F, I, L, O**) 9LDsRed gliomas only with GC treatment. *Source*: From Ref. 211 (*See Color Insert*).

distribution, normal or aberrant stem cell proliferation, extent and duration of transgene expression, response to therapy). To address this issue, Cao et al. (212) stably transduced murine embryonic stem (ES) cells with double or triple fusion reporter gene constructs expressing monomeric *rfp*, *Fluc*, and truncated HSV-1-*tk*, respectively, injected these cells subcutaneously into nude mice and tracked cell survival noninvasively by bioluminescence and PET imaging. This multimodality imaging approach was successful to monitor transplanted ES survival and

proliferation in vivo and to assess the efficacy of suicide gene therapy as a backup safety measure (death switch) against teratoma formation.

IMAGING-GUIDED GENE THERAPY

The treatment of cancer using gene therapy and the development of methods capable of imaging vector delivery and subsequent gene expression have received

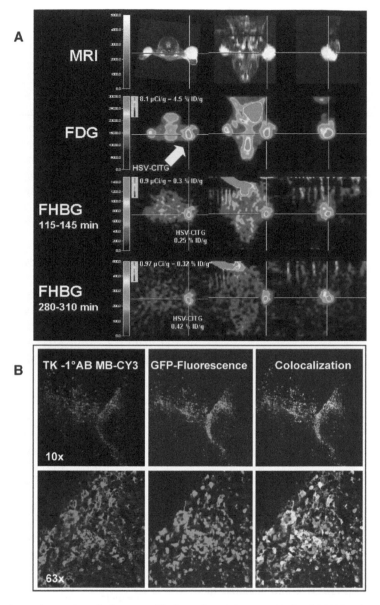

Figure 6 Multimodal imaging of gene-based therapy. (**A**) Experimental protocol for identification of viable target tissue and assessment of vector-mediated gene expression in vivo in a mouse model with three s.c. gliomas. Row 1, localization of tumors is displayed by MRI. Row 2, the viable target tissue is displayed by [^{18}F]FDG-PET; note the signs of necrosis in the lateral portion of the left-sided tumor (*arrow*). Rows 3 and 4, following vector application into the medial viable portion of the tumor (*arrow*), the tissue dose of vector-mediated gene expression is quantified by [^{18}F]FHBG-PET. Row 3, an image acquired early after tracer injection, which is used for coregistration; row 4, a late image with specific tracer accumulation in the tumor that is used for quantification. (**B**), good colocalization of the expression of both genetic components of the *tkgfp* fusion construct by thymidine kinase immunohistochemistry and GFP fluorescence microscopy in a tumor that had been injected with *tkgfp*-expressing HSV-1 amplicon vectors and imaged by [^{18}F]FHBG-PET. *Source*: From Ref. 215 (*See Color Insert*).

particular attention over the last few years. Several reporter gene systems have been developed for nuclear, optical, and MR imaging. Especially, HSV-1-*tk* has been studied extensively for gene therapy purposes because of the fact that it can serve as suicide gene and reporter gene simultaneously depending on the administered sub-strate (ganciclovir and FHBG or FIAU respiratory) (71,211,213). Furthermore, externally detectable labeled oligonucleotides hybridizing with the messenger RNA generated by the transferred gene has been proposed as a possibility to monitor successful gene delivery and serve as a means for therapy. Segura et al. (214) selected oligonucleotides capable of antisense binding to unique murine erythropoietin-mRNA sequences and labeled them with fluorescent and radioactive tags. After intravenous injection, these molecules preferentially accumulated in muscle cells previously transfected with the erythropoietin gene. Moreover, downregulation of newly expressed erythropoietin protein additionally confirmed the penetration and hybridizing properties of the selected labeled oligonucleotide and emphasized the possible therapeutic potential of the applied strategy.

Although gene therapy seems to be a highly promising approach for targeted treatment of tumors, its efficiency in clinical application has been disappointing and reported to be mostly due to the heterogeneity of tumor tissue and the limited transduction efficiency of current vectors. Our group (215) therefore aimed at the further characterization of these limiting factors by (*i*) identification of viable target tissue which might benefit from gene therapy; (*ii*) quantification of the transduction efficiency; and (*iii*) monitoring of therapeutic efficacy, all by means of molecular imaging technology. Employing a multimodal "imaging-guided" suicide gene therapy protocol we showed in a subcutaneous glioblastoma model a response rate of 68% of tumors in vivo transduced with an HSV-1 amplicon vector proportionally coexpressing *E. coli cd* as therapeutic gene and HSV-1-*tk* as combined PET marker and therapeutic gene. MRI was used for tumor localization. PET markers for endogenous gene expression, such as [^{18}F]FDG and [^{18}F]FLT for the expression of glucose and nucleoside transporters as well as for the expression of cellular hexokinase and thymidine kinase genes, respectively, and [^{11}C]MET for the expression of amino acid transporters were used to identify the actively proliferation tumor tissue. [^{18}F]FLT was also used to determine the gene therapy-induced inhibition of proliferative activity of the tumor. A marker for exogenously introduced therapeutic gene expression ([^{18}F]FHBG) could localize the transduced tissue dose of therapeutic gene expression. Most importantly, the primary transduction efficiency as measured by [^{18}F]FHBG-PET was correlated to the induced therapeutic effect as measured by [^{18}F]FLT-PET (Fig. 6).

Another problem of current gene therapy approaches is specific vector targeting. In an ideal gene therapy protocol, transgene expression must be strictly limited to the tissue of interest, mostly cancer cells, and spare surrounding normal cells. Numerous strategies have been developed to compensate this lack of specific targeting. By the use of inducible promoters or introduction of a suicide gene as "death switch" transgene expression can be controlled temporally and turned off when not desired any more. However, specific vector targeting can be realized by the use of tumor cell–specific promoters (122,123,216,217) or tumor cell–specific translation (218).

SUMMARY

With an increasing understanding of the molecular basis of disease, various new imaging targets have been identified allowing an early, sensitive, and disease-specific diagnosis and treatment monitoring. Molecular imaging allows the further exploration of the information coming out of genome sequencing to develop novel therapeutic drugs and imaging methods that are targeted at specific molecular features of the diseased tissue. Ultimately, molecular-genetic imaging will lead to improved understanding of disease kinetics with and without treatment intervention and hence, improved, more efficient and specific patient-tailored care.

ACKNOWLEDGMENTS

Our work is supported in part by the Deutsche Forschungsgemeinschaft (DFG-Ja98/1-2), Center for Molecular Medicine Cologne (CMMC-C5), 6th FW EU grants EMIL (LSHC-CT-2004-503569), DiMI (LSHB-CT-2005-512146), and CliniGene NoE (LSHB-CT-2006-018933).

REFERENCES

1. Blasberg RG, Gelovani-Tjuvajev J. In vivo molecular-genetic imaging. J Cell Biochem Suppl 2002; 39:172–183.
2. Weissleder R, Mahmood U. Molecular imaging. Radiology 2001; 219:316–333.
3. Massoud TF, Gambhir SS. Molecular imaging in living subjects: seeing fundamental biological processes in a new light. Genes Dev 2003; 17:545–580.
4. Townsend DW, Beyer T. A combined PET/CT scanner: the path to true image fusion. Br J Radiol 2002; 75 Spec No:S24–S30.
5. Beyer T, Townsend DW. Putting 'clear' into nuclear medicine: a decade of PET/CT development. Eur J Nucl Med Mol Imaging 2006; 33:857–861.
6. Pichler BJ, Judenhofer MS, Catana C, et al. Performance test of an LSO-APD detector in a 7-T MRI scanner for simultaneous PET/MRI. J Nucl Med 2006; 47:639–647.
7. Raylman RR, Majewski S, Lemieux SK, et al. Simultaneous MRI and PET imaging of a rat brain. Phys Med Biol 2006; 51:6371–6379.
8. Cizek J, Herholz K, Vollmar S, et al. Fast and robust registration of PET and MR images of human brain. Neuroimage 2004; 22:434–442.
9. Ray P, De A, Min JJ, et al. Imaging tri-fusion multimodality reporter gene expression in living subjects. Cancer Res 2004; 64:1323–1330.
10. Phelps ME. PET: the merging of biology and imaging into molecular imaging. J Nucl Med 2000; 41:661–681.
11. Acton PD, Kung HF. Small animal imaging with high-resolution single photon emission tomography. Nucl Med Biol 2003; 30:889–895.

12. Shah K, Jacobs A, Breakefield XO, et al. Molecular imaging of gene therapy for cancer. Gene Ther 2004; 11:1175–1187.

13. Contag CH, Bachmann MH. Advances in in vivo bioluminescence imaging of gene expression. Annu Rev Biomed Eng 2002; 4:235–260.

14. Blasberg RG, Tjuvajev JG. Molecular-genetic imaging: current and future perspectives. J Clin Invest 2003; 111:1620–1629.

15. Tavitian B. In vivo imaging with oligonucleotides for diagnosis and drug development. Gut 2003; 52(suppl 4): iv40–iv47.

16. Perez JM, Josephson L, Weissleder R. Use of magnetic nanoparticles as nanosensors to probe for molecular interactions. Chembiochem 2004; 5:261–264.

17. Perez JM, Josephson L, O'Loughlin T, et al. Magnetic relaxation switches capable of sensing molecular interactions. Nat Biotechnol 2002; 20:816–820.

18. Grimm J, Perez JM, Josephson L, et al. Novel nanosensors for rapid analysis of telomerase activity. Cancer Res 2004; 64:639–643.

19. Pickles MD, Lowry M, Manton DJ, et al. Role of dynamic contrast enhanced MRI in monitoring early response of locally advanced breast cancer to neoadjuvant chemotherapy. Breast Cancer Res Treat 2005; 91:1–10.

20. Turetschek K, Preda A, Floyd E, et al. MRI monitoring of tumor response following angiogenesis inhibition in an experimental human breast cancer model. Eur J Nucl Med Mol Imaging 2003; 30:448–455.

21. Checkley D, Tessier JJ, Kendrew J, et al. Use of dynamic contrast-enhanced MRI to evaluate acute treatment with ZD6474, a VEGF signalling inhibitor, in PC-3 prostate tumours. Br J Cancer 2003; 89:1889–1895.

22. Demetri GD, von Mehren M, Blanke CD, et al. Efficacy and safety of imatinib mesylate in advanced gastrointestinal stromal tumors. N Engl J Med 2002; 347:472–480.

23. Van den Abbeele AD, Badawi RD. Use of positron emission tomography in oncology and its potential role to assess response to imatinib mesylate therapy in gastrointestinal stromal tumors (GISTs). Eur J Cancer 2002; 38(suppl 5):S60–S65.

24. Pio BS, Park CK, Pietras R, et al. Usefulness of 3′-[F-18] fluoro-3′-deoxythymidine with positron emission tomography in predicting breast cancer response to therapy. Mol Imaging Biol 2006; 8:36–42.

25. Bogdanov A Jr., Weissleder R. The development of in vivo imaging systems to study gene expression. Trends Biotechnol 1998; 16:5–10.

26. Doubrovin M, Serganova I, Mayer-Kuckuk P, et al. Multimodality in vivo molecular-genetic imaging. Bioconjug Chem 2004; 15:1376–1388.

27. Jacobs A, Dubrovin M, Hewett J, et al. Functional coexpression of HSV-1 thymidine kinase and green fluorescent protein: implications for noninvasive imaging of transgene expression. Neoplasia 1999; 1:154–161.

28. Ponomarev V, Doubrovin M, Serganova I, et al. Cytoplasmically retargeted HSV1-tk/GFP reporter gene mutants for optimization of noninvasive molecular-genetic imaging. Neoplasia 2003; 5:245–254.

29. Ray P, Wu AM, Gambhir SS. Optical bioluminescence and positron emission tomography imaging of a novel fusion reporter gene in tumor xenografts of living mice. Cancer Res 2003; 63:1160–1165.

30. Wang Y, Yu YA, Shabahang S, et al. Renilla luciferase-Aequorea GFP (Ruc-GFP) fusion protein, a novel dual reporter for real-time imaging of gene expression in cell cultures and in live animals. Mol Genet Genomics 2002; 268:160–168.

31. Kummer C, Winkeler A, Dittmar C, et al. Multitracer positron emission tomographic imaging of exogenous gene expression mediated by a universal herpes simplex virus 1 amplicon vector. Mol Imaging 2007; 6:181–192.

32. Ray P, Tsien R, Gambhir SS. Construction and validation of improved triple fusion reporter gene vectors for molecular imaging of living subjects. Cancer Res 2007; 67:3085–3093.

33. Tjuvajev JG, Joshi A, Callegari J, et al. A general approach to the non-invasive imaging of transgenes using cis-linked herpes simplex virus thymidine kinase. Neoplasia 1999; 1:315–320.

34. Jacobs AH, Winkeler A, Hartung M, et al. Improved herpes simplex virus type 1 amplicon vectors for proportional coexpression of positron emission tomography marker and therapeutic genes. Hum Gene Ther 2003; 14:277–297.

35. Serganova I, Blasberg R. Reporter gene imaging: potential impact on therapy. Nucl Med Biol 2005; 32:763–780.

36. Serganova I, Doubrovin M, Vider J, et al. Molecular imaging of temporal dynamics and spatial heterogeneity of hypoxia-inducible factor-1 signal transduction activity in tumors in living mice. Cancer Res 2004; 64:6101–6108.

37. Gambhir SS, Barrio JR, Herschman HR, et al. Assays for noninvasive imaging of reporter gene expression. Nucl Med Biol 1999; 26:481–490.

38. Gambhir SS, Herschman HR, Cherry SR, et al. Imaging transgene expression with radionuclide imaging technologies. Neoplasia 2000; 2:118–138.

39. Herschman HR. PET reporter genes for noninvasive imaging of gene therapy, cell tracking and transgenic analysis. Crit Rev Oncol Hematol 2004; 51:191–204.

40. Serganova I, Ponomarev V, Blasberg R. Human reporter genes: potential use in clinical studies. Nucl Med Biol 2007; 34:791–807.

41. Saito Y, Price RW, Rottenberg DA, et al. Quantitative autoradiographic mapping of herpes simplex virus encephalitis with a radiolabeled antiviral drug. Science 1982; 217:1151–1153.

42. Tjuvajev JG, Stockhammer G, Desai R, et al. Imaging the expression of transfected genes in vivo. Cancer Res 1995; 55:6126–6132.

43. Tjuvajev JG, Finn R, Watanabe K, et al. Noninvasive imaging of herpes virus thymidine kinase gene transfer and expression: a potential method for monitoring clinical gene therapy. Cancer Res 1996; 56:4087–4095.

44. Gambhir SS, Bauer E, Black ME, et al. A mutant herpes simplex virus type 1 thymidine kinase reporter gene shows improved sensitivity for imaging reporter gene expression with positron emission tomography. Proc Natl Acad Sci U S A 2000; 97:2785–2790.

45. Tjuvajev JG, Doubrovin M, Akhurst T, et al. Comparison of radiolabeled nucleoside probes (FIAU, FHBG, and FHPG) for PET imaging of HSV1-tk gene expression. J Nucl Med 2002; 43:1072–1083.

46. Min JJ, Iyer M, Gambhir SS. Comparison of [18F]FHBG and [14C]FIAU for imaging of HSV1-tk reporter gene expression: adenoviral infection vs stable transfection. Eur J Nucl Med Mol Imaging 2003; 30:1547–1560.

47. Hackman T, Doubrovin M, Balatoni J, et al. Imaging expression of cytosine deaminase-herpes virus thymidine kinase fusion gene (CD/TK) expression with [124I]FIAU and PET. Mol Imaging 2002; 1:36–42.

48. Stegman LD, Rehemtulla A, Beattie B, et al. Noninvasive quantitation of cytosine deaminase transgene expression in human tumor xenografts with in vivo magnetic resonance spectroscopy. Proc Natl Acad Sci U S A 1999; 96:9821–9826.

49. Doubrovin M, Ponomarev V, Serganova I, et al. Development of a new reporter gene system–dsRed/xanthine phosphoribosyltransferase-xanthine for molecular imaging of processes behind the intact blood-brain barrier. Mol Imaging 2003; 2:93–112.

50. Conti PS, Alauddin MM, Fissekis JR, et al. Synthesis of 2′-fluoro-5-[11C]-methyl-1-beta-D-arabinofuranosyluracil ([11C]-FMAU): a potential nucleoside analog for in vivo study of cellular proliferation with PET. Nucl Med Biol 1995; 22:783–789.

51. Mangner TJ, Klecker RW, Anderson L, et al. Synthesis of 2′-deoxy-2′-[18F]fluoro-beta-D-arabinofuranosyl nucleosides, [18F]FAU, [18F]FMAU, [18F]FBAU and [18F]FIAU, as potential PET agents for imaging cellular proliferation. Synthesis of [18F]labelled FAU, FMAU, FBAU, FIAU. Nucl Med Biol 2003; 30:215–224.

52. Ponomarev V, Doubrovin M, Shavrin A, et al. A human-derived reporter gene for noninvasive imaging in humans: mitochondrial thymidine kinase type 2. J Nucl Med 2007; 48:819–826.

53. Neve KA, Cox BA, Henningsen RA, et al. Pivotal role for aspartate-80 in the regulation of dopamine D2 receptor affinity for drugs and inhibition of adenylyl cyclase. Mol Pharmacol 1991; 39:733–739.

54. Liang Q, Satyamurthy N, Barrio JR, et al. Noninvasive, quantitative imaging in living animals of a mutant dopamine D2 receptor reporter gene in which ligand binding is uncoupled from signal transduction. Gene Ther 2001; 8:1490–1498.

55. MacLaren DC, Gambhir SS, Satyamurthy N, et al. Repetitive, non-invasive imaging of the dopamine D2 receptor as a reporter gene in living animals. Gene Ther 1999; 6:785–791.

56. Ogawa O, Umegaki H, Ishiwata K, et al. In vivo imaging of adenovirus-mediated over-expression of dopamine D2 receptors in rat striatum by positron emission tomography. Neuroreport 2000; 11:743–748.

57. Umegaki H, Ishiwata K, Ogawa O, et al. In vivo assessment of adenoviral vector-mediated gene expression of dopamine D(2) receptors in the rat striatum by positron emission tomography. Synapse 2002; 43:195–200.

58. Sun X, Annala AJ, Yaghoubi SS, et al. Quantitative imaging of gene induction in living animals. Gene Ther 2001; 8:1572–1579.

59. Groot-Wassink T, Aboagye EO, Wang Y, et al. Noninvasive imaging of the transcriptional activities of human telomerase promoter fragments in mice. Cancer Res 2004; 64:4906–4911.

60. Zinn KR, Chaudhuri TR, Krasnykh VN, et al. Gamma camera dual imaging with a somatostatin receptor and thymidine kinase after gene transfer with a bicistronic adenovirus in mice. Radiology 2002; 223:417–425.

61. Zinn KR, Chaudhuri TR. The type 2 human somatostatin receptor as a platform for reporter gene imaging. Eur J Nucl Med Mol Imaging 2002; 29:388–399.

62. Boland A, Ricard M, Opolon P, et al. Adenovirus-mediated transfer of the thyroid sodium/iodide symporter gene into tumors for a targeted radiotherapy. Cancer Res 2000; 60:3484–3492.

63. Spitzweg C, Zhang S, Bergert ER, et al. Prostate-specific antigen (PSA) promoter-driven androgen-inducible expression of sodium iodide symporter in prostate cancer cell lines. Cancer Res 1999; 59:2136–2141.

64. Spitzweg C, Dietz AB, O'Connor MK, et al. In vivo sodium iodide symporter gene therapy of prostate cancer. Gene Ther 2001; 8:1524–1531.

65. Sieger S, Jiang S, Schonsiegel F, et al. Tumour-specific activation of the sodium/iodide symporter gene under control of the glucose transporter gene 1 promoter (GTI-1.3). Eur J Nucl Med Mol Imaging 2003; 30:748–756.

66. Huang M, Batra RK, Kogai T, et al. Ectopic expression of the thyroperoxidase gene augments radioiodide uptake and retention mediated by the sodium iodide symporter in non-small cell lung cancer. Cancer Gene Ther 2001; 8:612–618.

67. Axelrod J, Kopin IJ. The uptake, storage, release and metabolism of noradrenaline in sympathetic nerves. Prog Brain Res 1969; 31:21–32.

68. Moroz MA, Serganova I, Zanzonico P, et al. Imaging hNET reporter gene expression with 124I-MIBG. J Nucl Med 2007; 48:827–836.

69. Bonini C, Ferrari G, Verzeletti S, et al. HSV-TK gene transfer into donor lymphocytes for control of allogeneic graft-versus-leukemia. Science 1997; 276:1719–1724.

70. Verzeletti S, Bonini C, Marktel S, et al. Herpes simplex virus thymidine kinase gene transfer for controlled graft-versus-host disease and graft-versus-leukemia: clinical follow-up and improved new vectors. Hum Gene Ther 1998; 9:2243–2251.

71. Jacobs A, Voges J, Reszka R, et al. Positron-emission tomography of vector-mediated gene expression in gene therapy for gliomas. Lancet 2001; 358:727–729.

72. Penuelas I, Mazzolini G, Boan JF, et al. Positron emission tomography imaging of adenoviral-mediated transgene expression in liver cancer patients. Gastroenterology 2005; 128:1787–1795.

73. Ntziachristos V, Bremer C, Weissleder R. Fluorescence imaging with near-infrared light: new technological advances that enable in vivo molecular imaging. Eur Radiol 2003; 13:195–208.

74. Shah K, Tung CH, Chang CH, et al. In vivo imaging of HIV protease activity in amplicon vector-transduced gliomas. Cancer Res 2004; 64:273–278.

75. Bhaumik S, Lewis XZ, Gambhir SS. Optical imaging of Renilla luciferase, synthetic Renilla luciferase, and firefly luciferase reporter gene expression in living mice. J Biomed Opt 2004; 9:578–586.

76. Shah K, Tang Y, Breakefield X, et al. Real-time imaging of TRAIL-induced apoptosis of glioma tumors in vivo. Oncogene 2003; 22:6865–6872.

77. Shah K, Bureau E, Kim DE, et al. Glioma therapy and real-time imaging of neural precursor cell migration and tumor regression. Ann Neurol 2005; 57:34–41.

78. Kolb VA, Makeyev EV, Spirin AS. Co-translational folding of an eukaryotic multidomain protein in a prokaryotic translation system. J Biol Chem 2000; 275:16597–16601.

79. Thompson JF, Hayes LS, Lloyd DB. Modulation of firefly luciferase stability and impact on studies of gene regulation. Gene 1991; 103:171–177.

80. Day RN, Kawecki M, Berry D. Dual-function reporter protein for analysis of gene expression in living cells. Biotechniques 1998; 25:848–850, 852–854, 856.

81. Uhrbom L, Nerio E, Holland EC. Dissecting tumor maintenance requirements using bioluminescence imaging of cell proliferation in a mouse glioma model. Nat Med 2004; 10:1257–1260.

82. Vooijs M, Jonkers J, Lyons S, et al. Noninvasive imaging of spontaneous retinoblastoma pathway-dependent tumors in mice. Cancer Res 2002; 62:1862–1867.

83. Rehemtulla A, Hall DE, Stegman LD, et al. Molecular imaging of gene expression and efficacy following adenoviral-mediated brain tumor gene therapy. Mol Imaging 2002; 1:43–55.

84. Soling A, Theiss C, Jungmichel S, et al. A dual function fusion protein of Herpes simplex virus type 1 thymidine kinase and firefly luciferase for noninvasive in vivo imaging of gene therapy in malignant glioma. Genet Vaccines Ther 2004; 2:7.

85. Rehemtulla A, Stegman LD, Cardozo SJ, et al. Rapid and quantitative assessment of cancer treatment response using in vivo bioluminescence imaging. Neoplasia 2000; 2:491–495.

86. Tang Y, Shah K, Messerli SM, et al. In vivo tracking of neural progenitor cell migration to glioblastomas. Hum Gene Ther 2003; 14:1247–1254.

87. Michalet X, Pinaud FF, Bentolila LA, et al. Quantum dots for live cells, in vivo imaging, and diagnostics. Science 2005; 307:538–544.

88. Wu X, Liu H, Liu J, et al. Immunofluorescent labeling of cancer marker Her2 and other cellular targets with semiconductor quantum dots. Nat Biotechnol 2003; 21:41–46.

89. Gao X, Cui Y, Levenson RM, et al. In vivo cancer targeting and imaging with semiconductor quantum dots. Nat Biotechnol 2004; 22:969–976.

90. Akerman ME, Chan WC, Laakkonen P, et al. Nanocrystal targeting in vivo. Proc Natl Acad Sci U S A 2002; 99:12617–12621.

91. Gao X, Chung LW, Nie S. Quantum dots for in vivo molecular and cellular imaging. Methods Mol Biol 2007; 374:135–145.

92. Gilad AA, Winnard PT Jr., van Zijl PC, et al. Developing MR reporter genes: promises and pitfalls. NMR Biomed 2007; 20:275–290.

93. Blackstock AW, Lightfoot H, Case LD, et al. Tumor uptake and elimination of 2′,2′-difluoro-2′-deoxycytidine (gemcitabine) after deoxycytidine kinase gene transfer: correlation with in vivo tumor response. Clin Cancer Res 2001; 7:3263–3268.

94. Auricchio A, Zhou R, Wilson JM, et al. In vivo detection of gene expression in liver by 31P nuclear magnetic resonance spectroscopy employing creatine kinase as a marker gene. Proc Natl Acad Sci U S A 2001; 98:5205–5210.

95. Li Z, Qiao H, Lebherz C, et al. Creatine kinase, a magnetic resonance-detectable marker gene for quantification of liver-directed gene transfer. Hum Gene Ther 2005; 16:1429–1438.

96. Walter G, Barton ER, Sweeney HL. Noninvasive measurement of gene expression in skeletal muscle. Proc Natl Acad Sci U S A 2000; 97:5151–5155.

97. Weissleder R, Moore A, Mahmood U, et al. In vivo magnetic resonance imaging of transgene expression. Nat Med 2000; 6:351–355.

98. Moore A, Josephson L, Bhorade RM, et al. Human transferrin receptor gene as a marker gene for MR imaging. Radiology 2001; 221:244–250.

99. Funovics MA, Kapeller B, Hoeller C, et al. MR imaging of the her2/neu and 9.2.27 tumor antigens using immunospecific contrast agents. Magn Reson Imaging 2004; 22:843–850.

100. McAteer MA, Sibson NR, von Zur Muhlen C, et al. In vivo magnetic resonance imaging of acute brain inflammation using microparticles of iron oxide. Nat Med 2007; 13:1253–1258.

101. Sipkins DA, Gijbels K, Tropper FD, et al. ICAM-1 expression in autoimmune encephalitis visualized using magnetic resonance imaging. J Neuroimmunol 2000; 104:1–9.

102. Louie AY, Huber MM, Ahrens ET, et al. In vivo visualization of gene expression using magnetic resonance imaging. Nat Biotechnol 2000; 18:321–325.

103. Cui W, Otten P, Li Y, et al. Novel NMR approach to assessing gene transfection: 4-fluoro-2-nitrophenyl-beta-D-galactopyranoside as a prototype reporter molecule for beta-galactosidase. Magn Reson Med 2004; 51:616–620.

104. Kodibagkar VD, Yu J, Liu L, et al. Imaging beta-galactosidase activity using 19F chemical shift imaging of LacZ gene-reporter molecule 2-fluoro-4-nitrophenol-beta-D-galactopyranoside. Magn Reson Imaging 2006; 24:959–962.

105. Cui W LL, Adam A, Yu J, et al. Detection of beta-galactosidase activity in a human tumor xenograft by 1H MRI in vivo using S-Gal. Proc Int Soc Magn Reson Med 2005; 13:2593.

106. Koretsky A LY-J, Schorle H, Jaenisch R. Genetic control of MRI contrast by expression of the transferrin receptor. Proc Int Soc Magn Reson Med 1996; 4:69.

107. Weissleder R, Simonova M, Bogdanova A, et al. MR imaging and scintigraphy of gene expression through melanin induction. Radiology 1997; 204:425–429.

108. Alfke H, Stoppler H, Nocken F, et al. In vitro MR imaging of regulated gene expression. Radiology 2003; 228:488–492.

109. Cohen B, Dafni H, Meir G, et al. Ferritin as an endogenous MRI reporter for noninvasive imaging of gene expression in C6 glioma tumors. Neoplasia 2005; 7:109–117.

110. Genove G, DeMarco U, Xu H, et al. A new transgene reporter for in vivo magnetic resonance imaging. Nat Med 2005; 11:450–454.

111. Deans AE, Wadghiri YZ, Bernas LM, et al. Cellular MRI contrast via coexpression of transferrin receptor and ferritin. Magn Reson Med 2006; 56:51–59.

112. Hynes NE, Kennedy N, Rahmsdorf U, et al. Hormone-responsive expression of an endogenous proviral gene of mouse mammary tumor virus after molecular cloning and gene transfer into cultured cells. Proc Natl Acad Sci U S A 1981; 78:2038–2042.

113. Mayo KE, Warren R, Palmiter RD. The mouse metallothionein-I gene is transcriptionally regulated by cadmium following transfection into human or mouse cells. Cell 1982; 29:99–108.

114. Wurm FM, Gwinn KA, Kingston RE. Inducible overproduction of the mouse c-myc protein in mammalian cells. Proc Natl Acad Sci U S A 1986; 83:5414–5418.

115. Gossen M, Bujard H. Tight control of gene expression in mammalian cells by tetracycline-responsive promoters. Proc Natl Acad Sci U S A 1992; 89:5547–5551.

116. Christopherson KS, Mark MR, Bajaj V, et al. Ecdysteroid-dependent regulation of genes in mammalian cells by a Drosophila ecdysone receptor and chimeric transactivators. Proc Natl Acad Sci U S A 1992; 89:6314–6318.

117. No D, Yao TP, Evans RM. Ecdysone-inducible gene expression in mammalian cells and transgenic mice. Proc Natl Acad Sci U S A 1996; 93:3346–3351.

118. Wang Y, O'Malley BW Jr., Tsai SY, O'Malley BW. A regulatory system for use in gene transfer. Proc Natl Acad Sci U S A 1994; 91:8180–8184.

119. Delort JP, Capecchi MR. TAXI/UAS: a molecular switch to control expression of genes in vivo. Hum Gene Ther 1996; 7:809–820.

120. Yu YA, Szalay AA. A Renilla luciferase-Aequorea GFP (ruc-gfp) fusion gene construct permits real-time detection of promoter activation by exogenously administered mifepristone in vivo. Mol Genet Genomics 2002; 268:169–178.

121. Winkeler A, Sena-Esteves M, Paulis LE, et al. Switching on the lights for gene therapy. PLoS ONE 2007; 2:e528.

122. Iyer M, Wu L, Carey M, et al. Two-step transcriptional amplification as a method for imaging reporter gene expression using weak promoters. Proc Natl Acad Sci U S A 2001; 98:14595–14600.

123. Qiao J, Doubrovin M, Sauter BV, et al. Tumor-specific transcriptional targeting of suicide gene therapy. Gene Ther 2002; 9:168–175.

124. Wang W, El-Deiry WS. Bioluminescent molecular imaging of endogenous and exogenous p53-mediated transcription in vitro and in vivo using an HCT116 human colon carcinoma xenograft model. Cancer Biol Ther 2003; 2:196–202.

125. Doubrovin M, Ponomarev V, Beresten T, et al. Imaging transcriptional regulation of p53-dependent genes with positron emission tomography in vivo. Proc Natl Acad Sci U S A 2001; 98:9300–9305.

126. Ponomarev V, Doubrovin M, Lyddane C, et al. Imaging TCR-dependent NFAT-mediated T-cell activation with positron emission tomography in vivo. Neoplasia 2001; 3:480–488.

127. Gross S, Piwnica-Worms D. Real-time imaging of ligand-induced IKK activation in intact cells and in living mice. Nat Methods 2005; 2:607–614.

128. Ting AY, Kain KH, Klemke RL, et al. Genetically encoded fluorescent reporters of protein tyrosine kinase activities in living cells. Proc Natl Acad Sci U S A 2001; 98:15003–15008.

129. Zhang J, Ma Y, Taylor SS, et al. Genetically encoded reporters of protein kinase A activity reveal impact of substrate tethering. Proc Natl Acad Sci U S A 2001; 98:14997–15002.

130. Zhang GJ, Safran M, Wei W, et al. Bioluminescent imaging of Cdk2 inhibition in vivo. Nat Med 2004; 10:643–648.

131. Zhang L, Lee KC, Bhojani MS, et al. Molecular imaging of Akt kinase activity. Nat Med 2007; 13:1114–1119.

132. Carlsen H, Moskaug JO, Fromm SH, et al. In vivo imaging of NF-kappa B activity. J Immunol 2002; 168:1441–1446.

133. Magness ST, Jijon H, Van Houten Fisher N, et al. In vivo pattern of lipopolysaccharide and anti-CD3-induced NF-kappa B activation using a novel gene-targeted enhanced GFP reporter gene mouse. J Immunol 2004; 173:1561–1570.

134. Zhang W, Purchio AF, Chen K, et al. A transgenic mouse model with a luciferase reporter for studying in vivo transcriptional regulation of the human CYP3A4 gene. Drug Metab Dispos 2003; 31:1054–1064.

135. Lin AH, Luo J, Mondshein LH, et al. Global analysis of Smad2/3-dependent TGF-beta signaling in living mice reveals prominent tissue-specific responses to injury. J Immunol 2005; 175:547–554.

136. Zhang N, Ahsan MH, Purchio AF, et al. Serum amyloid A-luciferase transgenic mice: response to sepsis, acute arthritis, and contact hypersensitivity and the effects of proteasome inhibition. J Immunol 2005; 174:8125–8134.

137. Ohtani N, Imamura Y, Yamakoshi K, et al. Visualizing the dynamics of p21(Waf1/Cip1) cyclin-dependent kinase inhibitor expression in living animals. Proc Natl Acad Sci U S A 2007; 104:15034–15039.

138. Momota H, Holland EC. Bioluminescence technology for imaging cell proliferation. Curr Opin Biotechnol 2005; 16:681–686.

139. Green LA, Yap CS, Nguyen K, et al. Indirect monitoring of endogenous gene expression by positron emission tomography (PET) imaging of reporter gene expression in transgenic mice. Mol Imaging Biol 2002; 4:71–81.

140. Lee SY, Wang Z, Lin CK, et al. Regulation of intestine-specific spatiotemporal expression by the rat lactase promoter. J Biol Chem 2002; 277:13099–13105.

141. Zhang J, Tan X, Contag CH, et al. Dissection of promoter control modules that direct Bmp4 expression in the epithelium-derived components of hair follicles. Biochem Biophys Res Commun 2002; 293:1412–1419.

142. Zhang W, Feng JQ, Harris SE, et al. Rapid in vivo functional analysis of transgenes in mice using whole body imaging of luciferase expression. Transgenic Res 2001; 10:423–434.

143. Gross ME, Shazer RL, Agus DB. Targeting the HER-kinase axis in cancer. Semin Oncol 2004; 31:9–20.

144. Cai W, Niu G, Chen X. Multimodality imaging of the HER-kinase axis in cancer. Eur J Nucl Med Mol Imaging 2008; 35(1):186–208 [Epub 2007 September 11].

145. Niu G, Cai W, Chen X. Molecular imaging of human epidermal growth factor receptor 2 (HER-2) expression. Front Biosci 2008; 13:790–805.

146. Cai W, Chen K, He L, et al. Quantitative PET of EGFR expression in xenograft-bearing mice using 64Cu-labeled cetuximab, a chimeric anti-EGFR monoclonal antibody. Eur J Nucl Med Mol Imaging 2007; 34:850–858.

147. Sampath L, Kwon S, Ke S, et al. Dual-labeled trastuzumab-based imaging agent for the detection of human epidermal growth factor receptor 2 overexpression in breast cancer. J Nucl Med 2007; 48:1501–1510.

148. Villalobos V, Naik S, Piwnica-Worms D. Current state of imaging protein-protein interactions in vivo with genetically encoded reporters. Annu Rev Biomed Eng 2007; 9:321–349.

149. Ozawa T, Kaihara A, Sato M, et al. Split luciferase as an optical probe for detecting protein-protein interactions in mammalian cells based on protein splicing. Anal Chem 2001; 73:2516–2521.

150. Paulmurugan R, Gambhir SS. Monitoring protein-protein interactions using split synthetic renilla luciferase protein-fragment-assisted complementation. Anal Chem 2003; 75:1584–1589.

151. Luker GD, Sharma V, Pica CM, et al. Noninvasive imaging of protein-protein interactions in living animals. Proc Natl Acad Sci U S A 2002; 99:6961–6966.

152. Ray P, Pimenta H, Paulmurugan R, et al. Noninvasive quantitative imaging of protein-protein interactions in living subjects. Proc Natl Acad Sci U S A 2002; 99:3105–3110.

153. De A, Gambhir SS. Noninvasive imaging of protein-protein interactions from live cells and living subjects using bioluminescence resonance energy transfer. FASEB J 2005; 19:2017–2019.

154. Thornberry NA, Lazebnik Y. Caspases: enemies within. Science 1998; 281:1312–1316.

155. Schmitt CA, Lowe SW. Apoptosis and therapy. J Pathol 1999; 187:127–137.

156. Laxman B, Hall DE, Bhojani MS, et al. Noninvasive real-time imaging of apoptosis. Proc Natl Acad Sci U S A 2002; 99:16551–16555.

157. Messerli SM, Prabhakar S, Tang Y, et al. A novel method for imaging apoptosis using a caspase-1 near-infrared fluorescent probe. Neoplasia 2004; 6:95–105.

158. Blankenberg FG, Katsikis PD, Tait JF, et al. In vivo detection and imaging of phosphatidylserine expression during programmed cell death. Proc Natl Acad Sci U S A 1998; 95:6349–6354.

159. Mandl SJ, Mari C, Edinger M, et al. Multi-modality imaging identifies key times for annexin V imaging as an early predictor of therapeutic outcome. Mol Imaging 2004; 3:1–8.

160. Zhao M, Beauregard DA, Loizou L, et al. Non-invasive detection of apoptosis using magnetic resonance imaging and a targeted contrast agent. Nat Med 2001; 7:1241–1244.

161. Petrovsky A, Schellenberger E, Josephson L, et al. Near-infrared fluorescent imaging of tumor apoptosis. Cancer Res 2003; 63:1936–1942.

162. Schellenberger EA, Bogdanov A Jr., Petrovsky A, et al. Optical imaging of apoptosis as a biomarker of tumor response to chemotherapy. Neoplasia 2003; 5:187–192.

163. Chang J, Ormerod M, Powles TJ, et al. Apoptosis and proliferation as predictors of chemotherapy response in patients with breast carcinoma. Cancer 2000; 89:2145–2152.

164. Weissleder R, Tung CH, Mahmood U, et al. In vivo imaging of tumors with protease-activated near-infrared fluorescent probes. Nat Biotechnol 1999; 17:375–378.

165. Tung CH, Mahmood U, Bredow S, et al. In vivo imaging of proteolytic enzyme activity using a novel molecular reporter. Cancer Res 2000; 60:4953–4958.

166. Gondi CS, Lakka SS, Yanamandra N, et al. Adenovirus-mediated expression of antisense urokinase plasminogen activator receptor and antisense cathepsin B inhibits tumor growth, invasion, and angiogenesis in gliomas. Cancer Res 2004; 64:4069–4077.

167. Wunder A, Tung CH, Muller-Ladner U, et al. In vivo imaging of protease activity in arthritis: a novel approach for monitoring treatment response. Arthritis Rheum 2004; 50:2459–2465.

168. Bremer C, Bredow S, Mahmood U, et al. Optical imaging of matrix metalloproteinase-2 activity in tumors: feasibility study in a mouse model. Radiology 2001; 221:523–529.

169. Himmelreich U, Aime S, Hieronymus T, et al. A responsive MRI contrast agent to monitor functional cell status. Neuroimage 2006; 32:1142–1149.

170. Law B, Curino A, Bugge TH, et al. Design, synthesis, and characterization of urokinase plasminogen-activator-sensitive near-infrared reporter. Chem Biol 2004; 11:99–106.

171. Luker GD, Pica CM, Song J, et al. Imaging 26S proteasome activity and inhibition in living mice. Nat Med 2003; 9:969–973.

172. Gross S, Piwnica-Worms D. Monitoring proteasome activity in cellulo and in living animals by bioluminescent imaging: technical considerations for design and use of genetically encoded reporters. Methods Enzymol 2005; 399:512–530.

173. Sipkins DA, Cheresh DA, Kazemi MR, et al. Detection of tumor angiogenesis in vivo by alphaVbeta3-targeted magnetic resonance imaging. Nat Med 1998; 4:623–626.

174. Winter PM, Caruthers SD, Kassner A, et al. Molecular imaging of angiogenesis in nascent Vx-2 rabbit tumors using a novel alpha(nu)beta3-targeted nanoparticle and 1.5 tesla magnetic resonance imaging. Cancer Res 2003; 63:5838–5843.

175. Lanza GM, Winter PM, Caruthers SD, et al. Magnetic resonance molecular imaging with nanoparticles. J Nucl Cardiol 2004; 11:733–743.

176. Haubner R, Wester HJ, Weber WA, et al. Noninvasive imaging of alpha(v)beta3 integrin expression using 18F-labeled RGD-containing glycopeptide and positron emission tomography. Cancer Res 2001; 61:1781–1785.

177. Haubner R, Weber WA, Beer AJ, et al. Noninvasive visualization of the activated alphavbeta3 integrin in cancer patients by positron emission tomography and [18F] Galacto-RGD. PLoS Med 2005; 2:e70.

178. Kang HW, Josephson L, Petrovsky A, et al. Magnetic resonance imaging of inducible E-selectin expression in human endothelial cell culture. Bioconjug Chem 2002; 13:122–127.

179. Kang HW, Weissleder R, Bogdanov A Jr. Targeting of MPEG-protected polyamino acid carrier to human E-selectin in vitro. Amino Acids 2002; 23:301–308.

180. Neri D, Carnemolla B, Nissim A, et al. Targeting by affinity-matured recombinant antibody fragments of an angiogenesis associated fibronectin isoform. Nat Biotechnol 1997; 15:1271–1275.

181. Brower V. Tumor angiogenesis—new drugs on the block. Nat Biotechnol 1999; 17:963–968.

182. Pearson DA, Lister J, McBride WJ, et al. Thrombus imaging using technetium-99m-labeled high-potency GPIIb/IIIa receptor antagonists. Chemistry and initial biological studies. J Med Chem 1996; 39:1372–1382.

183. Bredow S, Lewin M, Hofmann B, et al. Imaging of tumour neovasculature by targeting the TGF-beta binding receptor endoglin. Eur J Cancer 2000; 36:675–681.

184. Anderson SA, Glod J, Arbab AS, et al. Noninvasive MR imaging of magnetically labeled stem cells to directly identify neovasculature in a glioma model. Blood 2005; 105:420–425.

185. Ferrari N, Glod J, Lee J, et al. Bone marrow-derived, endothelial progenitor-like cells as angiogenesis-selective gene-targeting vectors. Gene Ther 2003; 10:647–656.

186. Cai W, Chen X. Multimodality imaging of vascular endothelial growth factor and vascular endothelial growth factor receptor expression. Front Biosci 2007; 12:4267–4279.

187. Dove A. Cell-based therapies go live. Nat Biotechnol 2002; 20:339–343.

188. Gross S, Moss BL, Piwnica-Worms D. Veni, vidi, vici: in vivo molecular imaging of immune response. Immunity 2007; 27:533–538.

189. Koike C, Oku N, Watanabe M, et al. Real-time PET analysis of metastatic tumor cell trafficking in vivo and its relation to adhesion properties. Biochim Biophys Acta 1995; 1238:99–106.

190. Adonai N, Nguyen KN, Walsh J, et al. Ex vivo cell labeling with 64Cu-pyruvaldehyde-bis(N4-methylthiosemicarbazone) for imaging cell trafficking in mice with positron-emission tomography. Proc Natl Acad Sci U S A 2002; 99:3030–3035.

191. Hardy J, Edinger M, Bachmann MH, et al. Bioluminescence imaging of lymphocyte trafficking in vivo. Exp Hematol 2001; 29:1353–1360.

192. Kircher MF, Allport JR, Graves EE, et al. In vivo high resolution three-dimensional imaging of antigen-specific cytotoxic T-lymphocyte trafficking to tumors. Cancer Res 2003; 63:6838–6846.

193. Papierniak CK, Bourey RE, Kretschmer RR, et al. Technetium-99m labeling of human monocytes for chemotactic studies. J Nucl Med 1976; 17:988–992.

194. Gobuty AH, Robinson RG, Barth RF. Organ distribution of 99mTc- and 51Cr-labeled autologous peripheral blood lymphocytes in rabbits. J Nucl Med 1977; 18:141–146.

195. Koehne G, Doubrovin M, Doubrovina E, et al. Serial in vivo imaging of the targeted migration of human HSV-TK-transduced antigen-specific lymphocytes. Nat Biotechnol 2003; 21:405–413.

196. Dubey P, Su H, Adonai N, et al. Quantitative imaging of the T cell antitumor response by positron-emission tomography. Proc Natl Acad Sci U S A 2003; 100:1232–1237.

197. Kim YJ, Dubey P, Ray P, et al. Multimodality imaging of lymphocytic migration using lentiviral-based transduction of a tri-fusion reporter gene. Mol Imaging Biol 2004; 6:331–340.

198. Garbossa D, Fontanella M, Fronda C, et al. New strategies for repairing the injured spinal cord: the role of stem cells. Neurol Res 2006; 28:500–504.

199. Schouten JW, Fulp CT, Royo NC, et al. A review and rationale for the use of cellular transplantation as a therapeutic strategy for traumatic brain injury. J Neurotrauma 2004; 21:1501–1538.

200. Karussis D, Kassis I. Use of stem cells for the treatment of multiple sclerosis. Expert Rev Neurother 2007; 7: 1189–1201.

201. Parish CL, Arenas E. Stem-cell-based strategies for the treatment of Parkinson's disease. Neurodegener Dis 2007; 4:339–347.

202. Walczak P, Bulte JW. The role of noninvasive cellular imaging in developing cell-based therapies for neurodegenerative disorders. Neurodegener Dis 2007; 4:306–313.

203. Aboody KS, Brown A, Rainov NG, et al. Neural stem cells display extensive tropism for pathology in adult brain: evidence from intracranial gliomas. Proc Natl Acad Sci U S A 2000; 97:12846–12851.

204. Xu F, Zhu JH. Stem cells tropism for malignant gliomas. Neurosci Bull 2007; 23:363–369.

205. Hoehn M, Kustermann E, Blunk J, et al. Monitoring of implanted stem cell migration in vivo: a highly resolved in vivo magnetic resonance imaging investigation of experimental stroke in rat. Proc Natl Acad Sci U S A 2002; 99:16267–16272.

206. Modo M, Mellodew K, Cash D, et al. Mapping transplanted stem cell migration after a stroke: a serial, in vivo magnetic resonance imaging study. Neuroimage 2004; 21:311–317.

207. Kim DE, Schellingerhout D, Ishii K, et al. Imaging of stem cell recruitment to ischemic infarcts in a murine model. Stroke 2004; 35:952–957.

208. Sheikh AY, Lin SA, Cao F, et al. Molecular imaging of bone marrow mononuclear cell homing and engraftment in ischemic myocardium. Stem Cells 2007; 25:2677–2684.

209. Hung SC, Deng WP, Yang WK, et al. Mesenchymal stem cell targeting of microscopic tumors and tumor stroma development monitored by noninvasive in vivo positron emission tomography imaging. Clin Cancer Res 2005; 11:7749–7756.

210. Zhang Z, Jiang Q, Jiang F, et al. In vivo magnetic resonance imaging tracks adult neural progenitor cell targeting of brain tumor. Neuroimage 2004; 23:281–287.

211. Miletic H, Fischer Y, Litwak S, et al. Bystander Killing of Malignant Glioma by Bone Marrow-derived Tumor-Infiltrating Progenitor Cells Expressing a Suicide Gene. Mol Ther 2007; 15:1373–1381.

212. Cao F, Drukker M, Lin S, et al. Molecular imaging of embryonic stem cell misbehavior and suicide gene ablation. Cloning Stem Cells 2007; 9:107–117.

213. Rueger MAAM. (18F)FLT-PET for non-invasive monitoring of experimental gliomas during antiproliferative therapy with suicide genes in vivo 2007 (in preparation) 2007.

214. Segura J, Fillat C, Andreu D, et al. Monitoring gene therapy by external imaging of mRNA: pilot study on murine erythropoietin. Ther Drug Monit 2007; 29:612–618.

215. Jacobs AH, Rueger MA, Winkeler A, et al. Imaging-guided gene therapy of experimental gliomas. Cancer Res 2007; 67:1706–1715.

216. Yan C, Wen-Chao L, Hong-Yan Q, et al. A new targeting approach for breast cancer gene therapy using the human fatty acid synthase promoter. Acta Oncol 2007; 46: 773–781.

217. Maatta AM, Korja S, Venhoranta H, et al. Transcriptional targeting of virus-mediated gene transfer by the human hexokinase II promoter. Int J Mol Med 2006; 18:901–908.

218. Mathis JM, Williams BJ, Sibley DA, et al. Cancer-specific targeting of an adenovirus-delivered herpes simplex virus thymidine kinase suicide gene using translational control. J Gene Med 2006; 8:1105–1120.

29

Imaging Angiogenesis

AMBROS J. BEER and MARKUS SCHWAIGER

Department of Nuclear Medicine, Technische Universität München, Munich, Germany

INTRODUCTION

Angiogenesis is a fundamental process involved in a variety of physiological as well as pathological conditions. Physiologically, it is required for development, wound repair, reproduction, and response to ischemia. Pathologically, it is associated with disease conditions like arthritis, psoriasis, retinopathies, and cancer (1). Since Folkman in 1971 first articulated the concept that the growth of solid tumors remains restricted to 2 to 3 mm in diameter until the onset of angiogenesis, subsequent investigations have identified more than 20 angiogenic growth factors, their receptors, and signal transduction pathways. Moreover, endogenous angiogenesis inhibitors have been discovered and the cellular and molecular characterization of the angiogenic phenotype in human cancers has been achieved (2–4). As angiogenesis-dependent diseases afflict as many as 500 million patients in Western nations each year, most of them with oncological diseases, the concept of antiangiogenetic therapy has evolved over the last years as a therapeutic strategy in clinical oncology aimed at stopping cancer progression by suppressing the tumor blood supply (1). Recently, encouraging results have been achieved with the vascular endothelial growth factor (VEGF) antibody Avastin® in combination with standard cytotoxic chemotherapy in metastasized colorectal cancer, breast cancer, and non–small cell lung cancer (5,6). However, the results

of the first clinical trials using angiogenesis inhibitors were disappointing, although most of the applied substances were effective in preclinical trials (7,8). In part, this might be due to the difficulties in designing clinical trials for antiangiogenic drugs, which, unlike traditional chemotherapeutic agents, are not cytotoxic. This lack of cytotoxicity may be beneficial to the patient, but it poses challenges for selecting the most effective dose because with many of these new antiangiogenetic agents, a "dose limiting toxicity" is not reached. Therefore, the concept of looking for the maximum tolerated dose is not appropriate for most antiangiogenic drugs. But there is also the problem of defining tumor response with these new agents. Clinical trials with conventional cytotoxic chemotherapeutic agents mainly use morphological imaging to provide indices of therapeutic response, mostly computed tomography (CT) or magnetic resonance imaging (MRI). Simple linear measurements are mainly used to estimate changes in tumor mass in response to the investigational therapy as compared with a baseline measure. Through standardization of these measurements by introducing the RECIST (response evaluation criteria in solid tumors) criteria in the year 2000, considerable progress has been achieved (9). However, as antiangiogenetic agents lead to a stop of tumor progression rather than to tumor shrinkage, the approach of measuring tumor response by a reduction of tumor size is not applicable and might take months or years to assess. Therefore, there is great need to establish reliable biomarkers of early tumor response to noncytotoxic drugs, which predict subsequent clinical response (10). Such biomarkers would not only facilitate clinical trials of new drugs but could also be used to aid in the selection of optimal treatment for individual patients ("personalized medicine"). There is therefore great interest in imaging techniques that can be used as such a biomarker and which provide an early indicator of effectiveness at a functional or molecular level. Because antiangiogenic therapies are designed to affect the abnormal blood vessels found in tumors, changes in hemodynamic parameters such as blood flow, blood volume, or vessel permeability may be promising biomarkers for response evaluation. Current clinical trials employ various imaging techniques for this purpose, including dynamic contrast-enhanced MRI (DCE MRI), positron emission tomography (PET) (especially with [^{15}O]water), dynamic contrast-enhanced CT, and ultrasound (US) (11). However, in the future, markers at the molecular level might be used as well for response evaluation of antiangiogenic agents. PET tracers for assessment of glucose metabolism or proliferation like [^{18}F]FDG and [^{18}F]FLT have already shown promising results in clinical studies for response assessment of cytotoxic chemotherapies (12,13). In the same way, targeting specific molecular markers of angiogenesis might be used for response assessment of antiangiogenic therapies, like the VEGF pathway or cell surface markers like the integrin $\alpha_v\beta_3$.

In this chapter, the various methods for measurement of hemodynamic parameters of angiogenesis, such as blood flow, blood volume, or vascular permeability, will be discussed, with a focus on those technologies that are already in clinical use. Moreover, the different targets for assessment of angiogenesis at a molecular level as well as the approaches for imaging these targets will be presented.

BACKGROUND ON ANGIOGENESIS

Biology of Angiogenesis

The processes of angiogenesis are complex and only a short summary on this topic can be presented here. For more detailed information, see also the reviews in references (14) and (15).

All solid tumors start as small populations of transformed cells whose growth is controlled by a balance between apoptosis and tumor cell proliferation. Because early tumors lack a blood supply of their own, tumor growth is limited by the lack of access to circulating oxygen, growth factors, and nutrients. Tumors grow toward preexisting nearby blood vessels to overcome these limitations (16). Tumor cells may then infiltrate these blood vessels regionally and form vessels consisting of normal endothelial cells mixed with infiltrative tumor cells, called a "mosaic vessel." However, as this process mainly serves the tumor periphery, further tumor expansion leads to increasing central hypoxia. This initial phase of limited tumor growth may persist for months or even years.

The next phase of rapid phase of tumor growth occurs when the tumor switches to its angiogenic phenotype, a phenomenon also called the "angiogenic switch." Tumors produce a multitude of peptide angiogenic factors in response to tumor hypoxia, like the VEGF, the acidic and basic fibroblast growth factors (aFGF, bFGF), and platelet-derived endothelial cell growth factor (PD-ECGF) (17). The angiogenic switch occurs when the tumors produce these angiogenic factors in excess of local angiogenesis inhibitors like thrombospondin-1, endostatin, angiostatin, or antiangiogenic antithrombin III. Angiogenic growth factors diffuse toward nearby preexisting blood vessels and bind to receptors located on endothelial cells like receptors to VEGF (VEGFR-1/Flt-1, VEGFR-2/KDR/Flk-1, VEGFR-3/KDR, Flt-1, VEGF-R2, VEGF-R3/Flt-4, VEGF-R4/neuropilin-1) (18). The binding of ligands to their receptors leads to receptor dimerization and activation of various signal transduction pathways, like phosphorylation of tyrosine kinases, protein kinases, and mitogen-activated protein (MAP) kinases and consequently to activation of endothelial cells (19–25). Once endothelial cells become activated, the original vessels undergo characteristic morphological changes, like enlargement of the diameter and cross-sectional area. Thus, "mother vessels" are formed, which are characterized by basement membrane degradation, a thinned endothelial cell lining, increased endothelial number, decreased pericyte numbers, and pericyte detachment (26). These vessels not only have an enlarged diameter, they are also hyperpermeable compared with normal microvessel (27). This explains some of the earliest histopathological features of angiogenesis, which are microvascular dilatation, hyperpermeability, edema, and extravascular fibrin deposition. However, this is a transient process, lasting only a few days. In the next step, mother vessels undergo at least four divergent morphological transformations (28–31). They may retain their large diameter, and evolve into medium-sized arteries and veins by acquiring a smooth muscle and internal elastica. This process takes from a few days to several months. Alternatively, the endothelium of a mother vessel may form smaller separate well-differentiated vessel channels by projecting cytoplasmic structures into the lumen, which form translumenal bridges. This takes from several days to three weeks. A third process is called intussusception and involves focal invagination of connective tissue pillars from within the mother vessel, which takes from several days to several weeks. Finally, mother vessels may form daughter vessels by endothelial cell sprouting, which requires the focal dissolution of the basement membrane surrounding mother vessels (32). This is achieved by a number of proteolytic enzymes, including matrix metalloproteinases (MMPs) and plasminogen activator, which enable endothelial cells to exit the vessel ablumenally. Activated angiogenic endothelial cells proliferate rapidly and migrate into the extracellular matrix toward the angiogenic stimulus (33–35). They also express adhesion molecules known such as the $\alpha_v\beta_3$ and $\alpha_v\beta_5$ integrin that facilitate migration and vascular survival (36–39). At the sprouting tips of growing vessels, endothelial cells secrete MMPs that facilitate degradation of the extracellular matrix and cell invasion (40,41). In order to allow for the supply of nutrients and oxygen to the tumor via the circulation, a lumen within an endothelial cell tubule has to be formed. This requires interactions between the extracellular matrix and cell-associated surface proteins, among them are galectin-2, PECAM-1, and VE-cadherin (42,43). The formation of a vascular lumen also involves the comigration of three of endothelial cell populations as a single cord-like structure. An internal endothelial population is surrounded by a second cell population with multiple intracellular vacuoles. The internal population undergoes rapid apoptosis within 12 hours of formation and the vacuoles of the surrounding population fuse with the plasma membrane. This results in extensive remodeling of the center of a solid vascular cord into a lumen. The third endothelial population intersperses with the formed endothelial outer layer and thus expands the lumenal circumference. Finally, the newly formed vessels are stabilized through the recruitment of smooth muscle cells and pericytes. In this process, the angiopoietin family plays a major role, like angiopoietin-1 (Ang-1), which binds to the Tie-2 receptor on angiogenic endothelium (37). This consequently leads to promotion of vascular tubule formation and of endothelial survival and to secretion of PDGF and other chemokines that recruit smooth muscle cells and pericytes to the new vessel.

Antiangiogenic Therapeutic Strategies

Antiangiogenic drugs may be divided into three subgroups according to their main acting mechanism: first, true angiogenesis inhibitors; second, vascular targeting agents; and third, nonselective antiangiogenic agents, which include many conventional chemotherapeutic agents. True angiogenesis inhibitors do not destroy preexisting blood vessels within a tumor, but only stop neovascular formation. The expected effect of true angiogenesis inhibitors is thus disease stabilization rather than tumor regression.

Vascular targeting agents also destroy the preexisting tumor vasculature. Nonselective antiangiogenic agents show cytotoxic, antiproliferative, or anti-invasive effects on multiple cell types, including angiogenic endothelial cells. Several conventional cytotoxic chemotherapeutic drugs have shown antiangiogenic effects when administered at low concentrations. A multitude of antiangiogenic drugs targeting different steps in the angiogenic cascade have been or are currently studied in clinical trials, thus we can only present a short overview of the most important substances. For a detailed review see also references (44) and (45).

Growth Factor Antagonists and Endothelial Cell Signal Transduction Inhibitors

Several drugs, such as suramin, interferon-α, and angiozyme, suppress production of angiogenic growth factors. Monoclonal antibodies and soluble receptors have been developed against VEGF. The most promising agent in this group is Avastin (bevacizumab), which showed encouraging results in metastasized colorectal cancer, breast cancer, and non–small cell lung cancer (5,6). Small molecule drugs have been developed to inhibit the endothelial signal transduction caused by specific growth factor–receptor binding, most of them tyrosine kinase inhibitors. Both selective (against VEGF or PDGF) and nonselective agents are in clinical trial. Two of these nonselective small molecule tyrosine kinase inhibitors, SU11248 (Sutent®) and BAY-43-9006 (Nexavar®) have shown antitumor activity in clinical trials in patient with gastrointestinal tumor (GIST) refractory to Glivec® and in metastasized renal cell cancer. Consequently, these agents have recently been approved as monotherapy for kidney cancer (5,46).

MMP Inhibitors

Inhibition of MMPs activity interferes with both endothelial and tumor cell invasion into the extracellular matrix at primary and metastatic sites. The family of MMPs consists of at least 20 distinct enzymes, of which the gelatinases MMP-2 and MMP-9 are closely associated with angiogenesis. Selective and nonselective MMP inhibitors are in advanced clinical trial. Examples of these agents include marimastat, AG3340 (prinomastat), Col-3, neovastat, and BMS275291. Marimastat demonstrated a survival benefit in patients with metastatic gastric cancer and in patients with glioblastoma treated in combination with temozolomid. However, it is also one of the first antiangiogenic agents, which demonstrated dose-limiting side effects, mostly severe inflammatory polyarthritis (45).

Inhibitors of Endothelial Cell Proliferation

A variety of antiangiogenic agents inhibit endothelial cell proliferation. Examples of these types of agents include TNP-470, thalidomide, squalamine, and captopril.

Treatment with TNP-470 has been shown to be more effective in limiting the growth of micrometastases than the growth of established tumors. It has shown some disease stabilizing effects in clinical trials with Kaposi's sarcoma patients and patients with cervical cancer (45).

Inhibitors of Integrin Activation

Integrins are cell surface receptors that play an important role in cell-cell and cell-matrix interactions. The integrins $\alpha_v\beta_3$ and $\alpha_v\beta_5$ are especially well examined and are expressed on angiogenic endothelial cells and on some metastatic tumor cells, but not on quiescent endothelium. Disruption of the $\alpha_v\beta_3$ integrin by monoclonal antibodies or cyclic peptides leads to activation of p53 and endothelial cell apoptosis. Examples of drugs in clinical trial include Vitaxin® (humanized antibody to $\alpha_v\beta_3$ LM609) and EMD121974 (Cilengitide®), a cyclic pentapeptide with highly specific binding to $\alpha_v\beta_3$ and $\alpha_v\beta_5$. These agents are currently evaluated in phase I to III trials comprising patients with glioblastoma in combination with temozolomide, patients with irinotecan refractory colorectal cancer, and patients with Kaposi's sarcoma.

IMAGING MODALITIES FOR DETECTING ANGIOGENESIS

Imaging modalities used to detect angiogenesis include PET, single-photon emission computed tomography (SPECT), MRI, CT, US, and near-infrared optical imaging (NIR OI). For these modalities, methods have been developed to measure blood volume, blood flow, and several other semiquantitative and quantitative kinetic hemodynamic parameters like vascular permeability (47,48). Moreover, with MRI, PET, SPECT, US, and OI, characteristic molecular markers of angiogenesis can be visualized with the aid of molecular imaging agents, such as VEGFs or the $\alpha_v\beta_3$ integrin (49). However, none of these imaging modalities is ideal in every aspect. All have their strengths and weaknesses concerning their sensitivity, availability, reproducibility, the ability for quantitative measurements, the regions of the body that can be imaged, the availability of compatible intravascular contrast agents, and contrast agent toxicity.

PET and SPECT

Both PET and SPECT imaging have the advantage of being very sensitive to low concentrations of tracer molecules and having unlimited depth penetration. PET is approximately 10 times more sensitive than SPECT and is able to detect picomolar concentrations of tracer. At the moment, the high sensitivity of PET is only reached by optical imaging (OI) techniques, but not by MRI, CT, or

US. Moreover, both methods can be quantitative, especially with regard to PET. This is an advantage over MRI and conventional optical imaging techniques. However, with the introduction of fluorescence-mediated tomography (FMT), quantitative measurements are also possible with OI techniques (50). Both PET and SPECT are well suited to molecular imaging of angiogenesis using targeted tracers because of the generally low concentrations of target molecules. Moreover, quantitative measurements of blood flow, blood volume, and vascular permeability can be performed with tracers like [^{15}O]H$_2$O, [^{15}O]CO$_2$, and [^{68}Ga]Albumin (51). Because some of the radionuclides used in PET tracers have a very short half-life (e.g., 2 minutes for [^{15}O]), PET using these tracers can only be performed at facilities that have the necessary cyclotron and chemical laboratory for the preparation of the tracers. SPECT imaging is much more widely available than PET imaging, and the radionuclides used for SPECT are easier to prepare and usually have a longer half-life than those used for PET (6 hours for [^{99m}Tc], 67 hours for [^{111}In], and 13.2 hours for [^{123}I]). However, both PET and SPECT scanners used for clinical applications have a lower spatial resolution than clinical MRI, CT, and US scanners. With state-of-the-art clinical PET scanners, a resolution of 3 to 4 mm is possible (52). This does not apply to preclinical animal scanners, which allow for submillimeter resolutions even in small rodents (53).

Magnetic Resonance Imaging

MRI is a practical modality for assessing angiogenesis over time because it is already widely used clinically to assess tumor growth and for response evaluation. Anatomical information can be coregistered with functional and molecular information within a single imaging method. Moreover, MRI does not involve ionizing radiation and the commonly used contrast agent, gadolinium diethyltriamine pentaacetic acid (Gd-DTPA), has a low toxicity. Therefore, repeat imaging is mainly limited by instrument availability and cost factors (50). Its resolution depends on the exact protocol applied, but is usually higher than that of clinical PET scanners, and MRI also offers a good depth penetration. MRI contrast agents contain paramagnetic nuclei, such as gadolinium, which increase the rates of T1 recovery and T2 decay. Because the concentration of Gd-DTPA is initially high, first-pass $T2$-weighted imaging is, in general, sensitive to blood flow and blood volume and is currently widely used in clinical routine for measurement of cerebral perfusion in patients with acute stroke. $T1$-weighted imaging is very sensitive to low concentrations of Gd-DTPA, which permeate through capillary walls in angiogenic vasculature that makes MRI a good candidate for measuring parameters that are dependent on permeability (8). However,

MRI is not a fully quantitative method because the changes in signal strength in MRI are not linear over the range of concentrations of gadolinium. Moreover, MRI protocols and instrument performance have substantial effects on signal strength, making it difficult to compare data obtained with different instruments at different institutions. Therefore, estimates of angiogenic blood volume and flow are generally calculated relative to that of normal tissue. Intravascular MRI contrast agents, which are more accurate for measuring blood volume, may become available in the future and several of these agents are currently used in clinical trials (48). Another disadvantage of MRI is its lower sensitivity for the detection of targeted agents compared with PET, SPECT, and OI. Therefore, targeted molecular imaging agents for MRI have not entered clinical trials, except for the fibrin-specific contrast agent EP2140R (54). The problem of limited sensitivity might be overcome in the future by signal amplification strategies that generate higher target to background contrast (55).

Computed Tomography

In principal, CT has many advantages for imaging of angiogenesis, including high spatial resolution, good depth penetration, and wide availability at comparably low costs, when compared with MRI and PET. Moreover, hemodynamic data from CT imaging are quantitative because the change in CT image intensity due to the contrast agent is linearly related to its concentration (48). New macromolecular CT contrast agents have been developed and are currently evaluated preclinically. These might facilitate the assessment of blood volume with CT (56). However, the sensitivity of CT is limited, and relatively high concentrations of CT contrast agent are required. CT contrast agents have many well-known side effects, like allergic reactions in some patients and notably nephrotoxicity! As many patients in oncological trials with antiangiogenic agents will also receive cytotoxic chemotherapy, which also might impair renal function, the additional renal toxicity of CT contrast agents might be a serious problem. This toxicity, together with the relatively high doses of radiation needed, limits the use of CT for repeated scanning and for response evaluation (8). Moreover, due to its low sensitivity, molecular-targeted imaging agents have not been used for CT imaging up to now.

Ultrasound

Ultrasound imaging is inexpensive, widely available, and completely noninvasive, therefore it is a promising technique for evaluation of angiogenesis. Doppler US detects the frequency shifts of moving blood and can be used to estimate blood flow and blood volume. US enhanced with contrast agents containing microbubbles are true intravascular contrast agents and can be used for measuring blood volume and flow, although the calculated values obtained by using these agents are not absolute but relative to those in other tissues at similar depths (48). Microbubbles can be burst by high-intensity US, yielding a short but strong backscatter echo, known as stimulated acoustic emission, which reflects microvascular perfusion (57). In addition, microbubbles labeled with agents that bind to angiogenic markers, such as $\alpha_v\beta_3$, are useful for molecular imaging of angiogenesis (58). Limitations are the dependence on the skill of the operator and limited depth penetration. Moreover, adequate documentation for comparison of examinations at different time points is still problematic. However, the complete noninvasiveness of the method makes it ideally suited for repeat exams for assessment of therapeutic response.

Optical Imaging

Optical imaging and in particular, near-infrared fluorescence (NIRF) imaging, which makes use of photons emitted in the near-infrared and far-red range, has the advantage of being relatively inexpensive, highly sensitive, and noninvasive. Because of its limited depth penetration, it is mainly applied in preclinical animal studies and in superficial tissues or in combination with endoscopy. Near-infrared light penetrates tissue sufficiently well to allow one to obtain low-resolution images of tissues to a depth of a few centimeters, and the regional concentration of hemoglobin and oxygen saturation can be calculated from the absorption of hemoglobin and deoxyhemoglobin. Fluorescence imaging has been used for retinal angiography, cardiovascular surgery, and gastrointestinal endoscopy, using either indocyanine green, a clinically available contrast agent that fluoresces at near-infrared wavelengths or autofluorescence (50). Indocyanine green has also been used to image angiogenic vasculature in breast tumors (58,59). In addition, a vast array of sensitive molecular imaging agents associated with angiogenesis specific targets has been developed for OI techniques, such as agents sensitive for matrix metalloproteases (60). Limitations of OI include its limited depth penetration and the effects of blood absorption and autofluorescence. Moreover, conventional optical imaging does not allow for quantitative measurements. However, this has changed with the introduction of FMT, which allows for quantitative measurements of fluorochrome concentrations at different tissue depths (50).

IMAGING OF HEMODYNAMIC PARAMETERS

Imaging of hemodynamic parameters like blood flow, blood volume, and vascular permeability using PET, MRI or CT is currently of great importance for assessment of antiangiogenic therapies, and widely used in study trials as an imaging biomarker of angiogenesis (61). Up to now it is not clear, however, which parameters and which imaging modalities would be optimal in this context, as all have their inherent advantages and limitations.

Blood Flow

Blood Flow Measurements with PET and SPECT Tracers

In 1870, Fick described the central relationship between blood flow and tissue clearance of circulating tracers, which can be expressed as:

$$C_t = P \cdot \int (C_i - C_e)dt, \qquad (1)$$

where C_t = tissue concentration, mol/mL_{tissue};
$\qquad C_i$ = influx concentration, $mol/mL_{carrier}$;
$\qquad C_e$ = eflux concentration, $mol/mL_{carrier}$;
and P = perfusion, $mL_{carrier}/(min \cdot mL_{tissue})$

In literal terms, the amount of tracer cleared by the tissue over time t is the product of perfusion P and tracer extraction. Perfusion is calculated by rearranging equation (1) so that

$$P = \frac{C_t}{\int (C_i - C_e)dt}. \qquad (2)$$

A major advantage of the nuclear medicine techniques using radiotracers is that the tissue concentration C_t can be measured noninvasively. This mainly applies to PET, whereas SPECT is only rarely applied for blood flow measurements outside the brain, because of its limited spatial resolution and its limitations concerning true quantification and attenuation correction. One study showed a correlation between the change of $[^{201}Tl]$thallium uptake in SPECT in squamous cell carcinoma of the oral cavity after preoperative radiotherapy and tumor angiogenesis as determined by microvascular density (62).

Indicator Washout and Indicator Fractionation Methods

Some experimental designs such as indicator fractionation methods and indicator washout methods simplify the relationship such that C_i or C_e is equal to zero. Indicator washout studies rely on direct administration of tracer to the tissues or a large artery, e.g., the carotid artery for hemicerebral studies. For this purpose, $[^{133}Xe]$xenon can be used because effectively all tracer is exhaled at first pass through the lungs without recirculation. Therefore, C_a can be disregarded and C_i can be modeled as the concentration in tissue fluid (C_t) and C_e as regional venous concentration (C_v). However, this model is sensitive to assumptions including the profile of

lymphatic drainage and sequestration of the tracer in fat. Its main application in humans is the measurement of regional cerebral blood flow (63).

Indicator fractionation methods model C_i as arterial concentration (C_a) and C_e as the concentration in tissue fluid (C_t), which is equal to zero, because effectively all tracer is trapped in capillaries. This can be achieved by central arterial injection of radiolabeled $[^{11}C]$microspheres of approximately 10-μm diameter (64). $[^{11}C]$ Microspheres indicator methods are primarily of interest as "gold standard" for perfusion measurements or for validation of new imaging methods for perfusion measurement. A number of peripherally injected PET tracers also exhibit microsphere-like handling. The latter have the advantage of being more suitable for work in humans. Three candidate compounds have been evaluated primarily for the myocardial and brain perfusion, but only occasionally for peripheral tumors. $[^{13}N]$Ammonia is rapidly cleared from the vascular space by active transport and passive diffusion, and is metabolized in both normal and diseased cardiac myocytes by the glutamic acid–glutamine pathway. The half-life of 10 minutes is favorable and facilitates prolonged single-scan protocols with accurate signal counting, but the isotope requires synthesis in a cyclotron. Moreover, the fact that $[^{13}N]$ammonia is metabolized makes this tracer less robust for applications in oncology (65). $[^{62}Cu]$PTSM ($[^{62}Cu]$pyruvaldehyde-bis (N4-methylthiosemicarbazone) can be generated at distance from a cyclotron using a proprietary reaction kit and again has a favorable half-life of 9.3 minutes. However, it binds to serum albumin, leading to an underestimation of myocardial perfusion at high flow rates (66). Similarly, $[^{82}Rb]$rubidium has a 76-second half-life and does not require synthesis in a cyclotron as it can be produced in a column generator. Its limitation is emission of more energetic positrons that have a longer range in the tissues. This results in a poorer image resolution and in data more vulnerable to tissue heterogeneity. While this is of lesser importance for myocardial perfusion studies, where $[^{82}Rb]$ rubidium is mainly applied, it is less attractive for oncological work because most tumor tissues demonstrate marked heterogeneity (67).

Perfusion Imaging with $[^{15}O]$water

With a half-life of 123 seconds, $[^{15}O]$oxygen is the longest-lived positronic oxygen isotope. It can be further reacted with carbon or hydrogen to produce $[^{15}O]CO_2$, $[^{15}O]CO$, or $[^{15}O]H_2O$. $[^{15}O]H_2O$ satisfies all the requirements for a perfusion tracer in Fick's model because it is biologically and metabolically inert, and freely diffusible into and out of tissue water. Thus, "tissue water" can be modeled as a single compartment including both tissue and its draining fluids (lymphatics and veins).

In principal, two methods can be used for measuring perfusion with $[^{15}O]H_2O$, the steady-state method of Frackowiak and colleagues, and the $[^{15}O]$-dynamic water method by Lammertsma et al. The latter is currently used most often for perfusion studies due to improved PET scanner technology, but the steady-state method illustrates the basic model for perfusion imaging with $[^{15}O]H_2O$. Subjects inhale radioactive $[^{15}O]CO_2$, and this is converted in the lungs by carbonic anhydrase to $[^{15}O]H_2O$. An equilibrium is reached after five minutes, when $[^{15}O]H_2O$ arterial influx is balanced by efflux and isotope radiodecay. After this point, increasing accuracy of measurement can be achieved by prolonging data acquisition, typically for a further five minutes at each bed positions. The concentration of tissue radioactivity in the region of interest (ROI) can then be described as

$$C_t = \frac{C_a \cdot P}{\rho \cdot P + \lambda}, \tag{3}$$

where C_t = tissue radiotracer concentration, Bq/mL$_{tissue}$;
$\quad$ C_a = arterial radiotracer concentration, Bq/mL$_{blood}$;
$\quad$ P = perfusion, mL$_{blood}$/(min(mL$_{tissue}$));
$\quad$ ρ = partition coefficient for water: the proportionality constant for concentration when tracer equilibrates between tissue fluid and a unit volume of blood, mL$_{tissue}$/mL$_{blood}$; and
$\quad$ λ = radioactive decay constant for $[^{15}O]$, 0.338 Bq/(min·Bq).

In most accounts, however, equation (3) is rearranged so that

$$P = \frac{\lambda}{C_a/C_t - \rho} \tag{4}$$

or

$$P = \frac{\lambda}{C_a/C_t - 1} \tag{5}$$

since ρ is assumed to equal 1.

C_t can be measured from the image, and C_a can be measured by an arterial blood sample. When a large arterial pool such as the left atrium is in view, C_a can alternatively be measured from the image as well. The assumption about the proportionality constant for tissue-blood concentration ρ is the main limitation of the steady-state model. Especially in tumors many areas are likely to have low values of ρ, thus leading to underestimation of flow. Additionally, achieving and maintaining equilibrium requires prolonged administration of radiation resulting in approximately twice the systemic dose than is received with bolus administration. Moreover, due to spillover of radioactivity from inhaled $[^{15}O]CO_2$ gas in the lungs, intrathoracic tissues may be difficult to image (68).

More commonly used nowadays is the $[^{15}O]$dynamic water method. By this method, ρ can be measured directly

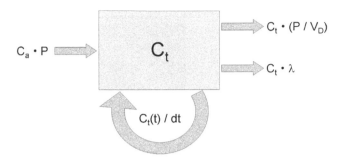

Figure 1 One compartment model of $[^{15}O]H_2O$ perfusion measurements. C_t = tissue tracer concentration in Bq/mL$_{tissue}$, C_a = arterial tracer concentration in Bq/mL$_{blood}$, P = perfusion in mL$_{blood}$/(min mL$_{tissue}$), λ = decay rate of $[^{15}O]$, 0.338 Bq/(min Bq), V_D = distribution volume in mL$_{tissue}$/mL$_{blood}$, $V_D = K_1/k_2 = C_t/C_a$; $V_D = 1/\rho$, and ρ = partition coefficient for water in mL$_{blood}$/mL$_{tissue}$.

and so it can be regarded as the current gold standard for imaging perfusion with $[^{15}O]H_2O$ (Fig. 1). The tracer is administered by inhalation or by peripheral venous bolus injection. Continuous arterial data are obtained either by image-based arterial input functions (AIFs) (a large vessel like the aorta or the left ventricle) or by peripheral sampling to a well counter device. In the case of peripheral sampling, a correction needs to be made for delay and dispersion of the recorded arterial curve, due to the length of the connecting tubes. The change in tissue concentration over time is modeled as

$$\frac{dC_t(t)}{dt} = P \cdot C_a(t) - (P/V_D + \lambda) \cdot C_t(t), \tag{6}$$

where V_D = "volume of distribution," the "proportion of the ROI in which the radioactive water is distributed," mL$_{blood}$/mL$_{tissue}$ = $1/\rho$;
$\quad$ $C_t(t)$ = instantaneous tissue concentration of $[^{15}O]H_2O$ at time t, Bq/mL$_{tissue}$; and
$\quad$ $C_a(t)$ = corrected instantaneous arterial concentration of $[^{15}O]H_2O$ at time t, Bq/mL$_{tissue}$.

The mathematics for solving P and V_D from the dynamic curves depends on convolution of the arterial and tissue datasets. The expression for tissue concentration at each time t is given by the convolution integral:

$$C_t(t) = \int P \cdot C_a(T) \cdot e^{-(P/V_D + \lambda) \cdot (t-T)} dT, \tag{7}$$

or

$$C_t(t) = P \cdot C_a(t) \otimes e^{-(P/V_D + \lambda) \cdot t}, \tag{8}$$

where $\otimes$ is the operation of convolution. $C_t(t)$ describes a biphasic curve with an initial peak followed by a longer tail of decay. P and V_D can be determined from this curve using nonlinear least-squares fitting. The dynamic method

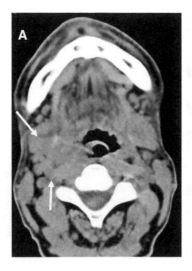
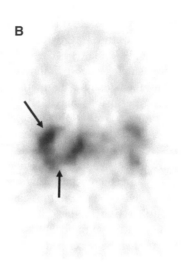

Figure 2 Large squamous cell carcinoma of the tonsillar area on the right side (*arrows*) in CT (**A**) and [^{15}O]H$_2$O PET (**B**). Note the increased perfusion in the tumor periphery, whereas the center remains cold.

has been shown to be less sensitive to tissue heterogeneity than the steady-state model. It is, however, more sensitive to assumptions about constancy of P and V_D and free and instantaneous diffusion of [^{15}O]H$_2$O out of arterial blood and through the tissues, because equilibrium is not reached (69). That means, it is assumed that tissues exhibit neither tracer binding nor concentration gradients and that the arterial extraction fraction is uniform. The exact physiological meaning of V_D still has to be evaluated. However, according to first results, V_D is expected to reflect tissue water composition. Thus, it should be high in water-secreting tissues, such as the renal cortex, and low in fatty tissues, such as breast tissues. Extremely low values for V_D are suggestive of ischemic or necrotic areas (Fig. 2). First results in patient studies corroborate these assumptions, as markedly lower V_D values were found in breast than in spleen or kidney (70). The validity and reproducibility of this method was initially assessed for the brain and myocardium, but subsequently also for tumors of pancreas, brain, breast, and liver. The data are compatible with those from diseases investigated with other methods, and the range of values reported by PET for tumors is within the reported range for PET in other tissues (71,72). However, the heterogeneity of tumor blood flow still is a major problem for interpretation of the data. The heterogeneity of tumor blood supply on microscopic scales, with such phenomena as ischemia, shunts, and necrosis makes it clear that the assumption of a single arterial input and equilibration of arterial and tissue water is not fully in accordance with the physiology of the tumor microcirculation. Ultimately, it has to be proven in patient studies that measurements of blood flow using PET provide relevant information for patient management, especially for response evaluation and dose optimization during chemotherapy. In locally advanced breast cancer, first results with dynamic [^{15}O]H$_2$O PET are promising, as blood flow decreased in the responder group after chemotherapy, whereas it increased in the nonresponder group (73). The role of dynamic [^{15}O]H$_2$O PET compared with other methods like DCE MRI still has to be evaluated.

Arterial Spin Labeling and BOLD Imaging

Arterial spin labeling is using the effect, that water molecules can be labeled by inverting the nuclear spin of their hydrogen atoms by a radiofrequency pulse directed at arterial blood before it enters the region of measurement. An absolute value for blood flow is determined by the change in the magnetic resonance signal as the labeled water in the arterial bloodstream arrives in the ROI. However, the signal-to-noise ratio of arterial spin labeling MRI is relatively low and the sensitivity and spatial resolution of this method are limited, especially if the rate of blood flow is low, because the spin label is very short-lived. Nevertheless, arterial spin labeling has been shown to be a reproducible method for measuring blood flow, e.g., by comparison with [^{123}I]iodoamphetamine SPECT in the brain (74). Moreover, it does not require the use of contrast agents or arterial blood sampling. Therefore, this method is completely noninvasive and well suited for repeat measurements.

Blood oxygen level dependent (BOLD) imaging can detect changes in the oxygen saturation of the blood. By measuring signal changes in response to hypercapnia and to hyperoxia, the vascular maturity can be detected, as only mature vessels react to hypercapnia (75). The underlying physiological processes giving rise to measured BOLD signal changes include contribution from changes in blood flow, blood volume, and metabolic rate of oxygen consumption. Because of the heterogeneity of tumors, the results are therefore hard to interpret and BOLD imaging is rarely used to image perfusion in tumors in patients. Some preclinical studies show no correlation between parameters derived from DCE MRI and BOLD MRI in a murine tumor xenograft. The authors conclude that the information from both techniques is complementary, but the exact physiological meaning of the BOLD signal in tumors remains complex and has to be further evaluated (76).

DCE CT and MRI Imaging

DCE imaging can be used to accurately measure blood flow, provided that no substantial amounts of tracer leak into the tissues. When small, low molecular weight imaging agents are used, like conventional iodinated CT contrast agents or Gd-DTPA, this only applies to the normal brain, due to the intact blood-brain barrier. In peripheral tumors, these contrast agents rapidly leak into the tissue, therefore exact measurements of blood flow are impaired and blood flow measurements using DCE CT or MRI are of limited use in oncology. However, various other hemodynamic parameters like capillary permeability and leakage can be derived, which will be discussed separately. An advantage of DCE CT or MRI is that it can be readily incorporated into routine conventional CT/MRI examinations. DCE CT

is simple, widely available, and reproducible and has been validated against $[^{15}O]H_2O$ PET in the brain (77,78). Quantification is simpler than for MRI, as the relationship between signal and contrast concentration is much more linear than that seen with MRI, although the sensitivity is less. The problem is that early clinical studies of antiangiogenic compounds require multiple imaging assessments of the tumor. As contrast-enhanced dynamic CT uses ionizing radiation, there is a limit to the number of studies that can be performed. Blood flow measurements in the brain with MRI mostly make use of the decrease in $T2$ signal early after start of contrast agent administration. This method requires high flow rates of 5 to 10 mL/sec and assumes an intact blood-brain barrier. It is widely applied in MRI stroke protocols but less so in oncological applications (79).

Ultrasound Using Doppler-Techniques and Contrast Agents

Ultrasound is one of the most widely used imaging modalities, it is relatively inexpensive and does not use ionizing radiation. Therefore, it is of great interest for repeat studies of tumor perfusion. Conventional Doppler imaging is able to directly image flow in vessels down to approximately the millimeter level (Fig. 3). Thus, it is mainly a tool for imaging the macrocirculation, rather than the microcirculation. Recently, several manufacturers

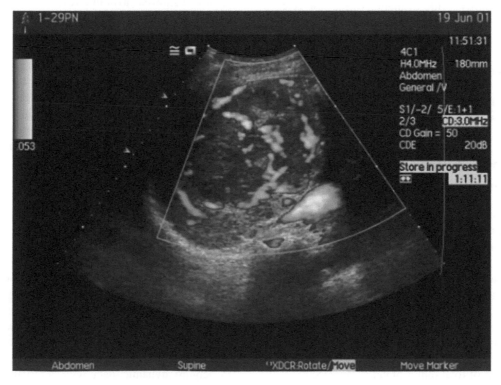

Figure 3 Power Doppler ultrasound of a hepatocellular carcinoma. Note the complex, tortuous vessel architecture. The smallest vessels that can be depicted are about a millimeter in diameter. *Source*: From Ref. 82.

have developed commercial real-time ultrasound systems, which can scan in Doppler modes at between 10 and 20 MHz with good tissue penetration (80). Such systems can detect flow even in submillimeter-sized vessels. Several studies have evaluated the relationship between histological indices of angiogenesis and indices derived from Doppler ultrasound. Current Doppler methods often perform relatively poorly when directly correlated with measures of tumor angiogenesis, such as microvessel density (81). One potential reason for this could be sampling errors in heterogeneous tumors. Intermittent ultrasound using microbubbles like the perfluoro gas filled agents (SonoVue) is a form of dynamic contrast imaging that is used to measure blood flow. It relies on the fragility of circulating microbubbles. A high-energy ultrasound pulse is applied to the ROI, destroying the microbubbles there. The refill of the ROI can then be monitored by low-power monitor frames, and the rate of increase in microbubble concentration is measured. Therefore, this is a negative bolus technique, which is unique to ultrasound because other contrast agents cannot be easily inactivated. There is a good correlation of blood flow derived from fitting the enhancement curve to an exponential model with absolute measures of blood flow in phantom studies and in ex vivo veins as well as with well-validated alternate methods, such as blood sampling of radiolabeled microspheres, in animal studies of blood flow in the myocardium and renal cortex (82). However, ultrasound, despite its popularity, wide availability, and low cost, is not as widely applied as other modalities such as MRI and PET in the functional assessment of response to therapy in oncology. One major problem is operator dependency of the study and the difficulty in obtaining images when flow rates are very low. Also, depth penetration is poor and many regions of the body are not accessible to ultrasound at all in adults, such as the lung, the brain, and bony structures.

Blood Volume and Vascular Permeability

PET and SPECT Techniques

The value of blood volume data are of great interest for response evaluation of some antiangiogenic therapies, because drugs such as combretastatin exert their main effect via collapse of blood vessels and not via reduced flow through isovolumetric vessels. So it is expected for this type of drug that blood flow will not be influenced, while blood volume should decrease in case of a drug response. For mainly capillary-directed antiangiogenic therapies, the value of blood volume measurements is less certain, because histological examinations show that capillaries account for only a minor part of total tumor blood volume (83).

Blood volume imaging with PET uses [^{15}O]CO or [^{11}C]CO carbon monoxide. The patient inhales a fixed dose of [^{15}O]CO through a loose-fitting mask and then breathes room air for approximately 90 seconds. [^{15}O]CO binds irreversibly with hemoglobin to form [^{15}O]CO-Hb carboxyhemoglobin. Because [^{15}O]CO-Hb remains exclusively within the vasculature it can be used as a tracer of vascular volume. A tissue concentration dataset is obtained over a further 5 to 6 min and an arterial [^{15}O]CO-Hb concentration curve is derived from a series of arterial blood samples over the same interval. Tissue vascular volume can be defined as

$$V_v = \frac{V_t \cdot \int C_t}{R \cdot \int C_a},\qquad(9)$$

where V_v = volume of vessels, mL$_{vessels}$;

$\quad V_t$ = volume of tissue within ROI on scan, mL$_{tissue}$;

$\quad R$ = ratio of small vessel to large vessel hematocrit (assumed to be 1 in tumors);

$\quad C_t(t)$ = tissue activity, Bq/(mL·min);

$\quad C_a(t)$ = arterial activity, Bq/(mL·min).

Another method for blood volume imaging is labeling red blood cells (RBCs) or albumin with radionuclides, because both are too large to leave normal blood vessels and are retained in the blood pool. In tumor vessels, leakage of these contrast agents into the tumor will occur, but this effect can be used to calculate the tumor vessel permeability when dynamic imaging is performed. For PET, the tracer [^{68}Ga]DOTA-albumin has been developed and showed favorable results in first animal studies (84). An advantage is that the radionuclide [^{68}Ga] is generator produced and is therefore continuously available even to centers lacking an in-house cyclotron.

For SPECT imaging of blood volume, the same principle is used. RBCs can be labeled with [^{99m}Tc] and used for steady-state measurements of blood volume, as can be [^{99m}Tc]-labeled human serum albumin (8,85). To our knowledge, no patient studies for response evaluation of antiangiogenic chemotherapies have been performed up to date with SPECT.

MRI and CT Techniques

Similar to PET and SPECT blood volume imaging, MR imaging with new, macromolecular contrast media (MMCM) has been reported to provide a more specific characterization of angiogenesis for tumors outside the CNS. Because dynamic image acquisition is necessary to calculate the permeability surface product, a series of images spanning at least 20 to 30 minutes after contrast medium administration, is required. However, short scan intervals are not necessary because the leakage of MMCM into tumors is a rather slow process. Usually it is sufficient to acquire dynamic data with intervals of one to two minutes. Various studies have shown that MMCM with the size of proteins, such as albumin with a molecular weight of 69000 Da, can detect and quantify blood volume and the increased microvessel hyperpermeability of tumors to macromolecules. Moreover, MMCM, but not the standard small molecular contrast agents, were able to grade malignancies, to differentiate benign and malignant tumors, and to predict tumor therapy response based on their microvascular permeability (48,86). The same principle applies to CT examinations with iodinated MMCM, which recently have been developed and evaluated preclinically (56). They allow for exquisite depiction of the macrovasculature and analysis of blood volume and vessel permeability. No reports about applications in humans are available up to date.

Another fascinating approach is using ultrasmall superparamagnetic iron oxide particles (USPIOs) as MMCM. The half-life of USPIO MCMM in the circulation is between 3 and 24 hours. The signal-to-noise ratio and the degree of enhancement correlate with the dose of USPIOs. However, at higher doses, $T2*$ effects can overwhelm the desired $T1$ effects (87). USPIOs are currently evaluated in patients for lymph node staging and thus could be readily used in studies evaluating antiangiogenic therapies as well. However, no reports about response evaluation in patients with USPIOs are available up to now.

Optical Imaging Techniques

As mentioned before, quantitative measurements of fluorochrome concentrations have been made possible by the introduction of FMT. By using a dual modality nanoparticle with both fluorescent and superparamagnetic properties called CLIO-Cy5.5 (cross-linked iron oxide–Cy5.5), blood volume could be determined in a murine tumor model, which correlated significantly with microvessel density (MVD) and results from SPECT using [^{99m}Tc]RBCs (88). Because of the limited depth penetration of FMT, this method is mainly of interest in preclinical tumor models.

Other Hemodynamic Parameters

Several other quantitative hemodynamic parameters have been established as standards in addition to blood flow and blood volume and vascular permeability, which can be measured by DCE imaging with either CT or MRI using small low molecular weight contrast agents, with CT having the advantage of being truly quantitative, as mentioned before. DCE MRI or CT imaging is used over a longer time course (in the first several minutes) to observe the extravasation of contrast agent from the vascular space to the interstitial space. The accumulation of contrast agent in the interstitium results in a signal increase on $T1$-weighted MRI or increase in Hounsfield units in CT. A subsequent washout effect can be observed if the vascular permeability is high and there is reflux of contrast agent back to the vascular space. The signal-intensity time curve can be quantified using either semiquantitative empirical measures such as peak enhancement, the initial area under the curve (AUC), time to peak enhancement, or signal enhancement ratio (SER). However, these parameters are not truly quantitative and might differ substantially in dependence of the protocols used at different institutions. Therefore, other more quantitative parameters are preferred to ensure reproducibility of the measurements.

These parameters are the volume transfer constant K^{trans} (min^{-1}), which describes the rate of flux of contrast agent into the extracellular extravascular space (EES) within a given volume; the volume of the EES per unit volume of tissue v_{e}; and the rate constant for the back flux from the EES to the vasculature κ_{ep} (min^{-1}). These terms are related to each other by the equation $\kappa_{\text{ep}} = K^{\text{trans}}/v_{e}$. Several other names have been used for these parameters in the literature. However, in a 1999 consensus publication, this set of terms was recommended by an international group of investigators developing DCE MRI methodologies. The authors proposed that this set of kinetic parameters and symbols be used universally to describe the uptake of low molecular weight gadolinium-based contrast agents that are in clinical use today and related them to previously published terms and symbols (89). K^{trans}, κ_{ep}, and v_{e} are currently the most commonly used hemodynamic parameters in clinical studies evaluating antiangiogenic therapies and are mainly derived by DCE MRI. However, the exact physiological meaning of these parameters is complex and not related to a single process such as blood flow or blood volume only. K^{trans} has several physiological interpretations, depending on the balance between capillary permeability and blood flow. When capillary permeability is very high, the flux of the contrast agent into the EES is limited by the flow rate. In this case, K^{trans} is equal to the blood plasma flow per unit volume of tissue. When tracer flux is very low and blood flow is high, the blood plasma can be considered as a single pool, in which the concentration of contrast agent does not change substantially during the scan. Therefore, any change in signal is due to the increase in the concentration of the contrast agent in the EES. In this case, K^{trans} is equal to the permeability surface area, which is the product of the permeability and the surface area of the capillary vascular endothelium. If blood flow as well as permeability is low and limiting, then the fractional reduction of capillary blood concentration of the contrast agent as it passes through the tissue must be considered as well. The rate of contrast agent flow out of the capillaries is initially high and then decreases over time as the backflow of the contrast agent increases (8). As discussed before, experimental macromolecular MRI and CT contrast agents (MCMM) that have lower permeability, such as albumin-Gd-DTPA, or USPIOs that remain confined within normal vasculature but not angiogenic vasculature, may be more useful than the commonly used contrast agents for monitoring changes in permeability.

The relationship of the different parameters K^{trans}, κ_{ep}, and v_e can be expressed by the equation

$$\frac{dC_t}{dt} = K^{trans} \cdot \left(C_p - \frac{C_t}{v_e} \right), \qquad (10)$$

or

$$\frac{dC_t}{dt} = K^{trans} \cdot C_p - \kappa_{ep} \cdot C_t, \qquad (11)$$

where C_t = the tracer concentration in tissue,
$\quad C_p$ = the tracer concentration in plasma,
and t = time (in seconds).

These parameters can be derived from the data by applying a two-compartment pharmacokinetic model to the MRI or CT enhancement time course (Fig. 4). Because there is no linear relationship of contrast agent concentration and signal intensity in MRI, measurements of the intrinsic $T1$ value and the AIF are needed for quantitation purposes and to ensure comparability of the results between institutions. It may not be possible to include a large vessel in the field of view (FoV) appropriate for measuring the AIF, but alternative approaches exist to derive the AIF by pixel analysis of the data. First, an algorithm selects those pixels with the highest signal intensity in the FoV, which represent arteries and veins. Next, only those pixels with a rapid and early peak enhancement are selected, which should only represent the arteries in the FoV (90). Instead of an individually measured AIF, average values measured in healthy control subjects from blood samples, are often used. The performance of alternative approaches like using global estimates of AIF, or of ignoring $T1$ effects, has not yet been established clinically (91).

Concerning the reproducibility of these hemodynamic parameters, the maximum enhancement and the AUC appear to be the most reproducible among the semiquantitative parameters. The slope or rate of enhancement

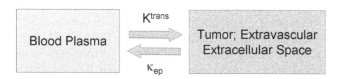

Figure 4 The two compartment kinetic model for DCE MRI using Gd-DTPA defines three parameters: the volume transfer constant K^{trans} between the blood plasma and the EES, the volume of the EES per unit volume of tissue v_e, and the flux rate constant between the EES and blood plasma $\kappa_{ep} = K^{trans}/v_e$. *Abbreviations*: DCE MRI, dynamic contrast-enhanced magnetic resonance imaging; Gd-DTPA, gadolinium diethyltriamine pentaacetic acid; EES, extracellular extravascular space.

appears to be the least reproducible, which may reflect the dependence of these measurements on the rate of injection of the contrast agent bolus as well as variations in cardiac input. Among the quantitative parameters, v_e seems to have the least variability, with interpatient variability being much greater than that intrapatient variability. However, K^{trans} and κ_{ep} also have sufficient reproducibility to be useful for measuring changes over time (92,93).

Since no simple noninvasive gold standard is available to directly verify the measurements made by DCE MRI or CT, the value of these techniques will be determined in the end by their clinical utility. DCE MRI has been used in many oncological applications to study cancers of the breast, prostate, cervix, liver, lung, and the rectum. The majority of studies have found associations between DCE MRI parameters and clinical outcome or other parameters, like markers of angiogenesis, such as MVD and VEGF expression (94–99). However, the ultimate test will be, if response assessment during antiangiogenic therapy or other forms of chemo- or radiotherapy will be feasible (Fig. 5). Results of recent studies are encouraging, but not uniformly so. DCE MRI was used to evaluate the effects of the VEGFR2 inhibitor SU5416, in a phase I study of patients with treatment refractory solid tumors, including soft tissue sarcoma, melanoma, renal cancers, and other entities. No changes in K^{trans} and v_e were seen in response to treatment, which might have been caused by several reasons. First, the potency of the agent at the doses studied might have been insufficient for detection with DCE MRI. Moreover, the wide range of tumor sites evaluated in a comparably small sample size with possibly very different physiological properties complicates interpretation of these results (100). In another study, patients with inflammatory and locally advanced breast cancer treated with Avastin alone for one cycle and subsequently in combination with chemotherapy were examined with DCE MRI at baseline and after cycles 1, 4, and 7. K^{trans}, κ_{ep}, and v_e showed significant decreases after treatment with Avastin alone, and continued to decrease after the start of chemotherapy. However, there was no significant correlation of any of these parameters with clinical response (101). One promising study evaluated DCE MRI in patients with colorectal cancer and metastatic liver lesions, receiving the VEGF receptor tyrosine kinase inhibitor PT787/ZK 222584. Twenty-six patients were evaluated at baseline and one or more time points during treatment. A significant negative correlation between the DCE MRI pharmacokinetic parameter K_i, which is related to K^{trans} and both the oral dose and plasma levels of PT787/ZK 222584 were found. Also, correct response evaluation was possible, as significantly greater reductions in K_i were found for responders with complete remission, partial remission, or stable disease according to the RECIST criteria than for nonresponders (102).

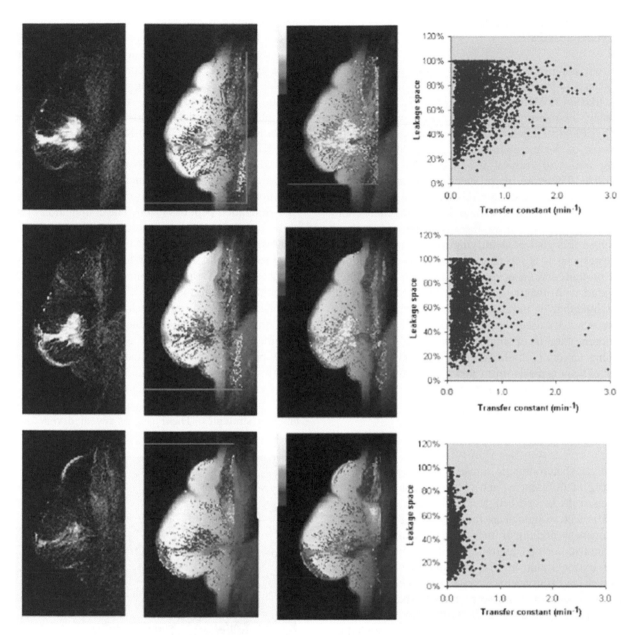

Figure 5 Monitoring chemotherapy response of breast cancer with DCE MRI. A 58-year-old postmenopausal woman with a recurrent infiltrating ductal carcinoma of the breast. Columns depict anatomic subtraction images (obtained by subtracting MR image acquired at 100 seconds after contrast agent administration from baseline image), corresponding transfer constant maps (color range, 0–1/min), leakage space (maximum ν_e value, 100%), and scatter plots showing individual pixel transfer constant and leakage space values. Rows show data before treatment and after two and six courses of FEC chemotherapy. With treatment, a reduction in the number of enhancing pixels is seen (first examination 4215, second examination 2080, third examination 1400). A stepwise reduction in kinetic parameter estimates is seen. Median transfer constant values: first examination 0.39/min, second examination 0.28/min, third examination 0.085/min. Median ν_e values: first examination 72%, second examination 61%, third examination 35%. *Abbreviation*: DCE MRI, dynamic contrast-enhanced magnetic resonance imaging. *Source*: From Ref. 86.

In conclusion, DCE CT and MRI using low molecular weight contrast agents are far from being ideal techniques for assessment of angiogenesis and the results are sometimes hard to interpret in their physiological meaning. However, the wide availability of MRI and CT and the use of clinically approved contrast agents make these techniques very attractive for patient studies. Moreover, the lack of ionizing radiation in DCE MRI and the low toxicity of Gd-DTPA are ideal prerequisites for repeat measurements for response evaluation in clinical trials.

IMAGING OF MOLECULAR MARKERS OF ANGIOGENESIS

While functional imaging of hemodynamic parameters of angiogenesis is possible with a variety of different techniques like DCE MRI and [^{15}O]H$_2$O PET, as discussed previously, the interpretation of the results with regard to their physiological meaning often remains difficult. Moreover, most of the methods applied are technically challenging and with regard to DCE MRI difficult to standardize. Therefore, more specific markers of angiogenetic activity in tumors are desirable and would facilitate pretherapeutic assessment of angiogenesis and response evaluation during therapy. One approach to accomplish this goal is identifying molecular markers of angiogenesis such as receptors, enzymes, or extracellular matrix proteins and using specific ligands to these targets conjugated with imaging probes for PET, SPECT, MRI, optical imaging, or ultrasound. All these methods have been successfully used for preclinical molecular imaging of different targets of angiogenesis. One of the most promising targets is the integrin $\alpha_v\beta_3$, which is the only marker of angiogenesis up to now, which has been successfully imaged in patients by using PET and SPECT techniques (103,104).

Integrin Expression

Integrins are heterodimeric transmembrane glycoproteins consisting of different α- and β-subunits, which play an important role in cell-cell and cell-matrix interactions. Especially well examined are the integrin $\alpha_v\beta_3$ and its role in angiogenesis and tumor metastasis by facilitating endothelial and tumor cell migration. It has been found that several extracellular matrix proteins like vitronectin, fibrinogen, and fibronectin interact with integrins via the amino acid sequence arginine-glycine-aspartic acid or RGD in the single letter code (105). On the basis of these findings, linear as well as cyclic peptides including the RGD sequence have been introduced. Kessler and coworkers developed the pentapeptide cyclo(-Arg-Gly-Asp-D-Phe-Val-), which shows high affinity and selectivity for $\alpha_v\beta_3$, which is the most prominent lead structure for the development of molecular imaging compounds for the determination of $\alpha_v\beta_3$ expression (106). For the first evaluation of this approach, radioiodinated RGD peptides have been synthesized, which showed comparable affinity and selectivity to the lead structure. In vivo they revealed receptor-specific tumor uptake but also predominantly hepatobiliary elimination, resulting in high activity concentration in the liver and intestine, which is unfavorable for patient studies (107). Several strategies to improve the pharmacokinetics of radiohalogenated peptides have therefore been developed, like conjugation with

sugar moieties, hydrophilic amino acids, and polyethylene glycol (PEG). The glycosylation approach is based on the introduction of sugar derivatives that are conjugated to the ϵ-amino function of a corresponding lysine in the peptide sequence. By conjugating the RGD-containing cyclic pentapeptide cyclo(-Arg-Gly-Asp-D-Phe-Val-) with glucose- or galactose-based sugar amino acids, [*I] Gluco-RGD and [^{18}F]Galacto-RGD have been developed for PET and SPECT imaging (Fig. 6). Both compounds showed improved pharmacokinetics with predominantly renal tracer elimination and increased activity uptake and retention in a murine tumor model compared with the first-generation peptides (108). The conjugation of hydrophilic D-amino acids was also used to improve the pharmacokinetics of peptide-based tracers (109). Again, tracer elimination could be shifted to the renal pathway, but tumor uptake of the compound [^{18}F]D-Asp3-RGD was lower than that found for [^{18}F]Galacto-RGD. However, tumor-to-background ratios calculated from small-animal PET images were comparable due to the even faster elimination. PEGylation is another way to improve many properties of peptides and proteins, like pharmacokinetics, plasma stability, and immunogenicity (110). Chen et al. conjugated RGD-containing peptides with PEG moieties of different sizes, using different radiolabeling strategies. These studies revealed very different

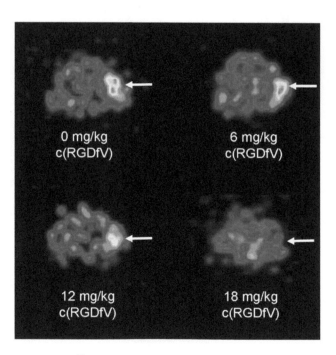

Figure 6 [^{18}F]Galacto-RGD small-animal PET of a A431 squamous cell carcinoma xenograft in the left flank: initially high tumor uptake, which continuously decreases with rising concentration of the unlabeled cyclic pentapeptide c(RGDfV). This demonstrates that receptor blockade can be successfully monitored (*See Color Insert*).

effects of PEGylation on the pharmacokinetics and tumor uptake and retention of RGD peptides, which seem to depend strongly on the nature of the lead structure and perhaps on the size of the PEG moiety (111).

Besides radiohalogenated RGD peptides, a variety of radiometallated tracers have been developed as well, including peptides labeled with [^{111}In], [^{99m}Tc], [^{64}Cu], [^{90}Y], and [^{188}Re]. Most of them are based on the cyclic pentapeptide and are conjugated via the ε-amino function of a lysine with different chelator systems, like DTPA, the tetrapeptide sequence H-Asp-Lys-Cys-Lys-OH, and DOTA. While all these compounds showed high receptor affinity and selectivity and specific tumor accumulation, the pharmacokinetics of most of them still have to be improved before a clinical application seems feasible (112).

In addition to monomeric RGD peptides, multimeric compounds presenting more than one RGD site have been introduced recently. A systematic study on the influence of multimerization on receptor affinity and tumor uptake was carried out by the groups of Wester and Kessler who synthesized a series of monomeric, dimeric, tetrameric,

and octameric RGD peptides. These compounds contain different numbers of c(RGDfE) peptides connected via PEG linker and lysine moieties, which are used as branching units. They found an increasing binding affinity in the series monomer, dimer, tetramer, and octamer in an in vitro binding assay, which was confirmed by small-animal PET studies. Moreover, PET studies comparing a tetrameric structure containing four c(RGDfE) peptides with a tetrameric compound containing only one c(RGDfE) and three c(RaDFE) peptides, which do not bind to the $\alpha_v\beta_3$ integrin, showed a threefold lower activity accumulation in the tumor for the pseudo monomeric tetramer than for the "real" tetramer, indicating that the higher uptake in the tumor really is due to multimerization and not based on other structural effects (Fig. 7) (113). Overall, the multimerization approach leads to increased binding affinity and tumor uptake as well as retention and can improve the pharmacokinetics of peptide-based tracers.

Besides radiolabeling, several other strategies for imaging $\alpha_v\beta_3$ expression have been successfully used in preclinical tumor models. Using RGD-Cy5.5, $\alpha_v\beta_3$

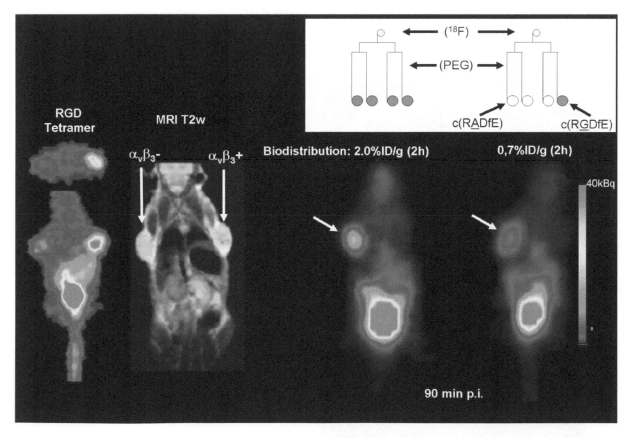

Figure 7 [^{18}F]-labeled multimeric RGD peptides in tumor xenografts. The MRI scan shows the subcutaneously implanted tumors, the $\alpha_v\beta_3$ positive M21 tumor on the left side, the $\alpha_v\beta_3$ negative tumor M21L on the right side. The positive tumor shows intense tracer uptake with the RGD multimer compared with the control tumor. Moreover, the RGD tetramer with four RGD binding sites clearly shows a much more intense accumulation in the tumor compared with the RGD tetramer with only one RGD binding site and three unspecific RAD (arginine, alanine, aspartate) sites (*See Color Insert*).

expression could be imaged in murine tumor models by NIR optical imaging (114). With FMT, even a quantification of $\alpha_v\beta_3$ expression similar to radiotracer techniques seems possible in the future. MRI using $\alpha_v\beta_3$ specific ligands has also been evaluated preclinically. Using $\alpha_v\beta_3$ specific perfluorocarbon nanoparticles conjugated with Gd-DTPA, Winter et al. imaged $\alpha_v\beta_3$ expression in murine tumor models as well as in animal models of atherosclerosis (115). Imaging based on T2 weighted sequences is also possible with iron-oxide based dual modality nanoparticles, like RGD-CLIO-Cy5.5, which allow both for MRI and fluorescence imaging. The long blood half-life of nanoparticles, depending on the actual size of the particle, does not allow for imaging at early time points after injection, because the signal mainly represents the nanoparticles concentration in the blood pool and is therefore unspecific. After approximately 24 hours, nanoparticles usually are cleared from the circulation and specific imaging is possible (116). Depending on the specific size and properties of the nanoparticles and the imaging time point, the signal mainly represents $\alpha_v\beta_3$ expression on endothelial cells, if the agent does not leave the circulation. If imaging at later time points is performed, even larger nanoparticles usually leak into tumor tissues and the signal also represents $\alpha_v\beta_3$

expressed on tumor cells, given that the specific tumor examined does express $\alpha_v\beta_3$. Finally, also microbubbles can be targeted to $\alpha_v\beta_3$ by conjugation with RGD-peptides and used for ultrasound molecular imaging of $\alpha_v\beta_3$ expression (117).

Up to now, the only approach of imaging $\alpha_v\beta_3$ expression, which has made the transition from bench to bedside, is the radiotracer approach (Fig. 8). [^{18}F]Galacto-RGD was the first substance applied in patients and could successfully image $\alpha_v\beta_3$ expression in human tumors with good tumor-to-background ratios (118). The biodistribution is favorable with predominantly renal tracer elimination and the effective dose is similar to [^{18}F]FDG (119). The correlation of tracer uptake and $\alpha_v\beta_3$ expression as determined by immunohistochemistry was significant in murine tumors as well as in patients (103,120). Recently, the SPECT tracer [^{99m}Tc]NC100692 was introduced by GE healthcare for imaging $\alpha_v\beta_3$ expression in humans and was first evaluated in breast cancer. Nineteen of 22 tumors could be detected with this agent, which was safe and well tolerated by the patients (104). It is therefore expected that commercial agents for $\alpha_v\beta_3$ imaging will soon be available. Future applications of [^{18}F]Galacto-RGD and similar compounds could be the assessment of angiogenic activity or the

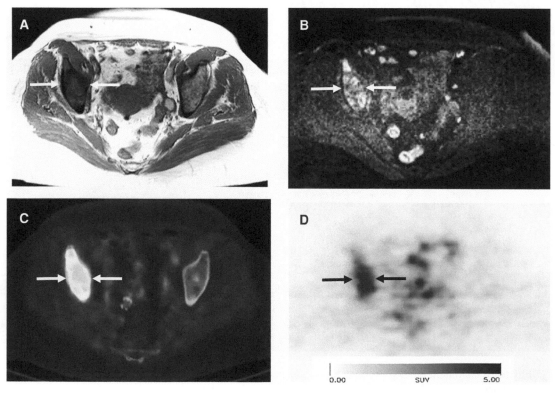

Figure 8 Patient with an osseous metastasis from non–small cell lung cancer in the right iliac bone (*arrows*). The (**A**) T1-weighted and (**B**) diffusion-weighted MRI scans clearly show the lesion. In the [^{18}F]FDG PET/CT scan (**C**) the lesion shows a high metabolic activity. The [^{18}F]Galacto-RGD PET (**D**) demonstrates intense $\alpha_v\beta_3$ expression in this lesion. Physiological uptake is seen in the intestine.

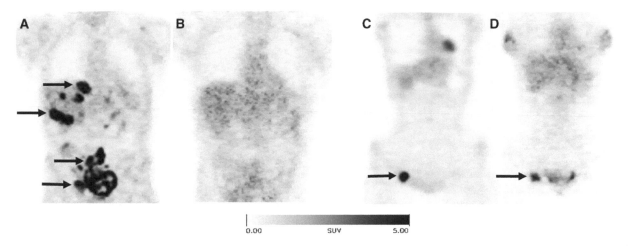

Figure 9 On the left side, a patient with diffuse metastasis from malignant melanoma (*arrows*); (**A**) [^{18}F]FDG PET and (**B**) [^{18}F] Galacto-RGD PET. On the right side, a second patient with a single lymph node metastasis from malignant melanoma in the right groin (*arrow*); (**C**) [^{18}F]FDG PET and (**D**) [^{18}F]Galacto-RGD PET. In both patients, the metastatic lesions are highly metabolic active, as demonstrated by [^{18}F]FDG PET. However, only the second patient shows $\alpha_v\beta_3$ expression in the lesion, as demonstrated by [^{18}F] Galacto-RGD PET. The information provided by [^{18}F]Galacto-RGD is more specific and could be used for patient selection before starting $\alpha_v\beta_3$ targeted therapies (Vitaxin, Cilengitide).

pretherapeutic selection of patients amenable for $\alpha_v\beta_3$-specific therapies, like with Cilengitide or Vitaxin (Fig. 9).

Extra Domain B of Fibronectin

Fibronectin is a large glycoprotein, which can be found physiologically in plasma and tissues. However, the extra domain B of fibronectin (EDB), consisting of 91 amino acids, is not present in the fibronectin molecule in normal conditions. In fact, except for the endometrium in the proliferative phase and some vessels of the ovaries, EDB is essentially undetectable in most normal adult tissues. It is typically inserted in the fibronectin molecules at sites of tissue remodeling by a mechanism of alternative splicing at the level of the primary transcript. What makes EDB interesting as a marker of angiogenesis is its expression in a variety of solid tumors, as well as in ocular angiogenesis and wound healing. The pattern of EDB expression in tumors either is predominantly perivascular or exhibits a diffuse staining of the tumor stroma (121). The human antibody fragment scFv(L19) binds with subnanomolar affinity to EDB and has been shown to efficiently localize on tumoral and nontumoral neovasculature both in animal models and in cancer patients. In a study with patients suffering from various solid tumors like lung cancer, metastases from colorectal cancer, and glioblastoma, 16 of 20 tumor lesions could be identified by SPECT using [^{123}I]scFv(L19). If the unidentified tumors were not detected because they were in a phase of slow growth with low levels of angiogenesis or due to the technical limitations of SPECT imaging is not clear

(122). No reports about PET tracers targeting EDB are available up to now.

Matrix Metalloproteinases

MMPs are zinc endopeptidases that are responsible for the enzymatic degradation of connective tissue and thus facilitate endothelial cell migration during angiogenesis. From the more than 18 members of the MMP family, the gelatinases MMP 2 and 9 are most consistently detected in malignancies and therefore interesting for assessment of angiogenesis (123). Many strategies have been used for radiolabeling of MMP-specific ligands. Via phage display techniques, the MMP-specific decapeptide H-Cys-Thr-Thr-His-Trp-Gly-Phe-Thr-Leu-Cys-OH was found and could be labeled via the Iodogene® method by adding a D-Tyr at the N-terminal end of this decapeptide. However, metabolic stability of the compound was low and lipophilicity was high, therefore this tracer has unfavorable characteristics for in vivo imaging. Another approach is labeling small molecule MMP inhibitors, which are also used as antiangiogenic drugs. Different [^{18}F] and [^{11}C] labeled MMP inhibitors have been synthesized and evaluated preclinically with mixed results (124). One of the more promising substances is based on a MMP inhibitor belonging to the family of *N*-sylfonylamino acid derivative. A [^{11}C] labeled analogue was synthesized, which showed favorable pharmacokinetics in mice and metabolic stability up to 30 minutes after injection (125). In murine tumor models, NIR optical imaging using fluorescent MMP substrates detected MMP activity in intact

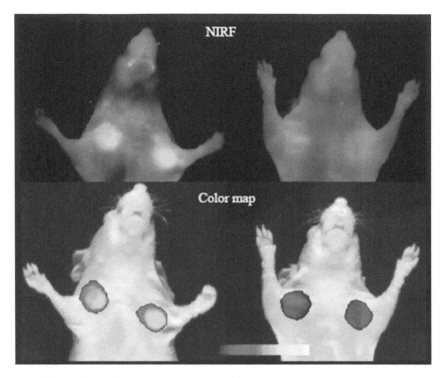

Figure 10 In vivo NIRF imaging of HT1080 tumor-bearing animals. The top row shows raw image acquisition obtained at 700-nm emission. Untreated animal on the left side, treated animal on the right side (150 mg/kg prinomastat, twice a day, i.p. for 2 days). The bottom row shows color-coded tumoral maps of MMP-2 activity superimposed onto white-light images [no treatment (*left*), prinomastat treatment (*right*)]. Note the decrease in signal intensity after therapy. *Abbreviations*: NIRF, near-infrared fluorescence; MMP, matrix metalloproteinase. *Source*: From Ref. 126 (*See Color Insert*).

tumors and could image the effect of MMP inhibition using the potent MMP inhibitor prinomastat (Fig. 10) (126). None of these compounds has been used in patient studies up to now.

VEGF and Its Receptors

The discovery of VEGFs as mediators of angiogenesis has stimulated interest in the use of VEGFs, VEGF receptors, and their complexes as antigens for the targeted delivery of imaging agents to the tumor neovasculature. However, the development of VEGF-based radiotracers is impaired by the fact that this fragile molecule is easily inactivated by conjugation with bifunctional chelators such as hydrazino nicotinate (HYNIC). A new approach has recently been presented by using a C-tagged, which could be successfully labeled with [^{99m}Tc]. The resulting compound [^{99m}Tc] HYNIC-VEGF could visualize murine mammary carcinoma models and uptake decreased during low-dose and high-dose chemotherapy (127). Whole-animal PET imaging studies with the human antibody VG76e that binds to VEGF, labeled with [^{124}I], showed high tumor-to-background ratios in VEGF overexpressing tumors (128). However, preliminary results in patients

with hepatic and pancreatic cancer and other solid tumors using radiolabeled VEGF165 and the VEGF antibody HuMV833 showed only very faint tumor uptake with very high activities in blood pool and in normal organs (129,130). Therefore, considerable improvements in the pharmacokinetic properties of these compounds have to be achieved before widespread use in patient trials.

Other Targets

There are many more molecular markers of angiogenesis, which have been labeled for molecular imaging in preclinical models, and even more possible targets, which have not yet been examined with molecular imaging. Two of these targets seem to be especially promising and warrant further evaluation as imaging markers of angiogenesis. One is magic roundabout (MR) or ROBO-4. Roundabouts are large transmembrane receptors for ligands known as slits. An endothelial-specific roundabout was discovered, which is highly restricted, as MR is absent from adult tissues except at sites of active angiogenesis, including tumors. This pattern of MR expression makes it ideally suited to vascular targeting (131). Biodistribution studies with radiolabeled ligands are eagerly awaited to assess the real potential of ROBO-4 as a target for imaging angiogenesis.

Other interesting targets are the tumor endothelial markers (TEMs) 1 to 8, which display elevated expression in endothelial cells isolated from colorectal carcinoma. Further studies showed that TEMs are also upregulated in endothelial cells undergoing physiological angiogenesis in humans and mice. TEM 5 belongs to a group of adhesion G-protein-coupled receptors (GPCRs), which are involved in cell-cell and cell-matrix interactions. It has recently been shown that a soluble fragment of TEM 5 (sTEM 5) is shed by endothelial cells upon activation by growth factors. When sTEM 5 is degraded by MMP 9, a cryptic RGD-containing binding site is revealed, which upon binding to $\alpha_v\beta_3$ mediates endothelial cell survival (132). Imaging studies with radiolabeled sTEM 5 are awaited in the near future.

OUTLOOK

A vast array of imaging techniques is available for assessment of angiogenesis on the functional level, as well as on a more specific molecular level. Whereas imaging of functional hemodyamic parameters like K^{trans}, blood flow, and blood volume is currently often used in the clinic for evaluation of antiangiogenic and cytotoxic chemotherapies, the role of molecular imaging strategies still has to be further evaluated in patient studies. Through the use of combined PET/CT scanners, the simultaneous acquisition of functional parameters by DCE CT and molecular parameters by PET with tracers like [^{18}F]Galacto-RGD in one examination is possible and will probably be more widely used in the future. Macromolecular MRI and CT contrast agents will become clinically available and will probably facilitate the assessment of hemodynamic parameters. Finally, by the introduction of combined PET/MR scanners for clinical use in the future, a thorough and complete assessment of the different aspects of angiogenesis at the functional and molecular level will hopefully become a reality and will be implemented in therapy planning and response evaluation as part of the concept of personalized medicine.

REFERENCES

1. Folkman J. Angiogenesis in cancer, vascular, rheumatoid and other disease. Nat Med 1995; 1:27–31.
2. Folkman J. Tumor angiogenesis: therapeutic implications. N Engl J Med 1971; 285:1182–1186.
3. Ribatti D, Vacca A, Dammacco, F. The role of the vascular phase in solid tumor growth: a historical review. Neoplasia 1999; 1:293–302.
4. Risau W. Mechanisms of angiogenesis. Nature 1997; 386:671–674.
5. Kerbel RS. Antiangiogenic therapy: a universal chemosensitization strategy for cancer? Science 2006; 312(5777):1171–1175.
6. Hurwitz H, Fehrenbacher L, Novotny W, et al. Bevacizumab plus irinotecan, fluorouracil, and leucovorin for metastatic colorectal cancer. N Engl J Med 2004; 350(23): 2335–2342.
7. Bergers G, Javaherian K, Lo KM, et al. Effects of angiogenesis inhibitors on multistage carcinogenesis in mice. Science 1999; 284:808–812.
8. Miller JC, Pien HH, Sahani D, et al. Imaging angiogenesis: applications and potential for drug development. J Natl Cancer Inst 2005; 97(3):172–187.
9. Jaffe CC. Measures of response: RECIST, WHO, and new alternatives. J Clin Oncol 2006; 24(20):3245–3251.
10. Tortora G, Melisi D, Ciardiello F. Angiogenesis: a target for cancer therapy. Curr Pharm Des 2004; 10(1):11–26.
11. Galbraith SM. Antivascular cancer treatments: imaging biomarkers in pharmaceutical drug development. Br J Radiol 2003; 76:83–86.
12. Pio BS, Park CK, Pietras R, et al. Usefulness of 3'-[F-18] fluoro-3'-deoxythymidine with positron emission tomography in predicting breast cancer response to therapy. Mol Imaging Biol 2006; 8:36–42.
13. Weber WA, Ott K, Becker K, et al. Prediction of response to preoperative chemotherapy in adenocarcinomas of the esophagogastric junction by metabolic imaging. J Clin Oncol 2001; 19:3058–3065.
14. Carmeliet P. Mechanisms of angiogenesis and arteriogenesis. Nat Med 2000; 6:389–395.
15. Auguste P, Lemiere S, Larrieu-Lahargue F. Molecular mechanisms of tumor vascularization. Crit Rev Oncol Hematol 2005; 54(1):53–61.
16. Holash J, Maisonpierre PC, Compton D, et al. Vessel cooption, regression, and growth in tumors mediated by angiopoietins and VEGF. Science 1999; 284:1994–1998.
17. Nguyen M. Angiogenic factors as tumor markers. Invest New Drugs 1997; 15:29–37.
18. Veikkola T, Karkkainen M, Claesson-Welsh L, et al. Regulation of angiogenesis via vascular endothelial growth factor receptors. Cancer Res 2000; 60:203–212.
19. Morabito A, De Maio E, Di Maio M, et al. Tyrosine kinase inhibitors of vascular endothelial growth factor receptors in clinical trials: current status and future directions. Oncologist 2006; 11(7):753–764.
20. Waltenberger J, Claesson-Welsh L, Siegbahn A, et al. Different signal transduction properties of KDR and Flt1, two receptors for vascular endothelial growth factor. J Biol Chem 1994; 269:26988–26995.
21. Landgren E, Schiller P, Cao Y, et al. Placenta growth factor stimulates MAP kinase and mitogenicity but not phospholipase C-gamma and migration of endothelial cells expressing Flt 1. Oncogene 1998; 16:359–367.
22. D'Angelo G, Struman I, Martial J, et al. Activation of mitogen-activated protein kinases by vascular endothelial growth factor and basic fibroblast growth factor in capillary endothelial cells is inhibited by the antiangiogenic factor 16-kDa N-terminal fragment of prolactin. Proc Natl Acad Sci U S A 1995; 92:6374–6378.

23. Nor JE, Christensen J, Mooney DJ, et al. Vascular endothelial growth factor (VEGF)-mediated angiogenesis is associated with enhanced endothelial cell survival and induction of Bcl-2 expression. Am J Pathol 1999; 154:375–384.

24. O'Connor DS, Schechner JS, Adida C, et al. Control of apoptosis during angiogenesis by survivin expression in endothelial cells. Am J Pathol 2000; 156:393–398.

25. Kim I, Kim HG, So JN, et al. Angiopoietin-1 regulates endothelial cell survival through the phosphatidylinositol 3′-kinase/Akt signal transduction pathway. Circ Res 2000; 86:24–29.

26. Paku S, Paweletz N. First steps of tumor-related angiogenesis. Lab Invest 1991; 65:334–346.

27. Pettersson A, Nagy JA, Brown L, et al. Heterogeneity of the angiogenic response induced in different normal adult tissues by vascular permeability factor/vascular endothelial growth factor. Lab Invest 2000; 80:99–115.

28. Djonov V, Schmid M, Tschanz SA, et al. Intussusceptive angiogenesis: its role in embryonic vascular network formation. Circ Res 2000; 86:286–292.

29. Patan S, Munn LL, Jain RK. Intussusceptive microvascular growth in a human colon adenocarcinoma xenograft: a novel mechanism of tumor angiogenesis. Microvasc Res 1996; 51:260–272.

30. Metzger RJ, Krasnow MA. Genetic control of branching morphogenesis. Science 1999; 284:1635–1639.

31. Ausprunk DH, Folkman J. Migration and proliferation of endothelial cells in preformed and newly formed blood vessels during tumor angiogenesis. Microvasc Res 1977; 14:53–65.

32. Pepper MS, Ferrara N, Orci L, et al. Vascular endothelial growth factor (VEGF) induces plasminogen activators and plasminogen activator inhibitor-1 in microvascular endothelial cells. Biochem Biophys Res Commun 1991; 181:902–906.

33. Denekamp J. Vascular attack as a therapeutic strategy for cancer. Cancer Metastasis Rev 1990; 9:267–282.

34. Zetter BR. Migration of capillary endothelial cells is stimulated by tumour-derived factors. Nature 1980; 285:41–59.

35. Asahara T, Chen D, Takahashi T, et al. Tie2 receptor ligands, angiopoietin-1 and angiopoietin-2, modulate VEGF-induced postnatal neovascularization. Circ Res 1998; 83:233–240.

36. Maisonpierre PC, Suri C, Jones PF, et al. Angiopoietin-2, a natural antagonist for Tie2 that disrupts in vivo angiogenesis. Science 1997; 277:55–60.

37. Friedlander M, Brooks PC, Shaffer RW, et al. Definition of two angiogenic pathways by distinct alpha v integrins. Science 1995; 270:1500–1502.

38. Brooks PC, Montgomery AM, Rosenfeld M, et al. Integrin alpha v beta 3 antagonists promote tumor regression by inducing apoptosis of angiogenic blood vessels. Cell 1994; 79:1157–1164.

39. Nelson AR, Fingleton B, Rothenberg ML, et al. Matrix metalloproteinases: biologic activity and clinical implications. J Clin Oncol 2000; 18:1135–1149.

40. Sang QX. Complex role of matrix metalloproteinases in angiogenesis. Cell Res 1998; 8:171–177.

41. Nangia-Makker P, Honjo Y, Sarvis R, et al. Galectin-3 induces endothelial cell morphogenesis and angiogenesis. Am J Pathol 2000; 156:899–909.

42. Gamble J, Meyer G, Noack L, et al. B1 integrin activation inhibits in vitro tube formation: effects on cell migration, vacuole coalescence and lumen formation. Endothelium 1999; 7:23–34.

43. Yang S, Graham J, Kahn JW, et al. Functional roles for PECAM-1 (CD31) and VEcadherin (CD144) in tube assembly and lumen formation in three-dimensional collagen gels. Am J Pathol 1999; 155:887–895.

44. Mousa SA, Mousa AS. Angiogenesis inhibitors: current and future directions. Curr Pharm Des 2004; 10:1–9.

45. Albo D, Wang TN, Tuszynski GP. Antiangiogenic therapy. Curr Pharm Des 2004; 10:27–37.

46. Morabito A, De Maio E, Di Maio M, et al. Tyrosine kinase inhibitors of vascular endothelial growth factor receptors in clinical trials: current status and future directions. Oncologist 2006; 11(7):753–764.

47. Brack SS, Dinkelborg L, Neri D. Molecular targeting of angiogenesis for imaging and therapy. Eur J Nucl Med Mol Imaging 2004; 31:1327–1341.

48. Daldrup-Link HE, Simon GH, Brasch RC. Imaging of tumor angiogenesis: current approaches and future prospects. Curr Pharm Des 2006; 12:2661–2672.

49. Haubner R, Wester HJ. Radiolabeled tracers for imaging of tumor angiogenesis and evaluation of anti-angiogenic therapies. Curr Pharm Des 2004; 10:1439–1455.

50. Jaffer FA, Weissleder R. Molecular imaging in the clinical arena. JAMA 2005; 293:855–862.

51. Weber WA. Positron emission tomography as an imaging biomarker. J Clin Oncol 2006; 24:3282–3292.

52. Matsumoto K, Kitamura K, Mizuta T, et al. Performance characteristics of a new 3-dimensional continuous-emission and spiral-transmission high sensitivity and high resolution PET camera evaluated with the NEMA NU 2-2001 standard. J Nucl Med 2006; 47:83–90.

53. Chatziioannou AF. Instrumentation for molecular imaging in preclinical research: micro-PET and micro-SPECT. Proc Am Thorac Soc 2005; 2:533–536.

54. Spuentrup E, Botnar RM. Coronary magnetic resonance imaging: visualization of vessel lumen and the vessel wall and molecular imaging of arteriotrombosis. Eur Radiol 2006; 16:1–14.

55. Jaffer FA, Weissleder R. Seeing within: molecular imaging of the cardiovascular system. Circ Res 2004; 94:433–445.

56. Simon GH, Fu Y, Berejnoi K, et al. Initial computed tomography imaging experience using a new macromolecular iodinated contrast medium in experimental breast cancer. Invest Radiol 2005; 40(9):614–620.

57. McDonald DM, Choyke PL. Imaging of angiogenesis: from microscope to clinic. Nat Med 2003; 9(6):713–725.

58. Ntziachristos V, Yodh A, Schnall M, et al. Concurrent MRI and diffuse optical tomography of breast after indocyanine green enhancement. Proc Natl Acad Sci U S A 2000; 97:2767–2772.

59. Cuccia DJ, Bevilacqua F, Durkin AJ, et al. In vivo quantification of optical contrast agent dynamics in rat tumors

by use of diffuse optical spectroscopy with magnetic resonance imaging coregistration. Appl Opt 2003; 42:2940–2950.

60. Bremer C, Bredow S, Mahmood U, et al. Optical imaging of matrix metalloproteinase-2 activity in tumors: feasibility study in a mouse model. Radiology 2001; 221:523–529.

61. Kothari M, Guermazi A, White D, et al. Imaging in antiangiogenesis trial: a clinical trials radiology perspective. Br J Radiol 2003; 76:92–96.

62. Suzuki A, Togawa T, Kuyama J, et al. Correlation between angiogenesis and reduction ratio measured using 201Tl chloride single photon emission computed tomography in patients with oral cavity squamous cell carcinoma. Ann Nucl Med 2004; 18(7):599–607.

63. Anderson RE. Cerebral blood flow xenon-133. Neurosurg Clin N Am 1996; 7:703–708.

64. Brooks DJ, Frackowiak RS, Lammertsma AA, et al. A comparison between regional cerebral blood flow measurements obtained in human subjects using 11C-methyl-albumin microspheres, the C15O2 steady-state method, and positron emission tomography. Acta Neurol Scand 1986; 73:415–422.

65. Schwaiger M, Muzik O. Assessment of myocardial perfusion by positron emission tomography. Am J Cardiol 1991; 67:35–43.

66. Okazawa H, Yonekura Y, Fujibayashi Y, et al. Measurement of regional cerebral blood flow with copper-62-PTSM and a three compartment model. J Nucl Med 1996; 37:1089–1093.

67. Saha GB, MacIntyre WJ, Go RT. Cyclotrons and positron emission tomography radiopharmaceuticals for clinical imaging. Semin Nucl Med 1992; 22:150–161.

68. Lammertsma AA, Jones T. Low oxygen extraction fraction in tumours measured with the oxygen-15 steady state technique: effect of tissue heterogeneity. Br J Radiol 1992; 65:697–700.

69. Blomqvist G, Lammertsma AA, Mazoyer B, et al. Effect of tissue heterogeneity on quantification in positron emission tomography. Eur J Nucl Med 1995; 22:652–663.

70. Wilson CB, Lammertsma AA, McKenzie CG, et al. Measurements of blood flow and exchanging water space in breast tumors using positron emission tomography: a rapid and noninvasive dynamic method. Cancer Res 1992; 52:1592–1597.

71. Anderson H, Price P. Clinical measurement of blood flow in tumours using positron emission tomography: a review. Nucl Med Commun 2002; 23:131–138.

72. Laking GR, Price PM. Positron emission tomographic imaging of angiogenesis and vascular function. Br J Radiol 2003; 76:50–59.

73. Tseng J, Dunnwald LK, Schubert EK, et al. 18F-FDG kinetics in locally advanced breast cancer: correlation with tumor blood flow and changes in response to neoadjuvant chemotherapy. J Nucl Med 2004; 45(11):1829–1837.

74. Arbab AS, Aoki S, Toyama K, et al. Quantitative measurement of regional cerebral blood flow with flow sensitive alternating inversion recovery imaging: comparison with [iodine123]-iodoamphetamin single photon emission CT. AJNR Am J Neuroradiol 2002; 23:381–388.

75. Neeman M, Dafni H, Bukhari O, et al. In vivo BOLD contrast MRI mapping of subcutaneous vascular function and maturation: validation by intravital microscopy. Magn Reson Med 2001; 45:887–898.

76. Baudelet C, Cron GO, Gallez B. Determination of the maturity and functionality of tumor vasculature by MRI: correlation between BOLD-MRI and DCE-MRI using P792 in experimental fibrosarcoma tumors. Magn Reson Med 2006; 56(5):1041–1049.

77. Gillard JH, Antoun NM, Burnet NG, et al. Reproducibility of quantitative CT perfusion imaging. Br J Radiol 2001; 74:552–555.

78. Gillard JH, Minhas P, Hayball MP, et al. Assessment of quantitative computed tomographic cerebral perfusion imaging with H215O positron emission tomography. Neurol Res 2000; 22:457–464.

79. Kidwell CS, Hsia AW. Imaging of the brain and cerebral vasculature in patients with suspected stroke: advantages and disadvantages of CT and MRI. Curr Neurol Neurosci Rep 2006; 6(1):9–16.

80. Goertz DE, Christopher DA, Yu JL, et al. High-frequency color flow imaging of the microcirculation. Ultrasound Med Biol 2000; 26:63–71.

81. Peters-Engl C, Medl M, Mirau M, et al. Color-coded and spectral Doppler flow in breast carcinomas—relationship with the tumour microvasculature. Breast Cancer Res Treat 1998; 47:83–89.

82. Cosgrove D. Angiogenesis imaging—ultrasound. Br J Radiol 2003; 76:43–49.

83. Anderson HL, Yap JT, Miller MP, et al. Assessment of pharmacodynamic vascular response in a phase I trial of combretastatin A4 phosphate. J Clin Oncol 2003; 21:2823–2830.

84. Hoffend J, Mier W, Schuhmacher J, et al. Gallium-68-DOTA-albumin as a PET blood pool marker: experimental evaluation in vivo. Nucl Med Biol 2005; 32:287–292.

85. Thakur ML, DeFulvio J, Tong J, et al. Evaluation of biological response modifiers in the enhancement of tumor uptake of technetium-99m labelled macromolecules. A preliminary report. J Immunol Methods 1992; 152:209–216.

86. Padhani AR. Dynamic contrast-enhanced MRI in clinical oncology: current status and future directions. J Magn Reson Imaging 2002; 16:407–422.

87. Turetschek K, Roberts TP, Floyd E, et al. Tumor microvascular characterization using ultrasmall superparamagnetic iron oxide particles (USPIO) in an experimental breast cancer model. J Magn Reson Imaging 2001; 13:882–888.

88. Montet X, Ntziachristos V, Grimm J, et al. Tomographic fluorescence mapping of tumor targets. Cancer Res 2005; 65(14):6330–6336.

89. Tofts PS, Brix G, Buckley DL, et al. Estimating kinetic parameters from dynamic contrast-enhanced T(1)-weighted MRI of a diffusable tracer: standardized quantities and symbols. J Magn Reson Imaging 1999; 10:223–232.

90. van Laarhoven HWM, Rijpkema M, Punt CJA, et al. Method for quantitation of dynamic contrast agent uptake in colorectal liver metastases. J Magn Reson Imaging 2003; 18:315–320.

91. Hylton N. Dynamic contrast-enhanced magnetic resonance imaging as an imaging biomarker. J Clin Oncol 2006; 24(20):3293–3298.

92. Galbraith SM, Lodge MA, Taylor NJ, et al. Reproducibility of dynamic contrast-enhanced MRI in human muscle and tumours: comparison of quantitative and semiquantitative analysis. NMR Biomed 2002; 15:132–142.

93. Padhani AR, Hayes C, Landau S, et al. Reproducibility of quantitative dynamic MRI of normal human tissues. NMR Biomed 2002; 15:143–153.

94. Oshida K, Nagashima T, Ueda T, et al. Pharmacokinetic analysis of ductal carcinoma in situ of the breast using dynamic MR mammography. Eur Radiol 2005; 15: 1353–1360.

95. Padhani AR, Gapinski CJ, Macvicar DA, et al. Dynamic contrast enhanced MRI of prostate cancer: correlation with morphology and tumour stage, histological grade and PSA. Clin Radiol 2000; 55:99–109.

96. Schlemmer HP, Merkle J, Grobholz R, et al. Can preoperative contrast-enhanced dynamic MR imaging for prostate cancer predict microvessel density in prostatectomy specimens? Eur Radiol 2004; 14:309–317.

97. Hara N, Okuizumi M, Koike H, et al. Dynamic contrast-enhanced magnetic resonance imaging (DCE-MRI) is a useful modality for the precise detection and staging of early prostate cancer. Prostate 2005; 62:140–147.

98. Hawighorst H, Knapstein PG, Weikel W, et al. Angiogenesis of uterine cervical carcinoma: characterization by pharmacokinetic magnetic resonance parameters and histological microvessel density with correlation to lymphatic involvement. Cancer Res 1997; 57:4777–4786.

99. Hawighorst H, Knapstein PG, Knopp MV, et al. Cervical carcinoma: standard and pharmacokinetic analysis of time-intensity curves for assessment of tumor angiogenesis and patient survival. MAGMA 1999; 8:55–62.

100. O'Donnell A, Padhani A, Hayes C, et al. A phase I study of the angiogenesis inhibitor SU5416 (semaxanib) in solid tumours, incorporating dynamic contrast MR pharmacodynamic end points. Br J Cancer 2005; 93:876–883.

101. Wedam SB, Low JA, Yang SX, et al. Antiangiogenic and antitumor effects of bevacizumab in inflammatory and locally advanced breast cancer patients. J Clin Oncol 2006; 24:769–777.

102. Morgan B, Thomas AL, Drevs J, et al. Dynamic contrast-enhanced magnetic resonance imaging as a biomarker for the pharmacological response of PTK787/ZK 222584, an inhibitor of the vascular endothelial growth factor receptor tyrosine kinases, in patients with advanced colorectal cancer and liver metastases: results from two phase I studies. J Clin Oncol 2003; 21:3955–3964.

103. Haubner R, Weber WA, Beer AJ, et al. Non-invasive visualization of the activated αvβ3 integrin in cancer patients by positron emission tomography and [18F]Galacto-RGD. PLoS Medicine 2005; 2:e70.

104. Bach-Gansmo T, Danielsson R, Saracco A, et al. Integrin receptor imaging of breast cancer: a proof-of-concept study to evaluate 99mTc-NC100692. J Nucl Med 2006; 47(9):1434–1439.

105. Ruoslahti E, Pierschbacher MD. New perspectives in cell adhesion: RGD and integrins. Science 1987; 238(4826): 491–497.

106. Haubner R, Finsinger D, Kessler H. Stereoisomeric peptide libraries and peptidomimetics for designing selective inhibitors of the αvβ3 integrin for a new cancer therapy. Angew Chem Int Ed Engl 1997; 36:1374–1389.

107. Haubner R, Wester HJ, Reuning U, et al. Radiolabeled αvβ3 integrin antagonists: a new class of tracers for tumor targeting. J Nucl Med 1999; 40:1061–1071.

108. Haubner R, Wester HJ, Weber WA, et al. Noninvasive imaging of αvβ3 integrin expression using 18F-labeled RGD-containing glycopeptide and positron emission tomography. Cancer Res 2001; 61:1781–1785.

109. Haubner R. αvβ3-Integrin imaging: a new approach to characterise angiogenesis? Eur J Nucl Med Mol Imaging 2006; 33:54–63.

110. Harris JM, Martin NE, Modi M. Pegylation: a novel process for modifying pharmacokinetics. Clin Pharmacokinet 2001; 40:539–551.

111. Chen X, Park R, Shahinian AH, et al. Pharmacokinetics and tumor retention of 125I-labeled RGD peptide are improved by PEGylation. Nucl Med Biol 2004; 31:11–19.

112. van Hagen PM, Breeman WA, Bernard HF, et al. Evaluation of a radiolabelled cyclic DTPA-RGD analogue for tumour imaging and radionuclide therapy. Int J Cancer 2000; 90:186–198.

113. Janssen MLH, Oyen WJG, Massuger LFAG, et al. Comparison of a monomeric and dimeric radiolabeled RGD-peptide for tumor imaging. Cancer Biother Radiopharm 2002; 17:641–646.

114. Chen X, Conti PS, Moats RA. In vivo near-infrared fluorescence imaging of integrin alphavbeta3 in brain tumor xenografts. Cancer Res 2004; 64(21):8009–8014.

115. Winter PM, Caruthers SD, Kassner A, et al. Molecular imaging of angiogenesis in nascent Vx-2 rabbit tumors using a novel alpha(nu)beta3-targeted nanoparticle and 1.5 tesla magnetic resonance imaging. Cancer Res 2003; 63(18):5838–5843.

116. Montet X, Montet-Abou K, Reynolds F, et al. Nanoparticle imaging of integrins on tumor cells. Neoplasia 2006; 8(3):214–222.

117. Ellegala DB, Leong-Poi H, Carpenter JE, et al. Imaging tumor angiogenesis with contrast ultrasound and microbubbles targeted to alpha(v)beta3. Circulation 2003; 108(3): 336–341.

118. Beer AJ, Haubner R, Goebel M, et al. Biodistribution and pharmacokinetics of the αvβ3 selective tracer 18F Galacto-RGD in cancer patients. J Nucl Med 2005; 46:1333–1341.

119. Beer AJ, Haubner R, Wolf I, et al. PET-based human dosimetry of 18F-galacto-RGD, a new radiotracer for imaging alpha v beta3 expression. J Nucl Med 2006; 47:763–769.

120. Beer AJ, Haubner R, Sarbia M, et al. Positron emission tomography using [18F]Galacto-RGD identifies the level of integrin {alpha}v{beta}3 expression in man. Clin Cancer Res 2006; 12:3942–3949.

121. Neri D, Carnemolla B, Nissim A, et al. Targeting by affinity matured recombinant antibody fragments of an angiogenesis associated fibronectin isoform. Nat Biotechnol 1997; 15:1271–1275.

122. Santimaria M, Moscatelli G, Viale GL, et al. Immunoscintigraphic detection of the ED-B domain of fibronectin, a marker of angiogenesis, in patients with cancer. Clin Cancer Res 2003; 9:571–579.

123. Hidalgo M, Eckhardt SG. Development of matrix metalloproteinase inhibitors in cancer therapy. J Natl Cancer Inst 2001; 93(3):178–193.

124. Furumoto S, Takashima K, Kubota K, et al. Tumor detection using 18F-labeled matrix metalloproteinase-2 inhibitor. Nucl Med Biol 2003; 30(2):119–125.

125. Fei X, Zheng QH, Liu X, et al. Synthesis of radiolabeled biphenylsulfonamide matrix metalloproteinase inhibitors as new potential PET cancer imaging agents. Bioorg Med Chem Lett 2003; 13(13):2217–2222.

126. Bremer C, Tung CH, Weissleder R. In vivo molecular target assessment of matrix metalloproteinase inhibition. Nat Med 2001; 7(6):743–748.

127. Blankenberg FG, Backer MV, Levashova Z, et al. In vivo tumor angiogenesis imaging with site-specific labeled (99m)Tc-HYNIC-VEGF. Eur J Nucl Med Mol Imaging 2006; 33(7):841–848.

128. Collingridge DR, Carroll VA, Glaser M, et al. The development of [(124)I]iodinated-VG76e: a novel tracer for imaging vascular endothelial growth factor in vivo using positron emission tomography. Cancer Res 2002; 62(20):5912–5919.

129. Li S, Peck-Radosavljevic M, Kienast O, et al. Imaging gastrointestinal tumours using vascular endothelial growth factor-165 (VEGF165) receptor scintigraphy. Ann Oncol 2003; 14:1274–1277.

130. Jayson GC, Zweit J, Jackson A, et al. Molecular imaging and biological evaluation of HuMV833 anti-VEGF antibody: implications for trial design of antiangiogenic antibodies. J Natl Cancer Inst 2002; 94(19):1484–1493.

131. Huminiecki L, Gorn M, Suchting S, et al. Magic roundabout is a new member of the roundabout receptor family that is endothelial specific and expressed at sites of active angiogenesis. Genomics 2002; 79:547–552.

132. Vallon M, Essler M. Proteolytically processed soluble tumor endothelial marker (TEM) 5 mediates endothelial cell survival during angiogenesis by linking integrin alpha v beta 3 to glycosaminoglycans. J Biol Chem 2006; 281(45):34179–34188.

30

Imaging Apoptosis

T. Z. BELHOCINE
Department of Diagnostic Radiology and Nuclear Medicine, St. Joseph's Hospital, London, Ontario, Canada

INTRODUCTION

A better understanding of carcinogenesis and tumor responsiveness to various anticancer therapies highlighted the importance of programmed cell death also called *apoptosis* (1,2). Inherited or acquired molecular alterations involving the apoptotic cascade have been documented in many cancer models (3,4). Accordingly, specific therapies are being developed to target one of the strategic checkpoints in the apoptotic signaling pathways (5,6). Conventional response criteria in solid tumors (RECIST criteria) based on morphological tumor changes cannot assess the biological effect of new therapies at the molecular level (7,8). Hence, there is a tremendous need for the introduction of biological criteria into the multiphase assessment of cancer as advocated by the National Institutes of Health (NIH), the Food and Drug Administration (FDA), and the European Organization for Research and Treatment of Cancer (EORTC) clinical trial cooperative group (9–11). This goal may be achieved in translational research by bridging basic sciences into clinical setting with the use of biotechnologies for a better assessment of cancer from genotype to phenotype (12–14). Accordingly, a new tracer was designed in nuclear medicine for the noninvasive imaging of apoptosis in preclinical and clinical research (15,16). Even though the imaging of apoptosis is still in the course of clinical validation, a large body of literature emphasized the perspectives opened by the radiolabeled annexin A5 as a biomarker of apoptotic changes in various oncological models (17,18).

THE APOPTOTIC MACHINERY

Despite the complexity of the apoptotic machinery, a number of molecules and intracellular elements have been well identified in the course of programmed cell death. Among them, cell death receptors (CD95 or IL-1), caspases-8, -9, -3, and mitochondria have been shown to play a key role from the initiation phase to the effective phase of apoptosis (1,2,4). In response to various stimuli, the apoptotic cascade is set up as a regulation system aimed at maintaining vital functions such as embryogenesis, homeostasis, and immunity (19,20). A contrario, a deficit of apoptosis is one of the hallmarks of cancers (21). Figure 1 illustrates current knowledge on the apoptotic pathways in a model of non–small cell lung cancer.

RADIOLABELED ANNEXIN A5

Mechanisms of Uptake

The externalization of phosphatidylserine (PS) from the inner leaflet to the outer leaflet of membrane cells undergoing programmed cell death has been used as a

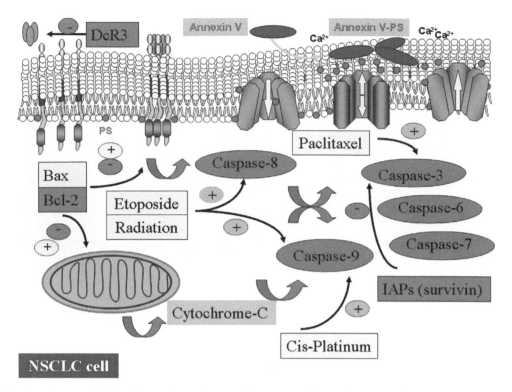

Figure 1 Activation of apoptotic signaling pathways in sensitive tumor cells. In the apoptotic cascade, key enzymes also called *caspases* (cysteinyl aspartate specific proteinases) are involved from the initiation phase (caspase-8 and caspase-9) to the effective phase (caspase-3, caspase-6, and caspase-7). In normal conditions, proapoptotic genes (Bax family) and antiapoptotic genes (Bcl-2 family) play a key role to maintain cell homeostasis. In a model of non–small cell lung cancer, cytotoxic drugs and radiation therapy have been shown to act by targeting different apoptotic signaling pathways. For instance, etoposide and cisplatin activate caspase-8 and caspase-9, respectively. Radiation therapy mainly acts on the capsase-9. On the other hand, paclitaxel directly activates caspase-3. Following the caspase activation, PS is exposed on the outer leaflet of the cell membrane and specifically binds to the annexin A5 in presence of Ca^{2+} ions; this early membrane event is a signal for removal of apoptotic bodies by activated macrophages. *Abbreviation*: PS, phosphatidylserine.

molecular target for the in vivo imaging of apoptosis. This early event in the apoptotic cascade occurs within 90 to 120 minutes after caspase activation, before membrane blebbing and DNA degradation (22).

Tracer Characteristics

The annexin A5 is a 36-kDa serum protein including 320 amino acids that binds specifically to the exposed PS in presence of calcium ions (23–25). This nanomolar affinity between annexin A5 and PS has been shown to be a specific signal for the phagocytosis of apoptotic bodies by macrophages (26).

Many attempts for the radiolabeling of annexin A5 have been experimented in vitro and in vivo with variable results (18,27,28). The most used radiolabeled form of annexin in preclinical and clinical settings has been the annexin A5 radiolabeled with [99mTc]-technetium, using the hydrazinonicotinamide (HYNIC) compound as linker (29). A recombinant human form of annexin A5

(rh-annexin A5) radiolabeled with 99mTc has been recently designed for clinical research purposes (30).

IMAGING OF APOPTOSIS

The radiolabeled annexin A5 has been shown to localize in normal and pathological structures. In oncology patients, increased uptake of radiolabeled annexin A5 within tumor sites was documented before and/or after therapy.

Normal Uptake Patterns

Biodistribution and dosimetry studies performed on healthy subjects with 99mTc-HYNIC-annexin A5 typically showed normal tracer uptake in the liver, the spleen, the kidneys, and the bladder (31). This physiological uptake pattern was consistent with protein biodistribution (Fig. 2). In the kidneys, increased tracer uptake was also

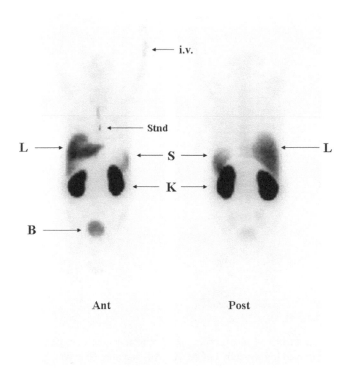

Figure 2 Normal distribution with ^{99m}Tc-HYNIC-annexin A5. Increased ^{99m}Tc-HYNIC-annexin A5 uptake is commonly observed in the liver, the spleen, the kidneys, and the bladder. No tracer uptake is noted in the bowels. *Abbreviations*: Stnd, standard used for tracer uptake quantification; i.v., intravenous injection. *Source*: Phase II/III study, North American Scientific 2020, Antwerp, Belgium.

related to the nephron PS–annexin A5 binding (15). Unlike ^{99m}Tc-BTAP-annexin A5, no tracer uptake was detected in the bowels with ^{99m}Tc-HYNIC-annexin A5 (32).

Spontaneous Apoptosis

A few number of oncology patients explored with the radiolabeled annexin A5 presented with increased tracer uptake within tumor sites immediately before the first course of chemotherapy and/or radiotherapy (16,33,34). Similarly, a faint tracer uptake was inconstantly observed in the salivary glands and the bone marrow (35). This imaging uptake pattern has been correlated to a certain degree of spontaneous apoptosis.

Induced Apoptosis

In oncology patients enrolled in clinical trials, increased uptake of radiolabeled annexin A5 was documented following naïve chemotherapy and/or radiation therapy (16,36–40). Comparative analyses between pretreatment and posttreatment annexin A5 studies revealed a significant

tracer uptake at tumor sites (i.e., primary tumor, lymph node metastases, bone metastases) as well as at nontumor sites (i.e., salivary glands, bone marrow). This annexin A5 uptake pattern was strongly consistent with a therapy-induced apoptosis (Fig. 3).

In summary, the annexin A5 imaging has the ability to detect an apoptotic signal, either spontaneous apoptosis or induced apoptosis, in normal and abnormal structures. Importantly, the radiolabeled annexin A5 uptake in normal and pathological structures was best detected by means of single-photon emission computed tomography (SPECT) and SPECT-CT fusion (17,34,38).

ONCOLOGICAL MODELS

Preclinical Applications

A large corpus of literature is nowadays available on the preclinical use of the radiolabeled annexin A5, particularly on animal models (41). For instance, the imaging of apoptosis with the radiolabeled annexin A5 was used to document qualitatively and quantitatively the proapoptotic effects of various cytotoxic drugs as early as 24 hours after treatment; examples include cyclophosphamide, cyclopentenylcytosine, paclitaxel, gemcitabine, doxorubicin, cycloheximide, and methylprednisolone (42–52). Similarly, apoptotic changes following radiation therapy have been documented with the radiolabeled annexin A5 on experimental and animal models (53). In these preclinical models, ^{99m}Tc-radiolabeled annexin A5 was most often used for the imaging of apoptosis and proofs of principles were obtained by means of histopathological correlations (TUNEL method, caspase-3 staining) and autoradiography studies (Fig. 4).

Table 1 summarizes current data on the use of radiolabeled annexin A5 on preclinical cancer models.

Clinical Applications

Although the radiolabeled annexin A5 is still in the process of clinical validation, the imaging of apoptosis by means of a noninvasive scintigraphy opens promising avenues for the assessment of treated and untreated cancers (54,55). In clinical research, emphasis was made on the annexin A5 applications in lung cancers, lymphomas, breast cancers, soft tissue sarcomas, and head and neck cancers (16,17,33–39). Available data from literature indicate the feasibility of radiolabeled annexin A5 to document apoptotic changes as early as 24 to 48 hours following the first course of chemotherapy. Increased uptake of ^{99m}Tc–annexin A5 into tumor sites was induced by various cytotoxic drugs such as mitomycin, ifosfamide, cisplatin, vepeside, cyclophosphamide, doxorubicin,

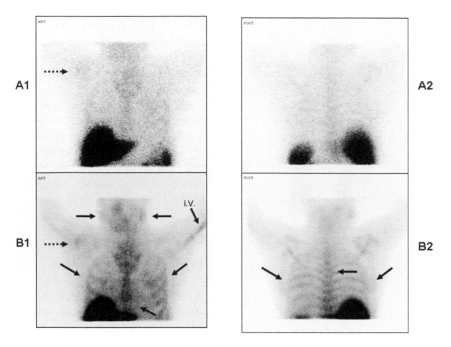

Figure 3 Radiolabeled annexin A5 uptake patterns. A patient with a non–small cell lung cancer and a right humerus metastasis was scheduled for a cisplatin-based chemotherapy. Annexin A5 imaging was performed immediately before (**A1**, **A2**) and after (**B1**, **B2**) the first course of chemotherapy. On planar views, baseline and posttherapy images showed increased tracer uptake in the liver and the spleen. After treatment, a significant tracer uptake was noted in the bone marrow (ribs, sternum, spine) and the salivary glands (*arrows*). A faint tracer uptake was detected in the right humerus head, which increased after treatment (*dashed arrow*). This uptake pattern was strongly suggestive of spontaneous apoptosis and induced apoptosis in normal and tumoral structures, respectively. *Source*: Phase II/III study, North American Scientific 2020, Antwerp, Belgium.

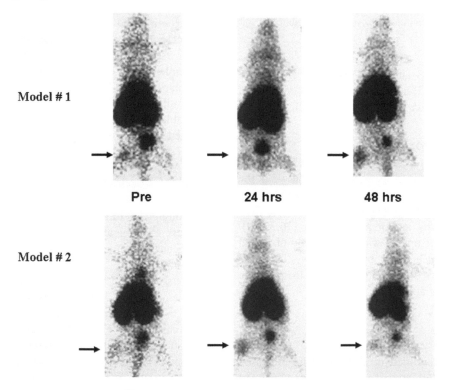

Figure 4 Preclinical imaging of apoptosis with ^{99m}Tc-HYNIC-annexin A5. A murine model of malignant melanoma (right flank) treated with doxorubicin. Assessment of treatment-induced apoptosis with ^{99m}Tc-HYNIC-annexin A5 at 24 hours and 48 hours compared to baseline. The model # 1 showed a significant increase of ^{99m}Tc-HYNIC-annexin A5 uptake 48 hours posttreatment (*arrows*), while the model # 2 presented with an increased tracer uptake 24 hours posttreatment (*arrows*). *Source*: Courtesy of Prof. F.G. Blankenberg, UCLA, Palo Alto, U.S.A.

Table 1 Imaging of Apoptosis on Oncological Models—Preclinical Data

Authors (references)	Animal models
Bennink et al. (48)	Cardiotoxicity induced by doxorubicin
Blankenberg et al. (43)	Intramedullary and splenic apoptosis induced by cyclophosphamide
Mochizuki et al. (47)	Lymphoma cell lines treated by cyclophosphamide
Lee et al. (45)	Lung cancer cell lines treated by gamma irradiation
Yang et al. (70)	Breast cancer cell lines treated by radiation and paclitaxel
Ke et al. (46)	Breast cancer cell lines treated by Taxol
Erba et al. (49)	Breast cancer cell lines treated by Taxol
Kuge et al. (44)	Hepatoma cell lines treated by cyclophosphamide
Takei et al. (42)	Hepatoma cell lines treated by gemcitabine
Yagle et al. (78)	Liver apoptosis treated by cycloheximide
Wang et al. (50)	Sarcoma cell lines treated by cyclophosphamide
Kumar et al. (51)	Thymoma cell lines treated by cyclophosphamide and radiation

Table 2 Imaging of Apoptosis on Oncological Models—Clinical Data

Authors (references)	N	Oncological models
Belhocine et al. (16)	15	NSCLC, SCLC, BC, NHL, HL treated by chemotherapy
Steinmetz et al. (36)	24	NSCLC, SCLC treated by chemotherapy
Van de Wiele et al. (39)	20	Primary staging of HNC treated by surgery
Vermeersch et al. (34)	18	Primary staging of HNC treated by surgery
Haas et al. (40)	11	Follicular lymphoma treated by radiation therapy
Kartachova et al. (38)	33	NHL, HL, Leukemia, NSCLC, HNC treated by radiation therapy and/or chemotherapy
Kartachova et al. (90)	16	NSCLC treated by chemotherapy
Rottey et al. (91)	23	HNC, SCLC, EC, BC, BLC, YSC, TTC, M, CUP, RCC, before radiotherapy and/or chemotherapy

Abbreviations: NSCLC, non–small cell lung cancer; SCLC, small cell lung cancer; BC, breast cancer; NHL, non-Hodgkin's lymphoma; HL, Hodgkin's lymphoma; HNC, head and neck cancer; EC, esophageal cancer; BLC, bladder cancer; YSC, Yolc sac tumour; TTC, teratocarcinoma; M, melanoma; CUP, cancer of unknown primary; RCC, renal cell carcinoma.

vincristine, prednisone, melphalan, cyclolal, adriamycine, bleomycin, carboplatin, and taxane. Similar results were also observed after radiation therapy (40). Interestingly enough, increased uptake of radiolabeled annexin A5 was also detected at tumor sites prior to any therapy (33–35). These different annexin A5 uptake patterns were correlated with partial or complete tumor response by using cytopathological gold standards or radiological RECIST criteria (41). Table 2 summarizes current data on the use of radiolabeled annexin A5 on clinical cancer models.

In oncology patients scheduled for conventional or new therapies, the imaging of apoptosis may be of particular clinical value for evaluating "the apoptotic reserve" in terms of spontaneous and induced apoptosis (6,56,57). The efficacy of many drugs relies on their ability to initiate apoptosis in sensitive tumor cells, which may be timely monitored by the radiolabeled annexin A5. Moreover, the early evaluation of tumor response to proapoptotic treatments (i.e., 2 to 3 days post chemotherapy or radiotherapy) may help reorient treatment strategies in patients with no evidence of induced apoptosis. Such an approach may avoid the costs and the side effects of heavy but ineffective therapeutic regimens. Figures 5 and 6 illustrate a negative study and a positive study with ^{99m}Tc-HYNIC-annexin A5, respectively. Figure 7 shows the potential of early annexin A5 imaging for predicting tumor response to chemotherapy.

Another field of clinical interest is the assessment of treatment-induced apoptosis in normal structures, especially in the salivary glands and the bone marrow (56–59). Because the chemotherapy and/or the radiation-induced toxicity is often the limiting factor for repeating and/or escalating doses, the accurate evaluation of apoptotic effects early after the first treatment, before a new course of chemoradiation, and then sequentially in the course of follow-up may help adjust the treatment-effect doses (35).

LIMITATIONS AND PERSPECTIVES

The merging of radiolabeled annexin A5 as a potential apoptosis tracer has raised considerable hopes for the noninvasive imaging of cell death (18,54). However, this new tracer requires further technical improvements in terms of signal-to-background ratio (28). Also important in clinical setting is the optimal timing for the imaging of apoptosis, which is a brief and transient phenomenon (42,60–62).

From this perspective, various isotopes (i.e., ^{18}F, ^{11}C, ^{68}Ga, ^{123}I, ^{124}I, ^{125}I, ^{111}In), different linkers (i.e., BTAP, IMB, EC, HYNIC, DOTA, MAG$_3$, PEG-DTPA), structurally modified annexins (i.e., annexin A117, annexin A128,

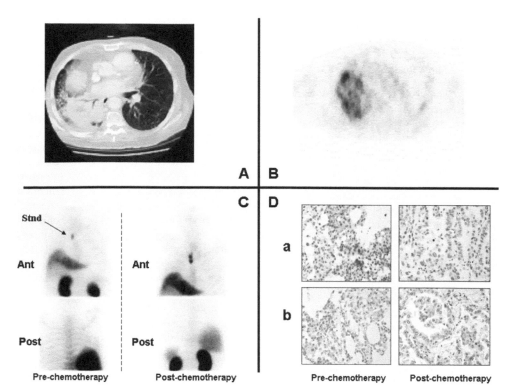

Figure 5 A negative study with ^{99m}Tc-HYNIC-rh-annexin. (Panel **A** and **B**) Conventional workup. A 77-year-old man with a stage IV non–small cell lung cancer underwent a pretreatment staging workup. A thoracic CT scan showed a large right lung tumor (**A**), which presented with an intense ^{18}FDG uptake on PET (**B**). (Panel **C**) Annexin A5 imaging. On annexin A5 images, no significant tracer uptake was detected within the lung tumor following the first course of chemotherapy when compared to baseline. This annexin A5 image pattern was suggestive of poor apoptotic tumor changes posttherapy. Pretreatment (day −2 and day −1) and posttreatment (day +1 and day +2) images were obtained at 4-hour and 24-hour posttracer injection. (Panel **D**) Pathological correlations. Pathologic analyses performed on the initial tumor biopsy (pretreatment) and after autopsy (posttreatment) revealed a low rate of spontaneous and induced apoptosis. No significant changes in the AI were observed before (AI = 0.5%) and after treatment (AI = 0.5%). TUNEL staining and caspase-3 immunostaining obtained on a tumor biopsy (a) and autopsy samples (b). *Abbreviations*: AI, apoptotic indices; TUNEL, terminal deoxyribonucleotidyl transferase-mediated dUTP nick end labeling (*See Color Insert*).

mini-annexin A5), and diverse radiolabeling methods (direct, indirect, pretargeting steps, site-specific targeting) have been tested in the few recent years (27,30–32,46,63–84). Further basic and clinical research studies are needed to select the most appropriate technique for the imaging of programmed cell death, particularly in terms of short or long-lived SPECT isotopes versus novel forms of annexin A5 versus PET-based annexin A5 (28,61).

Additionally, a better knowledge of the apoptotic phenomenon in treated and untreated cancers appears critical for designing appropriate research models and then translating the complexity of apoptosis into clinically suitable images.

Last but not least, the recent development of hybrid cameras, including SPECT-CT and PET-CT devices, may improve the annexin A5 imaging in terms of sensitivity and contrast resolution (85–89). Not only combined imaging provides exquisite anatomic and functional fused images in a "one-stop shop," it may also improve the quality of radiolabeled annexin A5 images by applying

dedicated iterative reconstruction algorithms aimed at correcting for image degrading factors, including attenuation correction, scatter correction, resolution recovery, and noise filters. In addition to a qualitative (visual) interpretation, standardized uptake values scores (SUV) dedicated to the annexin V hybrid imaging will be useful for a simple, reproducible, and standardized semi-quantification of apoptotic changes within tumor and non-tumor sites (39,90–93).

CONCLUSION

In many oncological models, the in vivo imaging of apoptosis is feasible with the radiolabeled annexin A5. This dedicated tracer may play a critical role for early prediction of tumor responsiveness; it may also help assess treatment-induced apoptosis into normal organs. As such, this new apoptosis agent is a valuable tool in preclinical and clinical research. Its implementation in

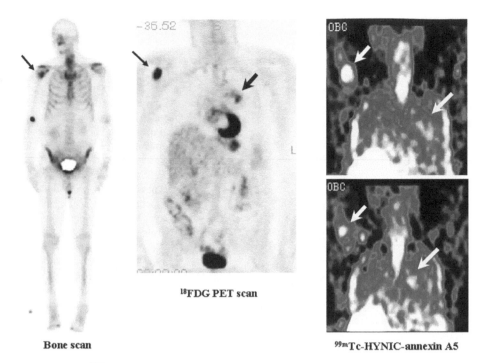

Bone scan　　　　　**¹⁸FDG PET scan**　　　　　**⁹⁹ᵐTc-HYNIC-annexin A5**

Figure 6 A positive study with ⁹⁹ᵐTc-HYNIC-rh-annexin. A 70-year-old man with a stage IV non–small cell lung cancer had a complete imaging workup before treatment. Left panel: Whole-body bone scan revealed an abnormal focus in the right humerus head (*small arrow*), which was strongly suspicious of bone metastasis. Middle panel: Whole-body PET confirmed the presence of an intense ¹⁸FDG-avid focus in the same bone localization (*small arrow*). In addition, a left lung tumor was clearly detected in the paramediastinal region (*large arrow*). Right panel: Immediately after the first course of chemotherapy (+24 hours), the annexin A5 imaging was performed for early prediction of tumor responsiveness. SPECT data showed increased tracer uptake in the right humerus, which corresponded to the documented bone metastasis (*large arrows*). In addition, a moderate but significant tracer uptake was asymmetrically detected in the left chest at the level of the primary lung tumor (*small arrows*). This uptake pattern was suggestive of significant apoptosis changes within both tumor sites including the primary lung tumor and its bone metastasis.

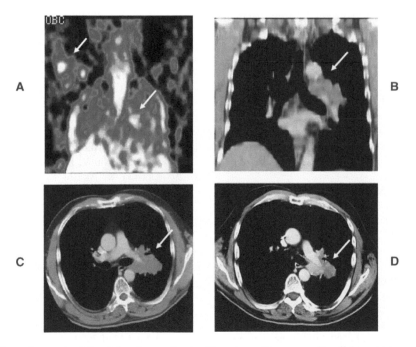

Figure 7 Predictive value of annexin A5 uptake. In a patient with a stage IV non–small cell lung cancer, the annexin A5 imaging revealed increased tracer uptake as early as 24 hours after the first course of chemotherapy within the left lung primary tumor and the right humerus metastasis (**A** and **B**; *arrows*). The CT evaluation performed one month after two courses of cisplatin-based chemotherapy showed a reduction of the lung tumor maximum diameter from 7.5 cm (**C**) to 6.5 cm (**D**), which was consistent with an apoptotic tumor response.

daily routine, however, will require further technical optimization and more clinical experience. The recent advent of hybrid imaging in nuclear oncology may timely prompt the refinement of the annexin A5 imaging for the noninvasive detection of cell death.

REFERENCES

1. Kerr JFR, Winterford CM, Harmon BV. Apoptosis—its significance in cancer and cancer therapy. Cancer 1994; 73(2):2013–2026.
2. Reed JC. Dysregulation of apoptosis in cancer. J Clin Oncol 1999; 17(9):2941–2953.
3. Hainault P, Hollstein M. p53 and human cancer: the first ten thousands mutations. Adv Cancer Res 2000; 77:81–137.
4. Reed JC. Regulation of apoptosis by bcl-2 family proteins and its role in cancer and chemoresistance. Curr Opin Oncol 1995; 7:541–546.
5. Los M, Burek CJ, Stroh C, et al. Anticancer drugs of tomorrow: apoptotic pathways as targets for drug design. Drug Discov Today 2003; 8:67–77.
6. Kaufmann SH, Earnshaw WC. Induction of apoptosis by cancer chemotherapy. Exp Cell Res 2000; 256:42–49.
7. Therasse P, Arbuck SG, Eisenhauer EA, et al. New guidelines to evaluate response to treatment in solid tumors. J Natl Cancer Inst 2000; 92:205–216.
8. Fox E, Curt GA, Balis FM. Clinical trial design for target-based therapy. Oncologist 2002; 7:401–407.
9. Biomarkers and surrogate endpoints: advancing clinical research and applications. Sponsored by the National Institutes of Health and Food and Drug Administration at Natcher Conference Center, Bethesda, MD, April 15–16, 1999
10. Zerhouni E. The NIH Roadmap. Science 2003; 302:63–72. Available at: http://nihroadmap.nih.gov.
11. Lehmann F, Lacombe D, Therasse P, et al. Integration of translational research in the european organization for research and treatment of cancer research (EORTC) clinical trial cooperative group mechanisms. J Transl Med 2003; 1:2. Available at: http://www.translational-medicine.com/content/1/1/2.
12. Sonntag KC. Implementations of translational medicine. J Transl Med 2005; 3:33. Available at: http://www.translational-medicine.com/content/3/1/33.
13. Workman P, Kaye SB. Translating basic cancer research into new cancer therapeutics. Trends Mol Med 2002; 4(suppl):S1–S9.
14. Colburn WA. Optimizing the use of biomarkers, surrogate endpoints, and clinical endpoints for more efficient drug development. J Clin Pharmacol 2000; 40:1419–1427.
15. Blankenberg FG, Katsikis PD, Tait JF, et al. In vivo detection and imaging of phosphatidylserine expression during programmed cell death. Proc Natl Acad Sc U S A 1998; 95:6349–6354.
16. Belhocine TZ, Steinmetz N, Hustinx R, et al. Increased uptake of the apoptosis-imaging agent (99m)Tc recombinant human annexin V in human tumors after one course of chemotherapy as a predictor of tumor response and patient prognosis. Clin Cancer Res 2002; 8:2766–2774.
17. Green AM, Steinmetz MD. Monitoring apoptosis in real time. Cancer J 2002; 8:82–92.
18. Boersma HH, Kietselaer BL, Stolk LM, et al. Past, present, and future of annexin A5: from protein discovery to clinical applications. J Nucl Med 2005; 46(12):2035–2050 (review).
19. Kerr JF, Wyllie AH, Currie AR. Apoptosis: a basic biological phenomenon with wide-ranging implications in tissue kinetics. Br J Cancer 1972; 26:239–257.
20. Hetts SW. To die or not to die: an overview of apoptosis and its role in disease. JAMA 1998; 279:300–307.
21. Israels LG, Israels ED. Apoptosis. Oncologist 1999; 4:332–339.
22. Martin SJ, Reutelingsperger CP, McGahon AJ, et al. Early redistribution of plasma membrane phosphatidylserine is a general feature of apoptosis regardless of the initiating stimulus: inhibition by over expression of Bcl-2 and Abl. J Exp Med 1995; 182:1545–1556.
23. Reutelingsperger CPM. Annexins: key regulators of haemostasis, thrombosis, and apoptosis. Thromb Haemost 2001; 86:413–419.
24. Huber R, Berendes R, Burger A, et al. Crystal and molecular structure of human annexin V after refinement. Implications for structure, membrane binding and ion channel formation of the annexin family of proteins. J Mol Biol 1992; 223:683–704.
25. Jin M, Smith C, Hsieh HY, et al. Essential role of B-helix calcium binding sites in annexin V-membrane binding. J Biol Chem 2004; 279:40351–40357.
26. Fadok VA, Voelker DR, Campbell PA, et al. Exposure of phosphatidylserine on the surface of apoptotic lymphocytes triggers specific recognition and removal by macrophages. J Immunol 1992; 148:2207–2216.
27. Lahorte CM, Vanderheyden JL, Steinmetz N, et al. Apoptosis-detecting radioligands: current state of the art and future perspectives. Eur J Nucl Med Mol Imaging 2004; 31:887–919.
28. Belhocine TZ, Tait JF, Vanderheyden JL, et al. Nuclear medicine in the era of genomics and proteomics: lessons from annexin V. J Proteome Res 2004; 3:345–349.
29. Ohtsuki K, Akashi K, Aoka Y, et al. Technetium-99m HYNIC-annexin V: a potential radiopharmaceutical for the in-vivo detection of apoptosis. Eur J Nucl Med 1999; 26:1251–1258.
30. Verbeke K, Kieffer D, Vanderheyden JL, et al. Optimization of the preparation of ^{99m}Tc-labeled HYNIC-derivatized annexin V for human use. Nucl Med Biol 2003; 30:771–778.
31. Kemerink GJ, Liu X, Kieffer D, et al. Safety, biodistribution, and dosimetry of ^{99m}Tc-HYNIC-annexin V, a novel human recombinant annexin V for human application. J Nucl Med 2003; 44:947–952.
32. Kemerink GJ, Boersma HH, Thimister PWL, et al. Biodistribution and dosimetry of ^{99m}Tc-BTAP-annexin-V in humans. Eur J Nucl Med 2001; 28:1373–1378.
33. Steinmetz N, Green A. Pre-treatment uptake of ^{99m}Tc-annexin V uptake is associated with an increased

platinum-based chemotherapy response rate in advanced non-small cell lung cancer. 2004 Annual Meeting, Society of Nuclear Medicine, Philadelphia, U.S.A. (abstr # 1173).

34. Vermeersch H, Loose D, Lahorte C, et al. ^{99m}Tc-HYNIC annexin-V imaging of primary head and neck carcinoma. Nucl Med Commun 2004; 25(3):259–263.

35. Kartachova MS, Valdes Olmos RA, Haas RL, et al. Mapping of treatment-induced apoptosis in normal structures: (99m)Tc-Hynic-rh-annexin V SPECT and CT image fusion. Eur J Nucl Med Mol Imaging 2006; 33(8): 893–899.

36. Steinmetz N, Green A. Chemotherapy-induced change in ^{99m}Tc-Hynic-rh-annexin V uptake as an early predictor of response to platinum therapy in advanced non-small cell lung cancer. 2004 Annual Meeting, Society of Nuclear Medicine, Philadelphia, U.S.A. (abstr # 105).

37. Kartachova MS, Haas RLM, Verheij M, et al. Correlation between in vivo imaging of apoptosis by ^{99m}Tc-Annexin V scintigraphy and tumour response in patients with malignant lymphoma. 2005 Annual Meeting, European Association of Nuclear Medicine, Istanbul, Turkey (abstr # 369).

38. Kartachova M, Haas RL, Olmos RA, et al. In vivo imaging of apoptosis by 99mTc-annexin V scintigraphy: visual analysis in relation to treatment response. Radiother Oncol 2004; 72:333–339.

39. van de Wiele C, Lahorte C, Vermeesch H, et al. Quantitative tumor apoptosis imaging using technetium-99m-HYNIC annexin V single photon emission computed tomography. J Clin Oncol 2003; 21:3483–3487.

40. Haas RL, de Jong D, Valdes Olmos RA, et al. In vivo imaging of radiation-induced apoptosis in follicular lymphoma patients. Int J Radiat Oncol Biol Phys 2004; 59:782–787.

41. Belhocine T. Radiolabeled recombinant human annexin A5: experimental use and clinical perspectives. Annexins 2004; 1(2):e13–e18.

42. Takei T, Kuge Y, Zhao S, et al. Time course of apoptotic tumor response after a single dose of chemotherapy: comparison with 99mTc-Annexin V uptake and histologic findings in an experimental model. J Nucl Med 2004; 45 (12):2083–2087.

43. Blankenberg FG, Katsikis PD, Tait JF, et al. Imaging of apoptosis (programmed cell death) with 99mTc Annexin V. J Nucl Med 1999; 40:184–191.

44. Kuge Y, Sato M, Zhao S, et al. Feasibility of (99m)Tc-Annexin V for repetitive detection of apoptotic tumor response to chemotherapy: an experimental study using a rat tumor model. J Nucl Med 2004; 45:309–312.

45. Lee TS, Chung HK, Woo KS, et al. Apoptosis imaging of lung cancer using ^{99m}Tc-Hynic-annexin V after gamma irradiation. 2004 Annual Meeting, Society of Nuclear Medicine, Philadelphia, U.S.A. (abstr # 423).

46. Ke S, Wen X, Wu QP, et al. Imaging taxane-induced tumor apoptotic using PEGylated, 111in-labeled annexin V. J Nucl Med 2004; 45:108–115.

47. Mochizuki T, Kuge Y, Zhao S, et al. Detection of apoptotic tumor response in vivo after a single dose of chemotherapy with ^{99m}Tc-annexin V. J Nucl Med 2003; 44:92–97.

48. Bennink RJ, van den Hoff MJ, van Hemert FJ, et al. Annexin V imaging of acute doxorubicin cardiotoxicity (apoptosis) in rats. J Nucl Med 2004; 45:842–848.

49. Erba PA, Lazzeri E, Giovacchini G, et al. Timing of taxol-induced apoptosis as assessed by ^{99m}Tc-annexin V biodistribution in mice with endogenous, virus-induced breast cancer. 2005 Annual Meeting, Society of Nuclear Medicine, Toronto, Canada (abstr # 454).

50. Wang F, Liu M, Zhang CL, et al. Study on tumor cell apoptosis imaging in vivo in mice bearing tumor. 2005 Annual Meeting, Society of Nuclear Medicine, Toronto, Canada (abstr # 453).

51. Kumar V, Wong E, Kumar D, et al. To Evaluate the potential of 99mTc-Hynic-annexin-V in detecting therapy induced apoptosis of thymoma (EL4) tumour in nude mice. 2005 Annual Meeting, European Association of Nuclear Medicine, Istanbul, Turkey (abstr # 368).

52. Kohanim S, Yang DJ, Bryant J, et al. Quantification of tumor apoptosis with ^{99m}Tc-annexin-V. 2005 Annual Meeting, Society of Nuclear Medicine, Toronto, Canada (abstr # 1270).

53. Yang DJ, Azhdarinia A, Wu P, et al. In vivo and in vitro measurement of apoptosis in breast cancer cells using 99mTc-EC-annexin V. Cancer Biother Radiopharm 2001; 16:73–83.

54. Blankenberg FG, Tait J, Strauss HW. Apoptotic cell death: its implications for imaging in the next millennium. Eur J Nucl Med 2000; 27:359–367.

55. Belhocine TZ, Blankenberg FG. 99mTc-Annexin A5 uptake and imaging to monitor chemosensitivity. Methods Mol Med 2005; 111:363–380.

56. Joseph B, Lewensohn R, Zhivothosky B. Role of apoptosis in the response of lung carcinomas to anti-cancer treatment. Ann N Y Acad Sci 2000; 926:204–216 (review).

57. Soini Y, Paakko P, Lehto VP. Histopathological evaluation of apoptosis in cancer. Am J Pathol 1998; 153(4): 1041–1053 (review).

58. Guchelaar HJ, Vermes A, Meerwaldt JH. Radiation-induced xerostomia: pathophysiology, clinical course and supportive treatment. Support Care Cancer 1997; 5(4): 281–288 (review).

59. Friesen C, Lubatschofski A, Kotzerke J, et al. Beta irradiation used for systemic radioimmunotherapy induces apoptosis and activates apoptosis pathways in leukaemia cells. Eur J Nucl Med Mol Imaging 2003; 30(9):1251–1261.

60. Blankenberg F. To scan or not scan, it is a question of timing: technetium-99m-annexin V radionuclide imaging assessment of treatment efficacy after one course of chemotherapy. Clin Cancer Res 2002; 8:2757–2758.

61. Belhocine T, Steinmetz N, Li C, et al. The Imaging of apoptosis with the radiolabeled annexin V: optimal timing for clinical feasibility. Technol Cancer Res Treat 2004; 3: 23–32.

62. Mandl SJ, Mari C, Edinger M, et al. Multi-modality imaging identifies key times for annexin V imaging as an early predictor of therapeutic outcome. Mol Imaging 2004; 3:1–8.

63. Lahorte C, Slegers G, Philippe J, et al. Synthesis and in vitro evaluation of 123I-labelled human recombinant annexin V. Bio Eng 2001; 17:51–53.

64. Ito M, Tomiyoshi K, Takahashi N, et al. Development of a new ligand, 11C-labeled annexin V, for PET imaging of apoptosis. Proc SNM 49th Annual Meeting, 2002; No. 1457.

65. Russell J, O'Donoghue JA, Finn R, et al. Iodination of Annexin V for imaging apoptosis. J Nucl Med 2002; 43:671–677.

66. Glaser M, Collingridge DR, Aboagye EO, et al. Iodine-124 labelled Annexin-V as a potential radiotracer to study apoptosis using positron emission tomography. Appl Radiat Isot 2003; 58:55–62.

67. Dekker B, Keen H, Zweit J, et al. Detection of cell death using 124I-Annexin V. Proc SNM 49th Annual Meeting, 2002, No. 256.

68. Keen H, Dekker B, Disley L, et al. Iodine-124 labelled Annexin V for PET imaging of in vivo cell death. Proc SNM 50th Annual Meeting, 2003, No. 586.

69. Watanbe H, Murata Y, Miura M, et al. In-vivo visualization of radiation-induced apoptosis using (125)I-annexin V. Nucl Med Commun 2006; 27(1):81–89.

70. Yang DJ, Azhdarinia A, Wu P, et al. In vivo and in vitro measurement of apoptosis in breast cancer cells using 99mTc-EC-annexin V. Cancer Biother Radiopharm 2001; 16(1):73–83.

71. Smith-Jones PM, Afroze A, Zanzonico P, et al. ^{68}Ga labelling of annexin-V: comparison to 99mTc-annexin-V and 67Ga-annexin. Proc SNM 50th Annual Meeting, 2003, No. 159.

72. Zijlstra S, Gunawan J, Burchert W. Synthesis and evaluation of a 18F-labelled recombinant annexin-V derivative, for identification and quantification of apoptotic cells with PET. Appl Radiat Isot 2003; 58:201–207.

73. Vaidayanathan G, Zalutsky MR. Labeling proteins with fluorine-18 using N-succinimidyl 4-[18F] fluorobenzoate. Int J Rad Appl Instrum B 1992; 19:275–281.

74. Boisgard R, Blondel A, Dolle F, et al. A new 18F tracer for apoptosis imaging in tumor bearing mice. Proc SNM 50th Annual Meeting, 2003, No. 157.

75. Mease RC, Weinberg IN, Toretsky JA, et al. Preparation of F-18 labeled Annexin V: a potential PET radiopharmaceutical for imaging cell death. Proc SNM 50th Annual Meeting, 2003, No. 1058.

76. Grierson JR, Yagle KJ, Eary JF, et al. Production of [F-18]-fluoroannexin for imaging apoptosis with PET. Bioconjug Chem 2004; 15:373–379.

77. Murakami Y, Takamatsu H, Taki J, et al. ^{18}F-labelled annexin V: a PET tracer for apoptosis imaging. Eur J Nucl Med Mol Imaging 2004; 31:469–474.

78. Yagle KJ, Eary JF, Tait JF, et al. Evaluation of 18F-annexin V as a PET imaging agent in an animal model of apoptosis. J Nucl Med 2005; 46:658–666.

79. Kemerink GJ, Boersma HH, Thimister PWL, et al. Biodistribution and dosimetry of ^{99m}Tc-BTAP-annexin-V in humans. Eur J Nucl Med 2001; 28:1373–1378.

80. Kemerink GJ, Liu X, Kieffer D, et al. Safety, biodistribution, and dosimetry of ^{99m}Tc-HYNIC-annexin V, a novel human recombinant annexin V for human application. J Nucl Med 2003; 44:947–952.

81. Tait JF, Brown DS, Gibson DF, et al. Development and characterization of Annexin V mutants with endogenous chelation sites for 99mTc. Bioconjug Chem 2005; 11: 918–925.

82. Tait JF, Smith C, Blankenberg FG. Structural requirements for in vivo detection of cell death with ^{99m}Tc-annexin V. J Nucl Med 2005; 46:807–815.

83. Subbarayan M, Häfeli UO, Feyes DK, et al. A simplified method for preparation of 99mTc-annexin V and its biologic evaluation for in vivo imaging of apoptosis after photodynamic therapy. J Nucl Med 2003; 44:650–656.

84. Tait JF, Smith C, Levashova Z, et al. Improved detection of cell death in vivo with annexin v radiolabeled by site-specific methods. J Nucl Med 2006; 47(9):1546–1553.

85. O'Connor MK, Kemp BJ. Single-photon emission computed tomography/computed tomography: basic instrumentation and innovations. Semin Nucl Med 2006; 36(4):258–266.

86. Liu RR, Erwin WD. Automatic estimation of detector radial position for contoured SPECT acquisition using CT images on a SPECT/CT system. Med Phys 2006; 33 (8):2800–2808.

87. Seo Y, Wong KH, Sun M, et al. Correction of photon attenuation and collimator response for a body-contouring SPECT/CT imaging system. J Nucl Med 2005; 46(5): 868–877.

88. Talbot JN, Petegnief Y, De Beco V, et al. Basics of PET and PET/CT imaging: instrumentation and radiopharmaceuticals for clinical diagnosis. Presse Med 2006; 35(9): 1331–1337 (French).

89. Beyer T, Townsend DW. Putting 'clear' into nuclear medicine: a decade of PET/CT development. Eur J Nucl Med Mol Imaging 2006; 33(8):57–61.

90. Kartachova M, van Zandwijk N, Burgers S, et al. Prognostic significance of 99mTc Hynic-rh-annexin V scintigraphy during platinum-based chemotherapy in advanced lung cancer. J Clin Oncol 2007; 25(18):2534–2539.

91. Rottey S, Loose D, Vakaet L, et al. 99mTc-HYNIC Annexin-V imaging of tumors and its relationship to response to radiotherapy and/or chemotherapy. Q J Nucl Med Mol Imaging 2007; 51(2):182–188.

92. Kartachova MS, Valdés Olmos RA, Haas RL, et al. 99mTc-HYNIC-rh-annexin-V scintigraphy: visual and quantitative evaluation of early treatment-induced apoptosis to predict treatsment outcome. Nucl Med Commun 2008; 29(1):39–44.

93. Seo Y, Mari C, Hasegawa BH. Technological development and advances in single-photon emission computed tomography/computed tomography. Semin Nucl Med 2008; 38 (3):177–198.

31

Imaging Cell Trafficking with MR Imaging

ASSAF A. GILAD, PIOTR WALCZAK, and JEFF W. M. BULTE

Russell H. Morgan Department of Radiology and Radiological Science, Division of MR Research, and Cellular Imaging Section, Institute for Cell Engineering, Johns Hopkins University School of Medicine, Baltimore, Maryland, U.S.A.

MICHAEL T. McMAHON,

Russell H. Morgan Department of Radiology and Radiological Science, Division of MR Research, Johns Hopkins University School of Medicine, Baltimore, Maryland, U.S.A. and F.M. Kirby Research Center for Functional Brain Imaging, Kennedy Krieger Institute, Baltimore, Maryland, U.S.A.

INTRODUCTION

Although the human body appears to be static, with defined and anatomically distinct organ systems, there are continuous dynamic processes of cell replacement, repair, and immune-mediated cell infiltrations. All these processes involve cell trafficking. Trafficking cells are cells navigating the body in response to different stimuli; some are chemoattractive and others are chemorepulsive. Perhaps the most pronounced example of cell trafficking is within the hematopoietic system, where cells traffic throughout the entire body. Leukocytes enter the circulation from the bone marrow, spleen, lymph nodes, or the thymus and travel to sites of inflammation and immune stimulation in a highly regulated fashion (1). Recently, it has been shown that circulating endothelial progenitor cells (EPCs) can be recruited from the blood and participate in angioneogenesis of infarcted heart (2). Even in an organ considered incapable of any regenerative activity, such as the postnatal brain, neurogenic regions (the hippocampus and the subventricular zone) remain active throughout life and generate a significant number of new neurons that participate in cell trafficking. Notably, in rodents, subventricular zone neurons migrate exten-

sively, navigating along the rostral migratory stream to reach their final destination, the olfactory bulb (3). Thus, even after full postnatal development, cell trafficking is a key biological phenomenon. In this chapter, we will illustrate how magnetic resonance (MR) imaging may be applied to obtain a deeper insight into the processes that govern cell migration, in particular as it relates to cancer.

CELL TRAFFICKING IN CANCER

Cell trafficking is of fundamental importance in cancer biology. On one hand, tumors utilize cell trafficking routes to metastasize, whereas, on the other hand, the local growth of tumors is largely dependent on the recruitment of stromal or endothelial precursors. Tumors are characterized by disrupted regulation of basic cytophysiological processes that are regulated by cytokines and growth factors. These molecules signal cells to proliferate, differentiate, and migrate. One example of disrupted regulation is the induction of angiogenesis, the formation of new blood vessels that nourish the tumor. The growth of new vessels in tumor tissue was already noted a century ago (4). Endothelial cells from existing vessels proliferate and form new capillaries that invade the tumor in response to cytokine stimulation

(5,6). Recently, it was shown that when these vessels are destroyed, the tumor periphery is replenished with EPC that migrate from the bone marrow via the circulation and are incorporated to the tumor vasculature (7). In addition to endothelial cells, stromal cells, such as pericytes and smooth muscle cells, migrate under the regulation of angiopoietins 1 and 2 and cover the endothelial capillaries (5,8). Another example of tumor-induced cell trafficking is a phenomenon observed in animal models, where transplanted neuronal progenitor (or stem) cells are attracted to brain tumors (9,10). Several stimuli have been posited to explain this phenomenon, such as cytokines produced by tumor-borne microglia (11) or vascular endothelial growth factor (VEGF) secreted by the tumor (12). However, most of the factors that promote this migration are still elusive and need to be understood thoroughly to use, for instance, stem cells to treat brain lesions.

MR IMAGING OF CELL TRAFFICKING

Basic Principles of MR Imaging

In contrast to other imaging modalities, MR imaging provides superior spatial resolution, ranging up to 50 to 100 μm, while the temporal resolution that can be provided is within hundreds of milliseconds. MR imaging utilizes the principle of "magnetization"—a sample (solution, cells, mouse, or human) is inserted into a magnetic field and irradiated with a short-radiofrequency pulse that affects a magnetic property of the sample. The energy absorbed from the radiofrequency pulse brings the magnetization to an excited, unstable state. When the irradiation is stopped, the magnetization returns to the basic non-excited state, followed by emission of energy in a form of a radiofrequency signal, through a process that is called "relaxation." The released radiofrequency signal is picked up by a detector, amplified, and then converted into a digital signal that can be further translated into an image.

Different nuclei (hydrogen-1, carbon-13, and fluorine-19) have different relaxation properties, and the relaxation is proportional to the concentration of the nuclei. It is also affected by the local microenvironment of the nuclei. Changing the power, duration, timing, and phase of the pulses is key in obtaining a change in signal intensity (or image contrast) for nuclei in different environments or tissues.

The goal in MR imaging of cell trafficking is to find conditions that will give the best contrast between the cells or tissues of interest and their surroundings. Contrast can be gained by either a decrease or an increase in the signal of the target relative to the background. This will result in hypointense regions (negative contrast) or hyperintense regions (positive contrast) on the MR images. This can be achieved by manipulating the major MR imaging relaxation parameters known as T_1, T_2, and T_2^*.

Labeling of Cells with "Negative" Contrast Agents

Relaxivity is the ability of magnetic compounds to increase the relaxation rates ($R_1 = 1/T_1$ and $R_2 = 1/T_2$) of the surrounding water proton spins. The relaxivities r_1 and r_2 are indicators of the efficacy of contrast agents and expressed in units of mM (metal ion)$^{-1}$ sec^{-1} at a given magnetic field and temperature. For contrast agents that have an $r_2/r_1 >> 1$, the agent produces a "negative" contrast, with hypointense pixels on all the images. If the ratio of $r_1/r_2 \approx 1$, the agent will in general produce a "positive" contrast (see below), resulting in a hyperintense pixels on the T_1-weighted image. The first demonstration of detection of circulating cells by MR imaging used endogenous contrast to discriminate circulating cells from their surroundings. Erythrocytes, which contain increased deoxygenated hemoglobin upon brain activation, can be imaged on the basis of the reduction in signal intensity on gradient echo images (13,14). In most cases, however, to track cell movements, it is necessary to label the cells with an exogenous rather than an endogenous contrast agent. Contrast agents can be defined as a molecular entity that generates contrast on an MR image. Studies in the early nineties demonstrated labeling of cells with superparamagnetic iron oxide (SPIO) particles. The cell-labeling procedure involved direct incubation of fetal brain tissue with lectin-conjugated magnetite, Fe_3O_4. It is not clear whether the particles entered the cells or just adhered to the membrane, although the cells remained labeled for a few weeks (15). Another example involved detecting a fetal brain tissue graft, labeled with viral envelopes containing dextran-coated superparamagnetic particles (16).

Tracking of iron oxide–labeled cells has also been applied to studying cancer. For instance, EPCs were isolated from bone marrow and labeled with Feridex® and a transfection agent. The cells were injected i.v. into an ortotopic model of R_2T rat glioma. Within several days, the labeled EPCs were observed in the tumor on T_2^*-weighted images, which was verified histologically (Fig. 1) (17). Dynamic trafficking and tumor homing of tumor antigen-specific cytotoxic T cells has been studied for OVA$^+$ (18) and HER2/neu$^+$ (19) tumors. Since iron oxide–labeled cells are demonstrated as hypointense regions on T_2/T_2^*-weighted images, it is sometimes difficult to distinguish these hypointensities from hemoglobin in blood, or pathological or experimentally induced artifacts, such as blood clots, hemorrhages, or necrosis. One attempt to differentiate iron oxide–labeled cells from blood vessels involved altering the inhaled oxygen levels to manipulate signal from deoxyhemoglobin (20). A more comprehensive discussion of the use of blood oxygenation modulation, as well as other methods for studying tumor vasculature, can be found in a recent review (21).

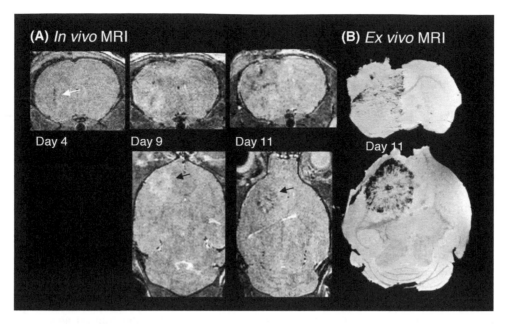

Figure 1 Serial MR imaging of mice that received magnetically labeled Sca1$^+$ bone marrow cells. (**A**) 3D RARE images showing evolution of hypointense regions within and around tumor due to incorporation of labeled cells into vascular structures or within the parenchyma of the tumor. Arrowheads indicate needle tract on day 4 after tumor implantation and growing tumor area on days 9 and 11. Hypointense areas in and around the tumor are evident at day 9, and a hypointense rim surrounding the tumor is observed on day 11. (**B**) Ex vivo gradient echo MRI of the same mouse at day 11. *Source*: From Ref. 17.

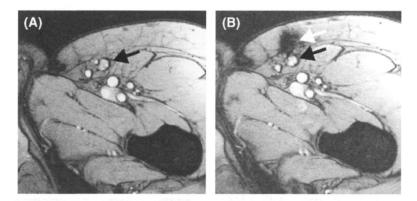

Figure 2 Monitoring of the accuracy of delivery of SPIO-labeled cells using MRI. (**A**) MRI before grafting; the inguinal lymph node to be injected is indicated by a black arrow. (**B**) MRI after grafting, demonstrating that the dendritic cells were not accurately delivered into the draining inguinal lymph node (*black arrow*) but instead into the perinodal, subcutaneous fat (*white arrow*). Accidental misinjection was found to have occurred in four out of eight patients. *Source*: From Ref. 22.

The emphasis on the importance of MRI for monitoring cell trafficking can be found in a study by de Vries et al. Injection of dendritic cells labeled with Feridex demonstrates the importance of the superior anatomical resolution of MRI. Using MRI, it was possible to distinguish between cells that were injected into the lymph nodes and cells that were misinjected and to monitor the migration of the former (Fig. 2) (22). The clinical study described above reported detection of as few as 1.5×10^5 cells, which is far below the therapeutic range of 2×10^6 cells (22). Encouraging as this finding is, it is still desirable to

detect a lower number of cells. Indeed, recently Shapiro and coworkers demonstrated detection of single-labeled cells in vivo in the rostral migratory stream (RMS) of the rat brain. This was achieved after direct injection of micron-sized particles ("Bang" particles) into the anterior horn of the right lateral ventricle. The particles were taken up by migrating neuroblast cells and carried along the RMS to their final location in the olfactory bulb (23). With improvements in particle properties and improved MRI hardware, imaging the migration of single cells in cancer research and therapy may become a reality.

Labeling of Cells with "Positive" Contrast Agents

Recently, gadolinium (Gd) complexes were suggested for obtaining cell labeling with positive contrast. EPCs were labeled with Gd-HPDO3A via incubation and showed contrast enhancement in T_1-weighted images. The Gd was substituted with another lanthanide, europium (Eu), for fluorescence microscopy verification (24).

Fibroblasts were also labeled by direct incubation with Gd-DTPA BSA (25) or by incubation with Gd-DTPA-fatty acid complex (26). In both cases, "positive" contrast was observed in vivo after transplantation. Labeling with gadolinium-rhodamine-dextran particles was used for tracking migration of transplanted neural stem cells toward stroke, which, however, resulted in a "negative" contrast in vivo (27). In general, cellular internalization reduces water exchange and inner sphere relaxation, reducing the R_1 of the contrast agent.

After gadolinium, manganese is probably the second most widely used T_1 contrast agent and its popularity is growing. Manganese-enhanced MRI is used for anatomical MR imaging, for example, to study neuronal activity and monitoring of neuronal tracts (28). Recently, manganese salt ($MnCl_2$) was used for efficient labeling of lymphocytes although it showed no decrease in T_1 in vitro for the first 24 hours (29).

Recently, manganese oxide (MnO) nanoparticles coated with polyethylene glycol (PEG)-phospholipid biocompatible shells have been developed. When conjugated with anti-EGFR (epidermal growth factor receptor) antibody, and targeted to tumors, these nanoparticles were able to produce "positive" contrast in vivo (30). To make a direct comparison between "positive" and "negative" contrast agents, we have labeled 9L rat glioma cells with either SPIO (Feridex) or MnO nanoparticles. Although the SPIO-labeled cells showed a more pronounced (negative) contrast, the MnO-labeled cells produced a good positive contrast, offering an alternative for tissues with a high occurrence of endogenous hypointensities. When SPIO- and MnO-labeled cells were each injected into the contralateral hemisphere, the two populations of cells could be distinguished from each other when simultaneously imaged in the same plane (31).

It should be mentioned that some alternative imaging methods have now been developed, such as the use of spectrally selective RF pulses that excite and refocus the off-resonance water surrounding the labeled cells (32), which can turn the SPIO-induced hypointensities into bright spots, but a clear advantage in vivo has not been demonstrated yet.

Labeling of Cells with (PARA)CEST Agents

A new class of MR contrast agents has been developed that relies on direct chemical exchange with bulk water to produce contrast. A variety of organic (33–37) and organometallic (38,39) compounds have a sufficient number of protons with suitable chemical exchange rates and chemical shifts to be detected sensitively. A radiofrequency pulse called a saturation pulse is applied on resonance with the exchangeable peak. This saturation or signal loss is then transferred via exchange to bulk water, producing a fractional reduction in the water signal (Fig. 3). As a result, these agents are called chemical exchange saturation transfer (CEST) contrast agents and are divided between compounds that are diamagnetic (Dia-CEST) and paramagnetic (PARACEST). Balaban and coworkers were the first group to demonstrate that this chemical exchange could be detected sensitively on endogenous metabolites ex vivo (40) or in vivo (41).

CEST contrast agents have two major advantages. First, they are switchable, that is, the contrast is detectable only when a radiofrequency pulse is applied at the specific frequency characteristic of an agent's exchangeable protons. Otherwise, the contrast agent is MR-invisible. The

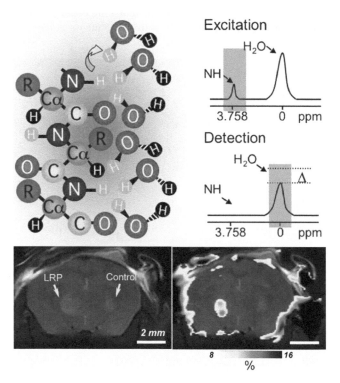

Figure 3 LRP as an MR-CEST reporter. (*Top*) Illustration of the CEST contrast mechanism. A frequency-selective radiofrequency pulse is used to label (*green*) the amide protons of the contrast agent. Only labeled protons exchange with water protons. This leads to a reduction in MR signal intensity (ΔSI). (*Bottom*) CEST ΔSI difference map (*right*) overlaid on an anatomical MR image (*left*). This map demonstrates that LRP-expressing xenografts can be distinguished from mock-transfected controls. *Source*: From Ref. 56 (*See Color Insert*).

second advantage is that different contrast agents with different excitation frequencies can be used simultaneously to label and track different population of cells, and image them, even on the same imaging plane.

One example of cell labeling with PARACEST contrast agents was reported by Aime and colleagues. In this study, the same cell line (rat hepatoma) was labeled by incubation for six hours with two different PARACEST contrast materials. One cell population was labeled with Eu-DOTAmGly, while the second population was labeled with Tb-DOTAmGly. Terbium (Tb) and europium (Eu) are both lanthanides. When the cells were imaged in vitro, each cell population was highlighted only after applying a pulse at its specific frequency (42), thus allowing "MR double labeling."

Labeling of Cells with ^{19}F Agents

The use of ^{19}F to label cells is a relatively new approach. The major advantage of this method is that ^{19}F has a negligible concentration in the body, resulting in the absence of background signal (43). In a pioneering study, dendritic cells—the antigen-presenting immune cells that migrate to lymph nodes—were labeled with perfluoropolyether (PFPE) agents ex vivo using transfection agents (Lipofectamine) (Fig. 4). Six hours after injection of 4×10^6 labeled dendritic cells into the footpad of the mouse, migration to the popliteal lymph nodes was visualized on MR images (44). Another fluorine compound, FITC poly-L-lysine-CF3, was used to directly label glial cells (45) and mouse cartilage stem cells (46). In all cases, the transplanted cells were successfully imaged in vivo.

The antitumor properties of modified neuronal progenitor cells (NPCs) were utilized in an experiment where ST14A, an immortalized NPC cell line, was engineered to express cytosine deaminase (CD). When the ST14A cells were co-injected in the brain, together with C6 rat glioma, a massive tumor cell death was observed upon injection of 5-fluorocytosine (5-FC) as measured histologically (47). In a similar experiment, the tumor-seeking and antitumor properties of engineered NPCs were demonstrated. CD-expressing mouse NPCs (C17.2) transplanted into mouse brain in a location distant from the glioma were shown to infiltrate the tumor and convert to a 5-FC prodrug, as confirmed by a reduction in tumor mass (47). It is highly desirable for monitoring anticancer therapy that 5-FU is detectable with noninvasive imaging, which is contingent upon improvements in MRI sensitivity.

Labeling of Cells Using MR Reporter Genes

For MR imaging, labeling of cells with exogenous contrast agents suffers from a few disadvantages. The label can be lost over time due to several mechanisms, for example, agents can be degraded or secreted by the cells. In addition, in the case of highly proliferative (tumor) cells or immortalized cell lines, with every division cycle, the contrast agent will be divided between the daughter cells, and thus, the contrast will be reduced by half. Another important disadvantage of cell labeling is that contrast agent excreted or released after cell death can be picked up by macrophages (48). One strategy to overcome this problem is to engineer the cells to produce their own contrast agent. In the last two decades, several MRI "reporter genes" have been developed. Here, we will review some of the highlights in the new and growing field of MR reporter genes; a more extensive review can be found in Ref. 31.

The fundamental requirement of a suitable MR reporter gene is that the translated protein (e.g., a membrane-bound receptor targeted for the contrast agent, a substrate-converting enzyme, or a metalloprotein) can produce detectable contrast with a sufficient signal-to-noise ratio.

Historically, the first MR reporter gene was designed for MR spectroscopy (MRS). Creatine kinase (CK), an enzyme that catalyzes ATP conversion to ADP, and its activity can be detected by ^{31}P MRS. The first demonstration of CK enzyme activity using MRS involved the transgenic expression of the enzyme derived from the mouse brain in *Escherichia coli* (49) and, subsequently, the transgenic overexpression of CK under a specific promoter in the liver (50). In both studies, high levels of phosphocreatine (PCr) were observed in the NMR spectra that were absent in control mice, due to the low to normal background expression of CK in the liver.

To date, the effort to develop MR reporter genes has been directed toward isolating proteins that are involved in iron transport and metabolism. Initially, this was accomplished by overexperssing the transferrin receptor (TfR) that binds the transferrin (Tf) protein containing two iron atoms. Upon binding of two iron-loaded transferrin molecules, the receptor internalizes rapidly, following which the TfR-Tf complex dissociates in acidic endosomes and the iron is released.

The application of TfR as a reporter gene was demonstrated in tumorigenic fibroblasts (51), and in gliomas engineered to overexpress human TfR, following the systemic injection of Tf-MION (52). In both cases, the TfR expression was demonstrated as a signal reduction that could be detected with T_2-weighted MRI.

More recently, a similar MR reporter system was proposed, which was based on ferritin expression. The heavy chain of murine ferritin was overexpressed in a C6 rat glioma cell line under a conditional tetracycline promoter, which allows "on and off" expression controlled by the presence of tetracycline in the cell culture media or drinking water. Xenografted C6 rat glioma expressing the

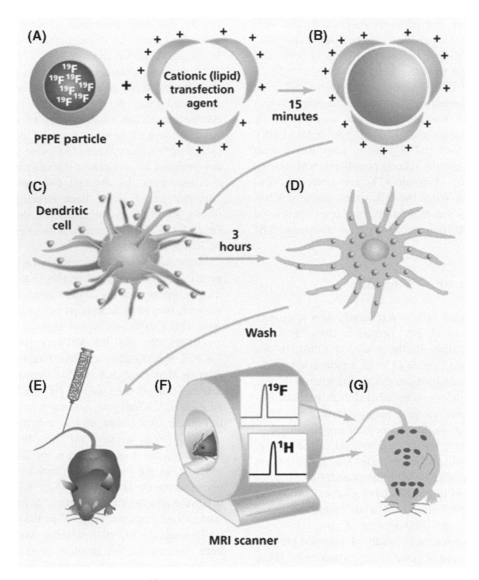

Figure 4 Use of fluorinated nanoparticles in ^{19}F MRI tracking of dendritic cells. Perfluoropolyether particles (**A**) surrounded by a cationic transfection agent (**B**) are combined with dendritic cells and rapidly bind to the cells' anionic surface (**C**). After several hours of incubation, the particles are efficiently internalized (**D**). Washed, labeled cells are injected into the animal (**E**), in this case intravenously, and subjects are imaged using conventional high-field animal scanners (**F**). As the endogenous ^{19}F background signal is negligible, the obtained "hot spots" of signal are specific for the labeled cells. When conventional ^{1}H images, which contain detailed soft tissue anatomical information, are acquired simultaneously, superimposition of the two scans (**G**) allows a precise determination of the location of labeled cells. *Source*: From Ref. 43.

transgene showed a significant reduction in both T_1 and T_2 values (53). Tetracycline-regulated ferritn expression was demonstrated as a cell type–specific marker gene in transgenic mice (54). The feasibility of using ferritin as a reporter gene was also demonstrated by injecting ferritin gene–encoding adenoviral vector into the mouse brain. After injection, the transfected cells showed a marked hypointensity on T_2- and T_2^*-weighted MR images, which correlated with the LacZ reporter gene used as a histological validation marker (55).

We have recently designed and expressed a new prototype of MR reporter based on CEST (Fig. 3). We cloned an artificial protein that encodes to a protein consisting of 200 lysines (77% of its amino acids), called a lysine-rich protein (LRP). Due to its high proton exchange rate, the new protein can provide MR contrast that can be switched "on" and "off" only by applying radiowave pluses. Xenografted 9L rat glioma overexpressing LRP can be visualized in vivo using CEST imaging and can be distinguished from control non-LRP expressing tumors (56). This is the first prototype of an MR reporter gene that, upon the development of new reporter proteins, provides the potential to label multiple cell populations with a CEST reporter that can be excited at different frequencies. This is important for studying the interactions of tumor and host tissue, including infiltration and recruitment of endothelial, stromal, and immune cells.

FUTURE DIRECTIONS—DEVELOPING CONTRAST AGENTS WITH IMPROVED SENSITIVITY

In molecular and cellular imaging, there is a need for improved sensitivity of contrast agents to detect the lowest possible number of cells, ideally single cells, and perhaps even measure changes in protein levels. There is definitely room for improvement of the sensitivity of MR contrast agents. Indeed, recently, there were several reports of new "ultra" sensitive contrast agents, such as MEIO (magnetism-engineered iron oxide) doped with different metals (Mn, Fe, Co, or Ni). MFe_2O_4 showed improved sensitivity. The $MnFe_2O_4$ derivative, with a relaxivity r_2 of 358 mM^{-1}sec^{-1}, in particular, showed contrast at 1.5 T that was superior to other agents. Improvement in tumor detection sensitivity was demonstrated with the use of this agent, conjugated to Herceptin and targeted to tumors expressing the HER2/neu receptor (57). In a different study, FeCo nanocrystals, with a single shell of graphitic/carbon with a relaxivity r_2 of 644 mM^{-1} sec^{-1} and r_1 of 70 mM^{-1} sec^{-1} at 1.5 T, demonstrated a positive contrast in vivo (58). Dextran-coated $GdPO_4$ nanocrystals (59) and Gd-fullerenes (60) have also been suggested as positive contrast agents. Contrast agents with improved sensitivity can help to detect lower cell numbers, or cells even after several division cycles.

SUMMARIZED PRACTICAL CONSIDERATIONS FOR TRACKING CELLS WITH MR IMAGING

There is no one general, universal method for tracking cells with MR imaging. In this section, a summary of currently available labeling methods is provided, and some practical considerations for choosing particles and labeling methods are suggested pending on the particular application.

Bang particles: These microspheres are the most sensitive agents available, with demonstrated single-cell imaging capabilities. One concern about these particles is their non-biodegradable character (they are coated with polystyrene), and it remains to be demonstrated whether their use is associated with long-term detrimental effects. As for now, its use is limited to animal studies.

Iron oxide nanoparticles (Feridex/Endorem®): These nanoparticles are the second most sensitive agents. The advantages include wide availability, FDA-approval, and in vivo cell detection sensitivity in the range of at least 10^3 to 10^4 cells using clinical imaging parameters and scanners. Currently, these are the most extensively used and best-characterized nanoparticles, offering good contrast, low toxicity, and full biocompatibility. They have been clinically used for MRI cell tracking (22).

MR reporter proteins: These reporter proteins offer sensitivity in the approximate range of 10^4 to 10^5 cells. Stable contrast is maintained in rapidly dividing cells, and the reporter can provide information about cell status, that is, cell survival and downstream cellular differentiation (in the case of stem cells). However, the labeling procedure is long (days to weeks) and involves complex genetic manipulation.

Positive contrast agents: These agents enable differentiation from hypointensities on images but are relatively new and still not widely in use. Their sensitivity for detection is low. At higher fields, positive contrast may diminish. One concern is clinical translation as free gadolinium ions, and at a certain level also manganese, is toxic unlike biocompatible iron; it is not clear how and when the paramagnetic chelates are excreted in the human body. In Table 1, an overview is given of the different strategies that are optimal for various MRI cell-tracking applications.

In summary, there are a variety of MRI contrast agent mechanisms and a variety of cell-labeling techniques. It is important to choose the appropriate methodology for a specific application to obtain the best possible information about tracking of labeled cells in vivo.

Table 1 Overview of Currently Available Strategies for MRI Cell Tracking

	Bang particles	Iron oxide (Feridex®)	Positive (Gd) agents	MR reporter proteins	PARACEST/ CEST agents	^{19}F agents
Detecting low cell number	+++	++	−	−	−	−
Differentiation of multiple cell types	−	−	−	++	+++	+
Clinically applicable	−	+++	+	?	?	+++
In vivo cell labeling	++	?	−	+++	−	?
Verification of accurate cell delivery	?	+++	+	?	?	?

REFERENCES

1. Luster AD, Alon R, von Andrian UH. Immune cell migration in inflammation: present and future therapeutic targets. Nat Immunol 2005; 6:1182–1190.

2. Numaguchi Y, Sone T, Okumura K, et al. The impact of the capability of circulating progenitor cell to differentiate on myocardial salvage in patients with primary acute myocardial infarction. Circulation 2006; 114:I114–I119.

3. Ghashghaei HT, Lai C, Anton ES. Neuronal migration in the adult brain: are we there yet? Nat Rev Neurosci 2007; 8:141–151.

4. Goldmann E. The growth of malignant disease in man and in the lower animal, with special reference to the vascular system. Lancet 1907; 2:1236–1240.

5. Hanahan D. Signaling vascular morphogenesis and maintenance. Science 1997; 277:48–50.

6. Hanahan D, Folkman J. Patterns and emerging mechanisms of the angiogenic switch during tumorigenesis. Cell 1996; 86:353–364.

7. Shaked Y, Ciarrocchi A, Franco M, et al. Therapy-induced acute recruitment of circulating endothelial progenitor cells to tumors. Science 2006; 313:1785–1787.

8. Gilad AA, Israely T, Dafni H, et al. Functional and molecular mapping of uncoupling between vascular permeability and loss of vascular maturation in ovarian carcinoma xenografts: the role of stroma cells in tumor angiogenesis. Int J Cancer 2005; 117:202–211.

9. Aboody KS, Brown A, Rainov NG, et al. Neural stem cells display extensive tropism for pathology in adult brain: evidence from intracranial gliomas. Proc Natl Acad Sci U S A 2000; 97:12846–12851.

10. Tang Y, Shah K, Messerli SM, et al. In vivo tracking of neural progenitor cell migration to glioblastomas. Hum Gene Ther 2003; 14:1247–1254.

11. Aarum J, Sandberg K, Haeberlein SL, et al. Migration and differentiation of neural precursor cells can be directed by microglia. Proc Natl Acad Sci U S A 2003; 100: 15983–15988.

12. Schmidt NO, Przylecki W, Yang W, et al. Brain tumor tropism of transplanted human neural stem cells is induced by vascular endothelial growth factor. Neoplasia 2005; 7: 623–629.

13. Ogawa S, Lee TM. Magnetic resonance imaging of blood vessels at high fields: in vivo and in vitro measurements and image simulation. Magn Reson Med 1990; 16:9–18.

14. Ogawa S, Lee TM, Nayak AS, et al. Oxygenation-sensitive contrast in magnetic resonance image of rodent brain at high magnetic fields. Magn Reson Med 1990; 14:68–78.

15. Norman AB, Thomas SR, Pratt RG, et al. Magnetic resonance imaging of neural transplants in rat brain using a superparamagnetic contrast agent. Brain Res 1992; 594:279.

16. Hawrylak N, Ghosh P, Broadus J, et al. Nuclear magnetic resonance (NMR) imaging of iron oxide-labeled neural transplants. Exp Neurol 1993; 121:181.

17. Anderson SA, Glod J, Arbab AS, et al. Noninvasive MR imaging of magnetically labeled stem cells to directly identify neovasculature in a glioma model. Blood 2005; 105:420–425.

18. Kircher MF, Allport JR, Graves EE, et al. In vivo high resolution three-dimensional imaging of antigen-specific cytotoxic T-lymphocyte trafficking to tumors. Cancer Res 2003; 63:6838–6846.

19. Daldrup-Link HE, Meier R, Rudelius M, et al. In vivo tracking of genetically engineered, anti-HER2/neu directed natural killer cells to HER2/neu positive mammary tumors with magnetic resonance imaging. Eur Radiol 2005; 15:4–13.

20. Himmelreich U, Weber R, Ramos-Cabrer P, et al. Improved stem cell MR detectability in animal models by modification of the inhalation gas. Mol Imaging 2005; 4:104–109.

21. Neeman M, Gilad AA, Dafni H, et al. Molecular imaging of angiogenesis. J Magn Reson Imaging 2007; 25:1–12.

22. de Vries IJ, Lesterhuis WJ, Barentsz JO, et al. Magnetic resonance tracking of dendritic cells in melanoma patients for monitoring of cellular therapy. Nat Biotechnol 2005; 23:1407–1413.

23. Shapiro EM, Gonzalez-Perez O, Manuel Garcia-Verdugo J, et al. Magnetic resonance imaging of the migration of neuronal precursors generated in the adult rodent brain. Neuroimage 2006; 32:1150–1157.

24. Crich SG, Biancone L., Cantaluppi V, et al. Improved route for the visualization of stem cells labeled with a Gd-/Eu-chelate as dual (MRI and fluorescence) agent. Magn Reson Med 2004; 51:938–944.

25. Granot D, Kunz-Schughart LA, Neeman M. Labeling fibroblasts with biotin-BSA-GdDTPA-FAM for tracking of tumor-associated stroma by fluorescence and MR imaging. Magn Reson Med 2005; 54:789–797.

26. Himmelreich U, Aime S, Hieronymus T, et al. A responsive MRI contrast agent to monitor functional cell status. Neuroimage 2006; 32:1142.

27. Modo M, Mellodew K, Cash D, et al. Mapping transplanted stem cell migration after a stroke: a serial, in vivo magnetic resonance imaging study. Neuroimage 2004; 21:311–317.

28. Silva AC, Lee JH, Aoki I, et al. Manganese-enhanced magnetic resonance imaging (MEMRI): methodological and practical considerations. NMR Biomed 2004; 17:532–543.

29. Aoki I, Takahashi Y, Chuang KH, et al. Cell labeling for magnetic resonance imaging with the T1 agent manganese chloride. NMR Biomed 2006; 19:50–59.

30. Na HB, Lee JH, An K, et al. Development of a T(1) contrast agent for magnetic resonance imaging using MnO nanoparticles. Angew Chem Int Ed Engl 2007; 46(28): 5397–5401.

31. Gilad AA, Winnard PT Jr., van Zijl PCM, Bulte JWM. MR reporter genes: Promises and pitfalls. NMR Biomed 2007; 20:275–290.

32. Cunningham CH, Arai T, Yang PC, et al. Positive contrast magnetic resonance imaging of cells labeled with magnetic nanoparticles. Magn Reson Med 2005; 53:999–1005.

33. Goffeney N, Bulte JW, Duyn J, et al. Sensitive NMR detection of cationic-polymer-based gene delivery systems using saturation transfer via proton exchange. J Am Chem Soc 2001; 123:8628–8629.

34. Snoussi K, Bulte JW, Gueron M, et al. Sensitive CEST agents based on nucleic acid imino proton exchange:

detection of poly(rU) and of a dendrimer-poly(rU) model for nucleic acid delivery and pharmacology. Magn Reson Med 2003; 49:998–1005.

35. Zhou J, Payen JF, Wilson DA, et al. Using the amide proton signals of intracellular proteins and peptides to detect pH effects in MRI. Nat Med 2003; 9:1085–1090.

36. Ward KM, Balaban RS. Determination of pH using water protons and chemical exchange dependent saturation transfer (CEST). Magn Reson Med 2000; 44:799–802.

37. Ward KM, Aletras AH, Balaban RS. A new class of contrast agents for MRI based on proton chemical exchange dependent saturation transfer (CEST). J Magn Reson 2000; 143:79–87.

38. Zhang S, Merritt M, Woessner DE, et al. PARACEST agents: modulating MRI contrast via water proton exchange. Acc Chem Res 2003; 36:783–790.

39. Aime S, Barge A, Delli Castelli D, et al. Paramagnetic lanthanide(III) complexes as pH-sensitive chemical exchange saturation transfer (CEST) contrast agents for MRI applications. Magn Reson Med 2002; 47:639–648.

40. Guivel-Scharen V, Sinnwell T, Wolff SD, et al. Detection of proton chemical exchange between metabolites and water in biological tissues. J Magn Reson 1998; 133:36–45.

41. Dagher AP, Aletras A, Choyke P, et al. Imaging of urea using chemical exchange-dependent saturation transfer at 1.5T. J Magn Reson Imaging 2000; 12:745–748.

42. Aime S, Carrera C, Delli Castelli D, et al. Tunable imaging of cells labeled with MRI-PARACEST agents. Angew Chem Int Ed Engl 2005; 44:1813–1815.

43. Bulte JW. Hot spot MRI emerges from the background. Nat Biotechnol 2005; 23:945–946.

44. Ahrens ET, Flores R, Xu H, et al. In vivo imaging platform for tracking immunotherapeutic cells. Nat Biotechnol 2005; 23(8):983–987 [Epub Jul 24, 2005].

45. Masuda C, Maki Z, Morikawa S, et al. MR tracking of transplanted glial cells using poly-L-lysine-CF3. Neurosci Res 2006; 56:224–228.

46. Maki J, Masuda C, Morikawa S, et al. The MR tracking of transplanted ATDC5 cells using fluorinated poly-L-lysine-CF3. Biomaterials 2007; 28:434–440.

47. Barresi V, Belluardo N, Sipione S, et al. Transplantation of prodrug-converting neural progenitor cells for brain tumor therapy. Cancer Gene Ther 2003; 10:396–402.

48. Weber R, Wegener S, Ramos-Cabrer P, et al. MRI detection of macrophage activity after experimental stroke in rats: new indicators for late appearance of vascular degradation? Magn Reson Med 2005; 54:59–66.

49. Koretsky AP, Traxler BA. The B isozyme of creatine kinase is active as a fusion protein in Escherichia coli: in vivo detection by 31P NMR. FEBS Lett 1989; 243: 8–12.

50. Koretsky AP, Brosnan MJ, Chen LH, et al. NMR detection of creatine kinase expressed in liver of transgenic mice: determination of free ADP levels. Proc Natl Acad Sci U S A 1990; 87:3112–3116.

51. Koretsky A, Lin Y-J, Schorle H, et al. Genetic control of MRI contrast by expression of the transferrin receptor. Proc Intl Soc Mag Res 1996; 4:69.

52. Weissleder R, Moore A, Mahmood U, et al. In vivo magnetic resonance imaging of transgene expression. Nat Med 2000; 6:351–355.

53. Cohen B, Dafni H, Meir G, et al. Ferritin as an endogenous MRI reporter for noninvasive imaging of gene expression in C6 glioma tumors. Neoplasia 2005; 7:109–117.

54. Cohen B, Ziv K, Plaks V, et al. MRI detection of transcriptional regulation of gene expression in transgenic mice. Nat Med 2007; 13:498–503.

55. Genove G, Demarco U, Xu H, et al. A new transgene reporter for in vivo magnetic resonance imaging. Nat Med 2005; 11:450–454 [Epub Mar 20, 2005].

56. Gilad AA, McMahon MT, Walczak P, et al. Artificial reporter gene providing MRI contrast based on proton exchange. Nat Biotechnol 2007; 25:217–219.

57. Lee JH, Huh YM, Jun YW, et al. Artificially engineered magnetic nanoparticles for ultra-sensitive molecular imaging. Nat Med 2007; 13:95–99.

58. Seo WS, Lee JH, Sun X, et al. FeCo/graphitic-shell nanocrystals as advanced magnetic-resonance-imaging and near-infrared agents. Nat Mater 2006; 5:971–976.

59. Hifumi H, Yamaoka S, Tanimoto A, et al. Gadolinium-based hybrid nanoparticles as a positive MR contrast agent. J Am Chem Soc 2006; 128:15090–15091.

60. Anderson SA, Lee KK, Frank JA. Gadolinium-fullerenol as a paramagnetic contrast agent for cellular imaging. Invest Radiol 2006; 41:332–338.

32

General Considerations for Labeling and Imaging of Cells

HISATAKA KOBAYASHI

Molecular Imaging Program, Center for Cancer Research, National Cancer Institute, NIH, Bethesda, Maryland, U.S.A.

INTRODUCTION

Live cell labeling and tracking in the living animal or tissue is an emerging robust technology, which has been enabled by the recent advanced development of the imaging hardware and signaling probes. The methods for cellular imaging should generally be considered in different ways as compared to the design of molecular imaging probes, such as contrast agents. In this chapter, we review the history, then give a gross current overview of cellular imaging methods, with a focus on the differences in molecular probe design. Additionally, practical techniques of live cell labeling are discussed. Then, finally, characteristics of the three modalities currently available for cell tracking imaging—nuclear medicine, magnetic resonance imaging (MRI), and optical imaging—will be introduced.

HISTORY OF CELL LABELING FOR IN VIVO USE

Cellular labeling/imaging is not a new technique. From the early era of nuclear medicine in 1950, cell labeling techniques already existed, and were even used in clinical practice. Gray and Sterling labeled red blood cells (RBCs) with radioactive chromium-51, in order to measure the blood volume and RBC count in human patients (1). Some time later, this method was also used for examining the

life span of RBCs in experimental animal models and in patients with erythrocyte disorders. The technique, although now more sophisticated, is still in use today. Briefly, RBCs were isolated and incubated with Cr(VI)-51 ions, which can freely permeate through the cell membrane. When Cr(VI)-51 ions enter the RBC, they are reduced to Cr(III)-51 ions. Cr(III)-51 ions then interact with hemoglobin or other intracellular proteins and stably stick within the cell (Fig. 1). However, any damage to the RBC causes Cr(III)-51 ions to be promptly released from the cell and excreted from the body mainly via the kidneys, enabling us to count the living cells either in vivo or in vitro. This method is still widely used for examining lifetime of RBC and blood volume in clinical practices, especially in patients with erythrocyte disorders, polycythemia rubra vera, or for cell killing experiments and quantifying the lifetime of cells in vivo in the laboratory.

SIZE ISSUES—CELLS Vs. IMAGING PROBES

In order to design a successful method of cell labeling, first, the size of cells and second, the labeling probes need to be taken into account (Fig. 2). Normal cells generally have diameters in the micron size range, for example, 2 μm for platelet, 8μm for RBC, 7 to 25 μm for white blood cell (WBC), and 7 to 100 μm for cancer cells; in terms of major intracellular organelles, cell membrane

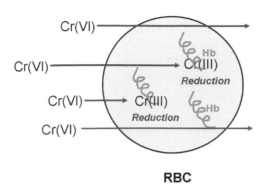

Figure 1 Scheme for cell labeling with Cr-51.

consists of a lipid bilayer, 6 to 10 nm in thickness, and endosomes and lysosomes, ~2 to 300 nm in diameter, but expandable to >1 μm with phagocytosis.

As regards imaging probes or contrast agents, those which are ≤1 nm in diameter are generally known as small molecular probes/contrast agents, that is, Gd–diethilenetriaminepentaacetic acid (DTPA), iodine contrast agents, nuclear medicine probes based on sugars or amino acids including ^{18}F-fluorodeoxyglucose (FDG). Agents that

are >2 nm in diameter are generally called macromolecular probes/contrast agents. Macromolecular agents, based on single molecules such as proteins and synthetic polymers, are relatively small, with size <20 nm in diameter. Conversely, macromolecular agents based on assembled multi-molecules such as liposomes, micelles, particles (including iron oxide particles and quantum dots), and bubbles are generally large, with a diameter of 20 nm to 1 μm.

This size information as well as the preferred modality are important considerations when designing the method of cell labeling for a specific imaging moiety, with each preferred modality.

PROBE CONCENTRATION Vs. CELL NUMBERS

In order to successfully detect cells in vivo or in tissue, sufficient concentrations of imaging moieties need to be incorporated into the cells. The concentration of imaging moieties (contrast agents) considered sufficient is dependent on the sensitivity of each modality. A general idea of the minimal concentration of imaging agent required for each of the major modalities is shown in Table 1. The nuclear medicine technique is the most sensitive of the imaging

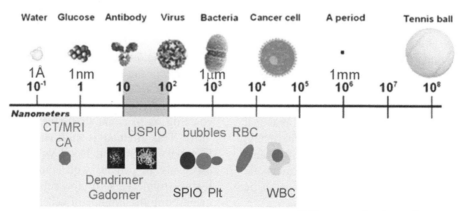

Figure 2 Scheme for gross ideas of the physical sizes of cells and probes.

Table 1 Sensitivity Comparison of Imaging Probes for Various Modalities

Imaging modalities	Signaling moieties	Detection limit as solution	Detection limit of labeled cell number
X-ray CT	Iodine	~10 mM	N/A
Nuclear medicine	Radionuclides	< 1 nM	10 to 100
MRI	Gadolinium	10 to 100 μM	100 to 1000
	Iron	10 to 100 μM	1
Ultrasound	Bubble	1 bubble	N/A?
Optical imaging	Fluorescence dyes	1 to 10 nM	~10
	Luciferin	N/A	~100

Abbreviations: CT, computed tomography; MRI, magnetic resonance imaging.

1-3 dendritic cells (SPIO)
(SPIO label with clinical 3T)

50-100 cancer cells in the SLN
(Bioluminescence imaging)

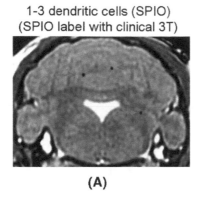

(A)

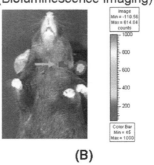

(B)

Figure 3 (A) Small iron oxide nanoparticles–labeled immature dendritic cell tracking with MR imaging using fast imaging employed steady-state acquisition at 3T is shown. Each spot contained one to three labeled dendritic cells. (B) Luciferase-labeled B16 melanoma cell tracking bioluminescence imaging is shown. Cervical lymph node contained 50 to 100 melanoma cells.

modalities available for in vivo diagnostic imaging, followed by optical imaging. Ultrasonography can detect a single micro-bubble of the contrast agent. However, these bubbles are inappropriate for cell labeling because of their large size and physical characteristics.

As for cellular imaging, the potential efficacy of cell labeling achievable by each probe is quite different. Therefore, in addition to the probe concentration, we should also be aware of the sensitivity of cell numbers for each modality. Since particles consist of large numbers of atoms, sensitivity of these particles can be very high. Single iron oxide particles of near micron size can be detected by MRI (2), enabling the detection of individual cells (3) (Fig. 3). In contrast, cells cannot be loaded with large nuclear medicine probes because the strong radiation may kill the labeled cells. Thus, even though the sensitivity of radioactivity is very high, it is impossible to detect a single cell using a nuclear medicine technique. Optical imaging with either bioluminescence or fluorescence method generally needs ~ 100 cells to allow detection, even in the most optimal setting for in vivo imaging (Fig. 3). Taken together, MRI has the highest potential to detect minimal numbers of cells for in vivo cellular imaging. An estimate of minimal cell numbers currently required for detection in each of the major modalities is also shown in Table 1.

IN VIVO CELLULAR IMAGING—HOW TO LABEL CELLS IN VIVO?

For in vivo cellular imaging, the methods can be categorized in two ways; exogenous or endogenous signaling probes for cell labeling, and ex vivo or in vivo cell labeling.

In terms of the former category, in order to produce signal in cells, one group of methods are to incorporate exogenous imaging moieties into the cell for labeling. Another method is to transfect genes into the target cells to label cells, which then code for endogenous signaling moieties such as fluorescence proteins or photo-activatable enzymes (Fig. 4).

In terms of the later category, in order to have cells producing signals in the body, one method is to remove target cells from the body, label them ex vivo, and then inject them back to the body, so called ex vivo labeling. Another method is to use target-specific labeling agents or targeted viral vector genes (encoding for signaling proteins or enzymes) injected into the body to label and image specific cells, termed in vivo labeling (Fig. 5).

Exogenous *vs* Endogenous probes

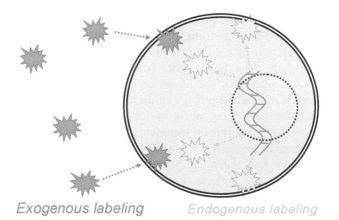

Exogenous labeling   Endogenous labeling

Figure 4 Scheme of exogenous signaling probes versus endogenous signaling probes.

Ex vivo labeling *vs In vivo* labeling

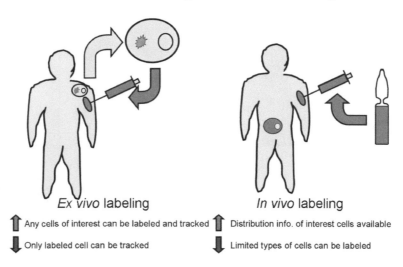

Figure 5 Scheme of ex vivo cell labeling versus in vivo labeling.

EXOGENOUS SIGNALING PROBES Vs. ENDOGENOUS SIGNALING PROBES

In order to perform exogenous labeling, various signaling moieties such as radioisotopes for nuclear medicine, iron oxide particles for MRI, and fluorescence dyes or quantum dots for optical imaging can be employed for the respective modalities. Cells labeled with either radioisotope (indium-111 or technetium-99m) or iron oxide particles have been used for imaging in clinical practice or trials. There are two technical problems with exogenous cell labeling. First, when the labeled cell proliferates, signaling moieties will be diluted and might become undetectable (usually after 5–6 divisions); secondly, when the labeled cell dies, signal can still be obtained from the dead cell, or in the worst case, signal can be transferred from the target cell to the macrophages, which clean up the dead cells.

In order to perform endogenous cell labeling, gene transfection of a signaling protein into the target cell is necessary. The fluorescence protein family for fluorescence imaging or the luciferase enzyme family for bioluminescence imaging can be employed for optical imaging. In future, nitrogen-rich proteins for chemical exchange saturation transfer (CEST) imaging may become available for in vivo MRI (4,5). Gene transfection methods have been well established in the experimental situation using electroporation, virus vectors, nonviral liposomes or macromolecules, etc. Endogenous cell labeling has technical advantages over exogenous labeling; all cells proliferated from the labeled cell are also labeled, and the dead cell is not visualized because it loses the ability to make signaling proteins. However, gene therapy

is yet to be approved in clinical practice because long-term safety for oncogenesis has not been proved. Therefore, although endogenous labeling, despite its inherent disadvantages, is technically a better method, exogenous cell labeling is a more feasible method for use in clinical practice.

EX VIVO LABELING Vs. IN VIVO LABELING

For ex vivo labeling, the target cells should be cultured, or collected and purified prior to labeling. Almost any kinds of cells are available for labeling. Once the cells are purified, the appropriate number of cells for labeling can be employed, if the modality is defined, although, the processing procedures may damage or change the character of target cells. After labeling, the cells can be administered to the appropriate places. Since only labeled cells can produce signal, clear images will be obtained with minimal background noise.

As regards in vivo labeling, only limited kinds of cells are currently available for cell labeling because specific cell labeling is not easy to achieve with high efficiency. The low signal from cells or high background meant that target cells were rarely visualized well. Macrophage family of cells can be successfully labeled via their phagocytic function. Injection of ultrasmall iron oxide nanoparticles (USPIO) has the ability to label tissue macrophages, and has been used to depict cancer metastasis in the lymph node (6) or migration of macrophages to the inflammatory lesion (7). An advantage of in vivo labeling is its ability to give information on the target cells' distribution. Summary of cell labeling methods are shown in Figure 6.

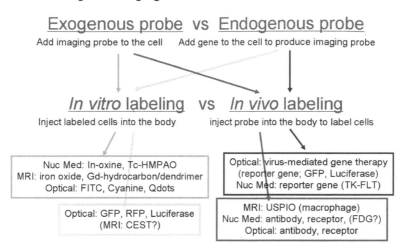

Figure 6 Schematic summary of cell labeling methods.

PRACTICAL METHODS FOR CELL LABELING IN WHICH CELLULAR COMPARTMENT IS THE PROBE LOCALIZED

Once the target cells of interest to be tracked are decided, there are three different cellular locations in which exogenous signaling probes can accumulate in the cell—cell membrane, endosomes and lysosomes, or cytosol (Fig. 7). If endogenous signaling probes are employed, signaling protein can be localized at any parts of cells by changing the genetic sequences of either the signal peptide or the protein itself.

Cell Membrane

The cell membrane can be labeled either on the cell surface proteins or within the lipid bilayer. The most popular way to label the cell surface proteins is to use antibodies targeted to surface antigens. The antibody binds with high specificity to its target, thus, this method is used for detecting or counting target cells in the experimental situation with radioimmuno-assay (RIA) or fluorescence-assisted cell sorter (FACS). Unfortunately, the binding affinity of an antibody to its antigen is generally not strong enough to enable in vivo imaging. Another effective method for in vivo imaging, although not targeting a specific protein, is to biotinylate cell surface proteins, and then follow this by labeling with the avidin-signaling moiety conjugate. The stability of cell labeling in this manner may be strong enough to use the labeled cells for in vivo imaging. However, immunogenicity of avidin may hamper the application of this method in clinical trials.

In order to label the lipid bilayer, hydrophobic compounds of signaling moieties, which are soluble in the lipid,

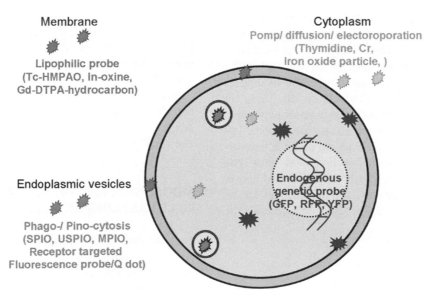

Figure 7 Scheme of probe localization in the cell.

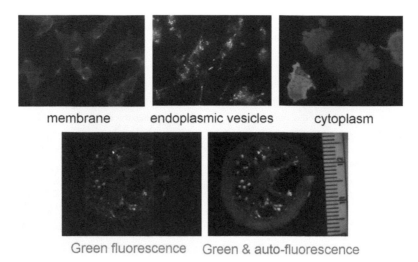

membrane   endoplasmic vesicles   cytoplasm

Green fluorescence   Green & auto-fluorescence

Figure 8 Microscopic images of cells labeled with membrane, endosomes and lysosomes, and cytoplasm are shown (*See Color Insert*).

can be used for cell labeling. This method can be performed by a relatively quick and easy process, and labeled cells remain stable in vivo for weeks. This method has been used in the clinical practice of nuclear medicine for decades as a means of tracking white blood cells to inflammatory lesions.

Endosomes and Lysosomes

Since all cells have phagocytic or pinocytic functions, cell labeling can be achieved by inducing endocytosis and delivering signaling moieties to the endosomes and lysosomes. One of the advantages of this labeling method is that endocytosis can deliver relatively large materials of up to micrometer size directly into the endosome or the lysosome. Therefore, this method is appropriate for cell labeling using particles such as iron oxide for MRI or quantum dots for fluorescence imaging. Macrophage or dendritic cells, which have high phagocytic activity, can be labeled simply by incubation with signaling particles. In order to label other cells, transfection agents can be employed for co-incubation to facilitate the access of particles to the cell surface by neutralizing the charge interaction or specific binding to antigens and induce pinocytosis/endocytosis (8). These are usually cationic molecules or polymers such as polylysine, polyamidoamine dendrimer, protamine sulfate, cationic liposome, or antibodies, which can bind and promote internalization. Using transfection agents or antibodies, most cells can be labeled by the signaling particles mentioned above. Cells labeled in this manner are stably labeled and can be tracked for weeks, unless the labeled cells die or the particles are digested.

Cytoplasm

Only ions or small molecules, which have specific pumps, are able to pass across the cell membrane, into the

cytoplasm of normal cells. Chromium ion, fluoroglucose, or thymidine can be used to label cells in the cytoplasm following simple incubation. However, for any larger molecules, it is necessary to use some additional methods to pass through the cell membrane.

Electroporation can physically loosen the cell membrane structure to facilitate the passage of large molecules through the cell membrane. This method is commonly used for plasmid transfection, and enables even submicron-size particles or nucleus delivery into the cytoplasm. Electroporation can sometimes kill or damage cells, but the damage can be minimized by optimizing the pulse/voltage condition. This method has reportedly been used for cell labeling with iron oxide particles for MRI (9).

In contrast, a biological way of cell labeling is the use of HIV Tat (transactivating regulatory protein), which can promote the transportation of extracellular proteins into the cell. Any extracellular protein can be delivered into the cell by adding the Tat sequence to any molecule. Since the Tat sequence lacks selectivity, signaling moieties conjugated with the Tat peptide can label virtually any cell.

The intracellular location of signaling moieties does not change the findings of in vivo imaging, therefore, a labeling method with higher efficiency would be a better choice (Fig. 8).

MODALITIES AND PRACTICAL METHODS FOR CELL LABELING AND CELL TRACKING IMAGING

Cell labeling and cell tracking imaging are currently performed with nuclear medicine, MRI, and optical imaging. In this section, established methods for cell labeling and cell tracking imaging in each modality are described.

Nuclear Medicine

Nuclear medicine techniques have the longest history, the most experience, and the greatest choice of methods amongst the three modalities, vide infra. Several nuclear medicine techniques have been used in clinical practice for decades. Cell tracking imaging using radiolabeled cells following ex vivo labeling method is a very low background and lacks information from the body, so anatomical location of signal is hard to be determined. The combination of an anatomical imaging modality such as X-ray computed tomography (CT) enables anatomical localization of the labeled cells.

Chromium-51 Red Blood Cell Labeling

This method has been described above. It has the longest history of all cell labeling methods. The labeled cells are used in the clinic for examining lifetime of RBC and blood volume in clinical practices especially in patients with erythrocyte disorders, polycythemia rubra vera, but not for imaging purposes because of long half-life and low energy emission of Cr-51.

Indium-111 Oxine or Technetium-99M Exametazime Cell Labeling

This is the most common method of ex vivo cell labeling using exogenous signaling probes. Just a short-time incubation of cells with either indium-111 oxine or technetium-99m exametazime (HMPAO) enables us to label cells with a high yield, usually >90%. Hydrophobic indium-111 oxine or technetium-99m HMPAO dissolves into the lipid bilayer of the cell membrane; no purification or washing is usually required. Any kind of cells can be labeled with this method. However, too high yield will damage or kill cells, especially when using indium-111 oxine, because of damage to the cell membrane and/or radiation toxicity.

Indium-111 oxine–labeled white blood cell scans for the detection of inflammatory lesions have the greatest experience of all cell labeling imagings used in clinical practice (Fig. 9).

Indium-111 Antibodies

The use of antibody/antigen system is the most common method of in vivo cell labeling with exogenous signaling probes. Antibody can target virtually any protein-expressing cells, provided enough copies of the antigen are exposed on the cell surface. Antibody labeling with indium-111 has been performed with bifunctional chelates such as DTPA- or 1,4,7,10-N,N′,N″,N‴, tetraazaciclododecane tetraacetic acid (DOTA)-derivatives. Radiolabeled antibodies are injected into the body to obtain the images. Because of

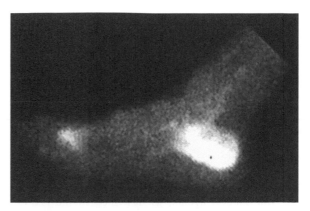

Chronic osteomyelitis of the calcaneus (white blood cell labeled with In-oxine)

Figure 9 ^{111}In-labeled cell tracking image of a patient with chronic osteomyelitis of the calcaneus.

slow clearance of antibodies, images usually have a high background signal from unbound antibody.

Indium-111-labeled anti-granulocyte monoclonal antibody has been used for tracking of granulocyte to detect inflammatory lesions in clinical trials and practices. A number of clinical trials have been performed in these 20 years (10). Other radiometals including positron emitters such as technetium-99 or technetium-94m, gallium-67 or gallium-68, and yttrium-90 or yttrium-88 are currently used for other purposes in clinical trials (11) that might be available for these cell labeling methods given above.

Expression of Reporter Proteins

The reporter method is a little different from those above. This method requires reporter gene transfection either ex vivo or in vivo. The thymidine kinase (enzyme), the sodium/iodine symporter (pump), and transferrin receptor (receptor) are currently used as reporter proteins. For cell tracking, the reporter gene is first transfected into the target cells, followed by injection of a reporter specific radiolabeled reagent, for example, I-123 or F-18 labeled thymidine analog for the thymidine kinase, I-123 or I-131 sodium iodide for the sodium/iodine symporter, In-111-labeled transferrin for the transferrin receptor. The reagent can accumulate in the cells, which express its specific reporter proteins. This method might become a good diagnostic method for the validation of gene delivery and expression at gene therapy (12).

MRI

Cell tracking techniques for MRI have recently been explored. MRI has emerged as the most sensitive method for in vivo cellular imaging among the three modalities in terms of detectable cell numbers. New methods for cell labeling have been explored as shown below. The sensitivity of cell tracking imaging is altered by the organ of interest, this is especially true for iron oxide particle–labeled cells, which produce negative signals on T2* images.

Iron Oxide Nano- or Micron-Sized Particles

Iron oxide particles are now used for both ex vivo and in vivo cell labeling. For ex vivo cell labeling, iron oxide particles are incubated with the cells either alone, or mixed with transfection agents, as described in the endosomes and lysosomes labeling section. Labeled cells can be injected into any places of interest. Iron oxide particle–labeled cells will appear as dark spots in the gradient echo T2* magnetic resonance (MR) images. Higher magnetic fields are more sensitive for the detection of labeled cells. Single-labeled cells can be detected in the mouse or rat (3). Actively proliferating cells are not appropriate for tracking by this method. After several divisions, either none or only one in ten of the cells can still produce a negative T2* signal. The sensitivity of cell tracking imaging is altered by the organ of interest because iron oxide particle–labeled cells produce negative signals on T2* images. Since air and bone show no signal on MRI, cell tracking imaging is easy in neurological system, muscle, and heart, but difficult in lung, abdominal organs, and soft tissue, in which scattered negative signals are found prior to contrast agent or labeled cells administration.

Gadolinium-Hydrocarbon Conjugate

Cell labeling methods, which can obtain positive MRI signals from labeled cells, have been proposed and investigated, but are yet to provide satisfactory in vivo MR imaging. Among them, an optimistic method is the use of gadolinium-hydrocarbon conjugates, whose hydrocarbon part can be integrated into the cell membrane whilst the Gd-chelate remains on the surface. The method may need some improvement and optimization to achieve successful in vivo imaging (13).

Chemical Exchange Saturation Transfer Imaging

Another possible new endogenous signaling method for cell labeling using MRI is the CEST method. Massive production of nitrogen-rich proteins by transfecting genes in target cells is necessary for obtaining the signal from target cells using the CEST method. The method may need some contrast agents of chelated lantanoid ions for enhancing the signal to achieve adequate in vivo MR imaging (4,5).

Optical Imaging

Both fluorescence and bioluminescence labeling of cells have been actively investigated ex vivo, especially for microscopic imaging (Fig. 10). Therefore, a number of cell labeling methods, using both exogenous and endogenous signaling moieties, have been explored and become available. Although none has yet been applied in clinical practice, a number of promising methods and probes for the clinical application exist, as described below. However, the general problem of optical imaging is that objects located deep within the body cannot be visualized because of absorption and scattering of the signal (light) along its path. Therefore, in spite of the great success of optical imaging in small-animal studies, clinical applications may be limited by the target depth, because of the size difference.

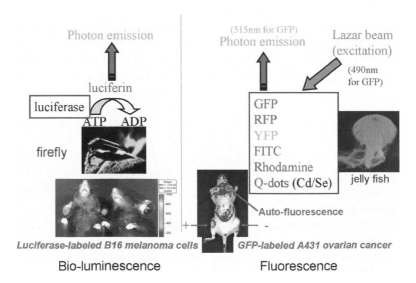

Figure 10 Scheme for methods of optical imaging.

Fluorescence Protein Families

Fluorescence protein families are the most commonly used endogenous signaling probes for cell labeling. Fluorescence proteins such as green, red, yellow, and cyan fluorescence proteins are mostly used for molecular imaging of the cell under the microscope in order to image a single molecule or analyze the functional interaction between molecules. The use of fluorescence proteins for in vivo imaging has recently increased for both ex vivo and in vivo labeling of cells, especially in cancer research. Ex vivo labeling of cancer cells with fluorescence proteins is used for various purposes such as monitoring tumor growth, observing drug response, and evaluating micrometastasis, etc. (14). Since plasmids for several standard fluorescence proteins are commercially available, the method for cell labeling is simple and straightforward, that is, transfection of plasmid followed by cloning labeled cells. The expressed location of fluorescence proteins in the cell can be controlled by modifying the gene sequence of signal peptides or making a fusion protein with other native proteins.

In vivo labeling of cells with fluorescence proteins is performed with virus vectors containing a gene encoding a fluorescence protein, similar to the paradigm of gene therapy. The method has been established in small-animal models, however, application to human studies has not been possible to date.

Fluorescence Dyes as Exogenous Signaling Probes

Numerous choices of fluorescence dyes have been synthesized and become available in the last couple of decades. Near-infrared (NIR) dyes for in vivo imaging can take advantage of greater-depth penetration and low-background autofluorescence of the body. As for cell labeling with ex vivo signaling probes, quantum dot particles can be employed by using phagocytic function to label endosomes and lysosomes. They have strong enough light emission for in vivo imaging and are resistant to photo-breaching. In the experimental situation, minimal toxicity of quantum dots has been observed. However, cadmium atoms contained in current NIR quantum dots might hamper their clinical application. Cyanine dye families can be alternative choices for NIR cell labeling, provided sufficient labeling yield can be achieved (15).

Fluorescence dyes with other emission lights of shorter wavelengths than NIR are not appropriate choices for imaging from outside of the body because of short penetration of both excitation and emission lights. However, fluorescence dyes with green to yellow range of emission lights may be a suitable choice for direct views of lesions under surgery or during endoscopy because of their high quantum yield (16).

Bioluminescence Imaging

The bioluminescence imaging method is an optical imaging version of the reporter gene method. This method consists of two parts similar to reporter gene method (see the nuclear medicine section); first, transfection of luciferase gene into target cells either ex vivo or in vivo to produce the enzyme luciferase; and secondly, injection of luciferin (a substrate working as a light source by the existence of luciferase and spending ATP as an energy source) into the animal to produce the signal (green light), thus imaging target cells. An advantage of the bioluminescence imaging over reporter strategy with the nuclear medicine technique is that luciferin does not have signal (light) without activation by luciferase, thus, there in no background signal produced by other cells. In contrast, all the nuclear medicine reporter system probes can produce signal even though the agent does not meet with the target, so unbound reagents will produce high background signal and compromise the quality of imaging.

SUMMARY

In this chapter, a general consideration of in vivo cellular imaging using various modalities and labeling methods has been broadly reviewed, with a particular focus on signaling probes and cell labeling methodology.

REFERENCES

1. Gray SJ, Sterling K. Determination of circulating red cell volume by radioactive chromium. Science 1950; 112:179–180.
2. Shapiro EM, Skrtic S, Sharer K, et al. MRI detection of single particles for cellular imaging. Proc Natl Acad Sci U S A 2004; 101:10901–10906.
3. Shapiro EM, Sharer K, Skrtic S, et al. In vivo detection of single cells by MRI. Magn Reson Med 2006; 55:242–249.
4. Ward KM, Aletras AH, Balaban RS. A new class of contrast agents for MRI based on proton chemical exchange dependent saturation transfer (CEST). J Magn Reson 2000; 143:79–87.
5. Gilad AA, McMahon MT, Walczak P, et al. Artificial reporter gene providing MRI contrast based on proton exchange. Nat Biotechnol 2007; 25:217–219.
6. Harisinghani MG, Barentsz J, Hahn PF, et al. Noninvasive detection of clinically occult lymph-node metastases in prostate cancer. N Engl J Med 2003; 348:2491–2499.
7. Jo SK, Hu X, Kobayashi H, et al. Detection of inflammation following renal ischemia by magnetic resonance imaging. Kidney Int 2003; 64:43–51.

8. Arbab AS, Yocum GT, Wilson LB, et al. Comparison of transfection agents in forming complexes with ferumoxides, cell labeling efficiency, and cellular viability. Mol Imaging 2004; 3:24–32.

9. Walczak P, Kedziorek DA, Gilad AA, et al. Instant MR labeling of stem cells using magnetoelectroporation. Magn Reson Med 2005; 54:769–774.

10. Goldenberg DM, Juweid M, Dunn RM, et al. Cancer imaging with radiolabeled antibodies: new advances with technetium-99m-labeled monoclonal antibody Fab′ fragments, especially CEA-Scan and prospects for therapy. J Nucl Med Technol 1997; 25:18–23; quiz 34.

11. De Jong M, Valkema R, Jamar F, et al. Somatostatin receptor-targeted radionuclide therapy of tumors: preclinical and clinical findings. 2002; 32:133–140.

12. Ray P, Bauer E, Iyer M, et al. Monitoring gene therapy with reporter gene imaging. Semin Nucl Med 2001; 31:312–320.

13. Anelli PL, Lattuada L, Lorusso V, et al. Mixed micelles containing lipophilic gadolinium complexes as MRA contrast agents. MAGMA 2001; 12:114–120.

14. Hoffman RM. The multiple uses of fluorescent proteins to visualize cancer in vivo. Nat Rev Cancer 2005; 5: 796–806.

15. Mahmood U, Weissleder R. Near-infrared optical imaging of proteases in cancer. Mol Cancer Ther 2003; 2:489–496.

16. Hama Y, Urano Y, Koyama Y, et al. A comparison of the emission efficiency of four common green fluorescence dyes after Internalization into cancer cells. Bioconjug Chem 2006; 17:1426–1431.

33

Molecular Imaging of the Extracellular Matrix and Lymphatic Phenomena in Tumors

ARVIND P. PATHAK and ZAVER M. BHUJWALLA

JHU ICMIC Program, Russell H. Morgan Department of Radiology and Radiological Science, and Sidney Kimmel Comprehensive Cancer Center, Johns Hopkins University School of Medicine, Baltimore, Maryland, U.S.A.

MOLECULAR IMAGING OF THE EXTRACELLULAR MATRIX

The tumor stroma comprising the extracellular matrix (ECM), mesenchymal cells, inflammatory cells, and a supporting network of blood vessels, lymphatic vessels, and nerves was traditionally believed to play a passive role in the regulation and development of cancer. However, discoveries in the past few decades have turned this paradigm on its head—the direct physical contact of tumor cells with stromal cells in conjunction with the effect of their growth factors transforms this quiescent stroma into an "activated" stroma, which facilitates the migration, invasion, survival, and proliferation of tumor cells (1,2). The two-way signaling between the ECM and cancer cells results in the continuous remodeling of the ECM via paracrine or autocrine actions of various growth factors and proteases (3). An understanding of this bidirectional exchange has resulted in the identification of several potential therapeutic targets in the tumor stroma (3) and a concurrent need for novel imaging techniques for probing such interactions noninvasively and in vivo.

Molecular imaging of the ECM or "extravascular" events occurring within the tumor stroma broadly consist of (*i*) imaging ECM-cellular interactions, (*ii*) imaging protease activity, and (*iii*) imaging the ECM in vivo.

Imaging ECM-Cellular Interactions

Several avant-garde techniques ranging from second harmonic generation microscopy to atomic force microscopy (AFM) have been harnessed to image the interaction between tumor cells and the ECM at spatial scales ranging from millimeters down to nanometers (Ref. 4 is an excellent summary of some of these techniques). For example, the macroscopic properties of type I collagen and interstitial ECM were evaluated and quantified using confocal reflection microscopy (5). In these studies, the backscattering of light combined with confocal microscopy provided reflection images at sequential focal planes that could be reconstructed for 3D visualization of collagen assemblies without necessitating any immunohistochemical (IHC) staining of the samples. Campagnola et al. initially proposed and developed the use of surface second harmonic generation (SHG) in laser scanning microscopy as a new contrast mechanism for live cell imaging (6). SHG is a nonlinear optical process that requires an environment without a center of symmetry, such as an interfacial region, to produce a signal. This contrast mechanism has been extended to image endogenous structural proteins within the collagen-rich dermis of the mouse ear (7). Nomarski differential interference contrast optics, wherein the optical path length gradients passing through a Nomarski prism produce image contrast (8), has also been used to dynamically track cell-induced matrix remodeling.

Fourier transform infrared (FTIR) microspectroscopy has also been used to generate infrared images of the proteolytic activity of matrix metalloproteinases (MMPs) produced by invasive cancer cells on collagen-based matrices (9). FTIR spectroscopy probes the vibration energy of chemical bonds that combined with microscopy provides a direct probe of chemical composition for imaging intact biological matrices at high spatial resolution (on the order of micrometers). More recently, ECM alterations in the pericellular microenvironment of cancer cells have been imaged and characterized at exquisite nanoscale resolution using AFM by Kusick et al. (10). Because AFM are surface-sensitive instruments capable of measuring forces in the pN range (11), both between and within single biomolecules, it is possible to create functional images at the subcellular level.

Imaging Proteases

Various proteases are involved in modulating, that is, degrading and remodeling the integrity of the ECM and basement membranes, thereby facilitating cancer cell invasion, metastasis, and angiogenesis. However, as mentioned earlier, by regulating growth factors and their receptors, cytokines, and a variety of enzymes, MMPs transform or "activate" the tumor ECM (1). In fact, MMPs such as MMP-2 (gelatinase) are overexpressed in several cancers and have been associated with the aggressive tumor phenotype and poor patient outcome (12). Therefore, being able to image the activity of proteases in cancer is a crucial step toward understanding their role in tumor progression and treatment outcome.

Imaging of protease activity in tumor models has been primarily performed using near-infrared (NIR) optical imaging of protease-activated probes. These probes are based on the principle that fluorophores in proximity to each other are quenched, and it is only after cleavage of the probe by an enzyme that the fluorophores are released from the carrier, and a fluorescent signal is detected. This approach has been used to detect MMP-2 (13) and for NIR imaging of cathepsin B-sensitive probes in breast cancer models (12). In the latter study, the fluorescence signal intensity was higher in the highly invasive metastatic tumor model consistent with higher cathepsin B protein activity compared with that in the well-differentiated tumors (12).

Lysosomes are cellular organelles that carry multiple proteases including cathepsins and play an important role in cancer invasion and metastasis (14). Noninvasive optical imaging of 6'-O-glucosamine-labeled fluorescent probes, which accumulate in lysosomal proteins due to their high degree of glycosylation, were recently developed to delineate the role of lysosomes and lysosomal trafficking in breast cancer invasion and metastasis (14). Lysosomal trafficking was found to be significantly altered under acidic pH conditions typically found in tumors (15).

Imaging The ECM In Vivo

A consequence of these innovative developments has led to their application for in vivo functional imaging of tumor-ECM interactions. The feasibility of imaging the motility and metastatic differences between carcinoma cells of differing metastatic potential in the same animal at subcellular resolutions was elegantly demonstrated in a recent study by Sahai et al. (16). In this study, to compare directly the behavior of cells with different metastatic potentials in the same tumor microenvironment in vivo, tumors were generated by injecting a mixed population of poorly metastatic cancer cells labeled with green fluorescent protein (GFP) and highly metastatic cancer cells labeled with cyan fluorescent protein (CFP). This was followed by simultaneously imaging GFP, CFP fluorescence, and collagen second harmonic imaging in vivo with multiphoton laser scanning microscopy. SHG imaging in tumors has also been applied to dynamically visualize the structure of fibrillar collagen, estimate relative diffusive hindrance, and the dynamics of enzymatic modification of tumor collagen with relaxin in vivo (17). In other studies, quantum dots, which are fluorescent semiconductor nanocrystals, were used to image and differentiate tumor vessels from the ECM and also track the recruitment of quantum dot-labeled bone marrow-derived precursor cells to the tumor vasculature (18).

More recently, innovative magnetic resonance imaging (MRI) methods have been developed to study interactions between cancer cells and the ECM. One such approach developed by us exploits the kinetics, that is, delivery and transport of a macromolecular MRI contrast agent through the ECM and supporting stroma of the tumor (Fig. 1) (19). Specifically, we developed a noninvasive imaging technique to characterize the delivery and interstitial transport of albumin-GdDTPA in an MCF-7 human breast cancer model in vivo, using MRI. The physiological parameters measured included vascular volume fraction, vessel permeability-surface area product, macromolecular fluid exudate volume, and drainage and pooling rates within the ECM. We were able to discern distinct pooling and draining regions within the ECM using MRI (Fig. 2). A few tumor-associated lymphatic vessels stained positively for LYVE-1 (Lymphatic Vessel Endothelial Receptor 1),

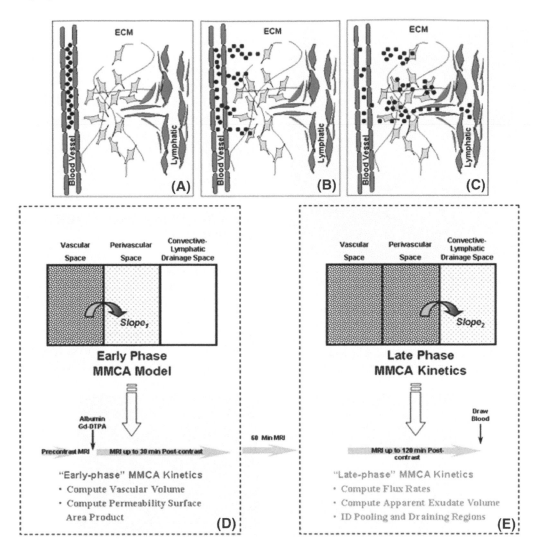

Figure 1 Schematic illustrating compartmentalization of the macromolecular contrast agent (MMCA) albumin-GdDTPA following intravenous administration. (**A**) During the early phase of the MRI protocol, the MMCA is confined to the vascular compartment, immediately followed by (**B**) extravasation from the hyperpermeable tumor vessels into the extravascular space, from which (**C**) it is cleared by convection and/or tumoral lymphatics, if present. Schematic illustrating the manner in which kinetics of the MMCA during the "early" and "late" phases of the MRI experiment were exploited to extract physiological information about the compartments described in **A–C**. (**D**) Assuming negligible reflux of the contrast agent and fast exchange for the duration of the MR experiment, uptake of the MMCA uptake was modeled as a linear function of time for the "early-phase," that is, the first 31 minutes of the MR acquisition. For this phase, the slope ($slope_1$) of the concentration-time curve provides the permeability-surface area product, PS (μL/g min), and the y-intercept the vascular volume, V_V (μL/g). During the early phase, we assume transport of MMCA from the vascular to the perivascular space is unidirectional, and that there is negligible transport (if any) of the MMCA from the perivascular to the drainage compartment. (**E**) Ninety to approximately 140 minutes after the administration of the MMCA, that is, for the "late-phase" of the MR experiment, MMCA uptake is also modeled as a linear function of time. During this phase, it was assumed that there was unidirectional transport of the MMCA from the perivascular to the slow drainage compartment with a flux rate, FR (μL/g min) given by the slope ($slope_2$) of the late phase concentration-time curve. *Source*: Adapted from Ref. 19.

but were primarily found to be collapsed and tenuous (Fig. 3). This suggested that lymphatic drainage played a minimal role, and that the bulk of drainage was due to convective transport through the ECM in this tumor model (19). In another dynamic contrast-enhanced MRI study, the effect of heparanase expression on lymph node metastasis,

in heparanase-overexpressing subcutaneous Eb mouse T-lymphoma tumors, and their draining lymph node was assessed using a fluorescently tagged version of the macromoleclar contrast agent, albumin-GdDTPA (20). Heparanase expression significantly increased contrast enhancement of the popliteal lymph node but not of the

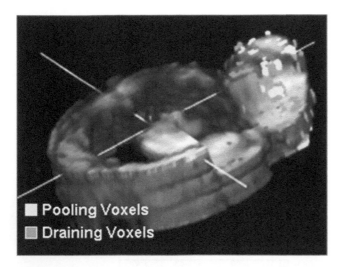

Figure 2 Three-dimensional cutaway of a post-contrast MR image of an MCF-7 tumor overlaid with a functional map showing the spatial distribution of the extravascular *draining* and *pooling* voxels, that is, voxels from which albumin-GdDTPA was either being cleared by convection/lymphatic drain, or voxels in which albumin-GdDTPA was found to be pooling. *Source*: Adapted from Ref. 19 (*See Color Insert*).

primary tumor, with changes in MR contrast enhancement preceding formation of pathologically detectable metastases. Finally, in a recent study the spatial distribution of tumor interstitial fluid pressure (IFP) in vivo was mapped using contrast-enhanced MRI (21). The MRI techniques described here bridge the gap between traditional intravital approaches and multiphoton laser-scanning microscopy (MPLSM) by providing relatively high spatial resolution (100–250 μm) for visualization of interstitial transport and drainage in deep-seated, optically nontransparent tumor tissue in vivo.

MOLECULAR IMAGING OF TUMOR-ASSOCIATED LYMPHATICS

The discovery of highly specific markers for the lymphatic endothelium has ushered in a new era in the field of lymphatic research and enabled the identification of novel pathways responsible for "lymphangiogenesis," that is, the de novo formation of lymphatic capillaries. Such markers include podoplanin, Prox-1, LYVE-1, and VEGFR-3 (22). The two new growth factors implicated in lymphangiogenesis

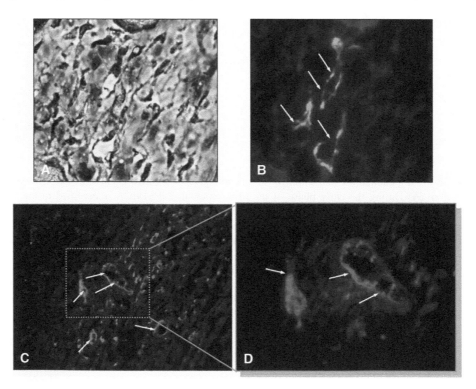

Figure 3 Photomicrographs from a 5-μm thick MCF-7 tumor section. (**A**) H&E stained MCF-7 tumor section (100×), and (**B**) the same section stained with LYVE-1, a lymphatic endothelial cell marker. Lymphatic vessels exhibiting green fluorescence (Alexa-Fluor® 488 secondary antibody) are clearly visible in the tumor margin (100×). Arrows in **A** and **B** indicate lymphatic vessel lumen punctuated by tumor cells. (**C**) Photomicrograph obtained at 40× from a 5-μm thick MCF-7 tumor section showing the intratumoral distribution of the MMCA biotin-albumin-GdDTPA. Blood vessels fluorescence red due to labeling with lectin-TRITC, and biotin-albumin-GdDTPA exhibiting blue fluorescence due to labeling with Streptavidin Marina Blue® conjugate. (**D**) Magnified (100×) image of the region in **C** outlined by the blue square illustrating the localization of the MMCA biotin-albumin-GdDTPA in the blood vessels. Arrows in each indicate blood vessel lumen. *Source*: Adapted from Ref. 19 (*See Color Insert*).

belong to the vascular endothelial growth factor (VEGF) family, and are VEGF-C and VEGF-D. A growing number of studies on human tumors reveal a clear relationship between the level of VEGF-C in tumors and the likelihood of metastases to the regional lymph nodes (23).

Although the significance of tumor-associated lymphatics in metastasis has been acknowledged for well over a century, several issues regarding their involvement in the metastatic cascade remain (24). This has resulted in a crucial need for techniques to dynamically image tumor-associated lymphatic function in vivo. Advances in optical imaging and modalities such as MRI, in conjunction with the synthesis of novel imaging probes, have begun to transform our understanding of the mechanisms underlying lymphangiogenesis and lymphatic metastases. To have an impact on the diagnosis and treatment of lymphogenous metastases, visualizing differences in lymphatic function between normal and tumor tissue in vivo is essential. A description of some of these novel molecular imaging approaches for probing the function of the tumor-associated lymphatics follows in the next section.

Since certain cancers like breast cancer first spread to the regional lymph node and then to the next tier of lymph nodes due to the unidirectional flow of lymph, initial studies on the functionality of lymphatic vessels were based on efforts to distinguish this sentinel node, that is, the first lymph node or group of nodes that would hypothetically be reached by metastasizing cancer cells (25,26). Colloidal proteins and dyes delivered into the interstitium, traverse the lymphatics and arrive at the draining lymph nodes, where they are accumulated by macrophages (27). The past few years have seen the development of a range of imaging techniques for characterizing fluid and macromolecule transport within the extravascular space of tumors that includes the interstitium and lymphatics. These techniques include the injection of fluorescently labeled macromolecules into the tumor interstitium followed by their eventual uptake into lymphatics, that is, microlymphangiography (28) and the use of fluorescence redistribution/recovery after photobleaching (FRAP) in situ. In FRAP, a fluorescent dye conjugated with a target macromolecule is bleached in the region of interest, and the recovery of fluorescence due to dye diffusion in the bleached portion is tracked (29). In one such study of a murine sarcoma model implanted in the tail, fluorescein isothiocyanate-labeled dextran (FITC-dextran) was used as a tracer for low-power in vivo fluorescent microscopy of tail lymphatics, in conjunction with a ferritin solution injected either into the tail tip or directly into the center of the tumor for microlymphangiography (30). The results of the combined in vivo lymphangiography and immunohistochemistry supported the hypothesis that the solid tumor was deficient in functional intratumoral lymphatics but surrounded by enlarged

peritumoral lymphatics that may be a sufficient avenue for tumor cell dissemination. Other studies employing a similar mouse tail-skin model in conjunction with fluorescent microscopy have also elegantly demonstrated how interstitial fluid flow not only guides but may also pave the way for lymphangiogenesis and lymphatic modeling (31).

The identification of VEGF-C and VEGF-D has significantly increased our understanding of lymphatic remodeling in normal tissues, although lymphatic remodeling in tumor tissue is still relatively unexplored. In a recent study, MPLSM was used to image deep-seated (>400 μm) tumoral lymphatic vessels (32), circumventing the disadvantages of traditional intravital microscopy techniques such as limited depth of penetration and phototoxicity. In this study in vivo visualization of the lymphatics in three dimensions at the level of individual cells was achieved, together with imaging of interactions between leukocytes and blood vessel endothelium at sub-second temporal resolutions. Recently, MPLSM was used for high-resolution imaging of functional lymphatics in a murine tumor model engineered to overexpress VEGF-C (28). Although overexpression of VEGF-C stimulated robust lymphangiogenesis in the tumor margins and increased metastasis, three independent assays for probing lymphatic function, that is, lymphangiography, epifluorescence microscopy, and MPLSM, revealed an absence of functional intratumoral lymphatic vessels in these tumors. Visualization of the initial invasion of tumor cells through the lymphatic system into the subcapsular sinuses and eventually into the parenchyma of the lymph nodes was recently demonstrated with in vivo fluorescence microscopy in an orthotopic human breast cancer model. These studies were performed in conjunction with measurements of IFP and suggest that intravasation of cancer cells into the lymphatic system may be mediated through IFP (33).

Despite major advances in intravital microscopy and optical imaging techniques, dynamic, noninvasive, in vivo investigations of the tumor-host tissue interface remain a challenge. Recent progress in MRI techniques and the synthesis of novel MRI contrast agents will help bridge the resolution gap between macroscopic lymphangiography approaches and intravital multiphoton microscopy. With MRI visualization of the tumor-host tissue interface in its entirety, including the lymphatics and extravascular transport through the ECM, can be achieved at relatively high spatial resolutions (100–250 μm) in vivo. This type of complete coverage of the entire tumor is not possible with the optical techniques currently available, especially for imaging deep-seated lymphatic-convective transport in tumor tissues that may be optically opaque.

In one recent study of the tumor-associated lymphatics, a biotinylated MR contrast agent (biotin-BSA-GdDTPA) was administered intravenously, and its extravasation from the leaky tumor vessels and eventual drainage via the peritumoral lymphatics was tracked in vivo using MRI. In this case, it was possible to image lymphatic uptake as the administration of the biotinylated MR contrast agent was followed by the administration of a "chaser" of avidin, which rapidly cleared away any residual contrast agent within the vascular space without affecting the extravasated contrast agent (34).

Understanding the various factors that influence delivery, movement, and clearance of macromolecules through the ECM of solid tumors is also important to understand cancer invasion and metastasis. In an extension of our initial study to characterize the delivery and interstitial transport of albumin-GdDTPA and determine the integrity of the tumor ECM in vivo, we conducted noninvasive in vivo MRI of two human breast cancer models with significantly different invasiveness (35). As before, we exploited the kinetics of the macromolecular contrast agent albumin-GdDTPA to characterize differences in vascularization (vascular volume, permeability-surface area product) and lymphatic-convective transport (macromolecular fluid transport rates/volumes, fraction of draining/pooling voxels) in vivo, with the goal of understanding their role in the regional spread of breast cancer to the axillary lymph nodes (Fig. 4). We found significant

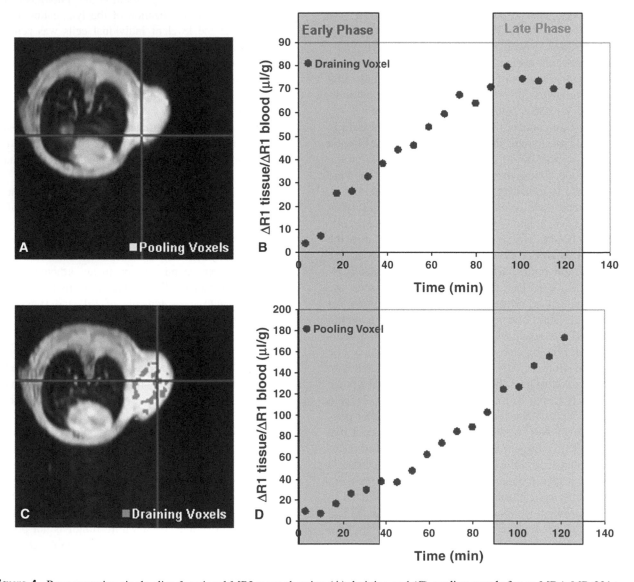

Figure 4 Representative single-slice functional MRI maps showing (**A**) draining and (**C**) pooling voxels for an MDA-MB-231 tumor (*arrows*) bearing animal. MMCA concentration-time curve typical of a (**B**) *draining* voxel (within cross-hairs in **A**) exhibiting slow uptake of the MMCA during the early phase followed by elimination of the MMCA during the late phase and (**D**) *pooling* voxel (within cross-hairs in **C**) exhibiting some uptake of the MMCA during the early phase followed by enhancement during the late phase. *Source*: Adapted from Ref. 35 (*See Color Insert*).

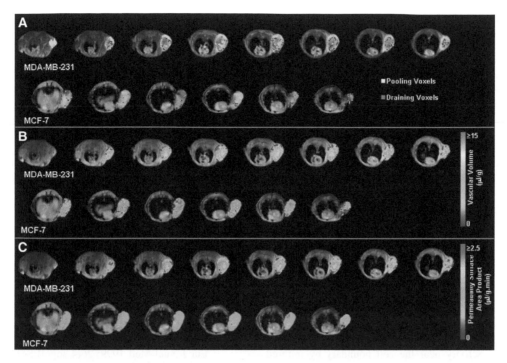

Figure 5 (**A**) Representative multislice functional MRI maps of pooling and draining voxels for an invasive MDA-MB-231 tumor xenograft bearing animal (*upper panel*), and a noninvasive MCF-7 tumor xenograft bearing animal (*lower panel*). (**B**) Corresponding multislice functional MRI maps of the vascular volume for the MDA-MB-231 bearing (*upper panel*) and MCF-7 bearing animals (*lower panel*) shown in **A**. (**C**) Corresponding multislice functional MRI maps of the permeability-surface area product for the MDA-MB-231 bearing (*upper panel*) and the MCF-7 bearing animals (*lower panel*) shown in **A**. This example nicely demonstrates our ability to noninvasively characterize differences in vascularization and ECM integrity in vivo, between two human breast cancer models with significantly different invasiveness, to quantify and understand the role of interstitial fluid transport, lymphatic-convective drain, and vascularization in the regional spread of breast cancer to the axillary lymph nodes. *Source*: Adapted from Ref. 35.

differences in vascular and extravascular transport parameters measured with MRI, as well as in lymphatic vessel morphology assessed with fluorescent microscopy, between the two breast cancer models. We also measured significant differences in lymph node and lung metastasis between the two tumor models. These data were consistent with the role of lymphatic drain in lymph node metastasis and suggested that increased lymph node metastasis may occur due to a combination of increased invasiveness and reduced ECM integrity. This remodeling of the ECM in turn allows increased pathways of least resistance for the transport of extravascular fluid and tumor cells. It was also possible that lymph node metastasis occurred via the cancer cell-bearing tumoral lymphatic vessels, and the congestion of these tumoral lymphatics with cancer cells may have precluded the entry and transport of macromolecules. A unique advantage of this MRI technique is the ability to characterize the spatiotemporal relationship between tumor angiogenesis and lymphatic-convective transport in vivo (Fig. 5).

Finally, the synthesis of dendrimer-based MRI contrast agents has enabled micro-magnetic resonance lymphangiography (MRL) methods to be developed. Such dendrimer-based MRI contrast agents enable the visualization of the entire murine lymphatic system, including lymph nodes. Abnormally enlarged lymph nodes in transgenic mice overexpressing interleukin-15 were easily identified by micro-MRL for eventual excision and analyses to demonstrate their cell type and receptor expression.

The dynamic, noninvasive, in vivo molecular and functional imaging approaches described in this chapter are transforming our understanding of both the role of the ECM and tumor-associated lymphatic phenomena in the process of tumor cell dissemination and the formation of metastases.

ACKNOWLEDGMENT

Support from P50 CA103175 is gratefully acknowledged.

BIBLIOGRAPHY

1. Stamenkovic I. Extracellular matrix remodelling: the role of matrix metalloproteinases. J Pathol 2003; 200(4): 448–464.

2. Tlsty TD, Coussens LM. Tumor stroma and regulation of cancer development. Ann Rev Pathol Mech Dis 2006; 1:119–150.

3. Mueller MM, Fusenig NE. Friends or foes - bipolar effects of the tumour stroma in cancer. Nat Rev Cancer 2004; 4(11):839–849.

4. Friedl P. Dynamic imaging of the immune system. Curr Opin Immunol 2004; 16(4):389–393.

5. Brightman AO, Rajwa BP, Sturgis JE, et al. Time-lapse confocal reflection microscopy of collagen fibrillogenesis and extracellular matrix assembly in vitro. Biopolymers 2000; 54(3):222–234.

6. Campagnola PJ, Wei MD, Lewis A, et al. High-resolution nonlinear optical imaging of live cells by second harmonic generation. Biophys J 1999; 77(6):3341–3349.

7. Campagnola PJ, Millard AC, Terasaki M, et al. Three-dimensional high-resolution second-harmonic generation imaging of endogenous structural proteins in biological tissues. Biophys J 2002; 82(1 Pt 1):493–508.

8. Petroll WM, Ma L. Direct, dynamic assessment of cell-matrix interactions inside fibrillar collagen lattices. Cell Motil Cytoskeleton 2003; 55(4):254–264.

9. Federman S, Miller LM, Sagi I. Following matrix metalloproteinases activity near the cell boundary by infrared micro-spectroscopy. Matrix Biol 2002; 21(7):567–577.

10. Kusick S, Bertram H, Oberleithner H, et al. Nanoscale imaging and quantification of local proteolytic activity. J Cell Physiol 2005; 204(3):767–774.

11. Allison DP, Hinterdorfer P, Han W. Biomolecular force measurements and the atomic force microscope. Curr Opin Biotechnol 2002; 13(1):47–51.

12. Bremer C, Tung CH, Bogdanov A Jr, et al. Imaging of differential protease expression in breast cancers for detection of aggressive tumor phenotypes. Radiology 2002; 222(3): 814–818.

13. Bremer C, Bredow S, Mahmood U, et al. Optical imaging of matrix metalloproteinase-2 activity in tumors: feasibility study in a mouse model. Radiology 2001; 221(2):523–529.

14. Glunde K, Foss CA, Takagi T, et al. Synthesis of 6'-O-lissamine-rhodamine B-glucosamine as a novel probe for fluorescence imaging of lysosomes in breast tumors. Bioconjug Chem 2005; 16(4):843–851.

15. Glunde K, Guggino SE, Solaiyappan M, et al. Extracellular acidification alters lysosomal trafficking in human breast cancer cells. Neoplasia 2003; 5(6):533–545.

16. Sahai E, Wyckoff J, Philippar U, et al. Simultaneous imaging of GFP, CFP and collagen in tumors in vivo using multi-photon microscopy. BMC Biotechnol 2005; 5:14.

17. Brown E, McKee T, di Tomaso E, et al. Dynamic imaging of collagen and its modulation in tumors in vivo using second-harmonic generation. Nat Med 2003; 9(6):796–800.

18. Stroh M, Zimmer JP, Duda DG, et al. Quantum dots spectrally distinguish multiple species within the tumor milieu in vivo. Nat Med 2005; 11(6):678–682.

19. Pathak AP, Artemov D, Ward BD, et al. Characterizing extravascular fluid transport of macromolecules in the tumor interstitium by magnetic resonance imaging. Cancer Res 2005; 65(4):1425–1432.

20. Dafni H, Cohen B, Ziv K, et al. The role of heparanase in lymph node metastatic dissemination: dynamic contrast-enhanced MRI of Eb lymphoma in mice. Neoplasia 2005; 7(3):224–233.

21. Hassid Y, Furman-Haran E, Margalit R, et al. Noninvasive magnetic resonance imaging of transport and interstitial fluid pressure in ectopic human lung tumors. Cancer Res 2006; 66(8):4159–4166.

22. Cao Y. Opinion: emerging mechanisms of tumour lymphangiogenesis and lymphatic metastasis. Nat Rev Cancer 2005; 5(9):735–743.

23. Pepper MS, Tille JC, Nisato R, et al. Lymphangiogenesis and tumor metastasis. Cell Tissue Res 2003; 314(1): 167–177.

24. Pepper MS. Lymphangiogenesis and tumor metastasis: more questions than answers. Lymphology 2000; 33(4): 144–147.

25. Haigh PI, Giuliano AE. Role of sentinel lymph node dissection in breast cancer. Ann Med 2000; 32(1):51–56.

26. Nieweg OE, Jansen L, Valdes Olmos RA, et al. Lymphatic mapping and sentinel lymph node biopsy in breast cancer. Eur J Nucl Med 1999; 26(4 suppl):S11–S16.

27. Wilhelm AJ, Mijnhout G, Franssen EJ. Radiopharmaceuticals in sentinel lymph-node detection - an overview. Eur J Nucl Med 1999; 26(4 suppl):S36–S42.

28. Padera TP, Kadambi A, di Tomaso E, et al. Lymphatic metastasis in the absence of functional intratumor lymphatics. Science 2002; 296(5574):1883–1886.

29. Netti PA, Berk DA, Swartz MA, et al. Role of extracellular matrix assembly in interstitial transport in solid tumors. Cancer Res 2000; 60(9):2497–2503.

30. Leu AJ, Berk DA, Lymboussaki A, et al. Absence of functional lymphatics within a murine sarcoma: a molecular and functional evaluation. Cancer Res 2000; 60(16):4324–4327.

31. Boardman KC, Swartz MA. Interstitial flow as a guide for lymphangiogenesis. Circ Res 2003; 92(7):801–808.

32. Padera TP, Stoll BR, So PT, et al. Conventional and high-speed intravital multiphoton laser scanning microscopy of microvasculature, lymphatics, and leukocyte-endothelial interactions. Mol Imaging 2002; 1(1):9–15.

33. Dadiani M, Kalchenko V, Yosepovich A, et al. Real-time imaging of lymphogenic metastasis in orthotopic human breast cancer. Cancer Res 2006; 66(16):8037–8041.

34. Dafni H, Landsman L, Schechter B, et al. MRI and fluorescence microscopy of the acute vascular response to VEGF165: vasodilation, hyper-permeability and lymphatic uptake, followed by rapid inactivation of the growth factor. NMR Biomed 2002; 15(2):120–131.

35. Pathak AP, Artemov D, Neeman M, et al. Lymph node metastasis in breast cancer xenografts is associated with increased regions of extravascular drain, lymphatic vessel area, and invasive phenotype. Cancer Res 2006; 66(10): 5151–5158.

34

Nuclear Imaging of Adoptive Cell Therapies

VLADIMIR PONOMAREV

Department of Radiology, Memorial Sloan Kettering Cancer Center, New York, New York, U.S.A.

INTRODUCTION

Recent developments in biotechnology have led to an increasing number of clinically available anticancer therapies that require administration of cells of different origins. These cellular therapies are based on the ex vivo manipulation of different therapeutically useful cell types (stem cells, lineage progenitors, mesenchymal cells, lymphocytes, dendritic cells, etc.) followed by local or systemic administration to patients (1–4). A promising role of cellular therapies in cancer treatment, especially minimal residual disease and micrometastases, is reflected by the constantly growing number of clinical trials with adoptively transferred cells (5).

Until recently, immunostaining of whole-body slices of small animals was the most straightforward, reliable, and traditional approach used for assessing the localization and targeting of adoptively transferred cells (6). However, the invasive nature of classical pathology precludes the repetitive monitoring of cellular trafficking in the same animal over time. For example, it is unclear if the adoptively transferred T-lymphocytes undergo substantial proliferation at the target site, or if the activation and proliferation occur at other sites (e.g., specific lymphoid organ sites) and are followed by migration and localization to the target site. The results obtained from multiple animals sacrificed at different time points may be flawed by individual variations, and a large number of animals

have to be studied to achieve statistical significance. Another major shortcoming of this method is that it cannot be applied in the clinical setting. Methods for noninvasive and repetitive evaluation of trafficking, homing, tumor targeting, differentiation, and persistence of adoptively transferred cells would significantly aid the development of progenitor or effector cell–based therapy approaches and facilitate their implementation in the clinic (6). These questions could potentially be answered by repetitive imaging using clinically applicable techniques, for example, nuclear imaging.

EX VIVO RADIOLABELING FOR NUCLEAR IMAGING

The marking of cells with radiolabeled tracers was first tested in the early 1970s. ^{3}H- and ^{14}C-labeled uridine was used to assess lymphocyte trafficking in a graft-versus-host disease (GVHD) model (7). Other earlier studies used ^{3}H-glycerol (8). A similar method, using ^{3}H-labeled glucose, was applied to patients to compare the kinetics of lymphocytes in normal and HIV-infected individuals (9). However, the use of β-emitting isotopes limits such studies to cellular kinetic studies based on sequential blood sampling.

Noninvasive imaging of lymphocyte trafficking dates back to the early 1970s, when the first experiments were performed with ^{51}Cr and ^{99m}Tc extracorporeal labeling of

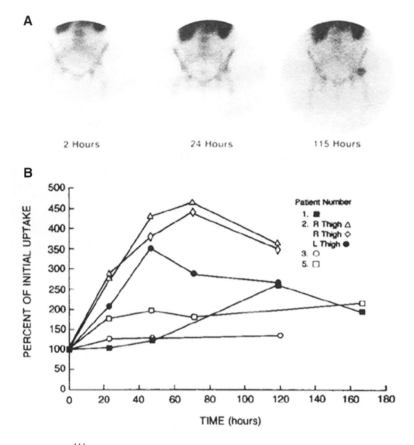

Figure 1 Gamma camera imaging of ^{111}In-labeled TILs in patients with malignant melanoma. (**A**) Areas of tumor enhancement in the left groin were observed in this anterior view of the pelvis as early as 24 hours after T-cell injection. Localization of ^{111}In shows a progressive increase in that same tumor five days later. (**B**) Serial changes in the concentration of ^{111}In for six individual tumor sites were calculated as percentage of the initial uptake at each site. Localization of ^{111}In increases in tumors with time with maximum uptake seen between 48 and 72 hours. *Abbreviation*: TILs, tumor-infiltrating lymphocytes. *Source*: From Ref. 15.

lymphocytes (10,11). These methods were applied to different immune cells using various radioisotopes for labeling (e.g., ^{111}In, ^{67}Co, ^{64}Cu) (10,11–14). ^{111}In, in particular, found a wide clinical application in oncology as an imaging agent for monitoring vaccination with tumor-infiltrating lymphocytes (15–17). In a study published by Fisher et al. (15), six patients with metastatic malignant melanoma who had multiple sites of subcutaneous, nodal, and/or visceral disease were treated with ^{111}In-labeled tumor-infiltrating lymphocytes (TILs). The patients received cyclophosphamide 36 hours before receiving the intravenous (i.v.) infusion of TILs (mean 8.4×10^9 labeled cells/patient) followed by i.v. administration of IL-2 every eight hours. The distribution and localization of the TILs were evaluated using serial whole-body gamma camera imaging, serial blood and urine samplings, and serial biopsies of tumor and normal tissue. ^{111}In-labeled TILs localized to lung, liver, and spleen within two hours after the infusion. Activity in the lung diminished within 24 hours. As early as 24 hours after injection of ^{111}In-labeled TILs, localization of TILs

to metastatic deposits was demonstrated in all six patients using either imaging studies or biopsy specimens or both (Fig. 1). ^{111}In activity in tumor tissue biopsies ranged from 3 to 40 times greater than activity in normal tissue. A progressive increase in the radioactive counts at sites of tumor deposits was seen. This study showed that labeled TILs can localize preferentially to tumor, and it provided information concerning the possible mechanism of the therapeutic effects of TIL administration.

In a similar study, Matera et al. (18) studied the migration of ^{111}In-oxine-labeled autologous natural killer (NK) cells to liver metastases in patients with colon carcinoma. NK cells were expanded ex vivo with IL-2, labeled with ^{111}In-oxine and injected intraarterially (i.a.) in the liver of three colon carcinoma patients. After 30 days, each patient had a new preparation of ^{111}In-NK cells injected intravenously. Migration of these cells to various organs was evaluated by pinhole single-photon emission computed tomography (SPECT) and their differential localization to normal and neoplastic liver was demonstrated after i.v. injection of 99mTc-phytate (^{99m}Tc phytate is transformed by chelation with serum calcium in vivo into a microcolloid, which is taken up by cells of the reticuloendothelial system, particularly Kupffer cells). When injected i.v., these cells localized to the lung before being visible in the spleen and liver. By contrast, localization of i.a. injected NK cells was virtually confined to the spleen and liver. Binding of NK cells to liver neoplastic tissues was observed only after i.a. injections.

Bennink et al. (19) evaluated a noninvasive scintigraphic technique able to assess ^{99m}Tc-hexamethylpropylene amine oxime (^{99m}Tc-HMPAO)–labeled neutrophil trafficking in a mouse model of dextran sulfate sodium (DSS)–induced colitis. SPECT of the abdomen was performed one hour after reinjection of 1.35 mCi of labeled neutrophils. Colonic uptake of ^{99m}Tc-HMPAO neutrophils was determined with dedicated animal pinhole SPECT in mice with DSS-induced colitis and correlated well with histological findings, wet colon weight, and clinical weight loss. The neutrophil uptake ratio was reduced significantly by blocking of neutrophil migration capacity with the CD97 antibody.

In another study, Olasz et al. (20) developed a novel method for labeling mouse bone marrow–derived dendritic cells (BMDC) with the positron-emitting radioisotope ^{18}F using N-succinimidyl-4-[^{18}F]fluorobenzoate, which covalently binds to the lysine residues of cell surface proteins. Based on the specific activity of ^{18}F, the cells were labeled with an average of 10^7 molecules/cell without BMDC activity compromised. Migration of ^{18}F-labeled BMDC after footpad injection was studied with whole-body gamma camera or positron emission tomography (PET) imaging. The authors found that four hours after injection of ^{18}F-labeled BMDC into the hind footpad, the majority of the injected dose remained at the site of injection in the footpad, but there was significant activity detected in the draining lymph node (DLN) as well as the liver, kidneys, and bladder. Unfortunately, because of the short half-life of ^{18}F (~ 109 minutes), repetitive imaging could not be performed in this study.

Imaging techniques that involve ex vivo labeling of lymphocytes or other adoptively transferred cells have several limitations. One of their major limitations is the relatively low attainable level of radioactivity per cell when cells are labeled with passively equilibrating radiotracers such as ^{111}In-oxine and ^{64}Cu-pyruvaldehyde-bis-(N^4-methylthiosemicarbazone) (PTSM). In a study described above by Fisher et al. (15), the mean concentration of radioactivity of 3.9 µCi/10^8 cells was achieved with a total of 283 µCi of ^{111}In activity injected. Significantly higher levels of radioactivity per cell could be obtained with tracers such as ^{18}F-fluorodeoxyglucose (FDG) that utilize facilitated transport and enzyme-amplified accumulation. However, both ^{64}Cu-PTSM and ^{18}F-FDG have been shown to gradually efflux out of the

labeled cells (14). Progressive loss of the radiolabel also occurs during cell division in vivo. More stable labeling of lymphocytes was achieved with ^{125}I-5-iodo-2′-deoxyuridine (IUDR), which is stably incorporated into the DNA of labeled cells (21). Although successful noninvasive imaging of tumors with ^{131}I-IUdR and ^{124}I-IUdR has been demonstrated with SPECT and PET, respectively (22,23), and could be applied to gamma camera and PET imaging of radiolabeled cells, such an approach has never been tested. Another shortcoming of the ex vivo radiolabeling approach is the limited period of monitoring, which is due to radiolabel decay, cell division, and biological clearance. The exposure of cells to higher doses of radioactivity during labeling may also be limited by radiotoxicity. In a study by Zanzonico et al. (24), human anti-Epstein-Barr virus (EBV)–specific T-lymphocytes genetically engineered to express herpes simplex virus type 1 thymidine kinase (HSV1-tk) were radiolabeled ex vivo with ^{131}I-2′-fluoro-2′-deoxy-1-β-D-arabinofuranosyl-5-iodouracil (FIAU) for two hours at concentrations between 1 and 50 µCi/ml. Because of the radiosensitivity of lymphocytes and the potentially high absorbed dose to the nucleus from intracellular ^{131}I (even at tracer levels), the nuclear absorbed dose [D(n)] and dose-dependent immune functionality were evaluated. At median nuclear absorbed doses up to 830 cGy, a ^{51}Cr-release assay against B-lymphoblastoid cells (BLCLs) showed no loss of immune cytotoxicity, thus demonstrating the functional integrity of genetically transduced, tumor-reactive T cells labeled at this dose level for in vivo cell trafficking and tumor targeting studies in the animals (Fig. 2A). These ^{131}I-FIAU ex vivo–labeled T-lymphocytes were used to target subcutaneous BLCL tumors in a mouse model and could be successfully visualized using a gamma camera up to four days after T-cell injection (25) (Fig. 2B).

GENETIC LABELING OF CELLS WITH REPORTER GENES FOR NUCLEAR IMAGING USING IN VIVO TRACER ADMINISTRATION

Stable genetic labeling of adoptively transferred cells with various reporter genes has been used to circumvent the temporal limitations of ex vivo radiolabeling or magnetic labeling. The effectiveness of cell-mediated gene therapy largely depends on efficient gene delivery to targeted cell populations and targeted transgene expression in an appropriate progeny of transduced cells. Retroviral-mediated transduction has proven to be one of the most effective means to deliver transgenes into mouse and human cells and results in high levels of sustained transgene expression (26,27). For example, long-term circulation of the EBV-specific cytotoxic donor-derived T cells has been shown to occur in patients treated for post–bone marrow

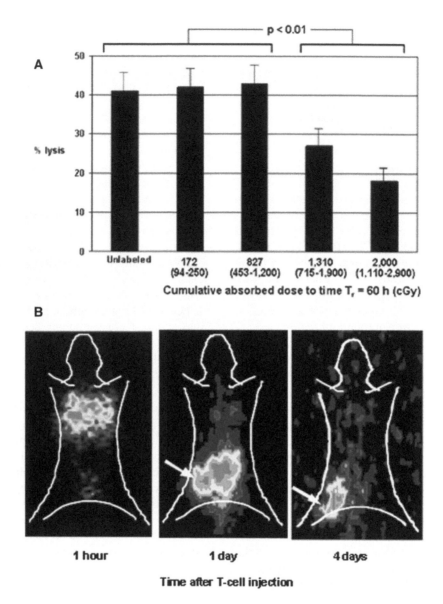

Figure 2 Radiotoxicity and gamma camera imaging studies using ex vivo–labeled anti-EBV-specific T cells. (**A**) Dose-dependent in vitro immune cytotoxicity of ^{131}I-FIAU-labeled HSV1-tk transduced T cells against B-lymphoblastoid cells determined by a ^{51}Cr-release cytotoxicity assay at a target-effector ratio of 20:1. Values indicated represent the calculated median cumulative absorbed doses to the effector cell nuclei projected to the reference time $T_\beta = 60$ hours after a 2-hour incubation in ^{131}I-FIAU-containing medium, that is, the absorbed doses, assuming 0.5 of the intracellular activity and cumulated activity is in the cytoplasm and 0.5 is in the nucleus. The values in parentheses represent the respective ranges of the calculated nuclear absorbed doses, with the lower limit corresponding to all of the intracellular activity in the cytoplasm and the upper limit corresponding to all of the intracellular activity in the nucleus. (**B**) Representative serial planar gamma camera images of SCID mice bearing a human EBV lymphoma xenograft at one hour, one day, and four days after tail vein injection of 3×10^7 autologous, EBV-specific T cells transduced with HSV1-tk, and labeled ex vivo with ^{131}I-FIAU. For anatomical orientation, manually drawn body contours of the mouse are shown. The arrows in the day 1 and day 4 images identify the tumor. *Abbreviations*: EBV, Epstein-Barr virus; HSV1-tk, herpes simplex virus type 1 thymidine kinase; SCID, severe combined immunodeficiency. *Source*: Courtesy of Refs. 24, 25 (*See Color Insert*).

transplantation (BMT) EBV-induced lymphoproliferative diseases. Retrovirally transduced with the neomycin resistance or low-affinity nerve growth factor receptor (LNGFR) and HSV1-tk genes, these T cells were detectable for prolonged periods of observation (years) in peripheral

blood samples from patients by polymerase chain reaction (PCR) or fluorescence-activated cell sorting (FACS) analysis (28–30).

HSV1-tk reporter gene has been used in the majority of seminal studies on imaging cell trafficking by nuclear techniques. The wild-type HSV1-tk and mutant herpes simplex virus type 1 (HSV1)-sr39tk are the most widely used reporter genes for nuclear imaging (31,32). The most widely used radiolabeled reporter probes for nuclear imaging of these reporter genes are FIAU, labeled with [131]I (33), [123]I (34), [124]I (35), and [125]I (36), its derivative [18]F-2′-fluoro-2′-deoxy-5-ethyl-1-β-D-arabinofuranosyl-uracil (FEAU) (37), and ^{18}F-9-[4-fluoro-3-(hydroxymethyl)butyl] guanine (FHBG) (38) (see molecular-genetic imaging section of the book). Initial clinical imaging studies published by Jacobs et al. (39) in 2001 for the first time reported a successful imaging of liposomal-mediated direct intratumoral HSV1-tk gene delivery and expression in human patients with glioblastoma with [124]I-FIAU and PET. Recently, Peñuelas et al. (40) demonstrated the feasibility of PET imaging with ^{18}F-FHBG to monitor reporter gene expression after intratumoral injection of HSV1-tk encoding adenovirus in patients with hepatocellular carcinoma.

Imaging of Immune Cell Therapies

Systemic administration of antigen-specific T-lymphocytes is one of the most studied and clinically applicable methods of adoptive anticancer cell therapy. Long-term trafficking and localization of T-lymphocytes is an important component of anticancer immune response, and in the elimination of abnormal cells and infectious agents from the body. Imaging could help to address several questions related to T-cell migration and homing to the tumor target, their long-term viability, and their subsequent activation and cytolytic activity. The ultimate aim of noninvasive imaging of T-cell persistence and function at the tumor target is to assess the cytolytic potential of tumor-infiltrating T cells and predict the tumorolytic efficacy early on during therapy in the clinical setting.

Koehne et al. (25) demonstrated the feasibility of long-term in vivo monitoring of adoptively transferred human EBV–specific cytotoxic T cells (CTLs) that were transduced to express a radionuclide-based reporter gene HSV1-tk for in vivo radiolabeling and PET imaging. In this study, human EBV–specific CTLs were obtained and stably transduced with a retroviral vector encoding for a constitutively expressed dual reporter gene (HSV1-tk/green fluorescent protein HSV1-tk/GFP fusion gene). Up to 50×10^6 transduced T cells were injected into EBV+/− autologous and allogeneic tumor-bearing severe combined immunodeficiency (SCID) mice. PET images were obtained as early as 28 hours after infusion of HSV1-tk/GFP expressing T cells and 4 hours after the first dose of [124]I-FIAU as well as after doses of [124]I-FIAU administered 8 and 15 days after T-cell infusion. PET images demonstrated high accumulations of the radiotracer in the human

leucocyte antigen (HLA)-A0201+ EBV+ autologous and allogeneic tumors (Fig. 3A,B). HLA disparate EBV+ tumors and HLA-A0201+ EBV− leukemia xenografts did not accumulate radiolabeled FIAU. Infusion of EBV-specific CTLs led to the elimination of subcutaneous autologous EBV-BLCL and HLA-A0201+ allogeneic EBV-BLCL tumor xenografts (Fig. 3D). This tumor rejection was abolished by administration of ganciclovir, which eliminated the HSV1-tk-transduced T cells. In contrast to a similar study, where HSV1-tk-expressing T cells were pre-labeled with ^{131}I-FIAU ex vivo, these studies demonstrated the feasibility of long-term (at least for several weeks) PET monitoring of targeting and migration of antigen-specific CTLs that are transduced to constitutively express a radionuclide-based reporter gene for in vivo labeling. This paradigm provides the opportunity for repeated visualization of transferred T cells within the same animal over time using noninvasive reporter gene PET imaging for continuous monitoring of T-cell localization and persistence, prediction of tumor response, and therapy outcome. The paradigm is potentially transferable to clinical studies in patients with EBV+ cancers.

Another study by Doubrovina et al. (41) showed the tumor-specific trafficking and tumoricidal activity of Wilms tumor (WT1) protein-specific T cells that were transduced with HSV1-tk/GFP fusion reporter gene and administered to animals bearing WT1-positive tumors. The WT1 protein is overexpressed in most acute and chronic leukemias. WT1 peptide–specific T cells after adoptive transfer into SCID mice bearing subcutaneous xenografts of WT1+ and WT1− HLA-A0201+ leukemias preferentially accumulated in and induced regressions of WT1+ leukemias that expressed the restricting HLA allele as shown by microPET imaging with ^{18}F-FEAU. Such cells are clinically applicable and may prove useful for adoptive cell therapy of WT1+ malignant diseases in humans.

Similar studies were conducted by Dubey et al. showing a specific targeting of murine sarcoma virus antigen-positive tumor by mouse antigen-specific T cells that were transduced with a PET reporter gene (42). Therapeutic antitumor immunity depends on a highly migratory CTL population capable of activation and trafficking between lymphoid and tumor-bearing microanatomic sites. In this study 5×10^6 splenic T cells from animals that had rejected a Moloney murine sarcoma virus/Moloney murine leukemia virus (M-MSV/M-MuLV)–induced tumor were stably marked with the HSV1-sr39tk reporter gene, injected into tumor-bearing mice and imaged in a microPET using ^{18}F-FHBG as an imaging probe. Specific localization of immune T cells to the antigen-positive tumor was detected over time by sequential imaging of the same animals for 10 days (Fig. 4). In a similar study (43), memory cells demonstrated early accumulation and apparent proliferation, with large T-cell numbers at the

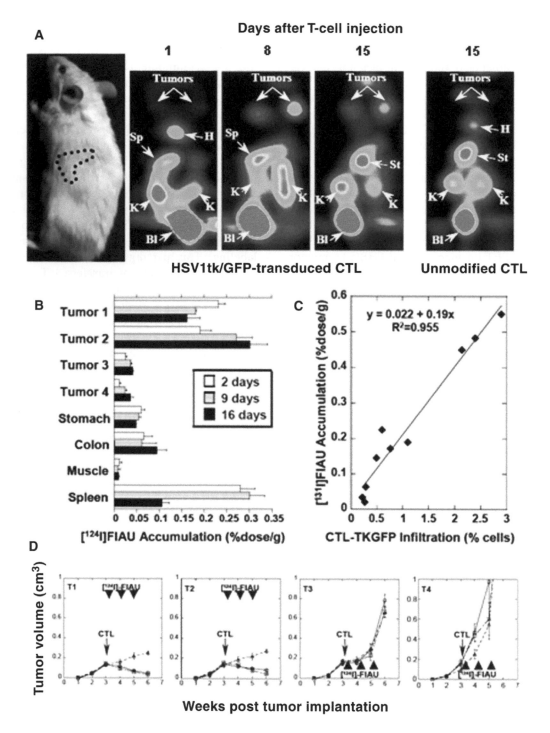

Figure 3 Long-term in vivo monitoring of adoptively transferred human CTLs that were transduced to express a radionuclide-based reporter gene HSV1-tk for in vivo radiolabeling and PET imaging. (**A**) Sequential oblique projections of summed coronal images at a 45° angle to visualize the spleen, targeted tumors, and other organs 4 hours after ^{124}I-FIAU injections on days 1, 8, and 15 after infusion of CTL-HSV1-tk/GFP. For comparison, PET image of a mouse treated with the same but non-transduced EBV-CTLs 4 hours after infusion of ^{124}I-FIAU on day 15 is shown. Accumulations of ^{124}I-FIAU were detected in the autologous and HLA-A0201$^+$ EBV$^+$ tumors and spleen of mice treated with CTL-HSV1-tk/GFP, but not mice treated with non-transduced CTLs. The activity in the kidneys, heart, stomach, and bladder four hours after infusion of ^{124}I-FIAU reflects the clearance of free ^{124}I-FIAU in mice treated with either transduced or non-transduced T cells. (**B**) Doses of radioactivity (% dose/g) accumulated in different tumors and tissues at three time points (days 2, 9, and 16) after EBV-specific CTL-HSV1-tk/GFP administration. Radioactivity was measured 24 hours after each [^{124}I]FIAU injection, by which time free ^{124}I-FIAU is almost completely cleared. (**C**) Mice bearing the same four tumors received either

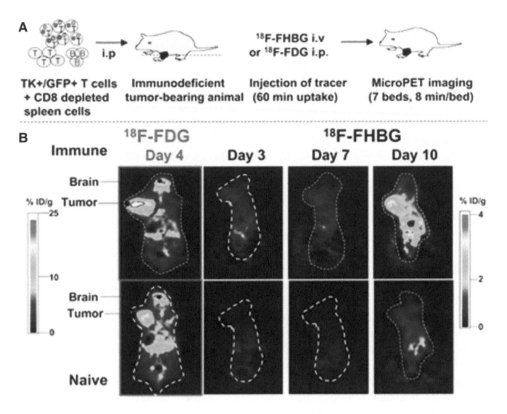

Figure 4 MicroPET imaging of specific targeting of murine sarcoma virus antigen-positive tumor by mouse antigen-specific T cells that were transduced with a HSV1-sr39tk PET reporter gene. (**A**) Immunodeficient CB-17[SCID/SCID] female mice were injected with M-MSV/M-MuLV. HSV1-sr39tk-marked T cells ($1.5-5 \times 10^6$) were injected i.p. when tumors measured at least 0.25 cm³. As a source of help, 1×10^7 CD8$^+$ T cell–depleted splenocytes (immune or naive) were also injected i.p. For microPET imaging, animals were injected i.v. with ^{18}F-FHBG for imaging of T cells and i.p. with ^{18}F-FDG for imaging of tumor progression. (**B**) ^{18}F-FHBG and ^{18}F-FDG scans were performed at least 24 hours apart. Immune but not naive lymphocytes migrated to the M-MSV/M-MuLV tumor. Data were reconstructed by using the filtered back projection for quantitation. *Abbreviations*: PET, positron emission tomography; HSV1, herpes simplex virus type 1; M-MSV/M-MuLV, Moloney murine sarcoma virus/Moloney murine leukemia virus; %ID/g, percent ID per gram of tissue. *Source*: Courtesy of Ref. 42.

antigen-positive tumor as early as day 1 after T-cell transfer. Naive T cells did not accumulate in the antigen-bearing tumor until day 8 and reached only 25% of the peak levels achieved by memory T cells. Both naive and memory cells eradicated the antigen-expressing tumor at a comparable density of intratumoral T cells ($2-4 \times$

10^6/g). However, because of the slower rate of T-cell expansion and continued tumor growth, naive cells required an approximately 10-fold higher antigen-specific precursor frequency to reach a tumoricidal cell density. This methodology can be used to assess the effects of immuno-modulatory agents intended to potentiate the immune

CTL-HSV1-tk/GFP or non-transduced CTLs and, 30 minutes thereafter, an infusion of 200 μCi ^{131}I-FIAU. On day 4, mice were imaged and killed. The doses of radioactivity (% dose/g) accumulated in autologous EBV-BLCL tumor, allogeneic HLA-A0201-homozygous EBV-BLCLs, HLA fully mismatched EBV-BLCLs, HLA-A0201$^+$EBV$^-$ B-ALL, and spleen were closely correlated with percentage of CTL-HSV1-tk/GFP infiltrating each site ($R^2 = 0.955$, $P < 0.001$), as determined by FACS analysis quantitating CD3$^+$ GFP$^+$ T cells in single-cell suspensions prepared from these tissues. (**D**) Tumor growth monitoring during adoptive T-cell therapy. The growth profiles of autologous EBV-BLCL (T1), HLA-A0201-matched EBV-BLCL (T2), HLA-mismatched BLCL (T3), and HLA-A0201$^+$EBV$^-$ ALL (T4) tumors are shown after treatment with EBV-specific unmodified CTLs (□), EBV-specific CTL-HSV1-tk/GFP labeled in vivo with ^{124}I-FIAU (○), and IL-2 injection only (Δ)—in the control group. Five mice were evaluated in each treatment group. In each mouse, transduced and non-transduced EBV-CTL induced selective regression of the autologous and allogeneic HLA-A0201$^+$EBV$^+$ tumors. Growth of the HLA-mismatched EBV$^+$ tumor and HLA-A0201$^+$, EBV$^-$ B-ALL xenograft was not affected by the EBV-specific HLA-A0201-restricted T cells infused. *Abbreviations*: CTL, cytotoxic T cell; HSV1-tk, TK herpes simplex virus type 1 thymidine kinase; PET, positron emission tomography; EBV, Epstein-Barr virus; BLCLs, B-lymphoblastoid cells; K, kidneys; H, heart; St, stomach; Sp, spleen; Bl, bladder. *Source*: Courtesy of Ref. 25.

response to cancer, and can also be useful for the study of other cell-mediated immune responses, including autoimmunity. Interestingly, in this study tumor growth was assessed by ^{18}F-FDG scans. By using two ^{18}F-based radiotracers with rapid clearance and a radioisotope with a short half-life, repetitive PET imaging of tumor progression and T-cell trafficking can be performed on daily basis, thus providing very accurate quantitative assessment of T-cell dynamics and tumor response in vivo.

In subsequent studies by the same group, in order to utilize multimodality in vivo imaging, a tri-fusion reporter gene containing HSV1-sr39tk, synthetic Renilla luciferase (hRluc), and enhanced green fluorescent protein (EGFP) was inserted into a lentiviral transfer vector and was used to transduce the lymphocytes that migrated to an immunogenic sarcoma site (44). In comparison to retrovirally transduced lymphocytes, the lentivirally transduced lymphocytes showed enhanced PET signal when equal numbers of transduced lymphocytes were transferred. Furthermore, using this adoptive transfer model, tumor-specific lymphocytic migration was detected by both microPET scans and bioluminescence imaging. Using the same genetic approach, bone marrow (BM) chimeric mice were generated by engraftment of hematopoietic stem and progenitor cells transduced with a tri-fusion reporter gene (45). Mice were challenged with the Moloney murine sarcoma and leukemia virus complex, and the induced immune response was monitored by using PET with ^{18}F-FHBG. Immune cell localization and expansion were seen at the tumor and DLNs. ^{18}F-FDG, which is sequestered in metabolically active cells, was used to follow tumor growth and regression. Elevated glucose metabolism was also seen in activated lymphocytes in the DLNs using the ^{18}F-FDG probe. When M-MSV/M-MuLV-challenged mice were treated with the immunosuppressive drug dexamethasone, activation and expansion of immune cell populations in the DLNs could no longer be detected. Therefore, PET imaging can be used to kinetically measure the induction and therapeutic modulations of cell-mediated immune responses.

Imaging of Stem and Mesenchymal Cell Therapies

Bone marrow transplantation (BMT) is one of the most radical and effective approaches in cancer treatment, not only in hematological malignancies, but also in solid tumor. It allows for successful displacement of affected BM of the recipient with donor hematopoietic cells. BMT can also serve as a support for high-dose chemotherapy and radiation, thus allowing more efficient dose regimens and prompt recovery from drug-induced anaplasia. Nuclear imaging can identify the initial skeletal engraftment sites after

BM-derived stem cells transplantation. Utilizing a standard mouse model of BMT, Doubrovin et al. (46) introduced a combined bioluminescence and PET imaging reporter gene, triple-fusion encoding for HSV1-tk, GFP, and Firefly luciferase (TGL) into mouse BM-derived stem cells. Bioluminescence imaging was used for monitoring serially the early in vivo stem cell engraftment/expansion every 24 hours. Significant cell engraftment/expansion was noted by greatly increased bioluminescence about one week posttransplant (Fig. 5A). Then PET was applied to acquire three-dimensional images of the whole-body in vivo biodistribution of the transplanted cells (Fig. 5B). To localize cells in the skeleton, PET was followed by computed tomography (CT) (Fig. 5C). Co-registration of PET and CT (Fig. 5D) mapped the sites of BM engraftment. Multiple, discrete stem cell engraftment sites were observed (Fig. 5E). These results allowed noninvasive, repeated imaging of the dynamics of engraftment and expansion in the bone following systemic transplantation of BM-derived stem cells. With noninvasive monitoring of stem cells engraftment using this multimodality approach, BMT can be tailored to the individual needs of patients, with minimal toxicity of conditioning regimens, sufficient numbers of transplanted cells, and adequate cytokine support.

Mesenchymal stem cell targeting of microscopic tumors and tumor stroma development was monitored by PET imaging in the study by Hung et al. (47). Human colon cancer cells of HT-29 Inv2 or CCS lines were implanted subcutaneously into immunodeficient mice, and three to four days later, "tracer" human mesenchymal stem cells (hMSCs) expressing HSV1-tk and enhanced EGFP reporter genes were systemically administered. Subsequently, these tumors were examined for specificity and magnitude of HSV1-tk(+), EGFP(+) stem cell engraftment and proliferation in tumor stroma by PET with ^{18}F-FHBG. In vivo PET images of tumors growing for four weeks showed the presence of HSV1-tk(+) tumor stroma. In vivo imaging results were validated by in situ correlative histochemical, immunofluorescent, and cytometric analyses, which revealed EGFP expression in vWF+ and CD31+ endothelial cells of capillaries and larger blood vessels in the germinal layer of the dermis and hair follicles proximal to the subcutaneous tumor site. The authors concluded that hMSCs can target microscopic tumors, subsequently proliferate and differentiate, and contribute to formation of a significant portion of tumor stroma. PET imaging should facilitate clinical translation of stem cell–based anticancer gene therapeutic approaches by providing the means for in vivo noninvasive whole-body monitoring of trafficking, tumor targeting, and proliferation of HSV1-tk-expressing "tracer" hMSCs in tumor stroma. Using this approach ganciclovir-mediated elimination of HSV1-tk-expressing "tracer" hMSCs in tumor stroma can be successfully monitored by PET.

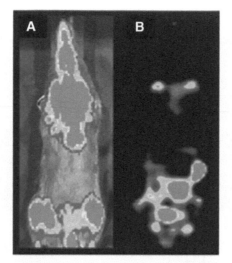

Luciferase Bioluminescence ^{18}F-FEAU microPET

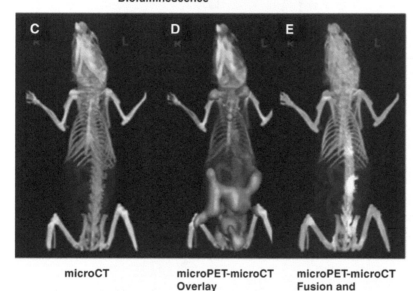

microCT   microPET-microCT Overlay   microPET-microCT Fusion and Segmentation

Figure 5 Multimodality imaging of autologous bone marrow–derived cells targeting bone. Multimodality imaging: bioluminescence (**A**); microPET (**B**); microCT (**C**); microPET-CT overlay (**D**); and microPET-CT registration, segmentation, and fusion (**E**). Bone marrow–derived cells were transduced with a constitutively expressing triple-modality reporter. The images show targeting of bone six days after intravenous administration. Note that the tomographic display (**E**) confirms the targeting of transduced cells to bone. (The image fusion and segmentation was performed by Dr. Luc Bidault, MSKCC). *Abbreviations*: PET, positron emission tomography; CT, computed tomography. *Source*: From Ref. 46 (*See Color Insert*).

FUNCTIONAL IMAGING OF CELLS

Recently, several groups have demonstrated that noninvasive reporter gene imaging of endogenous molecular genetic processes is feasible with PET (48,49). The simplest approach is based on the so-called *cis*-reporter system, in which the expression of a reporter gene is regulated by a target-specific enhancer/promoter element positioned upstream of the reporter gene, and therefore, a reporter gene is expressed whenever the endogenous genes are transcriptionally activated via similar enhancer/promoter elements. An essential component of the immune response in many normal and disease states is T-cell activation. Ponomarev et al. (50) have monitored and assessed T-cell receptor (TCR)–dependent activation in vivo using noninvasive PET imaging. TCR interactions with MHC-peptide complexes expressed on antigen-presenting cells initiate T-cell activation, resulting in transcription that is

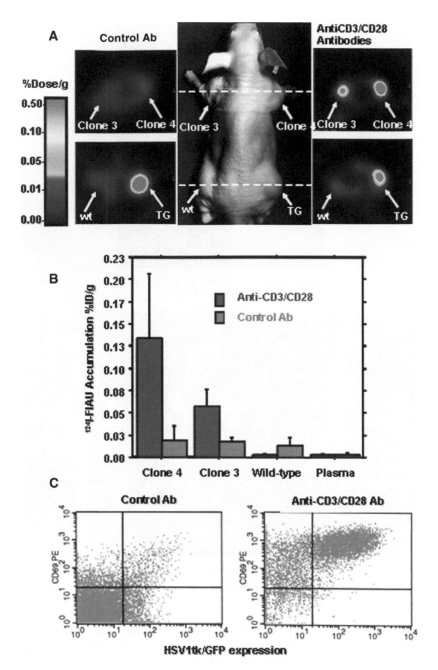

Figure 6 Imaging *cis*-NFAT-HSV1-tk/GFP reporter system activity with [124]I-FIAU and PET and assessments in tissue samples. (**A**) Photographic image of a typical mouse bearing different subcutaneous (s.c.) infiltrates (*middle*), transaxial PET images of HSV1-tk/GFP expression in a mouse treated with control antibody (*left*), and anti-CD3/CD28 antibodies (*right*) were obtained at the levels indicated by the dashed lines. Anti-CD28 was included in in vivo experiments in order to prolong Jurkat cell survival for better imaging results. (**B**) [124]I-FIAU accumulation in tissue samples of the Jurkat-NFAT-HSV1-tk/GFP clone 3 and 4 infiltrates, wild-type Jurkat infiltrates, and blood plasma, obtained after PET imaging. (**C**) FACS profiles of HSV1-tk/GFP and CD69 expression in a tissue sample from the same Jurkat-NFAT-HSV1-tk/GFP clone 4 infiltrate that was imaged with PET. *Abbreviations*: NFAT, nuclear factor of activated T cells; HSV1-tk, herpes simplex virus type 1 thymidine kinase; PET, positron emission tomography. *Source*: From Ref. 50 (*See Color Insert*).

mediated by several factors. These factors, including IL-2 and other cytokines, contribute to the regulation of a number of target genes through several activating pathways and involve several transcription factors such as the nuclear

factor of activated T cells (NFAT) (51). A retroviral vector was generated by placing the (HSV1-tk/GFP) fusion gene under control of the NFAT response element. The human T-cell leukemia Jurkat cell line that expresses a functional

TCR was transduced with the *cis*-NFAT-HSV1-tk/GFP retroviral reporter vector and used in these studies. Known activators of T cells, anti-CD3, and anti-CD28 antibodies produced significantly higher levels of HSV1-tk/GFP reporter gene expression in *cis*-NFAT-HSV1-tk/GFP+ Jurkat T cells than in non-treated or non-transduced cells. In mice with focal *cis*-NFAT-HSV1-tk/GFP+ Jurkat T-cell infiltrates, similar results were observed in the PET images obtained with [124]I-FIAU (Fig. 6). A strong correlation between HSV1-tk/GFP expression and upregulation of T-cell activation markers (CD69 and IL-2 production) was demonstrated both in vitro and in vivo (Fig. 6). It is very important to note that the *cis*-NFAT-HSV1-tk/GFP reporter system reflects only the process of TCR-mediated T-cell activation and is independent from the other co-stimulatory signaling. The *cis*-NFAT-HSV1-tk/GFP reporter system was very responsive, sufficiently sensitive, and specific for monitoring the processes of T-cell activation both in vitro and in vivo. The induction of signaling was observed at 16 hours and gradually decreased within 72 hours after stimulation. Furthermore, this activation can be arrested pharmacologically by the administration of clinically used calcineurin inhibitors such as cyclosporin A and FK506 (52). This circumstance makes this imaging approach clinically valuable, as it can be used in patients receiving immunosuppressive drugs after BM and organ transplantation. The results of the study by Ponomarev et al. demonstrated that PET imaging of T-lymphocyte activation in tumors following TCR engagement is feasible using the described *cis*-NFAT-HSV1-tk/GFP-based reporter system. When combined with imaging of NFAT-mediated activation of T cells, noninvasive PET imaging should allow monitoring of the trafficking, proliferation, and antigen-specific activation of T cells in antitumor clinical trials.

QUANTITATION OF ADOPTIVELY TRANSFERRED CELLS IN VIVO

The degree of PET signal in a region of anatomical interest (ROI) largely depends on the density of labeled cells in a volume of tissue and the level of reporter gene expression. The potential of PET imaging for quantifying cell signals in ROI provides a unique opportunity to estimate the absolute number of injected labeled cells at the target site. However, little is known about the constraints and parameters for using PET signal detection to establish cell numbers in different regions of interest. Su et al. (53) determined the correlation of PET signal to cell number and characterized the cellular limit of detection for PET imaging. These studies using human T cells transduced with HSV1-sr39tk reporter gene and PET imaging with ^{18}F-FHBG revealed a cell number–

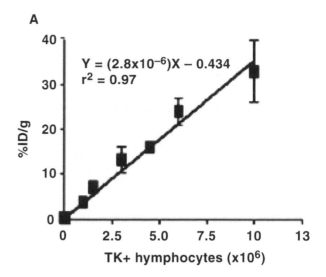

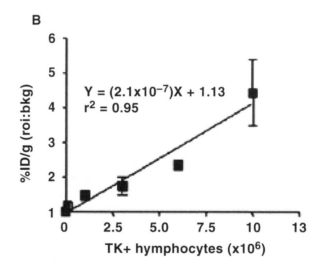

Figure 7 In vivo quantitative imaging of HSV1-sr39tk-transduced lymphocytes. (**A**) In vitro–labeled cells. Indicated numbers of wild-type and HSV1-sr39tk-transduced lymphocytes were labeled with ^{18}F-FHBG in vitro, transferred to the mouse shoulder region, and scanned by microPET. Signal (%ID/g) relative to cell number (linear scale). (**B**) In vivo–labeled cells. Wild-type and HSV1-sr39tk-transduced lymphocytes were injected intratumorally into mice, ^{18}F-FHBG was administered intravenously, and the animals were scanned by microPET one hour later. Signal relative to cell number (linear scale). *Abbreviations*: HSV1, herpes simplex virus type 1; PET, positron emission tomography; ID/g, injected dose per gram. *Source*: From Ref. 53.

dependent signal, with a limit of detection calculated as 10^6 cells in a region of interest of 0.1 mL volume (Fig. 7). Quantitatively similar parameters were observed with stably transduced primary T-lymphocytes and N2a glioma cells. These methods and findings provide a strategy for

Table 1 Reporter Genes Suitable for PET Imaging in Humans

Reporter gene	Origin	Reporter probe	Immunogenicity in humans	Suicidal function	Translational use
Herpes simplex virus type 1 thymidine kinase (HSV1-tk) (wild-type or sr39 mutant)	HSV-1	^{123}I-, ^{124}I-, ^{125}I-, ^{131}I-FIAU ^{18}F-FE(I)AU ^{18}F-FHBG	Yes	Yes	Yes
Mitochondrial thymidine kinase type 2 (hTK2)	Human	^{123}I-, ^{124}I-, ^{125}I-, ^{131}I-FIAU ^{18}F-FE(I)AU	No	Yes	Yes
Sodium iodide symporter (hNIS)	Human	^{123}I-, ^{124}I-, ^{99m}Tc-TcO4-^{94m}Tc-TcO4-	No	No	Yes
Norepinephrine transporter (hNET)	Human	^{123}I-, ^{124}I-, ^{125}I-, ^{131}I-MIBG	No	No	Yes
Dopamine receptor 2 (D2R)	Human	^{18}F-FESP, ^{11}C-FLB 457	No	No	Yes
Somatostatin receptor (hSSTr2)	Human	^{99m}Tc-, ^{188}Re- somatostatin-avid peptide P829	No	No	Yes

Abbreviations: FIAU, 2′-fluoro-2′-deoxy-1-ß-D-arabinofuranosyl-5-iodouracil; FEAU, 2′-fluoro-2′-deoxy-5-ethyl-1-ß-D-arabinofuranosyl-uracil; FHBG, 9-[4-fluoro-3-(hydroxymethyl)butyl]guanine; MIBG, meta-iodobenzylguanidine; FESP, 3-*N*-(2-Fluoroethyl)spiperone; FLB, 5-bromo-N-[(1-cyclopropylmethyl-2-pyrrolidinyl)methyl]-2,3-dimethoxybenzamide.

quantitation of cellularity using PET imaging that has implications for both experimental models and clinical diagnosis.

CONCLUSION AND FUTURE CONSIDERATIONS

Direct and indirect cell labeling for nuclear imaging of transferred cells have been proven a reliable method for imaging adoptive cellular therapies. Both methods show their advantages and limitations. Direct labeling is a relatively easy, inexpensive, and well-established methodology. High-contrast cell-to-media/tissue ratios can be archived easily. However, this approach is limited by a short period of monitoring (days), which is due to radiolabel decay, cell division, and biological clearance. High levels of radiolabel concentration can impair the biological functioning of the labeled cells.

Indirect labeling using a reporter gene imaging paradigm allows for reliable, stable, and harmless visualization of cellular trafficking, persistence, proliferation, and function at the target site. Genetically labeled cells can be repetitively imaged for a long period of observation (months). The genetic nature of this method (stable integration into the cell genome) permits in vivo labeling of the progeny of injected cells. Using inducible genetic reporter systems, functional imaging of cell activation, cytokine signaling, and proapoptotic events is feasible and can be performed in preclinical experiments and clinical settings. It is also important to mention that picomolar concentrations of radiotracer administered in vivo are harmless for the labeled cells as well as for the surrounding organs and tissues.

Indirect genetic labeling provides the opportunity to develop dual-reporter systems for genetic labeling of adoptively transferred cells; such dual-reporter systems contain a constitutive or "beacon" reporter gene for imaging the

location, magnitude, and duration of cell infiltration, and an inducible or "sensor" reporter gene for imaging the magnitude and duration of functional characteristics of the cell (e.g., T-cell activation). These dual-reporter systems could address several important questions that arise during development, optimization, and clinical implementation of various adoptive cell therapies.

The major impediment to the translation of viral- and bacterial-derived reporter gene imaging approaches into clinical practice is the immunogenicity of these nonhuman-derived reporter proteins. This is especially important when repetitive administration of a reporter gene or long-term monitoring of transgene expression is required, which could potentially be compromised by an immune reaction against this foreign protein. In order to circumvent this problem, a number of human-derived reporter genes have been proposed for nuclear imaging, including the dopamine receptor type 2 (hD2R) (54), somatostatin receptor (hSSTr2) (55), sodium iodide symporter (hNIS) (56), norepinephrine transporter (hNET) (57), and human mitochondrial thymidine kinase type 2 (hTK2) (58) (Table 1). It is expected that new human-derived reporter genes will be rapidly translated into clinical applications that require repetitive imaging for effective monitoring of various genetic and cellular therapies.

REFERENCES

1. Erlandsson A, Morshead CM. Exploiting the properties of adult stem cells for the treatment of disease. Curr Opin Mol Ther 2006; 8(4):331–337.
2. Keating A. Mesenchymal stromal cells. Curr Opin Hematol 2006; 13(6):419–425.
3. Rooney C, Smith CA, Ng CY, et al. Use of gene-modified virus-specific T lymphocytes to control epstein-barr-virus-related lymphoproliferation. Lancet 1995; 345(8941):9–13.

4. Buchsel PC, DeyMeyer ES. Dendritic cells: emerging roles in tumor immunotherapy. Clin J Oncol Nurs 2006; 10(5): 629–640.

5. Prados J, Melguizo C, Boulaiz H, et al. Cancer gene therapy: strategies and clinical trials. Cell Mol Biol 2005; 51(1):23–36.

6. Reinhardt R, Jenkins MK. Whole-body analysis of T cell responses. Curr Opin Immunol 2003; 15(4):366–371.

7. Atkins RC, Ford WL. Early cellular events in a systemic graft-vs.-host reaction. I. The migration of responding and nonresponding donor lymphocytes. J Exp Med 1975; 141(3):664–680.

8. Constantin G, Laudanna C, Butcher EC. Novel method for following lymphocyte traffic in mice using [3H]glycerol labeling. J Immunol Methods 1997; 203(1):35–44.

9. Hellerstein M, Hanley MB, Cesar D, et al. Directly measured kinetics of circulating T lymphocytes in normal and HIV-1-infected humans. Nat Med 1999; 5(1):83–89.

10. Gobuty AH, Robinson RG, Barth RF. Organ distribution of 99mTc- and 51Cr-labeled autologous peripheral blood lymphocytes in rabbits. J Nucl Med 1977; 18(2):141–146.

11. Papierniak C, Bourey RE, Kretschmer RR, et al. Technetium-99m labeling of human monocytes for chemotactic studies. J Nucl Med 1976; 17(11):988–992.

12. Korf J, Veenma-van der Duin L, Brinkman-Medema R, et al. Divalent cobalt as a label to study lymphocyte distribution using PET and SPECT. J Nucl Med 1998; 39(5):836–841.

13. Rannie GH, Thakur ML, Ford WL. An experimental comparison of radioactive labels with potential application to lymphocyte migration studies in patients. Clin Exp Immunol 1977; 29(3):509–514.

14. Adonai N, Nguyen KN, Walsh J, et al. Ex vivo cell labeling with 64Cu-pyruvaldehyde-bis(N4-methylthiosemicarbazone) for imaging cell trafficking in mice with positron-emission tomography. Proc Natl Acad Sci U S A 2002; 99(5):3030–3035.

15. Fisher B, Packard BS, Read EJ, et al. Tumor localization of adoptively transferred indium-111 labeled tumor infiltrating lymphocytes in patients with metastatic melanoma. J Clin Oncol 1989; 7(2):250–261.

16. Kasi LP, Lamki LM, Saranti S, et al. Indium-111 labeled leukocytes in evaluation of active specific immunotherapy responses. Int J Gynecol Cancer 1995; 5(3):226–232.

17. Dillman RO, Hurwitz SR, Schiltz PM, et al. Tumor localization by tumor infiltrating lymphocytes labeled with indium-111 in patients with metastatic renal cell carcinoma, melanoma, and colorectal cancer. Cancer Biother Radiopharm 1997; 12(2):65–71.

18. Matera L, Galetto A, Bello M, et al. In vivo migration of labeled autologous natural killer cells to liver metastases in patients with colon carcinoma. J Transl Med 2006; 14(4):49.

19. Bennink R, Hamann J, de Bruin K, et al. Dedicated pinhole SPECT of intestinal neutrophil recruitment in a mouse model of dextran sulfate sodium-induced colitis. J Nucl Med 2005; 46(3):526–531.

20. Olasz E, Lang L, Seidel J, et al. Fluorine-18 labeled mouse bone marrow-derived dendritic cells can be detected in vivo by high resolution projection imaging. J Immunol Methods 2002; 260(1-2):137–148.

21. Schelper RL, Adrian EK Jr. Monocytes become macrophages; they do not become microglia: a light and electron microscopic autoradiographic study using 125-iododeoxyuridine. J Neuropathol Exp Neurol 1986; 45(1):1–19.

22. Tjuvajev J, Macapinlac HA, Daghighian F, et al. Imaging of brain tumor proliferative activity with iodine-131-iododeoxyuridine. J Nucl Med 1994; 35(9):1407–1417.

23. Blasberg R, Roelcke U, Weinreich R, et al. Imaging brain tumor proliferative activity with [124I]iododeoxyuridine. Cancer Res 2000; 60(3):624–635.

24. Zanzonico P, Koehne G, Gallardo HF, et al. [(131)I]FIAU labeling of genetically transduced, tumor-reactive lymphocytes: cell-level dosimetry and dose-dependent toxicity. Eur J Nucl Med Mol Imaging 2006; 33(9):988–997.

25. Koehne G, Doubrovin M, Doubrovina E, et al. Serial in vivo imaging of the targeted migration of human HSV-TK-transduced antigen-specific lymphocytes. Nat Biotechnol 2003; 21(4):405–413.

26. Hagani AB, Riviere I, Tan C, et al. Activation conditions determine susceptibility of murine primary T-lymphocytes to retroviral infection. J Gene Med 1999; 1(5):341–351.

27. Gallardo HF, Tan C, Ory D, et al. Recombinant retroviruses pseudotyped with the vesicular stomatitis virus G glycoprotein mediate both stable gene transfer and pseudotransduction in human peripheral blood lymphocytes. Blood 1997; 90(3):952–957.

28. Rooney CM, Smith CA, Ng CY, et al. Use of gene-modified virus-specific T lymphocytes to control Epstein-Barr-virus-related lymphoproliferation. Lancet 1995; 345:9–13.

29. Verzeletti S, Bonini C, Marktel S, et al. Herpes simplex virus thymidine kinase gene transfer for controlled graft-versus-host disease and graft-versus-leukemia: clinical follow-up and improved new vectors. Hum Gene Ther 1998; 9(15):2243–2251.

30. Bonini C, Ferrari G, Verzeletti S, et al. HSV-TK gene transfer into donor lymphocytes for control of allogeneic graft-versus-leukemia. Science 1997; 276(5319):1719–1724.

31. Gambhir SS, Herschman HR, Cherry SR, et al. Imaging transgene expression with radionuclide imaging technologies. Neoplasia 2000; 2(1-2):118–138.

32. Gelovani Tjuvajev J, Blasberg RG. In vivo imaging of molecular-genetic targets for cancer therapy. Cancer Cell 2003; 3(4):327–332.

33. Tjuvajev J, Stockhammer G, Desai R, et al. Imaging the expression of transfected genes in vivo. Cancer Res 1995; 55:6126–6132.

34. Choi S, Zhuang ZP, Chacko AM, et al. SPECT imaging of herpes simplex virus type1 thymidine kinase gene expression by [(123)I]FIAU(1). Acad Radiol 2005; 12(7):798–805.

35. Tjuvajev J, Avril N, Oku T, et al. Imaging herpes virus thymidine kinase gene transfer and expression by positron emission tomography. Cancer Res 1998; 19:4333–4341.

36. Zinn K, Chaudhuri TR, Krasnykh VN, et al. Gamma camera dual imaging with a somatostatin receptor and thymidine kinase after gene transfer with a bicistronic adenovirus in mice. Radiology 2002; 223(2):417–425.

37. Serganova I, Doubrovin M, Vider J, et al. Molecular imaging of temporal dynamics and spatial heterogeneity of hypoxia-inducible factor-1 signal transduction activity

in tumors in living mice. Cancer Res 2004; 64(17): 6101–6108.

38. Yaghoubi S, Barrio JR, Dahlbom M, et al. Human pharmacokinetic and dosimetry studies of [(18)F]FHBG: a reporter probe for imaging herpes simplex virus type-1 thymidine kinase reporter gene expression. J Nucl Med 2001; 42(8):1225–1234.

39. Jacobs A, Voges J, Reszka R, et al. Positron-emission tomography of vector-mediated gene expression in gene therapy for gliomas. Lancet 2001; 358(9283):727–729.

40. Peñuelas I, Mazzolini G, Boan JF, et al. Positron emission tomography imaging of adenoviral-mediated transgene expression in liver cancer patients. Gastroenterology 2005; 128(7):1787–1795.

41. Doubrovina E, Doubrovin MM, Lee S, et al. In vitro stimulation with WT1 peptide-loaded epstein-barr virus-positive B cells elicits high frequencies of WT1 peptide-specific T cells with in vitro and in vivo tumoricidal activity. Clin Cancer Res 2004; 10(21):7207–7219.

42. Dubey P, Su H, Adonai N, et al. Quantitative imaging of the T cell antitumor response by positron-emission tomography. Proc Natl Acad Sci U S A 2003; 100(3): 1232–1237.

43. Su H, Chang DS, Gambhir SS, et al. Monitoring the antitumor response of naive and memory CD8 T cells in RAG1-/- mice by positron-emission tomography. J Immunol 2006; 176(7):4459–4467.

44. Kim Y, Dubey P, Ray P, et al. Multimodality imaging of lymphocytic migration using lentiviral-based transduction of a tri-fusion reporter gene. Mol Imaging Biol 2004; 6 (5):331–340.

45. Shu C, Guo S, Kim YJ, et al. Visualization of a primary antitumor immune response by positron emission tomography. Proc Natl Acad Sci U S A 2005; 102(48):17412–17417.

46. Doubrovin M, Serganova I, Mayer-Kuckuk P, et al. Multimodality in vivo molecular-genetic imaging. Bioconjug Chem 2004; 15(6):1376–1388.

47. Hung S, Deng WP, Yang WK, et al. Mesenchymal stem cell targeting of microscopic tumors and tumor stroma development monitored by noninvasive in vivo positron emission tomography imaging. Clin Cancer Res 2005; 11 (21):7749–7756.

48. Doubrovin M, Ponomarev V, Beresten T, et al. Imaging transcriptional regulation of p53 dependent genes with positron emission tomography in vivo. Proc Natl Acad Sci U S A 2001; 98(16):9300–9305.

49. Green LA, Yap CS, Nguyen K, et al. Indirect monitoring of endogenous gene expression by positron emission tomography (PET) imaging of reporter gene expression in transgenic mice. Mol Imaging Biol 2002; 4(1):71–81.

50. Ponomarev V, Doubrovin M, Lyddane C, et al. Imaging TCR-dependent NFAT-mediated T-cell activation with positron emission tomography in vivo. Neoplasia 2001; 3(6):480–488.

51. Li W, Handschumacher RE. Regulation of the nuclear factor of activated T cells in stably transfected Jurkat cell clones. Biochem Biophys Res Commun 1996; 219:96–99.

52. Kiani A, Rao A, Aramburu J. Manipulating immune responses with immunosuppressive agents that target NFAT. Immunity 2000; 12:359–372.

53. Su H, Forbes A, Gambhir SS, et al. Quantitation of cell number by a positron emission tomography reporter gene strategy. Mol Imaging Biol 2004; 6(3):139–148.

54. MacLaren D, Gambhir SS, Satyamurthy N, et al. Repetitive, non-invasive imaging of the dopamine D2 receptor as a reporter gene in living animals. Gene Ther 1999; 6(5): 785–791.

55. Zinn K, Buchsbaum DJ, Chaudhuri TR, et al. Noninvasive monitoring of gene transfer using a reporter receptor imaged with a high-affinity peptide radiolabeled with 99mTc or 188Re. J Nucl Med 2000; 41(5):887–895.

56. Groot-Wassink T, Aboagye EO, Glaser M, et al. Adenovirus biodistribution and noninvasive imaging of gene expression in vivo by positron emission tomography using human sodium/iodide symporter as reporter gene. Hum Gene Ther 2002; 13(14):1723–1735.

57. Buursma A, Beerens AM, de Vries EF, et al. The human norepinephrine transporter in combination with 11C-m-hydroxyephedrine as a reporter gene/reporter probe for PET of gene therapy. J Nucl Med 2005; 46(12):2068–2075.

58. Ponomarev V, Doubrovin M, Serganova I, et al. A novel non-immunogenic reporter gene for non-invasive imaging in humans: human thymidine kinase type 2. J Nucl Med 2002; 43(5 suppl S).

35

Optical Techniques for Imaging of Cell Trafficking

KHALID SHAH

Massachusetts General Hospital, Harvard Medical School, Boston, Massachusetts, U.S.A.

INTRODUCTION

Recent advances in molecular and cell biology techniques have helped us understand a number of human disorders that have ultimately led to the development of novel therapeutics and a changed clinical approach at patient level. One of the most critical issues for ensuring success of understanding diseases and developing new therapies is the development of noninvasive high-resolution in vivo imaging technologies. The in vivo monitoring of specific molecular and cellular processes, for example, gene expression, multiple simultaneous molecular events, progression or regression of cancer, and drug and gene therapy, are the major goals of this evolving technology. In recent years many advances have been made in high resolution, in vivo imaging methods, including radionuclide imaging, such as positron emission tomography (PET) and single photon emission tomography (SPECT), magnetic resonance (MR) imaging, and spectroscopy. Optical imaging techniques have used different physical parameters of light interaction with tissue and until recently a number of optical imaging approaches have been described. These techniques rely on fluorescence, absorption, reflectance, or bioluminescence as a source of contrast. The recently used optical imaging techniques that are gaining popularity include near-infrared fluorescence (NIRF) imaging, fluorescence mediated tomography, bioluminescence imaging (BLI) and intravital microscopy. These optical techniques impart molecular specificity to in vivo imaging technologies.

Optical imaging methods have been stimulated by the development of genetically engineered fluorescent and bioluminescent markers and new fluorescent probes. The most frequently used bioluminescence markers include the bacterial *lux* genes of terrestrial *Photorhabdus luminescens* and marine *Vibrio harveyi* bacteria, as well as eukaryotic firefly luciferase (Fluc) and *Renilla* luciferase (Rluc) genes from firefly species (*Photinus*) and the sea panzy (*Renilla reniformis*), respectively (1). Recently a new bioluminescent protein *Gaussia* luciferase (Gluc), has been cloned and shown to have a 200-fold higher signal intensity than Rluc in vivo (2). Fluorescent proteins are genetically encoded, easily imaged reporters crucial in biology and biotechnology (3,4). All the wild-type yellow-to-red fluorescent proteins reported so far are obligately tetrameric and often toxic or disruptive (5,6). Recently, next generation of monomers were reported (7), the latest red version matures more completely, is more tolerant of N-terminal fusions, and is over tenfold more photostable than mRFP1. Three monomers with distinguishable hues from yellow-orange to red-orange have higher quantum efficiencies. Based on the criterion of time, it takes for the emission to drop to 50% of its initial value, tdTomato and mCherry are the best among the generation of red shifted markers. Both are more than tenfold better than mRFP1 and nearly as good as EGFP (7).

The first fluorescent in vivo optical probes were based on fluorophores, such as the Alexa dyes and the cyanine dyes Cy5.5 and Cy7 (8). A large group of optical probes that consist of a fluorophore conjugated to a targeting moiety are represented by conjugates of a fluorophore with the ligand of $\alpha_v\beta_3$ integrin (9,10) for tumor detection and annexin V and Cy5.5 (11) probe for apoptosis detection. A modification to these probes is the activatable "smart" probes (12–14), which have a low signal-to-noise ratio and can be activated by upregled proteins. The large number of fluorophores in such close proximity results in the fluorescence quenching. Enzymatic cleavage of the backbone by selective proteases (PR) releases the fluorophore molecules from the quenched state in the polymer complex, permitting fluorescence for detection of the protease. Quantum dots (QDs) are emerging as a new class of fluorescent probe for in vivo biomolecular and cellular imaging. QD are based on semiconductor nanocrystals with a broad absorption spectrum, high extinction coefficient, extremely long fluorescence lifetime and a narrow symmetrical emission spectrum and practically negligible photobleaching (15). Recent advances have led to the development of multifunctional nanoparticle probes that are very bright and stable under complex in vivo conditions. Bioconjugated QDs have raised new possibilities for ultrasensitive and multiplexed imaging of molecular targets in living cells, animal models, and possibly in humans. The use of QDs for sensitive and multicolor cellular imaging has seen major recent advances, owing to significant improvements in QD synthesis, surface chemistry, and conjugation.

NEAR-INFRARED FLUORESCENCE REFLECTANCE IMAGING

Light in the visible-wavelength range is routinely used for conventional and intravital microscopy (16). Because hemoglobin (the principal absorber of visible light), water and lipids (the principal absorbers of infrared light) have their lowest absorption coefficient in the NIR region of approximately 650 to 900 nm (Fig. 1), the use of NIR light is ideal for imaging deeper tissues. Imaging in the near-infrared (NIR) spectrum (700–900 nm) maximizes tissue penetrance in addition to minimizing the autofluorescence from nontarget tissue. NIR fluorescence imaging relies on light with a defined band width as a source of photons that encounter a fluorescent molecule (optical contrast agent). This fluorescent molecule then emits a signal with different spectral characteristics that can be resolved with an emission filter and captured with an ultrasensitive CCD camera. Interpretation of NIR data and images generally requires advanced data processing techniques to account for the diffuse nature of photon propagation in tissue. The recent advances in NIRF imaging have been accelerated by the development of NIR fluorochromes coupled to quenching peptides, which are activated by specific PR at the target site (17). The NIRF probes typically consist of a delivery vehicle linked to the NIR fluorochromes via the enzyme-specific peptide substrates (Fig. 1B). The delivery vehicles are long-circulating, high molecular weight synthetic-protected graft copolymers that have already been tested in clinical trials (18). The underpinning hypothesis of this approach is that most disease processes have a molecular basis that can be exploited to detect disease earlier or to monitor novel therapies by imaging molecular biomarkers. In the

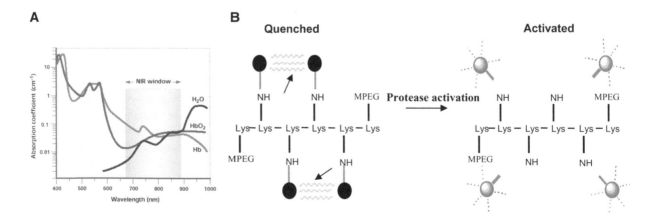

Figure 1 (**A**) Interaction of light with tissue. The absorption coefficient of light in tissue is dependent on wavelength and results from absorbers such as hemoglobins, lipids, and water. Given the decreased absorption of light in the near-infrared (NIR) region compared with visible light (∼400–650 nm) and infrared light (>900 nm), tissue penetration of NIR photons may be up to 10 to 15 cm. (**B**) Chemical structure of repeating graft copolymer segment indicating quenched and the activated state after the cleavage at the enzyme recognition sites indicated by arrows.

past few years NIRF imaging aided by activatable NIRF probes has been used, for example, in detecting tumors, imaging gene expression, and other molecular events in experimental models.

Imaging Tumor Detection and Targeting

A number of studies with NIRF probes, both in culture and in vivo, have shown that the nonactivated probes have a very-low background fluorescence and that protease activation of probes can increase the fluorescence over several hundredfold (19) with probes detectable in the nanomolar range and with no apparent toxicity (20). Autoquenched NIRF probes that become active after protease activation have been used in imaging tumors that have upregulated levels of certain PR, like cathepsins (14). Cathepsin B and cathepsin H protease activities have also been used to detect submillimeter-sized tumors using NIR fluorescent probes (14) and cathepsin D-positive tumors (21) have been imaged in mouse models (Fig. 2). In another study, cathepsin B activity has been used as a biomarker to readily identify dysplastic adenomatous polyps, which contrasts particularly well against normal adjacent mucosa (22). This detection technology can be adapted to endoscopy or tomographic optical imaging methods for screening of suspicious lesions and allows the potential for molecular profiling of protease activity in vivo. A number of different matrix metalloproteinase (MMP) inhibitors, which act as cytostatic and antiangiogenic agents are currently in clinical testing. One major hurdle in assessing the efficacy of such drugs

has been the inability to detect or image antiproteinase activity directly and noninvasively in vivo. Recent developments allow NIRF-MMP substrates to be used as activatable NIRF reporter probes to monitor MMP activity in intact tumors (12). These probes have the advantage of directly imaging MMP activity within hours after treatment with potent MMP inhibitors.

Integrins are a large family of heterodimeric transmembrane receptors that mediate cell-cell and cell-matrix interactions. They play key roles in tumor invasion, metastasis, and neovascularization. These proteins associate as $\alpha\beta$ heterodimers in native environment, where the α and β subunits control distinct but complementary physiological functions (23,24). Various tumor imaging agents (23,25,26) have been developed to target the $\alpha_v\beta_3$ integrin receptor (ABIR) because of its overexpression in a number of cancers (27–29). Biomolecules and synthetic compounds containing the arginine-glycine-aspartic acid (RGD) peptide sequence are known to bind ABIR and related integrin heterodimers with high affinity (25,30). Studies of hexa- and hepta-peptides labeled with a NIR fluorescent probe (cypate) showed that rearranging the glycine in a linear RGD peptide sequence to form the GRD analogue favored the uptake of the GRD compound by ABIR-positive A549 tumor cells and tissues (31). Recent studies by Bloch et al., (32) demonstrate that cypate-GRD peptide targets β_3 integrin, thereby providing a strategy to monitor drug-delivery efficacy, and physiopathological processes mediated by this protein. Very recently, RGD peptide-labeled QDs have been developed and used in vivo targeting and imaging of tumor vasculature. Mice with established subcutaneous U87MG human glioblastoma tumors were injected with QD705-RGD intravenously and the tumor fluorescence intensity was shown to reach the maximum at six hours postinjection with good contrast. These studies open up new perspectives for integrin-targeted NIR optical imaging and may aid in cancer detection and management including imaging-guided surgery.

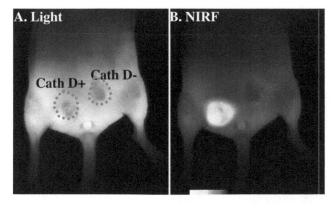

Figure 2 In vivo NIRF imaging of upregulated proteases. Representative optical images of the lower abdomen of a nude mouse implanted with cathepsin D-positive and -negative rat embryo (3Y1) tumors. (**A**) White light image 24 hours after intravenous (i.v.) injection of the cathepsin D–specific NIRF probe. (**B**) Identical imaging set-up as in A, except that NIRF fluorescence is shown at 700 nm. Note that the cathepsin D-positive tumor emits fluorescence, whereas the negative tumor has a significantly lower signal. *Source*: Adapted from Ref. 19.

Imaging Gene Expression

Imaging gene expression of targeted viral vectors in vivo is critical to assess their efficacy. Viral PR, which are not ubiquitously expressed in mammalian systems offer a possibility to develop such protease/substrate systems. In recent years, we have developed NIRF probes for HIV (human immunodeficiency virus)-1 and HSV (herpes simplex virus)-1 PR for imaging of gene delivery to tumors. We have shown specific fluorescence activation of this HIV-1 NIRF probe in human Gli36 gliomas injected with viral vector expressing HIV-1PR (33) demonstrating that viral PR can be imaged in live animals and can be used as transgene markers in tumor therapy in vivo. In order to develop regulatable therapeutic proteins whose regulation can be controlled by the imageable protease, we have coupled the regulation of a therapeutic protein, S-TRAIL (tumor necrosis factor-related apoptosis-inducing ligand), with the activation of HSV-1-specific NIRF probe using the HSV-1-specific protease (34). TRAIL is a type 2 transmembrane protein that induces apoptosis in tumor cells of diverse origins, by binding to death domain–containing receptors, DR4 (TRAIL-R1) and DR5 (TRAIL-R2) (35) on the tumor cell surface. We have engineered secretable form of TRAIL (S-TRAIL) and shown that this form of TRAIL is actively secreted from the cells and allows a "bystander effect" whereby trans-duced cells cause death of surrounding non-transduced tumor cells (36). We have developed means to control the secretion of S-TRAIL using a viral protease by engineer-ing endoplasmic reticulum (ER)-targeted TRAIL and

shown that it was inactively retained in the ER until selectively released by the HSV-1 viral protease. Expression of ER-targeted HSV-1 protease in the (ER)-targeted TRAIL-expressing cells resulted in the release of S-TRAIL from the ER and subsequent induction of apoptosis in glioma cells. The same HSV-1 protease was used to monitor gene delivery in vivo by systemic admin-istration of HSV-1 protease-specific NIRF probe activated by the protease (Fig. 3) (34). The mode of cancer therapy employed in this study has two important advantages: (i) control of the conversion of S-TRAIL from a non-apoptotic resident of the ER to a apoptosis-inducing pro-tein by selective protease activation, and (ii) in vivo imaging of protease activity using a NIRF probe. Release of S-TRAIL in tumors can be controlled by co-injection of viral vectors encoding ER-S-TRAIL and the viral pro-tease, and should be compatible with clinical trials for accessible tumor foci.

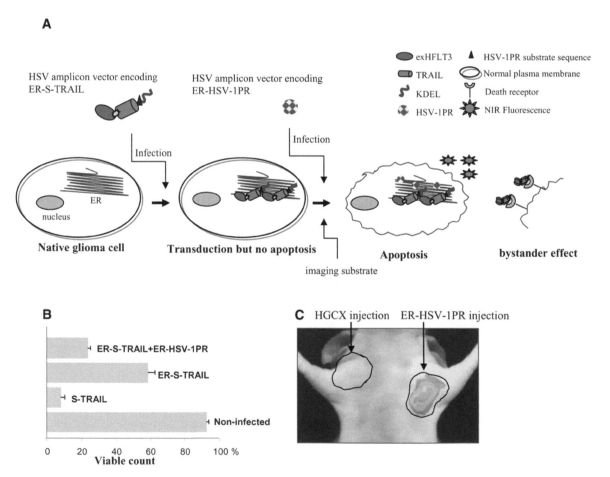

Figure 3 Regulation of apoptosis and in vivo imaging of HSV-1PR activity. (**A**) Schematic view of apoptosis and imaging after transduction of cells with vector encoding ER-S-TRAIL followed by vector encoding ER-HSV-1PR and incubation with HSV-1 protease-specific NIRF probe. (**B**) Gli36 glioma cells were left uninfected or infected with S-TRAIL, ER-S-TRAIL, or coinfected with ER-S-TRAIL and ER-HSVPR amplicon vectors and 24 hours later cell viability was assessed. (**C**) Mice were implanted with Gli36 glioma cells on both sides in the upper lateral abdomen and seven days later tumors were injected with 20 μL of 3.5 × 10^8 transducing units (tu)/mL of ER-HSV-1PR amplicon vector or HGCX control vector; 36 hours later mice were administered i.v. with 2.5 nanomoles of HSV-1PR-NIRF probe and imaged 24 hours later using a CCD camera. *Source*: Adapted from Ref. 34 (*See Color Insert*).

FLUORESCENCE MEDIATED TOMOGRAPHY

Fluorescence mediated tomography (FMT) has evolved as a tomographical method to overcome many of the limitations of planar imaging (reflectance and transillumination) and yield a robust and quantitative modality for fluorescent reporters in vivo. It uses a CW (continuous wave) laser source, and in contrast to reflectance fluorescence imaging methods, measures the intrinsic and fluorescence signals of the photons after they have diffused through the measured object immersed in "matching fluid" (37). FMT provides tomographical (3-D) information on the concentrations of the measured fluorophore in the imaged subject. Detection is based on the ability of probes to outline specific molecular processes and diseases and not on high resolution. The original FMT feasibility studies resolved PR in animal brains using circular geometry and fiber-based systems (38). Newer generation prototypes based on noncontact techniques have allowed superior imaging quality demonstrating sub-resolution imaging capacity (39) and sensitivity that reaches below a picomole of fluorescent dye (value reported for the Cy5.5 dye excited at 672 nm). Such advanced setups have been used for imaging PR (39) or the effects of chemotherapy on tumors (11). Multispectral FMT can further enhance the applications by simultaneously resolving multiple targets under identical physiological conditions. Montet et al. (40) has recently utilized long-circulating dextranated magento fluorescent nanoparticle containing long-circulating synthetic graft copolymers labeled with Cy5.5 or NIR dyes used in AngioSense™ 750 to image vasculature with FMT. They demonstrated correlation of tumor antiogenesis with microvessel density measured with intravital microscopy and enabled therapeutic evaluation of anti-VEGF antibody.

BIOLUMINESCENCE IMAGING

BLI has emerged as a useful and complementary experimental imaging technique for small animals. BLI exploits the emission of visible photons at specific wavelengths based on energy-dependent reactions catalyzed by luciferases. Luciferases comprise a family of photoproteins (Fluc, Rluc, and Gluc) that emit detectable photons in the presence of oxygen and ATP during metabolism of substrates such as luciferin into oxyluciferin. The light from these enzyme reactions typically has very broad emission spectra that frequently extend beyond 600 nm, with the red components of the emission spectra being the most useful for imaging by virtue of easy transmission through tissues. The light output per cell can be determined in culture as an a priori assessment of the sensitivity of detecting a signal in a given animal model, although there is a marked reduction of signal in vivo (41) Typical doses of luciferin are in large excess (120 mg/kg) and are injected immediately before data acquisition. Image acquisition times are on the order of minutes, depending on expression levels, depth, and photon flux and the light generated is detected and quantified using highly sensitive cooled charge-coupled device (CCD) cameras (42,43).

The predictions based on diffusion models and in vivo studies suggest that BLI can provide a sensitive and rapid assay for the study of oncogenesis and disease progression in living animal models. Furthermore, BLI in experimental animals complements other developments in the molecular imaging field allowing real-time information about complex pathophysiological processes in living organisms. This will lead to a better understanding of the underlying biology and thus result in improved disease prevention and treatment. Luciferases have been used for real-time, low-light imaging of gene expression in cell cultures, individual cells, whole organisms, and transgenic organisms. Sensitive imaging systems have been built to detect and quantitate small numbers of cells or organisms expressing luciferase as transgenes (44–46). BLI has been used to image transgene expression, develop imageable transgenic animal models, image immune response, and monitor the migration and fate of neural stem cells in real-time in vivo.

Imaging Tumor Models and Their Response to Therapy

Genetically engineered tumor cells with different luciferases allow for noninvasive, longitudinal quantitation of tumor growth in subcutaneous and orthotopic tumor models (Hoffman 2005). Imaging models follow tumor cells immediately after implantation and are well suited for quantitative evaluation of therapeutic efficacy. Metastatic models of cancer in which cancer cells stably express luciferase have been developed. For example, human prostate cancer cells PC-3M-luc-C6 when injected into mice via tail vein or intracardiac implantation develop experimental metastatic lesions in different organs (47). Luciferase imaging has revealed gene transfer to tumors followed by a decrease in transgene expression with tumor cell death over time. BLI has been employed to monitor tumor cell growth and regression to visualize the kinetics of tumor cell clearance by chemotherapeutics and to track gene expression (41,48–50). The ability to image two or more biological processes in a single animal can greatly increase the utility of luciferase imaging by offering the opportunity to distinguish the expression of two reporters biochemically. The luciferases from *Renilla* and firefly have different substrates, coelenterazine and D-luciferin, respectively, and can be imaged in tumors in

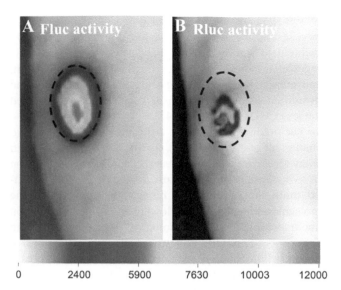

Figure 4 Dual imaging of amplicon vector delivery and glioma volumes. (**A**) Mice bearing subcutaneous Gli36fluc⁺ gliomas (Gli36 glioma cells stably expressing Fluc were injected i.p. with D-luciferin and imaged for Fluc activity. (**B**) HSV amplicon viral vector bearing Rluc was injected into the same tumor and 36 hours later, coelenterazine was injected into the tail vein and the mice were imaged for Rluc activity. Each image in A and B represents a scan time of one minute. The dashed circle around the tumor indicates the tumor periphery. *Source*: Adapted from Ref. 48 (*See Color Insert*).

the same living mouse with kinetics of light production being separable in time by separate injections of these two substrates (51). Dual BLI has been used to monitor gene delivery via a therapeutic vector and to follow the effects of the therapeutic protein TRAIL in gliomas (34). Glioma cells stably expressing Fluc were implanted subcutaneously into nude mice and the tumor growth was monitored in vivo over time by luciferin administration and BLI. HSV amplicon vectors bearing the genes for TRAIL and Rluc were injected directly into these Fluc-positive gliomas allowing super imposition of gene delivery to the tumor by coelentrazine administration and BLI (Fig. 4). This dual imaging approach has direct applications in studying the delivery of gene therapy vectors and simultaneously monitoring therapeutic effects in vivo.

Imaging Transgenic Animal Models

The development and optimization of successful cancer therapy strategies will require a detailed and specific assessment of biological processes in response to mechanistic intervention. A number of spontaneous transgenic animal model have been engineered by knocking out genes involved in cell proliferation. For example, PTEN-deficient mice develop metastatic prostate

carcinomas (52) whereas Rb knockout mice develop pituitary tumors, medullary thyroid carcinomas, and/or pheochromocytomas (53). The use of such transgenic models has extended our understanding of the mechanisms of pathogenesis and it is expected that these could more accurately predict response to novel anticancer drugs. The incorporation of optical imaging markers into such models has allowed to noninvasively image tumorigenesis, progression and metastases of spontaneous tumors and to evaluate therapeutic effects of potential anti-cancer drugs on those tumors. Vooijs et al. (54) generated transgenic mice that express luciferase and *Cre* recombinase in the pituitary gland under the control of intermediate lobe-specific POMC promoter. These mice were crossed with conditional RB knockout mice to develop mice with RB deletion solely in the pituitary gland. This model allowed noninvasive imaging of pituitary tumor development, progression, and therapeutic response in live animals via BLI. Similarly, a conditional luciferase transgenic mouse, in which loxP-luciferase, under the control of β-actin promoter, was crossed with a conditional oncogenic Kras2^{V12} mouse that develops lung adenocarcinomas after delivery of Ad-Cre to the lungs (55). The development of lung cancer in conditional Luc/Kras2^{V12} was visualized by BLI following intratracheal administration of Ad-Cre. The feasibility and the ease with which BLI can be used to monitor cell cycle in a genetically engineered model of glioma in vivo has been recently demonstrated (56). To image the loss of RB pathway function in tumor cells in vivo, Fluc gene under the control of human E2F1 promoter was used. E2F1 is negatively regulated by RB under normal conditions, and thus luciferase activity increases on loss of RB in tumors, regardless of mitotic status (57). Ef-Fluc transgenic mouse line was crossbred with the N–tv-a mouse strain that express the viral receptor tv-a from the nestin promoter and mice were injected intracranially with DF-1 cells producing RCAS-PDGFB retrovirus (58). The resulting spontaneous gliomogenesis and tumor progression was followed in real time by BLI. In such a model BLI also enables to analyze the potency and pharmacodynamics of drugs that interfere with tumor proliferation (56).

Visualizing Immune Responses

Until recently, much of our understanding of immune-cell trafficking and the factors that control this process has been obtained by using culture systems in which the influence of intact organ structure, circulation, endothelial barriers, and tissue effects have been removed. Insights into the specific locations and timing of immune-cell migration and proliferation that can be gained using imaging methods in living animals hold promise for providing new information on physiology and pathophysiology. BLI is an effective means of evaluating complex biological processes such as stem-cell engraftment, using use graft versus leukemia (GVL) reactions and graft-versus-host disease (GVHD) as examples. Transgenic L2G85 mice express a luciferase protein under the control of the chicken β-actin promoter in all hematopoietic cells, which provides a source of luciferase-positive donor cells for transplantation studies (59). In studies with cells from L2G85 mice, syngeneic or allogeneic recipient animals received lethal irradiation followed by injection of T-cell-depleted bone marrow cells from wild-type donor animals and splenocytes from L2G85 animals (to induce GVHD) (60). Serial BLI imaging showed striking differences between syngeneic and allogeneic recipients. In the syngeneic animals, a waxing and waning BLI signal from the transplanted luciferase-positive cells was observed, which ultimately resulted in bone marrow engraftment, probably from residual stem cells in the splenocyte preparations. By marked contrast, the transplanted cells in allogeneic recipients showed early (in the first 24–48 hours) infiltration of cervical lymph nodes and structures in the gut. At two to four days after transplantation, marked proliferation of the donor cells was observed at these lymph node and gut sites, indicated by the increase in BLI signal. This study identified the key target structures and organs involved in the induction of GVHD.

Tracking Neural Precursor Cells in Brain Tumor Models

The recognition that neural precursor cells (NPCs) can migrate and integrate appropriately throughout the mammalian central nervous system (CNS) following transplantation (61,62) has unveiled new roles for neural transplantation and gene therapy, and a new strategy for addressing CNS tumors. NPCs can become normal constituents of the host cytoarchitecture and are capable of disseminating bioactive molecules and virus vectors (63,64). The ability to noninvasively track the engraftment, migration and proliferation of NPCs has significant clinical and research implications. We have explored the macroscopic migratory capabilities of NPCs toward experimental tumors following implantation into nude mice at distant sites in the brain (65). A line of NPCs stably expressing Fluc was either implanted into the brain parenchyma or administered via intraparenchymal and intraventricular injections into mice bearing intracranial gliomas. Using serial BLI, migration of NPCs implanted in the brain was observed across the corpus callosum toward the tumor, with movement first being detected at one week and maximal density within the tumor site observed at two to three weeks after implantation (Fig. 5). This is in line with the histologically documented migratory capability of NPCs over considerable distances and their preferential

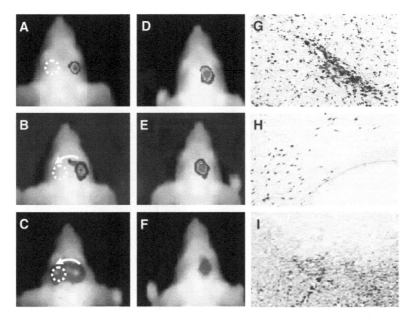

Figure 5 Parenchymal migration of NPC-LUCs expressing firefly luciferase (Fluc). NPC-LUC cells (NPCs stably expressing Fluc) were implanted into the right hemisphere of either mice bearing Gli36 tumors in the left hemisphere (**A, B, C**) or control mice, which did not have tumors (**D, E, F**). A, B, and C represents a time series of the same animal from the first group imaged at day 0 (A), 1 week (B), and 2 weeks (C). Migration toward the tumor (*dotted circle*) was first noted after one week (B; see faint bioluminescence signal along arrow) and migration across the midline was evident at two weeks. D, E, and F represent the time series of another animal representative of the non-tumor bearing group, in which no migration toward the contralateral side was observed. X-galactosidase staining of coronal sections shows the β-galactosidase-expressing cells in the injection site (**G**), the corpus callosum (**H**), and inside the tumor (**I**). *Source*: Adapted from 65.

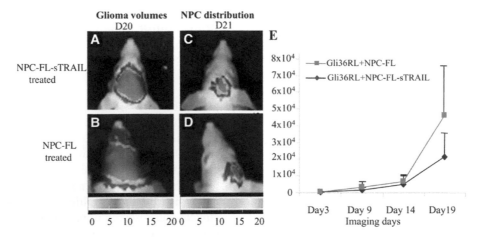

Figure 6 Dual imaging NPC migration and therapeutic effects of STRAIL expressing NPCs on glioma burden. Gli36 glioma cells stably expressing Rluc (Gli36-RL) were implanted into the right frontal lobe and NPC-FLs or NPC-FL-sTRAILs (NPCs stably expressing Fluc and S-TRAIL) were implanted into the close vicinity of mice bearing an established Gli36-RL glioma. Mice were followed for tumor progression by Rluc imaging and the images of mice injected with NPC-FL-sTRAILs (**A**) or NPC-FLs (**B**) after 20 days are shown. The presence of NPC-FL-sTRAILs (**C**) and NPC-FLs (**D**) in the tumor was followed by Fluc imaging on day 21. Color-coded maps of the photon intensities from Gli36-RL or NSC-FL-sTRAIL and NSC-FL cells are shown. (**E**) Rluc bioluminescence intensities of Gli36-RL tumors in mice implanted with either NPC-FL-sTRAILs or NPC-FLs over time. *Source*: Adapted from Ref. 36.

accumulation in brain tumors on CNS injection. Taking advantage of the extraordinary migratory properties of NPCs, we have engineered them with therapeutic protein, S-TRAIL (34) that specifically kills tumor cells while leaving the normal cells like NPCs behind (36). NPCs expressing S-TRAIL have the advantage of providing the extended release time of S-TRAIL and direct delivery to invasive tumor cells. To track the growth of highly malignant gliomas and migration of therapeutic NPCs, cell lines were also engineered with luminescent and fluorescent transgenes for fluorescence and dual BLI (36). Using a highly malignant human-glioma model expressing Rluc, intracranially implanted NPCs expressing both Fluc and S-TRAIL were shown to migrate into the tumors and have anti-tumor effects (Fig. 6). These studies demonstrate the potential of NPCs as therapeutically effective delivery vehicles for the treatment of gliomas, and also provide important tools to evaluate the migration of NPCs and changes in glioma-burden in vivo.

INTRAVITAL MICROSCOPY

IVM is a powerful optical imaging technique that allows continuous noninvasive monitoring of molecular and cellular processes in intact living tissue with 1 to 10 μm resolution. Intravital multiphoton microscopy (MPM) combines the advanced optical techniques to capture high-resolution, three-dimensional (3-D) images of living tissues that have been tagged with highly-fluorophores. The recent introduction of MPM (66,67) featuring infrared

pulsed laser excitation to generate optical sections of fluorescent signals, has allowed for much greater depth of penetration of tissue for imaging and has greatly decreased the amount of photobleaching and photodamage. The combination of MPM technology with IVM enables the analysis of cell migration in time-lapse recordings of 3-D tissue reconstructions (68). IVM has provided powerful insights into how carcinoma cells move within tumors, evaluating the responses to various therapies and following stem cell homing to tumors.

Imaging of Metastatic Cells

Intravital-imaging studies have been especially useful for characterizing primary-tumor properties, growth rates, and mechanisms of metastasis to target organs (69,70). Intravital imaging has identified several differences in which carcinoma cells move in tumors in live animals as compared with in-culture models of invasion. MPM has allowed a direct comparison of cell motility behavior in metastatic and nonmetastatic tumors. To identify important behavioral properties of metastatic cells within the primary tumor, the in vivo motility of cells of mammary tumors that are formed by the poorly metastatic MTC cell line with the highly metastatic MTLn3 carcinoma cell line (71) were compared. These cells were used to generate primary tumors in vivo and the motility of the cells in these tumors was observed. The comparison of the properties of these primary tumors highlights some intriguing aspects of the metastasis process. In MTC tumors, the cells move over each other, and the direction of motility is nonlinear and does not seem to be guided by collagen fibres (72,73). However, MTLn3 cells have no motility in areas where there are no vessels or collagen fibres, paradoxically making cell migration a rare event, even in the highly metastatic MTLn3 tumors. High-resolution time-lapse images of cell movement within MTLn3 tumors showed a linear and fiber-associated locomotion of carcinoma cells in vivo (72).

Imaging Therapeutic Response

The preclinical response to a new therapy, in general, is quantified in terms of reduction in (or stabilization of) tumor size) and survival time of the animal. However, the ability to monitor several parameters simultaneously with IVM has provided integrated insight into a tumor's response to various therapies. Tumor vasculature is an attractive alternative to targeting tumor cells because of (i) easy accessibility of blood-borne agents to endothelial cells, (ii) reliance of most tumor cells on vascular supply for survival, (iii) selective expression of proteins on tumor endothelial cells, and (iv) it is a prominent route for metastatic spread (reviewed in Iga et al., 2006). Vascular-disrupting agents (VDA) exploit the differences between tumor and normal endothelial cells to induce selective vascular dysfunction (74) by disrupting blood circulation in tumors. In vivo analysis of this intensely studied class of anticancer agents is invaluable for preclinical assessment of pharmacodynamical end points and effective therapeutic windows. Elucidation of the mechanism of action of various VDAs has been made possible through the use of intravital video microscopy (IVVM) (75,76), which allows dynamic observation of cancer cell activity in the microcirculation of intact organs and tissue in live animals. Hori et al. (75) showed that AC7700, a tubulin-binding agent, caused constriction of host arterioles, leading to narrowing of tumor vessels and hemolysis in tumor-draining vessels. The strength of IVVM lies in being able to quantify specific variables, such as vessel number, diameter, length, vascular density, permeability, and blood-flow velocity. The fact that IVVM requires no prior assumptions to be made about the likely effects of a particular VDA is a major advantage over other methods in preclinical assessment (77).

Of all the known angiogenic molecules, vascular epidermal growth factor (VEGF) appears to be the most critical (78). VEGF promotes the survival and proliferation of endothelial cells, increases the display of adhesion molecules on these cells, and increases vascular permeability. Blocking VEGF or its receptor VEGF-R leads to a decrease in vessel diameter and vessel density and a decrease in vascular permeability (79,80). Intravital imaging has revealed similar decrease in vascular density and

permeability following hormone withdrawal from a testosterone-dependent tumor (81) and following treatment of an HER2/neu overexpressing tumor with trastuzumab—a monoclonal antibody to ERBB2 (82). Intravital microscopy has been used to monitor the activity of the VEGF promoter in transgenic mice harboring enhanced GFP under control of this promoter (83). When subcutaneous pancreatic tumors in SCID mice were injected directly with adenovirus vectors encoding the soluble form of the VEGF flt-1 receptor (Adsflt) or control vectors (AdLacZ), intravital microscopy revealed that AdLacZ-infected cells prompted strong tumor angiogenesis, whereas Adsflt-infected cells secreting a decoy receptor failed to exert such an effect (84).

Tracking Bone Marrow–Derived Cells (Stroh and Jain Nature Medicine 2005)

The participation of local endothelial cells and the recruitment of circulating progenitor cells are important components of tissue neovascularization (85,86). Multiphoton intravital microscopy is well suited for tracking cells in vivo, but the relationship between single- and two-photon absorption spectra is not obvious, thus complicating the use of MPM with common dyes for cell tracking. Recently Stroh et al., (87) has exploited the optical properties of QDs to circumvent the limitation of common dyes. Primary bone marrow lineage-negative cells, a population enriched in progenitor and stem cells was labeled with QD590-TAT (encapsulated QD590-covalently coupled to the human immunodeficiency virus TAT protein). Mice bearing established intracranial tumors were infused with both QD470 micelles and the ex vivo–labeled lineage-negative cells through the carotid artery and the blood flow and rolling and adhesion of lineage-negative cells to tumor endothelium was imaged by multiphoton intravital microscopy. The ability to contemporaneously excite and monitor both QDs avoided difficulties with registration as a result of sequential monitoring with multiple wavelengths, and the bright, nonoverlapping QD emissions enabled clear differentiation of cell from plasma marker.

Tracking Human Neural Stem Cells

Transplantation of genetically manipulated cells of human origin to the CNS offers immense potential for the treatment of several neurological disorders. Monitoring the expression levels of transgenes and following cells at a cellular resolution in vivo is critical in assessing the efficacy of such therapies in vivo. We have engineered lentiviral vectors bearing fusions between fluorescent and bioluminescent marker proteins and employed BLI and intravital microscopy to study the fate of human neural

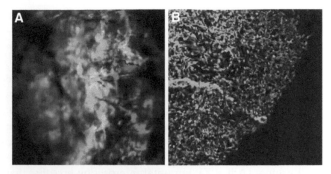

Figure 7 Human neural stem cell homing in response to glio-mas: Gli36-GFP-Rluc cells were implanted stereotactically into the right frontal lobe of SCID mice and two to three days later, Fluc-DsRed2 hNSC were injected 1 mm lateral to the glioma implan-tation. Mice were imaged by intravital microscopy on day 10 after hNSC implantation (**A**). Mice were sacrificed on day 10 after hNSC implantation and mice brains were sectioned and confocal microscopy was performed. hNSC (*red*) infiltrating the tumor (*green*) (**B**); 20× magnification. *Source*: Adapted from Ref. 88 (*See Color Insert*).

stem cells (hNSCs) in relation to gliomas in vivo. We used an GFP-Rluc expressing malignant human-glioma model and implanted hNSC expressing Fluc-DsRed2 intracrani-ally. Intravital microscopy revealed that transduced hNSC migrate extensively toward and into glioma tumors and survive longer in mice with gliomas than in normal brain (Fig. 7). These studies demonstrate the combined appli-cation of BLI and intravital microscopy in evaluating the fate of NSC and changes in glioma-burden in vivo, and provide a platform for accelerating cell and gene-based therapies for CNS disorders (88).

CONCLUSIONS

Noninvasive monitoring of both endogenous and deliv-ered gene expression offers numerous experimental ven-ues for research in animal models. With the development of new optical imaging technologies, investigators are poised to apply and extend current capabilities to assay the progression of diseases and the response to a variety of therapies. It is expected that clinical translation of optical molecular imaging technology will ultimately aid cancer diagnosis and the development of safe and efficient use of therapeutics.

REFERENCES

1. Greer LF III, Salary AA. Imaging of light emission from the expression of luciferases in living cells and organisms: a review. Luminescence 2002; 17(1):43–74.
2. Tannous BA, Kim DE, Fernandez JL, et al. Codon-optimized gaussia luciferase cDNA for mammalian gene expression in culture and in vivo. Mol Ther 2005; 11(3):435–443.
3. Tsien RY, Miyawaki A. Seeing the machinery of live cells. Science 1998; 280(5371):1954–1955.
4. Zhang J, Campbell RE, Ting AY, et al. Creating new fluorescent probes for cell biology. Nat Rev Mol Cell Biol 2002; 3(12):906–918.
5. Matz MV, Fradkov AF, Labas YA, et al. Fluorescent proteins from nonbioluminescent anthozoa species. Nat Biotechnol 1999; 17(10):969–973.
6. Baird GS, Zacharias DA, Tsien RY. Biochemistry, muta-genesis, and oligomerization of DsRed, a red fluorescent protein from coral. Proc Natl Acad Sci U S A 2000; 97(22) 11984–11989.
7. Shaner NC, Campbell RE, Steinbach PA, et al. Improved monomeric red, orange and yellow fluorescent proteins derived from discosoma sp. red fluorescent protein. Nat Biotechnol 2004; 22(12):1567–1572.
8. Berlier JE, Rothe A, Buller G, et al. Quantitative compar-ison of long-wavelength alexa fluor dyes to Cy dyes: fluorescence of the dyes and their bioconjugates. J Histo-chem Cytochem 2003; 51(12):1699–1712.
9. Chen X, Conti PS, Moats RA. In vivo near-infrared fluo-rescence imaging of integrin alphavbeta3 in brain tumor xenografts. Cancer Res 2004; 64(21):8009–8014.
10. Ye Y, Bloch S, Xu B. Design, synthesis, and evaluation of near infrared fluorescent multimeric RGD peptides for targeting tumors. J Med Chem 2006; 49(7):2268–2275.
11. Ntziachristos V, Schellenberger EA, Ripoll J, et al. Visu-alization of antitumor treatment by means of fluorescence molecular tomography with an annexin V-Cy5.5 conjugate. Proc Natl Acad Sci U S A 2004; 101(33):12294–12299.
12. Bremer C, Tung CH, Weissleder R. In vivo molecular target assessment of matrix metalloproteinase inhibition. Nat Med 2001; 7(6):743–748.
13. Mahmood U, Weissleder R. Near-infrared optical imaging of proteases in cancer. Mol Cancer Ther 2003; 2(5):489–496.
14. Weissleder R, Tung CH, Mahmood U, et al. In vivo imaging of tumors with protease-activated near-infrared fluorescent probes. Nat Biotechnol 1999; 17(4):375–378.
15. Zheng J, Nicovich PR, Dickson RM. Highly fluorescent noble-metal quantum dots. Annu Rev Phys Chem 2007; 58:409–431.
16. Brown EB, Campbell RB, Tsuzuki Y, et al. In vivo mea-surement of gene expression, angiogenesis and physiolog-ical function in tumors using multiphoton laser scanning microscopy. Nat Med 2001; 7(7):864–868.
17. Becker A, Hessenius C, Licha K, et al. Receptor-targeted optical imaging of tumors with near-infrared fluorescent ligands. Nat Biotechnol 2001; 19(4):327–331.
18. Callahan RJ, Bogdanov A Jr., Fischman AJ, et al. Preclin-ical evaluation and phase I clinical trial of a 99mTc-labeled synthetic polymer used in blood pool imaging. AJR Am J Roentgenol 1998; 171(1):137–143.
19. Tung CH, Bredow S, Mahmood U, et al. Preparation of a cathepsin D sensitive near-infrared fluorescence probe for imaging. Bioconjug Chem 1999; 10(5):892–896.
20. Weissleder R, Mahmood U. Molecular imaging. Radiology 2001; 219(2):316–333.
21. Tung CH, Mahmood U, Bredow S, et al. In vivo imaging of proteolytic enzyme activity using a novel molecular reporter. Cancer Res 2000; 60(17):4953–4958.

22. Marten K, Bremer C, Khazaie K, et al. Detection of dysplastic intestinal adenomas using enzyme-sensing molecular beacons in mice. Gastroenterology 2002; 122(2): 406–414.

23. Arnaout MA. Integrin structure: new twists and turns in dynamic cell adhesion. Immunol Rev 2002; 186:125–140.

24. Arnaout MA, Goodman SL, Xiong JP. Coming to grips with integrin binding to ligands. Curr Opin Cell Biol 2002; 14(5):641–651.

25. Haubner R, Wester HJ, Burkhart F, et al. Glycosylated RGD-containing peptides: tracer for tumor targeting and angiogenesis imaging with improved biokinetics. J Nucl Med 2001; 42(2):326–336.

26. van Hagen PM, Breeman WA, Bernard HF, et al. Evaluation of a radiolabelled cyclic DTPA-RGD analogue for tumour imaging and radionuclide therapy. Int J Cancer 2000; 90(4):186–198.

27. Gingras MC, Roussel E, Bruner JM, et al. Comparison of cell adhesion molecule expression between glioblastoma multiforme and autologous normal brain tissue. J Neuroimmunol 1995; 57(1–2):143–153.

28. Gruber G, Hess J, Stiefel C, et al. Correlation between the tumoral expression of beta3-integrin and outcome in cervical cancer patients who had undergone radiotherapy. Br J Cancer 2005; 92(1):41–46.

29. Wang X, Ferreira AM, Shao Q, et al. Beta3 integrins facilitate matrix interactions during transendothelial migration of PC3 prostate tumor cells. Prostate 2005; 63(1):65–80.

30. Kumar CC, Nie H, Rogers CP, et al. Biochemical characterization of the binding of echistatin to integrin alphavbeta3 receptor. J Pharmacol Exp Ther 1997; 283(2):843–853.

31. Achilefu S, Bloch S, Markiewicz MA, et al. Synergistic effects of light-emitting probes and peptides for targeting and monitoring integrin expression. Proc Natl Acad Sci U S A 2005; 102(22):7976–7981.

32. Bloch S, Xu B, Ye Y, et al. Targeting Beta-3 integrin using a linear hexapeptide labeled with a near-infrared fluorescent molecular probe. Mol Pharm 2006; 3(5):539–549.

33. Shah K, Tung CH, Chang CH, et al. In vivo imaging of HIV protease activity in amplicon vector-transduced gliomas. Cancer Res 2004; 64(1):273–278.

34. Shah K, Tung CH, Yang K, et al. Inducible release of TRAIL fusion proteins from a proapoptotic form for tumor therapy. Cancer Res 2004; 64(9):3236–3242.

35. Pan G, O'Rourke K, Chinnaiyan AM, et al. The receptor for the cytotoxic ligand TRAIL. Science 1997; 276(5309): 111–113.

36. Shah K, Bureau E, Kim DE, et al. Glioma therapy and real-time imaging of neural precursor cell migration and tumor regression. Ann Neurol 2005; 57(1):34–41.

37. Ntziachristos V. Fluorescence molecular imaging. Annu Rev Biomed Eng 2006; 8:1–33.

38. Ntziachristos V, Tung CH, Bremer C, et al. Fluorescence molecular tomography resolves protease activity in vivo. Nat Med 2002; 8(7):757–760.

39. Graves EE, Ripoll J, Weissleder R, et al. A submillimeter resolution fluorescence molecular imaging system for small animal imaging. Med Phys 2003; 30(5):901–911.

40. Montet X, Ntziachristos V, Grimm J, et al. Tomographic fluorescence mapping of tumor targets. Cancer Res 2005; 65(14):6330–6336.

41. Contag CH, Ross BD. It's not just about anatomy: in vivo bioluminescence imaging as an eyepiece into biology. J Magn Reson Imaging 2002; 16(4):378–387.

42. Honigman A, Zeira E, Ohana P, et al. Imaging transgene expression in live animals. Mol Ther 2001; 4(3):239–249.

43. Rice BW, Cable MD, Nelson MB. In vivo imaging of light-emitting probes. J Biomed Opt 2001; 6(4):432–440.

44. Contag CH, Jenkins D, Contag PR, et al. Use of reporter genes for optical measurements of neoplastic disease in vivo. Neoplasia 2000; 2(1–2):41–52.

45. Sweeney TJ, Mailander V, Tucker AA, et al. Visualizing the kinetics of tumor-cell clearance in living animals. Proc Natl Acad Sci U S A 1999; 96(21):12044–12049.

46. Wu JC, Sundaresan G, Iyer M, et al. Noninvasive optical imaging of firefly luciferase reporter gene expression in skeletal muscles of living mice. Mol Ther 2001; 4(4): 297–306.

47. Jenkins DE, Oei Y, Hornig YS, et al. Bioluminescent imaging (BLI) to improve and refine traditional murine models of tumor growth and metastasis. Clin Exp Metastasis 2003; 20(8):733–744.

48. Shah K, Tang Y, Breakefield X, et al. Real-time imaging of TRAIL-induced apoptosis of glioma tumors in vivo. Oncogene 2003; 22(44):6865–6872.

49. Rehemtulla A, Hall DE, Stegman LD, et al. Molecular imaging of gene expression and efficacy following adenoviral-mediated brain tumor gene therapy. Mol Imaging 2002; 1(1):43–55.

50. Shah K, Jacobs A, Breakefield XO, et al. Molecular imaging of gene therapy for cancer. Gene Ther 2004; 11(15):1175–1187.

51. Bhaumik S, Gambhir SS. Optical imaging of renilla luciferase reporter gene expression in living mice. Proc Natl Acad Sci U S A 2002; 99(1):377–382.

52. Wang S, Gao J, Lei Q, et al. Prostate-specific deletion of the murine Pten tumor suppressor gene leads to metastatic prostate cancer. Cancer Cell 2003; 4(3):209–221.

53. Jacks T, Fazeli A, Schmitt EM. Effect of an Rb mutation in a mouse. Nature 1992; 359(6393): 295–300.

54. Vooijs M, Jonkers J, Berns A. A highly efficient ligand-regulated Cre recombinase mouse line shows that LoxP recombination is position dependent. EMBO Rep 2001; 2(4):292–297.

55. Lyons SK, Meuwissen R, Krimpenfort P, et al. The generation of a conditional reporter that enables bioluminescence imaging of Cre/loxP-dependent tumorigenesis in mice. Cancer Res 2003; 63(21):7042–7046.

56. Uhrbom L, Nerio E, Holland EC. Dissecting tumor maintenance requirements using bioluminescence imaging of cell proliferation in a mouse glioma model. Nat Med 2004; 10(11):1257–1260.

57. Parr MJ, Manome Y, Tanaka T, et al. Tumor-selective transgene expression in vivo mediated by an E2F-responsive adenoviral vector. Nat Med 1997; 3(10): 1145–1149.

58. Uhrbom L, Holland EC. Modeling gliomagenesis with somatic cell gene transfer using retroviral vectors. J Neurooncol 2001; 53(3):297–305.

59. Cao YA, Wagers AJ, Beilhack A, et al. Shifting foci of hematopoiesis during reconstitution from single stem cells. Proc Natl Acad Sci U S A 2004; 101(1):221–226.

60. Beilhack A, Schulz S, Baker J, et al. In vivo analyses of early events in acute graft-versus-host disease reveal sequential infiltration of T-cell subsets. Blood 2005; 106 (3):1113–1122.

61. Aboody KS, Brown A, Rainov NG, et al. Neural stem cells display extensive tropism for pathology in adult brain: evidence from intracranial gliomas. Proc Natl Acad Sci U S A 2000; 97(23):12846–12851.

62. Ourednik J, Ourednik V, Lynch WP, et al. Neural stem cells display an inherent mechanism for rescuing dysfunctional neurons. Nat Biotechnol 2002; 20(11):1103–1110.

63. Herrlinger U, Woiciechowski C, Sena-Esteves M, et al. Neural precursor cells for delivery of replication-conditional HSV-1 vectors to intracerebral gliomas. Mol Ther 2000; 1(4):347–357.

64. Snyder EY, Deitcher DL, Walsh C, et al. Multipotent neural cell lines can engraft and participate in development of mouse cerebellum. Cell 1992; 68(1):33–51.

65. Tang Y, Shah K, Messerli SM, et al. In vivo tracking of neural progenitor cell migration to glioblastomas. Hum Gene Ther 2003; 14(13):1247–1254.

66. Helmchen F, Denk W. New developments in multiphoton microscopy. Curr Opin Neurobiol 2002; 12(5):593–601.

67. Williams RM, Zipfel WR, Webb WW. Multiphoton microscopy in biological research. Curr Opin Chem Biol 2001; 5(5):603–608.

68. Cahalan MD, Parker I, Wei SH, et al. Two-photon tissue imaging: seeing the immune system in a fresh light. Nat Rev Immunol 2002; 2(11):872–880.

69. Hoffman R. Green fluorescent protein imaging of tumour growth, metastasis, and angiogenesis in mouse models. Lancet Oncol 2002; 3(9):546–556.

70. Jain RK, Munn LL, Fukumura D. Dissecting tumour pathophysiology using intravital microscopy. Nat Rev Cancer 2002; 2(4):266–276.

71. Farina KL, Wyckoff JB, Rivera J, et al. Cell motility of tumor cells visualized in living intact primary tumors using green fluorescent protein. Cancer Res 1998; 58(12):2528–2532.

72. Condeelis J, Segall JE. Intravital imaging of cell movement in tumours. Nat Rev Cancer 2003; 3(12):921–930.

73. Wang W, Wyckoff JB, Frohlich VC, et al. Single cell behavior in metastatic primary mammary tumors correlated with gene expression patterns revealed by molecular profiling. Cancer Res 2002; 62(21):6278–6288.

74. Siemann DW, Rojiani AM. The vascular disrupting agent ZD6126 shows increased antitumor efficacy and enhanced radiation response in large, advanced tumors. Int J Radiat Oncol Biol Phys 2005; 62(3):846–853.

75. Hori K, Saito S. Microvascular mechanisms by which the combretastatin A-4 derivative AC7700 (AVE8062) induces tumour blood flow stasis. Br J Cancer 2003; 89(7):1334–1344.

76. Tozer GM, Prise VE, Wilson J, et al. Mechanisms associated with tumor vascular shut-down induced by combretastatin A-4 phosphate: intravital microscopy and measurement of vascular permeability. Cancer Res 2001; 61(17):6413–6422.

77. Tozer GM, Bicknell R. Therapeutic targeting of the tumor vasculature. Semin Radiat Oncol 2004; 14(3):222–232.

78. Dvorak HF. Vascular permeability factor/vascular endothelial growth factor: a critical cytokine in tumor angiogenesis and a potential target for diagnosis and therapy. J Clin Oncol 2002; 20(21):4368–4380.

79. Tsuzuki Y, Fukumura D, Oosthuyse B, et al. Vascular endothelial growth factor (VEGF) modulation by targeting hypoxia-inducible factor-1alpha–> hypoxia response element–> VEGF cascade differentially regulates vascular response and growth rate in tumors. Cancer Res 2000; 60(22):6248–6252.

80. Yuan F, Chen Y, Dellian M, et al. Time-dependent vascular regression and permeability changes in established human tumor xenografts induced by an anti-vascular endothelial growth factor/vascular permeability factor antibody. Proc Natl Acad Sci U S A 1996; 93(25): 14765–14770.

81. Jain RK, Safabakhsh N, Sckell A, et al. Endothelial cell death, angiogenesis, and microvascular function after castration in an androgen-dependent tumor: role of vascular endothelial growth factor. Proc Natl Acad Sci U S A 1998; 95(18):10820–10825.

82. Izumi Y, Xu L, di Tomaso E, et al. Tumour biology: herceptin acts as an anti-angiogenic cocktail. Nature 2002; 416(6878):279–280.

83. Lubiatowski P, Gurunluoglu R, Goldman CK, et al. Gene therapy by adenovirus-mediated vascular endothelial growth factor and angiopoietin-1 promotes perfusion of muscle flaps. Plast Reconstr Surg 2002; 110(1):149–159.

84. Hoshida T, Sunamura M, Duda DG, et al. Gene therapy for pancreatic cancer using an adenovirus vector encoding soluble flt-1 vascular endothelial growth factor receptor. Pancreas 2002; 25(2):111–121.

85. Carmeliet P, Jain RK. Angiogenesis in cancer and other diseases. Nature 2000; 407(6801):249–257.

86. Rafii S, Lyden D, Benezra R, et al. Vascular and haematopoietic stem cells: novel targets for anti-angiogenesis therapy? Nat Rev Cancer 2002; 2(11):826–835.

87. Stroh M, Zimmer JP, Duda DG, et al. Quantum dots spectrally distinguish multiple species within the tumor milieu in vivo. Nat Med 2005; 11(6):678–682.

88. Shah K, Hingtgen S, Kasmieh R, et al. Novel bimodal viral vectors and in vivo imaging reveal the fate of hNSCs in experimental glioma model 2008; 28(17):4406–4413.

36

Radiopharmaceutical Therapy of Cancer

DANIEL A. PRYMA and CHAITANYA R. DIVGI

Department of Radiology, Division of Nuclear Medicine and Clinical Molecular Imaging,
University of Pennsylvania, Philadelphia, Pennsylvania, U.S.A.

INTRODUCTION

Successful cancer therapy has long been among the greatest challenges in medicine. In the malignant transformation, cancer cells develop the ability to evade death and, given adequate nutrient and oxygent supplies, will continue to divide indefinitely. Therefore, curative therapy requires eradication of all malignant cells. Even a single remaining malignant cell can eventually repopulate.

Conventional chemotherapy exploits the elevated mitotic rates of cancer cells. These treatments are not specific, but target all cells in a specific stage of the cell cycle. Because cancer cells often cycle more rapidly than normal cells, they are more likely to be in the targeted stage at some point during therapy. Unfortunately, despite giving multiple cycles of therapy, conventional chemotherapy is unlikely to successfully eradicate all malignant cells, particularly in solid tumors. That is, while conventional therapy can induce marked treatment response, recurrent disease is common, even in the setting of high-dose chemotherapy requiring stem cell support.

Targeted therapies—those directed specifically at the malignant cells—can have greater success at complete eradication of all malignant cells in a given patient. Surgery, the quintessential targeted therapy, can successfully provide cancer cures in many patients, though curative surgery is generally limited to patients with localized disease. External beam radiotherapy is also a potent spatially targeted therapy that can provide curative therapy to patients with localized disease. While it sounds obvious, it is important to explicitly observe that surgery and external beam radiotherapy can only target disease that has been clinically detected and localized. Therefore, occult, micrometastatic disease cannot be reliably identified and targeted by surgery or external beam radiotherapy and remains an important source of treatment failures for both of these modalities. Furthermore, many patients have advanced disease at the time of diagnosis, which is not amenable to localized targeted therapy. For example, 30% of esophageal, 52% of pancreatic, 68% of ovarian, and 39% of lung cancer patients have distant disease on presentation (1).

For these reasons, there is a great clinical need for systemic targeted therapies, and unsealed source radiotherapy has properties ideal to fill this need. Targeted systemic radiotherapy can combine the excellent tumoricidal properties of external beam radiotherapy with exquisitely specific targeting of malignant cells. Furthermore, there is no need for localization of the metastatic deposits to allow for effective therapy. Targeted systemic radiotherapy can be used both in disease that is too small to detect with available imaging studies as well as with diseases that are difficult to accurately image (e.g., hepatocellular carcinoma in regenerative cirrhotic liver, osseous metastases from prostate or breast cancers).

In order to be effective, a targeted therapy must first localize to cancer cells and subsequently cause cell death. Localization can be accomplished by detecting an antigen or other receptor, which is overexpressed (or exclusively expressed) on the malignant cell, as is done with antibodies and some small peptides. Antigens can be nonfunctioning cell surface markers or receptors. Alternatively, various metabolic pathways are altered in malignancies and the substrates (or their analogs) of these processes can be used to localize malignant cells.

Once the malignant cell is targeted, cell killing can be caused by a variety of means. For example, the immune system may be activated by an antibody, causing T-cell or complement-mediated cytotoxicity. Cytotoxic chemotherapy can be conjugated to the targeting moiety, causing cell killing. However, this approach relies on internalization of the targeting substance. Furthermore, for immune activation or conjugated chemotherapy to be effective, each individual cell must be targeted. Cytotoxic radioactivity can be used either conjugated to the targeting agent [as in radiolabeled antibodies or samarium-153 ethylene diamine tetramethylene phosphonate (EDTMP)], or intrinsic to the agent (as in iodine-131 or radium-223). The great advantage of most radioactivity over other approaches is that the ionizing emissions will target not only a single cell, but, with most β-emitters, can also deliver cytotoxic radiation to nearby cells, obviating the need for targeting of each individual cell in order to achieve complete tumor eradication.

DOSIMETRY

In order to cause cell death, ionizing radiation must generally cause a double stranded DNA break in a given cell as single stranded breaks can be repaired. Ionizing radiation may be in the form of photons or particles (including β-particles, Auger electrons and α-particles). Each emission, whether particle or photon, has a characteristic energy and will deposit it over a defined path length. The energy deposited per unit path length is known as the linear energy transfer (LET). The greater the energy deposited within a tumor by an ionizing emission, the more likely it is to cause a double-stranded DNA break within a malignant cell.

Cytotoxicity is proportional to LET, and α-particle emission, which results in deposition of a large amount of energy within a few microns, is particularly lethal. Thus, if an α-particle is emitted within a cell, that cell is nearly certain to be killed by that particle. However, while the path length of an α-particle can extend somewhat beyond a single cell diameter, successful α-particle therapy approaches the same limitations of chemotherapy-conjugated targeted therapies: requiring internalization, or at least, targeting of each

individual malignant cell. Auger electrons have a similarly short path length and are subject to the same issues. At the other extreme, photons deposit their energy over a relatively large distance with consequent low LET. An individual γ-ray, then, is almost certain not to cause cell death.

Historically, the most successful systemic targeted radiotherapy has been with β-particles because they have a path length long enough to optimize the bystander effect, but retain an LET high enough to deliver tumoricidal radiation in many cases. Different β-particle-emitting isotopes each have a characteristic maximum energy and thus path length. β-particles thus have optimum tumor control sizes (2,3). If a β-particle emitter with a long path length targets a small metastatic deposit, much of the β-particle's energy will deposit outside the tumor; conversely, a β-particle emitter with a short path length in a very large tumor will irradiate only a small portion of that tumor. A combination of short and long path length β-particle emitters, or even a combination of β-particles and Auger or α-particle emitters could provide the most uniform tumor irradiation, particularly since patients have metastatic deposits of varying size (2,3).

Traditionally, administered doses for systemic radiotherapy have been fundamentally different from those for external beam radiotherapy. With external beam, the target is identified and the beams are designed to deliver a specific radiation dose to the target. The dose is designed to deliver what is expected to be a tumoricidal exposure to the target, while causing acceptable levels of damage to nearby normal tissues. On the other hand, systemic radiotherapy has generally delivered doses based on toxicity to normal tissues without any knowledge of dose to the malignant targets. Therefore, some patients receive far more radioactivity than would be necessary to eradicate their malignancy, while others receive futile treatments that cannot deliver tumoricidal exposure despite causing significant toxicity. While this is also true of conventional chemotherapy and is not a sufficient reason not to attempt therapy in patients who will otherwise die of their disease, choosing doses based on actual patient data would be advantageous. Using positron emission tomography (PET), it has been shown to be feasible to measure and characterize the radiation-absorbed dose to individual lesions, though the effect on clinical dose selection remains uncertain (4–7).

RADIOACTIVE SUBSTRATES

Differentiated Thyroid Cancer

Nuclear medicine was born as a specialty with the discovery that radioactive iodine localizes and can be detected in thyroid tissue, and subsequently that thyroid disorders can be both visualized and treated with radioactive iodine (8–10). These seminal investigations were the first, and for decades, the only examples of successful targeted systemic cancer radiotherapy. A key component of thyroid hormone is iodine and the thyroid gland relies on dietary iodine to provide the required substrate. When iodine is consumed, it is taken up from the stomach and enters the bloodstream. Sodium-iodide symporters (NIS) in the thyroid cell take up the iodine and it is subsequently organified and stored in colloid. Thereafter, in response to thyroid stimulating hormone (TSH), the iodinated thyroid hormone is cleaved from the colloid and released into the bloodstream.

While thyroid cancer cells behave abnormally in many ways, even after their malignant transformation, most-differentiated thyroid cancer cells maintain the ability to take up and organify iodine. This behavior can be exploited by giving oral radioactive iodine to visualize and treat malignant thyroid cells. Because of the exquisite specificity of iodine uptake, even widespread metastatic thyroid cancer can be successfully treated despite the fact that thyroid cells are inherently relatively radioresistant (Fig. 1). In order to optimize radioiodine uptake by thyroid cells, NIS function is optimized by insuring an elevated TSH, and the patient is deprived of dietary iodine. Traditionally, TSH elevation has been accomplished by establishing a hypothyroid state by thyroid hormone withdrawal. While reliable, hormone withdrawal can have a significant negative impact on quality of life (11). Administration of recombinant human TSH (12–14) obviates the adverse effects of thyroid hormone withdrawal. While there are no long-term data on the efficacy of this approach, it is clearly well tolerated by patients ranging from those with low risk disease through those with widespread metastatic disease.

Most centers utilize a standard dosing schema for radioactive iodine therapy. For example, a common approach is to administer 3.7 GBq of sodium iodine-131 to patients with low or moderate risk disease, 5.5 GBq of sodium iodine-131 to patients with high risk disease, including nodal involvement or extrathyroidal extension and 7.4 GBq of sodium iodine-131 to patients with metastatic disease (15). While this approach is certainly reasonable and appears to be efficacious, there is only modest supporting evidence and these doses can deliver excessive marrow burden to a subset of patients, particularly the elderly (16). A dosimetric approach to dose selection has also been used since described by Benua et al. in 1962 (17). Using this approach, multiple blood and whole body measurements are made after administration of a tracer dose of radioactive iodine and the clearance half times are extrapolated. The maximum dose is defined as that which delivers 2 Gray (Gy) to the blood and results in less than 2.96 GBq retained in the body at 48 hours after dosing (17). While this approach insures an

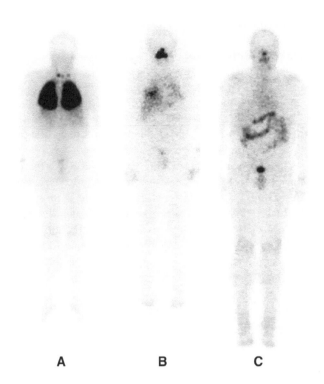

A   **B**   **C**

Figure 1 Metastatic thyroid cancer treated with sodium iodine-131. The patient is a 57-year-old male with cervical nodal metastases in addition to widespread pulmonary metastases. (**A**) Post-therapy scan seven days after administration of 14.8 GBq sodium iodine-131 demonstrates multifocal cervical uptake and extensive pulmonary uptake. (**B**) Post-therapy scan seven days after repeat therapy with 14.8 GBq sodium iodine-131. This treatment, done three years after the initial treatment in **A** demonstrates decreased pulmonary metastases with resolution of cervical metastases. (**C**) Two years after (**B**), diagnostic scan done three days after 185 MBq sodium iodine-131 demonstrates complete resolution of the previously seen malignancy. The patient remains without evidence of disease.

acceptable level of hematologic and pulmonary toxicity, as discussed above, it does not insure a tumoricidal radiation dose to the malignant cells. It does not fully adapt to difference in patient body size, as well, though it is used clinically in a number of centers.

Osseous Metastatic Disease

The osseous structures are a very common site of bone metastases in many cancers, most notably breast and prostate cancers. Because prostate and breast cancers account for 29% and 26% of new cancer cases in men and women, respectively, the number of patients with clinically significant osseous metastases is quite high (1). Osseous metastases are a source of significant morbidity in patients with metastatic disease including severe pain as well as pathologic fractures. Non-narcotic pain control has a marked positive effect on quality of life in patients with osseous metastatic disease, even in the absence of a significant impact on survival (18). Furthermore, in many patients, the osseous structures are the predominant or even sole site of metastases. Therefore, control of osseous metastases in these patients could have a significant impact on survival.

While the bones are seemingly rigid and fixed, there is a constantly ongoing process of remodeling wherein bone is destroyed by osteoclasts while new bone is formed by osteoblasts. While osseous metastases generally cause bone destruction, in many cases, this destruction results in a strong osteoblastic response of new bone formation. This osteoblastic response requires both calcium and phosphate in order to form new bone matrix, and this need for substrate can be exploited in order to treat osteoblastic metastatic disease. That is, administering a radioactive analog of either calcium or phosphate can result in decreased osteoblastic response as well as bystander effect on the adjacent malignant cells. While external beam radiotherapy is also efficacious in palliating bone metastases, its use is limited given the systemic nature of metastatic disease.

Strontium-89 is a β-emitter with a 50.5-day half-life that behaves in vivo as a calcium ion analog. It is administered intravenously as strontium chloride and is subsequently incorporated into new bone by osteoblasts. It has been shown to palliate pain in up to 80% of patients with painful prostate or breast cancer metastases (19–21). Toxicity is hematologic and generally mild and self-limiting (19–21). The major clinical concern with the use of strontium-89 is that while toxicity is mild, because of the long half-life, the toxicity can be prolonged, entailing potential delay in therapy with (other) hemato-toxic therapies.

Samarium-153 EDTMP is a radiolabeled phosphate analog. The phosphonate is taken up by osteoblasts; thus, its incorporation at metastatic sites is by being analogous to phosphate rather than calcium. Samarium-153 emits cytotoxic β-particles and a 103 keV photon; the photon permits gamma camera imaging. The 46.3-hour half-life of samarium-153 allows for a higher dose rate in addition to a shorter period of toxicity. Overall, bone pain palliation is achieved in 70% to 95% of patients after therapy with samarium-153 EDTMP (22–24). Similar to therapy with strontium-90, toxicity is hematologic, generally mild and reversible with recovery in most patients by five weeks (25).

Strontium-89 chloride and samarium-153 EDTMP are approved for use in Europe and the United States; clinical trials have explored other bone-seeking radiopharmaceuticals including rhenium-186 HEDP, rhenium-188 HEDP,

and radium-223 (26–32). Because the efficacy of the rhenium-labeled HEDP, samarium-153 EDTMP, and strontium-89 appear to be quite similar, the choice of which to use for palliation of bone pain falls to other issues, including toxicity, half-life, radiation safety, cost, and possibility of imaging (29,33). Radium-223, in contrast to the β-emitters discussed above, decays by the emission of multiple α-particles. As discussed earlier, α-particles have a much higher LET and thus, are far more lethal. However, the path length is quite short. Because bone-targeting radiopharmaceuticals rely on the osteoblastic response and do not directly target the malignant cells, there is a concern that a bone-seeking α-emitter will not cause sufficient tumor cell killing. Conversely, because of the short path length and the targeting of cortical bone, the marrow toxicity is expected to be lower than with the β-emitters. Indeed, recent phase I and phase II studies have shown radium-223 therapy to be safe and effective in patients with breast and prostate cancers and even showing a strong trend toward increased overall survival (32,34).

Many options exist for the palliative treatment of osseous metastases, both approved and experimental. The importance of pain palliation and decreased reliance on opioid analgesics on overall quality of life in individuals with metastatic cancer cannot be overstated. For poorly understood reasons, these bone-seeking radiopharmaceuticals are underutilized in most centers. While palliation is a noble and necessary goal, improving survival is the ultimate goal in cancer therapy.

There is evidence of improved survival in some studies with single-agent bone-seeking radiopharmaceuticals (32,35,36). However, it is more likely that bone-seeking radiopharmaceuticals may have their greatest effect on survival when used in combination with other treatments because not only do most patients have metastatic disease that is not entirely limited to the bones but also because most standard chemotherapeutic treatments have difficulty controlling osseous metastatic disease. There is encouraging evidence of the combination of bone-seeking radiopharmaceuticals with standard chemotherapy (37,38). Further investigation and optimization of combination therapy including bone-seeking radiopharmaceuticals in advanced malignancy is ongoing.

ANTIBODY: ANTIGEN TARGETING

Non-Hodgkin's Lymphoma

By far the most efficacious clinically used radiolabeled systemic cancer treatments have been the radiolabeled antibodies iodine-131 tositumomab and yttrium-90 ibritumomab tiuxetan. These antibodies target different epitopes on the CD20 antigen, which is ubiquitously expressed on B cells, including those involved in most non-Hodgkin's lymphomas. The success of these treatments is due to the ubiquity of this antigen expression on B cells (including malignant cells), its absence on other cells leading to acceptable toxicity and the relative radiosensitivity of lymphoma cells. Indeed, even in heavily pretreated patients, these radioimmunotherapies have shown previously unprecedented efficacy and durability of response (39–43).

While both antibodies are approved for use in non-Hodgkin's lymphoma, the details of their administration differ somewhat. Both regimens begin with an infusion of unlabeled antibody in order to saturate nonspecific binding sites. Tositumomab is given prior to iodine-131 tositumomab while rituximab (the chimeric form of ibritumomab) is given prior to ibritumomab tiuxetan. However, after this point, the procedures become different. For iodine-131 tositumomab, after the infusion of unlabeled antibody, approximately 185 MBq of iodine-131 tositumomab is infused intravenously. Whole body images and counts are performed over the course of a week to insure appropriate biodistribution as well as to determine the patient-specific radiopharmaceutical half-life. This half-life is used to calculate the iodine-131 tositumomab amount to deliver a whole body radiation absorbed dose no greater than 0.75 Gy for patients with platelet count at least 150,000 per mm^3 (0.65 Gy is prescribed for patients with platelets between 100 and 150,000/mm^3). The patient is then infused with unlabeled tositumomab immediately prior to the appropriate calculated therapeutic iodine-131 tositumomab amount.

While iodine-131 has both β and γ emissions allowing imaging, dosimetry, and therapy, yttrium-90 is a pure β-emitting transition metal. Therefore, a substitute transition metal with similar chelation chemistry (indium-111) must be used for imaging and is presumed to have similar in vivo behavior. In the United States, after infusion of rituximab (250 mg/m^2), 185 MBq of indium-111 ibritumomab tiuxetan is infused (imaging is not a requirement in Europe). Planar whole-body images are performed to insure appropriate biodistribution. Provided appropriate biodistribution (as manifest by adequate circulation of radioactivity and no evidence of excessive radioactivity in the reticuloendothelial system or kidneys) is present, a dose of 14.8 MBq/kg (with a maximum dose of 1184 MBq) yttrium-90 ibritumomab tiuxetan is prescribed for patients with at least 150,000 platelets/mm^3. For patients with between 100 and150,000 platelets per mm^3, the dose is reduced to 11.1 MBq/kg yttrium-90 ibritumomab tiuxetan. Again, the patient is infused with unlabeled rituximab immediately prior to the therapeutic yttrium-90 ibritumomab tiuxetan.

Both antibody regimens have hematologic dose-limiting toxicity, primarily neutropenia and thrombocytopenia, which is usually self-limited. At these dose levels in patients with recurrent or transformed non-Hodgkin's lymphoma, complete response rates range from 20% to 35% with overall response rate from 65% to 80% (40,44). These are impressive results given the heavily pretreated status of many of the patients in these studies. Furthermore, while the hematologic toxicity can be severe, it is less severe than most cytotoxic chemotherapeutic regimens and lacks almost entirely the nonhematologic toxicity common with cytotoxic chemotherapy.

Because these radioimmunotherapies are so well tolerated and efficacious in the patients with disease that is most difficult to treat (relapsed), there has been great interest in first-line treatment including radioimmunotherapy. A study by Kaminski et al. has shown complete and overall response rates of 75% and 95%, respectively, after first-line, single-agent iodine-131 tositumomab in patients with follicular non-Hodgkin's lymphoma (45). Furthermore, iodine-131 tositumomab included after first-line CHOP (cyclophosphamide, doxorubicin, vincristine and prednisolone chemotherapy regimen) chemotherapy was shown to improve remission status in 57% of those who achieved less than complete response after CHOP (46). Studies integrating radioimmunotherapy with first-line regimens are ongoing. Because radioimmunotherapy, particularly with the short β-particle range of iodine-131, will have its greatest success in small volume disease, volume reduction by other therapeutics immediately prior to radioimmunotherapy is likely to be more efficacious than radioimmunotherapy alone (47,48).

In addition to expanding radioimmunotherapy to first-line regimens, there has been exciting research, led by Oliver Press' group at the University of Washington in Seattle, using myeloablative radioimmunotherapy with peripheral stem cell support (39,43). Gopal et al. were able to demonstrate a complete or unconfirmed complete response rate of 57% with an overall response rate of 67% treating patients 60 years of age or older with myeloablative doses prescribed to deliver 25 to 27 Gy to the non-marrow organ (usually lung) receiving the highest radiation dose (43). Despite the fact that these doses are markedly higher than those used routinely, grade 4 non-hematologic toxicity was rare and there was no grade 4 infectious toxicity despite the myeloablation. These data suggest that further investigation of the role of myeloablative radioimmunotherapy is warranted.

Finally, because these two therapeutic regimens are relatively similar, questions arise as to which is best for a given patient. This question cannot be answered by prior studies that have provided evidence of each regimen's efficacy, as each study had somewhat different patient populations making their response rates incomparable. Jacene et al. attempted to cast light on the clinical aspects that may favor one regimen over another, specifically a slightly lower fractional decline in platelet counts post therapy with I-131 tositumomab, versus Y-90 anti CD20

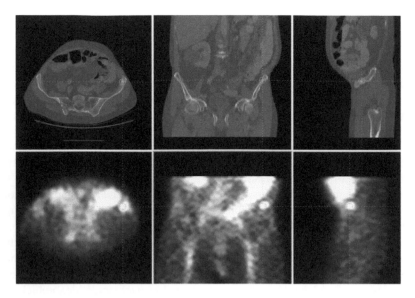

Figure 2 Lutetium-177 J591 therapy in prostate cancer. Coregistered axial, coronal, and sagittal computed tomography and lutetium-177 J591 SPECT images acquired three days after therapy with 740 MBq/kg lutetium-177 J591. SPECT images demonstrate antibody targeting of a left iliac crest osseous metastasis (*circle*).

(49). Other examples of clinical situations that may favor one regimen over another include a patient who would be expected to have a longer clearance time and compromised marrow function in whom the dosimetric approach of iodine-131 tositumomab might help to avoid severe hematologic toxicity. Furthermore, because ibritumomab tiuxetan and rituximab recognize the same epitope on CD20, iodine-131 tositumomab may be the better choice in patients who are heavily pretreated with or refractory to rituximab. On the other hand, because the yttrium-90 ibritumomab tiuxetan regimen requires fewer hospital visits, it may be preferred in patients who have difficulty with transportation or scheduling; yttrium-90 has theoretical advantages in bulky disease, and its pure β emissions minimize radiation safety concerns.

Other Radioimmunotherapies

The success of radioimmunotherapy for lymphoma has not yet been replicated in other malignancies, though there have been several promising studies. For example, the anti-CD33 antibody huM195 has been conjugated with iodine-131 as well as with the α-particle emitter bismuth-213 and used to assist with cytoreduction prior to stem cell transplant in patients with acute myeloid leukemias (50–52). The desire for complete myeloid cell killing while limiting nonhematologic toxicity is an ideal target for α-particle therapy, particularly since leukemic cells do not generally form solid clusters making the

shorter range of the bystander effect in α-therapy less of a limitation. Further study to evaluate the role of this therapy in the therapy of acute myeloid leukemia is continuing.

Successful radioimmunotherapy in solid tumors have been much more difficult to attain than with hematologic malignancies. This is largely due to the difficulties in achieving a uniform radiation dose throughout a large, solid tumor, most of which are more radioresistant compared with hematologic malignant cells. That is not to say that there have not been promising results in solid tumor radioimmunotherapy. The anti-prostate specific membrane antigen (anti-PSMA) antibody J591 has shown promising results in early stage trials conjugated to either lutetium-177 (Fig. 2) or yttrium-90 in patients both with prostate cancer as well as other advanced solid tumors that express PSMA on their vasculature (53,54). The antibody A33 targets an antigen ubiquitously expressed on lower gastrointestinal (GI) tract mucosa including colorectal cancers and, when radioiodinated, has shown some efficacy against advanced colorectal cancer in humans (55–57) with laboratory evidence of improved efficacy in combination with chemotherapy or external beam radiotherapy (58,59). Additionally, there is promising ongoing research involving radioimmunotherapy in other solid tumors, such as with cG250 in advanced clear cell renal cancer and hu3S193 in both papillary serous ovarian cancer (Fig. 3) and small cell lung cancer. Clearly, there is reason for optimism and further investigation into the optimum regimens and ideal clinical uses for radioimmunotherapy. Approaches in which

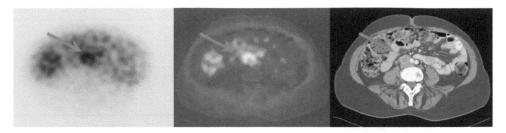

Figure 3 Indium-111 hu3S193 in advanced papillary serous ovarian cancer. The patient was imaged four days after intraperitoneal infusion of 185 MBq indium-111 hu3S193. Coregistered axial SPECT and enhanced CT images demonstrate antibody targeting of a right common iliac node. The patient subsequently received an intraperitoneal infusion of 370 MBq yttrium-90 hu3S193.

the absolute and/or the relative targeting of the radioantibody to tumor can be enhanced are no doubt going to help in the growth of this field. There can be no doubt that radioimmunotherapy could play a greater role in the therapy of patients with advanced solid malignancies, particularly in combination with other therapeutics.

SMALL MOLECULE–TARGETED RADIOTHERAPY

meta-Iodobenzylguanidine

Many malignancies of neural crest cell origin, such as neuroblastoma, pheochromocytoma, and paraganglioma, cause a great deal of morbidity and mortality, but because of their behavior are relatively insensitive to conventional chemotherapy. These malignancies generally retain their presynaptic amine and amine precursor transport into vesicles. This active transport can be exploited both for lesion detection as well as for therapy. Guanethidine is known to be avidly taken up via the amine transport system and the guanethidine analog *meta*-iodobenzylguanidine (mIBG) is readily taken up by these cells in addition to being iodinated, allowing for targeted therapy with iodine-131 (Fig. 4) in addition to imaging with iodine-123, iodine-131 and, potentially, the positron-emitting iodine-124 (60–69). With the iodine in the *meta* position, mIBG is very resistant to dehalogenation in vivo with approximately 90% excreted in the urine intact (70).

Many studies have evaluated the therapeutic potential of iodine-131 mIBG, though most have been with relatively small patient populations. The diseases for which mIBG therapy is likely to be useful are rare. Large randomized, controlled trials are thus very difficult to perform, but larger studies are ongoing. Furthermore, with the exception of neuroblastoma, most other malignancies of interest have a relatively indolent course making proof of prolonged survival a slow process. Despite these difficulties, studies have shown antitumoral efficacy utilizing various approaches ranging from multiple modest

doses of single agent iodine-131 mIBG causing little to no hematologic toxicity (71) to myeloablative doses requiring stem cell support (61,72) with many dosing protocols in between (60,62,63). The most common regimen in adults with neuroendocrine tumors is administering about 74 MBq/kg of iodine-131 mIBG, often as outpatient therapy, without dose-limiting toxicity. While objective responses are rare at this dose level, biochemical and symptomatic responses are common. Disease stabilization with repeated treatments is achievable in many patients. Increasing single doses are feasible with hematologic dose-limiting toxicity requiring stem cell support occurring at approximately 444 MBq/kg, though many patients have been treated with up to 703 MBq/kg with acceptable nonhematologic toxicity (61,62). Using high-dose therapy, there has been up to 25% complete response with 58% overall response rate in metastatic pheochromocytoma, and a 36% overall response rate in refractory or relapsed neuroblastoma (61,62), which are excellent responses in these very difficult-to-treat diseases.

There is also exciting research ongoing into variations of iodine-131 mIBG therapy. Extremely high specific activity (no carrier-added) preparations of iodine-131 mIBG have been postulated to have decreased toxicity as uptake into malignant cells can be saturated at lower-specific activities leading to nonspecific binding and, thus, toxicity. There is an ongoing phase I evaluation of high-specific activity iodine-131 mIBG with a planned phase II evaluation forthcoming. An alternative approach to improving mIBG therapy has been to synthesize a related compound, mABG, using the α-emitter astatine-211 (73). The high LET of α-particles from astatine-211 and its relatively short seven-hour half-life may markedly improve tumor cell killing and clinical investigations of this exciting compound are eagerly anticipated.

While most evaluations of therapeutic iodine-131 mIBG have been in pheochromocytoma, paraganglioma and neuroblastoma, mIBG is taken up by other neuroendocrine cancers, including pancreatic neuroendocrine cancers and gastrointestinal carcinoid tumors. Indeed,

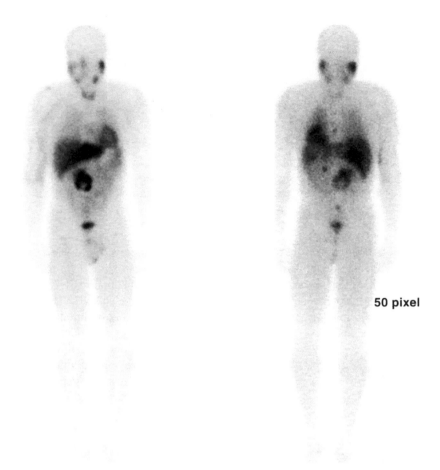

50 pixel

Figure 4 Iodine-131 mIBG in a patient with metastatic paraganglioma. Anterior and posterior planar images were acquired seven days following therapy with 5.5 GBq iodine-131 mIBG and reveal targeting of the large, centrally necrotic mid-abdominal paraganglioma in addition to hepatic and osseous metastases in the right shoulder, thoracic spine, sacrum, and left lower rib.

mIBG therapy has been shown to be effective in these cancers (74,75). However, the main limiting factor in the use of mIBG in these patients is that the pancreatic neuroendocrine cancers and gastrointestinal carcinoid tumors often demonstrate more somatostatin analog binding than mIBG binding (74). Thus, radiotherapy with labeled somatostatin analogs is likely a better approach in many of these patients.

Somatostatin Analogs

Somatostatin is a hormone whose receptors are overexpressed on the majority of neuroendocrine cancers such as pancreatic neuroendocrine cancers and carcinoid tumors. Additionally, many malignancies can have neuroendocrine features and overexpress somatostatin receptors, including malignant melanoma and small cell lung cancer. While somatostatin is a short-lived and potent hormone in vivo, many somatostatin analogs exist which are more stable in vivo. These analogs are commonly used in their

unlabeled forms for symptom palliation in carcinoid syndrome in addition to functioning pancreatic neuroendocrine cancers. While they may also provide disease stabilization, these analogs do not generally induce objective responses.

One such analog, octreotide, is an eight-amino acid peptide that binds to somatostatin receptors. It has been radiolabeled with the use of the chelator DTPA (diethylene triamine pentaacetic acid) and the radiometal indium-111. Indium-111-DTPA-octreotide is approved for use in the detection of somatostatin receptor overexpressing cancers. While indium-111 is a γ-emitter with favorable imaging properties, it also has a relatively high abundance of Auger electrons. These Auger electrons have a short path length (approximately 10 microns) and, thus, high LET. Indium-111-DTPA-octreotide has been used in large amounts as a therapeutic agent (74,76,77). While response rates were low, there was significant symptom control. As with most radiotherapy, hematologic toxicity is common with myelodysplastic syndrome, a concern after cumulative doses of 100 GBq or more. There is significant radiopharmaceutical retention in both the liver and kidneys, and hepatic and renal toxicity has been reported. The putative renoprotective effect from an infusion of positively charged amino acids (lysine and arginine) has been studied; the degree of renal protection must be considered in light of the toxicity of the amino acid infusion (78,79).

While indium-111-DTPA-octreotide does have some antitumoral activity, the short path length of the Auger electrons does likely limit the antitumor effect while the abundant γ-rays contribute a small, but significant, dose to normal tissues. Therefore, somatostatin analogs conjugated with other therapeutic isotopes have been investigated. The most commonly investigated are octreotide and octreotate using the chelator DOTA (known as DOTATOC and DOTATATE, respectively) and either yttrium-90 or lutetium-177. For example, after four cycles of therapy delivering a cumulative 7.4 GBq/m^2 yttrium-90 DOTA-TOC in patients with advanced neuroendocrine tumors, there was a 38% objective response rate with 63% of patients experiencing clinical benefit (80). Another study with yttrium-90 DOTATOC demonstrated a 57% rate of disease status improvement and 58% rate of performance status improvement (81), with improved overall survival compared with historical controls. A randomized, controlled study will be required to verify this finding.

There is evidence that the somatostatin analog octreotate may have better targeting of the somatostatin receptor subtype most common on neuroendocrine cancers (somatostatin receptor 2) with longer tumor retention compared with octreotide (82). There are no randomized, controlled evaluations of lutetium-177 DOTATATE; compelling evidence of its efficacy exists, both in neuroendocrine cancers as well as in other malignancies that overexpress somatostatin receptors (83,84). There was an overall response rate of 45% (including 3 patients with complete responses) in 130 patients with advanced pancreatic and gastric neuroendocrine cancers treated with cumulative doses up to 29.6 GBq of lutetium-177 DOTATATE (84). Among the 103 patients with at least stable disease, median time to progression was 36 months. In addition to the responses and disease stabilization, patients with progression of disease reported improved quality of life from therapy (85). The results were less striking in non-neuroendocrine cancers, though there was evidence of a possible role for lutetium-177 DOTATATE in combination with other treatments (83).

CONCLUSIONS

Targeted systemic cancer radiotherapies have been successful, notably in thyroid cancer, but the potential in still largely unrealized. There remains much to be done in terms of dose optimization as well as combination with

standard treatments (particularly radiosensitizing therapies) in order to achieve optimal synergy. Many innovations await clinical study. Antigen-binding constructs with improved tumor targeting and rapid serum clearance are being developed. Their small size may facilitate tumor penetration and enhance radiation dose delivery.

Bispecific constructs are fusion proteins that target more than one antigen. This can be a dimer of two Fv regions that recognize two distinct antigens. The choice of targets could potentially enhance the efficacy of treatment. Nonspecific binding occurs to some degree with all targeted molecules; by making a construct that targets two cancer antigens, one can optimize the targeting ratio (86,87). Bispecific targeting may also increase the residence time on the malignant cell (especially if the antigens are close enough to each other on the cell surface), allowing more time for therapeutic effect. Additionally, internalization could be optimized if a higher-affinity surface marker is used for initial cell targeting, bringing the construct into close proximity to a lower affinity antigen that mediates internalization.

In addition to nonspecific binding, another limitation of conventional radioimmunotherapy is the time to clearance from normal tissues and targeting of disease. This could be improved by making a bispecific construct that allows for the pre-targeting of malignant cells. Such a construct combines an antigen-binding protein against a malignant cell antigen with another that targets a molecule not normally present in the body. An interval of time after the construct is administered is allowed for tumor targeting and normal tissue clearance with, if necessary, an agent to bind and clear any construct that persists in the blood pool. Finally, the small molecule recognized by the bispecific construct is conjugated to an isotope and given intravenously. The small size of the molecule and its lack of nonspecific binding will potentially allow for very rapid targeting of the bispecific construct with minimal normal tissue exposure, greatly improving the therapeutic ratio. This has been shown to be feasible and promising in early phase trials (88–90).

However, the most important barriers to wider acceptance of targeted systemic radiotherapies are not necessarily scientific. There remains significant skepticism and fear of unsealed sources of radioactivity and the nuclear medicine physician must educate not only patients, but also the medical community at large regarding the safety and usefulness of targeted radiotherapy. Furthermore, while nuclear medicine has largely become a diagnostic imaging subspecialty, the nuclear medicine physician must provide clinical care for the toxicity associated with unsealed source radiotherapy; referring medical or surgical oncologists are reluctant to manage the toxicities caused by therapies not administered by them. Finally, the nuclear medicine physician must be an advocate for his or her patients to encourage the use of these safe, efficacious and underutilized treatments.

There is much cause for optimism for the future of targeted systemic radiotherapy of cancer. However, the road to greater acceptance and utilization of this modality will be long. While the best results to date have been in thyroid cancer, lymphoma and osseous metastatic disease, there is promising evidence of efficacious therapy for a wide range of other malignancies.

REFERENCES

1. Jemal A, Siegel R, Ward E, et al. Cancer statistics, 2007. CA Cancer J Clin 2007; 57(1):43–66.
2. Wheldon TE, O'Donoghue JA. The radiobiology of targeted radiotherapy. Int J Radiat Biol 1990; 58(1):1–21.
3. Wheldon TE, O'Donoghue JA, Barrett A, et al. The curability of tumours of differing size by targeted radiotherapy using 131I or 90Y. Radiother Oncol 1991; 21 (2):91–99.
4. Daghighian F, Pentlow KS, Larson SM, et al. Development of a method to measure kinetics of radiolabelled monoclonal antibody in human tumour with applications to microdosimetry: positron emission tomography studies of iodine-124 labelled 3F8 monoclonal antibody in glioma. Eur J Nucl Med 1993; 20(5):402–409.
5. Pentlow KS, Graham MC, Lambrecht RM, et al. Quantitative imaging of iodine-124 with PET. J Nucl Med 1996; 37(9):1557–1562.
6. Sgouros G, Chiu S, Pentlow KS, et al. Three-dimensional dosimetry for radioimmunotherapy treatment planning. J Nucl Med 1993; 34(9):1595–1601.
7. Sgouros G, Kolbert KS, Sheikh A, et al. Patient-specific dosimetry for 131I thyroid cancer therapy using 124I PET and 3-dimensional-internal dosimetry (3D-ID) software. J Nucl Med 2004; 45(8):1366–1372.
8. Hamilton JG, Soley MH, Eichorn KB. Deposition of radioactive iodine in human thyroid tissue. Univ Calif Publ Pharmacol 1940.
9. Keston AS, Ball RP, Frantz VK, et al. Storage of radioactive iodine in a metastasis from thyroid carcinoma. Science 1942; 95:362–363.
10. Seidlin SM, Marinelli LD, Oshry E. Radioactive iodine therapy: effect on functioning metastases of adenocarcinoma of the thyroid. JAMA 1946; 132:838–847.
11. Schroeder PR, Haugen BR, Pacini F, et al. A comparison of short-term changes in health-related quality of life in thyroid carcinoma patients undergoing diagnostic evaluation with recombinant human thyrotropin compared with thyroid hormone withdrawal. J Clin Endocrinol Metab 2006; 91(3):878–884.
12. Robbins RJ, Larson SM, Sinha N, et al. A retrospective review of the effectiveness of recombinant human TSH as a preparation for radioiodine thyroid remnant ablation. J Nucl Med 2002; 43(11):1482–1488.
13. Pacini F, Ladenson PW, Schlumberger M, et al. Radioiodine ablation of thyroid remnants after preparation with recombinant human thyrotropin in differentiated thyroid carcinoma: results of an international, randomized, controlled study. J Clin Endocrinol Metab 2006; 91 (3):926–932.
14. Robbins RJ, Driedger A, Magner J, Group USaCTCUPI. Recombinant human thyrotropin-assisted radioiodine therapy for patients with metastatic thyroid cancer who could not elevate endogenous thyrotropin or be withdrawn from thyroxine. Thyroid 2006; 16(11):1121–1130.
15. Karam M, Gianoukakis A, Feustel PJ, et al. Influence of diagnostic and therapeutic doses on thyroid remnant ablation rates. Nucl Med Commun 2003; 24(5):489–495.
16. Tuttle RM, Leboeuf R, Robbins RJ, et al. Empiric radioactive iodine dosing regimens frequently exceed maximum tolerated activity levels in elderly patients with thyroid cancer. J Nucl Med 2006; 47(10):1587–1591.
17. Benua RS, Cicale NR, Sonenberg M, et al. The relation of radioiodine dosimetry to results and complications in the treatment of metastatic thyroid cancer. Am J Roentgenol Radium Ther Nucl Med 1962; 87:171–182.
18. Porter AT, McEwan AJ, Powe JE, et al. Results of a randomized phase-III trial to evaluate the efficacy of strontium-89 adjuvant to local field external beam irradiation in the management of endocrine resistant metastatic prostate cancer. Int J Radiat Oncol Biol Phys 1993; 25(5): 805–813.
19. Dafermou A, Colamussi P, Giganti M, et al. A multicentre observational study of radionuclide therapy in patients with painful bone metastases of prostate cancer. Eur J Nucl Med 2001; 28(7):788–798.
20. Robinson RG, Preston DF, Baxter KG, et al. Clinical experience with strontium-89 in prostatic and breast cancer patients. Semin Oncol 1993; 20(3 suppl 2):44–48.
21. Silberstein EB, Williams C. Strontium-89 therapy for the pain of osseous metastases. J Nucl Med 1985; 26(4): 345–348.
22. Turner JH, Claringbold PG, Hetherington EL, et al. A phase I study of samarium-153 ethylene diamine tetramethylene phosphonate therapy for disseminated skeletal metastases. J Clin Oncol 1989; 7(12):1926–1931.
23. Farhanghi M, Holmes RA, Volkert WA, et al. Samarium-153-EDTMP: pharmacokinetic, toxicity and pain response using an escalating dose schedule in treatment of metastatic bone cancer. J Nucl Med 1992; 33(8):1451–1458.
24. Collins C, Eary JF, Donaldson G, et al. Samarium-153-EDTMP in bone metastases of hormone refractory prostate carcinoma: a phase I/II trial. J Nucl Med 1993; 34(11): 1839–1844.
25. Anderson PM, Wiseman GA, Dispenzieri A, et al. High-dose samarium-153 ethylene diamine tetramethylene phosphonate: low toxicity of skeletal irradiation in patients with osteosarcoma and bone metastases. J Clin Oncol 2002; 20(1):189–196.
26. de Klerk JM, van het Schip AD, Zonnenberg BA, et al. Phase 1 study of rhenium-186-HEDP in patients with bone metastases originating from breast cancer. J Nucl Med 1996; 37(2):244–249.
27. de Klerk JM, Zonnenberg BA, van het Schip AD, et al. Dose escalation study of rhenium-186 hydroxyethylidene

diphosphonate in patients with metastatic prostate cancer. Eur J Nucl Med 1994; 21(10):1114–1120.

28. Li S, Liu J, Zhang H, et al. Rhenium-188 HEDP to treat painful bone metastases. Clin Nucl Med 2001; 26(11): 919–922.

29. Liepe K, Franke WG, Kropp J, et al. [Comparison of rhenium-188, rhenium-186-HEDP and strontium-89 in palliation of painful bone metastases]. Nuklearmedizin 2000; 39(6):146–151.

30. Liepe K, Hliscs R, Kropp J, et al. Rhenium-188-HEDP in the palliative treatment of bone metastases. Cancer Biother Radiopharm 2000; 15(3):261–265.

31. Maxon HR III, Schroder LE, Thomas SR, et al. Re-186(Sn) HEDP for treatment of painful osseous metastases: initial clinical experience in 20 patients with hormone-resistant prostate cancer. Radiology 1990; 176(1):155–159.

32. Nilsson S, Franzén L, Parker C, et al. Bone-targeted radium-223 in symptomatic, hormone-refractory prostate cancer: a randomised, multicentre, placebo-controlled phase II study. Lancet Oncol 2007; 8(7):587–594.

33. Dickie GJ, Macfarlane D. Strontium and samarium therapy for bone metastases from prostate carcinoma. Australas Radiol 1999; 43(4):476–479.

34. Nilsson S, Larsen RH, Fossa SD, et al. First clinical experience with alpha-emitting radium-223 in the treatment of skeletal metastases. Clin Cancer Res 2005; 11(12): 4451–4459.

35. Buchali K, Correns HJ, Schuerer M, et al. Results of a double blind study of 89-strontium therapy of skeletal metastases of prostatic carcinoma. Eur J Nucl Med 1988; 14(7–8):349–351.

36. Palmedo H, Manka-Waluch A, Albers P, et al. Repeated bone-targeted therapy for hormone-refractory prostate carcinoma: tandomized phase II trial with the new, high-energy radiopharmaceutical rhenium-188 hydroxy ethylidene diphosphonate. J Clin Oncol 2003; 21 (15):2869–2875.

37. Sciuto R, Festa A, Rea S, et al. Effects of low-dose cisplatin on 89Sr therapy for painful bone metastases from prostate cancer: a randomized clinical trial. J Nucl Med 2002; 43(1):79–86.

38. Tu SM, Millikan RE, Mengistu B, et al. Bone-targeted therapy for advanced androgen-independent carcinoma of the prostate: a randomised phase II trial. Lancet 2001; 357 (9253):336–341.

39. Cremonesi M, Ferrari M, Grana CM, et al. High-dose radioimmunotherapy with 90Y-ibritumomab tiuxetan: comparative dosimetric study for tailored treatment. J Nucl Med 2007; 48(11):1871–1879.

40. Witzig TE, Gordon LI, Cabanillas F, et al. Randomized controlled trial of yttrium-90-labeled ibritumomab tiuxetan radioimmunotherapy versus rituximab immunotherapy for patients with relapsed or refractory low-grade, follicular, or transformed B-cell non-Hodgkin's lymphoma. J Clin Oncol 2002; 20(10):2453–2463.

41. Davies AJ, Rohatiner AZ, Howell S, et al. Tositumomab and iodine I 131 tositumomab for recurrent indolent and transformed B-cell non-Hodgkin's lymphoma. J Clin Oncol 2004; 22(8):1469–1479.

42. Fisher RI, Kaminski MS, Wahl RL, et al. Tositumomab and iodine-131 tositumomab produces durable complete remissions in a subset of heavily pretreated patients with low-grade and transformed non-Hodgkin's lymphomas. J Clin Oncol 2005; 23(30):7565–7573.

43. Gopal AK, Rajendran JG, Gooley TA, et al. High-dose [131I]tositumomab (anti-CD20) radioimmunotherapy and autologous hematopoietic stem-cell transplantation for adults > or = 60 years old with relapsed or refractory B-cell lymphoma. J Clin Oncol 2007; 25(11):1396–1402.

44. Kaminski MS, Zelenetz AD, Press OW, et al. Pivotal study of iodine I 131 tositumomab for chemotherapy-refractory low-grade or transformed low-grade B-cell non-Hodgkin's lymphomas. J Clin Oncol 2001; 19(19):3918–3928.

45. Kaminski MS, Tuck M, Estes J, et al. 131I-tositumomab therapy as initial treatment for follicular lymphoma. N Engl J Med 2005; 352(5):441–449.

46. Press OW, Unger JM, Braziel RM, et al. A phase 2 trial of CHOP chemotherapy followed by tositumomab/iodine I 131 tositumomab for previously untreated follicular non-Hodgkin lymphoma: Southwest Oncology Group Protocol S9911. Blood 2003; 102(5):1606–1612.

47. Connors JM. Radioimmunotherapy—hot new treatment for lymphoma. N Engl J Med 2005; 352(5):496–498.

48. Koral KF, Francis IR, Kroll S, et al. Volume reduction versus radiation dose for tumors in previously untreated lymphoma patients who received iodine-131 tositumomab therapy. Conjugate views compared with a hybrid method. Cancer 2002; 94(4 suppl):1258–1263.

49. Jacene HA, Filice R, Kasecamp W, et al. Comparison of 90Y-ibritumomab tiuxetan and 131I-tositumomab in clinical practice. J Nucl Med 2007; 48(11):1767–1776.

50. Jurcic JG, Caron PC, Nikula TK, et al. Radiolabeled anti-CD33 monoclonal antibody M195 for myeloid leukemias. Cancer Res 1995; 55(23 suppl):5908s–5910s.

51. Burke JM, Caron PC, Papadopoulos EB, et al. Cytoreduction with iodine-131-anti-CD33 antibodies before bone marrow transplantation for advanced myeloid leukemias. Bone Marrow Transplant 2003; 32(6):549–556.

52. Jurcic JG, Larson SM, Sgouros G, et al. Targeted alpha particle immunotherapy for myeloid leukemia. Blood 2002; 100(4):1233–1239.

53. Vallabhajosula S, Goldsmith SJ, Kostakoglu L, et al. Radioimmunotherapy of prostate cancer using 90Y- and 177Lu-labeled J591 monoclonal antibodies: effect of multiple treatments on myelotoxicity. Clin Cancer Res 2005; 11(19 pt 2):7195s–7200s.

54. Bander NH, Milowsky MI, Nanus DM, et al. Phase I trial of 177lutetium-labeled J591, a monoclonal antibody to prostate-specific membrane antigen, in patients with androgen-independent prostate cancer. J Clin Oncol 2005; 23(21): 4591–4601.

55. Chong G, Lee FT, Hopkins W, et al. Phase I trial of 131I-huA33 in patients with advanced colorectal carcinoma. Clin Cancer Res 2005; 11(13):4818–4826.

56. Welt S, Scott AM, Divgi CR, et al. Phase I/II study of iodine 125-labeled monoclonal antibody A33 in patients with advanced colon cancer. J Clin Oncol 1996; 14(6): 1787–1797.

57. Welt S, Divgi CR, Kemeny N, et al. Phase I/II study of iodine 131-labeled monoclonal antibody A33 in patients with advanced colon cancer. J Clin Oncol 1994; 12(8): 1561–1571.

58. Barendswaard EC, O'Donoghue JA, Larson SM, et al. 131I radioimmunotherapy and fractionated external beam radiotherapy: comparative effectiveness in a human tumor xenograft. J Nucl Med 1999; 40(10):1764–1768.

59. Tschmelitsch J, Barendswaard E, Williams C Jr., et al. Enhanced antitumor activity of combination radioimmunotherapy (131I-labeled monoclonal antibody A33) with chemotherapy (fluorouracil). Cancer Res 1997; 57(11): 2181–2186.

60. Howard JP, Maris JM, Kersun LS, et al. Tumor response and toxicity with multiple infusions of high dose 131I-MIBG for refractory neuroblastoma. Pediatr Blood Cancer 2005; 44(3):232–239.

61. Matthay KK, Yanik G, Messina J, et al. Phase II study on the effect of disease sites, age, and prior therapy on response to iodine-131-metaiodobenzylguanidine therapy in refractory neuroblastoma. J Clin Oncol 2007; 25(9): 1054–1060.

62. Rose B, Matthay KK, Price D, et al. High-dose 131I-metaiodobenzylguanidine therapy for 12 patients with malignant pheochromocytoma. Cancer 2003; 98(2): 239–248.

63. Safford SD, Coleman RE, Gockerman JP, et al. Iodine-131 metaiodobenzylguanidine is an effective treatment for malignant pheochromocytoma and paraganglioma. Surgery 2003; 134(6):956–962; discussion 962–953.

64. Takahashi H, Manabe A, Aoyama C, et al. Iodine-131-metaiodobenzylguanidine therapy with reduced-intensity allogeneic stem cell transplantation in recurrent neuroblastoma. Pediatr Blood Cancer 2008; 50(3):676–678.

65. Sisson JC, Shapiro B, Beierwaltes WH, et al. Radiopharmaceutical treatment of malignant pheochromocytoma. J Nucl Med 1984; 25(2):197–206.

66. Sisson J, Shapiro B, Beierwaltes WH, et al. Treatment of malignant pheochromocytoma with a new radiopharmaceutical. Trans Assoc Am Physicians 1983; 96:209–217.

67. Sisson JC, Frager MS, Valk TW, et al. Scintigraphic localization of pheochromocytoma. N Engl J Med 1981; 305(1):12–17.

68. Wieland DM, Brown LE, Tobes MC, et al. Imaging the primate adrenal medulla with [123I] and [131I] metaiodobenzylguanidine: concise communication. J Nucl Med 1981; 22(4):358–364.

69. Wieland DM, Wu J, Brown LE, et al. Radiolabeled adrenergi neuron-blocking agents: adrenomedullary imaging with [131I]iodobenzylguanidine. J Nucl Med 1980; 21(4):349–353.

70. Mangner TJ, Tobes MC, Wieland DW, et al. Metabolism of iodine-131 metaiodobenzylguanidine in patients with metastatic pheochromocytoma. J Nucl Med 1986; 27(1):37–44.

71. Basu S, Nair N. Stable disease and improved health-related quality of life (HRQoL) following fractionated low dose 131I-metaiodobenzylguanidine (MIBG) therapy in metastatic paediatric paraganglioma: observation on false "reverse" discordance during pre-therapy work up and its implication for patient selection for high dose targeted therapy. Br J Radiol 2006; 79(944):e53–e58.

72. Matthay KK, Tan JC, Villablanca JG, et al. Phase I dose escalation of iodine-131-metaiodobenzylguanidine with myeloablative chemotherapy and autologous stem-cell transplantation in refractory neuroblastoma: a new approaches to Neuroblastoma Therapy Consortium Study. J Clin Oncol 2006; 24(3):500–506.

73. Vaidyanathan G, Affleck DJ, Alston KL, et al. A kit method for the high level synthesis of [211At]MABG. Bioorg Med Chem 2007; 15(10):3430–3436.

74. Nguyen C, Faraggi M, Giraudet AL, et al. Long-term efficacy of radionuclide therapy in patients with disseminated neuroendocrine tumors uncontrolled by conventional therapy. J Nucl Med 2004; 45(10):1660–1668.

75. Sywak MS, Pasieka JL, McEwan A, et al. 131I-metaiodobenzylguanidine in the management of metastatic midgut carcinoid tumors. World J Surg 2004; 28(11): 1157–1162.

76. Valkema R, De Jong M, Bakker WH, et al. Phase I study of peptide receptor radionuclide therapy with [In-DTPA]-octreotide: the Rotterdam experience. Semin Nucl Med 2002; 32(2):110–122.

77. Anthony LB, Woltering EA, Espenan GD, et al. Indium-111-pentetreotide prolongs survival in gastroenteropancreatic malignancies. Semin Nucl Med 2002; 32(2):123–132.

78. Bodei L, Cremonesi M, Zoboli S, et al. Receptor-mediated radionuclide therapy with 90Y-DOTATOC in association with amino acid infusion: a phase I study. Eur J Nucl Med Mol Imaging 2003; 30(2):207–216.

79. Barone R, Pauwels S, De Camps J, et al. Metabolic effects of amino acid solutions infused for renal protection during therapy with radiolabelled somatostatin analogues. Nephrol Dial Transplant 2004; 19(9):2275–2281.

80. Waldherr C, Pless M, Maecke HR, et al. Tumor response and clinical benefit in neuroendocrine tumors after 7.4 GBq (90)Y-DOTATOC. J Nucl Med 2002; 43(5):610–616.

81. Valkema R, Pauwels S, Kvols LK, et al. Survival and response after peptide receptor radionuclide therapy with [90Y-DOTA0, Tyr3]octreotide in patients with advanced gastroenteropancreatic neuroendocrine tumors. Semin Nucl Med 2006; 36(2):147–156.

82. Esser JP, Krenning EP, Teunissen JJ, et al. Comparison of [(177)Lu-DOTA(0),Tyr(3)]octreotate and [(177)Lu-DOTA(0), Tyr(3)]octreotide: which peptide is preferable for PRRT? Eur J Nucl Med Mol Imaging 2006; 33(11):1346–1351.

83. van Essen M, Krenning EP, Kooij PP, et al. Effects of therapy with [177Lu-DOTA0, Tyr3]octreotate in patients with paraganglioma, meningioma, small cell lung carcinoma, and melanoma. J Nucl Med 2006; 47(10): 1599–1606.

84. Kwekkeboom DJ, Teunissen JJ, Bakker WH, et al. Radiolabeled somatostatin analog [177Lu-DOTA0,Tyr3]octreotate in patients with endocrine gastroenteropancreatic tumors. J Clin Oncol 2005; 23(12):2754–2762.

85. Teunissen JJ, Kwekkeboom DJ, Krenning EP. Quality of life in patients with gastroenteropancreatic tumors treated with [177Lu-DOTA0,Tyr3]octreotate. J Clin Oncol 2004; 22(13):2724–2729.

86. Gruaz-Guyon A, Janevik-Ivanovska E, Raguin O, et al. Radiolabeled bivalent haptens for tumor immunodetection and radioimmunotherapy. Q J Nucl Med 2001; 45(2): 201–206.

87. Dorvillius M, Garambois V, Pourquier D, et al. Targeting of human breast cancer by a bispecific antibody directed against two tumour-associated antigens: ErbB-2 and carcinoembryonic antigen. Tumour Biol 2002; 23(6):337–347.

88. Kraeber-Bodere F, Rousseau C, Bodet-Milin C, et al. Targeting, toxicity, and efficacy of 2-step, pretargeted radioimmunotherapy using a chimeric bispecific antibody and 131I-labeled bivalent hapten in a phase I optimization clinical trial. J Nucl Med 2006; 47(2):247–255.

89. Sharkey RM, Hajjar G, Yeldell D, et al. A phase I trial combining high-dose 90Y-labeled humanized anti-CEA monoclonal antibody with doxorubicin and peripheral blood stem cell rescue in advanced medullary thyroid cancer. J Nucl Med 2005; 46(4):620–633.

90. McBride WJ, Zanzonico P, Sharkey RM, et al. Bispecific antibody pretargeting PET (immunoPET) with an 124I-labeled hapten-peptide. J Nucl Med 2006; 47(10): 1678–1688.

37

Radioimmunodetection of Cancer: The Next Dimension

DAVID M. GOLDENBERG and ROBERT M. SHARKEY

Garden State Cancer Center, Center for Molecular Medicine and Immunology, Belleville, New Jersey, U.S.A.

INTRODUCTION

In order to respond to the question of the future of a technology, it is necessary to first determine the status of the technology and its clinical viability. If not currently successful, certain assumptions regarding improvements that are acceptable by the potential users will need to be made and tested. In the case of cancer radioimmunodetection (RAID), a term coined in 1980 to describe the use of radiolabeled antibodies for targeting and imaging of specific antigens present on abnormal tissues, such as cancers (1), more than a quarter of a century of efforts have been expended, several RAID products have achieved regulatory approval (2), and almost all have now been abandoned. In this chapter, we will attempt to convey our view as to why antibody imaging failed to fulfill its promise and why we also remain convinced that there will be a resurgence of interest and use, including new agents entering clinical practice.

The fundamental reason why RAID did not survive beyond about 10 years for most products lies in the images not providing what the clinicians required in terms of information about the disease being studied. Two principal gamma-emitting radionuclides were used, ^{99m}Tc and ^{111}In, for planar and single-photon emission computed tomography (SPECT). Although initial imaging studies were performed with purified polyclonal IgG and labeled with ^{131}I (3), murine monoclonal antibodies (mAbs) were adopted quickly and used as either intact IgG or IgG-Fab' fragments. The target antigens were surface markers on the cancer cells, mostly quantitatively increased as compared with normal tissues and sometimes not accessible by antibody targeting to normal tissues, and mostly glycoproteins integral to the cell membrane or elaborated on and within the cell. Even when elaborated into the circulation, such as for carcinoembryonic antigen (CEA) and other markers, binding to the injected antibody did not prevent tumor localization and imaging, apparently because the antibody was in excess or the binding avidity to circulating antigen was different from that to sessile tumor antigen (4,5). Although most were pancarcinoma antigens, the approved indications were for small cell lung, colorectal, ovarian, and prostatic cancers (2). Except for the prostate cancer–imaging agent, capromab pendetide, all have been removed from the market, being replaced by ^{18}F-fluorodeoxyglucose positron emission tomography (FDG-PET) imaging. FDG is a metabolic marker for cell proliferation, and therefore provided a means for distinguishing many cancerous lesions from the normal tissues where they were embedded. This sugar analogue is also retained after being taken up by the more metabolically active cells, which includes a number of normal tissues, most notably the brain, heart wall, and bone marrow (6). In contrast to the antibody imaging agents, FDG-PET provided a clearer image distinguishable over background, but importantly too, the registration process for approved clinical use partly circumvented the usual FDA process of proving efficacy by management change, which was required for the RAID products. Since FDG-PET is not reliable in the area of the prostate, the prostatic cancer–imaging agent has been sustained, but only with modest use. The use of 18-fluorine also ushered in the age of PET imaging, a technology within an innate enhanced sensitivity as compared with gamma-imaging systems.

The fact that FDG-PET provided a clear, unequivocal image is perhaps more important than how specific this is, because FDG-PET is certainly not specific for cancer. Yet in a patient with already diagnosed cancer, it can be very useful for staging and prognostication when combined with computed tomography (6–15). This invites the question of whether a PET radionuclide conjugated to the same antibodies and antibody fragments labeled previously with a gamma-emitting radionuclide would be more successful? Actually, some initial clinical results support this view, providing the specificity of a tumor-targeting antibody (16,17). However, it is not known yet what resolution can be achieved based on the relatively low targeting ratios of these antibodies as compared to background tissues, because these relatively large molecules distribute through most major organs via the blood until they clear, and only then can evidence of selective tumor accretion be seen. For the slow-clearing IgG, a positron-emitting radionuclide with a long physical half-life, such as ^{124}I, would need to be used (17). Smaller antibody fragments or modified constructs that clear more quickly from the blood could be adapted for use with shorter-lived radionuclides. Attempts to prepare ^{18}F-labeled antibody fragments for practical clinical use have largely failed because of poor labeling yields and inadequate uptake and contrast ratios within the one- to two-hour imaging window based on the short physical half-life of ^{18}F (18). However, there are a number of preclinical studies using ^{124}I and ^{64}Cu and early clinical studies with ^{124}I suggesting that directly labeled antibody constructs might provide the necessary favorable properties required for a successful imaging agent (17,19–31).

The prospects and problems of RAID are perhaps predicted by the experience with radiolabeled antibody therapy, or radioimmunotherapy (RIT or RAIT). Two RAIT products have been approved in the United States, tositumomab and ibritumomab tiuxetan, both for therapy of indolent and transformed non-Hodgkin lymphoma (NHL) (32). From the targeting and pretreatment imaging perspectives, they selectively image CD20-expressing lymphomas, with either ^{131}I or ^{111}In, and also show tumor regression even when low radiation doses are delivered with ^{131}I or ^{90}Y, respectively. But since FDG-PET has become accepted for diagnosing, staging, and prognosticating NHL lesions, especially after any therapy (33), a CD20 imaging agent has not been pursued. Early studies with a CD22 imaging antibody in NHL also showed promise (34–37), but lost favor when FDG-PET was introduced. With the increased interest in anticancer antibodies for solid tumor therapy, after the successful introduction of cetuximab and bevacizumab, it would seem that more specific antibody-based imaging methods for defining which tumors express the target antigens of such therapeutic antibodies would be of interest for qualifying patients.

The commercial RAID agents approved in the 1990s were all murine mAbs or their fragments. The intact IgG agents, such as satumomab pendetide (previously commercially marketed as "Oncoscint"), evoked anti-mouse antibodies (HAMA) that could affect future use of these mAbs because of altered pharmacokinetics as well as the risk of hypersensitivity reactions (38). Virtually all therapeutic antibodies are now either chimeric, humanized (CDR grafted), or fully human constructs, thus alleviating this problem (2,39). Therefore, future RAID agents will likely be quite different in their immunological makeup.

Another major issue is how to relate antibody imaging to clinical practice. In the case of FDG-PET, it was introduced by congressional legislation, review of retrospective and prospective clinical literature, and not the traditional regulatory process through the FDA. The reimbursement by government and insurance agencies came with increasing demonstrations of clinical utility in studies comparing and combining this functional test with anatomic-based imaging methods, such as computed tomography. RAID studies first started with an understanding with the FDA that if the test can correctly image cancer (as defined by other methods including histopathology), then it is a valid imaging method. Later, as agents progressed through clinical trials, the FDA determined that registration of such imaging agents required evidence of an impact on patient management. In the case of arcitumomab, which localized CEA-expressing cancers (marketed previously as CEA-Scan), it was required that it showed an improvement over CT, and the clinical trials were based on RAID being more sensitive than CT alone for determining the number of colorectal cancer metastases in the liver, which would qualify a patient for salvage surgical resection (40,41). Similar evidence of potential management change based on prospective trials was required also for the other antibody-based agents that won FDA approval. As mentioned, this bar was not the same for FDG-PET, whose role in affecting management was elucidated, in specific indications, after introduction in clinical practice, and continues even now in various disease settings. Given this experience, we wonder whether this can influence FDA requirements for the approval of future imaging agents. Clearly, if CT or ultrasound had to be proven in prospective trials that they could change clinical management, as contrasted to disclosing a pathological lesion, the practice of medicine would have been impeded significantly. But it appears that an instrument and a pharmaceutical are conceptually different from a regulatory perspective in terms of diagnostic impact. It also appears that the "bar" for new diagnostic agents to cross to achieve approval continues to rise, making it increasingly challenging to secure approval for new innovative diagnostic imaging agents.

FIRST RADIOLABELED ANTIBODIES

This section is intended only to review briefly the few RAID products approved in the United States, both from a historical perspective, as well as to emphasize that these need to be considered in their temporal setting. One product was approved for non–small cell lung cancer, two for colorectal cancer, of which one was also labeled for use in ovarian cancer and another for prostatic cancer imaging.

The first monoclonal antibody imaging agent to receive the FDA approval (1992) was satumomab pendetide (OncoScint) for imaging of colorectal cancer metastases and then later also for detection of ovarian cancer metastases (42–49). This is an intact IgG murine mAb against TAG-72 glycoprotein that is elaborated by a number of carcinomas and labeled with ^{111}In. Because IgG clears slowly from the blood, images were delayed several days to secure optimal tumor-background uptake ratios. More important to the diagnostic utility of this agent was the fact that because IgG is catabolized by the liver and because ^{111}In is retained inside the cells, the normal liver contained a higher level of ^{111}In activity than tumor, which meant that liver metastases would usually appear as negative lesions against a hot liver background. In 1996, arcitumomab (CEA-Scan) was also approved for use in conjunction with CT to identify colorectal cancer metastases. This agent was an IgG-Fab' against CEA (CEACAM5), which is expressed by a majority of carcinomas, and labeled with ^{99m}Tc. Since an IgG-Fab' clears more rapidly from the blood than an IgG, visualization was possible within a few hours, with 24-hour imaging feasible for verification. It clears from the body primarily through renal/urinary clearance, and thus liver metastases could be seen as hot lesions (except if they are very large, interfering with mAb penetration) (40). However, increased uptake by the kidneys and in the urine excreted into the bladder often required SPECT to disclose lesions in these regions. An intact IgG mAb against prostate-specific membrane antigen, labeled with ^{111}In, was approved in 1996 for imaging prostatic carcinoma patients suspected of having lymph node metastases presurgically and also in those suspected in having a postsurgical recurrence (50–57). In this case, the IgG form is preferred because there is less activity in the urinary bladder, an anatomic region of interest for prostate cancer. This product, capromab pendetide

(ProstaScint), is still in commercial use in the United States. In 1997, the FDA also approved a ^{99m}Tc-labeled anti-EGP1 (epithelial glycoprotein-1) mAb Fab' (nofetumomab or Verluma) for staging of small cell lung cancer (58). Except for the prostate cancer-imaging agent, the others have been removed from the market.

It should be noted that at the time these first RAID agents were studied and approved, older single-head gamma cameras were used, dual isotope blood-pool imaging with fusion was not practiced, and image fusion with CT or MRI was not yet available. Consequently, the imaging characteristics of these early products were probably underestimated compared with current nuclear medicine capabilities with more advanced imaging techniques. For example, many of these methods have been applied to prostatic cancer imaging with capromab pendetide, and since FDG-PET is not very reliable in this anatomic site, this RAID product still has some clinical use, albeit not as extensive as would be expected from the indications approved.

Would these agents, with advanced imaging equipment, more nuclear medicine experience reading such scans, and with fusion imaging with CT and MRI, be more accepted in clinical practice today? Perhaps with the use of PET radionuclides, they would have improved photon resolution and contrast in addition to the specificity of the antibodies for particular cancer markers, and would certainly permit the use of hybrid imaging systems involving PET and CT, as practiced with FDG-PET/CT. For example, the anti-carbonic-anhydrase-IX chimeric mAb, G250, was labeled with ^{124}I, permitting PET imaging, and showed positive presurgical imaging of 15 of 16 clear cell renal carcinomas (19).

It would be interesting to return to some of the other antibodies and antibody fragments with PET labels to assess how imaging, particularly when combined with CT fusion, would perform. In many academic centers, SPECT/CT fusion imaging is now available and is the preferred method for monoclonal antibody imaging, although this method was not widely available at the time these agents were in first use. However, even more interesting targeting constructs and modifications that enhance the ratios of antibody accretion in target tumors compared to background tissues, combined with PET, have stimulated a new interest in RAID, even using many of the standard tumor markers of the past and those of more recent interest.

CURRENT ADVANCES
Diverse Antibody Constructs

Once antibodies transverse the blood vessels into the tissue space, they generally bind with high affinity/avidity, which in turn determines their residence time in the tumor.

The vast majority of the injected antibody remains unbound and is processed by various organs in the body and eventually degraded. Slow blood clearance of IgG means it takes one or more days before a sufficient amount exits the circulation and concentrates in the tumor to produce a suitable signal to be distinguished from blood and adjacent tissue radioactivity. The slow clearance is in part due to the large size of IgG, ~ 150 kDa, which impedes its extravasation. Because a tumor's vasculature is leakier than most normal tissues (59) and its concentration in the blood remains high for a long period, the IgG is able to achieve the highest absolute concentration in tumors of all forms of antibodies. In mouse xenograft models, tumor uptake of a tumor targeting monoclonal antibody is typically between 10% to 30% of the injected activity per gram of tumor, but in humans, with a larger vascular and extravascular volume of distribution, this accretion is reduced to <0.1% per gram (60,61). As the molecular size of an antibody is reduced from a divalent F(ab')$_2$ fragment (~ 100 kDa) to the monovalent binding Fab' fragment (~ 50 kDa), there is a progressively faster clearance from the blood. Higher tumor-blood ratios are achieved with the smaller antibody forms and usually also a more rapid and uniform penetration within the tumor (62,63), but all these come at the cost of having proportionally less of the injected product reaching the tumor and with a commensurately shorter residence time. Smaller antibody structures, such as single-chain Fv (scFv, ~ 25 kDa), have been prepared using molecular engineering, and these clear even more rapidly from the blood with proportionally less uptake in tumors (64). However, the rapid clearance of these molecules from the blood and adjacent antigen-negative tissues can result in early high tumor-to-background ratios, achieving relatively strong signals compared to background (65,66). In addition, the faster renal clearance can result in renal accumulation of the antibody fragments with a relatively high renal radiation dose, which can limit the injected dose of radioactivity.

Although the monovalent fragments and constructs have favorable clearance properties, they lack the avidity of multivalent molecules. Innovative strategies have been undertaken to restore the multivalency of an antibody to enhance tumor retention, while also engineering the molecule for rapid clearance. For example, deleting the C_H2 sequence of an IgG results in a divalent construct of ~ 100 kDa that clears extraordinarily fast from the blood, resulting in high localization ratios within a short period (67). A number of new constructs, ranging from divalent diabodies, minibodies, (scFv)$_2$-Fc, and other assorted constructs, are essentially composed of multiple scFvs tethered in different ways, as illustrated in Figure 1 (64,68–70). An entirely different type of antibody, an affibody, has been described recently that has some promising properties for imaging as well as therapy. An affibody is not based on immunoglobulin structures, but instead is a novel scaffold protein prepared from a mutated variant of the B-domain of the *Staphylococcus aureus* protein A, known as the Z-domain. This 6.5-kDa molecule has been the basis for preparing targeting agents to HER2/*neu* labeled with ^{99m}Tc, ^{111}In, and even ^{177}Lu for therapy (71–75). Tolmachev et al. (72) have also described an affibody-albumin-binding domain fusion protein that allows the affibody to bind to a patient's own albumin on injection, which in turn favorably alters the pharmacokinetics and distribution properties of the labeled compound for improved imaging and therapy.

Pretargeting as a New Paradigm

Even with the great strides being made in reengineering antibodies and other targeting proteins, ultimately all directly radiolabeled products will be susceptible to problems associated with the retention of these compounds in unintended tissues. As mentioned, only a small portion of the total injected product localizes in the target, leaving the vast majority of the radioactivity to be either captured by some tissue in the body or eliminated. IgG is catabolized in the liver and antibody fragments <60 kDa in the kidney, resulting in elevated uptake within these tissues with the directly radiolabeled product. As in the example of capromab pendetide, where the IgG form is used with an agent intended to examine the pelvic region, and with arcitumomab that clears through the kidneys, yet is effective in disclosing hepatic lesions, an antibody-imaging agent can be effectively applied for a given region of the body while being more limited in other regions. The regional limitations imposed by these two agents are due primarily to the use of a radionuclide based on elements that are retained inside the cells after antibody catabolism. There are examples where improvements in chelation chemistry have significantly reduced normal tissue retention, but uptake can still interfere with interpretation. A radioiodinated product can circumvent this problem because its catabolic products are not retained by the cells but are removed by urinary and gastrointestinal excretion; however, thyroid uptake occurs even in patients who are premedicated with a thyroid-blocking agent. While there are forms of radioiodine for SPECT and PET imaging, commercial imaging agents have not been developed with these radionuclides, because their physical properties are not ideally matched to the antibody clearance properties or to the imaging system, as well as cost, availability, and handling issues. Another aspect to consider with directly radiolabeled agents is the possibility that the labeling procedure can alter the binding to the target antigen/receptor.

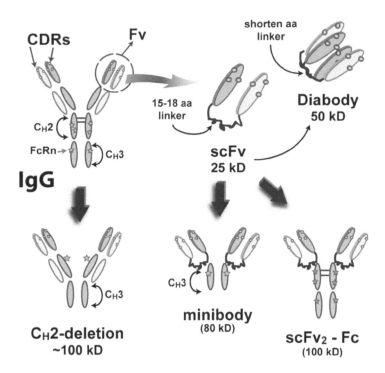

Figure 1 Examples of molecularly reengineered forms of antibody used for targeting radionuclides. Starting with the IgG (*upper left*), the separate portions of the Fv can be isolated and tethered together with an amino acid (aa) linker to form a scFv (single chain) construct. Shortening the length of the aa-linker can lead to the formation of homodimeric structures, such as diabodies, but other forms, such as tribodies and tetrabodies, have also been described. Larger constructs formed from scFv and various portions of the IgG's C_H3 and $C_H2 + C_H3$ have also been used. The scFv$_2$-Fc site specifically mutates FcRn residues in the heavy chain that control the pharmacokinetic behavior of the IgG. Another construct, the C_H2 deletion, also has accelerated clearance from the blood, but preserves divalent antigen binding. *Source*: From Ref. 39.

An ideal targeting compound would be easily adapted for use with a wide range of radionuclides, with the radionuclide tightly attached preferably to a small compound that has very limited and restricted binding to normal tissues, but can escape quickly into the extravascular space where it can interact with the tumor, yet be cleared rapidly from the blood and body. Its composition would have properties that preferentially allow the product to be cleared by urinary excretion, but with minimal renal retention. Most importantly, the compound would need to have appropriate selectivity, being able to bind to the target antigen/receptor. Receptor-binding peptides come close to meeting these criteria, but most often these peptides will have additional specificities for normal tissues, or because their structures must be more rigorously maintained to ensure receptor-binding affinity, their core structure will direct a sizeable portion of product to the liver or kidneys.

An alternative strategy, known as *pretargeting*, was conceived to overcome many of the deficiencies associated with directly radiolabeled antibodies. Pretargeting is a multistep process where the target antigen is first localized with a nonradioactive agent that has dual-binding specificity, one that enables it to bind to the target antigen and a second that allows it to bind to another compound. Three types of secondary binding systems have been examined, including antibody/hapten, streptavidin/biotin, and oligomers/complementary oligomers (76).

Pretargeting was first envisioned with a bispecific antibody (bsMAb) that would have specificity to a target antigen based on an antibody and a secondary ability to bind to a hapten using an anti-hapten antibody. The initial anti-hapten antibodies were prepared against a chelate preloaded with a metal that had a corresponding radiometal, e.g., indium and [111]In (77,78). Chelates are small, well-defined chemical structures that could be binding highly efficiently and tightly to a particular radiometal. Chelates had been used clinically to remove harmful metals from the body (e.g., lead poisoning), but also radiolabeled chelates, such as diethylenetriamine pentaacetic acid (DTPA)-indium, had already been examined clinically, so their favorable clearance and biodistribution properties were known. The pretargeting concept evolved to a procedure where the unlabeled bsMAb would be administered and given time to localize in the tumor and clear from the blood and tissues. The small size of the radiolabeled chelate allowed it to penetrate the tumor rapidly, where it would be bound to the anti-chelate binding arm of the prelocalized bsMAb, with the remaining product being cleared by the urinary system. For pretargeting to function optimally, the bsMAb needs to remain accessible within the tumor, but be removed from the blood and processed by the tissues. Clearing steps using an anti-antibody or other agent have been used to expedite the removal of excess bsMAb from the blood before the radiolabeled chelate is given.

Early clinical work based on this principle was promising and subsequently several other pretargeting methods were developed and applied, particularly involving biotin-

avidin (or streptavidin) binding, with encouraging results shown in certain situations (76). Two distinct methods for pretargeting with the avidin/streptavidin-biotin method have evolved (Fig. 2). Both use biotin as the radiolabeled carrier and both include a step to remove excess antibody conjugate from the blood, so that radiolabeled biotin can be administered one to two days after the conjugate's injection. Indeed, the ultrahigh affinity of streptavidin for biotin would require the concentration of an avidin-based conjugate to be reduced to very low levels in the blood before the radiolabeled agent could be given, and therefore this step is very important for those methods. In

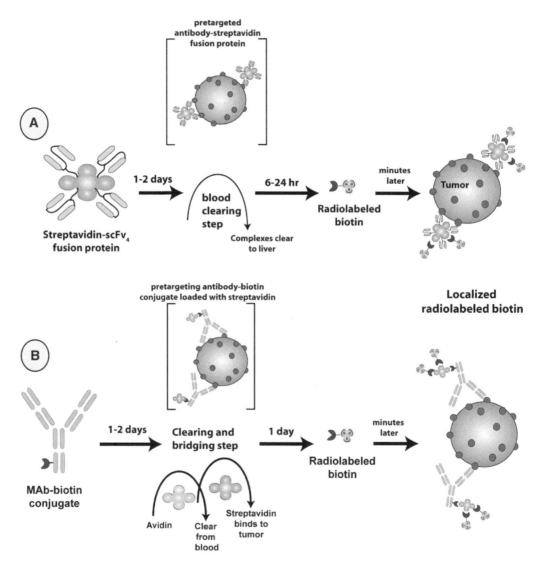

Figure 2 Schematic representation of two pretargeting methods based on streptavidin biotin. (**A**) "Two-step" approach uses a streptavidin-IgG conjugate (∼210 kDa) or more recently a scFv-streptavidin fusion protein (∼175 kDa) to pretarget the tumor. After one to two days, the conjugate is removed from the blood with a clearing agent, and then 6 to 24 hours later, radiolabeled biotin is given that will then very quickly bind to the available streptavidin. (**B**) "Three-step" approach pretargets a biotin-conjugated IgG and clears this product from the blood using avidin, which due to its glycosylation, is quickly removed in the liver. Streptavidin is then administered the same day, and this will localize to the prelocalized biotin conjugate establishing a bridge that will then bind to the subsequently administered radiolabeled biotin.

contrast, the binding affinity of the anti-hapten portion of the bsMAb is several logs lower, and therefore bsMAb pretargeting approaches have been used without relying on a clearing step. In avidin-biotin methods, radiolabeled biotin is strongly bound to streptavidin localized at the tumor site. bsMAb pretargeting relies on a radiolabeled effector that bears two haptens capable of binding to the anti-hapten binding arm of the bsMAb, thereby enhancing the binding avidity. This technique, called the affinity enhancement system (AES), improves the uptake and retention of the radiolabeled hapten-peptide (Fig. 3) (79–81). Although there is an affinity advantage for binding biotin to streptavidin in the tumor compared with the divalent hapten (i.e., 10^{-15} M vs. 10^{-9} M, respectively), ultimately these complexes are both held in the tumor by the association of the antitumor antibody to its antigen.

Since streptavidin has four binding sites for biotin, conceivably the pretargeted complex could bind more than one radiolabeled biotin. The major advantage for a bsMAb approach is the ability to use humanized antibodies that will have a lower immunogenicity than the foreign streptavidin or avidin proteins. Regardless of the pretargeting method used, each has been shown in animal models and in patients to be highly efficient targeting procedures, with improved imaging/therapeutic properties as a result of the enhanced tumor-blood ratios (76,82,83).

Except for some of the early studies performed when the technology was first being developed, pretargeting techniques have focused primarily on therapeutic applications. All of these studies were performed in relatively small numbers of patients and were intended primarily to illustrate the feasibility of this technique. For example, the

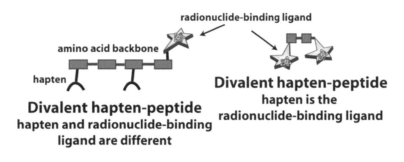

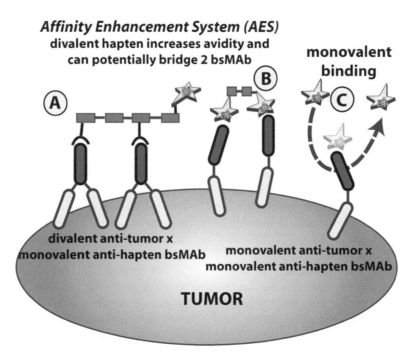

Figure 3 Modifications to the hapten-binding ligand used in bsMAb pretargeting for improved tumor uptake and retention. Initially, bsMAb were formed chemically by linking a Fab' of an antitumor antibody to the Fab' of an antibody binding to a chelate (i.e., hapten) (**C**). After pretargeting the bsMAb to the tumor, the radiolabeled chelate could bind, but this monovalent binding was not very stable. Linking two chelates together to make a divalent hapten improved uptake and retention by a process known as the AES (**B**). Additional improvements were made by separating the hapten-binding from the radionuclide-binding component, while maintaining the principles of AES (**A**). *Abbreviation*: AES, affinity enhancement system. *Source*: From Ref. 39.

first clinical testing of a bsMAb pretargeting method for cancer imaging reported successful localization of colon cancer metastases in the liver using an ^{111}In-chelate complex given five days after the administration of an unlabeled anti-CEA × anti-chelate bsMAb (84). This was a considerable advance at the time, since excessive amounts of ^{111}In in the liver frequently masked tumor targeting when using an ^{111}In-labeled antibody to colorectal cancer (85–88). Additional studies were reported using an anti-CEA × anti-DTPA(In) bsMAb pretargeting system paired with a divalent hapten that could be radiolabeled with either ^{111}In or ^{131}I (89–91). However, once ^{99m}Tc-Fab'-based imaging agents became available that allowed tumor visualization within a few hours, with minimal uptake in the liver, investigators turned to the simplicity of a single-step, direct targeting method, which was subsequently replaced by ^{18}F-FDG; however, recent results with pretargeted PET imaging agents suggest that this technique could set a new standard for molecular imaging. A number of advances have facilitated the potential for commercial development of the bsMAb pretargeting approach (92).

All of the early pretargeting antibody constructs were prepared chemically, but today, molecular engineering has facilitated the ability to produce streptavidin-scFv construct and a variety of bsMAb constructs more efficiently and reproducibly. At least for imaging applications, where multiple imaging sessions might be of interest, a bsMAb-based pretargeting system would have an advantage over the streptavidin-based systems primarily because of their reduced immunogenicity. The process of preparing bsMAb is efficiently performed through molecular engineering (92–94). Constructs as small as 50 kDa, with monovalent binding to the tumor target and to the hapten, have exceptionally fast blood clearance properties and perform well in pretargeting (94), but studies have indicated that a bsMAb with divalent binding to the tumor also has favorable pharmacokinetic properties and affords higher uptake and retention in tumors (94,95). More recently, a new, more modular, "dock and lock" (DNL) method for assembling bsMAbs has created highly stable, humanized bsMAb constructs with a molecular weight of ∼157 kDa and which have performed well in a pretargeting setting (92).

The radiolabeled hapten is another critical component of the bsMAb pretargeting system. Initially, the hapten was the radiolabeled chelate that bound to the anti-hapten arm of the bsMAb. To improve uptake and retention, two chelates were joined together (81,96). For example, DTPA was coupled to the epsilon-amino group of lysine that linked to tyrosine whose amino terminal end was joined to another DTPA. By using tyrosine as one of the amino acids, the di-DTPA-peptide could also be radioiodinated. Other di-DTPA-peptides containing ligands for binding ^{99m}Tc/^{188}Re have been prepared (97,98). While DTPA as

a hapten can be adapted for use with several radionuclides (i.e., ^{111}In, ^{131}I, ^{99m}Tc/^{188}Re), this system was not useful for binding other radionuclides of therapeutic interest, such as ^{90}Y or ^{177}Lu, which require a different chelate, such as DOTA (1,4,7,10-tetraazacyclododecane-N, N', N'', N'''-tetraacetic acid), for greater binding stability. Thus, there was a disadvantage for the hapten to also be the radiolabeled ligand, since not all radionuclides are optimally bound by a single ligand. Indeed, even the anti-hapten antibodies developed against a particular metal-loaded chelate might not bind with the same high affinity to the same chelate loaded with a different metal (99).

A more flexible solution is to build a structure where the hapten is used solely for binding to the anti-hapten antibody, allowing then for substitutions to be made with any type of binding ligand. In this regard, studies are now focused on the use of a hapten known as HSG (histamine-succinyl-glycine), showing that hapten-peptides can be prepared with ^{131}I/^{124}I/^{125}I, ^{111}In, ^{90}Y, ^{177}Lu, ^{67}Ga/^{68}Ga, and ^{99m}Tc/^{188}Re (100–102). The amino acid composition of the hapten-peptide can then be modified to provide properties that favor renal excretion over clearance through the hepatic-biliary pathway (102). This could have substantial advantages over directly radiolabeled peptide-based compounds, particularly when structural modifications affect the binding of a peptide to the target receptor. Unlike many radiometal-labeled peptides or small antibody fragments that in animal models have >50% of the injected dose per gram trapped in the kidneys, the hapten-peptides generally have only 2% to 4% of the injected dose bound in the kidneys a few hours after injection, and this level decreases by about 40% each day afterward (103,104). Animal studies (mice and rabbits) have indicated that in a properly optimized setting, 60% of the hapten-peptide activity is cleared into the urinary bladder within one hour, with >99% of the product removed from the whole body within six hours. Depending on the hapten-peptide and radionuclide used, the small amount of activity in the kidneys is the only residual activity remaining in any tissue. Dynamic imaging studies of human tumor-bearing nude mice showed selective uptake occurring in the tumor within 10 minutes of the radiolabeled hapten-peptide injection (105).

The uptake of the radiolabeled hapten-peptide appears to be highly efficient from a number of perspectives. Often, the hapten-peptide can be radiolabeled at higher specific activities than a directly radiolabeled antibody, which directs more radionuclide to the tumor per unit mass of hapten-peptide delivered. Unlike antibody fragments, where their rapid blood clearance results in a net loss of radioactivity in the tumor, the percentage of the injected dose bound to the tumor can equal that found with an IgG when pretargeting is properly adjusted (103,106). In this respect, pretargeting offers the best targeting properties of an IgG, namely high uptake, with the reduced blood and tissue uptake found with an antibody fragment, and normal tissue uptake for pretargeting is reduced even more. This has resulted in tumor-blood ratios that are 40-fold higher than a directly radiolabeled Fab' fragment, with tumor uptake that can be 10-fold higher, thereby providing a much stronger signal (105). When used in conjunction with PET, tumor localization with a pretargeting procedure provides a stronger signal in the tumor and less background in the normal tissues, making the images less ambiguous to read than ^{18}F-FDG (101). Indeed, PET imaging studies have even shown an ability to detect microdisseminated human tumor xenografts in nude mice as small as 0.3 mm in diameter that were not seen with ^{18}F-FDG (107) (Fig. 4).

The only drawback to using a pretargeting system is that the antigen marker being targeted must be accessible (i.e., on the cell surface or in the extracellular space within the target tissue microenvironment), and then the target-localized antibody needs to stay accessible in sufficient concentration to allow time for the untargeted material to clear from the blood. A targeted substance that internalizes quickly likely would not be a good candidate for a pretargeting application, and therefore direct targeting would be preferred. Because some antigens are more actively internalized when cross-linked, a good pretargeting signal potentially could be achieved if a monovalent binding construct were used instead of a divalent one. A divalent hapten-peptide could still be used in this situation, and may even improve the targeting system because its binding might trigger internalization, bringing the imaging or therapeutic payload inside the cell. In addition, with an internalizing target, a clearing step might be used to reduce the interval required between giving the pretargeting construct and the radiolabeled hapten-peptide, or a construct prepared in a manner to accelerate its blood clearance could be used. A 50-kDa bsMAb (i.e., 2 scFv) clears more quickly from the blood than a 100-kDa Fab' × Fab' chemical construct, and when used to pretarget an ^{111}In-hapten-peptide, tumor uptake reached similar levels, but tumor-nontumor ratios were significantly improved because the smaller construct also cleared from the normal tissues more efficiently (94). Pretargeting systems might also be less affected by antigen circulating in the blood. A directly radiolabeled antibody may form complexes with a circulating antigen, which would increase accretion of radioactivity in the liver or spleen. In pretargeting, as long as the unconjugated bsMAb-antigen complexes are effectively removed before the administration of the radiolabeled hapten-peptide, efficient targeting of the tumor occurs without additional localization of the liver or spleen. Problems associated with a large antigen sink in normal tissues (e.g., with anti-CD20 antibodies that would target normal

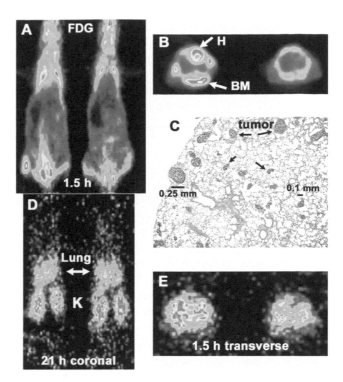

Figure 4 Localization of micrometastatic colon cancer in the lungs of nude mice using microPET. (**A**) Coronal cross-sections of two animals 1.5 hour after being given ^{18}F-FDG. No evidence of tumor involvement could be appreciated in the chest. Strong uptake in the bone marrow of the shoulder, ribs, skull, and pelvis are seen. (**B**) Transverse sections through the chest of these same animals again fail to reveal any evidence of tumor, but the heart wall was clearly seen. (**C**) Cross-section of the lungs taken from one of these animals at necropsy after this imaging session that illustrates multiple, yet very small, tumor nodules in lungs. (**D** and **E**) Representative coronal and transverse sections of animals bearing the same sized tumors in the lung, but had received an anti-CEA bsMAb followed one day later with an ^{124}I-labeled peptide. Strong uptake in the lungs was clearly evident in all imaging sessions from 1.5 to 21 hours after the ^{124}I-peptide injection. Uptake in the kidneys (K) was also seen as a result of the peptide clearing through the kidneys. *Source*: From Ref. 39 (*See Color Insert*).

and malignant B-cells) could be problematic for both directly radiolabeled antibodies and pretargeting systems, but innovative techniques that exploit differences in pharmacokinetics or other properties could further enhance the targeting specificity. Thus, for many targeting situations, a bsMAb pretargeting solution could have an advantage over a directly radiolabeled antibody.

With the DNL modular system for creating humanized bsMAbs and a more universal hapten-peptide binding system in the HSG-based peptides, pretargeting methods based on bsMAbs have advanced to a point where humanized recombinant bsMAb can be easily produced against other tumor antigens or even other disease markers. The technique can be applied for imaging or therapeutic applications with potentially a wide range of different compounds (108). As a multistep process, pretargeting will require minimally two injections separated by one or more days. For oncology applications, where it is often necessary to schedule imaging studies days or weeks in advance, the additional time required for completion of the study would not likely be an issue. The bsMAb infusion could be performed by the patient's oncologist, who would then coordinate this infusion with scheduling the injection of the radiolabeled hapten-peptide in a nuclear imaging facility.

What is the potential role of pretargeting for the molecular imaging of cancer? While pretargeting methods could be considered to be more complicated than a single-agent targeting method, once the optimal conditions are established, the injection sequence is straightforward. Imaging could be performed within a few hours of the radiolabeled hapten's injection. Thus, for a pretargeting procedure, it could require a few days before an image is acquired, while it may be possible with some of the smaller, directly radiolabeled antibody constructs to image in a shorter period. However, in our experience, preclinical data suggest that image quality with pretargeting is so superior to that of a directly radiolabeled antibody fragment that a two-step, delayed imaging procedure is justified (101,104,105).

FUTURE PROSPECTS

Since pretargeting methods are applicable to both imaging and therapy, they can be combined in a paradigm that allows imaging to qualify a patient for this specific targeted therapy and to also monitor disease response. Also, if the therapeutic radionuclide has gamma-imaging properties, such as for ^{131}I and ^{177}Lu, the patient can be monitored in terms of biodistribution and accretion of the radioactivity.

In terms of targets for imaging/therapy, these can be expanded to include virtually any marker or genetic product against which an antibody can be raised. Examples include HER2/*neu* (26,109), fibronectin and other vascular factors (110), P-glycoprotein and other multidrug-resistant proteins (111–114), carbonic anhydrase IX (19), infectious agents (115–118), and oncogene products (119). In the case of ED-fibronectin, a direct comparison of direct versus pretargeting has shown the advantage of the latter (110), so we propose that bsMab pretargeting will be a preferred method of any antibody-based imaging modality and will permit both SPECT and PET imaging combined with RAIT.

CONCLUSIONS

Antibody-based imaging methods have been researched for over 30 years, have resulted in commercial products a little over 10 years ago, and are now regaining interest because of the expanded use of antibody-based immunotherapy as well as the inclusion of PET radionuclides with RAID.

Highly specific and very sensitive images are possible with a bsMAb pretargeting, and both experimental and clinical studies have shown that pretargeting can have encouraging therapeutic effects. Although the studies indicate that PET imaging will likely outperform SPECT-based imaging systems, it is important to note that the strong signal and high tumor-tissue ratios produce excellent image contrast even with conventional gamma scintillation camera, and thus a pretargeting procedure based on a ^{99m}Tc-labeled peptide can be a useful and less expensive alternative to a PET-based system, which is an important consideration in societies that cannot afford multiple PET or PET/CT imaging equipment. There are also other positron-emitting radionuclides with better PET imaging properties, such as ^{64}Cu or ^{68}Ga, which might also improve image quality with pretargeting. Thus, humanized bsMAb pretargeting appears to offer new prospects for improved molecular imaging of cancer.

This also appears to be true for RAIT, where improved specific targeting and higher tumor radiation doses appear to be feasible. In medullary thyroid cancer, initial clinical results with a first-generation pretargeting method have shown evidence of improved survival (120). Therefore, there is a basis for combining pretargeted RAID with RAIT, where only the radionuclide is altered.

ACKNOWLEDGMENTS

We thank Professor J.-F. Chatal and Dr. J. Barbet of Nantes for participating in many studies conducted with our pretargeting agents; Drs. C.-H. Chang, E. Rossi, and W. McBride of Immunomedics and IBC Pharmaceuticals for reagent and technology development; Drs. S.M. Larson and P. Zanzonico of Memorial Sloan-Kettering Cancer Center and Drs. S. Goldsmith and S. Vallabhajosula of Weill Medical College of Cornell University for collaboration in microPET studies; and Dr. H. Karacay for conducting many of the preclinical studies reported herein. This work has been supported in part by NIH grant P01 CA103985, New Jersey Department of Health and Senior Services grant 06-1853-FS-N0, and the New Jersey Department of Treasury grant CDG-06103.

REFERENCES

1. Goldenberg DM. Introduction to the international conference on the clinical uses of carcinoembryonic antigen. Cancer 1978; 42(3 suppl):1397–1398.
2. Sharkey RM, Goldenberg DM. Targeted therapy of cancer: new prospects for antibodies and immunoconjugates. CA Cancer J Clin 2006; 56(4):226–243.

3. Goldenberg DM, DeLand F, Kim E, et al. Use of radio-labeled antibodies to carcinoembryonic antigen for the detection and localization of diverse cancers by external photoscanning. N Engl J Med 1978; 298(25):1384–1386.

4. Primus FJ, Bennett SJ, Kim EE, et al. Circulating immune complexes in cancer patients receiving goat radiolocalizing antibodies to carcinoembryonic antigen. Cancer Res 1980; 40(3):497–501.

5. Primus FJ, Goldenberg DM. Immunological considerations in the use of goat antibodies to carcinoembryonic antigen for the radioimmunodetection of cancer. Cancer Res 1980; 40(8 pt 2):2979–2983.

6. Kelloff GJ, Hoffman JM, Johnson B, et al. Progress and promise of FDG-PET imaging for cancer patient management and oncologic drug development. Clin Cancer Res 2005; 11(8):2785–2808.

7. Sun L, Wu H, Guan YS. Positron emission tomography/computer tomography: challenge to conventional imaging modalities in evaluating primary and metastatic liver malignancies. World J Gastroenterol 2007; 13(20):2775–2783.

8. Freudenberg LS, Rosenbaum SJ, Beyer T, et al. PET versus PET/CT dual-modality imaging in evaluation of lung cancer. Radiol Clin North Am 2007; 45(4):639–644, v.

9. Podoloff DA, Macapinlac HA. PET and PET/CT in management of the lymphomas. Radiol Clin North Am 2007; 45(4):689–696, vii.

10. Jadvar H, Connolly LP, Fahey FH, et al. PET and PET/CT in pediatric oncology. Semin Nucl Med 2007; 37(5):316–331.

11. Maldonado A, Gonzalez-Alenda FJ, Alonso M, et al. PET-CT in clinical oncology. Clin Transl Oncol 2007; 9(8):494–505.

12. Otsuka H, Morita N, Yamashita K, et al. FDG-PET/CT for cancer management. J Med Invest 2007; 54(3–4):195–199.

13. Benamor M, Ollivier L, Brisse H, et al. PET/CT imaging: what radiologists need to know. Cancer Imaging 2007; 7(spec no A):S95–S99.

14. Margolis DJ, Hoffman JM, Herfkens RJ, et al. Molecular imaging techniques in body imaging. Radiology 2007; 245(2):333–356.

15. Haug A, Tiling R, Sommer HL. FDG-PET and FDG-PET/CT in breast cancer. Recent Results Cancer Res 2008; 170:125–140.

16. Larson SM, Pentlow KS, Volkow ND, et al. PET scanning of iodine-124-3F9 as an approach to tumor dosimetry during treatment planning for radioimmunotherapy in a child with neuroblastoma. J Nucl Med 1992; 33(11):2020–2023.

17. Pentlow KS, Graham MC, Lambrecht RM, et al. Quantitative imaging of iodine-124 with PET. J Nucl Med 1996; 37(9):1557–1562.

18. Cai W, Olafsen T, Zhang X, et al. PET imaging of colorectal cancer in xenograft-bearing mice by use of an ^{18}F-labeled T84.66 anti-carcinoembryonic antigen diabody. J Nucl Med 2007; 48(2):304–310.

19. Divgi CR, Pandit-Taskar N, Jungbluth AA, et al. Preoperative characterisation of clear-cell renal carcinoma using iodine-124-labelled antibody chimeric G250 (^{124}I-cG250) and PET in patients with renal masses: a phase I trial. Lancet Oncol 2007; 8(4):304–310.

20. Li L, Bading J, Yazaki PJ, et al. A versatile bifunctional chelate for radiolabeling humanized anti-CEA antibody with In-111 and Cu-64 at either thiol or amino groups: PET imaging of CEA-positive tumors with whole antibodies. Bioconjug Chem 2008;19(1):89–96.

21. Kenanova V, Olafsen T, Crow DM, et al. Tailoring the pharmacokinetics and positron emission tomography imaging properties of anti-carcinoembryonic antigen single-chain Fv-Fc antibody fragments. Cancer Res 2005; 65(2):622–631.

22. Sundaresan G, Yazaki PJ, Shively JE, et al. ^{124}I-labeled engineered anti-CEA minibodies and diabodies allow high-contrast, antigen-specific small-animal PET imaging of xenografts in athymic mice. J Nucl Med 2003; 44(12):1962–1969.

23. Voss SD, Smith SV, DiBartolo N, et al. Positron emission tomography (PET) imaging of neuroblastoma and melanoma with ^{64}Cu-SarAr immunoconjugates. Proc Natl Acad Sci U S A 2007; 104(44):17489–17493.

24. Cai W, Chen K, He L, et al. Quantitative PET of EGFR expression in xenograft-bearing mice using ^{64}Cu-labeled cetuximab, a chimeric anti-EGFR monoclonal antibody. Eur J Nucl Med Mol Imaging 2007; 34(6):850–858.

25. Grunberg J, Novak-Hofer I, Honer M, et al. In vivo evaluation of ^{177}Lu- and $^{67/64}$Cu-labeled recombinant fragments of antibody chCE7 for radioimmunotherapy and PET imaging of L1-CAM-positive tumors. Clin Cancer Res 2005; 11(14):5112–5120.

26. Olafsen T, Kenanova VE, Sundaresan G, et al. Optimizing radiolabeled engineered anti-p185HER2 antibody fragments for in vivo imaging. Cancer Res 2005; 65(13):5907–5916.

27. Lewis MR, Wang M, Axworthy DB, et al. In vivo evaluation of pretargeted ^{64}Cu for tumor imaging and therapy. J Nucl Med 2003; 44(8):1284–1292.

28. Novak-Hofer I, Honer M, Ametamey S, et al. Imaging of renal carcinoma xenografts with ^{64}Cu-labelled anti-L1-CAM antibody chCE7. Eur J Nucl Med Mol Imaging 2003; 30(7):1066.

29. Lewis MR, Boswell CA, Laforest R, et al. Conjugation of monoclonal antibodies with TETA using activated esters: biological comparison of ^{64}Cu-TETA-1A3 with ^{64}Cu-BAT-2IT-1A3. Cancer Biother Radiopharm 2001; 16(6):483–494.

30. Philpott GW, Schwarz SW, Anderson CJ, et al. Radioimmuno PET: detection of colorectal carcinoma with positron-emitting copper-64-labeled monoclonal antibody. J Nucl Med 1995; 36(10):1818–1824.

31. Anderson CJ, Connett JM, Schwarz SW, et al. Copper-64-labeled antibodies for PET imaging. J Nucl Med 1992; 33(9):1685–1691.

32. Sharkey RM, Burton J, Goldenberg DM. Radioimmuno-therapy of non-Hodgkin's lymphoma: a critical appraisal. Exp Rev Clin 2005; 1(1):47–62.

33. Kelloff GJ, Sullivan DM, Wilson W, et al. FDG-PET lymphoma demonstration project invitational workshop. Acad Radiol 2007; 14(3):330–339.

34. Blend MJ, Hyun H, Kozloff M, et al. Improved staging of B-cell non-Hodgkin's lymphoma patients with

^{99m}Tc-labeled LL2 monoclonal antibody fragment. Cancer Res 1995; 55(23 suppl):5764s–5770s.

35. Murthy S, Sharkey RM, Goldenberg DM, et al. Lymphoma imaging with a new technetium-99m labelled antibody, LL2. Eur J Nucl Med 1992; 19(6):394–401.

36. Baum RP, Niesen A, Hertel A, et al. Initial clinical results with technetium-99m-labeled LL2 monoclonal antibody fragment in the radioimmunodetection of B-cell lymphomas. Cancer 1994; 73(3 suppl):896–899.

37. Gasparini M, Bombardieri E, Tondini C, et al. Clinical utility of radioimmunoscintigraphy of non-Hodgkin's lymphoma with radiolabelled LL2 monoclonal antibody, LymphoSCAN: preliminary results. Tumori 1995; 81(3):173–178.

38. Goldenberg DM, Larson SM. Radioimmunodetection in cancer identification. J Nucl Med 1992; 33(5):803–814.

39. Goldenberg DM, Sharkey RM. Novel radiolabeled antibody conjugates. Oncogene 2007; 26(25):3734–3744.

40. Moffat FL Jr., Pinsky CM, Hammershaimb L, et al. Clinical utility of external immunoscintigraphy with the IMMU-4 technetium-99m Fab' antibody fragment in patients undergoing surgery for carcinoma of the colon and rectum: results of a pivotal, phase III trial. The Immunomedics Study Group. J Clin Oncol 1996; 14(8):2295–2305.

41. Hughes K, Pinsky CM, Petrelli NJ, et al. Use of carcinoembryonic antigen radioimmunodetection and computed tomography for predicting the resectability of recurrent colorectal cancer. Ann Surg 1997; 226(5):621–631.

42. Collier BD, Abdel-Nabi H, Doerr RJ, et al. Immunoscintigraphy performed with In-111-labeled CYT-103 in the management of colorectal cancer: comparison with CT. Radiology 1992; 185(1):179–186.

43. Abdel-Nabi HH, Doerr RJ. Multicenter clinical trials of monoclonal antibody B72.3-GYK-DTPA ^{111}In (^{111}In-CYT-103; OncoScint CR103) in patients with colorectal carcinoma. Target Diagn Ther 1992; 6:73–88.

44. Neal CE, Meis LC. Correlative imaging with monoclonal antibodies in colorectal, ovarian, and prostate cancer. Semin Nucl Med 1994; 24(4):272–285.

45. Corman ML, Galandiuk S, Block GE, et al. Immunoscintigraphy with ^{111}In-satumomab pendetide in patients with colorectal adenocarcinoma: performance and impact on clinical management. Dis Colon Rectum 1994; 37(2):129–137.

46. Petersen BM Jr., Bass BL, Bates HR, et al. Use of the radiolabeled murine monoclonal antibody, ^{111}In-CYT-103, in the management of colon cancer. Am J Surg 1993; 165(1):137–142; discussion 142–133.

47. Surwit EA, Childers JM, Krag DN, et al. Clinical assessment of ^{111}In-CYT-103 immunoscintigraphy in ovarian cancer. Gynecol Oncol 1993; 48(3):285–292.

48. Bhatia M, Baron PL, Alderman DF, et al. False-positive imaging of In-111 labeled monoclonal antibody conjugate CYT-103 in a patient with metastatic colorectal carcinoma. Clin Nucl Med 1995; 20(11):979–980.

49. Dominguez JM, Wolff BG, Nelson H, et al. ^{111}In-CYT-103 scanning in recurrent colorectal cancer–does it affect standard management? Dis Colon Rectum 1996; 39(5):514–519.

50. Kahn D, Williams RD, Haseman MK, et al. Radioimmunoscintigraphy with In-111-labeled capromab pendetide predicts prostate cancer response to salvage radiotherapy after failed radical prostatectomy. J Clin Oncol 1998; 16(1):284–289.

51. Kahn D, Williams RD, Manyak MJ, et al. 111 Indium-capromab pendetide in the evaluation of patients with residual or recurrent prostate cancer after radical prostatectomy. The ProstaScint Study Group. J Urol 1998; 159(6):2041–2046; discussion 2046–2047.

52. Sodee DB, Ellis RJ, Samuels MA, et al. Prostate cancer and prostate bed SPECT imaging with ProstaScint: semiquantitative correlation with prostatic biopsy results. Prostate 1998; 37(3):140–148.

53. Elgamal AA, Troychak MJ, Murphy GP. ProstaScint scan may enhance identification of prostate cancer recurrences after prostatectomy, radiation, or hormone therapy: analysis of 136 scans of 100 patients. Prostate 1998; 37(4):261–269.

54. Sodee DB, Malguria N, Faulhaber P, et al. Multicenter prostaScint imaging findings in 2154 patients with prostate cancer. The ProstaScint Imaging Centers. Urology 2000; 56(6):988–993.

55. Raj GV, Partin AW, Polascik TJ. Clinical utility of indium 111-capromab pendetide immunoscintigraphy in the detection of early, recurrent prostate carcinoma after radical prostatectomy. Cancer 2002; 94(4):987–996.

56. Thomas CT, Bradshaw PT, Pollock BH, et al. Indium-111-capromab pendetide radioimmunoscintigraphy and prognosis for durable biochemical response to salvage radiation therapy in men after failed prostatectomy. J Clin Oncol 2003; 21(9):1715–1721.

57. Mohammed AA, Shergill IS, Vandal MT, et al. ProstaScint and its role in the diagnosis of prostate cancer. Expert Rev Mol Diagn 2007; 7(4):345–349.

58. Breitz HB, Tyler A, Bjorn MJ, et al. Clinical experience with Tc-99m nofetumomab merpentan (Verluma) radioimmunoscintigraphy. Clin Nucl Med 1997; 22(9):615–620.

59. Jain RK. Therapeutic implications of tumor physiology. Curr Opin Oncol 1991; 3(6):1105–1108.

60. Buchsbaum DJ. Experimental approaches to increase radiolabeled antibody localization in tumors. Cancer Res 1995; 55(23 suppl):5729s–5732s.

61. Siegel JA, Pawlyk DA, Lee RE, et al. Tumor, red marrow, and organ dosimetry for ^{131}I-labeled anti-carcinoembryonic antigen monoclonal antibody. Cancer Res 1990; 50(3 suppl):1039s–1042s.

62. Sharkey RM, Motta-Hennessy C, Pawlyk D, et al. Biodistribution and radiation dose estimates for yttrium- and iodine-labeled monoclonal antibody IgG and fragments in nude mice bearing human colonic tumor xenografts. Cancer Res 1990; 50(8):2330–2336.

63. Behr TM, Sharkey RM, Juweid ME, et al. Reduction of the renal uptake of radiolabeled monoclonal antibody fragments by cationic amino acids and their derivatives. Cancer Res 1995; 55(17):3825–3834.

64. Colcher D, Pavlinkova G, Beresford G, et al. Pharmacokinetics and biodistribution of genetically-engineered antibodies. Q J Nucl Med 1998; 42(4):225–241.

65. Wittel UA, Jain M, Goel A, et al. The in vivo characteristics of genetically engineered divalent and tetravalent single-chain antibody constructs. Nucl Med Biol 2005; 32(2):157–164.

66. Batra SK, Jain M, Wittel UA, et al. Pharmacokinetics and biodistribution of genetically engineered antibodies. Curr Opin Biotechnol 2002; 13(6):603–608.

67. Slavin-Chiorini DC, Horan Hand PH, Kashmiri SV, et al. Biologic properties of a CH2 domain-deleted recombinant immunoglobulin. Int J Cancer 1993; 53(1):97–103.

68. Wu AM. Engineering multivalent antibody fragments for in vivo targeting. Methods Mol Biol 2004; 248: 209–225.

69. Binz HK, Amstutz P, Pluckthun A. Engineering novel binding proteins from nonimmunoglobulin domains. Nat Biotechnol 2005; 23(10):1257–1268.

70. Kenanova V, Wu AM. Tailoring antibodies for radionuclide delivery. Expert Opin Drug Deliv 2006; 3(1):53–70.

71. Orlova A, Tolmachev V, Pehrson R, et al. Synthetic affibody molecules: a novel class of affinity ligands for molecular imaging of HER2-expressing malignant tumors. Cancer Res 2007; 67(5):2178–2186.

72. Tolmachev V, Orlova A, Pehrson R, et al. Radionuclide therapy of HER2-positive microxenografts using a ^{177}Lu-labeled HER2-specific affibody molecule. Cancer Res 2007; 67(6):2773–2782.

73. Nilsson FY, Tolmachev V. Affibody molecules: new protein domains for molecular imaging and targeted tumor therapy. Curr Opin Drug Discov Devel 2007; 10(2):167–175.

74. Orlova A, Rosik D, Sandstrom M, et al. Evaluation of [(111/114m)In]CHX-A"-DTPA-Z(HER2:342), an Affibody ligand conjugate for targeting of HER2-expressing malignant tumors. Q J Nucl Med Mol Imaging 2007; 51(4):314–323.

75. Orlova A, Feldwisch J, Abrahmsen L, et al. Update: affibody molecules for molecular imaging and therapy for cancer. Cancer Biother Radiopharm 2007; 22(5): 573–584.

76. Goldenberg DM, Sharkey RM, Paganelli G, et al. Antibody pretargeting advances cancer radioimmunodetection and radioimmunotherapy. J Clin Oncol 2006; 24(5): 823–834.

77. Goodwin DA, Meares CF, David GF, et al. Monoclonal antibodies as reversible equilibrium carriers of radiopharmaceuticals. Int J Rad Appl Instrum B 1986; 13(4): 383–391.

78. Reardan DT, Meares CF, Goodwin DA, et al. Antibodies against metal chelates. Nature 1985; 316(6025):265–268.

79. Boerman OC, Kranenborg MH, Oosterwijk E, et al. Pretargeting of renal cell carcinoma: improved tumor targeting with a bivalent chelate. Cancer Res 1999; 59(17):4400–4405.

80. Goodwin DA, Meares CF, Watanabe N, et al. Pharmacokinetics of pretargeted monoclonal antibody 2D12.5 and [88]Y-Janus-2-(p-nitrobenzyl)-1,4,7,10-tetraazacyclododecanetetraacetic acid (DOTA) in BALB/c mice with KHJJ mouse adenocarcinoma: a model for 90Y radioimmunotherapy. Cancer Res 1994; 54(22):5937–5946.

81. Le Doussal JM, Martin M, Gautherot E, et al. In vitro and in vivo targeting of radiolabeled monovalent and divalent haptens with dual specificity monoclonal antibody conjugates: enhanced divalent hapten affinity for cell-bound antibody conjugate. J Nucl Med 1989; 30(8):1358–1366.

82. Sharkey RM, Karacay H, Cardillo TM, et al. Improving the delivery of radionuclides for imaging and therapy of cancer using pretargeting methods. Clin Cancer Res 2005; 11(19 pt 2):7109s–7121s.

83. Boerman OC, van Schaijk FG, Oyen WJ, et al. Pretargeted radioimmunotherapy of cancer: progress step by step. J Nucl Med 2003; 44(3):400–411.

84. Stickney DR, Anderson LD, Slater JB, et al. Bifunctional antibody: a binary radiopharmaceutical delivery system for imaging colorectal carcinoma. Cancer Res 1991; 51(24):6650–6655.

85. Abdel-Nabi HH, Chan HW, Doerr RJ. Indium-labeled anti-colorectal carcinoma monoclonal antibody accumulation in non-tumored tissue in patients with colorectal carcinoma. J Nucl Med 1990; 31(12):1975–1979.

86. Abdel-Nabi HH, Schwartz AN, Higano CS, et al. Colorectal carcinoma: detection with indium-111 anticarcinoembryonic-antigen monoclonal antibody ZCE-025. Radiology 1987; 164(3):617–621.

87. Patt YZ, Lamki LM, Shanken J, et al. Imaging with indium111-labeled anticarcinoembryonic antigen monoclonal antibody ZCE-025 of recurrent colorectal or carcinoembryonic antigen-producing cancer in patients with rising serum carcinoembryonic antigen levels and occult metastases. J Clin Oncol 1990; 8(7):1246–1254.

88. Lamki LM, Patt YZ, Rosenblum MG, et al. Metastatic colorectal cancer: radioimmunoscintigraphy with a stabilized In-111-labeled F(ab')₂ fragment of an anti-CEA monoclonal antibody. Radiology 1990; 174(1):147–151.

89. Chetanneau A, Barbet J, Peltier P, et al. Pretargeted imaging of colorectal cancer recurrences using an ^{111}In-labelled bivalent hapten and a bispecific antibody conjugate. Nucl Med Commun 1994; 15(12):972–980.

90. Le Doussal JM, Chetanneau A, Gruaz-Guyon A, et al. Bispecific monoclonal antibody-mediated targeting of an indium-111-labeled DTPA dimer to primary colorectal tumors: pharmacokinetics, biodistribution, scintigraphy and immune response. J Nucl Med 1993; 34(10):1662–1671.

91. Peltier P, Curtet C, Chatal JF, et al. Radioimmunodetection of medullary thyroid cancer using a bispecific anti-CEA/anti-indium-DTPA antibody and an indium-111-labeled DTPA dimer. J Nucl Med 1993; 34(8):1267–1273.

92. Rossi EA, Goldenberg DM, Cardillo TM, et al. Stably tethered multifunctional structures of defined composition made by the dock and lock method for use in cancer targeting. Proc Natl Acad Sci U S A 2006; 103(18):6841–6846.

93. Rossi EA, Chang CH, Losman MJ, et al. Pretargeting of carcinoembryonic antigen-expressing cancers with a trivalent bispecific fusion protein produced in myeloma cells. Clin Cancer Res 2005; 11(19 pt 2):7122s–7129s.

94. Rossi EA, Sharkey RM, McBride W, et al. Development of new multivalent-bispecific agents for pretargeting tumor localization and therapy. Clin Cancer Res 2003; 9(10 pt 2):3886S–3896S.

95. Karacay H, Sharkey RM, McBride WJ, et al. Pretargeting for cancer radioimmunotherapy with bispecific antibodies: role of the bispecific antibody's valency for the tumor target antigen. Bioconjug Chem 2002; 13(5): 1054–1070.

96. Goodwin DA, Meares CF, McTigue M, et al. Pretargeted immunoscintigraphy: effect of hapten valency on murine tumor uptake. J Nucl Med 1992; 33(11):2006–2013.

97. Karacay H, McBride WJ, Griffiths GL, et al. Experimental pretargeting studies of cancer with a humanized anti-CEA × murine anti-[In-DTPA] bispecific antibody construct and a ^{99m}Tc-/^{188}Re-labeled peptide. Bioconjug Chem 2000; 11(6):842–854.

98. Gestin JF, Loussouarn A, Bardies M, et al. Two-step targeting of xenografted colon carcinoma using a bispecific antibody and ^{188}Re-labeled bivalent hapten: biodistribution and dosimetry studies. J Nucl Med 2001; 42(1): 146–153.

99. Feng X, Pak RH, Kroger LA, et al. New anti-Cu-TETA and anti-Y-DOTA monoclonal antibodies for potential use in the pre-targeted delivery of radiopharmaceuticals to tumor. Hybridoma 1998; 17(2):125–132.

100. Griffiths GL, Chang CH, McBride WJ, et al. Reagents and methods for PET using bispecific antibody pretargeting and ^{68}Ga-radiolabeled bivalent hapten-peptide-chelate conjugates. J Nucl Med 2004; 45(1):30–39.

101. McBride WJ, Zanzonico P, Sharkey RM, et al. Bispecific antibody pretargeting PET (ImmunoPET) with an ^{124}I-labeled hapten-peptide. J Nucl Med 2006; 47(10): 1678–1688.

102. Sharkey RM, McBride WJ, Karacay H, et al. A universal pretargeting system for cancer detection and therapy using bispecific antibody. Cancer Res 2003; 63(2):354–363.

103. Sharkey RM, Karacay H, Richel H, et al. Optimizing bispecific antibody pretargeting for use in radioimmunotherapy. Clin Cancer Res 2003; 9(10 pt 2):3897S–3913S.

104. Sharkey RM, Karacay H, McBride WJ, et al. Bispecific antibody pretargeting of radionuclides for immuno single-photon emission computed tomography and immuno positron emission tomography molecular imaging: an update. Clin Cancer Res 2007; 13(18 pt 2):5577s–5585s.

105. Sharkey RM, Cardillo TM, Rossi EA, et al. Signal amplification in molecular imaging by pretargeting a multivalent, bispecific antibody. Nat Med 2005; 11(11): 1250–1255.

106. Axworthy DB, Reno JM, Hylarides MD, et al. Cure of human carcinoma xenografts by a single dose of pretargeted yttrium-90 with negligible toxicity. Proc Natl Acad Sci U S A 2000; 97(4):1802–1807.

107. Sharkey RM, Karacay H, Vallabhajosula S, et al. Molecular imaging with pretargeted ImmunoSPECT and ImmunoPET in a model of metastatic colonic carcinoma. Radiology 2008; 246(2):497–507.

108. Chang CH, Rossi EA, Goldenberg DM. The dock and lock method: a novel platform technology for building multivalent, multifunctional structures of defined composition with retained bioactivity. Clin Cancer Res 2007; 13(18 pt 2):5586s–5591s.

109. Horak E, Heitner T, Robinson MK, et al. Isolation of scFvs to in vitro produced extracellular domains of EGFR family members. Cancer Biother Radiopharm 2005; 20(6): 603–613.

110. Moosmayer D, Berndorff D, Chang CH, et al. Bispecific antibody pretargeting of tumor neovasculature for improved systemic radiotherapy of solid tumors. Clin Cancer Res 2006; 12(18):5587–5595.

111. Shi T, Wrin J, Reeder J, et al. High-affinity monoclonal antibodies against P-glycoprotein. Clin Immunol Immunopathol 1995; 76(1 pt 1):44–51.

112. Scott AM, Rosa E, Mehta BM, et al. In vivo imaging and specific targeting of P-glycoprotein expression in multidrug resistant nude mice xenografts with [125I]MRK-16 monoclonal antibody. Nucl Med Biol 1995; 22(4):497–504.

113. Iwahashi T, Okochi E, Ariyoshi K, et al. Specific targeting and killing activities of anti-P-glycoprotein monoclonal antibody MRK16 directed against intrinsically multidrug-resistant human colorectal carcinoma cell lines in the nude mouse model. Cancer Res 1993; 53(22):5475–5482.

114. van Eerd JE, de Geus-Oei LF, Oyen WJ, et al. Scintigraphic imaging of P-glycoprotein expression with a radiolabelled antibody. Eur J Nucl Med Mol Imaging 2006; 33(11):1266–1272.

115. Goldenberg DM, Sharkey RM, Udem S, et al. Immunoscintigraphy of Pneumocystis carinii pneumonia in AIDS patients. J Nucl Med 1994; 35(6):1028–1034.

116. Casadevall A, Goldstein H, Dadachova E. Targeting host cells harbouring viruses with radiolabeled antibodies. Expert Opin Biol Ther 2007; 7(5):595–597.

117. Dadachova E, Bryan RA, Huang X, et al. Comparative evaluation of capsular polysaccharide-specific IgM and IgG antibodies and F(ab')2 and Fab fragments as delivery vehicles for radioimmunotherapy of fungal infection. Clin Cancer Res 2007; 13(18 pt 2):5629s–5635s.

118. Dadachova E, Casadevall A. Treatment of infection with radiolabeled antibodies. Q J Nucl Med Mol Imaging 2006; 50(3):193–204.

119. Hay RV, Cao B, Skinner RS, et al. Nuclear imaging of Met-expressing human and canine cancer xenografts with radiolabeled monoclonal antibodies (MetSeek). Clin Cancer Res 2005; 11(19 pt 2):7064s–7069s.

120. Chatal JF, Campion L, Kraeber-Bodere F, et al. Survival improvement in patients with medullary thyroid carcinoma who undergo pretargeted anti-carcinoembryonic-antigen radioimmunotherapy: a collaborative study with the French Endocrine Tumor Group. J Clin Oncol 2006; 24(11):1705–1711.

38

Diffusion Magnetic Resonance Imaging for Cancer Treatment Response Assessment

BRIAN D. ROSS, KUEI C. LEE, CRAIG J. GALBAN, CHARLES R. MEYER, and THOMAS L. CHENEVERT
Department of Radiology, University of Michigan, Ann Arbor, Michigan, U.S.A.

ALNAWAZ REHEMTULLA
Department of Radiation Oncology, University of Michigan, Ann Arbor, Michigan, U.S.A.

INTRODUCTION

Magnetic resonance imaging (MRI) can be used to obtain information related to biophysical, physiological, metabolical, anatomical, or functional properties of tissues. This chapter will highlight the application of diffusion MRI as a molecular imaging approach for oncological imaging. Applications of diffusion MRI range from assessment of cellular status (1), cellular density (2), diagnostic screening (3), and microstructural organization (4,5), all of which are used in clinical and research studies. Specific attention will be given to the application of this imaging approach for assessment of cancer treatment response. The overall concept for this application in cancer imaging is that diffusion MR can be used to quantify the mobility or diffusion of water molecules within tissue. Because the diffusion of individual water molecules relies on interactions which occur at the cellular level, subtle alterations in, for example, cellular density results in a corresponding change in the diffusion rate of water molecules which makes diffusion MRI a sensitive imaging biomarker (6,7). The goal of this chapter will be to provide the reader with an up to date

summary of the basic methods and applications of applying diffusion MRI in oncological research and clinical practice.

PRINCIPLES OF DIFFUSION MRI

Technical reviews of the topic of in vivo diffusion-weighted MR imaging have been published recently (8,9). In brief, molecular diffusion refers to the thermally driven, random translational motion of molecules in tissue, which is also called Brownian motion. MRI can be applied for quantification of water diffusion values spatially in vivo. Magnetic gradients are applied to the tissue region, which provide for "encoding" the initial locations of constituent water molecules within the tissue. For water molecules that experienced displacement from the initial location over short period of time, during the decoding process, these molecules will have a detectable loss of signal through spin de-phasing. The more mobile the water molecule is, the larger the net loss of signal will be relative to the corresponding immobile water molecules. Water signal loss is measured at several diffusion gradient values, which allows for determination of molecular mobility to be quantified in heterogeneous tissues such as tumors. Due to the fact that water is also located within different intra- and extracellular compartments, which are separated by semipermeable membranes, the measured diffusion values are reported as an apparent diffusion coefficient (ADC) (6,9).

Free water molecules at 37°C migrate 30 μm in 50 milliseconds, which is on the order of the typical MR time interval. Since the diameter of a tumor cell is a few to tens of micrometers, with other subcellular structures, such as membranes, organelles, and macromolecules having smaller dimensions, a given water molecule will encounter many interactions over the MRI measurement interval. Impediment of water diffusion via cellular/tissue interactions and restricted barriers reduces the overall mobility the lowering the measured ADC values, and, in fact, the greater the bulk density of structures within a region of tumor, the larger effect on impeding the water mobility will be, thus lowering the ADC value for that spatial region of the tumor mass. ADC can be considered to be able to follow the evolution of a tumor over time during treatment. Thus, the alterations of cellular structures due to therapeutic intervention impact the diffusion of water within those tumor regions sensitive to treatment thus providing for the application of diffusion MRI as an imaging biomarker of treatment response. Key aspects of using diffusion MRI in this context is that it is a quantifiable measurement, reproducible between scanner manufacturers, and magnetic field strength independent as comparable acquisition techniques are used.

PRECLINICAL DIFFUSION MRI FOR TUMOR RESPONSE ASSESSMENT

Treatment-induced volumetric changes occur relatively slowly following treatment. Preceding volumetric shrinkage, tumor cell death occurs resulting in changes in the tumor microenvironment, which can be detected using diffusion MRI. As these changes occur relatively early, this imaging biomarker can be used to detect early changes in tumor structure thus providing the possibility of using this imaging biomarker as an early response indicator in preclinical and clinical cancer studies. A specific goal of applying diffusion MRI in the clinical setting is that early response detection can provide for stratification of patient responders from nonresponders on an individual basis. As shown in Figure 1, current response assessment occurs following completion of treatment and is based on change in tumor volumes from treatment initiation. Typically volumetric assessment is made at 6 to 10 weeks following completion of treatment. If the patient was found to be a nonresponder, then enrollment into the next therapeutic line of intervention is undertaken followed again by volumetric

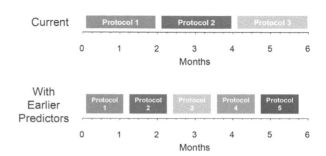

Figure 1 Schematic of current treatment paradigm wherein a patient undergoes treatment for six to eight weeks followed by response assessment using anatomical imaging (MRI or CT). Nonresponsive patients are entered into second-line therapy and the process is repeated. If an early imaging biomarker of treatment response were available, then stratification of nonresponders from responding patients could be achieved at a mid-point into treatment and the patient could be more rapidly entered into alternate treatments. This could in principle be repeated until a suitable treatment is identified.

assessment at the conclusion of therapy. If treatment response could be determined early on (i.e., at mid-treatment), then valuable time could be saved for individual patients and nonresponders could be more rapidly moved to second-line treatments.

The initial report showing the feasibility of detecting early changes in tumor water diffusion values following treatment was reported in an intracerebral 9L rat glioma wherein an increase in tumor diffusion values following treatment were found (10). Shown in Figure 2 are results from this study, which clearly reveal that an increase in tumor diffusion values occurred due to successful therapeutic intervention. This observation was confirmed by a variety of subsequent animal tumor studies where diffusion values were shown to increase as the tumor cells died during successful therapy supporting the hypothesis that diffusion MRI can be used to noninvasively quantify cellular changes associated with successful treatment in animal models (2,11–24). Key findings indicate that tumor diffusion values increased prior to tumor volume regression, diffusion changes were observed to be treatment independent and dose dependent, all supporting the claim that this imaging biomarker may indeed be used as a surrogate for treatment outcome. While studies are ongoing in both the preclinical and clinical settings, the data collected thus far provide for significant optimism.

An advantage for the application diffusion MRI relies on its excellent sensitivity to relatively small therapeutic effects, which can be utilized for studies involving evaluation and optimization of drug dosage and/or schedule. This is especially helpful if the test compound is in limited supply. An example of this application can be found in Figure 3. In this example, rats with 9L gliomas were treated with a chemotherapy administered in daily

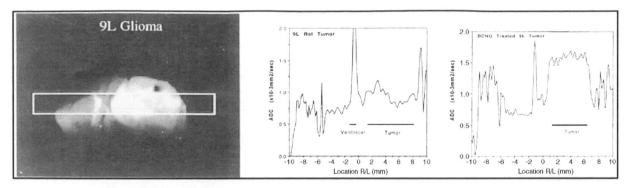

Figure 2 (*Left image*) T2-weighted MRI of a rat 9L glioma shown overlayed with the location of a column from which spatially derived diffusion measurements were acquired. (*Middle plot*) Diffusion values are shown corresponding to the locations on the adjacent image for the 9L glioma prior to treatment. Diffusion values within the tumor mass are shown to have an average value of about $0.5–1.0 \times 10^{-3}$ mm^2/sec. Following administration of a single dose of chemotherapy, the diffusion values within the tumor significantly increased to about 1.6×10^{-3} mm^2/sec. *Source*: From Ref. 10.

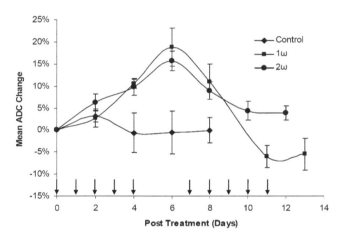

Figure 3 Mean ADC changes from serial acquisitions throughout therapy. Normalized ADC values from each group were plotted as a function of time. (*Arrows*) 2 mg/kg BCNU injections, where the first cycle was given from days 0 to 4, and animals receiving a second cycle were injected from days 7 to 11. Changes in mean ADC of control groups remained fairly constant, where as both BCNU-treated groups showed a significant rise in ADC after the initial cycle of BCNU therapy. Note that animals receiving a second cycle of BCNU therapy showed a progressive decrease in ADC throughout the second course of BCNU therapy. *Abbreviations*: ADC, apparent diffusion coefficient; BCNU, carmustine. *Source*: From Ref. 15.

fractionated doses for either one-week (1ω) or over a two-week period (2ω). As shown in Figure 3, increases in diffusion values for both treatment arms reached peak change at six days posttreatment initiation and fell back to baseline over the next four to five days. The fact that the diffusion changes were similar for both treatment groups indicated that the treatment effect (cell killing) reached its maximum following the first week of therapy, and that the

second week of treatment did not further impact on cell death. Follow-up animal survival studies and ex vivo chemosensitivity studies on excised cells revealed that this was in fact the case (15). Thus, diffusion MRI was able to reveal that a single week of treatment was optimal, and that the tumor had gained resistance to the treatment within the first week, thus the second course of treatment was ineffective (15). This study revealed that diffusion MRI can be effectively applied in the drug development stage for dose and/or schedule optimization for experimental therapeutics.

THE FUNCTIONAL DIFFUSION MAP

In order to facilitate the broad use and application of diffusion MRI in the context of tumor response monitoring, standardization of data analysis would assist in providing for cross comparison of data between different research and clinical sites. Furthermore, standardized analysis should provide for a more accurate and sensitive method for detection of treatment response. Initially, histogram analysis of ADC values from the entire tumor mass was used to quantify mean tumor ADC values or percentage change following treatment based upon the mean of the ADC histogram. This approach tended to work well in animal tumor studies where tumors responded in a relatively homogeneous fashion. One disadvantage of this approach was that the spatial information was not available to relate to the original anatomical location for the individual ADC values. Moreover, as shown in Figure 4A, cellular changes within a tumor following therapy may result in cell swelling and cell shrinkage in spatially distinct sites, thereby yielding decreases and increases in regional tumor diffusion values, respectively. The competing cell death pathways may

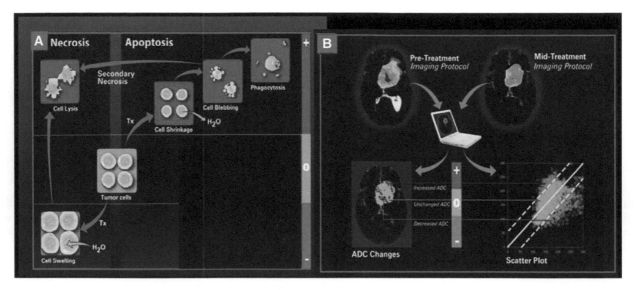

Figure 4 Cell death pathways involved in therapeutic-induced changes in tumor ADC values along with a pictorial description of the fDM analytical process. (**A**) Schematic of the two major cell death pathways associated with changes in tumor water diffusion values. Tumor cells within a range of image voxels may experience different fates during treatment. Cells may be resistant to therapy (unaltered ADC) or may undergo a necrotic death via transient cell swelling (decreased ADC). Cell swelling may also result from mitotic catastrophe or a focal ischemic event (decreased ADC). Progression to cell lysis and necrosis may occur resulting in an increased ADC value in that region. An apoptotic death pathway may also be activated by treatment leading to cell shrinkage and phagocytosis (increased ADC). (**B**) Analysis of diffusion MRI data via image coregistration of pretreatment images with images during treatment (mid-treatment). A three-color overlay is generated that represents regions of tumor ADC values, which remained unchanged during therapy, increased, or decreased. This data is summarized as a scatter plot wherein percentages assigned to the three defined ADC regions is accomplished allowing quantitative assessment of overall changes in tumor ADC values. *Abbreviations*: ADC, apparent diffusion coefficient; fDM, functional diffusion map. *Source*: From Ref. 25 (*See Color Insert*).

produce offsetting effects on the overall diffusion changes within a tumor mass, thereby underestimating the detected changes and reducing overall sensitivity when analysis is accomplished using a histogram-based, whole-tumor average diffusion measurement.

An analytical solution for optimizing the sensitivity of the diffusion imaging biomarker for assessment of treatment response in the presence of tumor diffusion heterogeneity has been proposed and is referred to as the functional diffusion map (fDM) (25). The fDM uses spatial registration of all three-dimensional image sets to provide for a common geometrical framework (Fig. 4B). This allows for treatment-induced changes in diffusion values to be assessed on a voxel-by-voxel basis from spatially aligned pre- and early posttreatment initiation image sets. Application of fDM to evaluate the treatment effects on several tumor types including human gliomas and metastatic prostate cancer to the bone have been reported (25,26). The fDM approach requires registration of early, posttreatment initiation images to the initial pretreatment T1- or T2-weighted images using an automated mutual information algorithm and affine transformation. After image registration, tumors are manually contoured and only voxels identified as "tumor" on

pretreatment and mid-treatment images are quantitatively compared. The tumor diffusion information is then segmented into three different categories representing voxels in which ADC increased by a specified threshold, voxels for which ADC decreased by the same magnitude, and voxels that did not change outside this threshold range (voxel-wise scatterplot of ADC pretreatment vs. at 3 weeks of treatment as illustrated in Fig. 4B). The fractional volume of tumor in these three categories can then be determined, which represent the relative percent volume of tumor that exhibits a significant increase, decrease or no change in ADC.

Recent examples of the application of fDM in animal studies have been reported (19,27). In one example, fDM was used to assess early treatment response using a preclinical model of metastatic prostate cancer. In this disease, the use of many multimodal imaging technologies for detection of treatment response has not been shown to be useful. Shown in Figure 5A is a schematic representation of a bone lesion undergoing therapy wherein loss of regional tumor cell viability within the tumor mass would be encoded by the fDM approach as red voxels, whereas regions not significantly affected by the treatment are displayed as green. Increased diffusion regions were

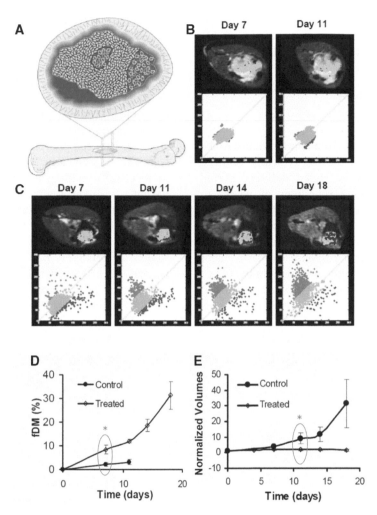

Figure 5 fDM analysis of metastatic prostate bone lesions in the tibia of mice. (**A**) Schematic drawing of a tumor residing in the bone with a pseudo-fDM overlay generated from registered diffusion MRI data pre- and posttreatment. Green voxels correspond to regions not responding to therapy, loss of cellularity within responsive regions are shown as red voxels. (**B**) fDM analysis including scatter plots from an untreated animal at 7 and 11 days post-initiation of sham treatment. (**C**) fDM analysis from a treated animal at days 7, 11, 14, and 18 post-initiation of docetaxel therapy. (**D**) Plot of mean percentage increased fDM values from the control ($n = 5$) and treated ($n = 7$) groups as a function of time post-initiation of therapy. (**E**) Mean-normalized tumor volumes from control ($n = 5$) and treated ($n = 7$) groups as a function of time. *Abbreviations*: fDM, functional diffusion map. *Source*: From Ref. 19 (*See Color Insert*).

detected early using fDM in docetaxel-treated versus untreated metastatic prostate bone tumors at seven days posttreatment initiation indicating loss of tumor cell viability, which increased further over time (Fig. 5B–E). Scatter plots (Fig. 5B) were also generated and the percentage of increased ADC was determined to be 1.2% and 2.5% on days 7 and 11, respectively for untreated tumors. However, for treated tumors, fDM analysis at days 7, 11, 14, and 18 post-initiation of docetaxel therapy revealed an increase in regions of red voxels (loss of cell density/viability) with time. Corresponding scatter plots revealed regions of increased ADC to be 4.0% (day 7), 13.1% (day 11), 30.0% (day 14), and 53.7% (day 18). Percent changes in tumor fDM values for control and treated groups are

plotted in Figure 5D. Statistically significant differences in fDM values between control and treated animals were achieved early from the initiation of therapy at as little as seven days. MRI measurements provided for tumor volume measurements to be made over time, which revealed untreated tumors increased in volume, whereas treated tumors did not increase in volume. This data correlated well with the fDM results and indicated docetaxel therapy was efficacious. In addition, differences in tumor volumes between the two animal groups reached significance at day 11 posttreatment initiation, which was much later than observed by fDM. These data reveal that fDM can serve as an early biomarker for treatment response. Validation of these fDM results was also accomplished by histological examination of excised tumor tissue. Overall, these results indicate that fDM may be useful as an imaging biomarker for assessment of treatment efficacy for metastatic cancer to the bone warranting clinical evaluation.

CLINICAL fDM Assessment of Tumor Response

Translation of diffusion indices from animal studies to the clinic can be hampered due to the typically reduced efficacy of treatments, the extended delivery period requiring fractionated dosage schedules of weeks to months, overlap in cytostructural treatment effects such as cellular necrosis, excess water, debris clearance, and cellular repopulation by disease progression. Thus, the overall heterogeneity of tumor response can be a major confounding factor in assigning a single indicator to patient's tumor response. However, the need for a non-invasive imaging biomarker for assessing tumor treatment response is urgently needed as at present, a comparison of sequential MRI or computed tomography scans is the method of choice for monitoring solid tumor response. Conventional anatomical imaging allows for comparison of parameters such as the change in maximal diameter, cross-sectional tumor area via the product of the maximal perpendicular tumor diameters, or a full tumor volume determination (28). These volumetric indices of response are made between pretreatment scans and images obtained weeks to months after the conclusion of a therapeutic protocol (29) yielding no opportunity to individualize a patient's treatment regimen.

Applications of diffusion MRI in the clinical setting for the purposes of treatment response assessment have been underway for some time. In summary, many of these studies are relatively preliminary with small numbers of patients and have utilized the traditional histogram analysis method limiting sensitivity (13,25,26,30–37). However, several recent studies have been undertaken with the

Week 2   Week 8

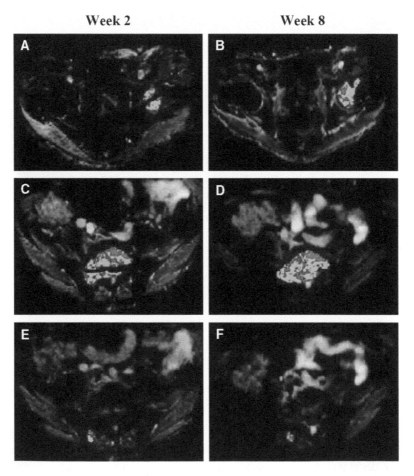

Figure 6 fDMs of a patient with multifocal metastatic prostate cancer to the bone. fDM analysis of the femoral head lesion at (**A**) two weeks and at (**B**) eight weeks after treatment initiation revealed distinct regions of red voxels signifying areas with significant increases in ADC ($>26 \times 10^{-6}$ mm^2/sec). fDM analysis of the sacral lesion at (**C**) two weeks and at (**D**) eight weeks after treatment revealed significant regions of increased ADC as depicted by the red voxels. fDM analysis of the ilium lesion at (**E**) two weeks and (**F**) eight weeks after treatment show large regions of increased ADC values (*red voxels*). *Abbreviations*: fDM, functional diffusion map; ADC, apparent diffusion coefficient. *Source*: From Ref. 38 (*See Color Insert*).

use of fDM for assessment of clinical tumor response in glioma patients (25,26), and a feasibility study with a patient with metastatic prostate cancer to the bone (38). Shown in Figure 6 are a series of fDMs of a patient with metastatic prostate cancer to the femoral head (Fig. 6A, B), sacrum (Fig. 6C, D), and ilium (Fig. 6E, F) at two and eight weeks following treatment initiation, respectively (38). This data reveals that significant detectable changes in spatial tumor diffusion values could be observed and quantified over time and at three different metastatic sites within a patient. The ability to conduct fDM measurements in multiple tumors is a single patient over time opens up interesting possibilities for applying the fDM biomarker to whole-body treatment assessment for multifocal metastatic disease in the future.

The use of fDM for assessment of treatment response in human gliomas (grade III/IV) have also been reported (25,26). These studies reported that treatment-induced alterations in fDM values could be observed as early as 3 weeks into treatment, which were predictive of the radiographic response measured at 10 weeks (25,26). An example of fDM measurements from a nonresponsive (Fig. 7A) and responsive patient (Fig. 7B) is provided. Note the increased amount of spatially varying regions in increased diffusion values within the tumor mass, which responded to ionizing radiation treatment (red voxels, Fig. 7B) compared with that obtained from a nonresponding patient (green voxels, Fig. 7A). Furthermore, glioma patient fDM measurements at three weeks posttreatment initiation provided an early indicator of the eventual clinical responses of disease time to progression and overall survival in patients with malignant glioma (25,26). Taken together, these data support the use of

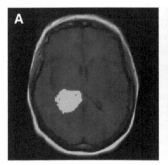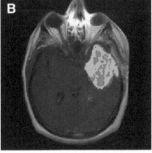

Figure 7 MRI of two patients with glioblastoma multiforme which were treated with six to seven weeks of fractionated ionizing radiation. fDM data shown is at three weeks posttreatment initiation. The regional spatial distributions of ADC changes (fDMs) in a single slice from each tumor are shown as color overlays for a progressive disease (**A**) and a partial response (**B**) patient. The red voxels indicate spatial regions of significantly increased diffusion values, whereas green voxels indicate regions of unchanged ADC. *Abbreviations*: fDM, functional diffusion map; ADC, apparent diffusion coefficient (*See Color Insert*).

fDM for quantification of tumor response and provide for a possible standardized approach for data analysis and reduction of tumor diffusion MR data warranting additional efforts to evaluate the use of diffusion MRI measurements as a biomarker for early treatment response in multicenter clinical trials for further validation.

REFERENCES

1. Warach S, Gaa J, Siewert B, et al. Acute human stroke studied by whole brain echo planar diffusion-weighted magnetic resonance imaging. Ann Neurol 1995; 37(2): 231–241.
2. Guo AC, Cummings TJ, Dash RC, et al. Lymphomas and high-grade astrocytomas: comparison of water diffusibility and histologic characteristics. Radiology 2002; 224(1): 177–183.
3. Takahara T, Imai Y, Yamashita T, et al. Diffusion weighted whole body imaging with background body signal suppression (DWIBS): technical improvement using free breathing, STIR and high resolution 3D display. Radiat Med 2004; 22(4):275–282.
4. Basser PJ, Pierpaoli C. Microstructural and physiological features of tissues elucidated by quantitative-diffusion-tensor MRI. J Magn Reson B 1996; 111(3):209–219.
5. Pierpaoli C, Basser PJ. Toward a quantitative assessment of diffusion anisotropy. Magn Reson Med 1996; 36(6): 893–906.
6. Le Bihan D, Breton E, Lallemand D, et al. Separation of diffusion and perfusion in intravoxel incoherent motion MR imaging. Radiology 1988; 168(2):497–505.
7. Sorensen AG, Buonanno FS, Gonzalez RG, et al. Hyperacute stroke: evaluation with combined multisection diffusion-weighted and hemodynamically weighted echo-planar MR imaging. Radiology 1996; 199(2):391–401.
8. Bammer R. Basic principles of diffusion-weighted imaging. Eur J Radiol 2003; 45(3):169–184.
9. Le Bihan D. Molecular diffusion nuclear magnetic resonance imaging. Magn Reson Q 1991; 7(1):1–30.
10. Ross BD, Chenevert TL, Kim B, et al. Magnetic resonance imaging and spectroscopy: application to experimental neuro-oncology. Q Magn Reson Biol Med 1994; 1:89–106.
11. Chenevert TL, McKeever PE, Ross BD. Monitoring early response of experimental brain tumors to therapy using diffusion magnetic resonance imaging. Clin Cancer Res 1997; 3(9):1457–1466.
12. Lyng H, Haraldseth O, Rofstad EK. Measurement of cell density and necrotic fraction in human melanoma xenografts by diffusion weighted magnetic resonance imaging. Magn Reson Med 2000; 43(6):828–836.
13. Ross BD, Moffat BA, Lawrence TS, et al. Evaluation of cancer therapy using diffusion magnetic resonance imaging. Mol Cancer Ther 2003; 2(6):581–587.
14. Hamstra DA, Lee KC, Tychewicz JM, et al. The use of 19F spectroscopy and diffusion-weighted MRI to evaluate differences in gene-dependent enzyme prodrug therapies. Mol Ther 2004; 10(5):916–928.

15. Lee KC, Hall DE, Hoff BA, et al. Dynamic imaging of emerging resistance during cancer therapy. Cancer Res 2006; 66(9):4687–4692.

16. Lee KC, Hamstra DA, Bhojani MS, et al. Noninvasive molecular imaging sheds light on the synergy between 5-fluorouracil and TRAIL/Apo2L for cancer therapy. Clin Cancer Res 2007; 13(6):1839–1846.

17. Lee KC, Hamstra DA, Bullarayasamudram S, et al. Fusion of the HSV-1 tegument protein vp22 to cytosine deaminase confers enhanced bystander effect and increased therapeutic benefit. Gene Ther 2006; 13(2):127–137.

18. Lee KC, Moffat BA, Schott AF, et al. Prospective early response imaging biomarker for neoadjuvant breast cancer chemotherapy. Clin Cancer Res 2007; 13(2 pt 1):443–450.

19. Lee KC, Sud S, Meyer CR, et al. An imaging biomarker of early treatment response in prostate cancer that has metastasized to the bone. Cancer Res 2007; 67(8):3524–3528.

20. Lyng HO, Haraldseth, Rofstad EK. Measurement of cell density and necrotic fraction in human melanoma xenografts by diffusion weighted magnetic resonance imaging. Magn Reson Med 2000; 43(6):828–836.

21. Galons JP, Altbach MI, Paine-Murrieta GD, et al. Early increases in breast tumor xenograft water mobility in response to paclitaxel therapy detected by non-invasive diffusion magnetic resonance imaging. Neoplasia 1999; 1(2):113–117.

22. Hakumaki JM, Poptani H, Puumalainen AM, et al. Quantitative 1H nuclear magnetic resonance diffusion spectroscopy of BT4C rat glioma during thymidine kinase-mediated gene therapy in vivo: identification of apoptotic response. Cancer Res 1998; 58(17):3791–3799.

23. Poptani H, Puumalainen AM, Grohn OH, et al. Monitoring thymidine kinase and ganciclovir-induced changes in rat malignant glioma in vivo by nuclear magnetic resonance imaging. Cancer Gene Ther 1998; 5(2):101–109.

24. Zhao M, Pipe JG, Bonnett J, et al. Early detection of treatment response by diffusion-weighted 1H-NMR spectroscopy in a murine tumour in vivo. Br J Cancer 1996; 73(1):61–64.

25. Moffat BA, Chenevert TL, Lawrence TS, et al. Functional diffusion map: a noninvasive MRI biomarker for early stratification of clinical brain tumor response. Proc Natl Acad Sci U S A 2005; 102(15):5524–5529.

26. Hamstra DA, Chenevert TL, Moffat BA, et al. Evaluation of the functional diffusion map as an early biomarker of time-to-progression and overall survival in high-grade glioma. Proc Natl Acad Sci U S A 2005; 102(46):16759–16764.

27. Moffat BA, Chenevert TL, Meyer CR, et al. The functional diffusion map: an imaging biomarker for the early prediction of cancer treatment outcome. Neoplasia 2006; 8(4): 259–267.

28. Sorensen AG, Patel S, Harmath C, et al. Comparison of diameter and perimeter methods for tumor volume calculation. J Clin Oncol 2001; 19(2):551–557.

29. Therasse P, Arbuck SG, Eisenhauer EA, et al. New guidelines to evaluate the response to treatment in solid tumors. European Organization for Research and Treatment of Cancer, National Cancer Institute of the United States, National Cancer Institute of Canada. J Natl Cancer Inst 2000; 92(3):205–216.

30. Chenevert TL, Stegman LD, Taylor JM, et al. Diffusion magnetic resonance imaging: an early surrogate marker of therapeutic efficacy in brain tumors. J Natl Cancer Inst 2000; 92(24):2029–2036.

31. Dzik-Jurasz A, Domenig C, George M, et al. Diffusion MRI for prediction of response of rectal cancer to chemoradiation. Lancet 2002; 360(9329):307–308.

32. Hayashida Y, Yakushiji T, Awai K, et al. Monitoring therapeutic responses of primary bone tumors by diffusion-weighted image: initial results. Eur Radiol 2006; 16(12): 2637–2643.

33. Kamel IR, Reyes DK, Liapi E, et al. Functional MR imaging assessment of tumor response after 90Y microsphere treatment in patients with unresectable hepatocellular carcinoma. J Vasc Interv Radiol 2007; 18(1 pt 1):49–56.

34. Mardor Y, Pfeffer R, Spiegelmann R, et al. Early detection of response to radiation therapy in patients with brain malignancies using conventional and high b-value diffusion-weighted magnetic resonance imaging. J Clin Oncol 2003; 21(6):1094–1100.

35. Pickles MD, Gibbs P, Lowry M, et al. Diffusion changes precede size reduction in neoadjuvant treatment of breast cancer. Magn Reson Imaging 2006; 24(7):843–847.

36. Theilmann RJ, Borders R, Trouard TP, et al. Changes in water mobility measured by diffusion MRI predict response of metastatic breast cancer to chemotherapy. Neoplasia 2004; 6(6):831–837.

37. Uhl M, Saueressig U, van Buiren M, et al. Osteosarcoma: preliminary results of in vivo assessment of tumor necrosis after chemotherapy with diffusion- and perfusion-weighted magnetic resonance imaging. Invest Radiol 2006; 41(8): 618–623.

38. Lee KC, Bradley DA, Hussain M, et al. A feasibility study evaluating the functional diffusion map as a predictive imaging biomarker for detection of treatment response in a patient with metastatic prostate cancer to the bone. Neoplasia 2007; 9(12):1003–1011.

39

Molecular Imaging of Breast Cancer

JEAN H. LEE

Department of Radiology, University of Washington and Seattle Cancer Care Alliance, Seattle, Washington, U.S.A.

LAVANYA SUNDARARAJAN

Department of Medicine, University of Washington and Seattle Cancer Care Alliance, Seattle, Washington, U.S.A.

WILLIAM B. EUBANK

Department of Radiology, University of Washington and Puget Sound VA Medical Center, Seattle, Washington, U.S.A.

DAVID A. MANKOFF

Departments of Radiology and Medicine, University of Washington and Seattle Cancer Care Alliance, Seattle, Washington, U.S.A.

INTRODUCTION

^{18}F-fluorodeoxyglucose positron emission tomography (FDG PET) has proven to be a useful clinical tool to help guide breast cancer treatment, and is increasingly used in the care of breast cancer patients, particular for staging of recurrent or metastatic breast cancer and monitoring response to treatment. While FDG is the dominant tracer for clinical PET imaging of breast cancer, the typical applications thus far represent what potentially is just a small part of what PET can do for breast cancer patients. More sophisticated analysis of FDG PET studies, and especially PET using tracers other than FDG, have yielded insights into the in vivo biology of breast cancer in early studies and are likely to contribute to breast cancer care in the future. Particularly as breast cancer treatment moves toward more individualized, targeted

therapy (1), the ability to characterize the in vivo tumor phenotype will play a key role in the selection of therapy and evaluation of it efficacy. PET imaging is well suited to guide targeted breast cancer therapy by evaluating the presence or absence of specific targets, identifying resistant phenotypes, and measuring early response to treatment. These applications are highlighted in this review. We first discuss recent data using more detailed analyses of FDG PET studies to gain insight into tumor response and resistance and then discuss PET imaging of breast cancer with radiopharmaceuticals other than FDG, with an emphasis on early studies in patients. The reader is referred to recent reviews of the use of FDG PET in breast cancer for more detailed discussion of the current role of FDG PET in clinical breast cancer management, including the chapter on clinical PET molecular imaging elsewhere in this text (2–4).

FDG PET OF BREAST CANCER: DETAILED ANALYSES

The scientific framework for FDG PET dates back to the work of Sokoloff and colleagues, who developed methods using ^{14}C-labeled deoxyglucose autoradiography to measure the regional cerebral glucose metabolic rate in animals (5). Subsequently, ^{18}F-fluorodexoyglucose (FDG) was developed to provide the same capability using PET imaging to quantify the regional concentration of the ^{18}F label in humans (6,7). FDG is transported into cells and phosphorylated in parallel to glucose; however, the presence of a fluorine atom, instead of a hydroxyl group, at the two-position prevents FDG from being a substrate for steps further down the glycolytic pathway (Fig. 1a). In most tissues, phosphorylated FDG (FDG-6P) is slowly, if at all, dephosphorylated, trapping the label in cells and providing an indication of metabolic rate.

In clinical practice, FDG PET scans are typically evaluated qualitatively and semiquantitatively using simple static uptake measures such as standardized uptake value (SUV). However, more detailed analysis of the kinetics of FDG obtained from dynamic PET imaging yields additional information on tumor biology. The most detailed method for quantifying regional glucose metabolism uses dynamic PET imaging to capture the tissue uptake curve from the time of injection until over 60 to 90 minutes postinjection, with blood sampling or imaging of a blood-pool structure such as the left ventricle to measure the blood-clearance curve (8,9). These data are applied to a compartmental model to estimate rate constants. The metabolic rate of glucose measured by FDG PET, sometimes termed the metabolic rate of FDG (MRFDG), is calculated from the flux of FDG from the blood to the phosphorylated state and calculated from individual rate constants as illustrated in Figure 1b (10). MRFDG is then estimated by the following:

$$MRFDG = [Glucose]K_i$$

where [Glucose] is the plasma glucose concentration (μmoles/mL), K_i is the flux constant from compartmental

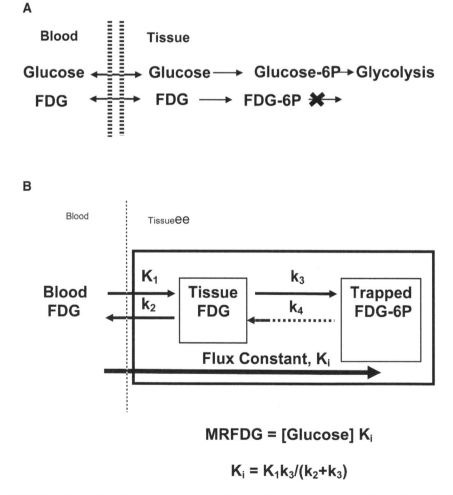

Figure 1 Diagram of FDG biochemical pathways compared to glucose (**A**) and compartmental model of FDG kinetics (**B**).

analysis (mL/min/g) and MRFDG is given in μmoles/min/g. This formulation does not assume a value for relative glycolytic flux of FDG and glucose, the so-called "lumped constant" used in the original Sokoloff formulation (5), but rather describes glucose metabolic rate as assessed using FDG (11).

The use of more rigorous analysis provides some insights not possible by simple measures such as SUV. Particularly for evaluating response, the added precision of more rigorous analysis of dynamic images may increase the ability to quantify response (12). While the MRFDG estimates the rate of FDG phosphorylation, SUV includes both phosphorylated FDG as well as non-phosphorylated FDG, whose presence is not necessarily related to glucose metabolism. Unincorporated FDG forms a background minimum value close to SUV = 1, which diminishes the ability to measure changes with response, especially for tumor with lower pre-therapy FDG uptake (8). Since cells accumulate FDG as long as it is present in the blood, SUV can change considerably with time, as much as 30% over 10 to 15 minutes (13,14). The variations in the injection to scan time in serial scans can confound response measurements. This is not the case for dynamic imaging and estimation of MRFDG.

In addition to more precise measurement of uptake, dynamic FDG PET with kinetic analysis provides information on the delivery and transport of FDG, in addition to its phosphorylation. Several studies have shown that the FDG blood-tissue transport constant, K_1, correlated with blood flow measured by ^{15}O-water (15,16). As changes in blood flow have been shown to be highly predictive of response and outcome in breast cancer treated with chemotherapy (17,18), dynamic FDG imaging and compartmental modeling may provide valuable insights into response not possible from simple static imaging. This may also be important in evaluating response to anti-vascular agents, such as bevacizumab (Avastin), which have shown promise in treating breast cancer (1).

Recent data using drugs targeted to growth factor pathways, such as imatinib in the treatment of gastrointestinal stromal tumor (GIST), suggests that alterations in glycolysis, and therefore, FDG uptake, occur within one to two days of starting treatment (19,20). Similar effects have been seen in early studies of animal models of mouse anti-neu therapy, the mouse equivalent of trastuzumab in humans from our center. The exact mechanism of this early change is unknown, with some recent studies implicating a rapid decline in glucose transporter expression (21); however, more studies are needed to elucidate the precise mechanism underlying these very interesting findings (22). Dynamic FDG and kinetic analysis may be able to address these interesting and important issues.

BEYOND FDG: PET IMAGING OF TUMOR BIOLOGY IN BREAST CANCER

As breast cancer treatment becomes more targeted, sophisticated, and individualized to each patient and her (or his) tumor's biologic characteristics, more specific PET radiopharmaceuticals may help guide treatment selection and evaluate treatment response (23). PET can help guide treatment selection by (i) quantifying the therapeutic target, (ii) identifying resistance factors and (iii) measuring early response to therapy. The most commonly exploited target in breast cancer is the estrogen receptor (ER) (24). Breast cancer can also express other targets such as HER2, EGFR, integrin, and angiogenic factors (1). Therefore, identifying the specific target will help determine treatment selection. However, even when a breast tumor expresses appropriate level of target, targeted therapy may fail if the tumor has characteristics that will render it resistant or ineffective to the chosen treatment. With many potentially effective treatments to choose from, detecting potential drug resistance factors before first-line chemotherapy or identifying ineffective treatment early after initiation would lead to more effective and successful treatment. The ability to measure the therapeutic target, specific resistance factors, and early response underlies the emerging role of PET in early drug testing (25). This section of review will discuss specific examples of how PET might be used in breast cancer for each task.

Quantifying Therapeutic Targets

Specific targeted treatment plays an increasing role in individualized breast cancer treatment, and imaging may play a role in target identification. Current examples of the PET imaging to measure target expression in addition to ER include HER2 imaging (26), imaging angiogenesis both nonspecifically by measuring blood flow (16,27) or by measuring specific components expressed in neovessels (28), and measuring novel targets such as matrix metalloproteins (MMPs) (29).

HER 2 Imaging

Some investigators have successfully imaged HER2 in breast cancer animal models and have shown that PET can quantify HER2 expression and predict early response after chemotherapy in animal studies (26,30). Smith-Jones and colleagues found that HER2 PET using ^{68}Ga-labeled trastuzumab fragments was able to measure pharmacodynamic changes in response to experimental treatment using HSP90 inhibitors (30). These drug target HSP90, a "chaperone" molecule important in membrane expression of HER2. With anti-HSP90 therapy, HER2 PET showed an early decline in HER2 expression in animal models, demonstrating the value of HER2 PET for measuring the pharmacodynamics of HER2-targeted therapy.

Imaging Blood Flow and Angiogenesis

Imaging of angiogenesis by several methods is under active investigation. One way to examine tumor vasculature indirectly is by measuring tumor perfusion. Based on the work of Beaney and colleagues (31) and Wilson and colleagues (27), several studies have used ^{15}O-water to measure breast cancer blood flow.

Measuring blood flow by ^{15}O-water PET can be used as a tool for monitoring treatment response. In serial ^{15}O-water PET studies over the course of neoadjuvant chemotherapy of locally advanced breast cancer, Mankoff and colleagues (18) found that change in midtherapy tumor blood flow was an excellent predictor of response and of patient outcome. Patients who responded to neoadjuvant chemotherapy had an average decline in tumor blood flow, whereas nonresponders had an average increase in blood flow. Furthermore, residual blood flow at midtherapy predicted both disease-free and overall survival; lower midtherapy blood flow was associated with better survival.

The comparison of tumor metabolism and blood flow using FDG and water PET has yielded additional insights. Metabolism and blood flow are generally coupled in normal tissues, and prior studies have shown some correlation between blood flow and metabolism in breast cancer (16). However, some recent studies have suggested that blood flow and metabolism are not always matched in breast cancer and that measuring blood flow provides tumor biologic information that is often independent of metabolism. Mankoff and coworkers found that a blood flow–metabolism mismatch, in form of high FDG metabolism relative to blood volume in locally advanced breast cancer, was an indicator of poorer response to neoadjuvant chemotherapy (32). Similar findings have been seen in comparisons of dynamic contrast enhanced MRI and FDG PET (33).

Imaging approaches that directly target specific components expressed in neovessels [e.g., integrins, vascular endothelial growth factor receptor (VEGF)] have been developed to image angiogenesis directly and to evaluate the efficacy of anti-angiogenic drugs (28). Molecules targeted for imaging are those that play a key role in angiogenesis and metastasis; therefore, in vivo identification of these targets will help facilitate new therapeutic and diagnostic strategies. Recently, Beer and colleagues have successfully demonstrated ability to visualize integrin alpha(v)beta3 expression in human by ^{18}F galacto-RDG PET (34). Cai and colleagues demonstrated the ability to visualize VEGF expression in vivo by VEGF-PET (35). This type of imaging may provide specific predictive value for therapy directed at tumor angiogenesis, such as bevacizumab (Avastin) (36).

Related to angiogenesis are imaging agents to more directly image tumor invasion. Methods for imaging MMPs (29,37,38), key factors in tissue invasion, are being developed. Overexpression of MMPs, particularly MMP-2 and MMP-9, has been correlated with poor prognosis in several cancer types including breast cancer. Detecting MMP expression may allow better selection of patients for more aggressive cancer therapy and may be useful for therapy directed against MMPs. Measuring these novel targets is under active research development (29,37,38).

Imaging ER Expression

Perhaps the best-studied, non-glycloytic target in breast cancer is the ER (24). The majority of breast cancers express ER (39). Clinical factors related to hormone sensitivity include a long disease-free interval, metastasis to non-visceral sites, and high quantitative levels of ER in the tumor (40). Although measures of ER expression by in vitro assay of biopsy material predict benefit from hormonal treatment in 30% to 70% of patients, objective response is seen in a smaller subset of patients, especially those with advanced disease or prior endocrine treatment failure (41–46). Furthermore biopsy to determine ER expression in metastatic breast cancer is associated with significant morbidity and sampling error. The need for decalcification of biopsy material from bone metastases, a common site of breast cancer spread, results in loss of ERs making it difficult to assess ER expression (41). Some tumors will alter ER expression over the course of treatment and progression, most typically losing ER expression in previously ER+ tumors (47,48). These considerations make the development of a method for assessing regional ER expression in breast cancer in vivo highly desirable.

A number of agents have been tested for PET ER imaging (49). Work with 16-alpha-^{18}F-fluoro-17-beta-estradiol (FES) has been the most promising to date (50). Radiation dosimetry studies show organ doses with FES PET are comparable to those associated with other commonly performed nuclear studies and potential radiation risks are well within accepted limits. The effective dose equivalent was 80 mrem/mCi and the organ that received the highest dose was the liver at 470 mrad/mCi (51).

FES has binding characteristics similar to estradiol for both the ER and its transport protein sex hormone–binding globulin (SHBG) or sex steroid–binding protein (SBP) (52). Blood-clearance curves and protein interactions of FES have been studied in humans and animals. FES is rapidly metabolized in the liver, largely to sulfate, and glucuronidate conjugates of FES (53). Typically in humans, about 45% of ^{18}F-FES in circulating plasma is bound to SHBG and is distributed between albumin and SHBG with equilibrium maintained under most circumstances (51,54). By 30 minutes after injection, blood clearance and washout of nonspecifically bound FES are sufficient to permit good quality ER imaging (53).

FES uptake has been validated as a measure of ER expression against in vitro assay of biopsy material in breast tumors. Mintun et al. (55) showed an excellent correlation between FES uptake within the primary tumor measured on PET images and the tumor ER concentration measured in vitro after excision in 13 patients with primary breast masses. FES uptake was seen at sites of primary carcinoma, axillary nodes, and one distant metastatic site. FES results in this study were reported qualitatively as positive or negative (55). They then extended the use of this radiopharmaceutical for imaging of metastatic breast cancer. Sixteen patients with metastatic disease underwent FES PET imaging with increased uptake seen on 53 of the 57 metastatic lesions resulting in a 93% sensitivity and only two apparent false positives (56). Imaging results were reported quantitatively as percentage uptake of injected dose per mL, ratio of lesion to soft tissue, ratio of lesion to uninvolved bone. These results were reproduced by the same group in a subsequent study of FES imaging in 21 patients with metastatic breast cancer with 88% overall agreement between in vitro ER assays and FES PET (57). In addition to subjective analysis, FES uptake in this study was reported quantitatively SUV (57). Using an SUV > 1 to determine hormone-sensitive disease, sensitivity of FES imaging was 76% with no false positives in 21 metastatic breast cancer patients (58).

Comparison of ER immunohistochemistry (IHC), now the method of choice for clinical determination of ER expression also shows good correlation between FES uptake and in vitro assay (59).

Heterogeneity of FES uptake as an indicator of heterogeneity of ER expression at metastatic sites has been well demonstrated (58,60). Mortimer et al. found that 4 of 17 patients with metastatic breast cancer had discordance in FES uptake (58). Mankoff et al. (60) found total absence of FES uptake in one or more metastatic sites in 10% of patients and calculated heterogeneity of FES uptake as coefficient of variation (COV). Thirteen percent of patients (6 of 47) with ER-positive primaries had one or more sites of FES-negative disease in a subsequent study by the same group (61).

Serial FES PET can measure the effect of endocrine therapy on estradiol binding to ER. In early studies, McGuire showed that tumor FES uptake decreased significantly after treatment with tamoxifen (56), a mixed ER agonist/antagonist. Mortimer showed that the early decline in FES uptake with tamoxifen therapy predicted response (40). Linden et al. showed differences in the effect on FES uptake for aromatase inhibitors (AIs), which reduce the concentration of the agonist, estradiol, versus

ER blockers like tamoxifen and fulvestrant (62). The decline in FES in SUV was greater for antagonists versus AIs. Posttreatment qualitative FES uptake showed complete blockage with tamoxifen but incomplete blockage with fulvestrant in 4 of the 5 patients. These studies show the potential benefit of imaging a therapeutic target to identify pharmacodynamic changes in response to targeted therapy.

Perhaps most relevant to clinical breast cancer practice, early studies have suggested that FES PET may be useful as a predictive assay for breast cancer endocrine treatment, in analogy to the accepted use of in vitro ER assays (63) (Fig. 3). Mortimer et al. showed that the level of FES uptake predicted response to tamoxifen in the locally advanced and metastatic setting (40). Forty women with biopsy proven ER-positive breast cancer had FES PET before and 7 to 10 days after initiation of tamoxifen therapy and tumor FES PET was assessed semiquantitatively with the SUV method. The level FES uptake pretherapy also predicted response to tamoxifen. The positive and negative predictive value for baseline FES uptake using a arbitrarily selected cutoff of SUV of 2.0 were 79% and 88%, respectively (40).

Linden et al. showed that initial FES uptake measurements in patients with ER-positive tumors correlated with subsequent tumor response to six months of hormonal therapy (64). Forty-seven heavily pretreated patients with ER-positive, metastatic breast cancer, were given predominantly salvage AI therapy. Objective response was seen in 11/47 patients or 23%. FES PET measurements were performed qualitatively and quantitatively using SUV and flux calculations as described previously. Qualitative FES PET results did not significantly predict response to hormonal therapy. However, in quantitative analysis, 0/15 patients with initial SUV < 1.5 responded to hormonal therapy as compared with 11/32 (34%) patients with initial SUV > 1.5. In patients with no HER2 over-expression, 11/24 (46%) of patients with SUV > 1.5 responded. Hypothetically using FES PET to select patients could have increased the response rate from 23% to 34% overall and from 29% to 46% in the subset of patients lacking HER2 over-expression.

Limitations of FES PET highlighted by these studies include difficulty in predicting stable disease in response to hormonal therapy. Stable disease includes patients with slow-growing disease independent of treatment and patients with rapidly progressive disease in whom the hormonal therapy slows but does not eradicate disease. FES PET cannot, at the current time, distinguish these two disease categories. Most studies on FES PET have not used uniform and rigorous eligibility criteria. Future trials, which are prospective, multi-institutional, and with uniform selection criteria and treatment regimens are warranted on the basis of currently available evidence.

Concomitant FES PET and hormonal treatment trials would also be beneficial. Such trials should be feasible with cooperative networks to test new diagnostic imaging agents.

Identifying Resistance Factors

If an individual tumor has biologic characteristics that render it resistant to therapeutic agents, the treatment, even if it is designed to target-specific molecular interactions, will be ineffective. Some of the known examples of resistance factors include tumor hypoxia for radiotherapy and cytotoxic chemotherapy (65,66) and the expression of P-glycoprotein (P-gp) for doxorubicin, taxanes, and other chemotherapeutic agents that are P-gp substrates (67).

Imaging Hypoxia

Tumor hypoxia imaging with PET has received considerable attention and has undergone preliminary human testing for a number of tumors, including breast cancer. Hypoxia results from an imbalance between the supply and consumption of oxygen. Major pathogenetic mechanisms for the hypoxia are (*i*) structural and functional abnormalities in the tumor microvasculature, (*ii*) an adverse diffusion geometry, and (*iii*) tumor-related and therapy-induced anemia leading to a reduced oxygen transport capacity of the blood (68). There are a number of consequences associated with tumor hypoxia including resistance to ionizing radiation, resistance to chemotherapy, and the amplification of mutated p53. In addition, tissue hypoxia has been regarded as a key factor for tumor aggressiveness and metastasis by activation of signal transduction pathways and gene-regulatory mechanisms (65,69). It is clear that hypoxia in solid tumors promotes a strong oncogenic phenotype and is a phenomenon that occurs in all solid tumors.

Although severe hypoxia is rare in small breast tumors, data from oxygen electrodes suggests that up to 30% of larger and more advanced breast cancers exhibit severe hypoxia in part of the cancer (70). Although hypoxia likely contributes to increased rate of glycolysis, a study in patients with a variety of tumor types, including breast cancer, showed that hypoxia could not be simply predicted by FDG uptake (71). Several PET agents specifically designed to image tumor hypoxia have been tested for hypoxia imaging. Of these, ^{18}F-fluoromisonidazole (FMISO) has the largest current body of preclinical validation studies and clinical experience (72). FMISO has nitro aromatic compounds that bind to hypoxic cells. It diffuses easily into hypoxic cells because of their high solubility and relative low metabolism (72). A preliminary study at our center that included large primary and

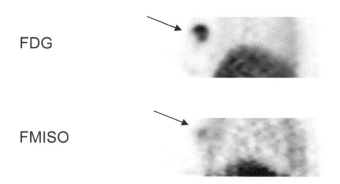

FDG

FMISO

Figure 2 Breast tumor hypoxia imaged by FMISO PET. A patient with a large, locally advanced right breast tumor underwent FDG and FMISO PET pre-therapy (*top and bottom*) Images are thick sagittal images, similar to MLO mammography views. The pre-therapy FDG study showed uniformly high FDG uptake throughout the tumor. FMISO PET showed uptake suggestive of tumor hypoxia, but only close to the center of the tumor. Residual viable tumor at the approximate location of the FMISO uptake was seen on the post-therapy FDG PET scan (not shown) and was found at surgery.

metastatic breast cancers showed that approximately one-third of tumors had one or more areas of severe hypoxia by ^{18}F-fluoromisonidazole PET (71). Other PET hypoxia tracers have been studied in patients (73). PET hypoxia imaging may provide a means for selecting alternate therapeutic strategies in tumors resistant to standard treatment on the basis of hypoxia (Fig. 2).

Imaging Drug Transport

Another area of active investigation is identifying mechanisms of drug resistance with drug efflux proteins, in particular, P-gp. P-gp is a membrane transport protein for which a number of xenobiotics (67) are substrates and may mediate enhanced efflux of a number of chemotherapeutic agents, including agents like doxorubicin and paclitaxel that are important in breast cancer treatment. P-gp is expressed on cell membranes of various organs (e.g., blood-brain barrier) and some solid tumors, including breast cancer. Therefore, it may cause drug resistance that could lead to chemotherapy failure in cancer treatment. Based on observations by Pinwica-Worms and others (74), Ciamello observed that enhanced washout of the SPECT agent, ^{99m}Tc-sestamibi (MIBI)-predicted resistance to epirubicin-based therapy (75). However, interpretation of MIBI images is confounded by blood flow, which is an important factor in MIBI's uptake and washout (76). Alternate PET tracers such as ^{11}C-verapamil have been developed as agents for imaging P-gp transport (77). We have recently shown that verapamil PET can be used to measure effect of P-gp inhibition on drug transport into the brain (78) and other agents have also been tested for use in tumors (79).

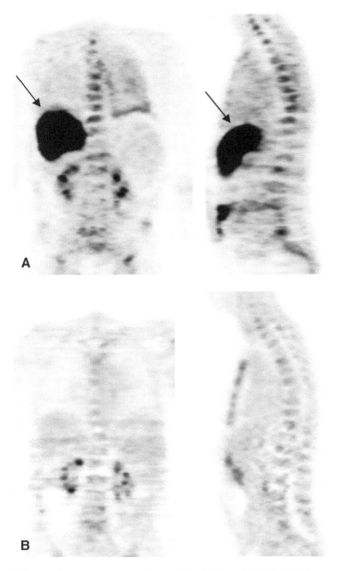

Figure 3 Breast cancer imaged by FES and FDG PET in a patient with progression on an aromatase inhibitor shows (**A**) diffusely increased FES uptake in bone disease in the axial skeleton corresponding to areas of diffusely, but mildly increased, uptake on FDG PET images and (**B**) suggesting strongly ER-expressing disease. Normal liver metabolism in the FES image is also seen (*arrows*). The patient subsequently responded to alternative endocrine therapy.

Measuring Early Response

As the choice of breast cancer treatments expands, there will be an increasing need to measure the efficacy of treatments early in the course of treatment. Therefore, identifying ineffective treatment early after initiation of therapy will play an important role in better care of the patient. However, this poses several challenges. A decrease in tumor size, the current standard for therapeutic monitoring, is a late event in response to treatment; it is,

therefore, desirable to measure response well before significant changes in tumor size. Additionally, some new therapies may be cytostatic rather than cytoreductive, in which case, successful treatment may not lead to a decrease in tumor size at all (1). Studies of FDG PET after a single dose of chemotherapy have supported ability of in vivo biochemical imaging to measure early response (80,81). It is likely that tracers more specifically designed to image tumor biology related to cell growth and cell death will provide even better early response measures.

Imaging Cellular Proliferation

Decreased tumor proliferation is an early event in response to successful treatment (82). This underlies the use of labeled thymidine and analogs to image cellular proliferation and early response to treatment (83). Thymidine is incorporated into DNA, but not RNA; therefore, thymidine uptake and retention in the tumor serves as a specific marker of cell growth (82). Studies using ^{11}C-thymidine and PET showed promise in assessing response, especially early response (83). Because of the short half-life of [11]C (approximately 20 minutes) and extensive metabolism of thymidine, ^{11}C-thymidine is not practical for routine clinical use outside of academic centers. This accelerated the development of ^{18}F-labeled, non-metabolized thymidine analogs to image tumor proliferation. The most promising thus far is ^{18}F-fluorothymidine (FLT) (84). Studies in several tumor types have shown that FLT uptake correlates with in vitro measures of proliferation performed on biopsy specimen (83). FLT has been preliminarily tested in breast cancer patients (85); FLT PET showed significant correlation with tumor marker levels, tumor size, and eventual treatment response (86). A recent study showed FLT to be effective in measuring response after a single cycle of chemotherapy and showed a high degree of reproducibility (10–15% difference or less) for repeat measures of FLT uptake (87). These early studies suggest great promise for FLT PET as a measure of early breast cancer response to treatment.

Imaging Cell Death

Besides an early decline in cell growth, effective therapy often leads to an early increase in cell death, typically by apoptosis (88). Radiolabeled annexin V is an ideal probe for in vivo apoptosis detection owing to its strong affinity for phosphatidylserine, the molecular flag on the surface of apoptotic cells (89). The SPECT agent ^{99m}Tc-annexin V has shown promise as a way to image apoptosis in vivo (90). Annexin tracers labeled for use in PET offer better image quality and quantification, and have undergone preliminary validation in animal model (91). The ability to image both changes in cell proliferation and cell death in response to treatment will be an effective means of characterizing how tumors respond to targeted therapy.

SUMMARY

FDG PET is currently clinically used for staging breast cancer and measuring response to therapy. As breast cancer treatment moves toward individualized, targeted therapy, other PET tracers such as FES, will help to better characterize tumor biology and more effectively measure response to therapy, even earlier than FDG PET. In addition, more detailed quantitative analysis of PET images for FDG and other tracers may yield additional insights and value in guiding therapy. The future use of PET radiopharmaceuticals other than FDG will help guide and monitor breast cancer therapy by the in vivo identification of therapeutic targets and resistance factors and by determining response early in the course of therapy.

ACKNOWLEDGMENT

Supported by NIH grants CA42005, CA 72064, CA 90771, and S10 RR17229.

REFERENCES

1. Kaklamani V, O'Regan RM. New targeted therapies in breast cancer. Semin Oncol 2004; 31(2 suppl 4):20–25.
2. Benard F, Turcotte E. Imaging in breast cancer: single-photon computed tomography and positron-emission tomography. Breast Cancer Res 2005; 7(4):153–162.
3. Eubank WB, Mankoff DA. Evolving role of positron emission tomography in breast cancer imaging. Semin Nucl Med 2005; 35(2):84–99.
4. Podoloff DA, Advani RH, Allred C, et al. NCCN task force report: positron emission tomography (PET)/computed tomography (CT) scanning in cancer. J Natl Compr Canc Netw 2007; 5(suppl 1):S1–S22; quiz S23–32.
5. Sokoloff L, Reivich M, Kennedy C, et al. The [14C]-deoxyglucose method for the measurement of local cerebral glucose utilization: theory, procedure, and normal values in the conscious and anesthetized albino rat. J Neurochem 1977; 28:897–916.
6. Phelps M, Huang S, Hoffman E. Tomographic measurement of local cerebral glucose metabolic rate in humans with (18F)2-fluoro-2-deoxy-D-glucose: validation of method. Ann Neurol 1979; 6(5):371–388.
7. Reivich M, Alavi A, Wolf A, et al. Glucose metabolic rate kinetic model parameter determination in humans: the lumped constant and rate constants for [18F]fluorodeoxy-glucose and [11C]deoxyglucose. J Cereb Blood Flow Metab 1985; 5:179–192.
8. Huang S-C. Anatomy of SUV. Nucl Med Biol 2000; 27:643–646.
9. Mankoff DA, Muzi M, Krohn KA. Quantitative positron emission tomography imaging to measure tumor response to therapy: what is the best method? Mol Imaging Biol 2003; 5(5):281–285.
10. Mankoff DA, Muzi M, Zabib H. Quantitative analysis of nuclear oncologic images. In: Zabib H, ed. Quantitative Analysis of Nuclear Medicine Images. Hingham, MA: Springer, 2004.
11. Spence AM, Muzi M, Graham MM, et al. Glucose metabolism in human malignant gliomas measured quantitatively with PET, 1-[C-11]glucose and FDG: analysis of the FDG lumped constant. J Nucl Med 1998; 39(3):440–448.
12. Hoekstra CJ, Paglianiti I, Hoekstra OS, et al. Monitoring response to therapy in cancer using [18F]-2-fluoro-2-deoxy-D-glucose and positron emission tomography: an overview of different analytical methods. Eur J Nucl Med 2000; 27:731–743.
13. Beaulieu S, Kinahan P, Tseng J, et al. SUV varies with time after injection in (18)F-FDG PET of breast cancer: characterization and method to adjust for time differences. J Nucl Med 2003; 44(7):1044–1050.
14. Thie JA, Hubner KF, Smith GT. Optimizing imaging time for improved performance in oncology PET studies. Mol Imaging Biol 2002; 4(3):238–244.
15. Tseng J, Dunnwald LK, Schubert EK, et al. 18F-FDG kinetics in locally advanced breast cancer: correlation with tumor blood flow and changes in response to neoadjuvant chemotherapy. J Nucl Med 2004; 45(11): 1829–1837.
16. Zasadny KR, Tatsumi M, Wahl RL. FDG metabolism and uptake versus blood flow in women with untreated primary breast cancers. Eur J Nucl Med Mol Imaging 2003; 30(2):274–280.
17. Dunnwald LK, Gralow JR, Ellis GK, et al. Residual tumor uptake of [99mTc]-sestamibi after neoadjuvant chemotherapy for locally advanced breast carcinoma predicts survival. Cancer 2005; 103(4):680–688.
18. Mankoff DA, Dunnwald LK, Gralow JR, et al. Changes in blood flow and metabolism in locally advanced breast cancer treated with neoadjuvant chemotherapy. J Nucl Med 2003; 44(11):1806–1814.
19. Gayed I, Vu T, Iyer R, et al. The role of 18F-FDG PET in staging and early prediction of response to therapy of recurrent gastrointestinal stromal tumors. J Nucl Med 2004; 45(1):17–21.
20. Stroobants S, Goeminne J, Seegers M, et al. 18FDG-Positron emission tomography for the early prediction of response in advanced soft tissue sarcoma treated with imatinib mesylate (Glivec). Eur J Cancer 2003; 39(14):2012–2020.
21. Su H, Bodenstein C, Dumont RA, et al. Monitoring tumor glucose utilization by positron emission tomography for the prediction of treatment response to epidermal growth factor receptor kinase inhibitors. Clin Cancer Res 2006; 12(19): 5659–5667.
22. Linden HM, Krohn KA, Livingston RB, et al. Monitoring targeted therapy: is fluorodeoxylucose uptake a marker of early response? Clin Cancer Res 2006; 12(19):5608–5610.
23. Mankoff DA, O'Sullivan F, Barlow WE, et al. Molecular imaging research in the outcomes era: measuring outcomes

for individualized cancer therapy. Acad Radiol 2007; 14(4):398–405.

24. Sledge GJ, McGuire W. Steroid hormone receptors in human breast cancer. Adv Cancer Res 1983; 38:61–75.

25. Aboagye EO, Price PM. Use of positron emission tomography in anticancer drug development. Invest New Drugs 2003; 21(2):169–181.

26. Gonzalez Trotter DE, Manjeshwar RM, Doss M, et al. Quantitation of small-animal (124)I activity distributions using a clinical PET/CT scanner. J Nucl Med 2004; 45(7):1237–1244.

27. Wilson CBJH, Lammertsma AA, McKenzie CG, et al. Measurements of blood flow and exchanging water space in breast tumors using positron emission tomography: a rapid and non-invasive dynamic method. Cancer Res 1992; 52:1592–1597.

28. Haubner R, Wester HJ, Burkhart F, et al. Glycosylated RGD-containing peptides: tracer for tumor targeting and angiogenesis imaging with improved biokinetics. J Nucl Med 2001; 42(2):326–336.

29. Zheng QH, Fei X, Liu X, et al. Synthesis and preliminary biological evaluation of MMP inhibitor radiotracers [^{11}C]-methyl-halo-CGS 27023A analogs, new potential PET breast cancer imaging agents. Nucl Med Biol 2002; 29(7):761–770.

30. Smith-Jones PM, Solit DB, Akhurst T, et al. Imaging the pharmacodynamics of HER2 degradation in response to Hsp90 inhibitors. Nat Biotechnol 2004; 22(6):701–706.

31. Beaney R, Jones T, Lammertsma A, et al. Positron emission tomography for in-vivo measurement of regional blood flow, oxygen utilisation, and blood volume in patients with breast carcinoma. Lancet 1984; 1(8369):131–134.

32. Mankoff DA, Dunnwald LK, Gralow JR, et al. Blood flow and metabolism in locally advanced breast cancer: relationship to response to therapy. J Nucl Med 2002; 43(4):500–509.

33. Semple SI, Gilbert FJ, Redpath TW, et al. The relationship between vascular and metabolic characteristics of primary breast tumours. Eur Radiol 2004; 14(11):2038–2045.

34. Beer AJ, Haubner R, Sarbia M, et al. Positron emission tomography using [^{18}F]Galacto-RGD identifies the level of integrin alpha(v)beta3 expression in man. Clin Cancer Res 2006; 12(13):3942–3949.

35. Cai W, Chen K, Mohamedali KA, et al. PET of vascular endothelial growth factor receptor expression. J Nucl Med 2006; 47(12):2048–2056.

36. Link JS, Waisman JR, Nguyen B, et al. Bevacizumab and albumin-bound paclitaxel treatment in metastatic breast cancer. Clin Breast Cancer 2007; 7(10):779–783.

37. Wagner S, Breyholz HJ, Faust A, et al. Molecular imaging of matrix metalloproteinases in vivo using small molecule inhibitors for SPECT and PET. Curr Med Chem 2006; 13(23):2819–2838.

38. Sprague JE, Li WP, Liang K, et al. In vitro and in vivo investigation of matrix metalloproteinase expression in metastatic tumor models. Nucl Med Biol 2006; 33(2):227–237.

39. Pujol P, Hilsenbeck SG, Chamness GC, et al. Rising levels of estrogen receptor in breast cancer over 2 decades. Cancer 1994; 74(5):1601–1606.

40. Mortimer JE, Dehdashti F, Siegel BA, et al. Metabolic flare: indicator of hormone responsiveness in advanced breast cancer. J Clin Oncol 2001; 19(11):2797–2803.

41. Briasoulis E, Karavasilis V, Kostadima L, et al. Metastatic breast carcinoma confined to bone: portrait of a clinical entity. Cancer 2004; 101(7):1524–1528.

42. Osborne CK, Yochmowitz MG, Knight WA 3rd, et al. The value of estrogen and progesterone receptors in the treatment of breast cancer. Cancer 1980; 46(12 suppl):2884–2888.

43. Bloom ND, Tobin EH, Schreibman B, et al. The role of progesterone receptors in the management of advanced breast cancer. Cancer 1980; 45(12):2992–2997.

44. Mouridsen H, Gershanovich M, Sun Y, et al. Superior efficacy of letrozole versus tamoxifen as first-line therapy for postmenopausal women with advanced breast cancer: results of a phase III study of the International Letrozole Breast Cancer Group. J Clin Oncol 2001;19(10):2596–2606.

45. Nabholtz JM, Buzdar A, Pollak M, et al., for the Arimidex Study Group. Anastrozole is superior to tamoxifen as first-line therapy for advanced breast cancer in postmenopausal women: results of a North American multicenter randomized trial. J Clin Oncol 2000; 18(22):3758–3767.

46. Buzdar A, Douma J, Davidson N, et al. Phase III, multicenter, double-blind, randomized study of letrozole, an aromatase inhibitor, for advanced breast cancer versus megestrol acetate. J Clin Oncol 2001; 19(14):3357–3366.

47. Spataro V, Price K, Goldhirsch A, et al., for the International Breast Cancer Study Group (formerly Ludwig Group). Sequential estrogen receptor determinations from primary breast cancer and at relapse: prognostic and therapeutic relevance. Ann Oncol 1992; 3(9):733–740.

48. Kuukasjarvi T, Kononen J, Helin H, et al. Loss of estrogen receptor in recurrent breast cancer is associated with poor response to endocrine therapy. J Clin Oncol 1996; 14(9):2584–2589.

49. Katzenellenbogen JA, Welch MJ, Dehdashti F. The development of estrogen and progestin radiopharmaceuticals for imaging breast cancer. Anticancer Res 1997; 17:1573–1576.

50. Sundararajan L, Linden HM, Link JM, et al. ^{18}F-Fluoroestradiol. Semin Nucl Med 2007; 37(6):470–476.

51. Mankoff DA, Peterson LM, Tewson TJ, et al. [^{18}F]fluoroestradiol radiation dosimetry in human PET studies. J Nucl Med 2001; 42(4):679–684.

52. Kiesewetter DO, Kilbourn MR, Landvatter SW, et al. Preparation of four fluorine-18-labeled estrogens and their selective uptakes in target tissue of immature rats. J Nucl Med 1984; 25:1212–1221.

53. Mankoff DA, Tewson TJ, Eary JF. Analysis of blood clearance and labeled metabolites for the estrogen receptor tracer [F-18]-16 alpha-fluoroestradiol (FES). Nucl Med Biol 1997; 24(4):341–348.

54. Tewson TJ, Mankoff DA, Peterson LM, et al. Interactions of 16alpha-[18F]-fluoroestradiol (FES) with sex steroid binding protein (SBP). Nucl Med Biol 1999; 26(8):905–913.

55. Mintun MA, Welch MJ, Siegel BA, et al. Breast cancer: PET imaging of estrogen receptors. Radiology 1988; 169(1):45–48.

56. McGuire A, Dehdashti F, Siegel B, et al. Positron tomographic assessment of 16ð-[^{18}F]fluro-17β-estradiol uptake in metastatic breast carcinoma. J Nucl Med 1991; 32(8): 1526–1531.

57. Dehdashti F, Mortimer JE, Siegel BA, et al. Positron tomographic assessment of estrogen receptors in breast cancer: a comparison with FDG-PET and in vitro receptor assays. J Nucl Med 1995; 36:1766–1774.

58. Mortimer JE, Dehdashti F, Siegel BA, et al. Positron emission tomography with 2-[^{18}F]Fluoro-2-deoxy-D-glucose and 16alpha-[^{18}F]fluoro-17beta-estradiol in breast cancer: correlation with estrogen receptor status and response to systemic therapy. Clin Cancer Res 1996; 2(6):933–939.

59. Peterson LM, Mankoff DA, Lawton T, et al. Quantitative imaging of estrogen receptor expression in breast cancer using PET and [^{18}F]-fluoroestradiol: comparison of tracer uptake and in vitro assay of ER expression by immunohistochemistry. J Nucl Med 2006; 49:367–374.

60. Mankoff DA, Peterson LM, Petra PH, et al. Factors affecting the level and heterogeneity of uptake [F-18] fluroestardiol [FES] in patients with estrogen receptor positive breast cancer. J Nucl Med 2002; 43:286–287.

61. Linden HM, Stekhova SA, Link JM, et al. Quantitative fluoroestradiol positron emission tomography imaging predicts response to endocrine treatment in breast cancer. J Clin Oncol 2006; 24(18):2793–2799.

62. Linden HM, Link JM, Stekhova S, et al. Serial ^{18}F-fluoroestradiol Positron Emission Tomography (FES PET) measures estrogen receptor binding during endocrine therapy. Breast Ca Res Treat 2005; 94S1: S237 (abstr).

63. Allred DC, Bustamante MA, Daniel CO, et al. Immunocytochemical analysis of estrogen receptors in human breast carcinomas. Evaluation of 130 cases and review of the literature regarding concordance with biochemical assay and clinical relevance. Arch Surg 1990; 125(1):107–113.

64. Linden HM, Stekhova SA, Link JM, et al. Quantitative fluoroestradiol positron emission tomography imaging predicts response to endocrine treatment. J Clin Oncol 2006; 24(18):2793–2799. [Epub 2006, May 8].

65. Sutherland R. Tumor hypoxia and gene expression. Acta Oncologica 1998; 37:567–574.

66. Teicher BA. Hypoxia and drug resistance. Cancer Metastasis Rev 1994; 13:139–168.

67. Kaye SB. Multidrug resistance: clinical relevance in solid tumours and strategies for circumvention. Curr Opin Oncol 1998; 10(suppl 1):S15–S19.

68. Vaupel P, Mayer A, Briest S, et al. Hypoxia in breast cancer: role of blood flow, oxygen diffusion distances, and anemia in the development of oxygen depletion. Adv Exp Med Biol 2005; 566:333–342.

69. Boyle RG, Travers S. Hypoxia: targeting the tumour. Anticancer Agents Med Chem 2006; 6(4):281–286.

70. Vaupel P, Hockel M. Oxygenation status of breast cancer: the Mainz experience. In: Vaupel P, Kelleher DH, eds. Tumor Hypoxia: Pathophysiology, Clinical Significance and Therapeutic Perspectives. Stuttgart, Germany: Wissenschaftliche Veragsgesellschaft mbH, 1999:1–11.

71. Rajendran JG, Mankoff DA, O'Sullivan F, et al. Hypoxia and glucose metabolism in malignant tumors: evaluation by [^{18}F]fluoromisonidazole and [^{18}F]fluorodeoxyglucose positron emission tomography imaging. Clin Cancer Res 2004; 10(7):2245–2252.

72. Rajendran JG, Krohn KA. Imaging hypoxia and angiogenesis in tumors. Radiol Clin North Am 2005; 43(1):169–187.

73. Dehdashti F, Grigsby PW, Mintun MA, et al. Assessing tumor hypoxia in cervical cancer by positron emission tomography with ^{60}Cu-ATSM: relationship to therapeutic response-a preliminary report. Int J Radiat Oncol Biol Phys 2003; 55(5):1233–1238.

74. Piwnica-Worms D, Chiu ML, Budding M, et al. Functional imaging of multidrug-resistant P-glycoprotein with an organotechnium complex. Cancer Res 1993; 53:977–984.

75. Ciarmiello A, Vecchio SD, Silvestro P, et al. Tumor clearance of technetium 99m-sestamibi as a predictor of response to neoadjuvant chemotherapy for locally advanced breast cancer. J Clin Oncol 1998; 16(5): 1677–1683.

76. Mankoff DA, Dunnwald LK, Gralow JR, et al. [Tc-99m]-sestamibi uptake and washout in locally advanced breast cancer are correlated with tumor blood flow. Nucl Med Biol 2002; 29(7):719–727.

77. Hendrikse NH, de Vries EG, Eriks-Fluks L, et al. A new in vivo method to study P-glycoprotein transport in tumors and the blood-brain barrier. Cancer Res 1999; 59(10): 2411–2416.

78. Sasongko L, Link JM, Muzi M, et al. Imaging P-glycoprotein transport activity at the human blood-brain barrier with positron emission tomography. Clin Pharmacol Ther 2005; 77(6):503–514.

79. Kurdziel KA, Figg WD, Carrasquillo JA, et al. Using positron emission tomography 2-deoxy-2-[^{18}F]fluoro-D-glucose, 11CO, and 15O-water for monitoring androgen independent prostate cancer. Mol Imaging Biol 2003; 5(2):86–93.

80. Schelling M, Avril N, Nahrig J, et al. Positron emission tomography using [^{18}F] fluorodeoxyglucose for monitoring primary chemotherapy in breast cancer. J Clin Oncol 2000; 18:1689–1695.

81. Smith I, Welch A, Hutcheon A, et al. Positron emission tomography using [^{18}F]-fluorodeoxy-D-glucose to predict the pathologic response of breast cancer to primary chemotherapy. J Clin Oncol 2000; 18:1676–1688.

82. Cleaver JE. Thymidine metabolism and cell kinetics. Frontiers Biol 1967; 6:43–100.

83. Mankoff DA, Shields AF, Krohn KA. PET imaging of cellular proliferation. Radiol Clin North Am 2005; 43(1): 153–167.

84. Grierson JR, Shields AF. Radiosynthesis of 3'-deoxy-3'-[(18)F]fluorothymidine: [(18)F]FLT for imaging of cellular proliferation in vivo. Nucl Med Biol 2000; 27(2):143–156.

85. Smyczek-Gargya B, Fersis N, Dittmann H, et al. PET with [^{18}F]fluorothymidine for imaging of primary breast cancer: a pilot study. Eur J Nucl Med Mol Imaging 2004; 31(5): 720–724.

86. Pio BS, Park CK, Pietras R, et al. Usefulness of 3′-[F-18]-fluoro-3′-deoxythymidine with positron emission tomography in predicting breast cancer response to therapy. Mol Imaging Biol 2006; 8(1):36–42.

87. Kenny L, Coombes RC, Vigushin DM, et al. Imaging early changes in proliferation at 1 week post chemotherapy: a pilot study in breast cancer patients with 3′-deoxy-3′-[(18)F]-fluorothymidine positron emission tomography. Eur J Nucl Med Mol Imaging 2007; 34(9):1339–1347.

88. Hockenbery D. Defining apoptosis. Am J Pathol 1995; 146(1):16–19.

89. Cauchon N, Langlois R, Rousseau JA, et al. PET imaging of apoptosis with (64)Cu-labeled streptavidin following pretargeting of phosphatidylserine with biotinylated annexin-V. Eur J Nucl Med Mol Imaging 2007; 34(2): 247–258.

90. Blankenberg F, Katsikis P, Tait J, et al. Imaging of apoptosis (programmed cell death) with ^{99m}Tc annexin V. J Nucl Med 1999; 40:184–191.

91. Yagle KJ, Eary JF, Tait JF, et al. Evaluation of ^{18}F-annexin V as a PET imaging agent in an animal model of apoptosis. J Nucl Med 2005; 46(4):658–666.

40

FDG PET/CT Imaging: Clinical Uses and Opportunities

OLEG M. TEYTELBOYM and RICHARD L. WAHL
Division of Nuclear Medicine, Department of Radiology and Radiological Sciences, Johns Hopkins University, Baltimore, Maryland, U.S.A.

INTRODUCTION

Positron emission tomography (PET) is a potent molecular imaging tool for research due to its ability to quantitatively assess and noninvasively spatially localize the distribution of radioactivity throughout the body. While PET remains a preeminent research tool for molecular imaging in man, it represents a superb example of the successful translation of molecular imaging techniques to clinical practice, in the form of 18-Fluorodeoxyglucose PET (FDG PET). Thus, over the last decade, PET imaging has moved from primarily being a research tool into the clinical mainstream, with an estimate of over 1.5 million exams performed in the United States in 2007. PET and PET/CT with FDG are being increasingly used for staging, restaging, and therapy monitoring of cancer patients. According to an extensive literature review combining 419 total articles and abstracts, performed in 2001 by Gambhir et al., the average FDG PET sensitivity and specificity across all oncology applications are estimated at 84% (based on 18,402 patient studies) and 88% (based on 14,264 patient studies), respectively (1). The average management change across all applications was estimated to be 30% (based on 5062 patients) (1). As the literature has matured and expanded with the use of PET/CT, even further improvements in results are being seen. Ongoing adoption of oncologic FDG PET/CT imaging has a potential to dramatically alter the current management protocols by offering "response adaptive" therapies in which results from PET imaging performed soon after treatments are initiated are used to make therapeutic management decisions. There is growing evidence that early or mid-therapy FDG PET/CT scans can be used to predict the outcome rather than waiting until the completion of therapy. This can lead to shorter regimens with reduced toxicity if therapy is successful or changing a chemotherapy regimen that is not working. There are already several ongoing studies that are evaluating these approaches. FDG PET and PET/CT are also being increasingly used for non-oncologic imaging. There is ever widening array of uses, including assessing dementia, cardiac perfusion, and viability assessment, and evaluations of inflammatory and infectious disease.

Clinical adoption of PET imaging took a significant step forward with appearance of commercially available clinical PET/CT scanners in 2001. This technology has evolved rapidly and there are already several vendors who are offering PET/CT scanners with the state-of-the-art 64-slice CT. At present, essentially all PET scanners now sold in the United States are PET/CT scanners. In addition to attenuation correction, anatomic information provided by CT imaging enables accurate lesion localization while avoiding potential misinterpretations related to physiologic FDG uptake. Furthermore, modern scanners combining state-of-the-art PET and CT technology provide capacity for "single-stop" comprehensive imaging, where the patient can receive an FDG PET and a contrast-enhanced CT scan as part of the same imaging session. At this point, most of the available FDG PET studies in the literature were performed on PET scanners only. However, there is growing evidence that combined FDG PET/CT provides yet another step forward with improved clinical accuracy compared with separately interpreted PET and CT. It is clear that technical advances will make PET even more clinically useful in the near future. PET/MRI scanners, now in very early phases of development, may provide unique opportunities for brain imaging that will likely advance our understanding of brain function and improve clinical problem solving. "Time-of-flight" PET technology is offering capacity for faster and or lower dose scanning, while potentially enhancing image quality in larger patients, but is computationally intensive, requires very "fast" detectors, and is early in its evolution as a clinical tool.

Performing clinical FDG PET or PET/CT is a complex task requiring extensive experience to avoid multiple potential pitfalls. First, FDG is not a tumor-specific tracer, but rather traces the distribution of glucose metabolism in vivo. Glucose metabolism is not specific for cancer, although most cancers do have elevated glucose metabolism. Other processes such as infections and inflammation can also have intense glycolytic signals, which possibly can be confused with tumor uptake. Potential sources of artifacts also include elevated glucose levels that can compete with FDG, misalignment between PET and CT data that can create attenuation or mislocalization artifacts, inappropriate attenuation correction due to the presence of oral or IV contrast, as well as many types of technical artifacts related to scanner performance. PET scan timing can also play a major role due to possible tumor stunning or flare that potentially can reduce or alter FDG uptake leading to a false-negative exam (or more intense uptake in response to effective hormonal therapy). Furthermore, a negative PET scan does not completely rule out the presence of viable tumor, given an inherent resolution of approximately 8 mm for a typical clinical protocol, translating into an approximately 10^8 cells detection threshold. While cautions are in order and the reader is referred to full texts on the topic of PET imaging, our task in this brief review is to summarize the major clinical uses of our most commonly applied clinical molecular imaging tool, FDG PET, and PET/CT.

BRAIN

PET was originally developed as a brain-imaging research tool. As PET has become more widely available due to its extensive clinical use in cancer imaging, brain applications have increased as well. Metabolic mapping of the brains' glycolytic activity provided by FDG PET has found multiple applications in imaging dementia, epilepsy, movement disorders, and brain tumors. Normal brain extensively utilizes glucose for its metabolism with intense FDG uptake in the cortical and deep gray matter, with gray matter activity typically three times higher than that of white matter. Fusion with anatomic imaging helps to localize activity seen on PET. Currently, virtually all of the clinical PET scanners are PET only or in the form of PET/CT; however, vendors are working on development of PET/MRI scanners. There are multiple commercially available software packages that enable fusion between separately obtained PET and MRI with good accuracy.

Dementia

Imaging of dementia is one of the most commonly used clinical applications of brain PET. In 2007, there are an estimated approximately 5 million patients in the United States with dementia and many additional patients in whom the diagnosis of dementia is raised, but uncertain. Furthermore, the number of patients is likely to dramatically escalate due to rapidly aging population in the industrialized nations, given estimates that dementia affects 5% of the population older than 65 years and up to 25% of the population older than 80 years (1). Alzheimer's disease (AD) is the most common type of dementia, accounting for approximately two-thirds of the cases. Other types include multi-infarct dementia, diffuse Lewy body disease, and mixed dementia due to a combination of underlying etiologies.

Currently, the diagnosis of AD is typically established on clinical grounds. However, FDG PET is in many studies highly accurate at establishing, or at least confirming, the diagnosis and distinguishing AD from other types of dementia, particularly frontotemporal dementia (2). In AD, FDG PET demonstrates diminished glucose metabolism in the bilateral posterior temperoparietal cortices (3) (Fig. 1). Other involved areas can also include anterior and mesial temporal lobes as well as associated frontal cortices. By contrast, frontal dementia typically disproportionately affects the frontal cortex. Hypometabolism can be asymmetric from side to side. Correlation of PET findings with cross-sectional imaging is essential to confirm that hypometabolism is out of proportion to degree of brain atrophy.

Development of new PET tracers focusing on β-amyloid-avid compounds holds significant promise for imaging of AD. Two compounds under investigation are 2-(4-methyl-amino)phenyl-6-hydroxy-benzothiozole (C-11 BTA or "Pittsburgh compound B") and 1-(1-(6((2-fluroethyl) (methyl)(amino))-2-naphyl-ethylidene)malonitrile

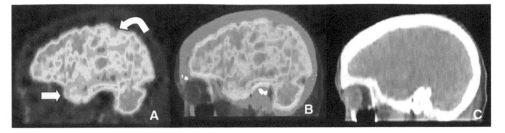

Figure 1 Alzheimer's dementia. (**A**) Sagital FDG PET, (**B**) PET/CT fusion, and (**C**) CT images demonstrate decreased FDG uptake in parietal (*curved arrow*) and anterior temporal (*straight arrow*) regions (*See Color Insert*).

(FDDNP) developed at UCLA. Both of these agents are currently undergoing clinical trials. However, it is likely that a fluorinated agent with uptake properties similar to the C-11 PIB, which appears to have higher amyoid/normal brain uptake ratios, would be highly desirable for imaging amyloid deposits, which may precede and perhaps cause dementia.

Other types of dementia also demonstrate specific patterns of FDG uptake enabling accurate and timely diagnosis. Diffuse Lewy body disease commonly demonstrates bilateral posterior temporoparietal hypometabolism similar to AD; however, the hypometabolism also frequently involves occipital lobes and does not involve anterior temporal lobes (4). Involvement of visual cortices may explain visual hallucinations commonly seen with this disorder. Frontotemporal dementias are characterized by decreased metabolism in both frontal and anterior temporal regions. Frontal lobe involvement frequently extends into sensorimotor and orbitofrontal regions (2).

Epilepsy

In the United States, epilepsy affects approximately 1.6 million patients (1). Most of these patients are managed medically; however, in the properly selected cases, particularly with mesial temporal lobe sclerosis, surgical therapy removing the epileptogenic focus can significantly improve or even cure the epilepsy (Fig. 2). Accurate localization of epileptogenic focus is of utmost importance for properly guiding the surgery. FDG PET should be used in combination with other tests that can include EEG, MRI, and ictal/interictal SPECT. Because of slow uptake of FDG, ictal PET is not practical, and FDG PET should be performed in the interictal state, which can be confirmed by EEG or clinical history/monitoring. Seizure foci are detected on interictal FDG PET by relative hypometabolism versus normal brain. This can be facilitated by comparison with the contralateral side, comparison with normal databases, and fusion with anatomic imaging, particularly MRI.

Brain Tumors

There are approximately 13,500 brain tumors diagnosed per year, accounting for approximately 2% of neoplasms in adults (2). Gliomas are the most common type arising from glial cells. FDG is the most commonly used PET tracer for imaging of these tumors, with FDG uptake correlating with tumor grade, with high uptake in highest grade gliomas. FDG PET is usually used as an adjunct to MRI for clinical problem solving. The most common clinical question is distinguishing postradiation necrosis from residual tumor since both of them can demonstrate contrast enhancement on MRI. FDG PET can resolve this dilemma by demonstrating increased uptake in residual or recurrent tumor and no increased uptake in areas of radiation-induced necrosis (5). Limitations of FDG PET include poor detection of low-grade brain tumors. PET is approximately 80% accurate in separating radiation necrosis from viable tumor.

Alternative PET tracers, particularly labeled amino acids, can provide clinically useful information and are complimentary to FDG, providing detectability for low-grade brain tumors. C-11-methionine is the most commonly used tracer and is U.S. Pharmacopeia listed. The

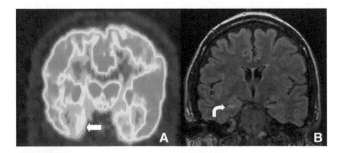

Figure 2 Mesial temporal lobe epilepsy. (**A**) Coronal FDG PET demonstrates decreased FDG uptake in right mesial temporal lobe (*straight arrow*), compared with contralateral side. PET findings are much more obvious than corresponding subtle increased signal (*curved arrow*) on (**B**) coronal FLAIR MRI image. *Abbreviation*: FLAIR MRI, fluid-attenuated inversion recovery magnetic resonance imaging (*See Color Insert*).

tumor is detected as the tracer is utilized in the tumor protein synthesis, although due to the short half-life of C-11, these images are mainly reflective of tumor amino acid transport. However, disadvantages include short half-life and tracer uptake in inflamed or ischemic tissues.

HEAD AND NECK

Squamous cell carcinoma (SCC), lymphoma, salivary gland tumors, and thyroid cancers are the most common tumors occurring in the head and the neck. FDG PET has been well established in imaging of SCC and will be the primary focus of this section. FDG PET imaging of lymphoma will be discussed in the later portion of the chapter. Role of FDG PET for evaluation of other head and neck malignancies is not as well defined, especially for salivary gland cancers where many are not particularly FDG avid.

Squamous Cell Carcinoma

Development of PET/CT technology has proven to be an essential milestone in confirming the clinical utility of FDG PET imaging for evaluation of SCC. Correlation and fusion with CT helps to avoid potential pitfalls due to physiologic uptake, including brown fat, muscle, and uptake due to atherosclerosis. In a study by Branstetter et al. (6), FDG PET/CT demonstrated 98% sensitivity and 92% specificity in evaluation of patients with known or suspected SCC. PET/CT was also compared with separately interpreted CT and PET, demonstrating better performance of PET compared with CT and superior performance of PET/CT compared with PET only. PET/CT was able to accurately characterize 62% of lesions equivocal on CT and 41% of lesions equivocal on PET. However, the accuracy of PET or PET/CT differs depending on the specific clinical question asked. In general, the smaller the tumor focus to be detected, the more challenging it will be for FDG PET/CT to detect the malignancy.

Initial diagnosis of SCC is usually made by direct inspection or endoscopy with only 1% to 5% of cancers presenting without a mucosal component (7). FDG PET can detect the unknown primary site in 25% to 35% of the cases with PET/CT, improving the detection rate to 33% to 57% (7). The role of FDG PET and PET/CT for primary staging remains somewhat controversial, since up to one-third of the tumors with metastasis at presentation have only micrometastasis, which is not detectable with any current noninvasive imaging exam. Therefore, all patients still require a neck dissection for definitive diagnosis and therapy. On the other hand, FDG PET/CT is likely the most accurate imaging modality for detecting metastatic disease, and presence of contralateral nodal metastasis or distant metastasis will result in significant management change.

FDG PET and PET/CT are superior to other imaging modalities for detection of recurrent disease and monitoring of therapy. Conventional cross-sectional imaging modalities are significantly limited by posttherapy changes that can result in distortion of normal anatomy. FDG PET/CT demonstrates 88% to 100% sensitivity and 75% to 100% specificity compared with 38% to 90% sensitivity and 38% to 85% specificity of CT and MRI (7).

Thyroid

Role of FDG PET in imaging of thyroid malignancies continues to be defined. Papillary thyroid cancer is the most common type, demonstrating correlation between the tumor grade and FDG uptake (Fig. 3). Low-grade papillary carcinomas show avidity for iodine, but typically are non-FDG avid. As the tumor becomes more dedifferentiated, the FDG uptake increases and iodine uptake diminishes. FDG PET may have a role in evaluation of patients with papillary thyroid cancer who have elevated serum thyroglobulin levels, but no detectable disease on radioiodine scan. Since thyroid-stimulating hormone (TSH) appears to stimulate thyroid cancer cell metabolism, FDG PET/CT should be performed when patients

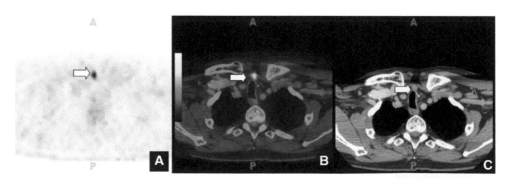

Figure 3 Metastatic papillary thyroid cancer. (**A**) Axial FDG PET, (**B**) PET/CT fusion, and (**C**) IV contrast-enhanced CT images demonstrate decreased FDG uptake in an enhancing thyroid bed lesion (*straight arrow*).

are withdrawn from thyroid hormone or have received recombinant TSH, although many thyroid cancers are detectable even when patients are taking thyroid hormone suppression. The most common indication for FDG PET in thyroid cancer is the rising serum thyroglobulin level in patients with a history of thyroid cancer who have negative I-131 scans. PET or PET/CT can help define tumor foci in order to guide subsequent biopsy and surgery.

FDG PET or PET/CT can sometimes detect an incidental primary thyroid cancer, which can appear as a hot focus in the thyroid of a patient having PET performed for another reason. In about half of such cases of FDG-avid thyroid nodules, there is a thyroid cancer present, so such a finding requires further evaluation with biopsy.

Other types of thyroid cancer are significantly less common and include medullary, Hurthle cell, and anaplasic carcinomas. The available literature is limited; however, it suggests that these cancers tend to be FDG avid.

LUNG

Lung cancer accounts for approximately 22% of all cancers in men and 8% of all cancers in women, with only five-year survival of 13% (1). FDG PET and PET/CT is a well-established modality for evaluation of thoracic malignancies. Almost all of the primary lung malignancies demonstrate increased FDG uptake, with FDG PET and PET/CT demonstrating superior performance to conventional anatomic imaging modalities. Non-FDG avid or only mildly avid lung cancers include bronchoalveolar carcinoma (BAC) and carcinoid tumors. Similar to other anatomic regions, development of PET/CT technology has improved the accuracy anatomic localization of FDG PET imaging.

Solitary Pulmonary Nodule

Evaluation of solitary pulmonary nodules is a very common clinical problem. The differential diagnosis of a pulmonary nodule is quite extensive with significant overlap in imaging appearance between benign and malignant lesions. Lung biopsies are technically difficult and are associated with significant morbidity due to a risk of pneumothorax and bleeding. While fine needle aspiration biopsy can be relatively safe, it can suffer in diagnostic accuracy due to sampling error issues. In a study by Yi et al., FDG PET/CT was significantly more accurate (93% vs. 85%; $p = 0.011$) than CT alone for evaluation of solitary pulmonary nodules (8). The authors concluded from their findings that PET/CT should be the test of choice for characterizing lung nodules. Potential pitfalls include increased FDG uptake on PET can be seen with both tumor and inflammation. False-negative PET can be seen on non-FDG avid, or only modestly FDG avid, tumors like BAC and carcinoid tumors. Another source of false-negative exams is small size of the nodule (8 mm is the typical clinical resolution of PET) and respiratory motion. However, recent developments of respiratory gating techniques and faster 3D acquisitions have improved evaluation of smaller lesions. Certainly, PET should be considered in the work up of pulmonary nodules 8 mm and larger in size and may be useful, if positive, in smaller lesions.

Non–Small Cell Lung Cancer

Non–small cell lung cancer (NSCLC) is the most common type of primary lung cancer and is the leading cause of cancer mortality worldwide. NSCLC includes adenocarcinoma, SCC, and large cell carcinoma. SCC and large cell carcinoma are strongly associated with smoking. Adenocarcinomas are not associated with smoking and most commonly tend to be peripheral (Fig. 4). BAC is a subtype or a precursor of adenocarcinoma, demonstrating only mild FDG uptake, perhaps in part due to its lipidic growth pattern leading to lower cellular density. BAC has the best prognosis compared with other types on NSCLC.

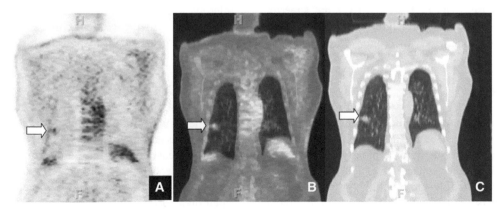

Figure 4 Non–small cell lung cancer discovered incidentally during follow-up after pancreatecomy for pancreatic adenocarcinoma. (A) Coronal FDG PET, (B) PET/CT fusion, and (C) CT images demonstrate modestly increased FDG uptake in right lower lobe nodule (*straight arrow*).

Accurate staging of NSCLC has important implications for therapy since early-stage disease is amendable to surgical therapy. FDG PET/CT is best available imaging modality for detecting advanced disease. In a meta-analysis by Silvestri et al. (9), sensitivity and specificity of CT scanning for identifying mediastinal lymph node metastasis were 51% (95% confidence interval [CI], 47–54%) and 85% (95% CI, 84–88%), respectively, confirming that CT scanning has limited ability either to rule in or exclude mediastinal metastasis. For FDG PET scanning, the sensitivity and specificity for identifying mediastinal metastasis were 74% (95% CI, 69–79%) and 85% (95% CI, 82–88%), respectively (9). Results with PET/CT have been superior to those of PET when directly compared; in addition to characterizing mass lesions and nodes for the presence of tumor, PET/CT is reported to have 89% sensitivity and 94% specificity for identification of malignant pleural effusion compared with only 50% accuracy of conventional CT (10), although these data are less well developed. FDG PET/CT is the best tool for detecting distant metastatic disease outside of the brain, finding occult metastasis in 10% to 20% of the patients that have been missed by other conventional imaging (11). Brain metastasis is often difficult to detect with FDG PET/CT due to high normal physiologic brain FDG uptake.

Small Cell Lung Cancer

Small cell lung cancer (SCLC) is the most aggressive type of primary lung cancer, accounting for approximately 20% of primary lung cancers (11). It is characterized by rapid growth and early metastasis, which are present in the majority of the patients at diagnosis. SLCL is classified as "limited" if it is confined to one hemithorax, the mediastinum, or supraclavicular nodes and can be targeted with one radiation field. Otherwise the tumor is classified as "extensive" disease. FDG PET and PET/CT are superior to conventional modalities for staging, treatment follow-up, and radiation planning.

Mesothelioma

Mesothelioma is the most common primary malignancy of the pleura and is strongly associated with remote asbestos exposure. Mesothelioma typically demonstrates increased FDG uptake, with FDG PET and PET/CT playing an important role in detecting lymph node and distant metastasis (11). Care must be taken to avoid confusing the treatment-related complications of talc pleurodesis of mesothelioma, which can result in intense radiotracer activity at sites of talc deposition, with active tumor.

BREAST

In the United States, breast cancer is the leading cause of cancer related mortality in women, after the lung cancer (1). It is the most common single cause of death for women between 35 and 50 years old (1). Cure is achievable if the cancer is detected early. Treatment options include surgery, radiation, hormonal therapy, and chemotherapy. Currently, FDG PET and PET/CT have no established role in breast cancer screening; however, this may change in the future with ongoing development of breast-specific PET scanners. PET with FDG can detect most primary breast cancers greater than 2 cm in diameter; however, smaller lesions may not be detected with current imaging equipment, so PET is not currently a reliable substitute for biopsy in patients with abnormal mammograms.

FDG PET has not proved to be useful in preoperative evaluation of early-stage breast cancer due to low sensitivity for detection of axillary micrometastasis. In early-stage disease, FDG PET has only 20% to 40% sensitivity compared with sentinel node biopsy (12–14). However, with more advanced disease, FDG PET and PET/CT can evaluate extra-axillary nodal regions and can detect distant metastatic disease (Fig. 5).

As to other cancers, FDG PET can play an important role in detection of recurrent or metastatic disease with sensitivity and specificity of up to 85% (15). Sclerotic bone metastasis has been reported to be an important cause of false-negative interpretations for FDG PET (16), despite being readily apparent on bone scans. However, FDG PET/CT may be able to detect the sclerotic metastasis (especially with the CT component of the study) and provide comprehensive staging exam (15). At present, lytic lesions are detected more clearly in bone than are sclerotic lesions.

There is growing evidence that FDG PET can accurately predict treatment response with neoadjuvant therapy at mid-therapy and even as early as three weeks into the therapy (17–21). FDG PET also appears useful for evaluation and follow-up of widespread systemic metastatic disease (15,21). This may be particularly important for patients with bone metastasis, given significant difficulties in assessing response with bone scans and CT. Thus, in breast cancer, the major clinical roles for FDG PET include detection of metastatic disease and treatment response assessment. As higher resolution dedicated breast PET instruments become available, a wider range of possibilities will become available for PET imaging.

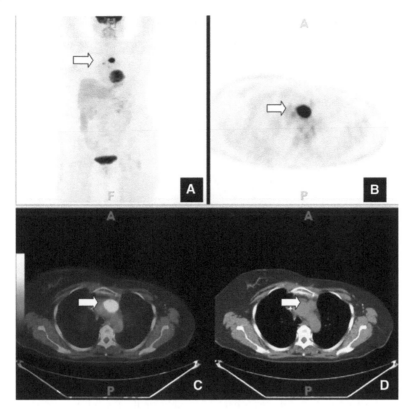

Figure 5 Metastatic breast cancer. (**A**) Coronal FDG PET MIP, (**B**) axial FDG PET, (**C**) PET/CT fusion, and (**D**) CT images demonstrate increased FDG uptake in enlarged mediastinal lymph nodes (*straight arrow*).

GASTROINTESTINAL TRACT

FDG PET and PET/CT has an important role for evaluation of many of gastrointestinal tract malignancies. However, while broadly useful, the results are tumor and disease location specific as some of the gastrointestinal malignancies are only minimally FDG avid.

Esophagus

Adenocarcinomas and SCCs account for most of esophageal cancers (1). The diagnosis is usually established by endoscopy with endoscopic ultrasound (EUS) providing local staging in many centers. FDG PET and PET/CT play an important role in providing comprehensive initial systemic staging. The esophagus lacks an enveloping fascia and has a rich lymphatic supply resulting in frequent nodal metastasis. FDG PET has been demonstrated to be more specific as compared with EUS, with PET specificity of 89% vs. 67% for EUS (22). A key role of FDG PET and PET/CT is the detection of nonlocoregional and distant disease, since local lymph node metastases do not alter the management because they are resected at the time of surgery. In a multicenter study by Meyers et al., FDG PET detected unsuspected distant disease in 14% of the patients (23). Thus, in many centers, FDG PET-CT is

performed at the time of the initial staging of esophageal carcinoma to determine if the disease is localized, and thus surgically resectable, or disseminated (Fig. 6).

There is growing evidence that FDG PET and PET/CT can accurately predict treatment response in esophageal cancer. In a study by Weber et al., a threshold of a 35% FDG uptake decrease after the first cycle of chemotherapy was able to predict clinical response with 93% sensitivity and 95% specificity (33%) (24). There is considerable evidence that PET/CT is superior to other imaging modalities in assessing response after completion of therapy. Patients who do not respond to chemoradiation are typically in a poor prognostic group compared with responders.

Stomach

FDG PET and PET/CT are not routinely used for screening or initial evaluation of gastric malignancies, since normal FDG uptake by the stomach can be highly variable and there is relatively easy access to the stomach for endoscopy. Gastric adenocarcinomas account for vast majority of primary gastric cancers with gastrointestinal stromal tumors (GIST) and lymphoma representing the majority of other malignancies.

Gastric adenocarcinomas are usually divided into intestinal and nonintestinal or signet ring types. FDG PET has

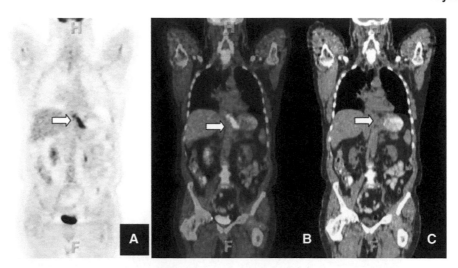

Figure 6 Esophageal carcinoma. (**A**) Coronal FDG PET, (**B**) PET/CT fusion, and (**C**) CT images demonstrate increased FDG uptake in the region of gastroesophageal junction (*straight arrow*).

83% sensitivity for detection of intestinal type and only 41% sensitivity for signet ring tumors (25). This lower detection rate is likely due to the large amounts of mucin present in the signet ring positive tumors. The role of FDG PET and PET/CT in initial staging is also limited by poor sensitivity for locoregional disease and for peritoneal carcinomatosis. However, similar to other malignancies, FDG PET and PET/CT can play a role in detecting distant metastasis or recurrent disease and in assessing chemotherapy response. In a study by Ott et al, in patients with locally advanced gastric cancer, FDG PET performed two weeks after the start of chemotherapy proved to be very accurate in predicting final response (26).

GIST are rare tumors likely arising from neuroenteric plexus and most commonly occurring in the stomach. Approximately one-third of these tumors are malignant and demonstrate intense FDG uptake. Nonmalignant GIST typically demonstrate only mild FDG uptake. Current therapeutic options include surgery and targeted therapies with tyrosine kinase inhibitors. FDG PET/CT has been demonstrated to be superior to PET or CT in detecting metastatic disease (27). There is also growing evidence that FDG PET can provide early and accurate assessment of response to tyrosine kinase inhibitors, with presence of residual FDG uptake implying a poor prognosis (27,28).

Colon and Rectum

Colorectal cancer is the third most common cancer in both men and women in the United States (1). Almost all colorectal cancers are adenocarcinomas, arising from adenomatous polyps that develop in the normal colonic mucosa. Colon cancers are usually discovered and diagnosed by colonoscopy, which may have been performed for routine screening or for blood discovered in the stool. Almost all the patients undergo surgical resection because of the tumor's potential to cause obstruction and bleeding. Local lymph nodes are typically resected during surgery allowing for accurate locoregional staging. Traditionally, additional staging is performed with contrast-enhanced CT. However, FDG PET and PET/CT can play an important role since it provides more accurate staging compared with anatomic imaging, with studies showing 15% to 42% management change with application of FDG PET (1). Similar to other tumors, FDG PET/CT has been shown to be superior to PET, by providing anatomic correlation and allowing detection of smaller lesions. In a comparison study, PET/CT was able to better characterize up to one-half of equivocal lesions (29).

FDG PET/CT is widely accepted as the modality of choice for restaging and detection of colorectal cancer recurrence. FDG PET/CT has been shown to have up to 90% sensitivity and 70% specificity (30). Overall, there is clear evidence that restaging by FDG PET and PET/CT can affect patient care, with reported changes in management in 32% of the patients (1). One important caveat is hepatic metastasis, where contrast-enhanced MRI is more sensitive per lesion, although FDG PET remains mores more specific (31). A notable caution is the lower sensitivity of FDG PET for detection of mucinous cancers than other types of colorectal cancers, possibly with 30% to 50% lower sensitivity due to lower cellular density and higher mucin content of these tumors.

FDG PET and PET/CT is also the modality of choice for evaluation of chemotherapy response. There is growing evidence that a significant decrease of FDG uptake in the tumor on PET early in the course of therapy can distinguish patients who are likely to respond to therapy and have better survival chances (32).

Thus, FDG PET/CT in colorectal cancer is most commonly performed when recurrence is suspected, including in the setting of a rising carcinoembryonic antigen (CEA) level in the serum, and before major surgical procedures are undertaken to remove metastatic colon cancer.

Pancreas

Pancreatic ductal adenocarcinoma is the most common type of pancreatic cancer, accounting for 5% of cancer-related deaths in the United States (33). Pancreatic adenocarcinoma is characterized by aggressive behavior with invasion into adjacent soft tissues, lymph node and hepatic metastasis, and a high mortality rate (Fig. 7). Early surgical resection offers the only opportunity for cure. The preoperative diagnosis, staging, and treatment of pancreatic adenocarcinoma remain challenging despite recent technical advances and multiple available imaging modalities. Dual-phase 3D CT is a leading modality for local tumor imaging as it can highly accurately define local tumor extension and particularly depicts vascular invasion well. FDG PET and PET/CT imaging is a useful adjunct to CT, by differentiating benign and malignant pancreatic masses as well as detecting CT-occult metastatic disease. FDG imaging is not superior to helical CT for N staging, but is more accurate than CT for M staging. In a study by Diederichs et al., FDG PET demonstrated a sensitivity of 49% and a specificity of 63% for lymph node staging, and sensitivity of 70% and a specificity of 95% for liver

metastases, with sensitivity decreasing as lesion size decreased (34). Detection of peritoneal carcinomatosis is a major challenge for all imaging modalities including PET. However, FDG PET/CT may improve the detection rate by providing anatomic correlation and allowing detection of smaller lesions.

FDG PET utility for monitoring of patients with pancreatic adenocarcinoma after surgical therapy, chemotherapy, and radiation has been confirmed in several studies (35–38). For example, Ruf et al. (37) evaluated 39 patients with subsequently confirmed recurrence after surgery, demonstrating that FDG-PET reliably detected local and nonlocoregional recurrences, whereas CT/MRI was more sensitive for the detection of hepatic metastases. Of 25 patients with local recurrences upon follow-up, initial imaging suggested relapse in 23 patients. Of these, FDG-PET detected 96% (22 of 23) and CT/MRI 39% (9 of 23). Among 12 liver metastases, FDG-PET detected 42% (5 of 12). CT/MRI detected 92% (11 of 12) correctly. Moreover, 7 of 9 abdominal lesions were malignant upon follow-up, of which FDG-PET detected 7 of 7 and CT/MR detected none. Additionally, FDG-PET detected extra-abdominal metastases in two patients.

There is growing evidence that FDG PET/CT can play an important role in evaluation of cystic pancreatic lesions. There is significant overlap between benign and malignant disease on both CT and MRI. Sperti et al. reported sensitivity, specificity, and positive and negative predictive values for FDG PET and CT scanning in

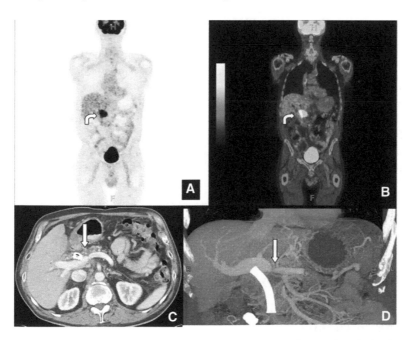

Figure 7 Locally advanced pancreatic adenocarcinoma. (**A**) Coronal FDG PET and (**B**) PET/CT fusion images demonstrate intensely FDG-avid tumor in the pancreatic head (*curved arrow*). (**C**) Venous phase axial CT and (**D**) coronal MIP CT images demonstrate a hypodense tumor in the pancreatic body, narrowing the portal confluence (*straight arrow*). This case illustrates complementarity of FDG PET and contrast-enhanced 3D CT.

detecting malignant tumors of 94%, 97%, 94%, and 97% and 65%, 87%, 69%, and 85%, respectively (39). A study by Tann et al. (40) demonstrated improved sensitivity of PET/CT in comparison to CT or PET only. Sensitivities of CT, PET, and combined PET/CT images were 67% to –71%, 57%, and 86%, respectively. Specificities of CT, PET, and combined PET/CT images were 87% to –90%, 65%, and 91%, respectively.

Hepatobiliary

Hepatocellular carcinoma (HCC) is the most common primary hepatic tumor arising from malignant transformation of hepatocytes. It typically occurs in the setting of chronic liver disease due to viral hepatitis, alcohol, or in patients exposed to carcinogens. HCC is fourth most common cause of cancer-related deaths in the world and is becoming increasingly common in the United States due to hepatitis C epidemic (41). Once cirrhosis is present, HCC develops in 1% to 4% of patients yearly (42). There are three patterns of uptake for HCC: FDG uptake higher than, equal to, or lower than liver background (55%, 30%, and 15%, respectively). FDG PET detects only 50% to 70% of HCCs but has a sensitivity of more than 90% for all other primaries (cholangiocarcinoma and sarcoma) and most other metastatic tumors of the liver (43,45). Delayed imaging at two or three hours after FDG injection may increase FDG PET sensitivity, with Lin et al. reporting 62.5% sensitivity for HCC detection on the two- and three-hour images compared with 56.3% on the one-hour image (45).

There is growing evidence that C-11-acetate PET is complementary to FDG in the detection of primary HCC (46–48). C-11-acetate is a metabolic substrate of β-oxidation, precursors of amino acid, fatty acid, and sterol, and is useful in evaluation for various malignancies. In a study, Ho et al. (47) showed value of dual-tracer PET/CT for evaluation of HCC metastasis demonstrating 98% sensitivity, 86% specificity, and 96% accuracy in the detection of HCC metastasis on per patient basis. The lesion-based and patient-based detection by both tracers was complementary, with 60% and 64% sensitivities by C-11-acetate, and 77% and 79% sensitivities by FDG. Since higher-grade HCCs tend to be more FDG avid, metastasis were more likely to be detected with FDG. The tracer uptake by the tumors is related to the tumor differentiation with preferential uptake of C-11-acetate by well-differentiated HCCs and FDG uptake by poorly differentiated tumors. C-11-Acetate was also highly specific for HCC, with no accumulation in cholangioadenocarcinoma or metastasis to the liver. C-11 acetate tracer availability is limited, however, due to it short, 20 minutes, half-life.

Cholangiocarcinomas account for approximately 30% of primary hepatic neoplasms and are often unresectable at the time of diagnosis (49). Adenocarcinoma is the most common histologic subtype, arising from intra- or extrahepatic bile duct epithelium. There are multiple reports confirming utility of FDG PET in evaluation of cholangiocarcinoma with reported sensitivity of 61% to 90% (50–54). In a study by Anderson et al. (52), FDG PET was more helpful in patients with nodular cholangiocarcinomas (85% sensitivity) than in those with the infiltrating variety (18% sensitivity). False-positive findings can be seen in patients with biliary stents, probably related to inflammatory changes, as well as in patients with acute cholangitis (50,51).

There is evidence that FDG PET imaging may be useful in the diagnosis and management of small cholangiocarcinomas in patients with primary sclerosing cholangitis (PSC) (50,51). Dynamic FDG-PET appears superior to conventional imaging techniques for both detection and exclusion of cholangiocarcinoma in advanced PSC, and may be useful for screening for cholangiocarcinoma in the pretransplant evaluation of patients with PSC. In a study by Prytz et al. (51), dynamic FDG PET was performed in 24 consecutive patients with PSC within two weeks after listing for liver transplantation and with no evidence of malignancy on CT, MRI, or ultrasound. Three patients had cholangiocarcinoma that was correctly identified by PET. Dynamic FDG PET was negative in one patient with high-grade hilar duct dysplasia and was false-positive in one patient with epithelioid granulomas in the liver.

Gallbladder carcinoma is the most common type of biliary cancer and is the fifth most common gastrointestinal malignancy accounting for approximately 6500 deaths per year in the United States (52). Adenocarcinoma is the most common histologic subtype representing approximately 90% of the tumors. FDG PET is not usually used for evaluation of primary gallbladder carcinoma since most patients are diagnosed incidentally after cholecystectomy (55). Therefore, FDG-PET is typically used for initial staging after cholecystectomy, or restaging when recurrence is suspected. Increased FDG uptake has been demonstrated in gallbladder carcinoma helping to identify recurrence in the area of the incision. In a study by Anderson et al. (56), the overall sensitivity of FDG PET for residual gallbladder carcinoma was 78% and the specificity was 80%. The sensitivity for detecting metastatic gallbladder carcinoma was 56% due to inability to detect carcinomatosis.

GENITOURINARY

FDG PET and PET/CT has an important role for evaluation of many of gynecologic and genitourinary malignancies. Development of PET/CT technology has resulted in significantly improved overall accuracy by reducing potential interpretation errors related to renal excretion of FDG.

Adrenal

Evaluation of adrenal nodules is becoming an increasing common clinical problem. Because of increasing prevalence of cross-sectional imaging, numerous adrenal lesions are discovered as incidentalomas. In patients without known or suspected malignancy, adrenal nodule is very unlikely to represent metastasis, and these incidentalomas are evaluated with CT or MRI to distinguish adrenal adenomas from other primary adrenal neoplasms like pheochromocytoma and adrenocortical carcinoma.

In patients with known or suspected malignancy, adrenal glands are a common site of metastatic disease. There is growing evidence that FDG PET/CT can reliably differentiate metastasis from benign adrenal lesions such as adenomas. In a study by Caoili et al. (57), all non-adenomas had a standardized uptake value (SUV) equal or higher to liver and very few adenomas had SUV above twice the level of the liver. Furthermore, combination of lesion density on noncontrast CT and lesion SUV to liver ratio provided definitive answer for almost all of the lesions.

Renal Cancers

The kidneys are normal sites of excretion of FDG and are also normally metabolically active. Radioactive urine in the collecting systems and renal cortex FDG uptake preclude reliable detection of primary renal cancers. In addition, renal cancers may sometimes have lower glycolytic rates than other types of cancer, causing false-negative exams in both primary and metastatic sites. Thus, FDG PET or PET/CT is not a robust test in evaluating primary renal masses, and false-negatives are sufficiently frequent so PET is not recommended in this setting. PET can be more sensitive for metastatic disease, but even then false-negative studies are not uncommon.

Bladder Cancer

Transitional cell carcinomas are the most common type of bladder cancers and typically have intense FDG uptake. Primary cancers can be hard to detect as they are in immediate contiguity with radioactive urine, which has sufficient intensity to make them very hard to detect. By contrast, transitional cell carcinoma metastases are typically quite FDG avid and within the size detection limitations of PET are quite reliably identified.

Prostate Cancer

The prostate is a challenging location for PET imaging with FDG, with the bladder in immediate physical contiguity. Thus, radiotracer in the bladder can degrade the quality of imaging of the prostate. FDG is not a reliable tool in detecting primary prostate cancers and can miss many nodal metastases due to poor avidity for FDG. While aggressive advanced metastases can be detected, a lower sensitivity is seen for metastatic prostate cancer than in many other types of cancer. Thus, while FDG may show metastases in a patient with a rising prostate-specific antigen level, it is by no means a robust tool in this setting, although it is applied in clinical practice in this difficult setting in some centers.

Gynecologic Malignancies

Gynecologic malignancies include ovarian, cervical, and endometrial carcinomas accounting for approximately one quarter of solid tumors in women. Prognosis and therapy of these cancers are highly dependent on extent of local and lymph node spread on presentation. FDG PET and PET/CT is an excellent modality for imaging of theses tumor since they intensely accumulate FDG. Development of PET/CT technology has significantly improved overall accuracy of gynecologic FDG PET imaging. Anatomic information provided by CT is a crucial aspect of the exam given highly variable FDG uptake of normal bowel, intense FDG uptake of normal endometrium, and urinary excretion of FDG. Also, precise lesion localization by PET/CT fusion allows detection of smaller lesions.

In patients with ovarian cancer, FDG PET and PET/CT are primarily used for detection of recurrent disease. In patients with rising CEA, FDG PET/CT has a higher sensitivity compared to purely cross-sectional anatomic imaging (58–61). FDG PET/CT has a reported accuracy of 82% for detection of ovarian cancer recurrence (61). For lesions larger than 1 cm, FDG PET/CT has been demonstrated to have 83% sensitivity and 94% positive predictive value (61). Micrometastasis and less FDG-avid histologic types of ovarian cancer are some of the potential sources of false-negative PET imaging.

Early stage cervical cancer is treated surgically, and the patients with metastatic lymphadenopathy are treated with radiation. FDG PET and PET/CT are widely used for staging, radiation planning, monitoring therapy, and detection of recurrent disease. FDG PET/CT has a reported sensitivity of 73% and specificity of 97% for detection of lymph nodes larger than 0.5 cm, which is superior to pelvic MRI (62,63). As for many other cancers, FDG PET/CT is the study of choice for detection of recurrent disease and provides important prognostic information with two year survival of 85% in patients with negative exam and survival of 11% with positive PET/CT. Patients identified as high risk on PET may also be candidates for more aggressive chemotherapy-containing trials.

In patients with endometrial cancer, FDG PET and PET/CT have been primarily used for detection of recurrent cancer. FDG PET has a reported sensitivity of 95% and specificity of 78% and has been reported to change patient management in up to a third of the patients (64). Similar to other cancers, FDG PET and PET/CT can be used for monitoring therapy response. Small tumor volumes, and diffuse large volumes of tumor with carcinomatosis, can be falsely negative on PET.

LYMPHOMA

Lymphomas represent a heterogenous group of lymphoproliferative malignancies with variable pattern of behavior and treatment response. The World Health Organization modification of the Revised European-American Lymphoma Classification recognizes three major categories of lymphoid malignancies based on morphology and cell lineage. These categories include Hodgkin's lymphoma, B-cell neoplasms, and T-cell/natural killer-cell neoplasms.

FDG PET and PET/CT are widely accepted as the modality of choice for imaging lymphoma (Fig. 8). Hodgkin's and most non-Hodgkin's lymphomas (NHL) accumulate FDG. Some of the lower-grade NHL, like mucosa-associated lymphoid tissue and marginal zone lymphomas, tend to have only low FDG uptake, reducing

utility of PET. However, in patients with low-grade lymphomas, FDG PET and PET/CT are capable of diagnosing transformation into a higher grade by identifying lesions with higher SUV compared with other tumor sites.

There is extensive evidence that FDG PET and PET/CT provide the most accurate staging information, outside of bone marrow involvement, which is probably better assessed by biopsy (1). Addition of FDG PET or PET/CT to staging has been demonstrated to alter patient management in 8% to 48% of the cases, sometimes because of upstaging the disease, leading to more aggressive therapy, but perhaps more commonly due to determinations by PET that masses which were large tumors have become FDG negative and are thus likely scars (1). Similar to other malignancies, FDG PET/CT has been shown to be superior to PET only by providing anatomic correlation and helping to avoid potential pitfalls due to physiologic uptake, including brown fat, muscle, and uptake due to atherosclerosis. In a study by Allen-Auerbach et al., FDG PET/CT had 94% accuracy compared with 84% for PET (65). PET/CT's increased diagnostic sensitivity is typically due to the detection of small tumor foci, which are otherwise considered normal by CT alone. Bone marrow biopsy remains the gold standard for detection of tumor involvement due to poor accuracy of FDG PET, particularly in patients with less than 30% involvement. Administration of hematopoetic growth factors or systemic illness can also result in errors of FDG PET and PET/CT interpretations as such administrations can markedly raise the FDG uptake in normal marrow, thus reducing detectability of tumor in marrow.

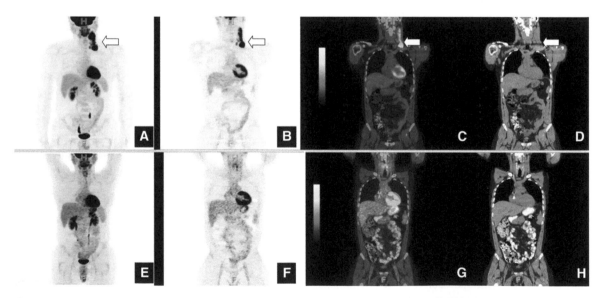

Figure 8 Hodgkin's lymphoma therapy follow-up. (**A**) Coronal FDG PET MIP, (**B**) FDG PET, (**C**) PET/CT fusion, and (**D**) CT images demonstrate increased FDG uptake in enlarged neck lymph nodes (*straight arrow*), representing recurrent disease. Following additional chemotherapy, (**E**) coronal FDG PET MIP, (**F**) FDG PET, (**G**) PET/CT fusion, and (**H**) CT images demonstrate complete response.

FDG PET or PET/CT is the modality of choice for assessing therapy response in the FDG-avid lymphomas. Enlarged nodes or masses may not completely resolve on anatomic imaging due to residual scarring, whereas FDG PET or PET/CT can assess for presence of viable tumor. There is increasing evidence that mid-therapy scan, which can be obtained as early as after one cycle, can predict and guide the therapy. There are multiple ongoing clinical trials that are assessing this "response-adaptive" therapy, where the regimen and its duration vary depending on response as it is judged by FDG PET/CT. The integration of PET into the management of lymphoma is quite well established by now, with new response criteria having been proposed that integrate the PET and CT data into an overall response, the International Workshop Criteria (IWC) + PET criteria. Thus, lymphoma represents one of the tumors in which the integration of PET into treatment response assessment is most complete and most well accepted.

CUTANEOUS MELANOMA

Melanoma is a potentially lethal type of skin cancer, with approximately 60,000 new cases diagnosed in the United States per year and accounting for over 8000 deaths (33). Mortality is dramatically dependent on the disease stage with five-year survival of 99% for localized disease, 65% for regional metastatic disease, and 15% in patients with distant metastasis. Given intense FDG avidity of melanoma FDG PET or PET/CT can be a valuable clinical tool in appropriate clinical settings. Melanoma is usually detected on clinical exam with subsequent excisional biopsy. Local staging is typically performed by sentinel node localization and excision. FDG PET or PET/CT is unlikely to improve local staging due to poor sensitivity for micrometastasis. While PET is able to detect lymph node metastases that may be occult on CT, sentinel lymph node localization/removal procedures are far more sensitive for detecting small tumor foci in lymph nodes.

In patients with suspected distant metastasis, FDG PET and particularly PET/CT are superior to other imaging modalities, outside of the brain. Reported sensitivity of FDG PET is up to 92% and specificity up to 94% (66). Although there is only limited literature evaluating role of FDG PET or PET/CT in therapy monitoring, similar to other tumors, PET/CT can probably provide better assessment of treatment response compared with only anatomic imaging. At present, the major role of PET/CT in melanoma is systemic staging and in following treatment response. If aggressive surgical procedures are planned, PET/CT is generally recommended before the surgery is undertaken, lest the planned surgical field not include all the known tumor.

Pediatric Neoplasms

PET has lagged in its utilization in pediatric patients, but has recently been shown to have considerable advantages compared with CT alone. PET can find small lesions missed on CT as well as can determine that cancer is not present in patients who have been treated for large tumors such as lymphoma or some sarcomas. PET/CT exhibited better diagnostic performance than CT and showed accurate findings in 90% (72 of 80) of lesions with discordant findings between them (67).

MYOCARDIAL IMAGING

Coronary artery disease (CAD) affects approximately 14 million people in the United States and is the most common cause of death in industrialized nations. Diagnosis and therapy of CAD are rapidly evolving. PET can provide quantitative information about perfusion, myocardial metabolism, neuronal, and receptor function. There is extensive evidence that PET can provide accurate diagnosis of obstructive CAD, superior to SPECT imaging (68). Furthermore, PET can quantify myocardial perfusion and can detect the presence of small vessel disease, providing a significant advantage over all other types of imaging.

Introduction of PET/CT technology and development of 64-slice PET/CT scanners, which are now available from multiple vendors, opens new exciting possibilities for providing comprehensive cardiac imaging. Anatomic characteristics of a lesion provided by coronary CT angiography (CTA) now can be combined with understanding of its functional significance as seen on perfusion pharmacologic stress PET.

The two most commonly used PET perfusion tracers are Rb-82 and N-13 ammonia. Rb-82 is most widely used tracer because it is produced by a generator, greatly simplifying its clinical use. It is a potassium analogue and has a physical half-life of 76 seconds. Myocardial uptake occurs via sodium/potassium adenosine triphosphate transporter, with absolute tracer uptake related to myocardial blood flow. In addition to its short half-life, the other main drawback of Rb-82 is comparatively higher kinetic energy of its emitted positron resulting in greater uncertainty of spatial localization (i.e., somewhat lower resolution images).

N-13 ammonia is a cyclotron product and has 9.96-minute physical half-life, requiring cyclotron proximity to the imaging center. The neutral form of ammonia molecule within the blood pool can rapidly diffuse into the cells, where it becomes trapped though incorporation into glutamine pool by glutamine synthase. The net tracer tissue extraction is linear for blood flow values of 2.5 mL/min/kg and therefore may underestimate blood flow at higher rates, which can occur at peak stress, unless a correction is made (68). Another drawback of this tracer is a nonuniform distribution within the myocardium, particularly reduced in the lateral wall by up to 10% versus the septum.

Cardiac FDG PET/CT can play an important role in management of patients with obstructive CAD by detecting hypoperfusion of myocardium that results in impaired contractile function. This "hibernating myocardium" is detected by observing preserved glycolytic metabolism in a dysfunctional/hypoperfused area. There is extensive evidence that FDG PET can reliably predict functional recovery after revascularization. Furthermore, there growing evidence that the presence of hibernating myocardium is a significant mortality risk factor, perhaps because it can serve as a source of arrhythmia.

Performing cardiac PET/CT is a complex task requiring extensive experience to avoid multiple potential pitfalls. Misalignment between PET and CT data, which are used for attenuation correction of PET, is one of the most common sources of potential artifacts. This occurs because PET is acquired over multiple breathing cycles, unlike the CT scan, which can be performed during any phase of the respiratory cycle with motion and breathing creating potential for misalignment. Multiple techniques have been developed to correct this potential problem including manual alignment of the data sets and cine CT sequences.

INFECTION AND INFLAMMATORY DISEASE

Application of FDG PET or PET/CT for imaging of inflammatory disease takes advantage of respiratory burst, which occurs during activation of both neutrophilic granulocytes in acute inflammation and mononuclear cells in chronic inflammation. This process is heavily glucose dependent, and therefore demonstrates intense FDG avidity. Combination of anatomic information from CT and metabolic information provided by PET makes FDG PET/CT an excellent modality for evaluation of suspected inflammation/infection.

FDG PET or PET/CT can play a major role in work up of fever of unknown origin (FUO), which has been defined as recurrent fever of 38.3°C or higher lasting for over three weeks. Common causes of FUO include infections (30–40%), malignancy (20–30%), and autoimmune diseases (10–20%). FDG PET can provide rapid whole-body imaging with reported ability to establish the diagnosis in 41% to 69% of the patients (69).

Evaluation for osteomyelitis of bone affected by prior trauma or surgery is another area where FDG PET or PET/CT appears to provide unique advantages over other imaging modalities. Since fibroblasts predominate in

normally healing bone, FDG uptake becomes normalized after four months of trauma or surgery (70), unlike bone scan that can remain abnormal for several years.

FDG PET or PET/CT appears to have a limited utility for work up of joint prosthesis infection, since FDG PET appears unable to distinguish infection from sterile inflammation caused by prosthesis loosening. The role of FDG PET or PET/CT remains controversial for examination of diabetic foot to differentiate neuropathic osteoarthropathy and osteomyelitis. Medicare in the United States has not yet approved the use of FDG PET for infection detection, but this area has grown rapidly and many already view FDG PET as a very viable alternative to cumbersome In-111 white cell imaging study.

CONCLUSION

Thus, in the past decade, the use of FDG PET in cancer and several benign diseases has grown markedly in frequency. This broadly useful molecular imaging agent is finding more applications on a regular basis, especially as response adaptive therapy grows in its application. While other PET tracers will evolve and no doubt be important, FDG represents an excellent example of a molecular imaging agent successfully translated to widespread, indeed worldwide, application.

REFERENCES

1. Gambhir SS, Czernin J, Schwimmer J, et al. A tabulated summary of the FDG PET literature. J Nucl Med 2001; 42: 1S–93S.
2. Van Heertum RL, Ichise M. PET and PET/CT brain imaging. In: Wahl RL, ed. Clinical PET and PET/CT Imaging. 2007 Syllabus. RSNA 2007.
3. Zakzanis KK, Graham SJ, Campbell Z. A meta-analysis of structural and functional brain imaging in dementia of the Alzheimer's type: a neuroimaging profile. Neuropsychol Rev 2003; 13(1):1–18.
4. Colloby S, O'Brien J. Functional imaging in Parkinson's disease and dementia with Lewy bodies. J Geriatr Psychiatry Neurol 2004; 17(3):158–163.
5. Kim EE, Chung SK, Haynie TP, et al. Differentiation of residual or recurrent tumors from post-treatment changes with F-18 FDG PET. Radiographics 1992; 12(2):269–279.
6. Branstetter BF IV, Blodgett TM, Zimmer LA, et al. Head and neck malignancy: is PET/CT more accurate than PET or CT alone? Radiology 2005; 235(2):580–586.
7. Blodgett TM. PET and PET/CT for the evaluation of head and neck cancer. In: Wahl RL, ed. Clinical PET and PET/CT Imaging. 2007 Syllabus. RSNA 2007.
8. Yi CA, Lee KS, Kim B-T, et al. Tissue characterization of solitary pulmonary nodule: comparative study between helical dynamic CT and integrated PET/CT. J Nucl Med 2006; 47:443–450.

9. Silvestri GA, Gould MK, Margolis ML, et al., and American College of Chest Physicians. Noninvasive staging of non-small cell lung cancer: ACCP evidenced-based clinical practice guidelines (2nd edition). Chest 2007; 132 (3 suppl):178S–201S.

10. Schaffler GJ, Wolf G, Schoellnast H, et al. Non-small cell lung cancer: evaluation of pleural abnormalities on CT scans with 18F FDG PET. Radiology 2004; 231(3): 858–865; [Epub April 22, 2004].

11. Steinert HC. Lung and esophageal cancer. In: Wahl RL, ed. Clinical PET and PET/CT Imaging. 2007 Syllabus. RSNA 2007.

12. Barranger E, Grahek D, Antoine M, et al. Evaluation of fluorodeoxyglucose positron emission tomography in the detection of axillary lymph node metastases in patients with early-stage breast cancer. Ann Surg Oncol 2003; 10(6): 622–627.

13. Wahl RL, Siegel BA, Coleman RE, et al. PET Study Group. Prospective multicenter study of axillary nodal staging by positron emission tomography in breast cancer: a report of the staging breast cancer with PET study group. J Clin Oncol 2004; 22(2):277–285.

14. Lovrics PJ, Chen V, Coates G, et al. A prospective evaluation of positron emission tomography scanning, sentinel lymph node biopsy, and standard axillary dissection for axillary staging in patients with early stage breast cancer. Ann Surg Oncol 2004; 11(9):846–853; [Epub August 16, 2004].

15. Mankoff DA. The application of PET and PET/CT to breast cancer. In: Wahl RL, ed. Clinical PET and PET/CT Imaging. 2007 Syllabus. RSNA 2007.

16. Cook GJ, Houston S, Rubens R, et al. Detection of bone metastases in breast cancer by 18FDG PET: differing metabolic activity in osteoblastic and osteolytic lesions. J Clin Oncol 1998; 16(10):3375–3379.

17. Wahl RL, Zasadny KR, MacFarlane D, et al. Iodine-131 anti-B1 antibody for B-cell lymphoma: an update on the Michigan phase I experience. J Nucl Med 1998; 39 (8 suppl):21S–27S.

18. Mankoff DA, Dunnwald LK, Gralow JR, et al. Changes in blood flow and metabolism in locally advanced breast cancer treated with neoadjuvant chemotherapy. J Nucl Med 2003; 44(11):1806–1814.

19. Mankoff DA, Dunnwald LK, Gralow JR, et al. Blood flow and metabolism in locally advanced breast cancer: relationship to response to therapy. J Nucl Med 2002; 43(4): 500–509.

20. Smith IC, Welch AE, Hutcheon AW, et al. Positron emission tomography using [(18)F]-fluorodeoxy-D-glucose to predict the pathologic response of breast cancer to primary chemotherapy. J Clin Oncol 2000; 18(8):1676–1688.

21. Dose Schwarz J, Bader M, Jenicke L, et al. Early prediction of response to chemotherapy in metastatic breast cancer using sequential 18F-FDG PET. J Nucl Med 2005; 46(7): 1144–1150.

22. Flamen P, Lerut A, Van Cutsem E, et al. The utility of positron emission tomography for the diagnosis and staging of recurrent esophageal cancer. J Thorac Cardiovasc Surg 2000; 120(6):1085–1092.

23. Meyers BF, Downey RJ, Decker PA, et al. American College of Surgeons Oncology Group Z0060. The utility of positron emission tomography in staging of potentially operable carcinoma of the thoracic esophagus: results of the American College of Surgeons Oncology Group Z0060 trial. J Thorac Cardiovasc Surg 2007; 133(3): 738–745.

24. Weber WA, Ott K, Becker K, et al. Prediction of response to preoperative chemotherapy in adenocarcinomas of the esophagogastric junction by metabolic imaging. J Clin Oncol 2001; 19(12):3058–3065.

25. Stahl A, Ott K, Weber WA, et al. FDG PET imaging of locally advanced gastric carcinomas: correlation with endoscopic and histopathological findings. Eur J Nucl Med Mol Imaging 2003; 30(2):288–295; [Epub November 8, 2002].

26. Ott K, Fink U, Becker K, et al. Prediction of response to preoperative chemotherapy in gastric carcinoma by metabolic imaging: results of a prospective trial. J Clin Oncol 2003; 21(24):4604–4610.

27. Goerres GW, Stupp R, Barghouth G, et al. The value of PET, CT and in-line PET/CT in patients with gastrointestinal stromal tumours: long-term outcome of treatment with imatinib mesylate. Eur J Nucl Med Mol Imaging 2005; 32(2):153–162; [Epub September 4, 2004].

28. Gayed I, Vu T, Iyer R, et al. The role of 18F-FDG PET in staging and early prediction of response to therapy of recurrent gastrointestinal stromal tumors. J Nucl Med 2004; 45(1):17–21; [Erratum in J Nucl Med 2004; 45(11): 1803].

29. Cohade C, Osman M, Leal J, et al. Direct comparison of (18)F-FDG PET and PET/CT in patients with colorectal carcinoma. J Nucl Med 2003; 44(11):1797–1803.

30. Delbeke D, Martin WH. PET and PET-CT for evaluation of colorectal carcinoma. Semin Nucl Med 2004; 34(3): 209–223 (review).

31. Bipat S, van Leeuwen MS, Comans EF, et al. Colorectal liver metastases: CT, MR imaging, and PET for diagnosis—meta-analysis. Radiology 2005; 237(1):123–131; [Epub August 11, 2005].

32. Guillem JG, Moore HG, Akhurst T, et al. Sequential preoperative fluorodeoxyglucose-positron emission tomography assessment of response to preoperative chemoradiation: a means for determining long-term outcomes of rectal cancer. J Am Coll Surg 2004; 199(1):1–7.

33. American Cancer Society. Cancer facts and figures 2002: year 2002 surveillance research from the American Cancer Society. Bethesda, MD: American Cancer Society, 2002.

34. Diederichs CG, Staib L, Vogel J, et al. Values and limitations of FDG PET with preoperative evaluations of patients with pancreatic masses. Pancreas 2000; 20:109–116.

35. Rose DM, Delbeke D, Beauchamp RD, et al. 18 Fluoro-deoxyglucose-positron emission tomography in the management of patients with suspected pancreatic cancer. Ann Surg 1999; 229:729–737.

36. Franke C, Klapdor R, Meyerhoff K, et al. 18-FDG positron emission tomography of the pancreas: diagnostic benefit in the follow-up of pancreatic carcinoma. Anticancer Res 1999; 19:2437–2442.

37. Ruf J, Lopez Hänninen E, Oettle H, et al. Detection of recurrent pancreatic cancer: comparison of FDG-PET with CT/MRI. Pancreatology 2005; 5(2–3):266–272; [Epub April 22, 2005].

38. Franke C, Klapdor R, Meyerhoff K, et al. 18-F positron emission tomography of the pancreas: diagnostic benefit in the follow-up of pancreatic carcinoma. Anticancer Res 1999; 19:2437–2442.

39. Sperti C, Pasquali C, Chierichetti F, et al. Value of 18-fluorodeoxyglucose positron emission tomography in the management of patients with cystic tumors of the pancreas. Ann Surg 2001; 234:675–680.

40. Tann M, Sandrasegaran K, Jennings SG, et al. Positron-emission tomography and computed tomography of cystic pancreatic masses. Clin Radiol 2007; 62(8):745–751; [Epub May 9, 2007].

41. El Serag HB, Davila JA, Petersen NJ, et al. The continuing increase in the incidence of hepatocellular carcinoma in the United States an update. Ann Intern Med 2003; 139: 817–823.

42. Fattovich G, Giustina G, Degos F, et al. Morbidity and mortality in compensated cirrhosis C a retrospective follow-up study of 384 patients. Gastroenterology 1997; 112: 463–472.

43. Khan MA, Combs CS, Brunt EM, et al. Positron emission tomography scanning in the evaluation of hepatocellular carcinoma. J Hepatol 2000; 32:792–797.

44. Delbeke D, Martin WH, Sandler MP, et al. Evaluation of benign vs. malignant hepatic lesions with positron emission tomography. Arch Surg 1998; 133:510–515.

45. Lin WY, Tsai SC, Hung GU. Value of delayed 18F-FDG-PET imaging in the detection of hepatocellular carcinoma. Nucl Med Commun 2005; 26(4):315–321.

46. Ho C-L, Yu SCH, Yeung DWC. C-11-Acetate PET imaging in hepatocellular carcinoma and other liver masses. J Nucl Med 2003; 44:213–221.

47. Ho CL, Chen S, Yeung DW, et al. Dual-tracer PET/CT imaging in evaluation of metastatic hepatocellular carcinoma. J Nucl Med 2007; 48(6):902–909.

48. Delbeke D, Pinson CW. C-11-acetate: a new tracer for the evaluation of hepatocellular carcinoma. J Nucl Med 2003; 44(2):222–223.

49. de Groen PC, Gores GJ, LaRusso NF, et al. Biliary tract cancers. N Engl J Med 1999; 341(18):1368–1378.

50. Keiding S, Hansen SB, Rasmussen HH, et al. Detection of cholangiocarcinoma in primary sclerosing cholangitis by positron emission tomography. Hepatology 1998; 28: 700–706.

51. Prytz H, Keiding S, Björnsson E, et al. Swedish Internal Medicine Liver Club. Dynamic FDG-PET is useful for detection of cholangiocarcinoma in patients with PSC listed for liver transplantation. Hepatology 2006; 44(6): 1572–1580.

52. Anderson CD, Rice MH, Pinson CW, et al. Fluorodeoxyglucose PET imaging in the evaluation of gallbladder carcinoma and cholangiocarcinoma. J Gastrointest Surg 2004; 8(1):90–97.

53. Widjaja A, Mix H, Wagner S, et al. Positron emission tomography and cholangiocarcinoma in primary sclerosing cholangitis. Z Gastroenterol 1999; 37:731–733.

54. Kluge R, Schmidt F, Caca K, et al. Positron emission tomography with [(18)F]fluoro-2-deoxy-D-glucose for diagnosis and staging of bile duct cancer. Hepatology 2001; 33:1029–1035.

55. Donohue JH, Stewart AK, Menck HR. The National Cancer Data Base report on carcinoma of the gallbladder, 1989–1995. Cancer 1998; 83(12):2618–2628.

56. Anderson CD, Rice MH, Pinson CW, et al. Fluorodeoxyglucose PET imaging in the evaluation of gallbladder carcinoma and cholangiocarcinoma. J Gastrointest Surg 2004; 8(1):90–97.

57. Caoili EM, Korobkin M, Brown RK, et al. Differentiating adrenal adenomas from nonadenomas using (18)F-FDG PET/CT: quantitative and qualitative evaluation. Acad Radiol 2007; 14(4):468–475.

58. Pannu HK, Cohade C, Bristow RE, et al. PET-CT detection of abdominal recurrence of ovarian cancer: radiologic-surgical correlation. Abdom Imaging 2004; 29(3): 398–403.

59. Pannu HK, Bristow RE, Cohade C, et al. PET-CT in recurrent ovarian cancer: initial observations. Radiographics 2004; 24(1):209–223 (review).

60. Bristow RE, del Carmen MG, Pannu HK, et al. Clinically occult recurrent ovarian cancer: patient selection for secondary cytoreductive surgery using combined PET/CT. Gynecol Oncol 2003; 90(3):519–528.

61. Nanni C, Rubello D, Farsad M, et al. (18)F-FDG PET/CT in the evaluation of recurrent ovarian cancer: a prospective study on forty-one patients. Eur J Surg Oncol 2005; 31(7): 792–797.

62. Sironi S, Buda A, Picchio M, et al. Lymph node metastasis in patients with clinical early-stage cervical cancer: detection with integrated FDG PET/CT. Radiology 2006; 238(1): 272–279; [Epub November 22, 2005].

63. Choi HJ, Roh JW, Seo SS, et al. Comparison of the accuracy of magnetic resonance imaging and positron emission tomography/computed tomography in the presurgical detection of lymph node metastases in patients with uterine cervical carcinoma: a prospective study. Cancer 2006; 106(4):914–922.

64. Belhocine T, De Barsy C, Hustinx R, et al. Usefulness of (18) F-FDG PET in the post-therapy surveillance of endometrial carcinoma. Eur J Nucl Med Mol Imaging 2002; 29(9): 1132–1139; [Epub June 19, 2002].

65. Allen-Auerbach M, Quon A, Weber WA, et al. Comparison between 2-deoxy-2-[18F]fluoro-D-glucose positron emission tomography and positron emission tomography/computed tomography hardware fusion for staging of patients with lymphoma. Mol Imaging Biol 2004; 6(6):411–416.

66. Rinne D, Baum RP, Hör G, et al. Primary staging and follow-up of high risk melanoma patients with whole-body 18F-fluorodeoxyglucose positron emission tomography: results of a prospective study of 100 patients. Cancer 1998; 82(9):1664–1671.

67. Tatsumi M, Miller JH, Wahl RL. 18F-FDG PET/CT in evaluating non-CNS pediatric malignancies. J Nucl Med 2007; 48(12):1923–1931.

68. Di Carli FM, Dorbala S, Meserve J, et al. Clinical myocardial perfusion PET/CT. In: Wahl RL, ed. Clinical PET and PET/CT Imaging. 2007 Syllabus. RSNA 2007.

69. Stumpe KD. PET and PET/CT imaging in infection and inflammation. In: Wahl RL, ed. Clinical PET and PET/CT Imaging. 2007 Syllabus. RSNA 2007.

70. Kaim AH, Gross T, von Schulthess GK. Imaging of chronic posttraumatic osteomyelitis. Eur Radiol 2002; 12(5): 1193–1202; [Epub December 15, 2001].

41

Molecular Imaging in Prostate Cancer

STEVE Y. CHO

Division of Nuclear Medicine, Russell H. Morgan Department of Radiology and Radiological Science, Johns Hopkins University School of Medicine, Baltimore, Maryland, U.S.A.

MARTIN G. POMPER

Division of NeuroRadiology, Russell H. Morgan Department of Radiology and Radiological Science, Johns Hopkins University School of Medicine, Baltimore, Maryland, U.S.A.

BIOLOGY AND CLINICAL MANAGEMENT OF PROSTATE CANCER

Prostate cancer (PCa) is the most common cancer among men in the United States. The American Cancer Society estimates 218,890 new cases of PCa in 2007, 29% of all sites in men, causing mortality in 27,050 or 9% of all male cancer deaths (1). The routine, widespread use of prostate-specific antigen (PSA) testing has resulted in a down-staging of PCa at diagnosis. The tumors detected today are smaller and of lower stage and grade than they were 20 years ago, but there remains a wide range of aggressive and advanced disease that continues to exist (2,3).

The paradigm of cancer care in the future will be a risk-adjusted patient-specific therapy designed to maximize cancer control while minimizing the risk of complications. In the management of PCa, patient care initially requires accurate tumor evaluation in order to select the optimal therapy from a growing array of alternatives including watchful waiting, androgen ablation, radical prostatectomy (radical retropubic or laparoscopic), radiation therapy (brachytherapy, external-beam radiation therapy, or combinations of these choices), and possibly focal

ablative therapies (cryoablation, radio frequency ablation, and focused ultrasound). PCa is currently characterized by its clinical tumor-node-metastasis (TNM) stage, Gleason grade, and PSA serum level (3). Algorithms or nomograms that combine stage, grade, and PSA level to predict pathologic stage or prognosis for individual patients have been developed and have demonstrated better performance than individual factors alone (4,5). Imaging has become increasingly important in the assessment of PCa management because of the need for help with treatment selection and planning (2).

Through early detection and improved local therapies, a large number of men will be cured; however, there will remain a significant number who experience disease relapse and will require continued surveillance and ongoing therapy. The minority of patients who present with advanced disease at the time of diagnosis will require systemic therapy as well as ongoing surveillance. PSA is the marker used for monitoring patients for recurrence. An estimated 50,000 new cases of so-called "biochemical" failure occur annually (6). When PSA becomes detectable after radical prostatectomy or the level increases above the nadir on three occurrences after radiation therapy, recurrence is suspected.

Patients who would benefit from salvage therapy include those who have a reasonable probability of localized disease. If distant disease is present, local salvage therapy is likely to have little if any impact on survival. The challenge is to identify those men in whom local salvage therapy would be appropriate and spare those with the greatest likelihood of metastasis from the toxic effects of local therapy, which would not likely be beneficial (3).

Autopsy studies indicate that the first site of metastatic PCa is the bone in 72% of patients, whereas soft tissue spread represents the first site of metastasis in the remaining 28%. Among 753 PCa cases that went to autopsy, which demonstrated metastasis, 476 (63%) had a lymph node metastasis whereas 277 (37%) did not. Two different lymph node metastatic patterns were observed: type 1, combined metastasis involving the pelvic and paraaortic lymph nodes, and type 2, metastasis to the paraaortic lymph nodes but not to those in the pelvis (7).

The clinical needs include early detection, accurate initial staging, and detection of local recurrence or metastases to permit application of the most appropriate therapy. Therapeutic monitoring and prognostic assessment are equally important. Imaging can play an important and crucial role in meeting these clinical needs, as detailed below.

THE ROLE OF SERUM BIOMARKERS

PCa screening is typically performed with a digital rectal examination and measurement of serum PSA level. Since the advent of PSA screening, the incidence of PCa has increased, but most prostate cancers are now diagnosed at an early stage. PSA is a kallekrein protein secreted by prostate epithelial cells and is a normal component of the ejaculate. Those epithelial cells are also the progenitor cells of prostate adenocarcinoma (6). PSA is not specific for PCa and can be elevated in other conditions, including benign prostatic hyperplasia, inflammation, trauma, and urinary retention. Although cancerous prostate tissue produces far more PSA in the serum than hyperplastic tissue, benign prostatic hyperplasia is the most common cause of elevated serum PSA concentration. Although PSA undoubtedly has positively impacted PCa detection, the problem of specificity remains (8).

Within the past decade advances in proteomics have stimulated a search for new biomarkers with increased specificity. A proteomics approach focused on profiling the nuclear structural elements of PCa cells identified two novel unrelated PCa biomarkers: early PCa antigen (EPCA) and EPCA-2 (9). An enzyme-linked immunosorbent assay to detect an epitope of the EPCA-2 protein, EPCA-2.22, was evaluated. Using a cutoff of 30 ng/mL,

the EPCA-2.22 assay had a specificity of 92% for healthy men and men with benign prostatic hyperplasia and sensitivity of 94% for overall PCa. The comparative specificity for PSA in these selected groups of patients was 65%. Additionally, EPCA-2.22 was highly accurate in differentiating between localized and extracapsular disease in contrast to PSA in this study.

CONVENTIONAL (ANATOMIC) IMAGING

Conventional anatomic imaging methods like computed tomography (CT), ultrasound (including transrectal), or magnetic resonance imaging (MRI) are insufficiently accurate for determination of the initial tumor stage because of their low sensitivities and specificities. The low rate of detection of lymph node involvement represents a major problem with conventional imaging. Therefore, laparoscopic or open dissection of pelvic lymph nodes is considered the gold standard (2). Transrectal ultrasound plays an important role in prostate biopsy guidance but has a limited role in the detection of PCa (10). With an accuracy of about 65%, CT is of limited clinical use for local staging of PCa (11), but may be helpful in detecting advanced disease within adjacent tissue and distant lymph node metastases (2). MRI detection of PCa and tumor localization for biopsy demonstrated sensitivities of 61% and 77% and specificities of 46% and 81%, respectively. (12). Like CT for assessment of lymph node metastases, MRI has low sensitivity due to its inability to detect metastases in normal-sized nodes (13).

MOLECULAR IMAGING AGENTS FOR PCa IN CLINICAL USE

Bone scintigraphy with [^{99m}Tc]Methylene Diphosphonate ([^{99m}Tc]MDP) remains the current standard of practice for the detection of osseous metastatic disease in PCa. In staging patients with newly diagnosed PCa, bone scans are considered for symptomatic patients or for those with PSA ≥ 20 μg/L, locally advanced disease, or Gleason score $\geq$ 8, who are at higher risk for bone metastases (14). This is based on two important studies evaluating [^{99m}Tc]MDP in a large number of patients. Evaluation of 521 newly diagnosed men with untreated PCa determined that patients with a PSA of <20 μg/L had a negative predictive value of 99.7% for bone scan findings (15). The second study of 852 patients with newly diagnosed PCa demonstrated that bone scans had a false-negative rate of 2% for a PSA cutoff level of <20 μg/L (16).

As stated above, an increasing PSA level in the follow-up of PCa can result from bone or soft tissue metastases. In a large prospective study in more than 400 patients, the negative predictive value of a PSA level <20 ng/mL for demonstration of metastases on a bone scan was 87%, while the positive predictive value of a PSA level > 100 ng/mL was 80% (17).

For patients undergoing follow-up or restaging for PCa, a bone scan is not generally warranted with a PSA level <10 μg/L unless there is a rapid PSA rise (PSA velocity > 5 μg/L per month) and clinical symptoms (14). The chance of a positive finding on serial bone scans is low when the follow-up PSA level is <15 μg/L (18).

Studies employing [18F]fluorodeoxyglucose positron emission tomography (FDG PET) have demonstrated mixed results in imaging PCa. These studies have led to varying results with low sensitivity for detection of primary disease and pelvic lymph node metastases, with false-positive findings often due to physiologic FDG urinary radioactivity (19–22). In a study evaluating patients with more advanced PCa, FDG PET/CT was reported to have a sensitivity of 83% for the detection of primary disease (23).

Chang et al. evaluated the role of FDG PET/CT in detecting recurrent PCa in the setting of elevated PSA after initial local therapy (24). Twenty-four patients were examined before pelvic lymph node dissection. At the sites with histopathologically proved metastases (66.7% or 16 of 24 patients), FDG uptake was found in 75% of patients with four cases representing false-negative results. No patient with a false-positive result on FDG PET images was seen. The calculated sensitivity, specificity, accuracy, positive predictive value, and negative predictive value of FDG PET in detecting metastatic pelvic lymph nodes were 75%, 100%, 83.3%, 100%, and 67.7%, respectively. They concluded that FDG PET may have utility in the staging of pelvic lymph nodes in

patients with PSA relapse after treatment of localized PCa in the setting of negative bone scintigraphy and equivocal pelvic CT.

More recently, Schoder et al. studied FDG PET/CT for detection of disease in the setting of biochemical relapse after radical prostatectomy and demonstrated that radiopharmaceutical uptake was truly positive in 31% (28 of 91) of patients with relatively high mean PSA (9.5 ± 2.2 ng/mL) (25). Although low PSA did not necessarily preclude FDG uptake, ROC analysis determined that a PSA level of >2.4 ng/mL and velocity of 1.3 ng/mL/yr was useful for deciding whether or not to use FDG PET/CT. Importantly, they emphasized the concept that FDG PET should not be used randomly to screen patients but to improve the likelihood for disease detection by incorporation of other aspects of the disease such as tumor burden and tumor biology combined with PSA levels. Figure 1 demonstrates an example of highly FDG-avid metastases in aggressive, recurrent PCa.

The role of FDG PET/CT imaging as an outcome measure during chemotherapy for metastatic PCa was studied by Morris et al. (26). FDG PET scans were performed in 23 patients with progressive metastatic disease despite castrate testosterone levels at baseline, 4, and 12 weeks during chemotherapy with a microtubule inhibitor. They applied the PSA Working Group Consensus Criteria guideline that a 25% increase in PSA constituted disease progression and that the FDG PET maximum standardized uptake value (SUV_{max}) would be averaged over the three scans. PET results identified the clinical status of 91% of the patients at 4 weeks and 94% of the patients at 12 weeks into therapy. They reported that the accuracy of PET could be further optimized if a >33%

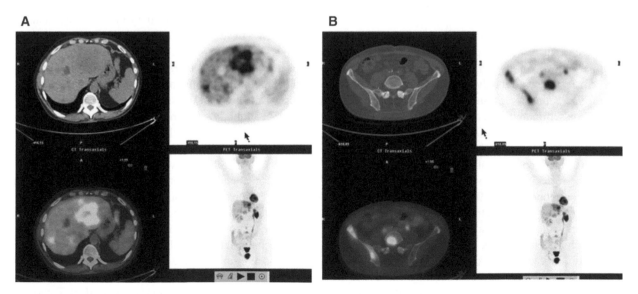

Figure 1 FDG PET/CT scan for patient with a history of metastatic, hormone refractory prostate cancer. Note abnormal FDG involving the liver, lumbar vertebral body, and pelvis. *Abbreviation*: FDG PET/CT, [18F]fluorodeoxyglucose positron emission tomography/computed tomography. *Source*: Division of Nuclear Medicine, Johns Hopkins Hospital.

increase in PSA and SUV_{max} average were used to define progression, optimally distinguishing disease progressors from nonprogressors on chemotherapy.

Prostate-specific membrane antigen (PSMA) is a type II membrane protein originally expressed on all types of prostate tissue and upregulated in higher grade, androgen-insensitive disease, and metastases (27–29). PSMA is also expressed by cells in the small intestine, proximal renal tubules, and salivary gland, although the expression levels of PSMA in these tissues is 100 to 1000 times lower than in prostate (30). A murine monoclonal antibody binding to PSMA, originally named 7E11 (31), has been used to detect PSMA in tissue, but was later developed as [^{111}In] capromab pendetide (ProstaScint™; Cytogen Corporation, Princeton, New Jersey, U.S.). In 1996, the FDA approved ProstaScint for use in the imaging of soft tissue metastatic PCa for staging prior to primary surgical resection or PSA relapse after local therapy (32).

Initial investigation of ProstaScint by Wynant et al. in 40 patients, with PCa and known distant metastases, detected bony metastases in 55% of patients (21 of 38) and soft tissue lesions in 67% (4 of 6) of patients (33). Manyak et al. evaluated prospectively 160 patients with PCa prior to pelvic lymph node dissection before or during definitive treatment with high risk of nodal involvement. Pathology demonstrated positive lymph nodes in 42% of the patients. ProstaScint scans demonstrated a sensitivity of 62%, specificity of 72%, a positive predictive value of 62%, a negative predictive value of 72%, and an overall accuracy of 68%. ProstaScint scans performed much better than CT, which had a sensitivity of 4% (specificity of 100%), or MRI with a sensitivity of 15% (specificity of 100%). In this early study, ProstaScint outperformed these standard diagnostic imaging techniques (34).

ProstaScint was also used to evaluate local versus systemic recurrent disease in patients with a PSA relapse after primary local therapy (35,36). The endpoint typically used is PSA response after salvage radiation therapy to the prostate fossa. Kahn et al. found that 28% of patients had detectable disseminated disease on Prosta-Scint scans, while 72% of the patients had either negative scans or their disease was limited to the prostatic fossa. Levesque et al. demonstrated that 73% of patients had uptake beyond the prostatic fossa, 6% of patients had activity in the prostatic fossa alone, and 23% of patients had uptake in abdominal and extrapelvic retroperitoneal nodes.

Subsequent studies evaluating ProstaScint suggested that the radiotracer was not fulfilling its promise and was of only limited or incremental value in selecting patients with local recurrence who may achieve PSA control (37,38). Deb et al. in a phase I trial of ProstaScint and [^{90}Y]7E11 for imaging and therapy reported that the known sites of disease were poorly imaged by ProstaScint

with about half of patients (5 of 12) without a detectable lesion and 45% (5 of 11) of patients with positive bone scans having no detectable uptake (37). Thomas et al. evaluated the prognostic significance of ProstaScint imaging in 30 patients with PCa who underwent salvage radiation therapy for recurrent disease after initial prostatectomy. The clinical interpretation of the scan results were compared with postradiation therapy PSA response. Positive scan findings outside the prostatic fossa were found not to be predictive of biochemical control after radiation therapy (38).

Initial studies suggested that ProstaScint scans could be used to distinguish patients with localized disease, and therefore benefit from local radiation therapy, from those with systemic disease. Wilkinson et al. evaluated ProstaScint scans of 42 patients with rising PSA levels after prostatectomy. Abnormal uptake was detected in 85.7% of patients. Forty-seven percent of patients with uptake isolated to the prostatic fossa showed a durable response to salvage radiation therapy. The authors concluded that a ProstaScint scan was not helpful (39).

A reason for the limited results of ProstaScint imaging may be due to the fact that it binds to a site on the cytoplasmic (intracellular) portion of PSMA rather than to an epitope on the extracellular portion of the protein (40). As a general rule, a protein such as an antibody cannot cross the cell membrane unless it first binds to an extracellular receptor and then becomes internalized. It has been suggested that the PSMA target epitope for ProstaScint imaging only becomes accessible on cell apoptosis or necrosis (41). Antibodies directed at the extracellular domain may increase the sensitivity of PSMA antibody imaging of PCa by recognizing surface epitopes on living cancer cells (32).

PSMA antibodies that bind to the extracellular domain of PSMA have been developed and bind to viable PSMA-expressing cells (42). The humanized antibody J591 has been evaluated for therapy in PCa (41,43–46). As part of these radioimmunotherapy trials, radiolabeled J591 imaging was conducted to assess the tumor targeting capability of the antibody. The results were compared with other radiologic studies including bone scan, CT, or MRI findings in patients with known metastatic disease. In a study imaging patients with radiolabeled J591, 98% (42 of 43) of evaluable patients had detectable bone and/or soft tissue lesions (43). Another study by Bander et al. with ^{111}In-labeled or ^{177}Lu-labeled J591 also demonstrated accurate targeting, delineating 98% of bone and/or soft tissue metastatic sites (Fig. 2) (47).

Sodee et al. reported improved performance of Prosta-Scint with the advent of SPECT/CT with the synergistic value of SPECT and CT images (48). SPECT and SPECT/CT image reconstruction techniques have been evaluated with ProstaScint images using an experimental algorithm,

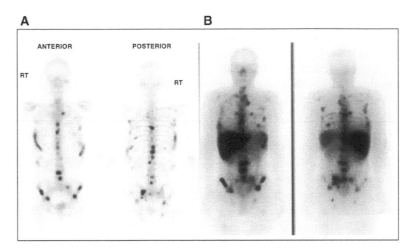

Figure 2 PSMA antibody imaging with [^{177}Lu]J591. Bone scan (**A**) and J591 scan (**B**) from the same patient. The bone scan shows excretion through kidneys and bladder as well as multiple areas of increased uptake in ribs, spine, and pelvis. The J591 scan, in addition to liver excretion of radiometal, shows superimposable areas of J591 accumulation/targeting. *Abbreviation*: PSMA, prostate-specific membrane antigen. *Source*: From Ref. 47.

which produced a subjective improvement in the interpretation confidence in 11 of 12 studies and changes in 4 of 12 interpretations (49). However, the changes to those interpretations were not sufficient to alter prognosis or the patient treatment plan. Another study investigated the use of SPECT iterative reconstruction with bladder suppression and blood pool subtraction to improve the interpretation and utility of ProstaScint SPECT scans for patient management (50).

Interestingly, PSMA is also known to be expressed on non-prostate tumor neovasculature (51). Milowsky et al. recently demonstrated in a phase I trial the ability of [^{111}In] J591 to target the extracellular domain of PSMA in patients with advanced solid tumor malignancies as a proof-of-principle evaluation of PSMA as a potential neovascular target. Seventy-four percent of 27 patients had one or more sites of known metastatic disease targeted by [^{111}In]J591 in patients with kidney, bladder, lung, breast, colorectal, and pancreatic cancers, and melanoma (52).

PROSTATE LYMPHOSCINTIGRAPHY

Prostate lymphoscintigraphy in combination with radiation-guided surgery with the use of gamma probes and lymphoscintigraphy for sentinel lymph node (SLN) identification has been described in PCa (53–55). A major limitation of PET or antibody-based imaging applied to PCa staging is the inability of detecting micrometastases. The identification of occult lymph node metastases has a significant impact on the outcome of patients with PCa with their presence significantly increasing the risk of tumor recurrence and death (56). The SLN technique is able to radiolabel the relevant lymph nodes prior to radical

prostatectomy, improving the diagnostic accuracy and limiting morbidity from lymph node dissection.

Joslyn et al. suggest that more extensive pelvic lymphadenectomy in patients undergoing radical prostatectomy could improve the accuracy of staging and improve disease-free survival and possibly overall survival (57). Wawroschek et al., using [^{99m}Tc]nanocolloid (Nanocoll^{TM}), were able to demonstrate the detection of at least one SLN in 335 out of 350 patients (55). The SLN concept might be the solution for accurate initial nodal staging in PCa patients (58). This method is currently widely accepted and utilized in other tumors such as breast cancer and melanoma.

EMERGING PCa MOLECULAR IMAGING AGENTS

Hara et al. introduced [methyl-^{11}C]choline ([^{11}C]choline) as a new PET radiotracer for imaging brain tumors (59). Choline is a natural blood constituent and penetrates cell membranes. In tumors, [^{11}C]choline is integrated into phospholipids. When [^{11}C]choline is taken up by tumor cells it undergoes phosphorylation and, after several biosynthetic steps, finally becomes integrated into lecithin, a major component of cell membrane phospholipids. The presence of choline transporters is likely also involved in [^{11}C]choline uptake in tumor cells, but this mechanism remains under investigation (60). [^{11}C]Choline has rapid blood clearance allowing for imaging to occur within five minutes after administration and is not confounded by muscle uptake, unlike FDG. However, it can be avidly taken up into benign lesions (61).

Biodistribution of [^{11}C]choline demonstrates prominent physiological uptake. Radiotracer was observed in the liver, renal cortex, and salivary glands. Less intense radiotracer uptake can also be seen in the lungs, spleen, skeletal muscles, and bone marrow. Other areas of variable uptake were observed in the pancreatic region, small intestine, thyroid gland, and minimally within brain. Mild uptake was also seen in the choroid plexus and pituitary gland. In two patients, accumulation of [^{11}C]choline in the bladder was observed (62).

PCa is often a low-grade tumor that demonstrates poor FDG uptake. [^{11}C]Choline is taken up by many different grades of PCa and only a relatively small amount of this radiotracer is excreted in the urine. Multiple studies have demonstrated that this radiotracer can be potentially useful in determining local, regional, and distant disease, and recurrence. However, the uptake of [^{11}C]choline in PCa can be variable and often cannot discriminate between carcinoma and dysplasia. Reports exist of false-positive lymph node uptake, and physiological gastrointestinal uptake has also hindered imaging (61).

Results of visualizing [^{11}C]choline accumulation within the prostate itself are somewhat controversial. In fact, [^{11}C]choline accumulation is present both in normal prostate and in PCa. Hara suggested that the [^{11}C]choline SUV is always higher in prostate tumor than in normal prostate or in benign disease such as prostatic hyperplasia (63). Conversely, Sutinen et al. showed that both cancerous and hyperplastic prostate were well visualized with [^{11}C]choline against low or moderate radiotracer accumulation in the bladder and rectal wall (64). However, the difference between the SUVs of PCa and benign prostate hyperplasia was not statistically significant [tumor—mean SUV was 5.6 ± 3.2 (range 1.9–15.5; $n = 15$); benign hyperplastic prostate—3.5 ± 1.0 (range 2.0–4.5; $n = 4$)] despite the fact that the highest SUVs were found in cancers. There was close association of the kinetic influx constant (K_i) and SUV using [^{11}C]choline. However, no correlation could be demonstrated between the tumor uptake of [^{11}C]choline and the histological grade, Gleason score, volume of the prostate or PSA (64). Kwee et al. evaluated dual-phase [^{18}F]fluorocholine PET (with imaging shortly after injection as well as at 1-hour postinjection) in a population of 26 men presenting at initial diagnosis or recurrence after therapy (65). On dual-phase imaging of the prostate, malignant regions demonstrated increasing uptake whereas benign tissue demonstrated decreasing uptake. A retrospective evaluation of the intraprostatic sextant localization of PCa with MRI, 3D MR spectroscopy, and [^{11}C]choline in 26 men with biopsy-proved PCa reported sensitivity, specificity, and accuracy of 55%, 86%, and 67%, respectively, with PET/CT; 54%, 75%, and 61% with MR imaging; and 81%, 67%, and 76% at 3D MR spectroscopy (66). The specificity of [^{11}C]choline for localizing PCa within the prostate was comparable to either 3D MR spectroscopy and MRI

or [^{11}C]choline PET/CT, although PET/CT has lower sensitivity compared with 3D MR spectroscopy alone or in combination with MRI.

[^{11}C]Choline PET has been evaluated for preoperative staging in PCa. In a large prospective study, de Jong et al. examined 67 consecutive patients with histologically proved PCa with [^{11}C]choline PET (67). The results of PET were compared with the results from histology of the pelvic lymph nodes and with the follow-up clinical data. The sensitivity, specificity, and accuracy of [^{11}C]choline PET in detecting lymph node neoplastic involvement from PCa was reported to be 80%, 96%, and 93%, respectively, suggesting that this radiotracer has a higher sensitivity than CT or MR imaging (67). More recently Scher et al. evaluated the utility of [^{11}C]choline PET and PET/CT in suspected PCa in 58 patients using SUV measurements, with disease confirmed by biopsy and histopathology (68). [^{11}C]Choline demonstrated a sensitivity of 86.5% and a specificity of 61.9% in the detection of the primary malignancy, and a per-patient sensitivity of 81.8% for detecting distant metastasis. Interestingly, using a qualitative image interpretation method they claimed to be able to differentiate between benign prostatic changes, benign prostatic hyperplasia or prostatitis, and PCa. False-positive results may occur due to focal bowel radioactivity or reactive lymph nodes and false-negative results are described in lymph node lesions smaller than 1 cm in diameter (69,70).

There have been several studies that have evaluated [^{11}C]choline for PCa staging. Rinnab et al. compared [^{11}C]choline PET and transrectal ultrasonography (TRUS) in the preoperative staging of 55 patients with clinically localized PCa (71). The overall accuracy of PET in defining local tumor stage, either limited to the prostate or with local invasion, was 70%; the overall accuracy by TRUS was 26%. PET was more sensitive than TRUS for detecting extracapsular extension and seminal vesicle invasion in advanced stages. The sensitivity and positive predictive value (95% confidence interval) for detection of local invasion for PET were 36 (17–59%) and 73 (39–89%). The sensitivity and positive predictive value for detection of local invasion for TRUS were 14 (3–35%) and 100 (29–100%). [^{11}C]Choline PET and TRUS tended to understage PCa. This series shows the current limited value of TRUS and PET for making treatment decisions in patients with clinically localized PCa. Eschman et al. compared [^{11}C]choline PET/CT and whole-body MRI for staging of PCa in 42 patients with untreated disease or increasing levels of PSA after local therapy (72). Overall sensitivity, specificity, and accuracy for [^{11}C] choline PET/CT were 96.6%, 76.5%, and 93.3%, respectively, and that for whole-body MRI were 78.4%, 94.1%, and 81.0%, respectively. Both [^{11}C]choline PET/CT and whole-body MRI demonstrated relatively high accuracy in the detection of bone and lymph node metastases.

In restaging of PCa after radical treatment, the ability of prostate cells to incorporate [11C]choline can be exploited diagnostically. In fact, as the prostate is the only organ in the pelvis to accumulate [11C]choline, pathologically increased radiotracer uptake in that area clearly indicates recurrence of disease. However, local recurrence can be missed by [11C]choline PET (73).

On the other hand, for the detection of lymph node and bone metastases, the usefulness of [11C]choline PET has been demonstrated definitively. [11C]Choline has also been evaluated in the detection of biochemical recurrence after initial local therapy (67,73–79). Picchio et al. reported a comparison of [11C]choline and FDG-PET in 100 patients referred for FDG restaging after prostatectomy or radiotherapy. Areas of abnormal focal radiopharmaceutical increases were noted in 47% of patients on [11C]choline PET and in 27% on FDG PET. Of the 100 patients, 49 had positive conventional imaging findings. All except 14 [11C]choline PET findings were concordant with conventional imaging, including six negative and eight positive conventional imaging results. All except one [11C]choline PET negative cases also had negative conventional imaging after one year. PSA at one year remained stable or decreased in 80% and 62% of [11C] choline PET negative and positive cases, respectively.

There have been a number of more recent studies evaluating [11C]choline PET in the setting of increasing PSA after primary treatment for PCa (75–77,79). They reported mixed results. Rinnab et al. demonstrated a sensitivity of 91% and specificity of 50% using a PSA level of <2.5 ng/mL. Krause et al. demonstrated a detection efficiency of 36% even of PSA values <1.0 ng/mL, showing a positive relationship with serum PSA levels in patients with biochemical recurrence after primary therapy. Reske et al. demonstrated that [11C]choline PET detected occult local relapse of PCa with focal uptake in the prostate bed with a sensitivity of 73% and specificity of 88%, identifying 71% of patients with a favorable biochemical response to local radiotherapy at two years (Fig. 3). Scattoni et al. evaluated [11C]choline PET lymph node recurrence in patients with biochemical relapse after prostatectomy. A lesion-based analysis demonstrated a sensitivity of 64%, specificity of 90%, positive predictive value of 86%, negative predictive value of 72%, and accuracy of 77%. Notably, the mean maximum diameter of true positive metastases was significantly larger (1.5 cm) than false-negative ones, providing evidence that the low negative predictive value is in part due to the limit of [11C] choline PET/CT to detect microscopic lesions. The high PPV, even with low PSA values, provides a basis for further treatment decisions.

De Jong et al. prospectively evaluated 36 patients with localized PCa, treated by either radical prostatectomy (n = 20) or by external beam radiotherapy (n = 16). [11C]Choline PET was performed in either previously treated patients with no biochemical evidence of disease

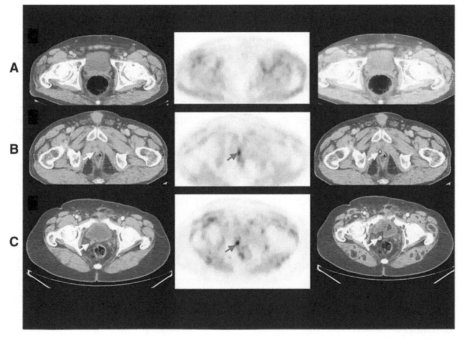

Figure 3 [11C]Choline PET/CT imaging of occult local relapse. CT, [11C]choline PET, and [11C]choline PET/CT fusion imaging. (**A**) Control with unremarkable findings, PSA 0.1 ng/mL. (**B**) Small perianastomotic relapse (*arrow*), PSA 1.05 ng/mL. (**C**) Right paramedian retrovesical relapse (*arrow*), PSA 1.9 ng/mL. *Abbreviations*: PET/CT, positron emission tomography/computed tomography; PSA, prostate-specific antigen. *Source*: From Ref. 76.

or in those with biochemical evidence of disease after radical prostatectomy, identified by a postoperative serum PSA > 0.2 ng/mL. [^{11}C]Choline PET imaging results were compared with the results of histology and with clinical follow-up. Fourteen patients had no biochemical failure after therapy and [^{11}C]choline PET was truly negative in 14 of 14 patients. In the 22 patient with biochemical failure in patients who underwent radical prostatectomy, [^{11}C]choline PET was truly positive in 5 of 13 (38%) cases. In the patients who underwent external beam radiotherapy, [^{11}C]choline PET was truly positive in 7 of 9 (78%) cases. The recurrent tumor was confirmed by biopsy or by bone scan in 11 of the 12 true positive patients. In 10 patients with biochemical recurrence but negative [^{11}C]choline PET scans, no recurrent tumor could be proved clinically, by biopsy or during variable periods of follow-up.

In restaging PCa, [^{11}C]choline PET has been shown to be complementary to conventional imaging techniques, but with the advantage that it can stage the disease in a single step (73). The main disadvantage of [^{11}C]choline is the short physical half-life of ^{11}C ($t_{1/2} = 20$ minutes), which limits its use to centers that have a cyclotron on-site.

The short physical half-life of ^{11}C was the reason why Hara et al. and DeGrado et al. developed ^{18}F-labeled analogs of choline (80). The behavior of these tracers is very similar to that of [^{11}C]choline; however, the fluorinated analogs demonstrate higher urinary excretion than [^{11}C]choline, which represents a disadvantage in imaging PCa.

There is some evidence to suggest that [^{18}F]choline may be avid at sites of infection—generating nonspecific uptake that can compromise tumor imaging. This was demonstrated in a rat model of intramuscular bacterial infection with [^{18}F]choline uptake in granulocytes and monocytes within the abscess wall determined by autoradiography and high-resolution small-animal PET imaging (81). That may explain prior studies demonstrating false-positive lymph node uptake.

[^{11}C]Choline is excreted to a minor extent by the kidney, while about 7.5% of injected [^{18}F]choline appears in urine (80). High urinary elimination limits the detection of local recurrence. By contrast, [^{11}C]acetate demonstrates no visible urinary excretion (82). However, the extent of urinary elimination of [^{18}F]acetate requires further investigation.

Recent evaluation of [^{18}F]choline for staging and restaging of PCa (43 initial, 68 restaging) demonstrated that initial N-staging results were discouraging, especially in terms of the inability of this radiopharmaceutical to detect small metastases. Histopathological workup was performed on 115 lymph nodes sampled from 25 patients. Only one of these lymph nodes showed pathological

[^{18}F]choline accumulation (see above) and was proved to be a metastasis measuring more than 1 cm. Four lymph nodes that did not show [^{18}F]choline accumulation turned out to contain metastatic cells, with an overall tumor load measuring less than 0.5 cm. All other lymph nodes did not contain malignant cells. Recurrent disease can be localized reliably in patients with PSA levels of >2 μg/L. Pathological [^{18}F]choline accumulation was seen in 57 of 68 patients who presented with biochemical recurrence of PCa and examined with [^{18}F]choline PET/CT. [^{18}F]Choline PET/CT was unable to demonstrate the site of recurrent disease in 11 patients, although a biochemical recurrence was present.

Other studies have evaluated [^{18}F]choline PET/CT for detection of PCa in the setting of elevated PSA after primary therapy (74,78). Cimitan et al. performed early and delayed [^{11}C]choline PET/CT scans in 100 patients with a persistent increase in serum PSA (>0.1 ng/mL) after various primary therapies (radical prostatectomy, radiotherapy, or hormonal therapy alone). [^{18}F]Choline PET/CT was unable to define local or distant tumor recurrence in 41 of 52 (79%) patients who had serum PSA levels <4 ng/mL, and performed particularly poorly in patients with well differentiated/moderately differentiated primary tumors with Gleason score ≤ 7. However, [^{18}F]choline PET/CT could be useful in a selected patient population with higher PSA levels and/or poorly differentiated prostate carcinoma to exclude distant metastases when salvage local treatment is intended. They demonstrated that 26 of 31 (84%) patients with PSA > 4 ng/mL and a Gleason score ≤ 7 and all (100%) patients with PSA > 4 ng/mL and a Gleason score > 7 were found to have positive uptake. Urinary activity reportedly did not interfere with image interpretation when using early and late PET/CT acquisition. Igerc et al. evaluated [^{18}F]choline PET/CT using a dual-phase protocol in 20 patients with elevated PSA and negative prostate needle biopsy. Qualitative analysis revealed focal uptake in 13 of 20 patients, with 5 patients confirmed to have PCa on repeat biopsy. However, semiquantitative analysis using SUV measurements was not helpful in discriminating malignancy from benign prostate disease.

[^{18}F]Choline PET/CT is not an ideal imaging modality for initial staging of PCa. In the case of biochemical recurrence, however, [^{18}F]choline PET/CT imaging can be very helpful. The sensitivity of 71% in localizing recurrent disease at PSA levels < 2 μg/L is not very high, but at the moment there is no other imaging modality that performs better (83).

Another promising PET radiotracer for imaging PCa is [^{11}C]acetate, used originally for heart studies. In vitro studies suggest that the high tumor-to-normal ratio of [1-^{14}C]acetate is mainly due to enhanced lipid synthesis, which reflects the high growth activity of neoplasms.

Tumor cells incorporated [1-^{14}C]acetate activity into the lipid-soluble fraction, mostly of phosphatidylcholine and neutral lipids, more prominently than did fibroblasts (84).

Although several studies on the use of [^{11}C]acetate in PCa are now available (70,82,85–89), this tracer has undergone less extensive evaluation in comparison to [^{11}C]choline. The above-mentioned studies evaluated patients with rising PSA after local therapy. [^{11}C]Acetate has been shown to be superior to FDG in defining prostate tumors and metastases (87), being similar to [^{11}C]choline (82). It has been suggested that [^{11}C]acetate enters the lipid pool of tumor tissue, although the metabolism of this agent and the mechanism for its incorporation into prostate tumors has not yet been definitively determined (90). As the biodistribution of [^{11}C]acetate and [^{11}C]choline differs while their degree of uptake within the tumor is similar, the relative amount of nonspecific binding of these compounds could determine which will ultimately prove successful.

In a report from Oyama et al., patients with rising PSA, after either prostatectomy or radiation therapy, were imaged with [^{11}C]acetate and FDG (86). The images demonstrated marked uptake of [^{11}C]acetate, with higher sensitivity for this tracer than for FDG. Limiting the analysis to studies considered at high probability of tumor recurrence (as confirmed by CT, bone scintigraphy, conventional radiography, or CT), 14 (30%) had disease identified by [^{11}C]acetate PET, whereas only 4 (9%) had disease identified by FDG PET. Thirteen of 22 patients (59%) with serum PSA > 3 ng/mL had positive [^{11}C] acetate PET findings, whereas only 1 of 24 patients (4%) with serum PSA levels ≤ 3 ng/mL had positive findings (85).

The most recent report from Albrecht et al. evaluated [^{11}C]acetate PET in 32 PCa patients with evidence of biochemical relapse after initial radiation therapy or prostatectomy. In the prostatectomy group using an SUV$_{max} \geq 2$, [^{11}C]acetate PET demonstrated local recurrences in 14 of 17 patients and two equivocal results. Distant metastasis was seen in six patients with one equivocal finding, and biopsy confirmed local recurrence in six of six (100%) patients. In the postradiation therapy group, 14 of the 17 patients had uptake in the residual gland, 6 of whom were biopsied and found to be positive. Fourteen of the 17 postradiation therapy patients had uptake in lymph nodes, 4 of 8 patients with positive bone scans were positive by PET, and a corpus cavernosum metastasis was documented.

[^{18}F]Fluoroacetate has been synthesized and evaluated in CWR22 PCa tumor-bearing mice and compared with [^{11}C]acetate (91). Rat biodistribution studies showed extensive defluorination, which was not observed in the baboon imaging studies. Prostate tumor uptake was higher with [^{18}F]fluoroacetate with a mean SUV of 4.01 ± 0.32

percent injected dose per gram of tissue (%ID/g) versus [^{11}C]acetate tumor uptake of 0.78 ± 0.06 %ID/g. For most organs, except blood, muscle, and fat, the tumor-organ ratios at 30 minutes after injection were higher with [^{18}F] fluoroacetate than with [^{11}C]acetate, whereas the tumor-to-heart and tumor-to-prostate ratios were similar (91). The first human images of [^{18}F]fluoroacetate were obtained showing high uptake in bone metastases in a patient with PCa (92).

The sensitivity of [^{14}C]choline uptake to proliferative activity was less than that of [1-^{14}C]acetate in an in vitro comparison of various cancer cell lines (93). Both radiotracers enter the normal prostate gland and its benign forms of hyperplasia (homogeneous distribution), as well as PCa (including local recurrence) and its metastases in lymph nodes, bone, and soft tissue. A study of interindividual variation of [^{11}C]choline and [^{11}C]acetate in the initial staging of 12 patients with PCa demonstrated a nearly identical pattern of uptake in the primary tumor and its metastases (82).

[^{11}C]Acetate appears to be equivalent to [^{11}C]choline in imaging PCa and its metastases. Currently, very few data are available to favor one tracer over the other. The limitations of both are similar regarding inability to detect microscopic lesions, the presence of nonspecific intestinal uptake, and uptake in inflammatory tissues. Neither radiotracer can replace SLN scintigraphy or bone scan, including [^{18}F]fluoride PET, in the workup of patients with PCa. Therefore, the most appropriate radiopharmaceutical for PCa depends on the clinical question, the availability of radiotracers, and individual experience (94).

A more recent comparison of [^{18}F]fluorocholine and [^{11}C]acetate by Vees et al. involved the detection of residual or progressive subclinical disease at very low PSA levels (<1 ng/mL) after radical prostatectomy (95). Both radiotracers were able to detect local residual or recurrent disease in about half of the patients.

Presently [^{11}C]choline PET does not present significant advantages over [^{11}C]acetate PET in patients with PCa, but larger, prospective studies are needed to define the role of each radiotracer for this indication.

[^{18}F]Sodium fluoride PET has been used to identify skeletal metastasis in patients with a range of primary tumors. Comparative studies have found [^{18}F]fluoride PET to be more accurate than [^{99m}Tc]MDP SPECT for identifying malignant as well as benign lesions of the skeleton (96,97). Prospective data from patients with newly diagnosed lung cancer indicate that [^{18}F]fluoride PET can detect skeletal involvement earlier than can conventional bone scan owing to the better resolution of PET (98).

Specifically with respect to PCa, Even-Sapir et al. compared detection of bone metastases by [^{99m}Tc]MDP planar bone scintigraphy, SPECT, [^{18}F]fluoride PET, and

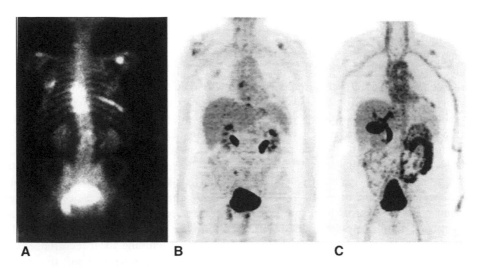

Figure 4 [^{18}F]FDHT androgen receptor imaging. Comparative whole-body images of a 75-year-old man with progressive prostate cancer metastatic to bones of the thoracic spine, left rib cage, and scapula: planar camera image of [^{99m}Tc]MDP (**A**); 1-pixel-thick coronal PET image of FDG (**B**); and 1-pixel-thick coronal PET image of [^{18}F]FDHT (**C**). *Abbreviations*: [^{18}F]FDHT, [^{18}F]6β-fluoro-5α-dihydrotestosterone; FDG, fluorodeoxyglucose; PET, positron emission tomography. *Source*: From Ref. 166.

[^{18}F]fluoride PET/CT in patients with high-risk PCa (99). Forty-four patients at high risk for bone metastases were prospectively evaluated in which 25 patients were newly diagnosed, with Gleason scores of $\geq$ 8, PSA levels $\geq$ 20 ng/mL, or nonspecific sclerotic lesions on CT. The remaining patients were referred for evaluation of suspected recurrence or progression later in the course of the disease. [^{18}F]Fluoride PET/CT was found to be the most sensitive and specific modality for detection of bone metastases in patients with high-risk PCa. The sensitivity, specificity, positive predictive value, and negative predictive value of [^{18}F]fluoride PET/CT was 100%, in comparison with planar bone scans, with 70%, 57%, 64%, and 55%, respectively, and of multi-field-of-view SPECT with 92%, 82%, 86%, and 90%, respectively. The added value of [^{18}F]fluoride PET/CT was thought to benefit the clinical management of patients with high-risk PCa. In another report [^{18}F]choline PET/CT was able to depict bone metastases, but [^{18}F]fluoride PET demonstrated greater sensitivity (100).

[^{11}C]Methionine accumulation in tumors is attributed to increased amino acid transport and metabolism (101,102). [^{11}C]Methionine has been compared with FDG in 12 patients with PCa and increasing PSA levels (21). The sensitivity of [^{11}C]methionine for detection of PCa was 72.1% compared to a sensitivity of 48% for FDG PET. A large fraction of lesions (26%) had no detectable metabolism of FDG or [^{11}C]methionine, which was attributed to necrotic or metabolically inactive tumor. A second study by Toth et al. evaluated 20 patients with recurrent PCa presenting with increasing serum PSA and negative repeat biopsies (103). [^{11}C]Methionine PET was positive in 75% of

the patients, of which 46.7% were found to have biopsy verified carcinoma. The overall detection rate was 35%.

16β-Fluoro-5α-dihydrotestosterone (FDHT) is a structural analog of 5α-dihydrotestosterone, the principle intraprostatic form of androgen. [^{18}F]FDHT has been evaluated in two PCa imaging studies to evaluate the concept of androgen receptor imaging (104,105). Larson et al. evaluated seven patients with recurrent PCa, with castrate levels of testosterone, and clinically progressive metastatic disease. The patients underwent both FDG and [^{18}F]FDHT PET scans (Fig. 4). Conventional imaging identified 59 lesions, of which [^{18}F]FDHT PET was positive in 78% with an average lesion SUV$_{max}$ of 5.28. By comparison, FDG PET was positive in 97% of lesions with an average lesion SUV$_{max}$ of 5.22. Dehdashti et al. evaluated 19 patients with advanced PCa. In comparison to lesions detected by conventional imaging, [^{18}F]FDHT PET was positive in 12 of 19 patients with a sensitivity of 63%, and detected 86% (24/28) of known lesions in the remaining 10 patients as well as 2 patients with innumerable metastases. Patients with a positive [^{18}F]FDHT PET study underwent a repeat examination after receiving flutamide, an oral antiandrogen, for one day and demonstrated an interval decrease in tumor uptake as measured by a significant decrease in SUV and tumor-muscle ratio. The tumor burden as measured by mean PSA in patients with positive [^{18}F]FDHT PET was significantly higher compared with those who had negative studies.

Radiolabeled synthetic amino acids demonstrate high uptake in tumors due to increased protein metabolism (102,106). A synthetic nonmetabolized L-leucine amino

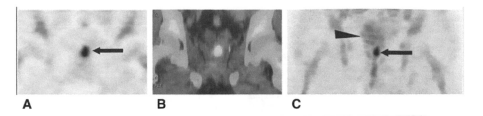

Figure 5 Anti-[^{18}F]FACBC imaging of prostate bed recurrence. Coronal PET (**A**) and CT fused (**B**) anti-[^{18}F]FACBC images in a 71-year-old patient with biopsy proved prostate bed recurrence extending toward left seminal vesicle (*arrow* in **A**). Maximum intensity projection image at 20 minutes (**C**) demonstrates uptake in the prostate bed (*arrow*) but little bladder uptake (*arrowhead*). *Abbreviations*: [^{18}F]FACBC, 1-amino-3-[^{18}F]fluorocyclobutane-1-carboxylic acid; PET, positron emission tomography. *Source*: From Ref. 108.

acid analog, anti-1-amino-3-[^{18}F]fluorocyclobutane-1-carboxylic acid (anti-[^{18}F]FACBC), demonstrated marked uptake in DU-145 prostate carcinoma cell lines and in an orthotopic mouse model of PCa (107). Schuster et al. reported an initial experience of anti-[^{18}F]FACBC in 15 patients with either newly diagnosed or suspected recurrent PCa (Fig. 5) (108). In the newly diagnosed patients, anti-[^{18}F]FACBC correctly diagnosed tumor in 40 of 48 prostate region sextants, and 7 of 9 patients had pelvic nodal uptake that was concordant with clinical follow-up (pathology, clinical, PSA, and imaging follow-up up to 1 year). Anti-[^{18}F]FACBC PET was positive in all four patients with proved recurrence. Interestingly, Prosta-Scint had no significant uptake in three of the four anti-[^{18}F]FACBC positive recurrences. Additionally, there was little renal excretion of radiotracer in comparison to FDG.

1-(2′-Deoxy-2′-fluoro-β-D-arabinofuranosyl)thymine (FMAU), an analog of thymidine, can incorporate into DNA and therefore image DNA synthesis and cell proliferation (109,110). Sun et al. evaluated the potential of [^{18}F]FMAU in 14 patients with various cancers (110). Three patients had PCa, one with locally advanced disease and two with bone metastases. One patient with bone metastasis previously had local radiation therapy and showed low uptake in the prostate bed. [^{18}F]FMAU PET demonstrated high uptake in prostate tumor with SUV_{max} of 2.89 and 4.49. Bone metastases also showed high radiopharmaceutical uptake with SUV_{max} of 2.41 and 3.34. Prostate tumor showed high tumor-to-background ratios of 2.26 to 6.31. A low level of radioactivity was seen in the bone marrow and low background levels of radioactivity were seen in the brain, thorax, and pelvis. There was renal excretion of this radiotracer but reportedly low urinary bladder radioactivity in 10 of 14 patients.

[^{18}F]Fluorothymidine ([^{18}F]FLT) is another PET agent for measuring cell proliferation. It has been studied in the CWR22 experimental model. [^{18}F]FLT tumor uptake was 0.69 ± 0.14 %ID/g, showing the most prominent activity in the tumor and reaching a tumor radioactivity plateau in 30 to 60 minutes (111). [^{18}F]FLT imaging in patients with PCa has not been published to date.

MRI-BASED TECHNIQUES

Although MRI is far less sensitive than the radiopharmaceutical-based techniques for detecting molecular species in vivo, its exquisite spatial resolution enables fine detail of imaging cells within tissues. Relevant to the molecular imaging of PCa, MR-based techniques include MR spectroscopic imaging (MRSI) and imaging with lymphotropic nanoparticles, sometimes referred to as lymphotropic nanoparticle-enhanced MRI (LNMRI).

MRSI, like anatomic MRI, requires excitation of tissue with a radio frequency pulse and interpretation of the effect of that pulse on the water protons within the tissue. The only difference is that Fourier transformation segregates the MR signal returning from tissue into individual frequencies. The signal intensities associated with the various frequencies are plotted on the x-axis of the MR spectrum, while the y-axis represents signal intensity, which is proportional to the concentration of the molecular species present at that resonant frequency. Those molecular species are substituents within certain key metabolites in tissue, which for prostate are choline, creatine, and citrate. Volumes of interest (VOIs) must be identified and encoded in the MR spectrum, and the methods for localizing VOIs must compromise between spatial resolution, spectral resolution, and signal-to-noise ratio. Pulsed field gradients are generally used for that localization and include sequences known as point resolved spectroscopy (PRESS) and stimulated echo acquisition mode (STEAM). Both of these techniques can be used for performing MR spectroscopy within a single volume element of tissue, or voxel, or for multi-voxel acquisition. The latter technique is referred to as MRSI and provides more global information about the prostate by evaluating nearly the entire gland at once. MRSI can detect and provide a parametric map of the concentration of protons or other atomic species with a magnetic moment, such as ^{13}C, as discussed below.

Because a limited, although growing (due to the availability of increasingly higher field strengths), number of metabolites can be measured, MRSI is considered a true

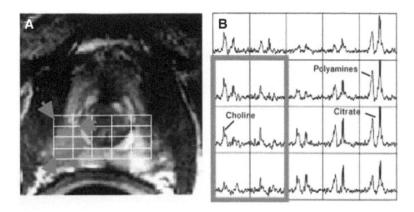

Figure 6 Multiparametric 3T image of prostate cancer. (**A**) T_2-weighted MRI showing a region of low signal intensity (*arrows*) in the right apex. (**B**) Corresponding spectral 0.16 cm^3 array showing abnormal spectra (*box*) in the same region as the suspicious region of low T_2 signal intensity. Note elevated choline and low citrate concentration, characteristic of prostate cancer. *Source*: From Ref. 113.

molecular imaging technique. For prostate MRSI (112–114), the important parameter is the ratio of [choline + creatine] to [citrate] (115). Knowledge regarding the physiological meaning of these species is increasing; however, traditionally choline has been thought of as a marker of membrane integrity and turnover, while creatine, ostensibly related to cellular energy status, is generally used as a relatively invariant constant against which to measure the other metabolites. Citrate is a metabolite that is distinctive for having prognostic implications in prostate as opposed to other tissues. While the concentration of choline tends to be elevated in PCa, that of citrate is diminished—perhaps a result of the increase in anaerobic metabolism and high energy demand of malignant tissue. Figure 6 shows a typical MR spectroscopic image of normal prostate and PCa.

The purpose of metabolic (or molecular) imaging of PCa with MRSI is to detect cancer in the peripheral zone, determine if there is extracapsular spread, for therapeutic monitoring, and perhaps even avoid the need for biopsy in patients with low tumor volume. The combination of anatomic MR and MRSI is highly sensitive and specific for PCa, with values for these parameters exceeding those of traditional sextant biopsy. The sensitivity and specificity of the combined anatomic and molecular techniques is 56% and 82%, respectively (115). The positive predictive value of combining these two modalities approaches 90%. This technique—and MR is always performed in conjunction with MRSI—is not used as a first-line approach to diagnosing PCa, but is used for presurgical staging and in radiotherapy planning. It is increasingly used to monitor patients with low volume (Gleason $\leq$ 6) disease who have opted for watchful waiting rather than prostatectomy (114).

MRSI for PCa has proved to be a successful advance for imaging of PCa. Only recently has it become widely

and commercially available. As more centers gain experience with this valuable technique and further correlation with clinical parameters and outcome become available, we will be able to realize the full potential of this safe radiation-free technique.

After many years of preclinical optimization, ultrasmall supraparamagnetic iron oxide (USPIO) particles have proved their utility in detecting metastatic involvement of PCa within pelvic lymph nodes (116–120). Knowledge of pelvic node involvement is critical to the management of PCa, and once demonstrated, will elevate the tumor grade. Demonstration of a positive node can mean the difference between local and systemic, or merely palliative, therapy. The USPIOs, e.g., ferumoxtran-10, used for this purpose are not actively targeted but are phagocytosed by peripheral macrophages after intravenous injection. The USPIOs are detected by virtue of the T_2-weighted signal intensity decrease they provide within macrophages as they aggregate in lymph nodes (Fig. 7). This technique has demonstrated extremely high sensitivity (100%) and specificity (96%) for involved lymph nodes that were between 5 mm and 1 cm in diameter (119). For nodes <5 mm, the sensitivity dropped to 41% (121), but the idea of a human imaging technique demonstrating metastatic involvement of lesions of <5 mm is nothing short of astounding. Neither the standard anatomic techniques (CT and MR) nor PET nor SPECT can provide the spatial resolution or contrast to enable detection of such small lesions. And those studies were performed at a field strength of 1.5 T. Studies at higher field (3.0 T, the new clinical standard) have been performed, enabling higher signal-to-noise ratio and therefore better spatial resolution (121). Such studies have demonstrated better delineation of lymph node borders. Other recent studies have attempted to improve image detection by comparing different T_2-weighted pulse sequences,

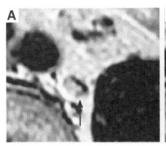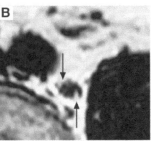

Figure 7 MRI nodal abnormality in a patient with prostate cancer. Conventional MRI shows high signal intensity in a node with micrometastasis (*arrow* in panel **A**). LNMRI demonstrates T_2 signal intensity decrease in regions accessible to macrophages but not where micrometastasis is present (*arrows* in panel **B**). *Abbreviations*: LNMRI, lymphotropic nanoparticle-enhanced MRI. *Source*: From Ref. 119.

concluding that the most sensitive sequence for this type of imaging is the gradient-refocused echo T_2^*-weighted (GRE-T_2^*) sequence (122). That is not surprising due to the exquisite sensitivity of that sequence to susceptibility artifact.

Although as of this writing it has not yet received approval by the U.S. Food and Drug Administration, LNMRI has proved safe and can be performed repeatedly in the same patient. That is significant because nanobiotechnology has seen few human applications to date, despite the vast promise of this field. Ferumoxtran-10 is a true nanoparticle and is genuinely inert, unlike most quantum dots and other nanoparticles with toxic metal cores, which will be useful in preclinical models but be unlikely to progress much further. As more experience is gained, as this technique has only been performed by a handful of physicians at a few centers, LNMRI may routinely complement other methods to seek metastatic node involvement. The technique has already been applied to diseases outside of the pelvis, and its first clinical use was to detect the margin of a recurrent brain tumor (123). Another obvious extension of this work is to use such particles for cell trafficking, which has been performed with striking success in the case of dendritic cells (124). Multifunctional versions of these nanoparticles have appeared in preclinical studies, and once refined for human use we may see their use in optical as well as MR and radiopharmaceutical-based applications (118). As nanoparticles, which can be developed to carry a toxic or genetic payload, they are also well-suited to serve as theranostic agents.

ON THE HORIZON

There are several techniques and radiotracers used for the molecular imaging of PCa that merit further mention, although most have not yet been administered to human

subjects. On the preclinical side, new highly relevant models for PCa are continually arising. This includes the transgenic adenocarcinoma mouse prostate (TRAMP) model (125), which recapitulates many aspects of the human disease. Researchers can now readily manipulate well-known cell lines to cause them to metastasize, for example, by inserting the vascular endothelial growth factor C (VEGF-C) gene, which promotes lymphangiogenesis (126). That could revolutionize the search for new imaging and therapeutic agents for PCa since existing metastatic models are inconsistent and difficult to use. Among the new, promising, primarily preclinical tracers and techniques are the radioiodinated phospholipid ethers (PLEs), hyperpolarized [^{13}C]pyruvate and ^{13}C MRSI, radiolabeled vasoactive intestinal peptide and pituitary adenylate cyclase-activating peptide receptor (VPAC) ligands, radiopharmaceuticals for imaging the PSMA, and molecular-genetic imaging of PCa.

Since the 1980s, Counsell et al. have been studying the potential of radioiodinated PLEs for tumor imaging—an effort that is now bearing fruit after many years of structural optimization (127,128). These agents work by virtue of the higher proportion of lipid within malignant relative to normal cells. That, in turn, has been attributed to the lower concentration of *O*-alkyl glycerol monooxygenase present within tumors (129). However, even compounds that are substrates of that enzyme are still able to be sequestered within the tumor cell membrane, so there must be some combination of lipophilicity and selective lack of metabolism/elimination that accounts for the mechanism of tumor accumulation of the PLEs. After many years of optimization two promising compounds have emerged, namely [^{131}I]NM324 and, in particular, the second generation compound [^{131}I]NM404 (129). The structure-activity relationships have revealed that chain length of the phospholipid moiety is critical, with longer chain lengths providing more tumor retention, but also increased nonspecific (liver and abdomen) binding. Compounds of short, e.g., C-7 length, hydrophobic chains tend not to demonstrate significant tumor uptake and are rapidly cleared. The C-18 compound NM404 provides the ideal scaffold for tumor imaging, demonstrating 9 %ID/g at one day and 15 %ID/g by eight days after administration. [^{131}I]NM404 is significantly cleared from nontarget organs, including abdomen, by day four. Because these compounds are metabolized through the gastrointestinal tract, they do not accumulate in the bladder, adding a further convenience for prostate tumor imaging (Fig. 8). Deiodination in vivo does occur, with 30 to 40 %ID/g of the radioactivity residing within thyroid. That should, however, be able to be overcome by pretreatment with suitable thyroid-blocking agents, such as potassium iodide (SSKI). Because imaging must be undertaken at least a day or so after intravenous injection, the PLEs must be labeled with radioiodine, specifically ^{124}I ($t_{1/2} = 4.2$ days),

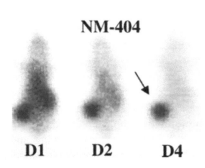

Figure 8 Scintigraphic images of [^{125}I]NM404 at one, two, and four days postinjection to a SCID mouse with a human prostate PC3 tumor implanted within the flank (*arrow*). Note the lack of background radioactivity at four days postinjection. *Source*: From Ref. 129.

for PET. More conventional and more readily available isotopes such as ^{18}F and ^{99m}Tc would not be applicable to PLE imaging. Nevertheless, the striking signal-to-noise ratio and high tumor uptake demonstrated in recent preclinical models make compounds of this series quite promising for radionuclide imaging and therapy.

Hyperpolarized [^{13}C]pyruvate takes advantage of the brief but significant retention of dynamic nuclear polarization of ^{13}C in solution, needed due to the low natural abundance and sensivity of imaging with ^{13}C compared with ^{1}H (130). Although images must be obtained within a minute of administration of [^{13}C]pyruvate, careful planning and attention to logistical detail make this a practical, new method for studying cellular bioenergetics in vivo. Similar attention to logistical detail was required in the early days of PET with [^{15}O]H$_2$O to study brain blood flow, before functional MR imaging largely replace the PET-based flow methods. Hyperpolarized [^{13}C]pyruvate allows the study of unique fluxes in metabolic processes such as glycolysis and the tricarboxylic acid cycle, both of which are altered in cancer. Because of the very high temporal resolution capable of MR instruments, those fluxes can be studied in real time in a tissue-specific fashion. A double spin echo sequence with a small-tip-angle excitation radio frequency pulse is applied to enable 10- to 14-second MRSI of [^{13}C]pyruvate and its metabolites at a nominal spatial resolution of 0.135 cm^3. That pulse sequence was designed to use the prepolarized magnetization quickly and efficiently. The hyperpolarized [^{13}C]pyruvate, with ^{13}C in C$_1$, produces similarly labeled alanine and lactate, which are the observed metabolites. Since tumors tend to have elevated anaerobic metabolism, they would be expected to have elevated lactate, which can be detected with this technique. This information complements that uncovered by MRSI, and more importantly, provides a more dynamic picture. This technique has recently been applied to the TRAMP model at 3 T

(130). As with most promising, new MR-based techniques, further improvements in coil design and the use of higher performance gradients should make the technique even more sensitive and provide a new facet of information to studying the bioenergetics of PCa in vivo.

VPAC1 receptor is reportedly expressed in 100% of prostate cancers, making it a highly desirable target for imaging (131). A modified version of the VIP$_{28}$ peptide was derivatized for PET imaging with ^{64}Cu ($t_{1/2}$ = 12.7 hours) ([^{64}Cu]TP3939) and tested in PCa xenografts and the TRAMP model (131). This compound demonstrated 4:1 tumor-muscle ratio at four hours that increased to 5:1 at 24 hours after injection in nude mice bearing PC3 tumors. At the first time point about 7 %ID/g was present within tumor. However, 15% of the radioactivity was transchelated to plasma proteins. This compound represents the latest in a series of promising peptide-based imaging agents for PCa, which includes the bombesins (132–135) among others (136), some of which have entered clinical use with "unconventional" isotopes such as ^{68}Ga (137).

As stated above, PSMA has abundant and restricted expression on the surface of prostate carcinomas, particularly in androgen-independent advanced and metastatic disease (138,139). The latter fact is important since almost all prostate cancers become androgen independent. PSMA possesses the criteria of an ideal target for immunotherapy, i.e., expression primarily restricted to the prostate, abundantly expressed as protein at all stages of the disease, presented at the cell surface but not shed into the circulation, and association with enzymatic or signaling activity (138). In normal prostate epithelium, PSMA is expressed primarily as PSM′, which resides in the cytoplasm (140), while in PCa, differential mRNA splicing leads to its expression as an integral membrane protein with a 19-aa cytoplasmic fragment, a 24-aa intramembrane domain, and a 707-aa extracellular region (138). The PSMA gene is located on the short arm of chromosome 11 and functions both as a folate hydrolase and a neuropeptidase. There are up to 10^6 PSMA molecules per cancer cell, making it an ideal target for imaging and therapy (141).

Although ProstaScint images are somewhat difficult to interpret (142–144), the target for this radiolabeled antibody, PSMA, has proved worthy of a radiosynthetic effort toward low molecular weight ligands for imaging. These compounds can be separated into two different classes, the phosphinic acids (145,146) and the ureas (147,148), but both can be thought of as metabolically stable "dipeptide" analogs. The primary indication for these compounds, like ProstaScint, will be for imaging metastatic disease in men who have undergone prostatectomy who present with a rising PSA level. While the phosphinic acids have shown promise in vitro (149), they have not yet demonstrated high binding selectivity to PSMA-expressing tissues in vivo. With the recent availability of a high-resolution crystal structure of PSMA (150–152), radiophamaceuticals of high affinity and in vivo selectivity of the urea series have been synthesized using a variety of radionuclides for PET and SPECT (153–156). Using SCID mice harboring a PC3 tumor that is naturally devoid of PSMA as well as another that has been transfected to express it, a ^{99m}Tc-based agent has achieved target-nontarget ratio of greater than 40:1 at two hours postinjection (156). Other compounds of that series, which use the single amino acid chelator (SAAC) concept, are fluorescent when chelated with rhenium. These compounds, being highly hydrophilic (each possesses three carboxylic acid groups), undergo little metabolism and undergo renal excretion. The proximal renal tubules contain PSMA, so at least a portion of the binding within kidney is specific (141,157). Because of that path of excretion and the low molecular weight of these agents, there is very little background radioactivity demonstrated on the preclinical images (Fig. 9). Whether these compounds will be useful for intraprostatic imaging remains to be seen; however, subtraction of bladder radioactivity using postprocessing methods may be possible. Interestingly, a compound in this series known as N-[N-[(S)-1,3-dicarboxypropyl]carbamoyl]-S-3-[^{125}I]iodo-L-tyrosine ([^{125}I]DCIT) has taken advantage of the neuropeptidase aspect of PSMA and has demonstrated the ability to distinguish between various groups of psychiatric patients in an in vitro autoradiography study (158).

Gene therapy has encountered several roadblocks. Although safety has been an important concern (159), the most significant roadblock has been the lack of efficacy of existing regimens. Molecular-genetic imaging

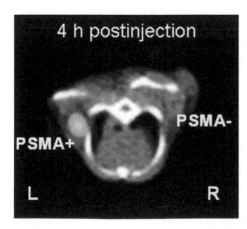

Figure 9 Axial prone SPECT image of a SCID mouse with PC3 PSMA+ and PC3 PSMA– tumors implanted within each flank. Imaging was performed four hours after injection of compound [^{99m}Tc]L1. *Abbreviation*: PSMA, prostate-specific membrane antigen (*See Color Insert*).

is among the best examples of performing imaging in the service of therapy because it is often coupled with gene therapy. By imaging expression of a therapeutic transgene, one may show that it is indeed being expressed and that the expression is located in expected target site(s). Molecular-genetic imaging of cancer generally requires the use of a reporter transgene (160,161). There have not been many clinical studies that employ molecular-genetic imaging, but one that has been undertaken has targeted PCa (see below).

Reporter genes can be thought of as pretargeting molecules (162). They are deliberately introduced into the cell of interest prior to administration of a tagged substrate or receptor-based imaging agent. They tend to be either intracellular, as with the herpes simplex 1 thymidine kinase (HSV1-*tk*), or they can be extracellular, as with the D_2 dopamine receptor. Higher sensitivity tends to be achieved through use of an enzymatic reporter (HSV1-*tk*) than of an extracellular receptor-based reporter due to an amplification effect. Reporter genes represent a method of indirect imaging—the reporter that is linked to the activity of the true gene of interest is what is actually imaged—and studies employing them can be divided into four categories, namely (*i*) imaging of gene marked cells, (*ii*) imaging gene therapy, (*iii*) imaging transgenic (reporter gene) animals, and (*iv*) imaging complex intracellular events such as protein interaction networks (162). Most of these items are covered elsewhere in this volume.

One group that has expended great effort attempting to optimize gene therapy for PCa has been that at the Henry Ford Health System. They have performed studies in preclinical models, including canine dosimetry, using the sodium-iodide symporter (NIS) as the reporter gene and ^{99m}TcO$_4$ as the reporter probe (163,164). The strategy they employ is to use a replication-competent oncolytic adenovirus in combination with radiation therapy (165). The vector they use is conveniently outfitted with an imaging reporter (NIS). The vector, Ad5-yCD/*mut*TK$_{SR39}$*rep*-hNIS, produces cytosine deaminase (for suicide gene therapy), a mutant form of the HSV1-TK, also for gene therapy—with ganciclovir—and the NIS for imaging. The HSV1-TK could also be used for imaging, with a suitably labeled TK substrate, such as 1-(2′-deoxy-2′fluoro-β-D-arabinofuranosyl)-5-[^{124}I]iodouracil ([^{124}I] FIAU) for PET, making this essentially a dual modality theranostic agent. The goals of clinical molecular-genetic imaging in PCa have been summarized by Freytag et al. as (*i*) to assess the quality of the adenovirus injection (although at more than one day after the injection), (*ii*) to determine the level and volume of therapeutic gene expression in the prostate, which can be correlated with clinical outcome, (*iii*) to optimize the deposition of adenovirus in the target organ, (*iv*) to determine the whole-body

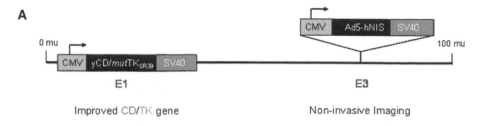

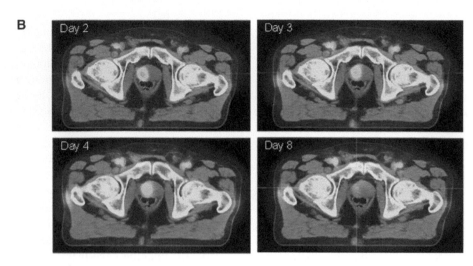

Figure 10 Kinetics of gene expression imaging in man. (**A**) Optimized theranostic vector used for imaging in (**B**), which depicts changes in expression of the gene within the right side of the prostate over time. The imaging agent is $^{99m}TcO_4$. *Source*: Courtesy of Svend Freytag, Henry Ford Health System (*See Color Insert*).

distribution of adenovirus, and (*v*) with serial imaging, to determine the persistence of therapeutic gene expression in the prostate, which can be correlated with clinical outcome. Kinetic studies such as that shown in Figure 10 have been performed, with changes in gene expression demonstrated long before any anatomic change in the tumor due to the oncolytic adenovirus are demonstrated. This study represents the first true molecular-genetic imaging study in PCa and is emblematic of the kinds of studies that will facilitate gene therapy for prostate and other cancers in the future.

REFERENCES

1. Jemal A, Siegel R, Ward E, et al. Cancer statistics. CA Cancer J Clin 2007; 57(1):43–66.
2. Hricak H, Choyke PL, Eberhardt SC, et al. Imaging prostate cancer: a multidisciplinary perspective. Radiology 2007; 243(1):28–53.
3. Walczak JR, Carducci MA. Prostate cancer: a practical approach to current management of recurrent disease. Mayo Clin Proc 2007; 82(2):243–249.
4. Kattan MW, Stapleton AM, Wheeler TM, et al. Evaluation of a nomogram used to predict the pathologic stage of clinically localized prostate carcinoma. Cancer 1997; 79(3): 528–537.
5. Kattan MW, Zelefsky MJ, Kupelian PA, et al. Pretreatment nomogram for predicting the outcome of three-dimensional conformal radiotherapy in prostate cancer. J Clin Oncol 2000; 18(19):3352–3359.
6. Thompson IM, Ankerst DP. Prostate-specific antigen in the early detection of prostate cancer. CMAJ 2007; 176(13): 1853–1858.
7. Saitoh H, Yoshida K, Uchijima Y, et al. Two different lymph node metastatic patterns of a prostatic cancer. Cancer 1990; 65(8):1843–1846.
8. Gretzer MB, Partin AW. PSA markers in prostate cancer detection. Urol Clin North Am 2003; 30(4):677–686.
9. Leman ES, Cannon GW, Trock BJ, et al. EPCA-2: a highly specific serum marker for prostate cancer. Urology 2007; 69(4):714–720.
10. Shinohara K, Wheeler TM, Scardino PT. The appearance of prostate cancer on transrectal ultrasonography: correlation of imaging and pathological examinations. J Urol 1989; 142(1):76–82.
11. Hricak H, Dooms GC, Jeffrey RB, et al. Prostatic carcinoma: staging by clinical assessment, CT, and MR imaging. Radiology 1987; 162(2):331–336.
12. Scheidler J, Hricak H, Vigneron DB, et al. Prostate cancer: localization with three-dimensional proton MR spectroscopic

imaging—clinicopathologic study. Radiology 1999; 213(2):473–480.

13. Tuzel E, Sevinc M, Obuz F, et al. Is magnetic resonance imaging necessary in the staging of prostate cancer? Urol Int 1998; 61(4):227–231.

14. Lawrentschuk N, Davis ID, Bolton DM, et al. Diagnostic and therapeutic use of radioisotopes for bony disease in prostate cancer: current practice. Int J Urol 2007; 14(2): 89–95.

15. Chybowski FM, Keller JJ, Bergstralh EJ, et al. Predicting radionuclide bone scan findings in patients with newly diagnosed, untreated prostate cancer: prostate specific antigen is superior to all other clinical parameters. J Urol 1991; 145(2):313–318.

16. Oesterling JE, Martin SK, Bergstralh EJ, et al. The use of prostate-specific antigen in staging patients with newly diagnosed prostate cancer. JAMA 1993; 269(1):57–60.

17. Bruwer G, Heyns CF, Allen FJ. Influence of local tumour stage and grade on reliability of serum prostate-specific antigen in predicting skeletal metastases in patients with adenocarcinoma of the prostate. Eur Urol 1999; 35(3): 223–227.

18. Yap BK, Choo R, Deboer G, et al. Are serial bone scans useful for the follow-up of clinically localized, low to intermediate grade prostate cancer managed with watchful observation alone? BJU Int 2003; 91(7):613–617.

19. Turlakow A, Larson SM, Coakley F, et al. Local detection of prostate cancer by positron emission tomography with 2-fluorodeoxyglucose: comparison of filtered back projection and iterative reconstruction with segmented attenuation correction. Q J Nucl Med 2001; 45(3):235–244.

20. Hofer C, Laubenbacher C, Block T, et al. Fluorine-18-fluorodeoxyglucose positron emission tomography is useless for the detection of local recurrence after radical prostatectomy. Eur Urol 1999; 36(1):31–35.

21. Nunez R, Macapinlac HA, Yeung HW, et al. Combined 18F-FDG and 11C-methionine PET scans in patients with newly progressive metastatic prostate cancer. J Nucl Med 2002; 43(1):46–55.

22. Shreve PD, Grossman HB, Gross MD, et al. Metastatic prostate cancer: initial findings of PET with 2-deoxy-2-[F-18]fluoro-D-glucose. Radiology 1996; 199(3):751–756.

23. Oyama N, Akino H, Suzuki Y, et al. Prognostic value of 2-deoxy-2-[F-18]fluoro-D-glucose positron emission tomography imaging for patients with prostate cancer. Mol Imaging Biol 2002; 4(1):99–104.

24. Chang CH, Wu HC, Tsai JJ, et al. Detecting metastatic pelvic lymph nodes by 18F-2-deoxyglucose positron emission tomography in patients with prostate-specific antigen relapse after treatment for localized prostate cancer. Urol Int 2003; 70(4):311–315.

25. Schoder H, Herrmann K, Gonen M, et al. 2-[18F]fluoro-2-deoxyglucose positron emission tomography for the detection of disease in patients with prostate-specific antigen relapse after radical prostatectomy. Clin Cancer Res 2005; 11(13):4761–4769.

26. Morris MJ, Akhurst T, Larson SM, et al. Fluorodeoxyglucose positron emission tomography as an outcome measure for castrate metastatic prostate cancer treated with antimicrotubule chemotherapy. Clin Cancer Res 2005; 11(9):3210–3216.

27. Chang SS. Overview of prostate-specific membrane antigen. Rev Urol 2004; 6(suppl 10):S13–S18.

28. Wright GL Jr., Grob BM, Haley C, et al. Upregulation of prostate-specific membrane antigen after androgen-deprivation therapy. Urology 1996; 48(2):326–334.

29. Silver DA, Pellicer I, Fair WR, et al. Prostate-specific membrane antigen expression in normal and malignant human tissues. Clin Cancer Res 1997; 3(1):81–85.

30. Sokoloff RL, Norton KC, Gasior CL, et al. A dual-monoclonal sandwich assay for prostate-specific membrane antigen: levels in tissues, seminal fluid and urine. Prostate 2000; 43(2):150–157.

31. Horoszewicz JS, Kawinski E, Murphy GP. Monoclonal antibodies to a new antigenic marker in epithelial prostatic cells and serum of prostatic cancer patients. Anticancer Res 1987; 7(5B):927–935.

32. Bander NH. Technology insight: monoclonal antibody imaging of prostate cancer. Nat Clin Pract Urol 2006; 3(4):216–225.

33. Wynant GE, Murphy GP, Horoszewicz JS, et al. Immunoscintigraphy of prostatic cancer: preliminary results with 111In-labeled monoclonal antibody 7E11-C5. 3 (CYT-356). Prostate 1991; 18(3):229–241.

34. Manyak MJ, Hinkle GH, Olsen JO, et al. Immunoscintigraphy with indium-111-capromab pendetide: evaluation before definitive therapy in patients with prostate cancer. Urology 1999; 54(6):1058–1063.

35. Kahn D, Williams RD, Haseman MK, et al. Radioimmunoscintigraphy with In-111-labeled capromab pendetide predicts prostate cancer response to salvage radiotherapy after failed radical prostatectomy. J Clin Oncol 1998; 16(1):284–289.

36. Levesque PE, Nieh PT, Zinman LN, et al. Radiolabeled monoclonal antibody indium 111-labeled CYT-356 localizes extraprostatic recurrent carcinoma after prostatectomy. Urology 1998; 51(6):978–984.

37. Deb N, Goris M, Trisler K, et al. Treatment of hormone-refractory prostate cancer with 90Y-CYT-356 monoclonal antibody. Clin Cancer Res 1996; 2(8):1289–1297.

38. Thomas CT, Bradshaw PT, Pollock BH, et al. Indium-111-capromab pendetide radioimmunoscintigraphy and prognosis for durable biochemical response to salvage radiation therapy in men after failed prostatectomy. J Clin Oncol 2003; 21(9):1715–1721.

39. Wilkinson S, Chodak G. The role of 111indium-capromab pendetide imaging for assessing biochemical failure after radical prostatectomy. J Urol 2004; 172(1):133–136.

40. Troyer JK, Beckett ML, Wright GL Jr. Location of prostate-specific membrane antigen in the LNCaP prostate carcinoma cell line. Prostate 1997; 30(4):232–242.

41. Milowsky MI, Nanus DM, Kostakoglu L, et al. Phase I trial of yttrium-90-labeled anti-prostate-specific membrane antigen monoclonal antibody J591 for androgen-independent prostate cancer. J Clin Oncol 2004; 22(13): 2522–2531.

42. Liu H, Moy P, Kim S, et al. Monoclonal antibodies to the extracellular domain of prostate-specific membrane

antigen also react with tumor vascular endothelium. Cancer Res 1997; 57(17):3629–3634.

43. Vallabhajosula S, Kuji I, Hamacher KA, et al. Pharmacokinetics and biodistribution of 111In- and 177Lu-labeled J591 antibody specific for prostate-specific membrane antigen: prediction of 90Y-J591 radiation dosimetry based on 111In or 177Lu? J Nucl Med 2005; 46(4): 634–641.

44. Vallabhajosula S, Goldsmith SJ, Hamacher KA, et al. Prediction of myelotoxicity based on bone marrow radiation-absorbed dose: radioimmunotherapy studies using 90Y- and 177Lu-labeled J591 antibodies specific for prostate-specific membrane antigen. J Nucl Med 2005; 46(5):850–858.

45. Vallabhajosula S, Goldsmith SJ, Kostakoglu L, et al. Radioimmunotherapy of prostate cancer using 90Y- and 177Lu-labeled J591 monoclonal antibodies: effect of multiple treatments on myelotoxicity. Clin Cancer Res 2005; 11(19 pt 2):7195s–200s.

46. Bander NH, Milowsky MI, Nanus DM, et al. Phase I trial of 177lutetium-labeled J591, a monoclonal antibody to prostate-specific membrane antigen, in patients with androgen-independent prostate cancer. J Clin Oncol 2005; 23(21):4591–4601.

47. Bander NH, Trabulsi EJ, Kostakoglu L, et al. Targeting metastatic prostate cancer with radiolabeled monoclonal antibody J591 to the extracellular domain of prostate specific membrane antigen. J Urol 2003; 170(5): 1717–1721.

48. Sodee DB, Sodee AE, Bakale G. Synergistic value of single-photon emission computed tomography/computed tomography fusion to radioimmunoscintigraphic imaging of prostate cancer. Semin Nucl Med 2007; 37(1):17–28.

49. Seo Y, Franc BL, Hawkins RA, et al. Progress in SPECT/ CT imaging of prostate cancer. Technol Cancer Res Treat 2006; 5(4):329–336.

50. Noz ME, Chung G, Lee BY, et al. Enhancing the utility of prostascint SPECT scans for patient management. J Med Syst 2006; 30(2):123–132.

51. Chang SS, O'Keefe DS, Bacich DJ, et al. Prostate-specific membrane antigen is produced in tumor-associated neovasculature. Clin Cancer Res 1999; 5(10):2674–2681.

52. Milowsky MI, Nanus DM, Kostakoglu L, et al. Vascular targeted therapy with anti-prostate-specific membrane antigen monoclonal antibody J591 in advanced solid tumors. J Clin Oncol 2007; 25(5):540–547.

53. Takashima H, Egawa M, Imao T, et al. Validity of sentinel lymph node concept for patients with prostate cancer. J Urol 2004; 171(6 pt 1):2268–2271.

54. Silva N Jr., Anselmi CE, Anselmi OE, et al. Use of the gamma probe in sentinel lymph node biopsy in patients with prostate cancer. Nucl Med Commun 2005; 26(12): 1081–1086.

55. Wawroschek F, Vogt H, Wengenmair H, et al. Prostate lymphoscintigraphy and radio-guided surgery for sentinel lymph node identification in prostate cancer. Technique and results of the first 350 cases. Urol Int 2003; 70(4): 303–310.

56. Pagliarulo V, Hawes D, Brands FH, et al. Detection of occult lymph node metastases in locally advanced node-negative prostate cancer. J Clin Oncol 2006; 24(18): 2735–2742.

57. Joslyn SA, Konety BR. Impact of extent of lymphadenectomy on survival after radical prostatectomy for prostate cancer. Urology 2006; 68(1):121–125.

58. Weckermann D, Goppelt M, Dorn R, et al. Incidence of positive pelvic lymph nodes in patients with prostate cancer, a prostate-specific antigen (PSA) level of < or =10 ng/mL and biopsy Gleason score of < or =6, and their influence on PSA progression-free survival after radical prostatectomy. BJU Int 2006; 97(6):1173–1178.

59. Hara T, Kosaka N, Shinoura N, et al. PET imaging of brain tumor with [methyl-11C]choline. J Nucl Med 1997; 38(6):842–847.

60. Roivainen A, Forsback S, Gronroos T, et al. Blood metabolism of [methyl-11C]choline; implications for in vivo imaging with positron emission tomography. Eur J Nucl Med 2000; 27(1):25–32.

61. Groves AM, Win T, Haim SB, et al. Non-[18F]FDG PET in clinical oncology. Lancet Oncol 2007; 8(9):822–830.

62. Pieterman RM, Que TH, Elsinga PH, et al. Comparison of (11)C-choline and (18)F-FDG PET in primary diagnosis and staging of patients with thoracic cancer. J Nucl Med 2002; 43(2):167–172.

63. Hara T. 11C-choline and 2-deoxy-2-[18F]fluoro-D-glucose in tumor imaging with positron emission tomography. Mol Imaging Biol 2002; 4(4):267–273.

64. Sutinen E, Nurmi M, Roivainen A, et al. Kinetics of [(11) C]choline uptake in prostate cancer: a PET study. Eur J Nucl Med Mol Imaging 2004; 31(3):317–324.

65. Kwee SA, Wei H, Sesterhenn I, et al. Localization of primary prostate cancer with dual-phase 18F-fluorocholine PET. J Nucl Med 2006; 47(2):262–269.

66. Testa C, Schiavina R, Lodi R, et al. Prostate cancer: sextant localization with MR imaging, MR spectroscopy, and 11C-choline PET/CT. Radiology 2007; 244(3): 797–806.

67. de Jong IJ, Pruim J, Elsinga PH, et al. 11C-choline positron emission tomography for the evaluation after treatment of localized prostate cancer. Eur Urol 2003; 44(1):32–38; discussion 8–9.

68. Scher B, Seitz M, Albinger W, et al. Value of 11C-choline PET and PET/CT in patients with suspected prostate cancer. Eur J Nucl Med Mol Imaging 2007; 34(1):45–53.

69. de Jong IJ, Pruim J, Elsinga PH, et al. Preoperative staging of pelvic lymph nodes in prostate cancer by 11C-choline PET. J Nucl Med 2003; 44(3):331–335.

70. Kotzerke J, Prang J, Neumaier B, et al. Experience with carbon-11 choline positron emission tomography in prostate carcinoma. Eur J Nucl Med 2000; 27(9):1415–1419.

71. Rinnab L, Blumstein NM, Mottaghy FM, et al. 11C-choline positron-emission tomography/computed tomography and transrectal ultrasonography for staging localized prostate cancer. BJU Int 2007; 99(6):1421–1426.

72. Eschmann SM, Pfannenberg AC, Rieger A, et al. Comparison of 11C-choline-PET/CT and whole body-MRI for

staging of prostate cancer. Nuklearmedizin 2007; 46(5): 161–168; quiz N47–N48.

73. Picchio M, Messa C, Landoni C, et al. Value of [11C] choline-positron emission tomography for re-staging prostate cancer: a comparison with [18F]fluorodeoxyglucose-positron emission tomography. J Urol 2003; 169(4): 1337–1340.

74. Cimitan M, Bortolus R, Morassut S, et al. [(18)F]fluorocholine PET/CT imaging for the detection of recurrent prostate cancer at PSA relapse: experience in 100 consecutive patients. Eur J Nucl Med Mol Imaging 2006; 33(12): 1387–1398.

75. Krause BJ, Souvatzoglou M, Tuncel M, et al. The detection rate of [(11)C]choline-PET/CT depends on the serum PSA-value in patients with biochemical recurrence of prostate cancer. Eur J Nucl Med Mol Imaging 2008; 35(1):18–23.

76. Reske SN, Blumstein NM, Glatting G. [(11)C]choline PET/CT imaging in occult local relapse of prostate cancer after radical prostatectomy. Eur J Nucl Med Mol Imaging 2008; 35(1):9–17.

77. Rinnab L, Mottaghy FM, Blumstein NM, et al. Evaluation of [11C]-choline positron-emission/computed tomography in patients with increasing prostate-specific antigen levels after primary treatment for prostate cancer. BJU Int 2007; 100(4):786–793.

78. Igerc I, Kohlfurst S, Gallowitsch HJ, et al. The value of (18)F-choline PET/CT in patients with elevated PSA-level and negative prostate needle biopsy for localisation of prostate cancer. Eur J Nucl Med Mol Imaging 2008; 35(5):976–983.

79. Scattoni V, Picchio M, Suardi N, et al. Detection of lymph-node metastases with integrated [11C]choline PET/CT in patients with PSA failure after radical retropubic prostatectomy: results confirmed by open pelvic-retroperitoneal lymphadenectomy. Eur Urol 2007; 52(2): 423–429.

80. DeGrado TR, Baldwin SW, Wang S, et al. Synthesis and evaluation of (18)F-labeled choline analogs as oncologic PET tracers. J Nucl Med 2001; 42(12):1805–1814.

81. Wyss MT, Weber B, Honer M, et al. 18F-choline in experimental soft tissue infection assessed with autoradiography and high-resolution PET. Eur J Nucl Med Mol Imaging 2004; 31(3):312–316.

82. Kotzerke J, Volkmer BG, Glatting G, et al. Intraindividual comparison of [11C]acetate and [11C]choline PET for detection of metastases of prostate cancer. Nuklearmedizin 2003; 42(1):25–30.

83. Husarik DB, Miralbell R, Dubs M, et al. Evaluation of [(18)F]-choline PET/CT for staging and restaging of prostate cancer. Eur J Nucl Med Mol Imaging 2008; 35(2): 253–263.

84. Yoshimoto M, Waki A, Yonekura Y, et al. Characterization of acetate metabolism in tumor cells in relation to cell proliferation: acetate metabolism in tumor cells. Nucl Med Biol 2001; 28(2):117–122.

85. Fricke E, Machtens S, Hofmann M, et al. Positron emission tomography with (11)C-acetate and (18)F-FDG in prostate cancer patients. Eur J Nucl Med Mol Imaging 2003; 30(4):607–611.

86. Oyama N, Miller TR, Dehdashti F, et al. 11C-acetate PET imaging of prostate cancer: detection of recurrent disease at PSA relapse. J Nucl Med 2003; 44(4):549–555.

87. Oyama N, Akino H, Kanamaru H, et al. 11C-acetate PET imaging of prostate cancer. J Nucl Med 2002; 43(2): 181–186.

88. Sandblom G, Sorensen J, Lundin N, et al. Positron emission tomography with C11-acetate for tumor detection and localization in patients with prostate-specific antigen relapse after radical prostatectomy. Urology 2006; 67(5): 996–1000.

89. Wachter S, Tomek S, Kurtaran A, et al. 11C-acetate positron emission tomography imaging and image fusion with computed tomography and magnetic resonance imaging in patients with recurrent prostate cancer. J Clin Oncol 2006; 24(16):2513–2519.

90. Dimitrakopoulou-Strauss A, Strauss LG. PET imaging of prostate cancer with 11C-acetate. J Nucl Med 2003; 44(4): 556–558.

91. Ponde DE, Dence CS, Oyama N, et al. 18F-fluoroacetate: a potential acetate analog for prostate tumor imaging—in vivo evaluation of 18F-fluoroacetate versus 11C-acetate. J Nucl Med 2007; 48(3):420–428.

92. Matthies A, Ezziddin S, Ulrich EM, et al. Imaging of prostate cancer metastases with 18F-fluoroacetate using PET/CT. Eur J Nucl Med Mol Imaging 2004; 31(5):797.

93. Yoshimoto M, Waki A, Obata A, et al. Radiolabeled choline as a proliferation marker: comparison with radiolabeled acetate. Nucl Med Biol 2004; 31(7):859–865.

94. Zophel K, Kotzerke J. Is 11C-choline the most appropriate tracer for prostate cancer? Against. Eur J Nucl Med Mol Imaging 2004; 31(5):756–759.

95. Vees H, Buchegger F, Albrecht S, et al. 18F-choline and/or 11C-acetate positron emission tomography: detection of residual or progressive subclinical disease at very low prostate-specific antigen values (<1 ng/mL) after radical prostatectomy. BJU Int 2007; 99(6):1415–1420.

96. Grant FD, Fahey FH, Packard AB, et al. Skeletal PET with 18F-Fluoride: Applying New Technology to an Old Tracer. J Nucl Med 2008; 49(1):68–78.

97. Even-Sapir E, Mishani E, Flusser G, et al. 18F-Fluoride positron emission tomography and positron emission tomography/computed tomography. Semin Nucl Med 2007; 37(6):462–469.

98. Schirrmeister H, Glatting G, Hetzel J, et al. Prospective evaluation of the clinical value of planar bone scans, SPECT, and (18)F-labeled NaF PET in newly diagnosed lung cancer. J Nucl Med 2001; 42(12):1800–1804.

99. Even-Sapir E, Metser U, Mishani E, et al. The detection of bone metastases in patients with high-risk prostate cancer: 99mTc-MDP Planar bone scintigraphy, single- and multi-field-of-view SPECT, 18F-fluoride PET, and 18F-fluoride PET/CT. J Nucl Med 2006; 47(2):287–297.

100. Langsteger W, Heinisch M, Fogelman I. The role of fluorodeoxyglucose, 18F-dihydroxyphenylalanine, 18F-choline, and 18F-fluoride in bone imaging with emphasis on prostate and breast. Semin Nucl Med 2006; 36(1):73–92.

101. Miyazawa H, Arai T, Iio M, et al. PET imaging of non-small-cell lung carcinoma with carbon-11-methionine: relationship between radioactivity uptake and flow-cytometric parameters. J Nucl Med 1993; 34(11): 1886–1891.

102. Kubota K, Yamada K, Fukada H, et al. Tumor detection with carbon-11-labelled amino acids. Eur J Nucl Med 1984; 9(3):136–140.

103. Toth G, Lengyel Z, Balkay L, et al. Detection of prostate cancer with 11C-methionine positron emission tomography. J Urol 2005; 173(1):66–69; discussion 9.

104. Dehdashti F, Picus J, Michalski JM, et al. Positron tomographic assessment of androgen receptors in prostatic carcinoma. Eur J Nucl Med Mol Imaging 2005; 32(3): 344–350.

105. Larson SM, Morris M, Gunther I, et al. Tumor localization of 16beta-18F-fluoro-5alpha-dihydrotestosterone versus 18F-FDG in patients with progressive, metastatic prostate cancer. J Nucl Med 2004; 45(3):366–373.

106. Jager PL, Vaalburg W, Pruim J, et al. Radiolabeled amino acids: basic aspects and clinical applications in oncology. J Nucl Med 2001; 42(3):432–445.

107. Oka S, Hattori R, Kurosaki F, et al. A preliminary study of anti-1-amino-3-18F-fluorocyclobutyl-1-carboxylic acid for the detection of prostate cancer. J Nucl Med 2007; 48(1):46–55.

108. Schuster DM, Votaw JR, Nieh PT, et al. Initial experience with the radiotracer anti-1-amino-3-18F-fluorocyclobutane-1-carboxylic acid with PET/CT in prostate carcinoma. J Nucl Med 2007; 48(1):56–63.

109. Mangner TJ, Klecker RW, Anderson L, et al. Synthesis of 2'-deoxy-2'-[18F]fluoro-beta-D-arabinofuranosyl nucleosides, [18F]FAU, [18F]FMAU, [18F]FBAU and [18F]FIAU, as potential PET agents for imaging cellular proliferation. Synthesis of [18F]labelled FAU, FMAU, FBAU, FIAU. Nucl Med Biol 2003; 30(3): 215–224.

110. Sun H, Sloan A, Mangner TJ, et al. Imaging DNA synthesis with [18F]FMAU and positron emission tomography in patients with cancer. Eur J Nucl Med Mol Imaging 2005; 32(1):15–22.

111. Oyama N, Ponde DE, Dence C, et al. Monitoring of therapy in androgen-dependent prostate tumor model by measuring tumor proliferation. J Nucl Med 2004; 45(3): 519–525.

112. Katz S, Rosen M. MR imaging and MR spectroscopy in prostate cancer management. Radiol Clin North Am 2006; 44(5):723–734, viii.

113. Kurhanewicz J, Vigneron D, Carroll P, et al. Multiparametric magnetic resonance imaging in prostate cancer: present and future. Curr Opin Urol 2008; 18(1):71–77.

114. Huzjan R, Sala E, Hricak H. Magnetic resonance imaging and magnetic resonance spectroscopic imaging of prostate cancer. Nat Clin Pract Urol 2005; 2(9):434–442.

115. Mueller-Lisse UG, Scherr MK. Proton MR spectroscopy of the prostate. Eur J Radiol 2007; 63(3):351–360.

116. Shen T, Weissleder R, Papisov M, et al. Monocrystalline iron oxide nanocompounds (MION): physicochemical properties. Magn Reson Med 1993; 29(5):599–604.

117. Weissleder R, Heautot JF, Schaffer BK, et al. MR lymphography: study of a high-efficiency lymphotrophic agent. Radiology 1994; 191(1):225–230.

118. Pittet MJ, Swirski FK, Reynolds F, et al. Labeling of immune cells for in vivo imaging using magnetofluorescent nanoparticles. Nat Protoc 2006; 1(1):73–79.

119. Harisinghani MG, Barentsz J, Hahn PF, et al. Noninvasive detection of clinically occult lymph-node metastases in prostate cancer. N Engl J Med 2003; 348(25):2491–2499.

120. Harisinghani MG, Barentsz JO, Hahn PF, et al. MR lymphangiography for detection of minimal nodal disease in patients with prostate cancer. Acad Radiol 2002; 9(suppl 2):S312–313.

121. Heesakkers RA, Futterer JJ, Hovels AM, et al. Prostate cancer evaluated with ferumoxtran-10-enhanced T2*-weighted MR Imaging at 1.5 and 3.0 T: early experience. Radiology 2006; 239(2):481–487.

122. Saksena M, Harisinghani M, Hahn P, et al. Comparison of lymphotropic nanoparticle-enhanced MRI sequences in patients with various primary cancers. AJR Am J Roentgenol 2006; 187(6):W582–588.

123. Enochs WS, Harsh G, Hochberg F, et al. Improved delineation of human brain tumors on MR images using a long-circulating, superparamagnetic iron oxide agent. J Magn Reson Imaging 1999; 9(2):228–232.

124. de Vries IJ, Lesterhuis WJ, Barentsz JO, et al. Magnetic resonance tracking of dendritic cells in melanoma patients for monitoring of cellular therapy. Nat Biotechnol 2005; 23(11):1407–1413.

125. Gingrich JR, Barrios RJ, Morton RA, et al. Metastatic prostate cancer in a transgenic mouse. Cancer Res 1996; 56(18):4096–4102.

126. Brakenhielm E, Burton JB, Johnson M, et al. Modulating metastasis by a lymphangiogenic switch in prostate cancer. Int J Cancer 2007; 121(10):2153–2161.

127. Meyer KL, Schwendner SW, Counsell RE. Potential tumor or organ-imaging agents. 30. Radioiodinated phospholipid ethers. J Med Chem 1989; 32(9):2142–2147.

128. Counsell RE, Schwendner SW, Meyer KL, et al. Tumor visualization with a radioiodinated phospholipid ether. J Nucl Med 1990; 31(3):332–336.

129. Pinchuk AN, Rampy MA, Longino MA, et al. Synthesis and structure-activity relationship effects on the tumor avidity of radioiodinated phospholipid ether analogues. J Med Chem 2006; 49(7):2155–2165.

130. Chen AP, Albers MJ, Cunningham CH, et al. Hyperpolarized C-13 spectroscopic imaging of the TRAMP mouse at 3T-initial experience. Magn Reson Med 2007; 58(6):1099–1106.

131. Zhang K, Aruva MR, Shanthly N, et al. PET Imaging of VPAC1 Expression in Experimental and Spontaneous Prostate Cancer. J Nucl Med 2008; 49(1):112–121.

132. de Visser M, Bernard HF, Erion JL, et al. Novel 111In-labelled bombesin analogues for molecular imaging of prostate tumours. Eur J Nucl Med Mol Imaging 2007; 34(8):1228–1238.

133. Zhang X, Cai W, Cao F, et al. 18F-labeled bombesin analogs for targeting GRP receptor-expressing prostate cancer. J Nucl Med 2006; 47(3):492–501.

134. Lin KS, Luu A, Baidoo KE, et al. A new high affinity technetium-99m-bombesin analogue with low abdominal accumulation. Bioconjug Chem 2005; 16(1):43–50.

135. Prasanphanich AF, Nanda PK, Rold TL, et al. [64Cu-NOTA-8-Aoc-BBN(7-14)NH2] targeting vector for positron-emission tomography imaging of gastrin-releasing peptide receptor-expressing tissues. Proc Natl Acad Sci U S A 2007; 104(30):12462–2467.

136. Line BR, Mitra A, Nan A, et al. Targeting tumor angiogenesis: comparison of peptide and polymer-peptide conjugates. J Nucl Med 2005; 46(9):1552–1560.

137. Maecke HR, Hofmann M, Haberkorn U. (68)Ga-labeled peptides in tumor imaging. J Nucl Med 2005; 46(suppl 1): 172S–178S.

138. Schulke N, Varlamova OA, Donovan GP, et al. The homodimer of prostate-specific membrane antigen is a functional target for cancer therapy. Proc Natl Acad Sci U S A 2003; 100(22):12590–2595.

139. Huang X, Bennett M, Thorpe PE. Anti-tumor effects and lack of side effects in mice of an immunotoxin directed against human and mouse prostate-specific membrane antigen. Prostate 2004; 61(1):1–11.

140. Su SL, Huang IP, Fair WR, et al. Alternatively spliced variants of prostate-specific membrane antigen RNA: ratio of expression as a potential measurement of progression. Cancer Res 1995; 55(7):1441–1443.

141. Tasch J, Gong M, Sadelain M, et al. A unique folate hydrolase, prostate-specific membrane antigen (PSMA): a target for immunotherapy? Crit Rev Immunol 2001; 21(1–3):249–261.

142. Lange PH. ProstaScint scan for staging prostate cancer. Urology 2001; 57(3):402–406.

143. Haseman MK, Rosenthal SA, Polascik TJ. Capromab pendetide imaging of prostate cancer. Cancer Biother Radiopharm 2000; 15(2):131–140.

144. Rosenthal SA, Haseman MK, Polascik TJ. Utility of capromab pendetide (ProstaScint) imaging in the management of prostate cancer. Tech Urol 2001; 7(1):27–37.

145. Jackson PF, Cole DC, Slusher BS, et al. Design, synthesis, and biological activity of a potent inhibitor of the neuropeptidase N-acetylated alpha-linked acidic dipeptidase. J Med Chem 1996; 39(2):619–622.

146. Majer P, Jackson PF, Delahanty G, et al. Synthesis and biological evaluation of thiol-based inhibitors of glutamate carboxypeptidase II: discovery of an orally active GCP II inhibitor. J Med Chem 2003; 46(10):1989–1996.

147. Kozikowski AP, Nan F, Conti P, et al. Design of remarkably simple, yet potent urea-based inhibitors of glutamate carboxypeptidase II (NAALADase). J Med Chem 2001; 44(3):298–301.

148. Zhou J, Neale JH, Pomper MG, et al. NAAG peptidase inhibitors and their potential for diagnosis and therapy. Nat Rev Drug Discov 2005; 4:1015–1026.

149. Humblet V, Lapidus R, Williams LR, et al. High-affinity near-infrared fluorescent small-molecule contrast agents for in vivo imaging of prostate-specific membrane antigen. Mol Imaging 2005; 4(4):448–462.

150. Barinka C, Rovenska M, Mlcochova P, et al. structural insight into the pharmacophore pocket of human glutamate carboxypeptidase II. J Med Chem 2007; 50(14): 3267–3273.

151. Barinka C, Starkova J, Konvalinka J, et al. A high-resolution structure of ligand-free human glutamate carboxypeptidase II. Acta Crystallogr Sect F Struct Biol Cryst Commun 2007; 63(pt 3):150–153.

152. Mlcochova P, Plechanovova A, Barinka C, et al. Mapping of the active site of glutamate carboxypeptidase II by site-directed mutagenesis. FEBS J 2007; 274(18):4731–4741.

153. Pomper MG, Musachio JL, Zhang J, et al. 11C-MCG: synthesis, uptake selectivity, and primate PET of a probe for glutamate carboxypeptidase II (NAALADase). Mol Imaging 2002; 1:96–101.

154. Foss CA, Mease RC, Fan H, et al. Radiolabeled Small molecule ligands for prostate-specific membrane antigen: in vivo imaging in experimental models of prostate cancer. Clin Cancer Res 2005; 11:4022–4028.

155. Mease RC, Dusich CA, Foss CA, et al. Synthesis of N-[N-[(S)-1,3-dicarboxypropyl]carbamoyl]-[18F]fluorobenzyl-L-cysteine, [18F]DCFBC, its biodistribution and use in imaging prostate cancer xenografts. Clin Cancer Res 2008; 14(10):3036–3043.

156. Banerjee SR, Foss CA, Mease RC, et al. Synthesis and evaluation of 99mTc/Re labeled PSMA inhibitors. J Nucl Med 2007; 48(suppl 2):18P.

157. Chang SS, Reuter VE, Heston WD, et al. Five different anti-prostate-specific membrane antigen (PSMA) antibodies confirm PSMA expression in tumor-associated neovasculature. Cancer Res 1999; 59(13):3192–3198.

158. Guilarte T, Hammoud DA, McGlothan JL, et al. Dysregulation of glutamate carboxypeptidase II in psychiatric disease. Schizophr Res 2008; 99(1–3):324–332.

159. Gottweis H. Gene therapy and the public: a matter of trust. Gene Ther 2002; 9(11):667–669.

160. Blasberg RG, Tjuvajev JG. Molecular-genetic imaging: current and future perspectives. J Clin Invest 2003; 111(11):1620–1629.

161. Gambhir SS, Herschman HR, Cherry SR, et al. Imaging transgene expression with radionuclide imaging technologies. Neoplasia 2000; 2(1–2):118–138.

162. Singh A, Massoud TF, Deroose C, et al. Molecular imaging of reporter gene expression in prostate cancer: an overview. Semin Nucl Med 2008; 38(1):9–19.

163. Siddiqui F, Barton KN, Stricker HJ, et al. Design considerations for incorporating sodium iodide symporter reporter gene imaging into prostate cancer gene therapy trials. Hum Gene Ther 2007; 18(4):312–322.

164. Freytag SO, Barton KN, Brown SL, et al. Replication-competent adenovirus-mediated suicide gene therapy with radiation in a preclinical model of pancreatic cancer. Mol Ther 2007; 15(9):1600–1606.

165. Freytag SO, Movsas B, Aref I, et al. Phase I trial of replication-competent adenovirus-mediated suicide gene therapy combined with IMRT for prostate cancer. Mol Ther 2007; 15(5):1016–1023.

166. Zanzonico PB, Finn R, Pentlow KS, et al. PET-based radiation dosimetry in man of 18F-fluorodihydrotestosterone, a new radiotracer for imaging prostate cancer. J Nucl Med 2004; 45(11):1966–1971.

42

Anticancer Drug Development with Optical Imaging

BOHUMIL BEDNAR, GUO-JUN ZHANG, and CYRILLE SUR

Imaging Department, Merck Research Laboratories, Merck & Co, Inc., West Point, Pennsylvania, U.S.A.

INTRODUCTION

The drug discovery process requires introduction of new paradigms that would qualitatively change development of new therapeutics. It has been demonstrated that the way to connect the large heterogeneity of information related to diseases is to define biomarkers of the disease as they manifest themselves in a particular technology or diagnostic method. The imaging biomarkers used for noninvasive reporting in clinical diagnostics as well as in the preclinical drug discovery process are becoming critical for future advancement in the development of new therapeutics. A leading example of the parallel use of several imaging biomarkers is oncology. For instance, biomarkers of tumor growth include the volume of a tumor detected by computed tomography (CT), the relaxation time of water molecules in the tumor detected by magnetic resonance imaging (MRI), positron emission generated by positron emission tomography (PET) probes, and optical signals generated by optical probes. Each of the individual modality biomarkers provides specific information on tumor growth in a different manner. Nevertheless, all of them help to characterize the cancer. Thus, high-throughput optical imaging accelerates preclinical development in mouse tumor models, while MRI, CT, and PET with high tissue penetration are used in clinical settings for human patients. Here we will provide some examples of the applications of optical imaging biomarkers in the preclinical drug discovery process of anticancer medicines.

Oncology is the research field where both endogenous and exogenous optical imaging biomarkers have found some of their first practical applications in drug target identification, validation, and testing of therapeutics (1). Both bioluminescence (BIL) generated by genetically encoded firefly luciferase and fluorescence of fluorescent proteins such as green fluorescent protein (GFP) and Discosoma sp. (DsRed) were extensively used as biomarkers of tumor growth (2,3). Although biomarkers based on genetically encoded probes play a pivotal role in the use of optical imaging in preclinical oncology, there are many applications, such as in clinical testing, where their use is experimentally difficult or for other reasons not possible. Thus, new exogenous probes with fluorescence in the far-red and near-infrared (NIR) area of the spectrum have been developed to provide fluorescence optical biomarkers for both preclinical as well as clinical applications. There is now a significant body of experimental evidence demonstrating clear correlation between endogenous and exogenous optical biomarkers for detection of cell growth (4,5).

A critical part of the drug discovery process is to evaluate the therapeutic potential of putative drugs in relevant animal models of cancer. It has been suggested that the disparity between preclinical and clinical activities of anticancer therapeutics is related to the treatment of advanced metastases in the clinic, whereas traditional subcutaneous xenograft models may not represent advanced metastatic disease. Thus, orthotopic and metastatic models have been developed to better recapitulate clinical disease and used to assess the efficacy of anticancer drugs (6). However, if therapeutic approaches to treating cancers according to their molecular characteristics are to be achieved, additional new models of human cancer are required that represent the genetic diversity that exists within tumor histology. One approach to this over the past twenty years, genetically engineered mouse (GEM) models, has made a significant contribution to the field of cancer research. GEM models have increased our understanding of the molecular pathways responsible for the initiation and progression of human cancers, and have recapitulated well-validated molecular/genetic changes [e.g., oncogene overexpression and tumor suppressor gene (TSG) mutations] in particular types of cancer. The choice of specific screening models is based primarily on response of the models to agents already identified as clinically active. Additionally, a new technology based on hollow fibers has found applications in target identification and validation (7).

EVALUATION OF ANTITUMOR ACTIVITY AND TARGET VALIDATION WITH OPTICAL IMAGING OF HOLLOW FIBERS

In comparison with the traditional xenograft tumor model, the advantages of the hollow fiber assay include shortened evaluation time and reduced compound consumption, capability of evaluating multiple cell lines in one mouse, and being able to isolate pure populations of tumor cells from retrievable hollow fibers for subsequent studies such as cell viability assays, flow cytometry, and/or western blot analysis. Its disadvantages are separation of the tumor cells from their surroundings by the fiber wall, growth of tumor cells being limited because of the geometric constraint of the fibers, necessity for mini-invasive surgery (implantation of hollow fibers), and lack of suitability of the approach for survival endpoints. The combination of optical imaging with hollow fibers not only allows rapid, repetitive, and longitudinal evaluation of anticancer drugs in animals but also enables to evaluate molecular pathways in vivo.

Growth Inhibition of Tumor Cells by Anticancer Drugs Assessed with Optical Imaging of Hollow Fibers

As reported by Zhang et al. (8), hollow fibers filled with reporter tumor cells are visualized with bioluminescence imaging and have been used to evaluate cyclin-dependent

kinase-2 (cdk2) activity in vivo. Thus, hollow fibers can be a tool to follow the tumor cell growth with noninvasive optical imaging. A previous study by Hollingshead's group (9) demonstrated that hollow fibers filled with U251-pGL3 cells in vivo can be imaged with bioluminescence imaging. In this preliminary study, however, Hollingshead has not used the hollow fiber technology to follow growth of tumor cells. In order to evaluate antitumor activities of known anticancer drugs, hollow fibers filled with MCF7-Luc cells (an estrogen receptor–positive human breast cancer cell line stably expressing luciferase) were incubated with Taxotere (an anticancer drug to stabilize microtubule and to arrest cell cycle in M phase) and Camptosar (topoisomerase inhibitor). Proliferation of MCF7-Luc cells was inhibited as evidenced by bioluminescence imaging (Fig. 1A). The proliferation of MCF7-Luc cells in hollow fibers in vivo is significantly inhibited after i.p. administration of Taxotere and Camptosar (Fig. 1B, C). Similarly, Mat B III rat mammary adenocarcinoma cells stably expressing luciferase have also been imaged in hollow fiber models using bioluminescence (data not shown). A noninvasive longitudinal imaging study confirmed the proliferation of Mat B III cells in the hollow fiber model. These results demonstrated that the hollow fiber model allows for monitoring tumor growth with noninvasive imaging and an accurate evaluation of antitumor activities of novel anticancer drugs. Given the fact that microvessels have been proved to form around hollow fibers by visualization of morphological appearance (10), medium to relatively long-term monitoring of tumor growth in the hollow fiber model would provide additional and helpful insight of antitumor activity.

Target Validation with Optical Imaging of Hollow Fibers

A big challenge in drug discovery is to expedite in vivo evaluation of in vitro leads, that is, to investigate whether a compound capable of acting on a target in vitro will also hit the target in vivo. Optical molecular imaging permits visualization of a specific molecular target in a live animal and validating the drug's action on the target. The in vivo hollow fiber assay enables us to evaluate molecular pathways quickly in combination with optical imaging.

The transcription factor nuclear factor-κB (NFκB) plays an important role in tumor development and progression. NFκB and the signaling pathways involved in its activation are therefore attractive targets for therapeutics and cancer prevention. To investigate whether NFκB induction can be imaged in the hollow fiber model, tumor necrosis factor α (TNF-α) was administrated i.p. into nude mice harboring hollow fibers filled with MAT B III-NFκB-Luc cells (NFκB reporter cell line stably transfected with luciferase driven by the NFκB responsive element). After administration of TNF-α, bioluminescence of NFκB reporter cells increased sixfold during 8 hours, while the NFκB activity dropped significantly after 24 hours (Fig. 2A, B). The study demonstrated that optical imaging of cancer cells in hollow fibers can serve as a tool for the evaluation of the drug actions on NFκB pathway.

Cdk2 is a potential anticancer drug target, and several pharmaceutical companies are developing cdk2 inhibitors as anticancer agents (11). In a previous study, Zhang et al. (8) have utilized bioluminescence imaging of hollow fibers to validate cdk2 inhibition in vivo. A p27-luciferase fusion protein was generated, based on the phosphorylation-dependent (i.e., cdk2-dependent) ubiquitination and

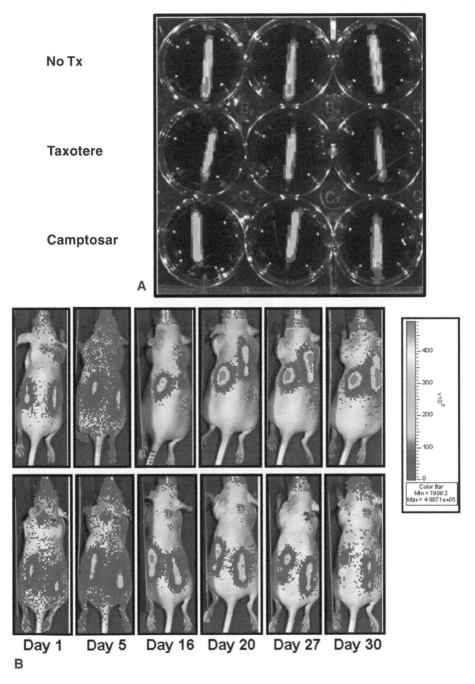

Figure 1 Growth inhibition of MCF7-Luc cells in vitro and in vivo. (**A**) Hollow fibers filled with MCF7-Luc cells cultured in 12-well tissue plates were treated in vitro with Taxotere or Camptosar. The image shows bioluminescence acquired at 48 hours after treatment (acquisition time, 1 minute). (**B**) Nude mice bearing hollow fibers filled with MCF7-Luc cells were either vehicle-treated (top row) or treated with Taxotere (20 mg/kg) starting from day 14 after implantation of hollow fibers. (**C**) Data points show the means of bioluminescent photons of six hollow fibers from three mice (each bearing two hollow fibers, error bars represent standard error of mean (SEM)) (*See Color Insert*).

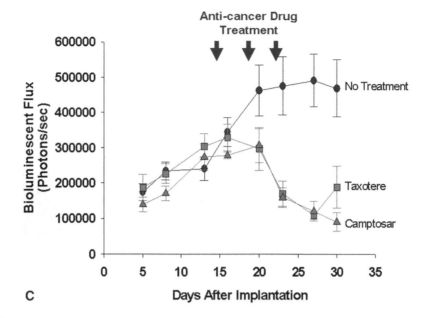

Figure 1 (*Continued*)

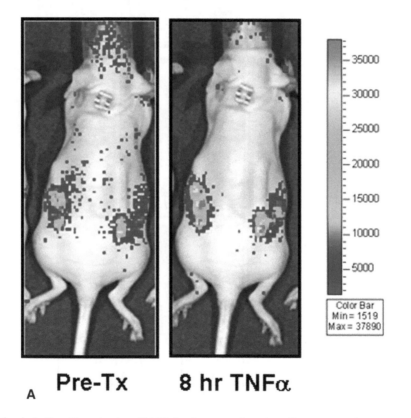

Figure 2 Target validation in hollow fibers in vivo. (**A**) Bioluminescence imaging of a representative mouse pre- and posttreatment with TNF-α. Nude mice harboring hollow fibers with MAT B III-NFκB-Luc cells were administered TNF-α (2 μg/mouse, i.p.). (**B**) Time course of treatment effect on in vivo hollow fibers. Data points show a mean bioluminescent flux (photons/sec) of six hollow fibers from three mice before and after TNF-α treatment (each bearing two hollow fibers, error bars represent SEM). (**C**) Nude mice harboring U2OS cells stably expressing wild-type luciferase (Luc) of cdk2 reporter luciferase (p27Luc) were treated with flavopiridol. Bioluminescence imaging was acquired before and 48 hours after treatment. *Abbreviations*: TNF-α, tumor necrosis factor α; NFκB, nuclear factor-κB.

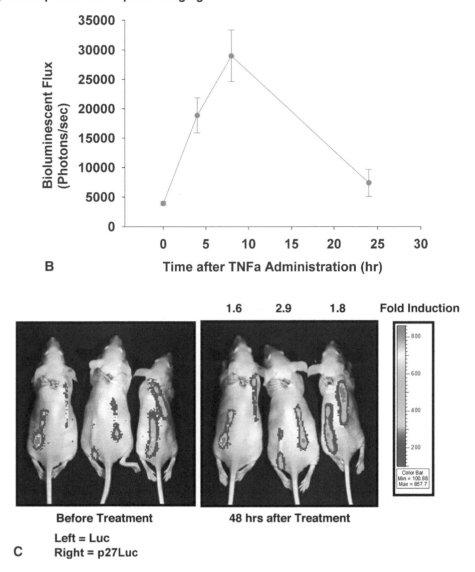

Figure 2 *(Continued)*

degradation of p27 protein, to measure cdk2 inhibition in vitro and in vivo. Two commercially available cdk2 inhibitors, flavopiridol and roscovitine, were administrated i.p. in nude mice harboring hollow fibers filled with U2OS cdk2 reporter cell line. Both cdk2 inhibitors stimulated bioluminescence of cdk2 reporter cells in hollow fibers (Fig. 2C).

With any cell line that is genetically engineered with a pathway-dependent optical reporter, the hollow fiber model can be utilized to monitor molecular pathways in animals as part of the drug development process. In particular, implantation of multiple fibers (each bearing one pathway-specific reporter cell line) will allow visualization of multiple molecular pathways in one mouse. Thus, the specificity of one compound for several targets can be evaluated in one experiment.

MOUSE TUMOR MODELS BASED ON CANCER CELL LINES WITH GENETICALLY ENCODED REPORTERS

Subcutaneous Xenograft Model

Mouse xenograft tumor models based on implantation of human or rodent cancer cells into experimental animals have been a critical component of the drug development process of cancer therapeutics for over 45 years. These in vivo efficacy measurements have historically relied upon determination of tumor growth either by measuring the size of the tumor or by following the life span of experimental animals. More relevant models of human cancers are orthotopic models where the human tumor cells are implanted into the same organ (area) where the experimental tumor cells originated. However, in many cases, this has been very difficult to achieve. Therefore, the most frequent rodent model used for testing of cancer therapeutics is the subcutaneous xenograft model, where the cancer cells are implanted on the flanks of the animal. This model, besides being too far from clinical conditions for many tumor types, suffers from variability in caliper measurements. Newly developed cancer cell lines with the genetically encoded reporters such as luciferase, GFP, and DsRed allow for noninvasive, longitudinal quantitation of tumor growth in subcutaneous and orthotopic tumor models. Imaging models follow tumor cells immediately after implantation and are well suited for quantitative evaluation of therapeutic efficacy. Although both

bioluminescence and fluorescence have been successfully used in these models, the inherent limitations of the reflectance fluorescence measurements of GFP or DsRed limit the practical use of these probes.

An example of subcutaneous xenograft tumor model based on rat mammary adenocarcionoma cells with the genetically encoded optical probe luciferase, MAT B III-luc-3h9, is shown in Figure 3A. Tumor growth in an athymic mouse implanted subcutaneously on the left and right flanks with cancer cells was followed using bioluminescence and caliper to measure the size of the tumors. In the course of the experiment (Fig. 3B), the animals were treated at different periods of time after cell implantation with the commercially available cancer

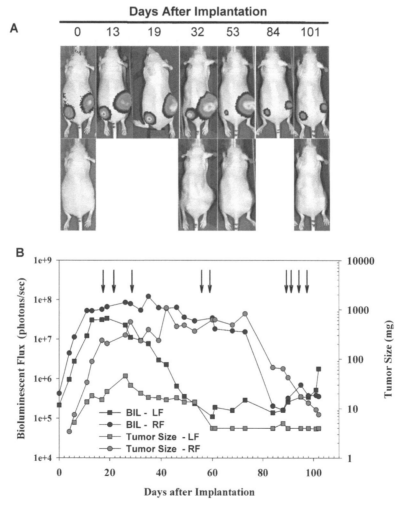

Figure 3 Subcutaneous xenograft tumor model of rat adenocarcinoma cells with the genetically encoded probe luciferase, MAT B III-luc-3H9. MAT B III-luc-3h9 rat adenocarcinoma cells were implanted (1×10^5 cells/100 μL, in PBS) on left and right flanks of an athymic female mouse. (**A**) Top row depicts overlay of photo- and bioluminescence images obtained using IVIS 200 and software Living Image 2.5. Bottom row depicts selected photo images of the mouse from top overlaid images. (**B**) Plots of bioluminescent flux as a biomarker of tumor growth and the tumor size measured by caliper for the tumor on the left and right flanks of the animal. Arrows mark the day of treatment with Taxotere (20 mg/kg). *Abbreviation*: PBS, phosphate buffered saline.

therapeutic Taxotere (20 mg/kg). Bioluminescence as a biomarker of tumor growth indicates the expected time increase of tumor cell number until the first administration of Taxotere. After the third drug administration (28 days after implantation), bioluminescence of the smaller (left) tumor started to decrease precipitously, and by 60 days after implantation, the number of tumor cells detected by bioluminescence was close to the limit of detection. At the same time, the size of the tumor went from ∼50 mg at the maximum to a size not detectable by caliper. Between day 60 and the end of the experiment, the bioluminescence of this tumor started to increase again, while the size of the tumor was below the limit of detection by caliper. Further drug administration had no effect on bioluminescence of this tumor. The bioluminescence of bigger tumor on the right flank started to decrease slowly after first three administrations, while the size of the tumor measured by caliper was still increasing, reaching the maximum of ∼1000 mg 72 days after implantation. Drug administration on day 56 and day 59 had no immediate effect on either bioluminescence or the size of the tumor. However, both bioluminescence as well as the size of the tumor dropped precipitously between day 72 and day 84 after cell implantation. The last four drug administrations (day 90–day 98) had no effect on the bioluminescence, which started in this period of time to increase again, while the size of the tumor continued to decrease below detection level by caliper. Thus, at the end of the study, caliper measurements indicated that both tumors were eliminated, while bioluminescence of both tumors was increasing, indicating continuing cancer cell growth. Results of this experiment demonstrate clear benefits of using bioluminescence as a biomarker of tumor growth over classical size measurements by caliper.

Metastatic Models

In order to stimulate metastatic development, researchers frequently use direct implantation of cancer cells into the circulation by tail vein or by intracardiac injection. However, analysis of such metastatic models has relied only on survival curves and postmortem histological evaluations of tumor distribution within the experimental animals. Although these models have served reasonably well, their limitations and the development of new imaging technologies have stimulated significant progress in animal tumor models.

Many cancer cell lines developed with stably expressed luciferase have allowed the development and noninvasive longitudinal monitoring of metastatic models using several different methods of cell implantation (12–14). As an example of metastatic tumor model based on tail vein injection of cancer cells with the genetically encoded optical probe luciferase, we present data here for two

cohorts (10 animals in each cohort) of athymic mice injected with rat adenocarcinoma cells, Mat B III-luc-3H9. As depicted in Figure 4A, cancer cells are detected by bioluminescence in the lungs of mice right after the cell injection. As the lesions develop, bioluminescence detects growth of tumors noninvasively in different organs and tissues of the mice. Mice in the vehicle-treated cohort develop metastases much faster than the cohort of mice treated with Taxotere (four doses of 20 mg/kg as shown in Fig. 4A). To quantitatively describe the growth of metastases, we have used three regions of interest (ROIs) in the areas of head, thorax, and abdomen on both dorsal and ventral images of the mouse, as depicted in Figure 4B. Thus, there are six time-dependent plots of bioluminescence plus two plots representing sums of three ROIs on the ventral and dorsal sides of the mouse that describe the longitudinal development of metastases (Fig. 4B). If there is interest to follow longitudinally only one of the metastatic lesions, acquired images are always available for additional, more detailed analysis. The final summary of the study may be represented, for example, by the plot depicted in Figure 4C. It shows that the four doses of Taxotere significantly slowed down tumor growth in this model of metastasis.

An experimental model that is technically more challenging is the intracardiac injection of tumor cells, which is used to avoid development of tumors in lungs (which leads to early death of animals before metastasis in other organs can develop). An intracardiac injection into the left ventricle results in the distribution of cancer cells in the whole body without accumulating in any particular organs as shown in Figure 5A for human prostate cancer cells PC-3M-luc-C6 (Xenogen-Caliper Company). Images of the ventral side of the animal at the selected time points of the experiment indicate development of tumors in different organs and tissues of the animal. The longitudinal plot of bioluminescence in Figure 5A describes the growth of metastatic lesions in the head area. The details of the bone lesions are documented by two inserts of co-registered X-ray and bioluminescence images. The application of the intracardiac mouse tumor model for testing of cancer therapeutics is described in Figure 5B. Animals in the three cohorts (10 animals in each cohort) were inoculated by intracardiac injection with 3×10^6 human prostate cancer cells PC-3M-luc-C6, and the longitudinal development of tumors was followed by measuring luminescence in IVIS 200 (Xenogen-Caliper Company). One cohort of animals was treated with four doses (20 mg/kg) of Taxotere, another cohort with the commercially available drug zoledronic acid (15 µg/kg once a week), and there was a control cohort. As documented in Figure 5B, Taxotere almost completely blocked the growth of tumors, while zoledronic acid only slowed down the tumor development. This example demonstrates the power of optical imaging in measuring noninvasively

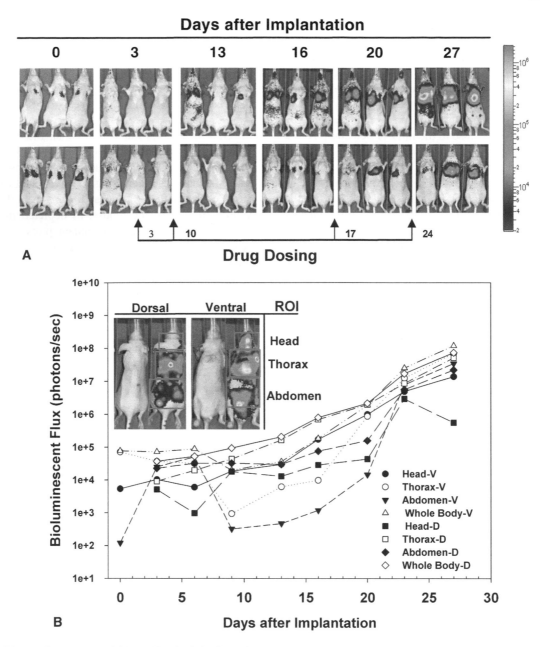

Figure 4 Metastatic tumor model by tail vein injection of rat adenocarcinoma cells MAT B III-luc-3h9. MAT B III-luc-3h9 rat adenocarcinoma cells were implanted by tail vein injection (2×10^5 cells/100 μL, in PBS) into athymic female mice. Development of metastasis was followed using bioluminescence imaging in IVIS 200 and software Living Image 2.5. (**A**) Overlay of photo and bioluminescence images for three mice from the vehicle (top row) and treatment cohort at the selected periods of time after cell implantation. Arrows mark the dates of treatment with Taxotere (20 mg/kg). (**B**) Mouse images with the selected ROIs for the quantitation of bioluminescence and time-dependent plots of bioluminescent flux at the selected ROIs and periods of time after cell implantation for both sides of the animal (V and D). (**C**) Average ± standard error values of whole-body bioluminescence for vehicle and treated animals as a function of time after cell implantation. There were ten animals in each cohort. Arrows mark the day of treatment with Taxotere (20 mg/kg). *Abbreviations*: ROIs, regions of interest; V, ventral; D, dorsal.

the effect of cancer therapeutics on longitudinal development in a model of metastasis, thus providing relatively high throughput testing of drugs in animal models with close physiological relevance to cancer development in humans.

It has been documented in the literature that the metastases of different types of cancer show an organ-specific pattern of spread. In breast cancer, for example, metastases develop in the lymph nodes, bone, and lungs, and less

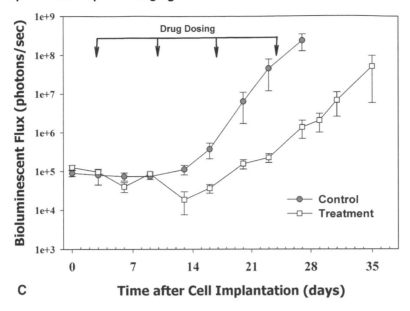

Figure 4 (*Continued*)

frequently in other organs (15). Thus, it would be beneficial for the development of new cancer therapeutics to have organ-specific tumor models. This can be achieved by repeated implantation and collection from specific metastatic lesions of cancer cells stably expressing luciferase (16,17).

TRANSGENIC ANIMALS

The introduction of GEM models of human diseases has extended our understanding of the mechanism of pathogenesis by placing target genes and processes in the appropriate physiological milieu. A number of important

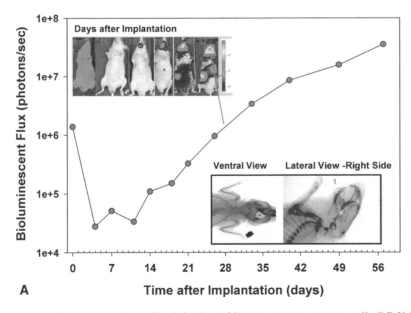

Figure 5 Metastatic tumor model based on intracardiac injection of human prostate cancer cells PC-3M-luc-C6. Human prostate cancer cells PC-3M-luc-C6 (Xenogen-Caliper Company) were implanted into male athymic mice by intracardiac injection into left ventricle. (**A**) Top set of images are overlays of photo- and bioluminescence images of one mouse at selected periods of time after cell implantation. The plot represents longitudinal changes in the bioluminescence of the head area. Images in the lower right corner are overlayed X-ray and bioluminescence images of tumors in the head area of the animal. (**B**) Time-dependent plots of average ± standard error values of whole-body bioluminescence on the ventral side of the animal for control cohort and cohorts of animals treated with Taxotere (20 mg/kg) and zoledronic acid.

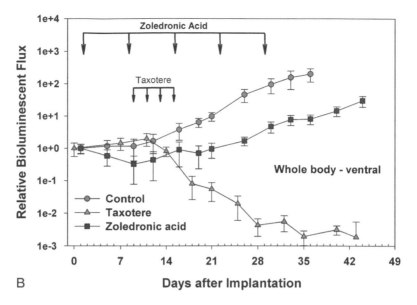

Figure 5 (*Continued*)

genes such as retinoblastoma (Rb), p53, APC, VHL, and PTEN have been knocked out by homologous recombination to recapitulate human tumors in mice (18–21). For example, Rb knockout mice developed pituitary tumors, medullary thyroid carcinomas, and/or pheochromocytomas (18), p53-null mice developed osteosarcomas and myelomas (19), while PTEN-deficient mice developed metastatic prostate carcinomas (21). It is expected that GEM models will more accurately predict responses to novel anticancer drugs in clinical trials.

Imaging of Tumorigenesis and Tumor Progression with Luciferase Reporter

A simple approach to image GEM models is to construct a targeting vector with a reporter gene. This strategy allows expression of luciferase in the same cells/tissues that have been targeted for oncogenic transgene or TSG knockout. For instance, in a doxycycline-inducible bitransgenic mouse model for HER2/neu-induced mammary carcinomas (MMTV-rtTA/TetO-NeuNT), an IRES-luciferase cassette was constructed in the TetO-NeuNT transgene so that both luciferase and Neu are conditionally expressed in the mammary glands in the presence of doxycycline. The model allowed monitoring tumor progression and regression longitudinally in the Neu-induced mammary carcinomas as well as Neu expression (22).

A more general approach has been used to generate a mouse for monitoring tumorigenesis and tumor progression, that is, crossing a reporter mouse (luciferase or GFP) with a preexisting conditional tumor-susceptible mouse (i.e.,

TSG KO or oncogene transgene). For example, Vooijs et al. (23) generated transgenic mice that express luciferase and *Cre* recombinase in the pituitary gland under the control of intermediate lobe–specific pro-opio melanocortin (POMC) promoter. These mice were crossed with conditional RB knockout mice to develop mice with RB deletion solely in the pituitary gland. This model allowed for noninvasive imaging of pituitary tumor development, progression, and therapeutic response in live animals via bioluminescence imaging. A similar mouse model was developed from a conditional *lox*-P-luciferase transgenic mouse by crossing with a conditional oncogenic Kras2^{V12} mouse. The offspring of this cross developed lung adenocarcinomas after delivery of Ad-Cre to the lungs (24). The development of lung cancer in conditional Luc/Kras2^{V12} was visualized by bioluminescence imaging following intratracheal administration of Ade-Cre. The tumor types detected with optical imaging in GEM mice have been greatly expanded, including those in prostate (25), breast (22), lung (24), and brain (26).

A conditional Rosa26 knock-in reporter mouse has been generated by Safran et al. (27), where firefly luciferase is placed downstream of loxP-stop-loxP cassette and is activated after delivery of Cre recombinase. This conditional Rosa26 luciferase mouse can be used for detecting tumor development, and metastases in tumor-prone GEM mice that are mediated by Cre-recombination. For example, this mouse strain could be crossed with a mouse that harbors a conditional oncogene transgene or a TSG knockout. Then, an additional cross with a Cre mouse strain or administration of Ad-Cre would deliver Cre recombinase to a certain organ/tissue, and it would allow for imaging of

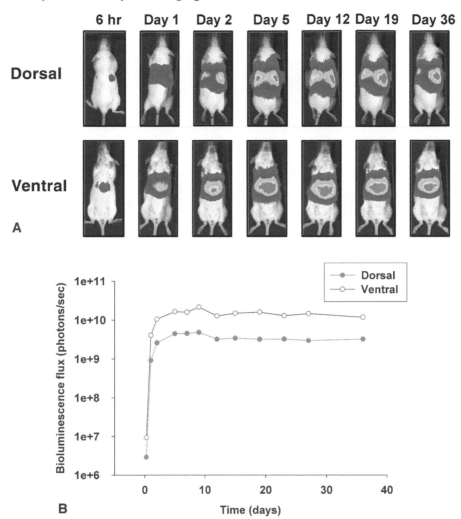

Figure 6 Luciferase expression in the liver in Rosa26-LSL-Luc mouse by tail vein injection of Ade-Cre. (**A**) Longitudinal bioluminescence imaging was acquired for both dorsal and ventral positions after administration of Ade-Cre by tail vein injection. (**B**) Quantitative images showed luciferase expression after Cre-recombination.

tumor formation and tumor cell migration. By local or systemic administration of Ad-Cre, one can generate a mouse with an organ/tissue-specific luciferase expression. For example, the tail vein injection of Ad-Cre generates dominant expression of luciferase in the liver (Fig. 6A, B), and such reporter mice can be potentially used to evaluate autochthonous liver tumors as well as targeted delivery of novel therapeutic vectors such as siRNA.

Imaging Therapeutic Effects in GEM Models

As discussed above, optical imaging of tumor development in GEM mice is mainly based on changes of cell number and tumor size. Uhrbom et al. (26) developed a reporter mouse capable of imaging cell proliferation by monitoring E2F activity. As E2F activity is strictly regulated

during cell cycle progression, a vector in which the firefly luciferase is driven by multiple E2F consensus sequence (Ef-Luc) was used to generate transgenic mice for the detection of S-phase fraction. The Ef-Luc transgenic mice were then crossed with N-tv-a transgenic mice, which express the viral receptor tv-a, allowing retroviral transduction to glial progenitor cells. The double Ef-Luc/N-tv-a transgenic mice have been used to monitor oligodendrogliomas induced with RCAS-PDGFB (platelet-derived growth factor B) vector. In this GEM model, longitudinal bioluminescence imaging was applied to follow the inhibition of PDGFB-induced tumors with a PDGFR (PDGF-receptor) inhibitor, PTK787/ZK222584, and an mTOR inhibitor, CCI-779 (Fig. 7). Significant inhibition of tumor proliferation was detected by bioluminescence observed in the groups treated with PDGFR-specific inhibitors and confirmed by PCNA

PDGFR inhibition

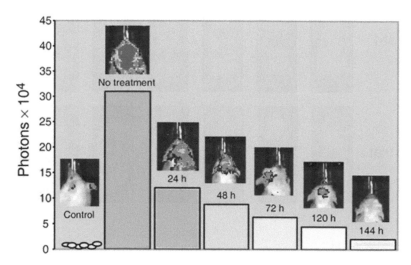

Figure 7 Longitudinal imaging of PDGFB-induced glioma. PDGFB-induced glioma-bearing mouse treated with PTK787/ZK222584, a PDGFR inhibitor, daily for six days (*See Color Insert*).

immunostaining (32). So far, there are only a few reports available to monitor therapeutic effects of anticancer drugs with optical imaging in GEM models (26,28).

Despite their potential for higher drug efficacy predictability, GEM models have some limitations. One limitation of GEM models is that a particular genetic alteration, although it leads to tumor development in mice, may not mimic exact genetic alterations in human cancers. For example, deletion of TSGs by homologous recombination is not equal to mutation in the same genes occurring in humans. The tumors developed in mice may lack the environmental influences as well as genomic instability associated with human cancers. More preclinical work as well as feedback from future clinical trials is required to more fully evaluate the predictive value of GEM models for cancer therapeutic efficacy and assess the value of their contribution to the drug development process. Moreover, efficient integration of GEMs in the drug discovery process poses some challenges, such as the relatively long time required for tumors to develop compared to the xenograft model, the necessity to establish imaging-based enrollment criteria for drug efficacy studies (as most of the autochthonous tumors are not palpable), and specific imaging protocols to follow tumor growth in GEM not engineered with a reporter system like luciferase. One approach in facilitating the use of GEM in drug development while retaining a significant throughput screening is to use exogenous fluorescent probes.

Exogenous Probes

The limitations of reflectance fluorescence for tumor detection using genetically encoded fluorescent probes GFP and DsRed are compensated when using exogenous probes such as the NIR fluorescent $\alpha_V\beta_3$ ligand (29,30), the protease-activated probe ProSense™, and the blood pool probe AngioSense™ (31–33). Applications of such probes for detection of tumor growth are independent of any genetically encoded fluorophores, allowing use of a much wider spectrum of tumor cell lines as well as making possible the detection of tumor growth in transgenic animals of cancer (34).

A parallel detection of tumor growth as well as the effect of drug treatment using both genetically encoded luciferase and the fluorescence probe AngioSense™ is depicted in Figure 8. Similar to the model described previously, athymic mice were inoculated subcutaneously on left and right flanks with rat cancer cells MAT B III-luc-3H9. As shown in the control plot in Figure 8A, fluorescence of the AngioSense™ probe detected tumor growth similar to that of the bioluminescence of the genetically encoded probe luciferase shown in the control plot of Figure 8B. Both plots correlate well with the tumor size measured by caliper. Treatment of another animal with four doses (20 mg/kg) of Taxotere inhibited tumor growth as detected by both bioluminescence of the luciferase (Fig. 8B) as well as fluorescence of AngioSense™ (Fig. 8A). Thus, the fluorescence of exogenous optical

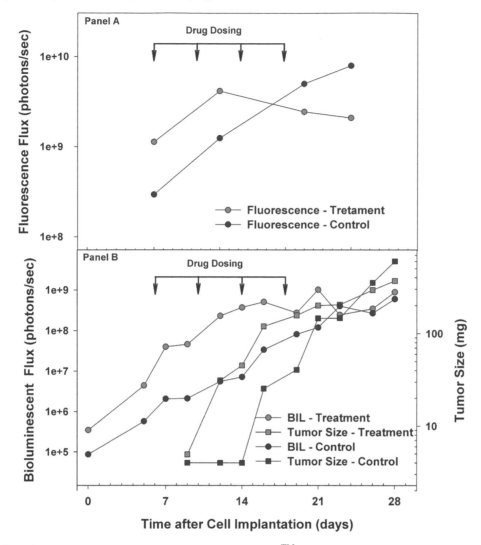

Figure 8 Detection of tumor growth by an exogenous probe AngioSense™. Athymic female mice were implanted by subcutaneous injection with rat adenocarcinoma cells MAT B III-luc 3h9 (2×10^5 cell/100 μL in PBS) on the flanks of the animals. Tumor growth was followed using bioluminescence, caliper, and fluorescence of exogenous probe AngioSense™ 750 (~ 1 nmol/animal). (**A**) The longitudinal changes in the fluorescence of AngioSense™ probe for the treated (Taxotere 20 mg/kg/dose) and control animal. (**B**) The longitudinal changes in bioluminescence (BIL) and tumor size as measured by caliper for treated and control animals, respectively.

probe AngioSense™ serves as a biomarker of tumor growth similar to the bioluminescence of genetically encoded probe luciferase. Recently, AngioSense™ 750 has been successfully used for detection of tumors in NeuNT transgenic mice (Dr. W. Zhang, personal communication).

SUMMARY

In summary, optical imaging has been incorporated into all available tumor mouse models for oncology drug discovery with either genetically engineered reporters or injectable optical probes. In the future, reporter mice capable of imaging specific cancer pathways (i.e., hypoxia, angiogenesis) when crossed with tumor-prone mice should provide the ability not only to image spontaneous

tumorigenesis but also to image biological/pathological changes associated with tumor formation and progression, allowing detection of tumorigenesis at earlier times and with greater sensitivity.

Optical imaging has started and will continue to impact all aspects of drug discovery in preclinical development, such as target validation, biomarker discovery, lead optimization, and drug efficacy study. It has been proven to have advantages over the clinical imaging modalities (PET, MRI, CT) in preclinical development, including intermediate throughput and lower cost. However, one of its weaknesses is that genetically engineered reporters cannot easily be translated into clinical use in humans. NIR-labeled probes under investigation may overcome this weakness in the future.

REFERENCES

1. Bednar B, Zhang GJ, Williams DL, et al. Optical molecular imaging in drug discovery and clinical development. Expert Opin Drug Discov 2007; 2:65–85.
2. Gelovani Tjuvajev J, Blasberg RG. In vivo imaging of molecular-genetic targets for cancer therapy. Cancer Cell 2003; 3(4):327–332.
3. Hoffman R. Green fluorescent protein imaging of tumour growth, metastasis, and angiogenesis in mouse models. Lancet Oncol 2002; 3(9):546–556.
4. Achilefu S. Lighting up tumors with receptor-specific optical molecular probes. Technol Cancer Res Treat 2004; 3(4):393–409.
5. Gross S, Piwnica-Worms D. Spying on cancer: molecular imaging in vivo with genetically encoded reporters. Cancer Cell 2005; 7(1):5–15.
6. Hoffman RM. Orthotopic metastatic (MetaMouse) models for discovery and development of novel chemotherapy. Methods Mol Med 2005; 111:297–322.
7. Zhang GJ, Chen TB, Bednar B, et al. Optical imaging of tumor cells in hollow fibers: evaluation of the antitumor activities of anticancer drugs and target validation. Neoplasia 2007; 9(8):652–661.
8. Zhang GJ, Kaelin WG Jr. Bioluminescent imaging of ubiquitin ligase activity: measuring Cdk2 activity in vivo through changes in p27 turnover. Methods Enzymol 2005; 399:530–549.
9. Hollingshead MG, Bonomi CA, Borgel SD, et al. A potential role for imaging technology in anticancer efficacy evaluations. Eur J Cancer 2004; 40(6):890–898.
10. Phillips RM, Pearce J, Loadman PM, et al. Angiogenesis in the hollow fiber tumor model influences drug delivery to tumor cells: implications for anticancer drug screening programs. Cancer Res 1998; 58(23):5263–5266.
11. Shapiro GI. Cyclin-dependent kinase pathways as targets for cancer treatment. J Clin Oncol 2006; 24(11):1770–1783.
12. Jenkins DE, Hornig YS, Oei Y, et al. Bioluminescent human breast cancer cell lines that permit rapid and sensitive in vivo detection of mammary tumors and multiple metastases in immune deficient mice. Breast Cancer Res 2005; 7(4):R444–R454.
13. Jenkins DE, Oei Y, Hornig YS, et al. Bioluminescent imaging (BLI) to improve and refine traditional murine models of tumor growth and metastasis. Clin Exp Metastasis 2003; 20(8):733–744.
14. Scatena CD, Hepner MA, Oei YA, et al. Imaging of bioluminescent LNCaP-luc-M6 tumors: a new animal model for the study of metastatic human prostate cancer. Prostate 2004; 59(3):292–303.
15. Kang Y, Siegel PM, Shu W, et al. A multigenic program mediating breast cancer metastasis to bone. Cancer Cell 2003; 3(6):537–549.
16. Minn AJ, Gupta GP, Siegel PM, et al. Genes that mediate breast cancer metastasis to lung. Nature 2005; 436 (7050):518–524.
17. Minn AJ, Kang Y, Serganova I, et al. Distinct organ-specific metastatic potential of individual breast cancer cells and primary tumors. J Clin Invest 2005; 115(1): 44–55.
18. Jacks T, Fazeli A, Schmitt EM, et al. Effects of an Rb mutation in the mouse. Nature 1992; 359(6393):295–300.
19. Donehower LA, Harvey M, Slagle BL, et al. Mice deficient for p53 are developmentally normal but susceptible to spontaneous tumours. Nature 1992; 356(6366):215–221.
20. Gnarra JR, Ward JM, Porter FD, et al. Defective placental vasculogenesis causes embryonic lethality in VHL-deficient mice. Proc Natl Acad Sci U S A 1997; 94(17):9102–9107.
21. Wang S, Gao J, Lei Q, et al. Prostate-specific deletion of the murine Pten tumor suppressor gene leads to metastatic prostate cancer. Cancer Cell 2003; 4(3):209–221.
22. Moody SE, Perez D, Pan TC, et al. The transcriptional repressor Snail promotes mammary tumor recurrence. Cancer Cell 2005; 8(3):197–209.
23. Vooijs M, Jonkers J, Lyons S, et al. Noninvasive imaging of spontaneous retinoblastoma pathway-dependent tumors in mice. Cancer Res 2002; 62(6):1862–1867.
24. Lyons SK, Meuwissen R, Krimpenfort P, et al. The generation of a conditional reporter that enables bioluminescence imaging of Cre/loxP-dependent tumorigenesis in mice. Cancer Res 2003; 63(21):7042–7046.
25. Lyons SK, Lim E, Clermont AO, et al. Noninvasive bioluminescence imaging of normal and spontaneously transformed prostate tissue in mice. Cancer Res 2006; 66(9): 4701–4707.
26. Uhrbom L, Nerio E, Holland EC. Dissecting tumor maintenance requirements using bioluminescence imaging of cell proliferation in a mouse glioma model. Nat Med 2004; 10(11):1257–1260.
27. Safran M, Kim WY, Kung AL, et al. Mouse reporter strain for noninvasive bioluminescent imaging of cells that have undergone Cre-mediated recombination. Mol Imaging 2003; 2(4):297–302.
28. Seethammagari MR, Xie X, Greenberg NM, et al. EZC-prostate models offer high sensitivity and specificity for noninvasive imaging of prostate cancer progression and androgen receptor action. Cancer Res 2006; 66(12):6199–6209.
29. Ye Y, Bloch S, Xu B, et al. Design, synthesis, and evaluation of near infrared fluorescent multimeric RGD peptides for targeting tumors. J Med Chem 2006; 49(7):2268–2275.
30. Chen X, Conti PS, Moats RA. In vivo near-infrared fluorescence imaging of integrin alphavbeta3 in brain tumor xenografts. Cancer Res 2004; 64(21):8009–8014.
31. Weissleder R, Tung CH, Mahmood U, et al. In vivo imaging of tumors with protease-activated near-infrared fluorescent probes. Nat Biotechnol 1999; 17(4):375–378.
32. Bremer C, Tung CH, Weissleder R. In vivo molecular target assessment of matrix metalloproteinase inhibition. Nat Med 2001; 7(6):743–748.
33. Mahmood U, Weissleder R. Near-infrared optical imaging of proteases in cancer. Mol Cancer Ther 2003; 2(5):489–496.
34. Bremer C, Ntziachristos V, Weitkamp B, et al. Optical imaging of spontaneous breast tumors using protease sensing 'smart' optical probes. Invest Radiol 2005; 40(6):321–327.

43

Drug Development with Radiopharmaceuticals

HENRY F. VANBROCKLIN

Department of Radiology and Biomedical Imaging, University of California, San Francisco, California, U.S.A.

INTRODUCTION

Our understanding of cancer as a disease has significantly improved over the last decade as genomics and proteomics have provided key insights into the genetic and molecular "hallmarks" of cancer (1–3). The further definition of the molecular landscape and cellular circuitry has enhanced the development of specific molecular therapeutics, targeting specific pathways in cancer as presented in the individual patient. Thus, identifying the molecular basis for cancer is leading toward personalized diagnosis and therapy.

Genomics and proteomics continue to provide a wealth of new drugable targets. This coupled with combinatorial chemistry for small molecule and peptide library synthesis, phage display techniques for targeted peptide and single chain antibody fragment library production, and improved techniques for preparation of immunogenic monoclonal antibodies as well as molecular modeling and high-throughput screening has greatly expanded the chemical space that is searchable for new chemical entities. Evaluating the interaction of the new drugs with the drugable targets is the daunting and challenging task undertaken largely by the pharmaceutical industry to produce a pipeline of new drugs. The successful emergence of effective therapeutics from this pipeline is slowed by the ability to critically evaluate the interaction of the drug with the target and fully assess their toxicity and safety profiles.

Molecular nuclear imaging permits the visualization of the distribution of labeled compounds in living systems. Imaging probes may be used to define the pharmacokinetic (PK) properties of labeled compounds or assess the pharmacodynamic (PD) properties of new drugs. Molecular imaging's role in drug discovery and development has grown over the last decade, and it will have a significant impact on the assessment and profiling of new drugs in the foreseeable future. This chapter is devoted to describing the many ways that molecular nuclear imaging techniques may be applied to increase the efficiency of the drug discovery and development process.

THE COST OF DEVELOPING NEW DRUGS

The timeline and expense for developing new drugs present a significant barrier to success. On the basis of a survey of 68 drugs, the cost associated with the new drug discovery and development has been estimated to be between $1 and $2 billion (4). While this figure has been debated (5,6), it is evident that both the financial and timeline constraints of the current drug development process will force a change in the way new drugs are developed. Under the current paradigm, it will be nearly impossible to produce effective new drugs that will improve quality of life as well as meet the challenges of minimizing health care costs.

In a study undertaken by the Tufts Center for the Study of Drug Development (CSDD), it was noted that the timeline for discovery and development of a new chemical entity from lead identity through the clinical trial phases to an approved new drug application (NDA) had increased by nearly 75% from an average 7.9 years in the 1960s to an average 12.8 years in the mid 1990s (7,8). The study separated out the investigational new drug (IND) portion of the process from the NDA-approval phase and found that nearly all of the increased time was in the IND phase. This is not surprising, given the increased regulatory requirements and the clinical trial complexities (4,7–10). Obviously, the length of the timeline and the multifaceted clinical trials add significantly to the cost of new drug development. DiMasi noted that 16% cost savings could be gained by reducing the clinical phase timelines by 25%. Molecular imaging approaches have the potential to realize these timeline reductions without compromising safety.

The cost of drug development is also impacted by rate of compound attrition from the development pipeline. Of 5 to 10,000 compounds produced in the early discovery phase, only 5 survive to enter the clinical phases, and only one of those becomes a fully approved drug (10). This number corresponds well with the data recently reported by DiMasi and Grabowski (11), where 25% of all drugs entering phase I trials receive NDA approval. DiMasi also noted that increasing the phase I NDA approval rate to 33% would translate into a cost reduction of nearly 50%. Thus, it is necessary to develop better screening tools that will select the best compounds to emerge from the preclinical testing. Also, effective use of the exploratory IND (phase 0) will reduce the number of compounds that are likely to fail in the clinical trials. Molecular imaging approaches will be crucial for effective screening of compounds prior to entering the clinical phases. In order to support go-no-go decisions, imaging biomarkers must be reliable, validated, and reproducible with minimal intra- and intersubject variability. The cost savings will only be realized when the strength of the selection tools is enhanced.

One of the benefits of introduction of imaging bio-markers early in the drug development schema is the ability to assess potential efficacy. In the current para-digm, therapeutic efficacy is evaluated in late phase II and phase III of the process. The ability to confidently inter-pret the PK data early in humans is critical to making the difficult decision to halt a clinical trial. Validated imaging biomarkers may provide that data and the confidence necessary to make those key decisions.

Efficacy is an important criterion for new chemical entity (NCE) approval. It is not uncommon to find targeted oncologic therapeutic agents with reported response rates of 10% to 20%, even when the target is overexpressed in the patient as shown by biopsy. For example, ErbB2 receptors are overexpressed in 25% to 30% of breast tumors. One of the current treatments, trastuzamab (Herceptin), is only effective as a frontline therapy in 25% of patients with elevated ErbB2 levels and as a secondary therapy in 15% of ErbB2-positive tumors (12). Therefore, even though the receptor has been identified in these patients, this is not a predictive biomarker for response to targeted therapy. Molecular imaging may be able to improve the odds of therapeutic efficacy by select-ing those patients that not only possess the desired target but also accumulate the desired therapeutic into those tissues containing the target. Preselecting patients may improve patient quality of life by eliminating the need for testing therapeutics in patients and waiting for a response that may never come. Monitoring treatment is also another way to improve patient management. In some cases, diseases become resistant to a therapy, and it is necessary to make a mid-course correction in dose or drug. Molecular imaging tools and radiolabeled probes provide valuable information for making informed decisions.

The World Health Organization (WHO) established and published a set of objective response criteria in the late 1970s/early 1980s that would be used worldwide to commonly describe cancer therapeutic intervention (13). Four categories of criteria—complete response, partial response, stable disease, and progressive disease—were defined largely on the measurement of tumor size and tumor burden. According to the established guidance, a responding tumor must decrease by 50%. For 20 years, these criteria were used to characterize tumoral changes in response to therapy. During those years, anatomic imaging (MRI and CT) became widely available. As a result of the availability of the noninvasive imaging measures of tumor size and tumor burden as well as other shortcomings of the original definitions, a new set of criteria, known as the RECIST (Response Evaluation Criteria In Solid Tumors) guidelines, was established in 2000 (14). These guidelines have retained the four original categories and are based on morphological measurement of tumor burden and tumor size using MRI and CT imaging. The response metric was also reduced to 30% change in tumor size. While these guidelines do provide some measure of tumor responsive-ness to therapeutic intervention, they may not be able to keep pace with the new molecular medicines being developed now and in the future. There are many cases where the response to a therapeutic is slow and may not necessarily result in the immediate regression of the tumor burden or change in tumor size. The degree of response may depend on the length of the phase III trial (often only 1–1.5 years) or even the type of drug under evaluation. Many of the new drugs today are cytostatic rather than cytocidal, which means that the loss of cell volume may never be manifested. There are also flare responses, metabolic and osteoblastic, to treatment that complicate the assessment using the RECIST criteria. A recent publication reported the case of a 43-year-old diagnosed with gastric adenocarcinoma (15). Six weeks after initiating treatment: the lymph nodes demonstrated a 43% decrease, a partial response; and pulmonary nodules were gone, a complete response. However, bone lesions from an osteoblastic flare were noted, which confounds the overall response; in this case, it might be considered progressive disease. Thus, a strict interpretation of the RECIST criteria might alter treatment or adversely influence clinical trials. Metabolic and osteoblastic flare have been seen by positron emission tomography (PET) imaging and should be incorporated into the treatment response criteria (16). Metabolic flare has been identified by [^{18}F]fluorodeoxyglucose (FDG) imaging and 16α-[^{18}F]fluoro-17β-estradiol imaging following tamoxifen therapy (17,18). Similarly, osteoblastic flare has been observed in up to 75% of breast cancer patients (19–21). The flare phenomena are often linked to successful outcome rather than disease progression that highlights the need to establish response criteria using molecular imaging assessments so that the correct response is attributed to the therapeutic under evaluation.

Radiolabeled molecular imaging probes such as those discussed herein may show evidence of response within the first 24 hours of treatment. A response that fast is unlikely to be concomitant with an immediate decrease in tumor burden or tumor size. Therefore, the response criteria need to be updated to reflect molecular imaging and measurement of functional response. New criteria incorporating molecular imaging methods of response may further decrease the unnecessary waiting period to see if a new therapeutic has beneficial effects (22). The objective is to assess the therapeutic response early with molecular imaging so that nonbeneficial, expensive, and potentially toxic treatment is replaced with alternative therapies, thereby increasing the likelihood of a good outcome.

FINDING AND FOLLOWING THE "CRITICAL PATH"

There has been a significant reduction in the number of applications submitted to the Food and Drug Administration (FDA) for approval since 1995. The data for the total submissions and the approval by submission type are shown in Figure 1. Submissions of the total number of new molecular entities (NMEs), typically small-molecule drugs, and biological license applications (BLAs), amino acid-based agents (e.g. antibodies), have decreased from a high of approximately 85 in 1995 to 30 to 40 in 2003–2004. Concomitantly, the approvals have alarmingly dropped to 20 per year for 2005 and 2006. These approval

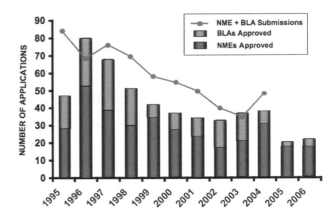

Figure 1 Annual number of NME applications and BLAs received and approved by the FDA. *Abbreviations*: NME, new molecular entity; BLA, biologic license applications; FDA, Food and Drug Administration. *Source*: From Ref. 68.

numbers are 25% of the peak year on this graph, 1996. This precipitous drop in submissions and approvals was a wakeup call for the agency. In 2004, the FDA published a critical report on the state of new drug development and the approval process, titled "Innovation or Stagnation: Challenge and Opportunity on the Critical Path to New Medical Products" (23). In this report, the agency outlined a new paradigm called the "Critical Path Initiative" (CPI), which might hasten approvals and encourage new submissions (24).

The CPI is a framework for a new approach to drug approvals. The FDA wanted to reduce the time it takes to approve new applications and stimulate the submission of new applications by encouraging the use of enabling technologies such as genomics, proteomics, bioinformatics, material science, and medical imaging. Out of this process came a reexamination of the IND process and the pathway for first-in-human studies. Under the original IND process, new chemical entities had to go through extensive toxicity testing, costing upward of $1 million, before initial human studies would be allowed. This process is inefficient as first-in-human studies are in the critical path and where many new drugs fail. In concert with the drug industry, the concept of microdosing was accepted as a means of early testing in humans. With minimal toxicity requirements, several compounds may be brought forward for microdosing studies in humans. This process was captured in guidance documentation by the FDA and became known as the "exploratory investigational new drug" application or phase 0 clinical trials (25). While this process was largely developed to evaluate multiple new drug compounds in humans, a section of the new guidance was devoted to requirements for radiotracer first-in-human studies. Like the drug entities, the toxicity data required for new radiotracers are significantly reduced compared with a full IND application. This lower barrier to initial human testing has already stimulated the evaluation of several new drugs (26) and radiotracers in humans.

RADIOLABELED MOLECULAR IMAGING PROBES AND THEIR ROLE IN THE DRUG DEVELOPMENT PARADIGM

Radiolabeled molecular imaging agents are emerging as major tools for the drug discovery and development paradigm (27). Many of the large pharmaceutical manufacturers have expanded their radiolabeling operations from what was once mainly tritium and carbon-14 labeling for preclinical distribution and metabolism studies to include single photon (e.g., technetium-99m and iodine-123) as well as positron (e.g., fluorine-18 and carbon-11) labeling for more comprehensive preclinical functional imaging and translational studies. Additionally, the proliferation of small animal equipment has made it feasible for pharmaceutical companies to develop their own small animal imaging facilities. Availability of longer-lived PET isotopes (e.g., fluorine-18, copper-64) permits the preparation of radiotracers in-house for preclinical evaluation of new therapeutics.

Molecular imaging provides valuable information at nearly every stage of the process. Figure 2 shows the various stages of discovery and development flanked by the types of information that may be garnered from imaging with radiolabeled tracers throughout the process. In the following sections, the applications of nuclear molecular imaging at the various stages of drug development are highlighted.

Target Identification/Validation

In the early discovery phase, the evaluation of target expression and function related to a particular disease leads to important target identification, the key to the

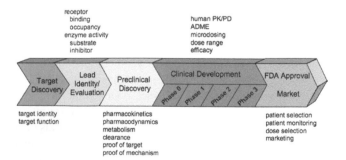

Figure 2 Drug discovery and development pathway flanked by the molecular imaging information that may be obtained at each stage.

downstream discovery of a target-modulating drug. Target validation involves positively linking the target expression to the particular disease as well as demonstrating that modulation of the target has a positive impact on the disease phenotype (28,29). Receptor-based agents or radiotracers that target cell surface proteins are examples of probes that may be used to establish a disease-associated target. Central nervous system imaging agents targeting neurotransmitter systems, specifically receptor subtypes and transporters, are among the earliest examples of proof of target studies. Measuring receptor occupancy by a therapeutic agent provides proof that one is hitting the desired target. For these studies, PET scans are obtained following administration of varying concentrations of test drug. A curve of receptor occupancy as measured by PET versus concentration administered or plasma concentration measured is generated to determine the effective dose. Farde and colleagues (30) followed the loss of [^{11}C]raclopride, a dopamine D_2 receptor-imaging agent, to assess D_2 occupancy by classic and atypical antipsychotics given to schizophrenic patients. They found that the receptor occupancy ranged from 65% to 85%. Receptor occupancy alone does not constitute a suitable validation of the target. One may also wish to correlate the occupancy with a measure of PD information. In a recent example, a fluorine-18-labeled NK1 receptor agent [^{18}F]SPA-RQ demonstrated the 80% to 90% receptor occupancy of NK1 receptors by the aprepiant, a NK1 receptor antagonist. In spite of the high receptor occupancy, aprepiant was not found to be an effective treatment of depression; however, at these receptor occupancy levels, aprepiant did prevent chemotherapy-induced nausea and vomiting (31). This information provided valuable feedback for halting the continuation of the development of aprepiant as an antidepressant.

Lead Identification/Lead Optimization

Lead identification is largely accomplished by traditional synthetic and high-throughput medicinal chemistry strategies. Imaging does not have a direct role to play in identifying a lead compound. However, once a lead compound has been selected, imaging may be incorporated into lead optimization studies. Lead optimization involves the expanding evaluation of lead compound analogs to find optimal candidates for preclinical testing. Imaging probes may be applied to assess receptor binding or occupancy as well as measuring functional parameters such as enzyme inhibition related to the selected leads and analogs. Early PK studies involving the labeled lead compound or analogs may be integrated into the iterative optimization process. Likewise, initial definition of the metabolic fate and clearance properties of the new drugs may be explored with labeled compounds. Imaging provides some powerful tools for lead optimization that may also provide a window to view how probes may be used throughout the remainder of the development process, including validation studies.

In vitro evaluation in cultured tumor cells may provide early assessment of potential response to new lead cancer therapeutics. In a study designed by Dittmann and colleagues (32), squamous cells were cultured with various antineoplastic agents [5-fluorouracil (5-FU), methotrexate, cisplatin, and gemcitabine]. Fluorine-18-labeled fluorothymidine (FLT) and FDG were added to the cells following a recovery period. The cellular uptake of the labeled probes was assayed as a function of time post-removal of treatment and dose of therapeutic. They found that fluorouracil, methotrexate, and gemcitabine increased FLT cellular accumulation as a result of the increased DNA salvage pathway activation rather than increased proliferation. FLT accumulation in the cisplatin-treated decreased drastically indicative of a reduction in cellular proliferation. This assay is an example of the types of experiments that may be carried out during the lead optimization phase to evaluate proof of therapeutic potential in vivo and also to provide insight on how labeled tracers may respond to various treatments.

Preclinical Discovery

Once lead compounds have been identified, the molecules advance into the preclinical evaluation phase. In this phase, a critical analysis of the in vivo-targeting properties of new drugs is conducted. Additionally, the first studies of in vivo metabolism and toxicity are performed. Here, the selective use of radiotracer imaging may provide significant feedback on the targeting, selectivity, metabolic fate, and mechanism of action of the new drug.

Depending on the nature of the compound under study, a decision must be made at this point to use either a labeled probe or the labeled drug. The labeled drug will provide largely PK information, while a labeled probe will afford evidence of the drug effect on the target and downstream systems (i.e., PD information). The labeled drug candidate may not necessarily make a suitable radiotracer as its selectivity or affinity for the target may not be sufficiently high to demonstrate focal uptake at the target site. Typical receptor-targeted pharmaceuticals possess μM to sub-μM receptor binding affinities, whereas the target to background ratio for imaging agents is optimal with nM to sub-nM affinities. The labeled drug may, however, be applied to determine the absorption, distribution, metabolism, and excretion (ADME) properties of the drug, including whole body distribution, metabolism, and clearance. An example of the synthesis and evaluation of a radiolabeled, known cancer therapeutic was recently reported (33). Imatinib (Gleevec) has been shown to be effective in the treatment of gastrointestinal stromal tumors (GIST)

as well as chronic myeloid leukemia. Imatinib was labeled with the 20-minute half-life carbon-11 and evaluated in normal nonhuman primates using PET. The radiolabeled drug distributed throughout the body as expected. Organ uptake (heart, lung, kidney, and spleen) was unchanged after administration of a dose of nonradioactive imatinib. On the basis of this preclinical assessment of the labeled imatinib, this tracer may be useful for PK studies in humans as well as for treatment planning or measuring therapeutic response (33). Since the toxicity of imatinib in humans was already known, clinical PK research studies using [^{11}C]imatinib may be conducted under Radioactive Drug Research Committee (RDRC) approval.

Alternatively, labeled probes may be used to assess changes related to the drug effect that includes proving the drug is hitting the desired target or proving its mechanism of action. In many cases, especially where the drug is itself a receptor-targeted entity, the labeled drug will not be able to directly measure its own efficacy as the nonradioactive drug will effectively block the binding sites. Labeled receptor imaging agents may be applied to quantify receptor occupancy. Validation of these receptor probes may prove useful to determine dose-occupancy curves in future human studies. An example of an oncologic receptor-based probe that has been applied to preclinically assess receptor occupancy of the hormone-based drug tamoxifen is fluorine-18-labeled fluoroestradiol (FES) (34), a marker of estrogen receptor density. A study in rats revealed that specific targeting of tamoxifen at the estrogen receptors was measurable using FES. On the basis of the dose-occupancy studies in this model, the ability to quantitatively measure estrogen receptor content in humans was predicted (35).

Probes such as those listed in Table 1, including FDG (glucose metabolism), [^{18}F]fluorothymidine (FLT; proliferation), [^{18}F]fluoromisonidazole (FMISO; hypoxia), or [^{11}C]choline (cell membrane synthesis), are markers of cellular processes that may be altered relative to the administration of a therapeutic dose of the drug. Many of these tracers have been used to evaluate therapeutic response in preclinical models and validate their ultimate potential as a biomarker for therapeutic intervention in humans (36).

Clinical Development

Imaging studies are increasingly being used in humans to assess PK and PD of new therapeutics. This is the most costly stage of the drug development schema with each phase becoming increasingly expensive. Phase 0 provides exploratory first-in-human PK information, phase I involves safety and dose-escalation studies, phase II encompasses the initial evaluation of efficacy with an eye on potential side effects, and phase III entails large

Table 1 PET/SPECT Imaging Probes Available for Cancer Imaging in Human Subjects

Cancer	Probe	Target	References
Various	[^{18}F]fluorodeoxyglucose (FDG)	Glucose metabolism	69,70
Various	[^{18}F]fluoropaclitaxel (FPAC)	Binding to β-tubulin, potential predictor of paclitaxel PK and response, MDR substrate	71–73
Various	[^{18}F]fluorouracil (5-FU)	Inhibit thymidylate synthase, enzyme for DNA synthesis	49
Various	[^{18}F]fluoromisonidazole (FMISO), [^{18}F]fluoroazomycin arabinoside (FAZA), [^{123}I]iodoazomycin arabinoside (IAZA), [^{60,64}Cu]ATSM	Hypoxic tissue	74–78
Various	[^{18}F]fluorothymidine (FLT)	Cell proliferation	79
Various	[^{11}C]choline, [^{18}F]fluorocholine	Cell membrane synthesis	80,81
Various	[^{11}C]PK11195	Inflammation/macrophage	82
Prostate	[^{11}C]acetate	Acetate metabolism	83
Prostate	[^{111}In]PSMA antibody Prostascint®	PSMA	84
Prostate	[^{18}F]fluorodihydrotestosterone (FDHT)	Androgen receptors	85
Breast	[^{18}F]fluoroestradiol (FES)	Estrogen receptors	34
Breast	[^{111}In]EGF, [^{99m}Tc]anti-EGF	EGF receptor	86,87
Breast	[^{99m}Tc]sestamibi, [^{11}C]verapamil	P-glycoprotein substrate MDR	88,89
Breast	[^{99}mTc] or [^{64}Cu]somatostatin	Somatostatin receptors	91,92

Abbreviations: PK, pharmacokinetic; MDR, multidrug resistance; PSMA, prostate-specific membrane antigen; EGF, epidermal growth factor; ATSM, diacetyl-bis(N^4-methylthiosemicarbazone).

multicenter trials to verify efficacy and side effects associated with longer-term use. Molecular imaging will have its greatest impact on accelerating the clinical process or assisting with the decision to remove a drug from further evaluation. In the early phases of clinical development, monitoring response for signs of clinical efficacy is important for making decisions about continuing the development program. In the following section, examples of the application of labeled drugs and labeled probes for the assessment of new drug PK and PD are provided.

Pharmacokinetics in Humans

The current assessment of the tumoral delivery of cytostatic agents is largely based on plasma, urine, or cerebral spinal fluid analysis and occasionally a biopsy sample (37,38). These methods of PK analysis do not provide a suitable temporal profile of the delivery and accumulation of the agent nor do they fully address the lack of uptake in resistant tumors. Over the last two decades, there have been several studies involving both PET- and single photon emission computed tomography (SPECT)-labeled cytostatic agents to assess the potential therapeutic PK and/or to study the effects of either drug formulation or cofactors that may alter the metabolism and/or the distribution of the drug. These agents have been summarized in Table 2.

An intra-arterial injection of [^{11}C]BCNU (nitrosourea) demonstrated a 50-fold increase in glioma accumulation compared with the conventional IV administration (39). Labeled BNCU also clears faster from brain tissue than

Table 2 Radiolabeled Cancer Chemotherapeutics Evaluated in Preclinical and Clinical Studies

Drug	Labeled tracer	Summary of preclinical/clinical assessment	References
5-fluorouracil (5-FU)	5-[^{18}F] FU	Tumor uptake a strong predictor of therapeutic response.	48–52
Temozolomide (TEM)	[^{11}C]TEM	Revealed metabolic mechanism of action. Tumor concentration higher than surrounding brain tissue.	45–47
N-[2-(dimethylamino) ethyl]acridine- 4-carboxamide (DACA)	[^{11}C]DACA	Rapid metabolism in preclinical and human studies. Tumor uptake proportional to blood flow.	43,44
Nitrosourea (BCNU)	[^{11}C]BCNU	Intra-arterial route of administration increases uptake in glioma over IV administration. Normal brain clears faster than tumor.	39
Cisplatin	[^{13}N]cisplatin	Intra-arterial route of administration increases uptake in glioblastoma over IV administration.	40
Bleomycin	[^{57}Co]bleomycin	Higher uptake in primary tumors	41,42

the glioma. This same PK phenomenon versus route of administration was seen with $[^{13}N]$cisplatin (40). Cobalt-57-labeled bleomycin was used to assess the temporal concentration of bleomycin in tumors. While higher uptake was associated with primary tumors relative to metastases, no correlation was found between tumor concentration of the tracer and the blood concentration (41,42). Preclinical studies with $[^{11}C]$DACA (*N*-[2-(dimethylamino)ethyl]acridine-4-carboxamide) in rats demonstrated rapid metabolism. The metabolic profile was similar in humans (43). The studies in humans also revealed that DACA crossed the blood-brain barrier and tumor uptake was proportional to blood flow (44). Temozolomide, labeled with carbon-11 in the 3 position (3-TEM) and 4 position (4-TEM), was used to evaluate drug PK and metabolic activation in patients with glioma (45). Temozolomide is metabolically degraded to methyldiazonium ion, which in turn alkylates DNA. This process occurs rapidly in environments with basic pH, as seen in gliomas. The imaging study in glioma patients with 3-TEM and 4-TEM confirmed this metabolic pathway, as higher amounts of $[^{11}C]CO_2$ were seen following 4-TEM injection into patients (46,47). PK assessment of 3-TEM demonstrated greater tumor uptake of the tracer compared with normal tissue. Together, the PET studies revealed the metabolic mechanism of action of this drug and confirmed tumor PK.

The most widely studied and applied labeled cytostatic agent is 5-$[^{18}F]$fluorouracil. As a common antineoplastic chemotheraputic agent, 5-FU is used to treat a variety of tumors of various organ systems either alone or in combination with other therapeutic agents. 5-FU, a purine base, is taken up by cells phoshorylated and converted into 2′-deoxy-5-fluorouridine monophosphate (FdUMP). FdUMP is an inhibitor of thymidylate synthetase-blocking DNA synthesis. Several tumor lines have been found to be resistant to 5-FU treatment.

5-FU labeled with fluorine-18 was first prepared in 1973 by Fowler and colleagues (48). Subsequently, this tracer has been used to provide a means of determining which tumors would respond well to 5-FU therapy. Initially, 5-$[^{18}F]$FU demonstrated a fivefold increase in accumulation in drug-sensitive versus drug-resistant lymphocytic leukemia tumors in mice (49). Subsequently, 5-$[^{18}F]$FU accumulation was shown to be a strong predictor of therapeutic response in patients with liver mataseses from colorectal cancer (50,51). This tracer is still being evaluated as a predictor of therapeutic outcome and a model for treatment planning (52).

Pharmacodynamics in Humans

Similar to the preclinical PK studies, the PD measures have provided valuable information in humans relative to the evaluation of new drugs. These studies have demonstrated proof of mechanism and proof of efficacy even within 24 hours of the initial dose of therapeutic agent. Treatment planning and monitoring strategies have also been derived from these studies. Table 1 lists the various imaging agents that have been or may be used for clinical phase imaging in new therapeutic studies.

FDG is the most widely used PET imaging agent in the world. FDG-PET imaging has been broadly applied to monitor therapeutic response in many tumor types, especially breast and non–small cell lung cancer. Most cancer cells rely on the glycolysis metabolic pathway for energy. Therefore, any therapeutic that effectively shuts down the cellular processes will significantly reduce the reliance on glucose. A recent review thoroughly covers the application of FDG-PET in the assessment and management of cancer patients as well as FDG-PET in the development of cancer therapy (53). One of the most widely cited and striking examples of rapid response to therapeutic intervention is the use of FDG-PET to image the treatment of GISTs with imatinib mesylate (Gleevec) (54,55). There was a significant loss of glucose uptake in the GIST within 24 hours of administration of imatinib that corresponded with eventual tumor regression in patients responding to imatinib treatment.

While FDG is one of the most widely used and powerful imaging agents in the oncologic arsenal, there are other agents that have and may also be applied for the assessment of therapeutic outcomes (56,57). FDG has some shortcomings, including its uptake in tissue in response to inflammation. Additionally, changes in glucose metabolism may not always rapidly correlate with response to treatment. Also, FDG does not directly measure the density of cell surface proteins and receptors that are altered or occupied as a result of pharmaceutical administration.

Preselecting patients that may respond to treatment would enhance not only the efficacy of therapeutics but also a patient's quality of life by eliminating unnecessary treatment with drugs that have no effect yet have significant side effects. Linden and colleagues (58) have shown the utility of FES uptake in breast tumors as means of selecting breast cancer patients who respond to hormone treatment. Up to one-third of the patients with elevated uptake responded to the treatment. When the patient pool was further selected by eliminating those overexpressing HER2, up to 50% responded to the treatment. Thus, imaging may play a role in the selection of patient populations that are more likely to respond to treatment.

Approval and Marketing

Once a drug has been approved for use in humans, the development process does not terminate. Often titled "phase IV" in the clinical trials stage of drug development, the postapproval stage involves further evaluation of the drug for long-term side effects and additional indications. Imaging may continue to play a role in several capacities. First, the molecular imaging agent may be used to validate or evaluate other targets or indications for the drug. Second, it may be used for patient selection, identifying those who may benefit from the targeted therapeutic. Third, the agent may monitor therapeutic efficacy highlighting any changes in the response that may indicate drug resistance. Finally, the images produced during the course of drug evaluation may be applied as educational/ promotional material to market the new drug and show the potential therapeutic benefit (59).

RADIOTRACER DEVELOPMENT

Radiotracer development follows the same pathway as therapeutic drug development (Fig. 2). Similar to new drug development, the cost of radiotracer development for agents that will be used as diagnostic radiopharmaceuticals has been estimated to be between $150 and $200 million (60), and the length of time for full approval is about nine years, only 25% shorter than conventional drugs. Given the market size for most diagnostic agents, the production of the potential diagnostic would be cost prohibitive and would not be supported by future sales. Thus, new tracer development and application will largely be relegated to the biomarker market with a significantly lower regulatory burden to apply for an IND.

Most of the radiolabeled biomarkers in use today are well-known and established tracers (Table 1). The use of tracers in the clinical phases of drug development requires that the tracer be validated in humans. Only a small number of tracers have been validated in humans, especially in the area of oncologic imaging. In order to keep pace with the development of new drugs and the expected need for biomarkers as a result of the changes instituted for the CPI and new validated targets, new radiotracer development must occur in parallel with drug development.

The development of new tracers for drug or diagnostic applications can take a page from the current drug development paradigm (61). The key to finding new successful tracers will be their validation as a marker of a particular biochemical pathway that directly relates to a particular disease or modification of the pathway following therapeutic intervention. Also, important for new tracer validation is the development of animal models for evaluation. Knockout mice provide a suitable platform for the rapid assessment of new radiotracers (62). This combined with in vitro and in vivo evaluation of metabolic properties and PK measures will advance tracer development so that it may ultimately be used in the clinical phases of drug development (63).

Several Institutes within the National Institutes of Health (NIH), notably the National Cancer Institute (NCI), the National Institute of Mental Health (NIMH), and the National Institute of Biomedical Imaging and BioEngineering (NIBIB), have supported the development of new molecular imaging agents. The NCI provides several programs to facilitate the development of new radiotracers for ultimate use in humans. The NCI DCIDE program (Development of Clinical Imaging Drugs and Enhancers), in particular, provides resources to move molecular imaging agents through the IND stage (64). This includes synthesis of nonradioactive compound for pharmacological and toxicological evaluation along with support to prepare the IND for FDA submission. Programs such as these have been developed to foster new radiotracer development as biomarkers and diagnostic agents.

RESOURCES FOR RADIOTRACER DEVELOPMENT AND APPLICATION IN DRUG DEVELOPMENT

There are several organizations and consortia that promote and support the use of imaging in clinical trials. Two relatively new organizations, the Biomarkers Consortium (BC) and the Radiotracer Clearinghouse (RCH), have been created to facilitate the discovery of new imaging biomarkers and their application to therapeutic development. These organizations will help to eliminate the repeated production of imaging agents for the same targets by facilitating the sharing of these tracers among pharmaceutical companies, government agencies (e.g., NIH), and academic institutions.

Biomarkers Consortium

The BC is a public-private partnership under the Foundation for the National Institutes of Health (FNIH), launched in October 2006. Partners in this organization include the Pharmaceutical Research and Manufacturers of America (PhRMA), FDA, the Center for Medicare and Medicaid Services (CMS), and nonprofit organizations as well as academic, government, and industry sponsors (65,66). The objectives of the BC are "to facilitate the discovery and development of biomarkers; validate their ability to diagnose disease, predict therapeutic response, and modify medical practice; identify patient groups who are better suited for a particular intervention; speed approval of new therapeutic entities; and make consortium project results broadly available" (67).

There are currently two radiotracer projects under the BC umbrella. The first is a multicenter trial to establish FDG PET as a biomarker for therapeutic outcomes and measures of response to cytotoxic drugs. The second is an approved project concept—the NIH Intramural radiopharmaceutical program for the production of new tracers. The projects established under the BC are collaborative with partners contributing to their success.

Radiotracer Clearinghouse

One of the challenges, as described above, to the use of radiotracers in drug development is tracer availability. Many groups are actively developing tracers for preclinical and clinical assessment of new drugs, especially in the pharmaceutical industry. Most radiotracers will never be carried through the full development process nor marketed as diagnostic radiopharmaceuticals. Many of these tracers, produced as part of a drug development program, are proprietary. Disclosure of these compounds may compromise a class of compounds being explored as new drugs. While many of the tracers will be validated in humans, their intended use may only be to evaluate the PK or PD of new drugs not intended to be developed as diagnostic tracers. Many of these may not even make it into the peer-reviewed public literature, and if they do, only a fraction of the information known about the compound may be published. The question arises—how may these compounds be accessed and shared such that new tracers do not have to be produced every time a new drug needs to be assessed in vivo? This inefficiency will have a negative impact on the use of imaging in drug development.

To address this issue, members of the American College of Neuropsychopharmacology (ACNP) led by Dr. Dean Wong and members of the Society of Noninvasive Imaging in Drug Development, a council of the Academy of Molecular Imaging (SNIDD/AMI), led by Dr. Henry VanBrocklin have partnered to establish the RCH, a nonprofit organization (66). The RCH is designed to serve as a network facilitator for the transfer of information between two member parties (e.g., industrial, academic, or government laboratory). Radiotracers from any party (party A) for any conceivable target will be accepted by the RCH. The data for these tracers will remain with the holder of the intellectual property. When another party (party B) is interested in using the tracer held by party A, they come to the RCH and search for their target of interest. If a tracer for the target exists in the RCH then the RCH will facilitate an agreement between parties A and B to share the information. It is envisioned that there will be a spectrum of interactions among the parties that are sharing information, covering the full spectrum of disclosure from total privacy to full public disclosure. The RCH will provide a secure environment for the member parties to share information without compromising their internal drug development programs.

Another of the goals of the RCH is to foster collaboration among the tracer development community and the pharmaceutical industry to support the preparation of new tracers for drug development applications. To this end, the RCH will provide a mechanism for precompetitive collaboration among members. The ultimate goal for all tracers in the RCH is to make the information widely accessible for future drug development applications. It is envisioned that the RCH and many other organizations including the BC will enhance the availability of biomarkers for new drug development.

PERSPECTIVE

Molecular imaging using radiolabeled probes has evolved over the last 60 years into a powerful tool not only for the diagnosis of a variety of diseases and disorders but also for the definition of the molecular basis for the disease/disorder. In addition, the evaluation of drug distribution and metabolic fate in living systems, selection of patient subpopulations that may benefit from a particular treatment, and monitoring patients following therapy have been enabled by development of molecular imaging technologies. Advances in PET and SPECT instrumentation, including higher spatial resolution, higher sensitivity, dual modality imaging (PET/CT, SPECT/CT, and MR/PET), and sophisticated reconstruction and kinetic modeling techniques have made preclinical imaging more accessible and available for the evaluation of therapeutic efficacy. A complementary set of small animal instruments (PET, SPECT, MR, CT, and Optical) has facilitated translation of imaging protocols from small animals to humans. Broader availability of radionuclides, especially short-lived positron emitting radioisotopes, and advances in radiochemistry, including automated synthesis, has paved the way for development of sensitive labeled probes for drug development applications. Further, the establishment of good laboratory and manufacturing practices at many imaging centers permits the evaluation of new biomarkers or monitoring therapy in multicenter trials. New regulatory mechanisms, including the expanded scope of investigational drug applications through the exploratory IND, allow earlier first-in-human studies for both new therapeutics and new radiotracers. Finally, the establishment of the BC and the RCH, among many other organizations, fosters the collaborative development of new biomarkers and efficient use of biomarker probes in the drug development paradigm.

Taken together, all these components comprise a molecular imaging armamentarium that supports the future advancement of drug discovery and development.

REFERENCES

1. Hanahan D, Weinberg RA. The hallmarks of cancer. Cell 2000; 100:57–70.
2. Fearon ER. Human cancer syndromes: clues to the origin and nature of cancer. Science 1997; 278:1043–1050.

3. Vogelstein B, Kinzler KW. Cancer genes and the pathways they control. Nat Med 2004; 10:789–799.

4. DiMasi JA, Hansen RW, Grabowski HG. The price of innovation: new estimates of drug development costs. J Health Econ 2003; 22:151–185.

5. Drug costs: research and development costs: the great illusion. Prescrire Int 2004; 13:32–36.

6. Adams CP, Brantner VV. Estimating the cost of new drug development: is it really 802 million dollars? Health Aff (Millwood) 2006; 25:420–428.

7. Dickson M, Gagnon JP. Key factors in the rising cost of new drug discovery and development. Nat Rev Drug Discov 2004; 3:417–429.

8. DiMasi JA. Trends in drug development costs, times and risks. Drug Info Assoc J 1995; 29:375–384.

9. Reichert JM. Trends in development and approval times for new therapeutics in the United States. Nat Rev Drug Discov 2003; 2:695–702.

10. Seddon BM, Workman P. The Role of functional and molecular imaging in cancer drug discovery and development. Br J Radiol 2003; 76(spec no 2):S128–S138.

11. DiMasi JA, Grabowski HG. Economics of new oncology drug development. J Clin Oncol 2007; 25:209–216.

12. McKeage K, Perry CM. Trastuzumab: a review of its use in the treatment of metastatic breast cancer overexpressing Her2. Drugs 2002; 62:209–243.

13. Miller, A.B.; Hoogstraten, B.; Staquet, M.; Winkler, A., Reporting Results of Cancer Treatment. Cancer, 1981, 47, 207–14.

14. Therasse P, Arbuck SG, Eisenhauer EA, et al. New guidelines to evaluate the response to treatment in solid tumors. European Organization for Research and Treatment of Cancer, National Cancer Institute of the United States, National Cancer Institute of Canada. J Natl Cancer Inst 2000; 92:205–216.

15. Amoroso V, Pittiani F, Grisanti S, et al. Osteoblastic flare in a patient with advanced gastric cancer after treatment with pemetrexed and oxaliplatin: implications for response assessment with Recist criteria. BMC Cancer 2007; 7:94.

16. Basu S, Alavi A. Defining co-related parameters between 'metabolic' flare and 'clinical', 'biochemical', and 'osteoblastic' flare and establishing guidelines for assessing response to treatment in cancer. Eur J Nucl Med Mol Imaging 2007; 34:441–443.

17. Dehdashti F, Flanagan FL, Mortimer JE, et al. Positron emission tomographic assessment of "metabolic flare" to predict response of metastatic breast cancer to antiestrogen therapy. Eur J Nucl Med 1999; 26:51–56.

18. Mortimer JE, Dehdashti F, Siegel BA, et al. Metabolic flare: indicator of hormone responsiveness in advanced breast cancer. J Clin Oncol 2001; 19:2797–2803.

19. Hamaoka T, Madewell JE, Podoloff DA, et al. Bone imaging in metastatic breast cancer. J Clin Oncol 2004; 22:2942–2953.

20. Koizumi M, Matsumoto S, Takahashi S, et al. Bone metabolic markers in the evaluation of bone scan flare phenomenon in bone metastases of breast cancer. Clin Nucl Med, 1999, 24, 15–20.

21. Vogel CL, Schoenfelder J, Shemano I, et al. Worsening bone scan in the evaluation of antitumor response during hormonal therapy of breast cancer. J Clin Oncol 1995; 13:1123–1128.

22. Kelloff GJ, Sigman CC. New science-based endpoints to accelerate oncology drug development. Eur J Cancer 2005; 41:491–501.

23. Food and Drug Administration. Innovation or stagnation: challenge and opportunity on the critical path to new medical products, HHS, Editor 2004:31. Available at: http://www.fda.gov/oc/initiatives/criticalpath/whitepaper.html. Accessed August 5, 2007.

24. FDA's Critical Path Initiative. Available at: http://www.fda.gov/oc/initiatives/criticalpath/. Accessed August 5, 2007.

25. Office of New Drugs in the Center for Drug Evaluation and Research (CDER), FDA, Department of Health and Human Services. Guidance for Industry, Investigators, and Reviewers. Exploratory IND Studies. Available at: http://www.fda.gov/cder/guidance/7086fnl.htm. Accessed August 5, 2007.

26. Lappin G, Kuhnz W, Jochemsen R, et al. Use of microdosing to predict pharmacokinetics at the therapeutic dose: experience with 5 drugs. Clin Pharmacol Ther 2006; 80:203–215.

27. Smith JJ, Sorensen AG, Thrall JH. Biomarkers in imaging: realizing radiology's future. Radiology 2003; 227:633–638.

28. Lindsay MA. Target discovery. Nat Rev Drug Discov 2003; 2:831–838.

29. Lindsay MA. Finding new drug targets in the 21st century. Drug Discov Today 2005; 10:1683–1687.

30. Farde L, Wiesel FA, Jansson P, et al. An open label trial of raclopride in acute schizophrenia. Confirmation of D2-dopamine receptor occupancy by PET. Psychopharmacology (Berl) 1988; 94:1–7.

31. Bergström M, Hargreaves RJ, Burns HD, et al. Human positron emission tomography studies of brain neurokinin 1 receptor occupancy by aprepitant. Biol Psychiatry 2004; 55; 1007–1012.

32. Dittmann H, Dohmen BM, Kehlbach R, et al. Early changes in [18f]Flt uptake after chemotherapy: an experimental study. Eur J Nucl Med Mol Imaging 2002; 29:1462–1469.

33. Kil KE, Ding YS, Lin KS, et al. Synthesis and positron emission tomography studies of carbon-11-labeled imatinib (Gleevec). Nucl Med Biol 2007; 34:153–163.

34. Kiesewetter DO, Kilbourn MR, Landvatter SW, et al. Preparation of four fluorine-18-labeled estrogens and their selective uptakes in target tissues of immature rats. J Nucl Med 1984; 25:1212–1221.

35. Katzenellenbogen JA, Mathias CJ, VanBrocklin HF, et al. Titration of the in vivo uptake of 16 alpha-[^{18}F]fluoroestradiol by target tissues in the rat: competition by tamoxifen, and implications for quantitating estrogen receptors in Vivo and the use of animal models in receptor-binding radiopharmaceutical development. Nucl Med Biol 1993; 20:735–745.

36. Barthel H, Cleij MC, Collingridge DR, et al. 3'-Deoxy-3'-[^{18}F]fluorothymidine as a new marker for monitoring

tumor response to antiproliferative therapy in vivo with positron emission tomography. Cancer Res 2003; 63: 3791–3798.

37. Langer O, Muller M. Methods to assess tissue-specific distribution and metabolism of drugs. Curr Drug Metab 2004; 5:463–481.

38. Brunner M, Muller M. Microdialysis: an in vivo approach for measuring drug delivery in oncology. Eur J Clin Pharmacol 2002; 58:227–234.

39. Tyler JL, Yamamoto YL, Diksic M, et al. Pharmacokinetics of superselective intra-arterial and intravenous [^{11}C]BCNU evaluated by PET. J Nucl Med 1986; 27:775–780.

40. Ginos JZ, Cooper AJ, Dhawan V, et al. [^{13}N]cisplatin PET to assess pharmacokinetics of intra-arterial versus intravenous chemotherapy for malignant brain tumors. J Nucl Med 1987; 28:1844–1852.

41. Front D, Israel O, Even-Sapir E, et al. The concentration of bleomycin labeled with Co-57 in primary and metastatic tumors. Cancer 1989; 64:988–993.

42. Front D, Israel O, Iosilevsky G, et al. Spect quantitation of cobalt-57 bleomycin delivery to human brain tumors. J Nucl Med 1988; 29:187–194.

43. Osman S, Luthra SK, Brady F, et al. Studies on the metabolism of the novel antitumor agent [N-methyl-11c]-N-[2-(dimethylamino)ethyl]acridine-4-Carboxamide in rats and humans prior to phase I clinical trials. Cancer Res 1997; 57:2172–2180.

44. Harte RJA, Matthews JC, Flavin A, et al. Prephase I tracer kinetic studies in humans can contribute to new drug evaluation. In: Proceedings of the 9th NCI/EORTC Symposium on New Drugs in Cancer Therapy; 1996.

45. Brown GD, Luthra SK, Brock CS, et al. Antitumor imidazotetrazines. 40. radiosyntheses of [4-11c-carbonyl]- and [3-N-11c-methyl]-8-carbamoyl-3-methylimidazo[5,1-D]-1,2,3,5-tetrazin-4(3h) -one (temozolomide) for positron emission tomography (PET) studies. J Med Chem 2002; 45:5448–5457.

46. Saleem A, Brown GD, Brady F, et al. Metabolic activation of temozolomide measured in vivo using positron emission tomography. Cancer Res 2003; 63:2409–2415.

47. Saleem A, Osman S, Brown G, et al. Evaluation of the in vivo mechanism of action of temozolomide. Proc Am Soc Clin Oncol 2001; 20:114a.

48. Fowler JS, Finn RD, Lambrecht RM, et al. The synthesis of 18 F-5-fluorouracil. vii. J Nucl Med 1973; 14:63–64.

49. Shani J, Wolf W. A model for prediction of chemotherapy response to 5-fluorouracil based on the differential distribution of 5-[18f]fluorouracil in sensitive versus resistant lymphocytic leukemia in mice. Cancer Res 1977; 37: 2306–2308.

50. Dimitrakopoulou-Strauss A, Strauss LG, Schlag P, et al. Intravenous and intra-arterial oxygen-15-labeled water and fluorine-18-labeled fluorouracil in patients with liver metastases from colorectal carcinoma. J Nucl Med 1998; 39:465–473.

51. Dimitrakopoulou-Strauss A, Strauss LG, Schlag P, et al. Fluorine-18-fluorouracil to predict therapy response in liver metastases from colorectal carcinoma. J Nucl Med 1998; 39:1197–1202.

52. Dimitrakopoulou-Strauss A, Strauss L. Quantitative studies using positron emission tomography (PET) for the diagnosis and therapy planning of oncological patients. Hell J Nucl Med 2006; 9:10–21.

53. Kelloff GJ, Hoffman JM, Johnson B, et al. Progress and promise of FDG-PET imaging for cancer patient management and oncologic drug development. Clin Cancer Res 2005; 11:2785–2808.

54. Stroobants S, Goeminne J, Seegers M, et al. 18FDG-positron emission tomography for the early prediction of response in advanced soft tissue sarcoma treated with imatinib mesylate (Glivec). Eur J Cancer 2003; 39:2012–2020.

55. Van den Abbeele AD, Badawi RD. Use of positron emission tomography in oncology and its potential role to assess response to imatinib mesylate therapy in gastrointestinal stromal tumors (GISTs). 2002; 38:S60–S65.

56. Hicks RJ, Beyond FDG: novel PET tracers for cancer imaging. Cancer Imaging 2003; 4:22–24.

57. Hicks RJ. The role of PET in monitoring therapy. Cancer Imaging 2005; 5:51–57.

58. Linden HM, Stekhova SA, Link JM, et al. Quantitative fluoroestradiol positron emission tomography imaging predicts response to endocrine treatment in breast cancer. J Clin Oncol 2006; 24:2793–2799.

59. Berridge MS, Lee Z, Heald DL. Regional distribution and kinetics of inhaled pharmaceuticals. Curr Pharm Des 2000; 6:1631–1651.

60. Nunn AD. The cost of developing imaging agents for routine clinical use. Invest Radiol 2006; 41:206–212.

61. Eckelman WC, Rohatagi S, Krohn KA, et al. Are there lessons to be learned from drug development that will accelerate the use of molecular imaging probes in the clinic? Nucl Med Biol 2005; 32:657–662.

62. Eckelman WC. The use of PET and knockout mice in the drug discovery process. Drug Discov Today 2003; 8: 404–410.

63. Bergstrom M, Awad R, Estrada S, et al. Autoradiography with positron emitting isotopes in positron emission tomography tracer discovery. Mol Imaging Biol 2003; 5:390–396.

64. National Cancer Institute. Cancer Imaging Program. Development of Clinical Imaging Drugs & Enhancers (DCIDE). Available at: http://imaging.cancer.gov/programsandresources/specializedinitiatives/dcide. Accessed August 5, 2007.

65. The Biomarkers Consortium Vision. Available at: http://www.biomarkersconsortium.org/index.php?option=com_content&task=view&id=26&Itemid=47. Accessed August 5, 2007.

66. McCormick T, Martin K, Hehenberger M. The evolving role of biomarkers: focusing on patients from research to clinical practice. IBM (Imaging) Biomarker Summit III, 2007.

67. The Biomarkers Consotrium Vision. Available at: http://www.biomarkersconsortium.org/index.php?option=com_content&task=view&id=26&Itemid=47. Accessed August 5, 2007.

68. VanBrocklin HF. Radiopharmaceuticals for drug development: United States regulatory perspective. Current Radiopharmaceuticals 2008; 1:2–6.

69. Ido T, wan CN, Cassela V, et al. Labeled 2-deoxy-D-glucose analogs. 18f-labeled 2-deoxy-2-fluoro-D-glucose, 2-deoxy-2-fluoro-D-manose and 14c-2-deoxy-2-fluoro-D-glucose. J Labelled Comp Radiopharm 1978; 14:175–183.

70. Som P, Atkins HL, Bandopadhyay D, et al. A fluorinated glucose analog, 2-fluoro-2-deoxy-D-glucose (F-18): nontoxic tracer for rapid tumor detection. J Nucl Med 1980; 21:670–675.

71. Kurdziel KA, Hirsch JI, Kalen JD, et al. Human biodistribution of F-18 paclitaxel (FPAC): a potential pet tracer for evaluating multidrug resistance (MDR). Mol Imaging Biol 2006; 8:72.

72. Kurdziel KA, Kalen JD, Hirsch JI, et al. Imaging multidrug resistance with 4-[(18)F]fluoropaclitaxel. Nucl Med Biol 2007; 34:823–831.

73. Kurdziel KA, Kiesewetter DO, Carson RE, et al. Biodistribution, radiation dose estimates, and in vivo Pgp modulation studies of 18F-paclitaxel in nonhuman primates. J Nucl Med 2003; 44:1330–1339.

74. Jerabek PA, Patrick TB, Kilbourn MR, et al. Synthesis and biodistribution of 18f-labeled fluoronitroimidazoles: potential in vivo markers of hypoxic tissue. Int J Radiat Appl Instrum [A] 1986; 37:599–605.

75. Laforest R, Dehdashti F, Lewis JS, et al. Dosimetry of 60/61/62/64cu-atsm: a hypoxia imaging agent for PET. Eur J Nucl Med Mol Imaging 2005; 32:764–770.

76. Mannan RH, Somayaji VV, Lee J, et al. Radioiodinated 1-(5-iodo-5-deoxy-beta-D-arabinofuranosyl)-2-nitroimidazole (iodoazomycin arabinoside: iaza): a novel marker of tissue hypoxia. J Nucl Med 1991; 32:1764–1770.

77. McQuade P, Martin KE, Castle TC, et al. Investigation into 64cu-labeled bis(selenosemicarbazone) and bis(thiosemicarbazone) complexes as hypoxia imaging agents. Nucl Med Biol 2005; 32:147–156.

78. Reischl G, Ehrlichmann W, Bieg C, et al. Preparation of the hypoxia imaging PET tracer [18f]Faza: reaction parameters and automation. Appl Radiat Isot 2005; 62:897–901.

79. Grierson JR, Shields AF. Radiosynthesis of 3'-deoxy-3'-[(18)F]fluorothymidine: [(18)F]FLT for imaging of cellular proliferation in vivo. Nucl Med Biol 2000; 27:143–156.

80. DeGrado TR, Coleman RE, Wang S, et al. Synthesis and evaluation of 18f-labeled choline as an oncologic tracer for positron emission tomography: initial findings in prostate cancer. Cancer Res 2001; 61:110–117.

81. Rosen MA, Jones RM, Yano Y, et al. Carbon-11 choline: synthesis, purification, and brain uptake inhibition by 2-dimethylaminoethanol. J Nucl Med 1985; 26:1424–1428.

82. Shah F, Hume SP, Pike VW, et al. Synthesis of the enantiomers of [N-methyl-11c]Pk 11195 and comparison of their behaviours as radioligands for Pk binding sites in rats. Nucl Med Biol 1994; 21:573–581.

83. Ishiwata K, Ishii S-I, Sasaki T, et al. A distillation method of preparing C-11 labeled acetate for routine clinical use. Appl Radiat Isot 1993; 44:761–763.

84. Jana S, Blaufox MD. Nuclear medicine studies of the prostate, testes, and bladder. Semin Nucl Med 2006; 36:51–72.

85. Liu A, Dence CS, Welch MJ, et al. Fluorine-18-labeled androgens: radiochemical synthesis and tissue distribution studies on six fluorine-substituted androgens, potential imaging agents for prostatic cancer. J Nucl Med 1992; 33:724–734.

86. Ramos-Suzarte M, Rodriguez N, Oliva JP, et al. 99mtc-labeled antihuman epidermal growth factor receptor antibody in patients with tumors of epithelial origin: Part III. Clinical trials safety and diagnostic efficacy. J Nucl Med 1999; 40:768–775.

87. Reilly RM, Kiarash R, Cameron RG, et al. 111in-labeled egf is selectively radiotoxic to human breast cancer cells overexpressing EGFR. J Nucl Med 2000; 41:429–438.

88. Piwnica-Worms D, Chiu ML, Budding M, et al. Functional imaging of multidrug-resistant P-glycoprotein with an organotechnetium complex. Cancer Res 1993; 53:977–984.

89. Piwnica-Worms D, Holman BL. Noncardiac applications of hexakis(alkylisonitrile) technetium-99m complexes. J Nucl Med 1990; 31:1166–1167.

90. Elsinga PH, Franssen EJ, Hendrikse NH, et al. Carbon-11-labeled daunorubicin and verapamil for probing P-glycoprotein in tumors with PET. J Nucl Med 1996; 37:1571–1575.

91. Anderson CJ, Pajeau TS, Edwards WB, et al. In vitro and in vivo evaluation of copper-64-octreotide conjugates. J Nucl Med 1995; 36:2315–2325.

92. Vallabhajosula S, Moyer BR, Lister-James J, et al. Preclinical evaluation of technetium-99m-labeled somatostatin receptor-binding peptides. J Nucl Med 1996; 37:1016–1022.

44

NIH Funding Sources for Molecular Imaging in Oncology

ANNE E. MENKENS, BARBARA Y. CROFT, and DANIEL C. SULLIVAN
Cancer Imaging Program, National Cancer Institute, National Institutes of Health, Bethesda, Maryland, U.S.A.

INTRODUCTION

The National Institutes of Health (NIH) is the primary federal agency for conducting and supporting medical research. The NIH is composed of 27 Institutes and Centers (ICs), each of which has a defined scientific mission, and most of which support imaging research. Each NIH Institute and Center has unique scientific priorities and ways of funding those priorities. Imaging in oncology is supported through a number of different ICs. The understanding of a few basic elements common to all NIH grant funding will provide a firm foundation for obtaining NIH support for cancer imaging research.

NIH FUNDING CYCLE OVERVIEW

The NIH funding cycle from the applicant's point of view is shown below. The cycle is one that typically starts with the applicant considering an idea for an application, consulting colleagues and mentors, and writing a grant application. Investigators will need to be aware of three things. First, they will need to consider how their research ideas and preliminary data align with an appropriate grant mechanism. Second, they will need to find an NIH Institute or Center whose scientific mission encompasses the specific research being planned. Third, applicants will also need to consider and to monitor the assignment of their application to a scientific review group, commonly

referred to as a study section (Fig. 1). It is a good idea to consult a program director of the relevant institute and program, or the person named on an initiative of interest, well ahead of the submission to clarify points and issues surrounding the application.

GRANT FUNDING MECHANISMS

The majority of NIH extramural dollars support investigator-initiated research. However, the ICs of NIH each have processes through which they identify and prioritize unique scientific opportunities that merit additional attention and/or targeted funding. These identification and prioritization processes typically involve significant input from the extramural community, including recommendations generated through NIH-sponsored workshops and formal NIH Advisory Committees. The implementation of recommendations may result in the availability of an NIH Funding Opportunity Announcement (FOA) to support research on that area of scientific opportunity.

Funding Opportunity Announcements

The *NIH Guide for Grants and Contracts* is the official publication for NIH research grant policies, guidelines, and FOAs. It is published on a weekly basis, and investigators should routinely monitor this publication for

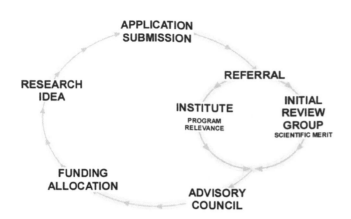

Figure 1 A schematic drawing of the NIH grant funding process. Starting with a research idea, proceeding through application submission to referral and review, as well as institute assignment, to consideration for funding by an advisory council, to funding if the score is satisfactory. Otherwise the investigator begins the cycle again with a revised application.

current opportunities. There are many types of FOAs. The primary types are referred to as Requests for Application (RFAs) and Program Announcements [PAs (Table 1)].

Requests for Applications

RFAs are initiatives with narrowly defined scientific areas. The intent of an RFA is to attract new talent and expertise to an emerging or underemphasized discipline or to fund a specific kind of program. To emphasize the importance of the scientific area supported by an RFA, one or more NIH institutes set aside funds for awarding grants. RFAs usually have a single receipt date (specified in the RFA announcement), and are usually reviewed by a review panel convened specifically for that group of applications.

Program Announcements

PAs identify areas of increased priority for a specific area of science. Unlike RFAs, PAs are not usually associated with set-aside funds. Applications submitted in response to a PA generally are subject to existing NIH paylines for funding. PAs are usually accepted three times a year on standard receipt dates.

Program Announcements With Special Referral Guidelines

Program Announcements with Special Referral guidelines (PARs) are very similar to PAs, except that there are additional guidelines for reviewers. These guidelines highlight topics or emphasis areas within the PAR to which reviewers are expected to give additional consideration when assessing the merit of an application.

Program Announcements With Set-Aside Funds

Program announcements with set-aside funds (PASs) are also similar to PAs, except that there are funds set aside for the successful applications. This is described in the announcement, along with the funding mechanism and the programmatic priorities that are being addressed by the PAS.

NIH Grant Mechanisms for Molecular Imaging in Oncology

The ICs of NIH utilize many different types of grant mechanisms to support research and training in molecular imaging. Each NIH Institute and Center has flexibility in the way in which it utilizes these mechanisms. The following sections summarize some of the mechanisms that are particularly useful for cancer imaging investigators. All applications must be made in response to FOA. As of the time of this writing, applications for most of the mechanisms described below must be made electronically. The current exceptions are T: Training Programs, F: Fellowship Programs, K: Research Career Programs, D: Training Projects, P: Research Program Projects and Centers, and U: Cooperative Agreements; be aware that these mechanisms will transition to electronic submission as well.

Research Support

R01

Almost all NIH ICs support R01 (Research Project) grants. The R01 grant is defined as an award made to support a discrete, specified, circumscribed project to be performed by the named investigator(s) in an area representing the investigator's specific interest and competencies, based on the mission of the NIH. Any eligible investigator may submit a health-related R01 application to the NIH.

Table 1 Types of funding initiative announcements.

	RFA/PAS	PA	PAR
Set-aside funding	Yes	No	No
Receipt dates	Often single	Usually multiple	Usually multiple
Review	Ad hoc review group	Chartered CSR study sections	Either ad hoc or chartered CSR study sections

R21

The R21 grant mechanism is designed to support the early and conceptual stages of exploratory/developmental research projects. There are a wide variety of R21 initiatives available at NIH at any given time. For example, an R21 initiative has been available through the Cancer Imaging Program (CIP) at the NCI that specifically supports the entire spectrum of in vivo cancer imaging research, from basic discovery of new cancer imaging agents and technologies, through preclinical testing and validation, to the early feasibility testing of those novel agents and technologies in small clinical trials. Investigators with ideas for exploratory/developmental in molecular imaging should consult NIH Staff to find an appropriate FOA.

P01

Many, but not all, NIH Institutes support Program Project (P01) grants. Because P01 grants support integrated, multi-project research programs involving a number of independent investigators, they tend to be much larger in scope and budget than an R01 grant. A P01 grant typically includes several individual, interrelated projects that are expected to generate scientific synergy. Importantly, P01 grants also support research core facilities that are expected to provide services to more than one of the research projects. Each NIH Institute establishes its own P01 policies. Investigators interested in submitting a P01 application should find the relevant policy and consult the program director to whom the application will be directed well in advance of putting the application together.

S10

Historically, the National Center for Research Resources (NCRR) of NIH has supported the purchase of commercially available and technologically sophisticated instruments through the S10 grant mechanism. Commonly referred to as "shared instrumentation" grants, NCRR has supported the purchase of both moderate and high-end instrumentation. This mechanism has been an important source of equipment for molecular imaging investigators. The shared instrumentation purchased through this program must support the ongoing research funded by NIH grants.

SBIR (R43, R44) and STTR (R41, R42)

Small Business Innovation Research (SBIR) grants and Small Business Technology Transfer (STTR) grants are very useful mechanisms for funding molecular imaging research being conducted at a small business (SBIR) or in collaboration with a small business (STTR). There is a small business set-aside of 2.5% of an institute or center's extramural budget for SBIR grants and 0.3% for STTR grants.

Training Support

R25

The R25T institutional training grant mechanism is available through the National Cancer Institute (NCI). This is particularly a useful mechanism for the support and training of young molecular imaging investigators. The R25T supports interdisciplinary and collaborative cancer research through the development and implementation of predoctoral/postdoctoral programs with specific core didactic and research requirements. Imaging has been an area of emphasis within the NCIs R25T initiative, and has been utilized with success by molecular imaging groups.

K99/R00

The NIH Pathway to Independence (PI) Award is an exciting new mechanism designed to support new investigators as they transition from postdoctoral research positions to an independent academic positions. These phased awards support one to two years of mentored support during postdoctoral training, followed by up to three years of independent support contingent on securing an independent research position.

NIH INSTITUTES AND CENTERS

NIH ICs are responsible for the funding and monitoring of research projects. Many NIH ICs fund imaging-related research. Examples of those funding Institutes are provided here.

National Cancer Institute

The NCI is the primary support for imaging research and other activities focused on the cause, diagnosis, prevention, and treatment of cancer. In 1997, the NCI identified molecular imaging as an "extraordinary opportunity," and made a strategic decision to increase the funding for oncologic imaging research. That decision led to the establishment of the CIP in 1997. Since then, NCI has committed more than $1.2 billion toward extramural oncologic imaging research (Fig. 2).

The research supported by CIP/NCI covers the entire spectrum of in vivo cancer imaging research, from basic discovery of new cancer imaging agents and technologies, through preclinical testing and validation, to testing of those novel agents and technologies in clinical trials. As the field of molecular oncologic imaging has matured,

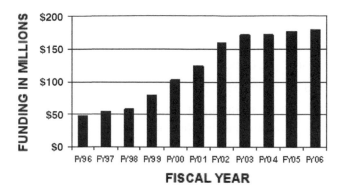

Figure 2 NCI Cancer Imaging Program grant funding by fiscal year.

increasing emphasis has been placed on the translation of basic discoveries into clinical practice.

National Institute of Biomedical Imaging and Bioengineering

The National Institute of Biomedical Imaging and Bioengineering (NIBIB) funds research that integrates the physical and biological sciences to develop new health-related technologies. Increasing the pace of discovery and speed the development of biomedical technologies that prevent or treat illnesses is a major priority.

Although the NIBIB does not support disease-specific imaging research, it does fund the development of many platform technologies that will fundamentally improve the diagnosis, treatment, and prevention of cancer.

Trans-NIH Activities

As medical research has become increasingly multidisciplinary, the NIH has responded to the needs of the community. A number of trans-NIH activities focus on the support of imaging in general, and many are applicable to the support of oncologic imaging.

NIH Roadmap

In 2002, the director of NIH, Dr. Elias A. Zerhouni, MD, instituted the NIH "Roadmap." Through the NIH Roadmap process, ideas are solicited from the broad scientific community for projects that cut across multiple IC missions. The first round of selection included a number of projects that were specifically targeted to imaging. The availability of future funding opportunities will be published in the *NIH Guide to Grants and Contracts*.

APPLICATION PROCESS

Over the past couple of years, the NIH has transitioned the grants application process from the submission of paper grants to the submission of an electronic document through the individual applicant's institutional grants and contracts office. The institution (termed the Applicant Organization) completes a one-time registration with Grants.gov, which applies for applications to all federal agencies. The institution must also register with the NIH eRA Commons. The applicant must also register with the NIH eRA Commons. This process takes some time, so it is wise to start well ahead of the deadline for submitting the application, to be sure all the registrations are in place.

The application, made on the SF424 form, is prepared using special software. The information supplied must include the name and number of the chosen FOA.

The application process involves 2 steps. The application is submitted by the Applicant Institution to Grants.gov in pieces. It is checked there, and either passed along to the chosen funding agency such as the NIH and eRA Commons or rejected, in e-mail messages sent to the Authorized Organizational Representative, from the grants and contracts office. Once the application has been passed to the NIH eRA Commons, it is assembled and checked again. It may be accepted or warnings and errors may result; e-mail messages are sent to the Authorized Organizational Representative and to the investigator.

APPLICATION REVIEW

Initial Review Group or Study Section

Applications submitted to the NIH undergo rigorous peer review of the proposed scientific research. On receipt of an application at NIH, the application is assigned to a funding institute, and to an Initial Review Group (IRG) (referred to as the study section) for scientific review. It is very important for investigators to monitor these assignments. The scientific expertise of the members of the study section should closely match the research being proposed in the application. The rosters of many study sections are available on the NIH website. If an investigator of an application has questions about the study section assignment, the investigator should contact the NIH Program Director or Scientific Review Officer to discuss the situation.

Following the study section meeting, investigators will receive a written review that includes the priority score, a percentile rating for many grant funding mechanisms, and comments from the reviewers. About half of the applications considered by any study section are not scored. It is very typical for applications to require revision and

Table 2 Useful internet URLs for grant applications.

NIH Home Page: http://www.nih.gov
Cancer Imaging Program—NCI: http://imaging.cancer.gov/
NIBIB: http://www.nibib.nih.gov/
NIH New Investigators Program: http://grants2.nih.gov/grants/new_investigators/index.htm
NIH Guide for Grants and Contracts: http://grants.nih.gov/grants/guide/index.html
CSR Study Section Roster Index: http://www.csr.nih.gov/Committees/rosterindex.asp
NIH Research Training Opportunities: http://grants.nih.gov/training/
NCI - Extramural Training Funding: http://www.cancer.gov/researchandfunding/training
NIH Commons: https://commons.era.nih.gov/commons/index.jsp
NIH Grant Writing Tips Sheets: http://grants1.nih.gov/grants/grant_tips.htm
NIH Award Data and Trends: http://grants.nih.gov/grants/award/award.htm
NCI Grants Process Book: http://www3.cancer.gov/admin/gab/index.htm
Computer Retrieval of Information on Scientific Projects: http://crisp.cit.nih.gov/
Molecular Imaging and Contrast Agent Database (MICAD): http://micad.nih.gov/
NIH Roadmap for Medical Research: http://opasi.nih.gov/
DCIDE (Development of Preclinical Drugs and Enhancers): http://imaging.cancer.gov/programsandresources/specializedinitiatives/dcide

---

resubmission in response to these critiques. Investigators are advised to carefully read the summary statement and respond respectfully and thoroughly to the reviewers' comments.

Advisory Council

After the study sections score the applications, the results are sent to the assigned institute for consideration for funding. Each institute has a presidentially appointed council or board that decides which grant applications may be funded. The decisions may be made in a series of en bloc votes or specifically by application, depending on the operation of a particular council. The council passes on whether the grant could be funded, but it may or may not decide whether it should be funded.

FUNDING ALLOCATION

After an institute's council has made its decisions, the funding decisions are ultimately made by each NIH Institute and Center, taking into consideration many factors, but especially how much money they have budgeted for paying grants. It is necessary that an institute have a budget before the funding decisions can be made and such budgets are often delayed depending on the timing of Congressional appropriations. Each IC sets its own priorities and funding lines. Investigators should contact their Program Directors to discuss the outcome of an application's review and its possibility for funding. There are special considerations for new investigators and for scores and percentiles that are just above the funding line.

OTHER PROGRAMS FOR FUNDING MOLECULAR IMAGING RESEARCH

The NCI CIP became concerned about the number of molecular imaging agents that did not seem to transition into use in patients. There seemed to be a need for funding of the toxicology studies and other preclinical efforts to move the compounds into clinical use. The DCIDE (Development of Preclinical Drugs and Enhancers) program was created for this purpose. Typically it funds the pharmacology/toxicology studies and returns to the requesting investigator if necessary for submission of an Investigative New Drug Application (IND) to the FDA. There are special procedures for requesting this assistance, which are described on the CIP web site. Consult with a CIP Program Director for information.

ONLINE RESOURCES

The NIH provides numerous online resources for investigators. There are links to those of particular interest to the molecular imaging community in Table 2.

SUMMARY

NIH funding is a very competitive process. It requires excellent grantsmanship skills and, for new investigators, it requires mentoring by experienced NIH-funded scientists. To succeed, investigators should understand the process and take advantage of as many sources of information as possible.

45

Drug Development with Magnetic Resonance Imaging

JEFFREY L. EVELHOCH

Imaging Sciences, Medical Sciences, Amgen, Inc., Thousand Oaks, California, U.S.A.

INTRODUCTION

Over the past decade, biomarkers [objectively measured indicators of a biological/pathobiological process or pharmacologic response to treatment (1)] have been recognized as a critical element to improve predictability and efficiency in the process of developing more effective, more affordable, and safer therapeutics for patients (2). Biomarkers can be used to establish presence of target, determine target coverage, assess treatment effect on biological pathways, select patients most likely to benefit from treatment and evaluate treatment impact on clinical outcome. This information provides critical input to both internal decision-making (e.g., committing additional resources to develop a given molecule and/or additional molecules for a given target, dose selection for later phase trials) and establishing efficacy and/or safety for regulatory approval when the biomarker is established as a surrogate endpoint (i.e., substitute for a clinical characteristic or variable reflecting patient feeling, function, or survival).

Prior to use for decision making at any level, a biomarker must be established as suitable for its intended use through a graded evidentiary process linking it with pertinent biological processes and clinically relevant endpoints (3). This process, known as biomarker "qualification," should not be confused with "validation," which focuses on performance characteristics of the biomarker assay (such as sensitivity, specificity, limit of detection, etc.) and does not fully describe the qualification process (4). The evidence used to qualify a biomarker for its intended use includes a combination of preclinical development, biomedical literature, technical performance, clinical trials, and consensus expert panels—the amount of evidence required depends on the intended use (3). When biomarkers are used for internal decision-making, individual companies might consider a biomarker qualified based on their own experience, even before the broader drug development community generally accepts it. However, qualification of a biomarker for regulatory licensure decisions (i.e., use as a surrogate endpoint) requires results from several clinical trials and evaluation by an independent panel advising the regulatory bodies (5,6).

Imaging offers a number of biomarkers that can provide information about genetic, biochemical, physiological, and anatomic processes in the tissue of interest (7). Although most of the biomarker literature focuses on "omic"-based biomarkers and their validation/qualification (8–11), many of the same principles apply to imaging even though the analytical methodologies differ considerably. In oncology, the ability of imaging biomarkers to directly assess the tumor often provides an advantage over proteomic, genomic, or metabonomic biomarkers that rely on samples of bodily fluids or biopsies. Moreover, in many instances the information from imaging biomarker studies in preclinical cancer models can be translated directly to the clinic to provide a framework for interpreting clinical results. In this chapter, we will consider the use of one imaging modality, magnetic resonance imaging (MRI), as a biomarker for drug development with a focus on MRI biomarkers that have been translated successfully between preclinical and clinical studies.

MRI BIOMARKERS

Biomarkers that provide information on the expression and coverage of molecular targets are often referred to as target biomarkers. Because of the intrinsically low sensitivity of magnetic resonance, it is not ideally suited to quantify most molecular targets that are present in sub-micromolar levels. As described in several chapters within this book, a number of creative approaches to increase the sensitivity of MR for detection of molecular targets are being explored. While the initial results are very promising, they have not yet been successfully translated to the clinic, so will not be considered further in this chapter.

Biomarkers that provide a measure of the impact of treatment on the course of disease are commonly referred to as outcome biomarkers. Typically, tumor burden is assessed using either computed tomography (CT) or MRI data and the Response Evaluation Criteria in Solid Tumors (RECIST) are used to evaluate clinical effect (12). Since CT is the imaging modality of choice for most cancers outside the brain and chapter 47 focuses on brain tumors, we will not consider this use of MRI to measure changes in tumor burden in this chapter. However, as noted by the International Cancer Imaging Society, one of the weaknesses of using the RECIST criteria is the lack of information regarding tumor function (13). Some MR biomarkers may provide insight into tumor response independent of tumor burden due to their sensitivity to the effects of treatment distal to the therapeutic target and indicative of tumor function. The apparent diffusion coefficient (ADC) of water, which is influenced by the restriction of diffusion due to the limited permeability of cell membranes to water, reflects tumor cellularity (14) and shows dose-dependent changes in response to effective therapy in preclinical tumor models (15–17). Because of the technical challenges in applying diffusion MRI in the body (18), most clinical studies have been in brain tumors (19). Although a few diffusion MRI studies have been conducted in tumors in the body (20,21), the development of methods to minimize motion artifact (22) and for whole-body diffusion MRI (22,23) will facilitate broader application and a critical evaluation of the utility of this biomarker.

A third general category of biomarkers, commonly referred to as mechanism biomarkers, assess treatment effect on a biological pathway proximally related to the therapeutic target. Dynamic contrast-enhanced MRI (DCE-MRI) assessment of tumor vasculature correlates well with independent measures of functional angiogenesis (24). It has been used to quantify the effects of vascular targeting agents on the tumor blood supply starting as early as hours to days after the start of treatment in both preclinical and clinical studies (25). Consequently, the remainder of this chapter will focus on DCE-MRI and its use as a mechanism biomarker for anticancer drugs targeting the tumor blood supply.

DCE-MRI

Background

Effect of Contrast Agent on MR Signal

Characterization of tumor vasculature with MR contrast agents most commonly uses low molecular weight (<1000 g) paramagnetic gadolinium (III) chelates that extravasate in the absence of a blood-brain barrier, but cannot permeate viable cell membranes (26). These contrast agents, which are extensively used in clinical radiology, alter the MR signal due to their effect on the relaxation processes of tissue water protons. The unpaired electrons in these contrast agents provide an efficient mechanism for spin-lattice relaxation of water protons when the water molecule binds in the first or second coordination sphere of the contrast agent complex (27). As a consequence, the spin-lattice relaxation rate (R_1, the reciprocal of the first-order time constant for spin-lattice relaxation, T_1) is decreased in proportion to the contrast agent concentration (28). The decreased R_1 leads to an increase in MRI signal intensity, which, if the MRI acquisition parameters are selected judiciously, increases linearly in proportion to the contrast agent concentration. This effect of low molecular weight Gd(III)-based contrast agents on R_1 is the basis for DCE-MRI, the most commonly used method for clinical assessment of the effects of anticancer treatment on tumor vasculature. DCE-MRI involves acquisition of a series of T_1-weighted images before, during, and after bolus intravenous injection of contrast agent.

Relation to Physiology

The change in signal over time measured by DCE-MRI reflects the exchange of contrast agent between the vasculature and, since the contrast agent does not penetrate viable cells, interstitial (extravascular-extracellular) space. That exchange depends on the capillary blood flow (F), capillary permeability–surface area product (PS), contrast agent distribution volume [V_d, which is commonly assumed to equal the fractional volume of extravascular-extracellular space, V_e (29)], and the blood contrast agent concentration as a function of time (30). The tumor (and blood) contrast agent concentration is inferred from the magnitude of the signal change and parameters reflecting the underlying vascular physiology are derived using various analytical approaches (31). The two primary endpoints recommended for early phase trials of anticancer therapeutics (31) are the transfer constant [K^{trans} (29)] and the initial area under the (contrast agent concentration–time) curve [IAUC (32)]. K^{trans}, which requires fitting the contrast-time curve to a two-compartment model, reflects contrast delivery (F) and transport across the vascular endothelium (PS). The relative influence of F and PS depends on the specific values of F and PS unless F is much greater than PS (tissue-blood exchange is permeability limited, K^{trans} reflects PS only) or vice versa (tissue-blood exchange is flow limited, K^{trans} reflects only F). Fitting the contrast concentration–time curve also provides a measure of V_d. IAUC, which does not require a model, reflects V_d in addition to F and PS (Fig. 1).

It should be noted that the assumption V_d is equivalent to V_e has not been tested. For measurements of V_e with radio-labeled ethylene diamine tetraacetic acid (EDTA) (e.g., ^{51}Cr-EDTA, note the extravascular-extracellular space is also referred to as interstitial space in the physiology literature), at least 30 to 60 minutes are allowed for the EDTA to distribute throughout interstitial space (33). Moreover, additional procedures such as constant infusion (34) or, in animals, renal ligature (35) are often used to ensure radio-labeled EDTA distributes throughout the interstitial space. Given the similarity of the chelating agents EDTA and diethylene triamine pentaacetic acid (DTPA), contrast agent may only reach tumor extravascular-extracellular space in proximity to the vasculature during data acquisition in

typical DCE-MRI experiments (<10 minutes). Hence, in regions with low vascular density, V_d may underestimate the true V_e. This is consistent with the two- to threefold lower V_e reported for rodent tumor core than in the (better perfused) rim (36).

Input Function

The importance of accounting for differences in the blood contrast concentration–time curve (commonly referred to as the input function) between DCE-MRI measurements is widely recognized (32). In 2001, an approach to identify pixels within the imaged volume reflecting the input function was used to demonstrate its impact experimentally (37). Test-retest data from 11 patients with different types of tumor demonstrated a clear improvement in the reproducibility when individual input functions were used rather than an assumed general input function. Although the test-retest data were not reported in terms of the root mean square coefficient of variability (rms CV), extracted data from the figures suggest a threefold improvement (from 25% rms CV with a general input function, which is comparable to other reports where individual input functions were not measured (38), to 8% rms CV with individual input functions). Also, it should be noted that normalization of the tumor IAUC with a reference tissue (32), preferably blood (39), also accounts for variations in the input function.

Transcytolemmal Water Exchange

With respect to the relationship between signal change and contrast agent concentration, it is commonly assumed that the linear relationship observed between R_1 and contrast agent concentration in homogeneous solutions also applies to biological tissues. However, since contrast agent does not enter viable cells, most tissue water is intracellular and water molecules must be in direct contact with the contrast agent to alter R_1, this assumption may not be valid (40). The exchange between intracellular and extracellular water would have to be much faster than the difference in R_1 in the presence and absence of contrast agent for all water molecules in the tissue to have equal access to the contrast agent (i.e., equivalent to a homogeneous solution) (40). This is generally not the case after a bolus injection of contrast agent (41), resulting in underestimation of contrast agent concentration, which is greatest at highest concentrations (42). As a result, there is a K^{trans}-dependent underestimation of K^{trans} if the rate of exchange between intra- and extracellular spaces is not taken into account. A "shutter-speed" model to account for the effect of transcytolemmal water exchange was introduced in 1999 (40) and extended to include a blood compartment in 2005 (43). Of particular interest, when the shutter-speed model is applied to DCE-MRI data from

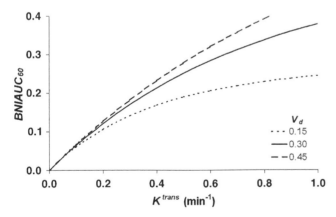

Figure 1 Relationship between IAUC and K^{trans} also depends on the volume of contrast agent distribution (V_d). The initial area under the tissue contrast–time curve for the first 60 seconds after bolus arrival normalized to the initial area under the blood contrast–time curve over that same time (BNIAUC$_{60}$) increases with K^{trans} over the range likely to be observed in tumors. However, that relationship also depends on V_d, which is particularly evident at low V_d.

patients with breast lesions (44), K^{trans} in an invasive ductal carcinoma increased threefold compared with the standard model (from 0.41/min to 1.22/min, while K^{trans} in a fibroadenoma remained constant (0.023/min and 0.024/min). Thus, use of the shutter-speed model appears to increase the dynamic range of DCE-MRI considerably.

It should be noted that this approach has been used almost exclusively by the investigators who have developed this model and has not, to the author's knowledge, been applied to data acquired in the context of treatment monitoring. If the data from such studies are of sufficient quality to account for transcytolemmal water exchange and the shutter-speed model can be included routinely, the sensitivity of DCE-MRI to treatment effects could be enhanced by the increased dynamic range.

Change Measurement

In consideration of the relation to physiology discussed in the "Background" section, treatment-induced changes in K^{trans} can reflect changes in F and/or PS, while changes in IAUC can reflect changes in V_d as well as F and/or PS. Given the lack of a direct relationship between IAUC and any of the underlying physiological variables (45), there is some concern that only changes in K^{trans} are interpretable on a physiologic basis (46). Although there are a limited number of studies reporting both K^{trans} and IAUC, some insight into the relative information content of both

measures can be gained by comparing those results. A comparison of the time- and dose-dependent changes in K^{trans}, IAUC, and F [measured using the freely diffusible radiotracer, iodoantipyrene (47)] induced by the vascular targeting agent combretastatin A-4 3-O-phosphate (CA-4-P) investigated the relationship of both K^{trans} and IAUC to F in rodent tumors (48). Dose- and time-dependent changes in K^{trans} and IAUC were very similar to that measured in independent animals for F, but as expected from the dual dependence of K^{trans} and IAUC on both F and PS, the magnitudes of the changes were less for these parameters than that for F.

A sense of the relative importance of changes in factors other than F and PS for both vascular targeting and antiangiogenic therapy in humans can be gained by comparing treatment-induced changes in K^{trans} and IAUC observed in two phase 1 studies (49,50). As evident in Figure 2, there is a strong correlation between $\%\Delta\,K^{trans}$ and $\%\Delta$ IAUC for CA-4-P at both 4 hours and 24 hours after therapy and for AG-012736 48 hours after therapy (p value for correlation is <0.001 for all cases). Moreover, there is no significant difference between $\%\Delta\,K^{trans}$ and $\%\Delta$ IAUC ($0.4 <$ paired Student's t-test; p value < 0.9 for all cases) and, with the exception of two subjects studied 24 hours after CA-4-P where $\%\Delta\,K^{trans}$ is $\geq +94\%$ and more than twofold greater than $\%\Delta$ IAUC, the points are evenly distributed about the line corresponding to an equal effect for both measures. These results suggest that the

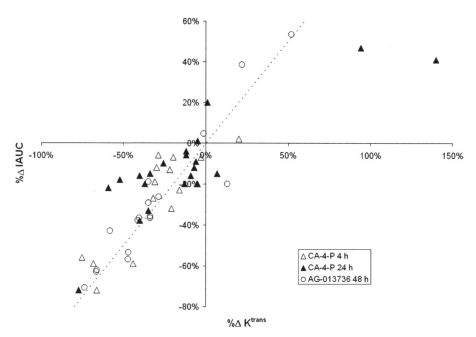

Figure 2 Relationship between changes measured by IAUC and K^{trans} in response to a multi-tyrosine kinase inhibitor. Relationships between change in IAUC and K^{trans} four hours after treatment with CA-4-P ($N = 14$; Pearson product-moment correlation coefficient, $r = 0.858$; p value for 2-tailed paired Student's t-test $= 0.4$); 24 hours after treatment with CA-4-P ($N = 21$; $r = 0.860$; p value $= 0.9$); and 48 hours after treatment with AG-013736 ($N = 17$; $r = 0.943$; p value $= 0.6$). The dashed line corresponds to a 1:1 relationship.

primary effects observed are due to changes in F and/or PS and supports the consensus recommendation that both $\%\Delta \ K^{trans}$ and $\%\Delta$ IAUC are appropriate endpoints for assessing treatment effects on tumor vasculature.

DCE-MRI Protocol

The oncology DCE-MRI community has established and updated consensus recommendations for acquisition and analysis of DCE-MRI data for oncology applications in general (51), and more recently for early clinical trials of anticancer therapeutics affecting tumor vascular function (31,52,53). The most pertinent aspects of the consensus recommendations include the following.

- Entry criteria should include tumors in a fixed superficial location at least 2 cm in diameter, with other tumors at least 3 cm in diameter.
- The entire tumor should be imaged (3D measurements are preferred because single-slice measurements may be prone to sampling error) with the best possible spatial and temporal resolution (trade-offs among coverage, spatial, and temporal resolution depend on the specific application), while specification of the field of view (FOV) should be flexible. Orientation should be adjusted so that motion is in-plane when motion effects cannot be avoided (e.g., liver, lungs).
- Prior to injection, T_1 should be measured using the same resolution and FOV used for acquisition of dynamic data, if possible.
- A power injector should be used for contrast agent injection to minimize variation and a saline flush (at least 20 cc) should always be used. Injection dose should be standardized by body weight with 15 to 30 seconds for total injection.
- For first 150 seconds after bolus injection, use fastest sampling possible consistent with spatial resolution/anatomic coverage requirements, but not slower than 20-second temporal resolution (note: the arterial input function cannot be sampled and K^{trans} will be artificially lowered with 20-second temporal resolution unless the contrast injection is slowed). Data should be acquired out to at least eight minutes (continual sampling is optional).
- The input function (preferably arterial) should be measured with no inflow effect.
- Dynamic image datasets should be spatially registered before analysis.
- The region of interest (ROI) should be constant in position and size for each image in the series under analysis. Ideally the early subtraction images may guide the position for ROI placement (may not apply in some region, e.g., liver), which should also take account of nonenhanced images (i.e., include nonenhancing

tumor). Adjacent blood vessels or regions with other sources of artifact should be excluded.
- Measurements of K^{trans} or IAUC should be made voxel-wise to evaluate tumor heterogeneity. In the event of significant motion, it may be necessary to adjust the ROI position on each image, measuring only a mean value. The "vascularized" tumor volume can be obtained by summing voxels with values above a predetermined threshold (definition of threshold should be reported).

DCE-MRI Applications

There are multiple reviews of the applications of DCE-MRI to measure tumor perfusion and vascularity (54–58). Hence, we will focus on its use as a mechanism biomarker to evaluate the impact of vascular targeted therapies (59,60) on the tumor blood supply. Two types of vascular targeting agents have been studied using DCE-MRI thus far, vascular disrupting agents and vascular endothelial growth factor (VEGF) targeted agents. Vascular disrupting agents seek to compromise the existing tumor blood supply by directly damaging already established tumor endothelium (61). A biomarker capable of reliably assessing treatment effects on the tumor vasculature is of considerable interest for development of these agents because several of them work best in combination with antiproliferative chemotherapy agents (62) or radiation (62,63), showing little activity as monotherapy. VEGF-targeted agents belong to a broader class of agents commonly referred to as antiangiogenic agents (60). VEGF-targeted agents can target VEGF or its receptors, which are tyrosine kinases, and often target other tyrosine kinases associated with angiogenesis (e.g., platelet-derived growth factor receptor, FMS-like tyrosine kinase 3). These agents have exhibited activity as monotherapy generating interest in identifying biomarkers to facilitate their use clinically (64).

DCE-MRI has been used to assess the effects of several vascular disrupting agents in preclinical studies and in early phase clinical trials. DCE-MRI studies were conducted in rodent tumor models prior to phase 1 studies for both CA-4-P (50,65) and ZD6126 (66,67). For CA-4-P, K^{trans}, and IAUC in P22 carcinosarcomas implanted subcutaneously on the flank of male rats decreased by greater than 50% at one hour and six hours after 10 mg/kg, 30 mg/kg, or 100 mg/kg doses. At 24 hours after treatment, K^{trans} and IAUC remained decreased in the 30 mg/kg and 100 mg/kg groups, but returned to pretreatment levels in the 10 mg/kg group. In phase 1 clinical studies (50,68,69), K^{trans} and/or IAUC decreased by more than 50% four to six hours after treatment with CA-4-P at doses greater than 50 mg/m^2 in a third of the patients studied. In the one study where K^{trans} and IAUC were also measured 24 hours after treatment in 14 patients (50), the decrease was less than at four to six hours after treatment in two-thirds of the subjects (and 75% of the subjects with a decrease greater than 50% at 4–6 hours after treatment). Thus, the preclinical and clinical data were consistent and considered to provide proof that this drug has tumor antivascular activity. Preclinical studies of ZD6126 (66,67) showed a dose-dependent decrease in IAUC 24 hours after treatment with decreases as large as 90% at the highest doses. The dose-dependent decrease in IAUC correlated with the extent of treatment-induced necrosis, but there was little or no delay in tumor growth (66). In the phase 1 clinical study (66), IAUC decreased by more than 50% in a third of the patients treated at 56 mg/m^2 or higher. Similar to the case for CA-4-P, preclinical studies translated well to the clinic and DCE-MRI was considered to provide a useful endpoint for quantifying ZD6126 antivascular effects in human tumors.

In the case of VEGF-targeted agents, the widespread use of DCE-MRI in clinical trials has raised awareness of the potential to use it as a biomarker in clinical practice (64,70). A seminal paper (71) on the clinical use of DCE-MRI as a mechanism biomarker for a multi-tyrosine kinase inhibitor, PTK 787 (vatalanib), found that reductions in K^{trans} of 40% or more are associated with lesion size reduction. Subsequent studies with this and other multi-tyrosine kinase inhibitors showed an early (within days) dose-response effect on DCE-MRI measures of vascularity (49,71–80). These data provide considerable support for the supposition that a substantial decrease in F and/or PS is necessary, but not sufficient for a significant reduction in tumor size after treatment with VEGF-targeted agents. In light of the robustness of these observations, the antiangiogenic drug development community is considering the potential that DCE-MRI could function as a marker of early benefit and could help to choose the most appropriate dose of drug (64). The most data to address this possibility are in renal cell cancer (RCC). In 17 patients participating in a phase 2 study of RCC patients treated with sorafenib (70), the reduction in K^{trans} significantly correlated with prolonged time to progression (TTP) but not with the amount of tumor regression determined by CT. Also, in the RCC patients, elevated (>3 mL/mL/min) K^{trans} at baseline was significantly correlated with TTP, with the median TTP greater than 500 days compared with a median TTP of less than 200 days for baseline $K^{\text{trans}} < 3$ mL/mL/min. While these data support the use of DCE-MRI in RCC patients treated with a VEGF-targeted multi-tyrosine kinase, these results need to be confirmed and their applicability to other tumors evaluated. It should also be noted that, given the complexity and costs associated with using DCE-MRI routinely in the clinic, there is considerable effort ongoing to establish serum-based biomarkers

(e.g., VEGF or placental growth factor) that provide similar information (64,70).

Summary

DCE-MRI, which employs a commonly used contrast agent (gadopentetate dimeglumine), has been implemented in preclinical and clinical studies to quantify the effects of antivascular agents on the tumor blood supply within hours to days after the start of treatment. Various analytic approaches have been used to quantify variables reflecting F, PS, and the contrast distribution volume (generally assumed to reflect extravascular-extracellular space) from DCE-MRI data and treatment-induced changes in these variables generally reflect changes in F and/or PS. Since many of these studies were conducted before the DCE-MRI community reached a consensus on methods for acquisition and analysis of data, standardized methods have not been used. Nonetheless, the outcomes of these studies are surprisingly consistent and, taken as a whole, qualify DCE-MRI for use as a mechanism biomarker to assess treatment-induced vascular effects.

Substantial decreases in F and/or PS are induced by both vascular targeting agents and VEGF-targeted agents. For VEGF-targeted agents, it appears that a substantial (40–50%) decrease in F and/or PS is necessary, but not sufficient for a significant reduction in tumor size. In some instances, it appears that tumor vascularization before treatment and/or the magnitude of the treatment effect on tumor vasculature may be indicative of clinical outcome. Interestingly, for vascular targeting agents a similar reduction in F and/or PS is not associated with a reduction in tumor size. This clearly illustrates that the relationship between the effects of antivascular therapy on tumor vasculature quantified by DCE-MRI and clinical outcome depends on mechanism of action (and may depend on the type of tumor). Thus, while it is reasonable to interpret DCE-MRI data as evidence for a treatment effect on tumor vasculature, as drugs are developed for other antiangiogenic targets such as $\alpha_v\beta_3$ integrin, VE-cadherin, or Tie-2/angiopoietin (63), it is important to realize that the association of that vascular effect and clinical activity may vary for each target.

REFERENCES

1. Atkinson AJ, Colburn WA, DeGruttola VG, et al. Biomarkers and surrogate endpoints: Preferred definitions and conceptual framework. Clin Pharmacol Ther 2001; 69(3):89–95.
2. Food and Drug Administration. Innovation or Stagnation? Challenge and opportunity on the critical path to new medical products. 2004; Available at: http://www.fda.gov/oc/initiatives/criticalpath/whitepaper.pdf. Accessed August 30, 2007.

3. Wagner JA, Williams SA, Webster CJ. Biomarkers and surrogate end points for fit-for-purpose development and regulatory evaluation of new drugs. Clin Pharmacol Ther 2007; 81(1):104–107.

4. Food and Drug Administration. Guidance for Industry: Bioanalytical Method Validation, 2001. Available at: http://www.fda.gov/cder/guidance/4252fnl.htm. Accessed August 30, 2007.

5. Lesko LJ, Atkinson AJ. Use of biomarkers and surrogate endpoints in drug development and regulatory decision making: criteria, validation, strategies. Annu Rev Pharmacol Toxicol 2001; 41(1):347–366.

6. Katz R. Biomarkers and surrogate markers: an FDA perspective. NeuroRx 2004; 1(2):189–195.

7. Frank R, Hargreaves R. Clinical biomarkers in drug discovery and development. Nat Rev Drug Discov 2003; 2(7): 566–580.

8. Wagner JA. Overview of biomarkers and surrogate endpoints in drug development. Dis Markers 2002; 18(2): 41–46.

9. Rolan P, Atkinson AJ, Lesko LJ. Use of biomarkers from drug discovery through clinical practice: report of the Ninth European Federation of Pharmaceutical Sciences Conference on Optimizing Drug Development. Clin Pharmacol Ther 2003; 73(4):284–291.

10. Colburn WA. Biomarkers in drug discovery and development: from target identification through drug marketing. J Clin Pharmacol 2003; 43(4):329–341.

11. Lee J, Devanarayan V, Barrett Y, et al. Fit-for-purpose method development and validation for successful biomarker measurement. Pharm Res 2006; 23(2):312–328.

12. Therasse P, Arbuck SG, Eisenhauer EA, et al. New guidelines to evaluate the response to treatment in solid tumors. European Organization for Research and Treatment of Cancer, National Cancer Institute of the United States, National Cancer Institute of Canada. J Natl Cancer Inst 2000; 92(3):205–216.

13. Husband JE, Schwartz LH, Spencer J, et al. Evaluation of the response to treatment of solid tumours—a consensus statement of the International Cancer Imaging Society. Br J Cancer 2004; 90(12):2256–2260.

14. Gupta RK, Sinha U, Cloughesy TF, et al. Inverse correlation between choline magnetic resonance spectroscopy signal intensity and the apparent diffusion coefficient in human glioma. Magn Reson Med 1999; 41(1):2–7.

15. Charles-Edwards EM, deSouza NM. Diffusion-weighted magnetic resonance imaging and its application to cancer. Cancer Imaging 2006; 6:135–143.

16. Chenevert TL, McKeever PE, Ross BD. Monitoring early response of experimental brain tumors to therapy using diffusion magnetic resonance imaging. Clin Cancer Res 1997; 3(9):1457–1466.

17. Zhao M, Pipe JG, Bonnett J, et al. Early detection of treatment response by diffusion-weighted 1H-NMR spectroscopy in a murine tumour in vivo. Br J Cancer 1996; 73(1):61–64.

18. Koh D-M, Collins DJ. Diffusion-weighted MRI in the body: applications and challenges in oncology. Am J Roentgenol 2007; 188(6):1622–1635.

19. Chenevert TL, Sundgren PC, Ross BD. Diffusion imaging: insight to cell status and cytoarchitecture. Neuroimaging Clin N Am 2006; 16(4):619–632, viii–ix.

20. Theilmann RJ, Borders R, Trouard TP, et al. Changes in water mobility measured by diffusion MRI predict response of metastatic breast cancer to chemotherapy. Neoplasia 2004; 6(6):831–837.

21. Dzik-Jurasz A, Domenig C, George M, et al. Diffusion MRI for prediction of response of rectal cancer to chemoradiation. Lancet 2002; 360(9329):307–308.

22. Deng JMS, Miller FHMD, Salem RMD, et al. Multishot diffusion-weighted PROPELLER magnetic resonance imaging of the abdomen. Invest Radiol 2006; 41(10): 769–775.

23. Mürtz P, Krautmacher C, Träber F, et al. Diffusion-weighted whole-body MR imaging with background body signal suppression: a feasibility study at 3.0 Tesla. Eur Radiol 2007; 17(12):3031–3037.

24. Hawighorst H, Weikel W, Knapstein PG, et al. Angiogenic activity of cervical carcinoma: assessment by functional magnetic resonance imaging-based parameters and a histomorphological approach in correlation with disease outcome. Clin Cancer Res 1998; 4(10):2305–2312.

25. Galbraith SM. MR in oncology drug development. NMR Biomed 2006; 19(6):681–689.

26. Mitchell DG. MR imaging contrast agents—what's in a name? J Magn Reson Imaging 1997; 7(1):1–4.

27. Springer CS Jr. Physico-chemical principles influencing magnetopharmaceuticals. In: Gillies RJ, ed. NMR in Physiology and Biomedicine. Orlando, FL: Academic Press, Inc., 1994:75–99.

28. Donahue KM, Burstein D, Manning WJ, et al. Studies of Gd-DTPA relaxivity and proton exchange rates in tissue. Magn Reson Med 1994; 32(1):66–76.

29. Tofts PS, Brix G, Buckley DL, et al. Estimating kinetic parameters from dynamic contrast-enhanced T(1)-weighted MRI of a diffusable tracer: standardized quantities and symbols. J Magn Reson Imaging 1999; 10(3):223–232.

30. Kety SS. Theory and application of the exchange of inert gas at the lungs and tissues. Pharmacol Rev 1951; 3:1–41.

31. Leach MO, Brindle KM, Evelhoch JL, et al. The assessment of antiangiogenic and antivascular therapies in early-stage clinical trials using magnetic resonance imaging: issues and recommendations. Br J Cancer 2005; 92(9): 1599–1610.

32. Evelhoch JL. Key factors in the acquisition of contrast kinetic data for oncology. J Magn Reson Imaging 1999; 10(3):254–259.

33. Levitt DG. The pharmacokinetics of the interstitial space in humans. BMC Clinical Pharmacol 2003; 3:3.

34. Larsson M, Johnson L, Nylander G, et al. Plasma water and 51Cr EDTA equilibration volumes of different tissues in the rat. Acta Physiol Scand 1980; 110:53–57.

35. Reed RK, Lepsoe S, Wiig H. Interstitial exclusion of albumin in rat dermis and subcutis in over- and dehydration. Am J Physiol 1989; 257:H1819–1827.

36. Zhou R, Pickup S, Yankeelov TE, et al. Simultaneous measurement of arterial input function and tumor pharmacokinetics in mice by dynamic contrast enhanced imaging:

effects of transcytolemmal water exchange. Magn Reson Med 2004; 52(2):248–257.

37. Rijpkema M, Kaanders JH, Joosten FB, et al. Method for quantitative mapping of dynamic MRI contrast agent uptake in human tumors. J Magn Reson Imaging 2001; 14(4):457–463.

38. Galbraith SM, Lodge MA, Taylor NJ, et al. Reproducibility of dynamic contrast-enhanced MRI in human muscle and tumours: comparison of quantitative and semi-quantitative analysis. NMR Biomed 2002; 15(2):132–142.

39. Redman BG, Esper P, Pan Q, et al. Phase II trial of tetrathiomolybdate in patients with advanced kidney cancer. Clin Cancer Res 2003; 9(5):1666–1672.

40. Landis CS, Li X, Telang FW, et al. Equilibrium transcytolemmal water-exchange kinetics in skeletal muscle in vivo. Magn Reson Med 1999; 42(3):467–478.

41. Landis CS, Li X, Telang FW, et al. Determination of the MRI contrast agent concentration time course in vivo following bolus injection: effect of equilibrium transcytolemmal water exchange. Magn Reson Med 2000; 44(4):563–574.

42. Yankeelov TE, Rooney WD, Huang W, et al. Evidence for shutter-speed variation in CR bolus-tracking studies of human pathology. NMR Biomed 2005; 18(3):173–185.

43. Li X, Rooney WD, Springer CS Jr. A unified magnetic resonance imaging pharmacokinetic theory: intravascular and extracellular contrast reagents. Magn Reson Med 2005; 54(6):1351–1359.

44. Li X, Huang W, Yankeelov TE, et al. Shutter-speed analysis of contrast reagent bolus-tracking data: Preliminary observations in benign and malignant breast disease. Magn Reson Med 2005; 53(3):724–729.

45. Walker-Samuel S, Leach MO, Collins DJ. Evaluation of response to treatment using DCE-MRI: the relationship between initial area under the gadolinium curve (IAUGC) and quantitative pharmacokinetic analysis. Phys Med Biol 2006; 51(14):3593–3602.

46. Roberts C, Issa B, Stone A, et al. Comparative study into the robustness of compartmental modeling and model-free analysis in DCE-MRI studies. J Magn Reson Imaging 2006; 23(4):554–563.

47. Sakurada O, Kennedy C, Jehle J, et al. Measurement of local cerebral blood flow with iodo[14C]antipyrine. Am J Physiol 1978; 234:H59–H66.

48. Maxwell RJ, Wilson J, Prise VE, et al. Evaluation of the anti-vascular effects of combretastatin in rodent tumours by dynamic contrast enhanced MRI. NMR Biomed 2002; 15:89–98.

49. Liu G, Rugo HS, Wilding G, et al. Dynamic contrast-enhanced magnetic resonance imaging as a pharmacodynamic measure of response after acute dosing of AG-013736, an oral angiogenesis inhibitor, in patients with advanced solid tumors: results from a phase I study. J Clin Oncol 2005; 23(24):5464–5473.

50. Galbraith SM, Maxwell RJ, Lodge MA, et al. Combretastatin A4 phosphate has tumor antivascular activity in rat and man as demonstrated by dynamic magnetic resonance imaging. J Clin Oncol 2003; 21(15):2831–2842.

51. Evelhoch J. Consensus recommendation for acquisition of dynamic contrasted-enhanced MRI data in oncology. In: Dynamic Contrast-Enhanced Magnetic Resonance Imaging in Oncology, Jackson A, Buckley DL, and Parker GJM, eds. Berlin: Springer, 2005:109–114.

52. Evelhoch J, Garwood M, Vigneron D, et al. Expanding the use of magnetic resonance in the assessment of tumor response to therapy: workshop report. Cancer Res 2005; 65(16):7041–7044.

53. Recommendations for MR measurement methods at 1.5-Tesla and endpoints for use in phase 1/2a trials of anticancer therapeutics affecting tumor vascular function, 2004; Dynamic contrast MRI (DCE-MRI) guidelines resulted from the NCI CIP MR Workshop on Translational Research in Cancer—Tumor Response, Bethesda, MD, November 22–23, 2004. Available at: http://imaging.cancer.gov/clinicaltrials/guidelines. Accessed August 30, 2007.

54. Choyke PL, Dwyer AJ, and Knopp MV. Functional tumor imaging with dynamic contrast-enhanced magnetic resonance imaging. J Magn Reson Imaging 2003; 17(5):509–520.

55. Hylton N. Dynamic contrast-enhanced magnetic resonance imaging as an imaging biomarker. J Clin Oncol 2006; 24(20):3293–3298.

56. Jackson A, O'Connor JP, Parker GJ, et al. Imaging tumor vascular heterogeneity and angiogenesis using dynamic contrast-enhanced magnetic resonance imaging. Clin Cancer Res 2007; 13(12):3449–3459.

57. Martincich L, Montemurro F, De Rosa G, et al. Monitoring response to primary chemotherapy in breast cancer using dynamic contrast-enhanced magnetic resonance imaging. Breast Cancer Res Treat 2004; 83(1):67–76.

58. Padhani AR, Leach MO. Antivascular cancer treatments: functional assessments by dynamic contrast-enhanced magnetic resonance imaging. Abdom Imaging 2005; 30(3):324–341.

59. Siemann DW, Bibby MC, Dark GG, et al. Differentiation and definition of vascular-targeted therapies. Clin Cancer Res 2005; 11(2 pt 1):416–420.

60. Siemann DW, Bibby MC, Dark GG, et al. Differentiation and definition of vascular-targeted therapies. Clin Cancer Res 2005; 11(2):416–420.

61. Thorpe PE. Vascular targeting agents as cancer therapeutics. Clin Cancer Res 2004; 10(2):415–427.

62. Siemann DW, Rojiani AM. Antitumor efficacy of conventional anticancer drugs is enhanced by the vascular targeting agent ZD6126. Int J Radiat Oncol Biol Phys 2002; 54(5):1512–1517.

63. Siemann DW, Rojiani AM. The vascular disrupting agent ZD6126 shows increased antitumor efficacy and enhanced radiation response in large, advanced tumors. Int J Radiat Oncol Biol Phys 2005; 62(3):846–853.

64. Jubb AM, Oates AJ, Holden S, et al. Predicting benefit from anti-angiogenic agents in malignancy. Nat Rev Cancer 2006; 6(8):626–635.

65. Maxwell RJ, Wilson J, Prise VE, et al. Evaluation of the anti-vascular effects of combretastatin in rodent tumours by dynamic contrast enhanced MRI. NMR Biomed 2002; 15(2):89–98.

66. Evelhoch JL, LoRusso PM, He Z, et al. Magnetic resonance imaging measurements of the response of murine and human tumors to the vascular-targeting agent ZD6126. Clin Cancer Res 2004; 10(11):3650–3657.

67. Robinson SP, McIntyre DJ, Checkley D, et al. Tumour dose response to the antivascular agent ZD6126 assessed by magnetic resonance imaging. Br J Cancer 2003; 88(10): 1592–1597.

68. Stevenson JP, Rosen M, Sun W, et al. Phase I trial of the antivascular agent combretastatin A4 phosphate on a 5-day schedule to patients with cancer: magnetic resonance imaging evidence for altered tumor blood flow. J Clin Oncol 2003; 21(23):4428–4438.

69. Dowlati A, Robertson K, Cooney M, et al. A phase I pharmacokinetic and translational study of the novel vascular targeting agent combretastatin A-4 phosphate on a single-dose intravenous schedule in patients with advanced cancer. Cancer Res 2002; 62(12):3408–3416.

70. Flaherty KT. Sorafenib in renal cell carcinoma. Clin Cancer Res 2007; 13(2 pt 2):747s–752s.

71. Morgan B, Thomas AL, Drevs J, et al. Dynamic contrast-enhanced magnetic resonance imaging as a biomarker for the pharmacological response of PTK787/ZK 222584, an inhibitor of the vascular endothelial growth factor receptor tyrosine kinases, in patients with advanced colorectal cancer and liver metastases: results from two phase I studies. J Clin Oncol 2003; 21(21):3955–3964.

72. Drevs J, Siegert P, Medinger M, et al. Phase I clinical study of AZD2171, an oral vascular endothelial growth factor signaling inhibitor, in patients with advanced solid tumors. J Clin Oncol 2007; 25(21):3045–3054.

73. Thomas AL, Morgan B, Horsfield MA, et al. Phase I study of the safety, tolerability, pharmacokinetics, and pharmacodynamics of PTK787/ZK 222584 administered twice daily in patients with advanced cancer. J Clin Oncol 2005; 23(18):4162–4171.

74. O'Donnell A, Padhani A, Hayes C, et al. A phase I study of the angiogenesis inhibitor SU5416 (semaxanib) in solid tumours, incorporating dynamic contrast MR pharmacodynamic end points. Br J Cancer 2005; 93(8):876–883.

75. Mross K, Drevs J, Muller M, et al. Phase I clinical and pharmacokinetic study of PTK/ZK, a multiple VEGF receptor inhibitor, in patients with liver metastases from solid tumours. Eur J Cancer 2005; 41(9):1291–1299.

76. Dowlati A, Robertson K, Radivoyevitch T, et al. Novel Phase I dose de-escalation design trial to determine the biological modulatory dose of the antiangiogenic agent SU5416. Clin Cancer Res 2005; 11(21):7938–7944.

77. Xiong HQ, Herbst R, Faria SC, et al. A phase I surrogate endpoint study of SU6668 in patients with solid tumors. Invest New Drugs 2004; 22(4):459–466.

78. Peterson AC, Swiger S, Stadler WM, et al. Phase II study of the Flk-1 tyrosine kinase inhibitor SU5416 in advanced melanoma. Clin Cancer Res 2004; 10(12):4048–4054.

79. Medved M, Karczmar G, Yang C, et al. Semiquantitative analysis of dynamic contrast enhanced MRI in cancer patients: variability and changes in tumor tissue over time. J Magn Reson Imaging 2004; 20(1):122–128.

80. Wedam SB, Low JA, Yang SX, et al. Antiangiogenic and antitumor effects of bevacizumab in patients with inflammatory and locally advanced breast cancer. J Clin Oncol 2006; 24(5):769–777.

46

Industrial-Academic Collaboration

RAYMOND E. GIBSON

Imaging Department, Merck Research Laboratories, West Point, Pennsylvania, U.S.A.

CYNTHIA J. ZARSKY

Technology and Acquisition and Outlicensing, Merck Research Laboratories, Rahway, New Jersey, U.S.A.

INTRODUCTION

The goal of research is not necessarily to make money, but biomedical research is an expensive proposition regardless of whether this is conducted in an academic environment, government laboratory, or pharmaceutical company, and therefore successful funding is a prerequisite for any scientific advancement. Academic research is largely funded through government agencies, such as the National Institutes of Health (see Menkin et al., Chapter 44). Funding by this mechanism makes most academics feel comfortable since they are pursuing research, which they have initiated, and consequently falls within their own interests. This perception may not be strictly true since the research conducted under such funding is usually tailored to requests offered by agencies such as the NIH (RFA/PA mechanisms). In addition to government funding agencies, industry represents an opportunity to obtain funding as long as the research to be conducted falls within the range of interest of the company. This is less surprising than it sounds since pharmaceutical companies by nature do conduct biomedical research. In the area of imaging sciences, there has been growth in interest by big pharma in which imaging modalities are seen as unique oppor-tunities to develop novel biomarkers and methods for conducting proof-of-concept studies of drugs under investigation (1–6). This, therefore, presents an opportunity for academic imaging scientists to collaborate with scientists in the pharmaceutical industry—and provides a means by which academicians can obtain funding for projects, which are of mutual interest.

While there have been several very good reviews of the potential/actual issues in collaborations between academia and industry, these tend to focus on issues of academic freedom, pure versus applied research, and conflicts that arise in these interactions (7–13). Largely, these represent concerns over intellectual property (IP). The ability of academic researchers to patent their inventions should advance their interests, since Industry prefers dealing with IP that is clearly defined, and would rather engage in research in which there is a clear opportunity to license in methods, technologies, or leads of interest that have good patent protection. This presentation is clearly the point of view of the authors. While most comments will be generally applicable, variations on these themes will likely be encountered in interactions with different pharmaceutical companies and different academic institutions.

JUSTIFICATION FOR COLLABORATION

Inasmuch as many (most) targets for pharmaceutical development originate outside a company, this is particularly so in the fields of imaging sciences. Imaging is either new to or not extensively utilized by most pharmaceutical companies. The extensive experience in the academic community therefore offers levels of experience and expertise not available within the industry. Take for example, radiotracers for oncologic imaging. Academic institutions have been exploring the use of various radiotracers in the diagnosis and staging of cancer for several decades. This effort has led to the development of a number of interesting radiopharmaceuticals for imaging tumor metabolism (14–17), proliferation (18–21), hypoxia (22), and angiogenesis (23,24) associated with tumors. These agents were developed primarily for diagnosis and the application as oncology "biomarkers" became apparent with the successful application of FDG imaging to the effect of Gleevec treatment of gastrointestinal stromal tumors (GIST) (25–27). From the point of view of the pharmaceutical industry, all the diagnostic agents that now fall under the rubric of "molecular imaging agents" hold the potential as imaging "biomarkers." The question can then be posed—who will demonstrate this utility?

Herein is the first opportunity for collaboration—to demonstrate in a preclinical model that a particular treatment leads to a useful change in a measure of a particular radiotracer. Similarly, experimental medicine (clinical) studies can be pursued to demonstrate the use of a biomarker, which circumvent questions of the applicability of preclinical models. Therapies, which may lead to increased rates of apoptosis, may be detected early and efficiently by agents that measure apoptosis or hypoxia. Since PET or SPECT facilities are not common in most pharmaceutical companies, these studies may be most conveniently accomplished in collaborations.

Merck Research Laboratories provide a different challenge to potential collaborators since they have extensive internal imaging capabilities for preclinical studies, covering not only all imaging modalities (PET, SPECT, MRI, Optical, CT, and Ultrasound) represented by both clinical and so-called microinstrumentation, but also has extensive capabilities in the development of new, novel radiotracers biomarkers (3–6). Nonetheless, academic colleagues have generated novel imaging platforms and/or agents, or have come to the company with novel ideas for the development of potentially valuable biomarkers. So, even as a company with extensive imaging capability and expertise, we are consistently interested in the opportunities for interactions with our academic colleagues.

OPPORTUNITIES FOR ACADEMIC-INDUSTRIAL INTERACTION

In addition to collaborative opportunities, there are several other potential interactions, which we will briefly outline: information transfer, materials transfer, fee for service, collaboration, and license.

Information Transfer

Information transfer may or may not be of a confidential nature. For example, an academic scientist may be invited to present a seminar on his/her work. In the absence of a confidentiality agreement, this visit is clearly circumscribed and topics other than that presented in the seminar or in the public domain are not discussed. This is for the protection of both parties. If, however, either or both parties are interested in exploring possible interactions (e.g., fee for service or collaboration), this may require open discussions of specific IP. A confidentiality agreement will be established, usually two-way, so free discussion on a desired topic is possible. This will, however, be circumscribed to specific areas of mutual interest. If, during discussions, other areas of mutual interest outside the confidentiality agreement become apparent, these cannot be discussed without expansion of the agreement. Furthermore, *any information shared during these discussions cannot be used or acted on outside of the specific use and purpose of the CDA.* An extension of information transfer, which allows the pharmaceutical company to act on the information is the consultant agreement. In this case, the academic partner is being paid specifically to provide advice to the company for its own use. Consultant agreements are, again, usually well circumscribed to cover specific topics, for example, uses of metabolic or proliferative radiotracers as biomarkers for drug efficacy trials.

Material Transfer Agreements

Material transfer agreements usually allow provision of unique and proprietary compounds to an academic center for studies of specific interest to the academic partner, or material provided to the pharmaceutical company for evaluation. If an academic colleague requests a compound, specifics of the study to be done are required. Additionally, these materials cannot be used for human studies. We also request the right to review any publication or presentation containing data generated using one of our compounds prior to its submission to ensure that IP is protected.

Study Agreements

The study agreement is probably the best-known mechanism by which industry conducts studies in academic institutions. Frequently, an academic center has developed a specific model or technology (imaging modality or new radiotracer), which is of interest for the evaluation of compounds under development. The more complex or expensive a technique is, the more likely we would want to have the work conducted externally. A clear work plan is established with a budget for the single study. Industry provides whatever material is required for the study to the academic center, and, of course, the funds for the study. Industry will also usually stipulate a time line for completion and availability of study results. While we understand that the academic institution must preserve its right to publish the study results, we will need to preserve our right to review the proposed publication prior to its submission to ensure that IP is protected and that confidential information of the company is not inadvertently disclosed.

Collaborative Agreement

The most interesting approach to conducting research in which mutual parties have substantial contributions to make to the effort is the collaboration. Collaborations between academic colleagues are frequent, and usually, not complicated. One investigator has access to a technique or instrument that can provide unique information on pharmacology, physiology, or pathology available to a primary investigator, which leads to a collaborative study, coauthorship, etc. By contrast, collaborative agreements between academic and industry partners can be quite complicated to arrange because of concerns with IP. The academic partner needs to ensure that they have filed a patent on any technology being brought to the collaboration with industry; our interest in the collaboration will be determined, in part, by the presence of good patent protection. This patent protection not only protects the IP of the academic partner, but may also lead to licensing agreements in which clear IP is required. In some cases, we may be interested in developing a particular technology for the public good. For example, the FNIH Consortia for validating FDG as a biomarker in multicenter trials (http://www.biomarkersconsortium. org/index.php?option=com_content&task=view&id= 51&Itemid=61) is viewed as providing advantage not only to companies involved but also to the medical community in general.

The structure of collaborative agreements may vary considerably, depending on the nature of the work to be done. The essentials are similar to the "study agreement"

in that a specific work plan is established, the difference being that the work to be conducted is shared between the academic and industrial partners. When the IP resides with the academic partner, the results may lead to licensing opportunities. As before, most academic partners will need to reserve rights regarding publication of results from the collaboration, and the industrial partner will need to balance that with a right to review, delay publication for weeks to a few months to file patents to protect IP, and also remove any confidential information of the company.

License

Research conducted within a collaborative agreement or brought to a company with substantial results demonstrating potential utility to the company may lead to licensing of the technology or further development by the company. We will not deal in this discussion with these opportunities, which may be structured in a variety of ways. Needless to say, the technology needs to be viewed by the company as key to the development of a particular program, and the information thus obtained not easily available by any other means. Thus, the justification for academics patenting good ideas as early as possible.

ISSUES

Before entering an agreement with industry, academicians need to be aware of several concerns of the pharmaceutical industry. The first of these is, obviously, protecting the company's IP. Agreements that have potential for compromising the company IP will obviously not be pursued. A second consideration is the timeliness of results generated through a study or collaborative project. The pace of academic research and that within the pharmaceutical industry may differ considerably. One of the advantages of the academic environment is that funding from government sources allows freedom to generate data as the investigator sees fit—with the obvious requirement that something needs to be provided in progress reports by end-of-year to insure continued funding. When entering a project with an industrial partner, results are needed as quickly as reasonably possible. Those in industry function under constrained timelines, where results are often needed within weeks of proposing a particular study. If a study is conceptualized with an estimated time to completion of six weeks, it is not acceptable to provide the company results in six months.

Time constraints in academic research are often very difficult to negotiate, particularly in imaging, since these facilities are usually part of a clinical environment and scheduling of either preclinical or experimental clinical studies need to allow for the clinical requirements of the imaging facility. The primary reason Merck has invested significantly in preclinical imaging within the company, and in dedicated clinical imaging sites are that prolonged delays are not acceptable. Tasks that may require several months of effort by academic colleagues may be done within several weeks using dedicated preclinical imaging capability, or established clinical imaging centers foremost to the projects and requirements of the company. Pharmaceutical company–established clinical imaging centers have been adopted by several pharmaceutical companies.

While this discussion has focused primarily on concerns of the pharmaceutical industry, there are several issues, which may be of concern to the academic partner. For example, study agreements are limited in scope providing funds for a particular study, and may not be sufficient to provide additional staff—or of duration sufficient to justify additional hires. Of more value, collaborative projects may be longer in duration and provide sufficient funding to help support students or technicians. Projects with durations longer than a year may be rare, however, and other mechanisms may be pursued for longer-term support (e.g., grants to support training). Finally, academic careers rise and fall on publications. Companies will require review of manuscripts prior to submission as previously described.

CONTACTS

If you have a good idea, and you think it may be of value to a pharmaceutical company, what do you do? Most companies will have technology assessment committees or external scientific development departments, which can be contacted with ideas. Such ideas brought to a company are directed to appropriate investigators for evaluation. The alternatives are to contact individuals who are conducting research in the area of interest. For example, a new radiotracer for imaging in oncology can be directed to individuals within oncology research department of a pharmaceutical company. As part of the departments of imaging and technology acquisitions, we are frequently contracted with regards to potential collaborative development or licensing opportunities. This latter approach may generate a champion for the concept, which will help move request through the machinery of the company. Equally problematic for those in the pharmaceutical industry is to know what opportunities are available/under development in the academic community. As much as we consider ourselves to be well informed, the field of imaging is too broad and too rapidly advancing for the industrial researcher to be able to keep abreast of all exciting developments. It is, therefore, highly likely that new ideas will first be brought to industry attention by the academic community.

CONCLUSION

As mentioned in the introduction, the contents of this discussion are the point of view of the authors. Nonetheless, variations across the pharmaceutical industry will likely be in the details, not in the overview. Within the constraints described, collaborative investigations provide advantage and opportunity for both the academic and industrial partners. For the academic institution, this may be seed funding for ideas that can be obtained more rapidly than through granting agencies. The best case is that such interactions will lead to further collaborations and licensing opportunities, which again, provide funding for research. Efforts to bring about agreements between industry, academic laboratories, and government laboratories to increase access to propriety compound information are ongoing. How likely these may be, this writer does not want to speculate, but a collaborative development project for a new imaging radiotracer, for example, may well lead to knowledge of structure-activity relationships available within a company, which are not otherwise available. The advantage of collaborative efforts for the pharmaceutical industry are that (*i*) we cannot do everything, and (*ii*) many of the best ideas come from our academic colleagues. It thus behooves the industry to keep the channels open for collaborative studies whenever possible.

REFERENCES

1. Frank R, Hargreaves R. Clinical biomarkers in drug discovery and development. Nat Rev Drug Discov 2003; 2(7): 566–580.
2. Hietala J, Nyman MJ, Eskola I, et al. Visualization and quantification of neurokinin-1 (NK1) receptors in the human brain. Mol Imaging Biol 2005; 7(4):262–272.
3. Yasuno F, Sanabria SM, Burns D, et al. PET imaging of neurokinin-1 receptors with [F-18]SPA-RQ in human subjects: assessment of reference tissue models and their test-retest reproducibility. Synapse 2007; 61(4):242–251.
4. Burns HD, Van Laere K, Sanabria-Bohorquez S, et al. [^{18}F] MK-9470, a positron emission tomography (PET) tracer for in vivo human PET brain imaging of the cannabinoid-1 receptor. Proc Natl Acad Sci 2007; 104(23):9800–9805.
5. Addy C, Rothenberg P, Burns D, et al. Clinical evaluation of brain CB-1 receptor occupancy of a novel CB1R inverse agonist using CB-1R PET. Diabetes 2007; 56(suppl 1): A693–A693.
6. Erondu N, Gantz I, Musser B, et al. Neuropeptide Y5 receptor antagonism does not induce clinically meaningful weight loss in overweight and obese adults. Cell Metab 2006; 4(4):275–282.
7. Cooper T, Galligan JE. The anomaly as a necessity. Academic-industrial collaboration in research. Int J Cardiol 1982; 1:449–458.

8. Culliton BJ. The academic-industrial complex. Science 1982; 216:960–962.

9. Ferguson RK, Vlasses PH, Abrams WB. Academic-industrial clinical pharmacology: a working model. J Clin Pharmacol 1985; 25:4–7.

10. Frankel MS. Perception, reality, and the political context of conflict of interest in university-industry relationships. Acad Med 1996; 71(12):1297–1304.

11. Martin JB. Academic-industrial collaboration: the good, the bad, and the ugly. Trans Am Clin Climatol Assoc 113; 2002:227–240.

12. Gelijns AC, Thier SO. Medical innovation and institutional interdependence. Rethinking university-industry connections. J Am Med Assoc 2878; 2002:72–77.

13. Evans GR, and Packham DE. Ethical issues at the university-industry interface: a way forward? Sci Eng Ethics 2003; 9:2–16.

14. Kole AC, Nieweg OE, Pruim J, et al. Detection of unknown occult primary tumors using positron emission tomography. Cancer 1998; 82(6):1160–1166.

15. Alavi JB, Alavi A, Chawluck J, et al. Positron emission tomography in patients with glioma—a predictor of prognosis. Cancer 1988; 62(6):1074–1078.

16. Hiesgler EM, Fowler J, Brodie JD, et al. Human-brain tumor imaging by positron emission tomography (pet) using [1-c-11] putrescine (c-11-pu) and [1-c-11] 2-deoxy-d-glucose (c-11-2dg). Neurology 1986; 36(4):335–335.

17. Kubota K, Matsuzawa T, Ito M, et al. Lung-tumor imaging by positron emission tomography using [C-11] l-methionine. J Nucl Med 1985; 26(1):37–42.

18. Shields AF. Positron emission tomography measurement of tumor metabolism and growth: its expanding role in oncology. Mol Imaging Biol 2006; 8(3):141–150.

19. Alexander S, Varaha ST, John G, et al. FLT: measuring tumor cell proliferation in vivo with positron emission tomography and 3′-Deoxy-3′-[F-18]Fluorothymidine. Semin Nucl Med 2007; 37:429–439.

20. Chen W, Delaloye S, Silverman DHS, et al. Predicting treatment response of malignant gliomas to bevacizumab and irinotecan by imaging proliferation with [F-18] fluorothymidine positron emission tomography: a pilot study. J Clin Oncol 2007; 25:4714–4721.

21. Kenny L, Coombes RC, Vigushin DM, et al. Imaging early changes in proliferation at 1 week post chemotherapy: a pilot study in breast cancer patients with 3′-deoxy-3′-[F-18] fluorothymidine positron emission tomography. Eur J Nucl Med Mol Imaging 2007; 34(9):1339–1347.

22. Serganova I, Humm J, Ling C, et al. Tumor hypoxia imaging. Clin Cancer Res 2006; 12(18):5260–5264.

23. Beer AJ, Grosu AL, Carlsen J, et al. [F-18]Galacto-RGD positron emission tomography for imaging of alpha v beta 3 expression on the neovasculature in patients with squamous cell carcinoma of the head and neck. Clin Cancer Res 2007; 13:6610–6616.

24. Choe YS, Lee KH. Targeted in vivo imaging of angiogenesis: present status and perspectives. Curr Pharm Des 2007; 13(1):17–31.

25. Van den Abbeele AD, Badawi RD, Cliche J, et al. Response to Imatinib mesylate (GleevecTM) therapy in patients with advanced gastrointestinal stromal tumors (GIST) is demonstrated by F-18-FDG-PET prior to anatomic imaging with CT. Radiology 2002; 225(suppl. S): 424.

26. Gayed I, Vu T, Iyer R, et al. The role of F-18-FDG PET in staging and early prediction of response to therapy of recurrent gastrointestinal stromal tumors. J Nucl Med 2004; 45(1):17–21.

27. Heinicke T, Wardelmann E, Sauerbruch T, et al. Very early detection of response to imatinib mesylate therapy of gastrointestinal stromal tumours using (18)fluoro-deoxyglucose-positron emission tomography. Anticancer Res 2005; 25(6C): 4591–4594.

47

The Future of Molecular Imaging

STEVEN M. LARSON

Memorial Sloan-Kettering Cancer Center, New York, New York, U.S.A.

INTRODUCTION

Molecular imaging is a multimodality approach that brings together advances in biology with advances in the technology of imaging. During the preceding chapters of this book, many brilliant examples have been quoted of molecular imaging in the laboratory with fewer but a still substantial number of methods that have been translated to humans. Molecular imaging has vast potential, and one day I have no doubt that we will be able to noninvasively image key elements of the proteome and genome in man. This brief overview, is not well suited to this grand vision and so is confined to nuclear approaches, and molecular imaging with potential for clinical imaging in cancer. I have chosen to emphasize the near horizon that molecular imaging will have a great impact in the near future in improving treatment of the oncology patient. This will be done primarily by better biomarkers and improved treatment response assessment. Treatment response will be carried out by metabolic biomarkers, like 2-[18F]-fluoro-2-D-deoxyglucose (FDG) and [18F]-F-L-thymidine (FLT) as well as methods, which selectively image biomolecules of key importance to individual tumors, such as androgen receptor (AR) and the growth factor receptor, Her 2, as well as antibody-targeted molecules.

Molecular imaging of cancer can be thought of as imaging the key molecules or molecularly based events, which are fundamental to the process of oncogenesis and tumor pathophysiology. Advances in cancer biology provided us with numerous molecules that may serve as effective targets for imaging. Of course from the standpoint of nuclear imaging, we depend on the tracer principle, that is, we use a radioactive form a key biomolecule or element, to trace the in vivo behavior, through imaging of like molecules in vivo. By definition, when used as a radiotracer, the chemical concentration of the radiolabeled form is below pharmacologic effect.

CANCER BIOLOGY OF IMPORTANCE TO MOLECULAR IMAGING

Hanahan and Weinberg (1) have provided a useful description of distinctions between cancer and the tissue from which they arise, for use as a summary of the cancer biology which is relevant to molecular imaging (Fig. 1). A fundamental feature of cancer is that process of oncogenesis confers on cancer cells' specific properties that make the cell malignant: resistance to apoptosis, immortality, the ability to proliferate indefinitely without dying, the ability to a ignore signals which would otherwise stop growth of normal cells, self-sufficiency in growth signals, the ability to invade and metastasize, and sustained angiogenesis (Fig. 1A). A second critical feature involves the tumor mass itself, which is not simply a collection of cancer cells, but consists of the numerous cells of different biology, which are essentially recruited by the cancer cells to help sustain growth. In addition to the mass may also contain inflammatory cells, which represent the response of the host to the cancer (Fig. 1B). A third critical feature is disordered communication within the cell, because this has been shown to be the proximate cause of the malignant state for some types of cancer cells. A genetic mutation occurs which results in an aberrant protein, which is a component of the communications apparatus, and which takes over the cell to drive proliferation and to participate in an oncogenesis for the cell. In this case the mutated gene is called an oncogene. Numerous cancers have been associated with an identified oncogene, for example, chronic myelogenous leukemia (Bcr/Abl), gastrointestinal stromal tumor (c-kit), lung cancers, especially in never smokers (EGFR tyrosine kinase mutations).

ADVANTAGES OF NUCLEAR APPROACHES FOR MOLECULAR IMAGING

All these distinctive properties of cancer are associated with fundamental molecular changes, which in principle could be a reached with the appropriate radiotracer and imaging instrument. There is a huge diversity of radiotracers available for studying numerous properties of cancer and is likely that this list will grow further (2) (Table 1 for selected radiotracers as examples).

A second advantage of the nuclear approach for molecular imaging is the availability of high-resolution imaging units adapted for animals, and high-resolution human units, which are practical for clinical imaging. Thus, a radiotracer can be developed and studied in the laboratory in animals, and then using the same tracer translated to human studies, which over time may be developed into clinical tests (Fig. 2).

Disordered Communication

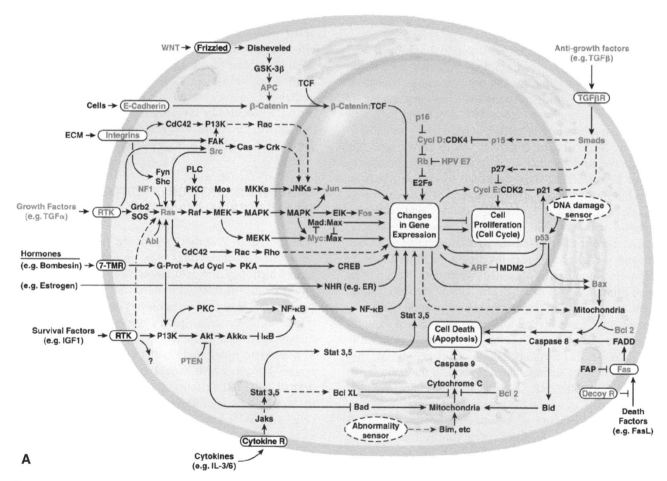

Figure 1 (**A**) Illustrates what is perhaps the most important hallmark of cancer cover and that is disordered communication within the cell. (**B**) Demonstrates that with the tumor mass, there are many different cell types with distinct properties and a heterotypic biology. (**C**) Summarizes the distinctions between cancer cells and the cells from which they arise. *Source*: From Ref. 1

The Tumor as a Community of Cells

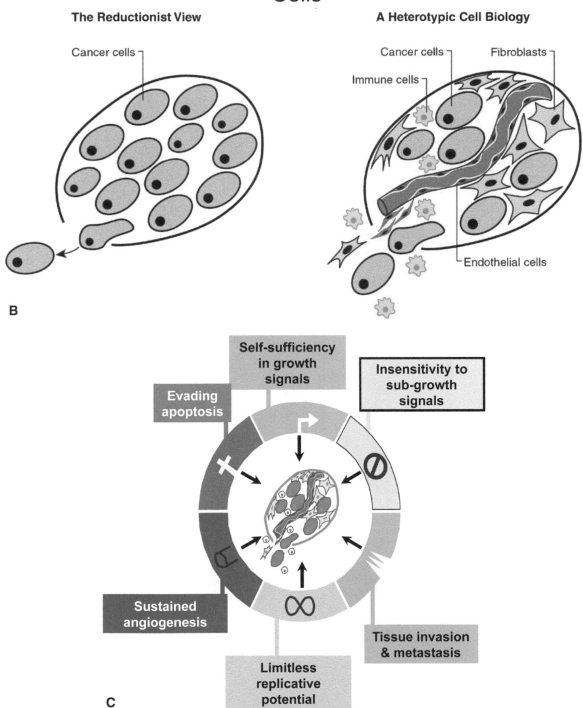

Figure 1 *(Continued)*

Table 1 Selected Radiopharmaceuticals in Common Use for Clinical Research

Radiopharmaceutical	Target molecule	Biochemical process imaged
FDG	Glucose 6-kinase	Glycolysis
11C-methionine	Amino acid transporters	Amino acid uptake
[F-18]-F-ion	Hydroxyapatite crystal	Bone turnover
[F-18]-F-L-thymidine	Thymidine kinase	Proliferation
[F-18]-fluoromisonidazole	Reduced macromolecules	Hypoxia
[Ga-68]-octreotide	Somatostatin receptor II	Stasis of growth
[F-18]-RGD peptide	Integrins	Neovascularity
[C-11]-CO	Hemoglobin	Blood volume
[F-18]-fluorodopa	Dopa decarboxylase	Storage of biogenic amines

Abbreviations: FDG, 2-[18F]-fluoro-2-D-deoxyglucose; RGD, arginine-glycine-aspartate.

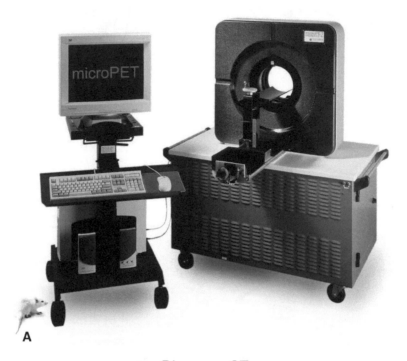

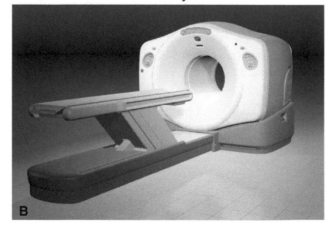

Figure 2 (**A**) Example of a microPET Focus high-resolution scanner (Concord, Oak Ridge, Tennessee, U.S.) and (**B**) PET/CT, the General Electric Discovery STE 16.

MOLECULAR IMAGING IN CURRENT CLINICAL PRACTICE

The clinical practice of nuclear medicine is in large part radiotracer-based functional imaging, in the sense that it is imaging of the dynamic process of in vivo physiology as the basis for clinical scanning. The "bread and butter" procedures, such as cardiac perfusion imaging, bone scanning, lung perfusion and aerosol studies, renal studies, and lymphoscintigraphy, are a vital part of medical practice and are likely to remain so for the foreseeable future. About 20 million procedures are being performed per year in the United States that are dependent on the radionuclide technetium-99m (Tc 99m). Growth in these procedures is projected at 5% to 7% per year. For single-photon radionuclides such as Tc 99m, single-photon emission computed tomography (SPECT) is a highly useful tool. Although SPECT is evolving into a quantitative imaging tool with high resolution, there is considerable development yet required before the clinically available instruments, which are based on standard gamma cameras, can overcome the inherent limitations of scatter correction to become a truly quantitative molecular-imaging tool. For this reason, I will confine my remarks largely to positron emission tomography (PET), which because of inherent superiorities of physics of decay of the positron and the way that this facilitates detection by the instrument (well-discussed in previous chapters of this book). PET is the current "poster child" for the translation of molecular imaging to clinical practice.

PET studies in cancer performed clinically with full reimbursement are pretty much exclusively performed with FDG. More than one million procedures have been performed in the United States on an annual basis, predominantly in oncology. There are nine tumor types that are reimbursed routinely. These include non-small cell lung cancer (NSCLC), breast cancer, head and neck cancer (including thyroid), colorectal, cervical, esophageal cancers; melanoma, lymphoma (Hodgkin's disease and non-Hodgkin's lymphoma), for diagnosis, staging tumor extent, and restaging recurrent tumor. Monitor of treatment response is permitted only in breast cancer although restaging is allowed in the Hodgkin's and non-Hodgkin's lymphoma. The interested reader is referred to a review by Kelloff, which is a particularly erudite discussion about the use of FDG PET as the molecular imaging (3). Currently, the CMS, "PET Registry," is allowing reimbursement for PET scans performed in other cancers, under a coverage with evidence development approach.

In the United States today, PET is largely performed with combination instruments that include high-resolution CT (4). In the last five years, this technology was enthusiastically embraced by the major instrument manufacturers, and dedicated PET has been largely abandoned in favor of combined instruments. Although technically

more demanding, it is likely that PET/MRI will also become popular particularly for some applications such as brain imaging. Successful animal images have been recorded on PET/MRI machines (5), and prototype clinical units are under investigation in several centers. Benefits from the combined PET/MRI will include reductions in radiation exposure to patients versus PET/CT, particularly for pediatric patients, as well as the ability to have both temporal and spatial image fusion for the PET and MRI signals.

AREAS OF FUTURE DEVELOPMENT FOR MOLECULAR IMAGING

In the near term, perhaps the greatest area of development will be in drug discovery. The focus will be the use of metabolic markers, to monitor treatment response, and on the pharmacokinetics of cancer drugs.

Molecular Imaging as Biomarkers

There is growing recognition of the need for improving the evaluation of the effects of drugs and other treatments in human disease (6,7). Accordingly, the National Cancer Institute (NCI), the FDA, and the CMS have developed a memorandum of understanding in which they propose a new initiative: the oncology biomarker qualification initiative (OBQI). For the purposes of this program, "Biomarkers are indicators of disease or therapeutic effects, which can be measured through dynamic imaging tests, as well as tests on blood, tissue, and other biologic samples" (http://www.fda.gov/oc/mous/domestic/FDA-NCI-CMS .html). The rationale for biomarkers is then with the clinical trials is to help reduce the growing cost of obtaining the drug approvals and dissatisfaction with the class for the current anatomic-based imaging methods for assessing treatment response such as RECIST. In regard to clinical trials, it is envisioned that there will be numerous potential benefits of biomarkers to determine if patient's tumor is likely to respond at all to specific treatments; to assess shortly after the treatment is initiated or at completion, which can be challenging if done only by size; to determine which patients are at higher risk for recurring after surgery or radiotherapy.

BIOMARKERS BASED ON METABOLIC RESPONSE OF TUMOR TO TREATMENT

The combination of PET/CT with FDG would seem to be ideally suited as an imaging biomarker, as it does provide information about the biochemistry of the patient's tumor from PET with anatomic correlates from CT.

Furthermore, PET plus CT is now widespread in its availability, both in academic institutions and in the private sector. So, there are now more than 2000 PET/CT units available for patient use throughout the United States.

As a starting point for these efforts, NCI has convened several workshops intended to serve as roadmap for standardization of pet imaging with FDG (8). In addition, NCI has sponsored direct efforts to systematize data collection for certain key tumors where success is considered likely, such as lymphoma (9).

APPLICATION OF FDG PET TO GASTROINTESTINAL STROMAL TUMOR

Gastrointestinal stromal tumor (GIST) is an uncommon tumor of mesenchymal cells that surround the intestine. The oncogene c-kit, is responsible for much of the growth and proliferation of this tumor. The development of imatinib, a tyrosine kinase inhibitor drug, has revolutionized the treatment of this tumor type. FDG PET is a powerful tool for monitoring treatment response, as well as a potential for recurrence in GIST (10,11).

Patient Example of the Role of FDG PET in a GIST

The patient is a middle-aged male with a two-month history of abdominal swelling. A peritoneal mass was biopsied and was shown to be GIST. FDG PET images were performed immediately before and at four months after beginning therapy with imatinib. A profound reduction in metabolic activity is seen in the lesion (Fig. 3).

THE ROLE OF FDG PET IN CASTRATE-RESISTANT PROSTATE CANCER

Clinical studies in prostate cancer show that prostate cancer is often hormone responsive, but eventually the tumor cells become resistant to hormones, and from that point, progression to patient death from progressive tumor is practically inevitable. The clinical states model of Scher and Heller provide a roadmap for the progression of prostate cancer. We have found that FDG PET is useful for monitoring treatment response of tumors during the castrate resistant stage of the disease (12).

Patient Example of FDG PET in Castrate-Resistant Prostate Cancer

The patient is a middle-aged man with a five-year history of prostate cancer, who after a two-year response to hormone therapy has developed a progressive increase in serum prostate-specific antigen (PSA). The patient was treated with a Taxol-based regimen, the results are shown in Figure 4.

RADIOTRACERS FOR MONITORING TREATMENT RESPONSE

As can be seen from the examples cited in Figures 3 and 4, the response of tumors in terms of FDG uptake, a measure of glucose metabolism, can vary widely, and still be indicative of response. In general, the response of GIST to imatinib is very rapid and a measurable change in metabolism can be seen within days. For most other types

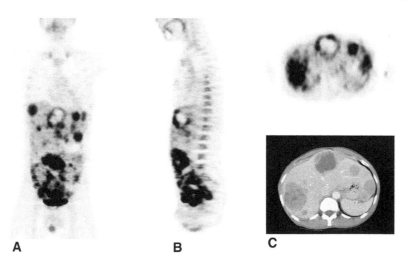

A   **B**   **C**

Figure 3 Baseline study at one hour after intravenous injection of 15 mCi of FDG. The uptake is proportional to the black intensity of the scan. (**A**) Coronal image, (**B**) Saggital image, (**C**) Transaxial image, PET above, CT below. There are numerous-metabolic masses throughout the peritoneal cavity and involving the parenchyma of the liver. After one month of treatment with Gleevec, most of the patient's tumor had responded, except for region in the left lobe of liver, which grew larger and continued to be hypermetabolic.

of tumors, there maybe a longer period of response, where the remaining FDG metabolism is proportional to the remaining viable tumor mass, which may differ from the total tumor mass.

FLT as a Biomarker for Targeted Therapy Response

In some circumstances, FDG is not a very good biomarker, and other radiotracers will undoubtedly be introduced for these specific tumor types. Perhaps the most likely radiotracer to compete with FDG in the near term will be 2F-18-L-thymidine, a thymidine analogue, which is phosphorylated by a thymidine kinase and retained in the

cell in proportion to the rate of proliferation of the cell (13–15). The FLT phosphate is not incorporated into DNA. FLT has been used in humans on numerous occasions; a tracer uptake appears to be reasonably well correlated with markers of proliferation such as Ki-67.

Activating mutations of BRAF occur in approximately 7% of all human tumors and in the majority of melanomas. These tumors are very sensitive to pharmacologic inhibition of mitogen-activated protein kinase (MEK)/ extracellular signal-regulated kinase, which causes a G1 arrest. Growth arrest may or may not lead to cell death and is more likely to result in "stable disease". In patients with cancer, this can be difficult to distinguish from indolent tumor growth. A series of experiments were performed at

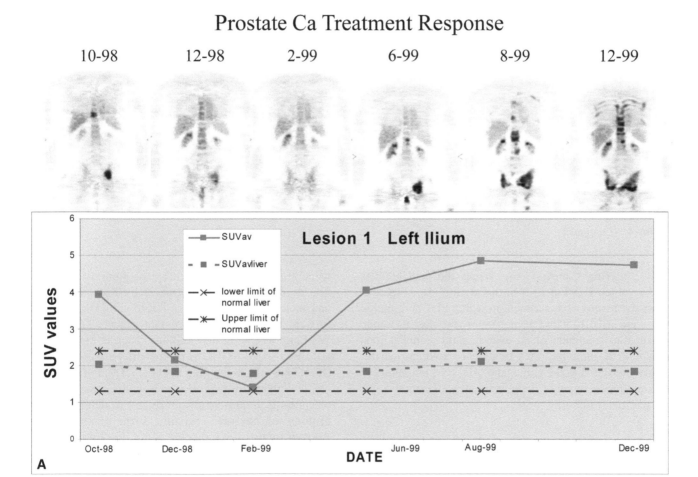

Figure 4 Eight separate images are shown during the time of the priest patients treatment with a regimen that included Taxol estramustine and carboplatin. Two different ways of plotting the results include an SUV and the TLG. (**A**) Attention is directed to the left sarcoiliac (SI) joint, where there is a hypermetabolic site on the PET scan. The patient gets an objective metabolic response with marked reduction in metabolism over the first few months, but thereafter, the patient's tumor escapes from treatment control and begins to progress. It should be noted that the SUV value dropped more than 60%, well below the limit of 25%, which has been proposed as a limit by European authorities (20). Because the SUV value is a per gram measure, it reaches a maximum and does not increase even though the tumor is expanding in volume. (**B**) The same series of patients scales, but this time the parameter plotted is the total lesion glycolysis or TLG. The TLG is a combination of the mean SUV across the tumor, and the volume of the tumor in this case determined from a thresholding technique. The interested reader is referred to Ref. 21. *Abbreviations*: SUV, standardized uptake value; TLG, total lesion glycolysis.

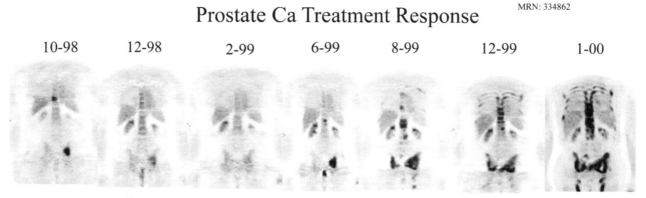

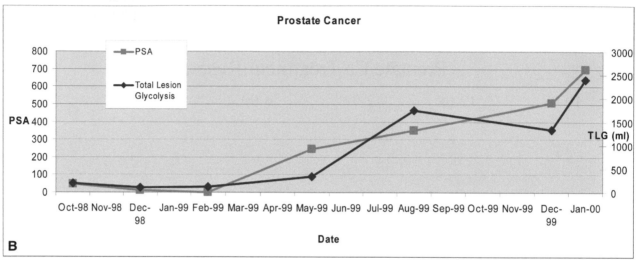

Figure 4   (*Continued*)

Sloan-Kettering Cancer Center using the standardized uptake value (SUV) of FLT in this setting (16). Figure 5 shows the results of experiment in which FLT and micro-PET were used to show a very rapid response in tumor uptake after treatment of an experimental animal tumor with a MEK inhibitor. This treatment paradigm can be readily translated to the clinic, and offers the potential for very rapid assessment of the effectiveness of drug therapy in a particular tumor.

MONITORING TREATMENT RESPONSE BASED ON CHANGES IN SPECIFIC BIOMOLECULES

Changes in specific biomarkers maybe more rapid than overall changes in the metabolic pathway, like glycolysis or DNA substrate phosphorylation. In castrate resistant prostate cancer, the ARs of great interest because changes in the sensitivity of AR to androgenic signals may be an important mechanism for inducing the castrate resistant state. Also, since many of the treatments are hormone based, it is important to know

whether the AR is saturated by the administered drugs. The development of radiotracers by Katzenellenbogen and Welch, which can image AR in vivo, is a major step forward in the study of prostate cancer. The group at Washington University, and our group at MSKCC have studied 16β-[18F]fluoro-5α-dihydrotestosterone (FDHT) as a PET imaging agent (17,18). Further studies are underway to explore the role of other hormonal receptors in treatment response and in determining the biology of castrate-resistant form of the disease. Another interesting molecule is the Her 2 growth receptor, which is important to the proliferation of some forms of breast cancer. We have developed the gallium 68 Her 2 F(ab')$_2$ radiotracer that permits study of rapid changes of Her 2 receptor in response to inhibition of the human heat-shock protein (HSP) 90. In animal models, within 24 hours of treatment with the HSP 90 inhibitor, there is more than 80% drop in the protein expression as measured by uptake of radiotracer in vivo, and Western blots of excised tumor confirm these quantitative changes. Also of interest in the treatment response is that these single molecular changes to Her 2

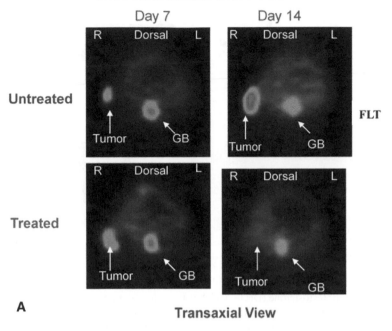

FLT images of Mel-28 SQ tumor-bearing mice untreated/treated with PD901

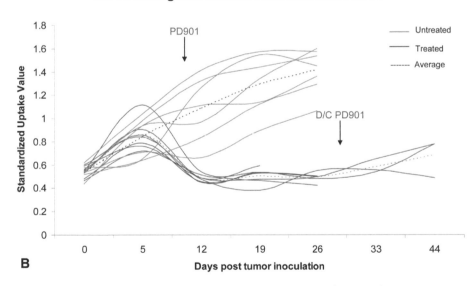

Figure 5 (**A**) Transaxial image showing uptake in control and treated animal of (3′-deoxy-3′-[(18)F]fluorothymidine ([(18)F]FLT) performed with the positron emission tomography (PET) imaging. In SKMEL-28 tumor xenografts, MEK inhibition completely inhibited tumor growth and induced differentiation with only modest tumor regression. (**B**) Comparison curves of treated animals and control. There is rapid response in the treated group with inhibition during therapy. When therapy is stopped, some of the tumors begin to grow again (*See Color Insert*).

protein are much more rapid than changes in glycolysis, suggesting that the Her 2 receptor changes would be a better biomarker than FDG uptake in monitoring treatment effects with HSP 90 inhibitors. Figure 6 illustrates the use of these two tracers showing study benefits in animals and man.

Molecular Imaging with Antibodies Finally Begins to Fulfill Its Promise

Radiolabeled antibodies have been extensively studied in nuclear medicine. By and large, especially for diagnosis, these monoclonal antibodies have been a disappointment.

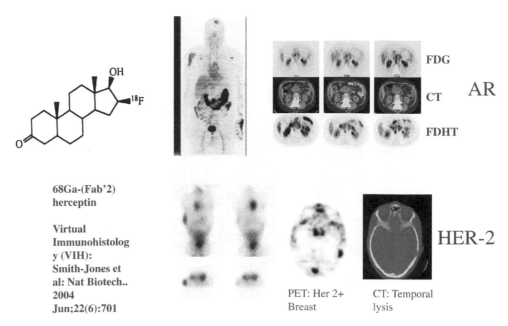

Figure 6 Examples of potential biomarkers which image individual biomolecules. Upper Panel showing AR tracer FDHT chemical structure. FDHT is an analog of dihydrotestosterone (DHT), which is the active androgen at the cellular level in vivo. In the center panel on the upper row is an image obtained at one hour after intravenous injection of 9 mCi of FDHT. There is clear-cut uptake in the skull, and in the right upper arm, as well as to bilateral ribs, and biopsy confirmed uptake in the prostate bed. The pattern of metabolism is well shown, with residual uptake in the vascular pool in which FDHT metabolites are bound to sex-binding globulin. These radiolabeled forms are rapidly taken out of the blood by the liver and excreted into the intestine. The far right panel in the upper row shows treatment response in a patient who progressed showing increasing expression of AR and FDG despite treatment. The lower panel shows the gallium 68 Her 2 imaging agent, with a microPET image of Her 2 expressing breast cancer before and 24 hours after treatment with the HSP 90 inhibitor drug 17 AAG. There has been no change in mass in other tumor over this interval, and FDG uptake (not shown) was unchanged. Her 2 positive breast cancer patient was imaged with gallium 68 Her 2 and there was uptake noted in a lytic skull lesion (*lower panel, right inside*).

These wonderfully specific high-affinity biomolecules, were never intended by nature to have very high target to background ratios between tumorous and surrounding tissue. It is my opinion that the advent of PET and the extensive use of positron labels for antibodies will be a very significant aid in characterizing and rendering a diagnosis of a specific tumor tissue type tumors in patients with metastatic disease. This is not really a new idea, PET imaging with radiolabelled antibodies was performed in humans to image neuroblastomas more than 15 years ago (19). It has only been recently that advances in technology have allowed PET-antibody imaging to become practical. As an example, the recent development of 124 G250 and antibody that binds to carbonic anhydrase IX promises to improve characterizing the renal mass for better patient selection for surgical treatment. Figure 7 shows an example of PET imaging in a patient with colorectal cancer.

THE CLOUD ON THE HORIZON

From a scientific and technical point of view, the nuclear aspect of molecular imaging is moving very rapidly with many advances in biology, the development of new radiotracers, and the prospect for major beneficial changes in patient management. The versatility of this technique with the ability to radiolabel many biomarkers, and the strength of the tracer principle are likely to carry this field very far.

There is a cloud on the horizon. The uncertainties about the regulatory climate for molecular imaging radiotracers and whether or not it will be possible to obtain reimbursement in a timely way for the advances of molecular imaging. Discussion of this is outside the scope of this review, but the interested reader is referred to it excellent article recently published by Hoffman et al. (9). Clearly, molecular imaging has a very bright future, but only if we can make common cause with regulators to develop innovative ways in which effective molecular-imaging techniques can be introduced more rapidly in clinical research and in patient care.

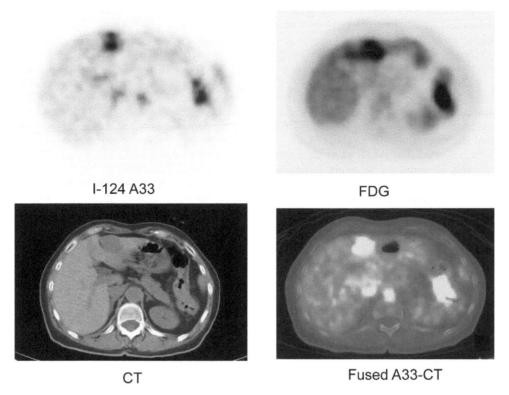

Figure 7 Imaging with radio antibodies using PET. The sample showed is an image of a patient with colorectal cancer, imaged at five days after intravenous injection of 124 A33 in which there is uptake both within a hepatic lesion and in the primary splenic flexure of the colon. The intense uptake of the antibody indicates that the mass in the liver and the mass of the splenic flexure are expressing the antigen target. In this way, this is a kind of virtual immunohistology in which the PET camera replaces the microscope.

REFERENCES

1. Hanahan D, Weinberg RA. The hallmarks of cancer. Cell 2000; 100:57–70.
2. Kelloff GJ, Krohn KA, Larson SM, et al. The progress and promise of molecular imaging probes in oncologic drug development. Clin Cancer Res 2005; 11:7967–7985.
3. Kelloff GJ, Hoffman JM, Johnson B, et al. Progress and promise of FDG-PET imaging for cancer patient management and oncologic drug development. Clin Cancer Res 2005; 11:2785–2808.
4. Beyer T, Townsend DW, Blodgett TM. Dual-modality PET/CT tomography for clinical oncology. Q J Nucl Med 2002; 46:24–34.
5. Pichler BJ, Judenhofer MS, Catana C, et al. Performance test of an LSO-APD detector in a 7-T MRI scanner for simultaneous PET/MRI. J Nucl Med 2006; 47:639–647.
6. Kelloff GJ, Bast RC Jr., Coffey DS, et al. Biomarkers, surrogate end points, and the acceleration of drug development for cancer prevention and treatment: an update prologue. Clin Cancer Res 2004; 10:3881–3884.
7. Larson SM, Schwartz LH. 18F-FDG PET as a candidate for "qualified biomarker": functional assessment of treatment response in oncology. J Nucl Med 2006; 47:901–903.
8. Shankar LK, Hoffman JM, Bacharach S, et al. Consensus recommendations for the use of 18F-FDG PET as an indicator of therapeutic response in patients in National Cancer Institute Trials. J Nucl Med 2006; 47:1059–1066.
9. Hoffman JM, Gambhir SS, Kelloff GJ. Regulatory and reimbursement challenges for molecular imaging. Radiology 2007; 245:645–660.
10. Van den Abbeele AD, Badawi RD. Use of positron emission tomography in oncology and its potential role to assess response to imatinib mesylate therapy in gastrointestinal stromal tumors (GISTs). Eur J Cancer 2002; 38(suppl 5): S60–S65.
11. Holdsworth CH, Badawi RD, Manola JB, et al. CT and PET: early prognostic indicators of response to imatinib mesylate in patients with gastrointestinal stromal tumor. AJR Am J Roentgenol 2007; 189:W324–W330.
12. Morris MJ, Akhurst T, Larson SM, et al. Fluorodeoxyglucose positron emission tomography as an outcome measure for castrate metastatic prostate cancer treated with antimicrotubule chemotherapy. Clin Cancer Res 2005; 11:3210–3216.
13. Grierson JR, Shields AF. Radiosynthesis of 3'-deoxy-3'-[(18)F]fluorothymidine: [(18)F]FLT for imaging of cellular proliferation in vivo. Nucl Med Biol 2000; 27:143–156.

14. Shields AF. Positron emission tomography measurement of tumor metabolism and growth: its expanding role in oncology. Mol Imaging Biol 2006; 8:141–150.

15. Shields AF, Grierson JR, Dohmen BM, et al. Imaging proliferation in vivo with [F-18]FLT and positron emission tomography. Nat Med 1998; 4:1334–1336.

16. Solit DB, Santos E, Pratilas CA, et al. 3′-deoxy-3′-[18F] fluorothymidine positron emission tomography is a sensitive method for imaging the response of BRAF-dependent tumors to MEK inhibition. Cancer Res 2007; 67:11463–11469.

17. Dehdashti F, Picus J, Michalski JM, et al. Positron tomographic assessment of androgen receptors in prostatic carcinoma. Eur J Nucl Med Mol Imaging 2005; 32:344–350.

18. Larson SM, Morris M, Gunther I, et al. Tumor localization of 16beta-18F-fluoro-5alpha-dihydrotestosterone versus 18F-FDG in patients with progressive, metastatic prostate cancer. J Nucl Med 2004; 45:366–373.

19. Larson SM, Pentlow KS, Volkow ND, et al. PET scanning of iodine-124-3F9 as an approach to tumor dosimetry during treatment planning for radioimmunotherapy in a child with neuroblastoma. J Nucl Med 1992; 33:2020–2023.

20. Young H, Baum R, Cremerius U, et al. Measurement of clinical and subclinical tumour response using [18F]-fluorodeoxyglucose and positron emission tomography: review and 1999 EORTC recommendations. European Organization for Research and Treatment of Cancer (EORTC) PET Study Group. Eur J Cancer 1999; 35: 1773–1782.

21. Larson SM, Erdi Y, Akhurst T, et al. Tumor treatment response based on visual and quantitative changes in global tumor glycolysis using PET-FDG imaging. The visual response score and the change in total lesion glycolysis. Clin Positron Imaging 1999; 2:159–171.

Index

Absorbed dose, 220–221
Academic-industrial interaction
　contacts for, 690
　issues for, 689–690
　opportunities for, 688–689
　　collaborative agreement, 689
　　information transfer, 688
　　license, 689
　　material transfer agreements, 688
　　study agreements, 689
Acetate, in cell membrane synthesis,
　　298–299
Acetylpromazine, 380
ACNP. *See* American College
　　of Neuropsychopharmacology
　　(ACNP)
Acoustic impedance, ultrasound, 110
Acoustic radiation force, 112
　accumulation of contrast
　　agents and, 115
　adhesion enhancement, 115
ADC. *See* Apparent diffusion coefficient
　　(ADC)
Adeno-associated virus (AAV), 429
Adenomatous polyposis coli
　　(APC), 9–10
Adenovirus vectors, 429
Adrenergic compounds, 194
Aerobic glycolysis, 22–23
Affinity enhancement system (AES), 577
AFM. *See* Atomic force microscopy
　　(AFM)
Agency for the Evaluation of Medicinal
　　Products (EMEA), 340

Albumin-GdDTPA, 528
Allophycocyanin, 249
α—melanoma stimulating hormone
　　(α-MSH) receptors, radiotracers,
　　317–318
American College of Neuropsychophar-
　　macology (ACNP), 667
Amide proton transfer (APT) imaging,
　　239–240
Amino acids
　PET, protein synthesis using, 298
　radiolabeled, 632
　　as tracers, 193–194
5-aminolevulinic acid (ALA), 251
Anatomic imaging, of PCa, 624
Anesthesias
　assessing level of, 378
　cardiac monitoring, using ECG
　　electrodes, 385–386
　inhalational anesthesia
　　isoflurane, 378–379
　injectable drugs, 379–380
　respiratory-depressive effects of, 381
Aneuploidy, 12
Angiogenesis, 469, 596
　angiogenic switch, 470
　antiangiogenic drugs
　　endothelial cell proliferation
　　　inhibitors, 471–472
　　growth factor antagonists and
　　　endothelial cell signal transduc-
　　　tion inhibitors, 471
　　integrin activation inhibitors, 472
　　MMP inhibitors, 471

[Angiogenesis]
　imaging
　　CT, 473
　　hemodynamic parameters, 473–481
　　molecular markers, 482–487
　　MRI, 472–473
　　optical, 473
　　PET and SPECT, 472
　　ultrasound, 473
　intussusception, 470
　mosaic vessel, 470
　mother vessels, 470–471
　in murine transgenic model of prostate
　　cancer, 146–147
　processes of, 470–471
　sustained, 20–21
Angiopoietin-1 (Ang-1), 471
Angiozyme, 471
Animal PET scanners, 80–82
Annexin, 298, 494
Annihilation coincidence detection,
　　PET, 68–70
Anoikis, 19
　resistance to, 21–22
Antibodies
　catabolism, 574
　molecular imaging with, 701–702
　radiolabeled. *See* Radiolabeled
　　antibody therapy
Antigrowth signals, in cancer, 19
Antineoplastic agents, 663
Antitumor activity, 646–649
α-particle emitters, radiolabeled
　　antibody therapy, 222

705